Orofacial Pain
And Headache

EDITED BY

Professor Yair Sharav
Department of Oral Medicine
Hebrew University Faculty of Dental Medicine
Hadassah Medical Centre
Jerusalem
Israel

Professor Rafael Benoliel
Chairman
Department of Oral Medicine
Hebrew University Faculty of Dental Medicine
Hadassah Medical Centre
Jerusalem
Israel

FOREWORD BY

Professor Barry J. Sessle
Canada Research Chair
Faculty of Dentistry and Centre
for the Study of Pain
University of Toronto
Toronto
Canada

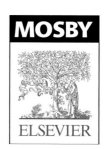

Edinburgh   London   New York   Oxford   Philadelphia   St Louis   Sydney   Toronto   2008

MOSBY
ELSEVIER
An imprint of Elsevier Limited

First published 2008

ISBN–13: 9780723434122
ISBN–10: 0723434123

British Library Cataloguing in Publication Data
A catalogue record for this book is available from the British Library

Library of Congress Cataloging in Publication Data
A catalog record for this book is available from the Library of Congress

ELSEVIER
your source for books, journals and multimedia in the health sciences

www.elsevierhealth.com

Working together to grow libraries in developing countries

www.elsevier.com | www.bookaid.org | www.sabre.org

ELSEVIER | BOOK AID International | Sabre Foundation

The publisher's policy is to use **paper manufactured from sustainable forests**

Printed in China

Contents

Foreword

Orofacial Pain and Headache is a timely and comprehensive addition to the important area of the diagnosis and treatment of craniofacial pain. It is true to state that the diagnosis and management of acute pain conditions are readily achieved; this is one of the characteristic features of the practice of dentistry. However, this is sadly not the case for many chronic pain conditions. A patient with chronic orofacial pain can represent a significant challenge to the clinician, leading to repeated and usually unsuccessful interventions. Why is this? Unfortunately, the curriculum of most dental and medical schools has only a limited emphasis on pain mechanisms, diagnosis and management. Additionally, there is at present only an incomplete understanding of the mechanisms underlying the aetiology and pathogenesis of chronic orofacial pain conditions. Furthermore, chronic orofacial pain can take many forms, with a wide variety of apparently successful treatment options; many of these do not have a strong scientific or evidence basis. To further complicate matters, pain is a multidimensional experience involving physical, cognitive and emotional aspects and chronic pain in particular recruits active involvement of these dimensions. An important related factor is that the orofacial region has special meaning to each of us since we communicate with and express our feelings to others through this body region. We recognize our acquaintances by their facial features, and from the moment of birth, we sustain our life through the intake of air, fluids and foodstuffs through orofacial structures.

The trigeminal system provides most of the craniofacial sensory innervation, and is associated with specific physiological qualities and pain conditions. For example, pain syndromes such as trigeminal neuralgia or migraine are specific to the area, and trigeminal nerve injury responses differ from those in spinal nerves. Furthermore, the trigeminal nerve innervates anatomically related but functionally diverse organs such as the meninges, the craniofacial vasculature, the eyes, the ears, the teeth, oral soft tissues, muscles and the temporomandibular joint. In the brainstem, the trigeminal sensory nucleus overlaps with upper cervical dermatomes. Taken together, these features account for the complex and extensive pain referral patterns that often make clinical diagnosis so difficult.

The philosophy and design of this book make it a timely and instructive addition to the pain literature.

Management of orofacial pain demands the services of clinicians from various specialties due to the anatomical density of the region. Based on their extensive clinical experience and a thorough understanding of pain mechanisms specific to the trigeminal system, the editors, Professors Yair Sharav and Rafael Benoliel, are well equipped to integrate knowledge across the various disciplines. They have written the major part of this comprehensive textbook and have successfully integrated knowledge from the areas of headache and craniofacial pain. In particular, they have succinctly explained common mechanisms involved in the two regions, with important implications for pain diagnosis and management.

The anatomy and neurophysiology relevant to orofacial pain are covered in Chapter 2, and this provides a solid basic science underpinning for subsequent chapters that present current knowledge of aetiologic and pathophysiologic mechanisms. The book emphasizes the four major clinical entities of orofacial pain: acute dental (Chapter 5), neurovascular (Chapters 9, 10), musculoskeletal (Chapters 7, 8) and neuropathic (Chapter 11). Diagnostic and management strategies are emphasized in these chapters and in Chapter 1, supplemented by expert contributions on otolaryngology and facial pain (Chapter 6) and neurosurgical procedures (Chapter 12), pharmacotherapy for acute and chronic pain (Chapters 15, 16), complementary and alternative medicine (Chapter 17) and psychologically based interventions (Chapter 4). Novel in its approach is the chapter on the occurrence of craniofacial pain in systemically complex patients (Chapter 14). The clinical chapters are complemented by several informative case reports that offer insight into the complexity of orofacial pain diagnosis and management.

As such, this book should be an invaluable resource for dental or medical students, dental practitioners, pain specialists from all fields and basic and clinical pain scientists who are interested in an up-to-date and comprehensive review of the diagnostic and management issues in the orofacial pain field.

Barry J. Sessle
Professor and Canada Research Chair
Faculty of Dentistry and Centre for the Study of Pain
University of Toronto

Preface

For many years the area of orofacial pain was completely dominated by the concept that most facial pains were due to 'disturbed function of the temporomandibular joint'. This was an approach established by an otolaryngologist named Costen who linked aetiology to derangements of the dental occlusion; facial pain was thus handed over to dentistry. As a profession we enthusiastically adopted the treatment of facial pain but have for many years concentrated our efforts on a mechanistic approach to treatment. These events essentially segregated facial pain from headache, and in effect from mainstream medicine. As a result ideal conditions were established in each of the two disciplines for the development of different approaches to the understanding of mechanisms and therapy of craniofacial pain. However, as our understanding of pain mechanisms, and in particular chronic pain, developed, it became clear that facial pain has underlying neurophysiological mechanisms common to headaches and other body areas. Masticatory muscle pain was examined in light of other regional muscle pains, and management of the temporomandibular joint was related to, and brought in line with, basic orthopaedic principles. Most importantly, features of some facial pain entities are very similar to those of some headaches. Examples include masticatory myofascial pain and tension-type headache and a facial equivalent of migraine.

The dental profession has been slow in adopting medically based classification and approaches to therapy. In a similar fashion the medical profession has been very resistant to incorporating established facial pains into current classifications; temporomandibular disorders are a prime example and currently unrecognized by the International Headache Society.

One may correctly claim that toothache is unique, but is it really? On a mechanistic level pulpitis is an inflammatory process within a confined space—not very different from the inflammatory process of migraine confined within the skull. Indeed we believe that migraine-like mechanisms exist within the pulp chamber mimicking pulpitis, in the paranasal sinuses imitating sinusitis and in other confined cranial structures causing atypical symptomatology. In each of these cases anti-migraine medications are the correct treatment.

Clearly the task required is integration of knowledge in this anatomically dense region, traditionally divided between many medical disciplines. Based on our extensive clinical experience with patients suffering from orofacial pain and headache, and our thorough understanding of pain mechanisms specific to the trigeminal system, we feel that we are well equipped to fulfil this task. This textbook therefore deals with oral and facial pain as well as with headaches, and aims to integrate the knowledge across these disciplines. We hope we have succeeded.

We appreciate the contribution of our teachers, colleagues and students. Throughout our professional lives we have interacted with many professionals worldwide, and each has enriched our understanding of pain mechanisms and our clinical knowledge. Being in the 'business' of teaching, both undergraduates and residents, we have been consistently challenged by curious students with difficult questions. These have kept us up to date and enabled us to re-examine and reassess the way orofacial pain is understood and taught.

Last but not least, our warm gratitude and appreciation to our families for bearing with us through the long process of preparing, writing, editing and publishing this book.

Yair Sharav
Rafael Benoliel
Jerusalem 2007

Contributors

Donald S Ciccione PhD
Associate Professor
Department of Psychiatry
UMDNJ—New Jersey Medical School
Newark
USA
Psychological aspects of chronic orofacial pain

Marshall Devor PhD
Professor & Chairman
Department of Cell & Animal Biology
Institute of Life Sciences, and
Center for Research on Pain
Hebrew University of Jerusalem
Jerusalem
Israel
Anatomy and neurophysiology of orofacial pain

Franklin M Dolwick DMD PhD
Professor and Associate Chair
Oral & Maxillofacial Surgery Department
University of Florida College of Dentistry
Gainesville
USA
Pain and dysfunction of the temporomandibular joint

Sharon Elad DMD MSc
Lecturer
Department of Oral Medicine
Hebrew University Faculty of Dental Medicine
Hadassah Medical Center
Jerusalem
Israel
Orofacial pain in the medically compromised patient

Ron Eliashar MD
Senior Lecturer
Department of Otolaryngology, Head & Neck Surgery
Hebrew University Faculty of Medicine
Hadassah Medical Center
Jerusalem
Israel
Otolaryngological aspects of orofacial pain

Eli Eliav DMD PhD
Professor, Robert & Susan Carmel Endowed Chair in Algesiology
Director, Division of Orofacial Pain
UMDNJ—New Jersey Medical School
Newark
USA
Measuring and assessing pain; Neuropathic orofacial pain; Referred and secondary orofacial pain syndromes

Joel Epstein DMD MSD FRCD(c)
Professor & Head
Department of Oral Medicine and Diagnostic Sciences
Chicago
USA
Orofacial pain in the medically compromised patient

Richard H Gracely PhD
Professor
Departments of Internal Medicine—Rheumatology and Neurology
University of Michigan
Ann Arbor
USA
Measuring and assessing pain

Menachem Gross MD
Lecturer
Department of Otolaryngology, Head & Neck Surgery
Hebrew University Faculty of Medicine
Hadassah Medical Center
Jerusalem
Israel
Otolaryngological aspects of orofacial pain

Gary M Heir DMD
Clinical Associate Professor
Department of Oral Medicine
Orofacial Pain Services
UMDNJ—New Jersey Medical School
Newark
USA
Pain and dysfunction of the temporomandibular joint; Neuropathic orofacial pain

Gary D Klasser DMD
Assistant Professor
Department of Oral Medicine and Diagnostic Sciences
Chicago
USA
Orofacial pain in the medically compromised patient

Dorrit W Nitzan DMD
Professor
Department of Oral and Maxillofacial Surgery
Hebrew University Faculty of Dental Medicine
Hadassah Medical Center
Jerusalem
Israel
Pain and dysfunction of the temporomandibular joint

Karen Raphael PhD MS
Associate Professor
Departments of Psychiatry and Diagnostic Sciences
UMDNJ—New Jersey Medical School
Newark
USA
Psychological aspects of chronic orofacial pain

Z Harry Rappaport MD
Professor and Director
Department of Neurosurgery, Rabin Medical Center, Petah Tiqva
Sackler School of Medicine, Tel Aviv University
Israel
Neurosurgical aspects of orofacial pain

Herve Sroussi DMD PhD
Assistant Professor
Department of Oral Medicine and Diagnostic Sciences
Chicago
USA
Orofacial pain in the medically compromised patient

Michael Tal DMD MS
Professor, Chair Neurobiology Unit
Department of Anatomy and Cell Biology
Hebrew University
Jerusalem
Israel
Anatomy and neurophysiology of orofacial pain

CHAPTER 1

The diagnostic process

Yair Sharav and Rafael Benoliel

1. The Problem

Diagnosis and treatment of orofacial pain is a complex process compounded by the density of anatomical structures and the prominent psychological significance attributed to this region. Management of orofacial pain thus demands the services of clinicians from various specialties, such as dentistry, otolaryngology, ophthalmology, neurology, neurosurgery, psychiatry and psychology. Complex referral patterns to adjacent structures are common in orofacial pain and, indeed, one man's headache is another man's facial pain. In clinical practice, they are often intimately related. Consequently, the patient with orofacial pain may wander from one specialist to the other in order to get adequate help.

There are excellent textbooks available on orofacial pain or headache; each with its own individual emphasis, aimed at specific reader groups. Do we need another textbook? A textbook that integrates orofacial pain with headache based on contributions by various disciplines, all with extensive clinical experience and a thorough understanding of pain mechanisms specific to the trigeminal system, is indeed required. These, in essence, are the foundations for writing this book. Accordingly, we relate to *all regional craniofacial pains* and aim at presenting the wider picture of orofacial pain syndromes, including the overlap between primary headaches and primary orofacial pain entities. Many of the patients with chronic orofacial pain are primary headache variants, present in the orofacial region, and a lack of familiarity with these syndromes probably underlies misdiagnosis by dental practitioners as well as by medical specialists. Other patients that remain unclassified by the International Headache Society (IHS) and are unknown to neurologists, otolaryngologists, other medical practitioners and even to dentists are probably primary orofacial pain entities (Benoliel *et al* 1997; Czerninsky *et al* 1999; Sharav and Benoliel 2001; Benoliel and Sharav 2006). We believe the integration between headache and orofacial pain classifications to be of paramount importance, especially since about half of patients in tertiary care craniofacial pain clinics are still labelled as 'idiopathic' or 'undiagnosable' under IHS classification (Zebenholzer *et al* 2005, 2006; Benoliel and Sharav 2006). Moreover, there is considerable overlap in the clinical presentation of headaches such as tension type, with regional myofascial pains of the face and generalized pain syndromes such as fibromyalgia (Chapter 7). There is also a growing patient population with chronic craniofacial pain due to trauma associated with traffic accidents (Benoliel *et al* 1994) and with invasive dental procedures such as dental implants, which demands a multidisciplinary approach. We hope that by applying this approach the gap between medically trained headache specialists and dentally trained orofacial pain specialists will be bridged. Additionally we have attempted to compile a book that will be useful to readers at different stages of their careers: undergraduate students, residents and practitioners, as well as dental and medical pain specialists. The chapters are clearly subdivided to allow quick navigation through the text and selection of relevant sections. Although each chapter is independent, we have no doubt that working through the book will serve the reader best.

1.1. The Scope

The diagnosis and management of orofacial pain, both acute and chronic, have become important subjects in dentistry (Sharav 2005). Additionally orofacial pain is quite prevalent in the general population: around 17–26%, of which 7–11% are chronic (Goulet *et al* 1995; Riley *et al* 1998; Macfarlane *et al* 2002a; Ng *et al* 2002; McMillan *et al* 2006). Naturally therefore, the emphasis of this book is on the four major clinical families of orofacial pain: acute dental, neurovascular, musculoskeletal and neuropathic (Chapters 5, 7–11). In these chapters, we review current aetiology, diagnosis and treatment. Although the many case presentations included are largely 'virtual', i.e. created from integrated data, the cases are real in that they reliably duplicate the type seen in orofacial pain clinics, and any resemblance to specific cases is purely coincidental. However, as any experienced clinician will attest, the 'typical' textbook cases are rare and we relate to the changes in presentation that may cause diagnostic confusion under each relevant section. Atypical cases may be difficult to manage; many have superimposed traum and consequent neuropathic pain. Some of these cases often have a history of misdiagnosed acute pains in the orofacial region leading to repeated and unsuccessful interventions that slowly escalate and result in dental extractions and surgeries. Accurate diagnosis of acute dental and orofacial conditions is therefore essential and covered in Chapter 5. The importance of acute and chronic otolaryngological syndromes in the differential diagnosis of facial pain is paramount and our colleagues cover this area in Chapter 6. The growing number of older, often medically compromised, patients with orofacial pain deserves special attention: Is orofacial pain in these patients related to their medical condition? The answer is found in Chapter 14.

One of the mainstays of pain management is indisputably pharmacotherapy. Because many of the drugs used are common to many of the syndromes, we have included two separate chapters on pharmacotherapy: acute and chronic (Chapters 15 and 16). The management of pain relies on accurate diagnosis and on reliable follow-up that demonstrates objective improvement. Chapter 3 covers the important area of pain measurement as well as the assessment of peripheral nerve function. Unfortunately, we are a long way from optimal patient care and some of the best drugs will offer substantial relief (not absolute) for only about 75% of patients, many with disturbing side effects. Many patients therefore enquire about neurosurgical options; see Chapter 12. In parallel, there is rising popularity and demand among orofacial pain patients for complementary and alternative medicine (CAM), and we must know the available treatment options in this field (Chapter 17). No diagnosis and treatment of orofacial pain is complete without understanding its emotional undercurrents or having a thorough knowledge of its psychological aspects and treatment possibilities, which are covered in Chapter 4. Although this is essentially a clinical book, anatomy and neurophysiology are covered in a manner specifically relevant to the topic of orofacial pain (Chapter 2).

1.2. The Philosophy

The need to base our therapeutic approaches on evidence-based medicine (EBM) is obvious, and we wholeheartedly agree with this approach. The book cites state-of-the-art research to support statements whenever this is possible. However, EBM is a tasteless science, unless peppered by clinical experience and judgment, careful appraisal of drug side effects and complications

(especially in the medically compromised), the patients' individual variability, and a respectful approach to the patient's autonomy. We have therefore also encouraged enrichment of the text with 'expert opinion'.

As in most other medical textbooks, the presentation of knowledge here is done in a 'linear', disease-based, manner. We describe pain syndromes and outline their signs, symptoms and associated features, which is very different to the 'circular' process of clinical data collection and indeed how patients present with complaints rather than diseases. Knowledge of a disease does not automatically guarantee the ability to identify it from a given set of signs and symptoms. The process of accumulating clinical data in order to reach a diagnosis is as much a science as it is an art, and part of this chapter is devoted to the understanding and application of this process.

The great strength of classification systems, especially if they have been field-tested, lies in their ability to predefine into a recognizable and universally accepted entity the sign and symptom complex that patients present. We employ criteria published by the IHS (Olesen *et al* 2004), the American Academy of Orofacial Pain (AAOP) (Okeson 1996) and the International Association for the Study of Pain (IASP) (Merskey and Bogduk 1994). None of these are perfect, nor are they individually comprehensive. Therefore, we integrate all these systems according to their strengths in the following manner. For headaches the IHS classification reigns supreme and is used throughout this book for all 'headache' entities. However, it is not detailed enough for orofacial pain entities and so we have used the AAOP's criteria. For temporomandibular disorders (TMDs), the Research Diagnostic Criteria for TMD (RDC-TMD) are often referred to (Dworkin and LeResche 1992). The IASP's strength lies in its regional and systems approach to pain classification (e.g. musculoskeletal, neurovascular pain) and its excellent approach to neuropathic pain entities. The integration of such internationally accepted systems into pain clinics and research papers is essential, and ultimately an enriching endeavour.

2. The Revolution: Pain as a Disease

Pain is a multifaceted experience involving physical, cognitive and emotional aspects (see Table 1.1). There are three mechanistically distinct types of pain: nociceptive, inflammatory and neuropathic. Nociceptive pain is the baseline defence mechanism that protects us from potential harm. Inflammatory and neuropathic pain are characterized by altered and often aberrant function of the nervous system as a result of persistent pathology or plastic changes in the nervous system.

Thus, although we tend to term any sensation that hurts 'pain', many types of pain exist that subserve various biological functions. For example, acute pain from extreme heat initiates a reflex withdrawal and ensures minimal tissue damage (nociceptive pain). This type of

Table 1.1	Definition of Pain Terms	
Term	**Definition**	**Clinical Implication**
Pain	An unpleasant sensory and emotional experience associated with actual or potential tissue damage, or described in terms of such damage.	Some patients may be unable to communicate verbally. Pain is an individually subjective experience.
Allodynia	Pain due to a stimulus which does not normally provoke pain (e.g. touch, light pressure, or moderate cold or warmth).	Associated with neuropathy, inflammation and certain headache states; see Chapters 5, 9 and 11. A lowered threshold where the stimulus (e.g. light touch) and response mode (pain) differ from the normal state.
Hyperalgesia	An increased response to a stimulus which is normally painful.	Associated with neuropathy or inflammation—reflects increased pain on suprathreshold stimulation. The stimulus and response modes are basically the same.
Hyperaesthesia	Increased sensitivity to stimulation, excluding the special senses. Includes both allodynia and hyperalgesia.	Associated with neuropathy or inflammation. See Chapter 11
Hyperpathia	A painful syndrome characterized by an abnormally painful reaction to a stimulus, especially a repetitive stimulus, as well as an increased threshold.	Typical of neuropathic pain (Chapter 11)
Hypoalgesia	Diminished pain in response to a normally painful stimulus.	Typical of neural damage. Raised threshold: stimulus and response mode are the same but with a lowered response.
Analgesia	Absence of pain in response to stimulation which would normally be painful.	Commonly observed after complete axotomy or nerve block. Not unpleasant.
Hyperpathia	A painful syndrome characterized by an abnormally painful reaction to a stimulus, especially a repetitive stimulus, as well as an increased threshold. May occur with allodynia, hyperaesthesia, hyperalgesia or dysaesthesia.	Typical of neuropathic pain syndromes (Chapter 11). Faulty identification and localization of the stimulus, delay, radiating sensation, and after-sensation may be present, and the pain is often explosive in character.
Paraesthesia	An abnormal sensation, whether spontaneous or evoked.	Typical of neuropathic pain syndromes; see Chapter 11.
Hypoaesthesia	Decreased sensitivity to stimulation, excluding the special senses.	
Dysaesthesia	An unpleasant abnormal sensation, whether spontaneous or evoked. Hyperalgesia and allodynia are forms of dysaesthesia.	

pain is a survival mechanism termed 'good' pain (Iadarola and Caudle 1997). Consequently, if tissue has been damaged, the local inflammatory response in the injured tissue causes increased sensitivity in peripheral nociceptors (peripheral sensitization) and in dorsal horn neurons (central sensitization) associated with pain transmission. As a result, the hand is sensitive to touch and more sensitive to pain (allodynia and hyperalgesia, Table 1.1) so that the individual protects and immobilizes the limb to aid rapid healing. Essentially the system has been altered to behave differently. In most cases, tissue injury followed by a healing period associated with ongoing pain resolves with no residual problems for the individual (still good pain).

In contrast, pain with no biological advantage to the organism is 'bad' pain. For example, chronic pain not associated with ongoing tissue damage, that inflicts severe physical and emotional suffering on the individual, offers no survival value. Such chronic pain syndromes are typical of neuropathic pain but also include other

syndromes, for instance chronic orofacial pain syndromes and headaches. Chronic pain is often the result of primary or reactive changes in the nervous system associated with neuronal plasticity, which are unable to modulate and actually serve to perpetuate the sensation of pain (see post-traumatic neuropathic pain, Chapters 2 and 11); the system has malfunctioned and maladaptive pain remains. Chronic pain is, therefore, a disease in its own right and often not a symptom. Additionally chronic pain responds to therapy differently from acute pain and is associated with emotional and social behavioural changes (see Chapter 4). Acute and chronic pains differ from each other in many respects, and some of the major differences are presented in Table 1.2.

Patients, and sometimes physicians, find it hard to distinguish between pain as a disease and pain as a symptom. The latter signifies an expression of a pathological process that if treated will cause the pain to disappear. Unfortunately, the inability to perceive pain as a *disease*

Table 1.2 Major Features of Acute and Chronic Pain

Features	Acute Pain	Chronic Pain
Time course	Short (Hours to days)	Long (months to years)
Aetiology	Peripheral mechanisms	Central mechanisms
Behavioural response	Anxiety, 'guarding'	Depression, 'illness behaviour'
Response to treatment:		
Local intervention	Good	Poor
Analgesic drugs	Good	Poor
Psychotropic drugs	Poor	Moderate to good

may result in repeated and unsuccessful interventions, all in an attempt 'to eradicate the cause of pain'.

3. The Process: Diagnosis of Orofacial Pain

Faced with a patient with a pain complaint we must answer three major questions: Where, What and Why; and if possible in the order presented. The first, *where*, is concerned with the location, such as the anatomical structure or system affected. The second, *what*, deals primarily with the pathological process. The third, *why*, is about the aetiology. The patient's decision to seek medical help is the first step in the diagnostic chain; surprisingly not all patients with significant pain seek treatment. Based mostly on the pain *location* patients will *choose* which specialist to consult. Naturally, if it is a 'toothache' the patient decides to consult the dentist, and most times the choice will be correct. However, suppose that the patient's pain is referred to the oral cavity from a remote organ (such as the heart, see Chapter 13), or is associated with migraine-like mechanisms (Chapter 9) and he consults his dentist. The patient has clearly, and understandably, missed or misinterpreted the 'where' or the 'what'. It is the responsibility of the clinician to analyse the patient's complaints and to reach the correct diagnosis. In other words, the clinician must rigorously apply the diagnostic process in order to accurately define the location, identify the pathological process and ideally establish the aetiology of the pain.

Our natural starting point is a comprehensive gathering of information. We routinely start with history taking, the strongest tool when it comes to the diagnosis of pain. Pain symptoms should specify location, duration, pain characteristics and other pertinent data (see below). In addition, a thorough personal history should include

details on medical, drug and psychosocial history, occupation, stress and a family history relating to marital status, recent events (e.g. bereavement) and any history of familial disorders (e.g. migraine, diabetes). We proceed with the physical examination, supplemented by other tests as needed. Once we have gone through this process, we then generate a working hypothesis, namely a diagnosis. Gathering information is a starting point, but on its own does not make a diagnosis! We will describe in the following the process of utilizing the patient's clinical data to generate diagnostic hypotheses.

3.1. The Methodology

Patients are normally willing to tell their 'story' or pain history, but there is usually a need to supplement this information with specific questions concerning the location, temporal behaviour, intensity and relation to function and to sensory modalities. We find that a structured intake for the clinical interview and examination findings is useful (Boxes 1.1 and 1.2 and Fig. 1.1), particularly for teaching and training. The intake systematically records the basic information needed in a pain history (Box 1.3) and practitioners can design their own forms based on these principles. Additionally the structured intake, or 'form', presents questions and examination procedures vital to the diagnosis of the more common clinical conditions (see Chapters 7–11)—for this, we draw on accepted classification systems such as those of the IHS, the AAOP and the IASP.

3.1.1. The Pain History

Location. Precisely identifying location is a complex issue when specifically dealing with orofacial or craniofacial pain; the region is compact, with many important structures close together (brain, eyes, nose, sinuses and teeth), so pain spread is common. Notwithstanding, certain craniofacial pain syndromes have a propensity for particular areas and specific referral patterns. In order to record location patients should point to the area where they feel the pain. Pain should also be marked on pre-prepared drawings of extra-oral and intraoral regions (Fig. 1.1); these are very helpful for communicating with the patient, and serve as an important reference at a later stage. Pain can be unilateral, meaning on one side of the face, head or mouth, or bilateral, on both sides. Often pain is unilateral but may change sides from attack to attack (migraine) whereas in others it may predominantly affect one side or even be side-locked (always on the same side). The patient should describe, and outline by finger pointing, whether the pain is localized or diffuse. Diffuse implies a large area with ill-defined borders and is usually outlined by patients with the whole hand rather than by finger pointing. Pain may radiate, which means that the pain felt in a certain point spreads in a vector-like fashion or it may spread in all directions. Pain radiation and pain spread are usually associated with severe

Box 1.1 Pain History

1. **Patient's details:** Name.....................................
   Age..................
   Sex: Male/Female Marital status........................
   Occupation..
2. **Medical status** – Summary of relevant medical conditions, medications, etc *(patient must complete a detailed medical questionnaire, not shown here)*
   ....
   ....
3. **Pain complaint:**
   a. Pain location (also marked on pre-prepared drawing, see Fig. 1.1) ....
   b. Pain onset and duration ....
   c. Age at onset of pain attacks ....
   d. Pain attack frequency (mark continuous if no pain free periods) ....
   e. Pain attack duration ....
   f. Pain severity- mark on scale below (10cm line)

   ☺ 0 ▭▭▭▭▭▭▭▭▭▭ 10 ☹

   No Pain   Worst Pain
   g. Factors that precipitate/aggravate pain ....
   h. Pain is eased by ....
   i. Pain quality: pressing/piercing/throbbing/burning/ electric/sharp/other ....
4. **Accompanying signs and symptoms:**
   a. Systemic: nausea/vomiting/photophobia/phonophobia/ dizziness
   b. Local: tearing/rhinorrhea/swelling/redness
5. **History of trauma yes/no** (if yes): date...................
   Description...
6. **Pain history summary** *(additional details including response to previous treatments)* ....
7. **Pain in other body regions** (also mark on Fig. 1.1)
   ....
8. **How does your pain affect your quality of life?**

   ☺ 0 ▭▭▭▭▭▭▭▭▭▭ 10 ☹

   No effect   Extremely
9. **How well do you sleep?**

   ☺ 0 ▭▭▭▭▭▭▭▭▭▭ 10 ☹

   Very well   Extremely badly
10. **Does the pain wake you? Yes/No Frequency: /night**
    Comment: ....

pain; see Chapter 5 (Sharav *et al* 1984). When the source of pain is in one location but felt in another, remote location, the pain is called referred. In many such cases, the patient is usually aware only of the pain in the area of referral and the primary source or location is identified by the clinician at a later stage (e.g. myofascial trigger points; see Chapter 7). The craniofacial symptoms may be associated with other body pains and these are best recorded on a body drawing.

Temporal behaviour. Another valuable descriptor is the behaviour of pain in relation to time. The temporal behaviour of the pain, once established, may be crucial in diagnosis. One of the essential features of many craniofacial pains is the age of onset; migraine typically begins early in life whilst trigeminal neuralgia affects older subjects.

Pain may occur at specific times of the day, such as the morning or evening. Moreover pain onset may be associated with weekly (e.g. weekends), monthly (e.g. menstruation) or even yearly (e.g. seasonal) events. Pain can be *intermittent*, such as in pulpitis, or *continuous*, as in muscular pain. Episodic pain, also termed *periodic*, appears during certain periods; otherwise the patient is pain-free. For example, pain appears for a day or two a couple of times in a month, as in migraine, or for a couple of weeks once a year, as in cluster headache (see Chapters 9, 10). Pain may become inactive for prolonged periods and be in *remission*, such as observed in cluster headache and in trigeminal neuralgia. Of diagnostic significance is whether the pain *wakes* the patient from sleep since this is common in neurovascular-type pain or pulpitis; see section on sleep disruption below.

Pain *duration* is often included in the classification of orofacial pain syndromes. Masticatory myofascial pain, for example, may last from some hours to the best part of a day with a mean of about 5-6 hours (see Chapter 7). Very short pain attacks—from a few seconds to 2 minutes—characterize trigeminal neuralgia. At the other end of the spectrum tension-type headaches may last a few days and in the chronic form are often continuous. Overlap in pain duration is common among related facial pain syndromes such as the trigeminal autonomic cephalalgias (see Chapter 10, Fig. 10.9A).

A further temporal aspect of pain behaviour relates to the *frequency* of pain attacks. Frequency is the number of attacks over a defined period; per day, week, month or months and in very frequent attacks in units of minutes to hours. As described below pain may be evoked or initiated by external stimuli, in which case the frequency of pain is related to the frequency of the stimulus application. Although specific entities are associated with a characteristic frequency of attacks there may be significant overlap (for example see Chapter 10, Fig. 10.9B). Frequency of attacks is easily obtained from conscientiously kept pain diaries (see below and Box 1.4).

3.1.1.1. Modes of Onset
When strong pain develops very rapidly in an aggressive fashion such as in pulpitis or trigeminal neuralgia, it is termed *paroxysmal*. Pain is *evoked* when it occurs only after stimulation, e.g. cold application to a tooth with a carious lesion; *spontaneous* when it occurs on its own with no external stimulus (e.g. pulpitis); or *triggered* when the pain response is out of proportion to the stimulus, such as is typical for trigeminal neuralgia. Pain is termed *progressive* when it becomes more severe, or stronger, over time.

Pain intensity. Pain intensity is of valuable diagnostic information, and we ask patients to evaluate how strong their pain feels. A simple and quick way is to ask the

Box 1.2 Physical Examination

(Continued from Box 1.1, pain history)
(Including, diagnostic considerations and treatment plan)

1. **Extra-oral examination**
   a. **Head and Neck** (mark any asymmetry, change in color, swellings, etc.) ....
   b. **Lymph nodes** ....
2. **TMJ and masticatory muscles examination** (mark tenderness to palpation on a scale from: 0 = no tenderness, to 3 = very tender)

Muscles	Right	Left	TMJ	Right	Left	Opening	In mm
Masseter			Lat. tenderness			Max. open	
Temporalis			Ext. Miatus Tend.			Deviation (R, L)	
Med. Pterygoid			Right Occ loading			Lat. Move (R)	
Lat. Pterygoid			Left Occ loading			Lat. Move (L)	
Sub-occipital			Click*				
SC mastoid			Reciprocal click*				
Trapezius			Crepitation				

*mark presence and the interincisal opening at which click occurs; SC, sternoeleido; Occ, occsulal

3. **Cranial nerves** *(mark if examined and intact; findings to be summarized under 'remarks')*
   Corneal reflex ... Pupillary reflex ... III, IV, VI eye movements ... Vth sensory ... Vth motor...
   Facial (VII) ... IX ... XI ... XII ...
   Remarks: ....
4. **Intra-oral examination (summary)**
   ....
5. **Ancillary tests, X-rays** (modality and summary of findings)
   ....
6. **Discussion of findings and suggested diagnosis**
   ....
7. **Treatment plan** (medications, other treatment modalities, follow-up planning):
   ....

patient to assess pain intensity on a scale of 0–10 (verbal analogue scale, where 0 means no pain at all, and 10 the most excruciating pain imagined). The use of a visual analogue scale (VAS), where the patient can mark the pain intensity, is also useful and there are a number of such scales available. Chapter 3 gives detailed descriptions of the methods that can be used to evaluate and measure pain intensity and unpleasantness. It is important to note, however, that there is tremendous overlap between intensities reported for craniofacial pain syndromes (Fig. 1.3).

Pain quality. Patients suffering from particular pain syndromes more often employ certain descriptive terms. Trigeminal neuralgia presents with pain that is sharp or electric, whereas other neuropathies have burning pain (Fig. 1.2). Neurovascular pain is usually throbbing in character, although some forms of dental pathologies also possess this quality (Fig. 1.4). We therefore try to elucidate specific descriptions from pain patients by verbal interview or by employing established questionnaires such as the McGill Pain Questionnaire (see Chapter 3).

Aggravating or alleviating factors. We attempt to elucidate if the pain is aggravated by specific factors. These may be local factors such as chewing, ingestion of cold or hot drinks or more generalized stimuli such as exposure to cold air, bending down, physical activity, stress or excitement. Certain syndromes are characterized by

what alleviates or reduces the pain severity: rest or sleep often alleviates pain for patients with migraine. The response to simple analgesics or specific medications may often aid in diagnosis (see, for example, Chapters 10, 11).

Impact on daily function and quality of life. Pain often interferes with basic orofacial functions such as chewing, speaking or even tooth brushing. Secondary results may include detrimental dietary changes, social isolation and dental neglect with ensuing pathology. Additionally most chronic pain states induce an increasingly negative impact on the patient's general physical function and quality of life. This may reduce the patient's work capacity and affect the function of the surrounding family members.

Sleep disruption. Pain-related sleep disorders are very common and underlie many of the affective and cognitive problems in chronic pain patients (Moldofsky 2001a). Prolonged periods of disturbed sleep induce daytime fatigue, sleepiness, difficulties with concentration and reduced coping abilities (Lavigne *et al* 1999; Brousseau *et al* 2003). Additionally disturbed sleep per se may induce generalized muscle pain and reduced pain thresholds and endurance (Moldofsky 2001a). These are important factors to consider in the management of chronic orofacial pain.

Sleep disorders may occur directly because of pain or medical comorbidity (Nicholson and Verma 2004;

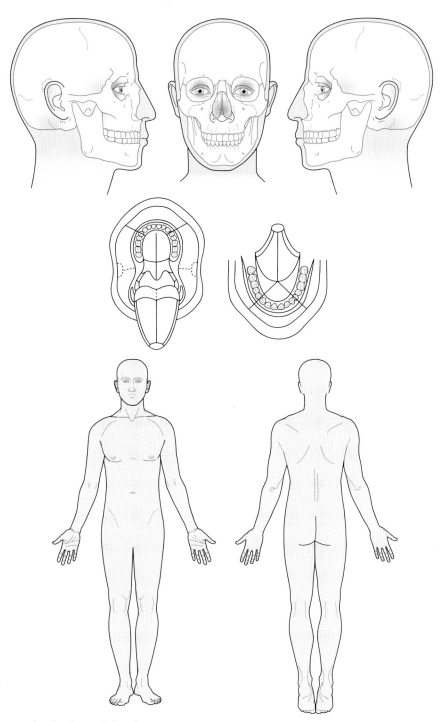

Fig. 1.1 • Suggested diagram for drawing pain location.

Sabatowski *et al* 2004; Kelman and Rains 2005; Zelman *et al* 2006). Acute dental conditions such as irreversible pulpitis or acute dentoalveolar abscess may cause disturbed sleep. The association between such dental conditions and sleep is based on the intensity of pain and not a specific diagnosis (Sharav *et al* 1984). Certain pain syndromes such as the trigeminal autonomic cephalgias (Chapter 10) and fibromyalgia (Chapter 7) may be pathophysiologically related to specific sleep disorders (Moldofsky 2001b; Rains and Poceta 2005). Pain diaries, where the patients record nighttime pain, are often the first sign that patients suffer from disturbed sleep.

However, patients may often report getting a full night's sleep but awaken feeling not rested or unrefreshed. This pattern of unrefreshing sleep may itself aggravate the pain condition and a vicious cycle is set up. Referral for a sleep study will determine the nature of the sleep disorder and help formulate a more comprehensive management approach. The orofacial pain specialist must be cognizant of the structure, control and function of normal sleep and the effects of pain- or stress-related disruption (Vgontzas and Chrousos 2002; Hirshkowitz 2004; Harris 2005).

Associated features. A number of local or general features often consistently accompany pain attacks. These

Box 1.3 Essentials of an Orofacial Pain History

- Location
  - Local: Head, neck, intra oral
  - Other body regions
- Attack Onset
  - Time of day; morning, midday, evening.
  - Month- menstrual
  - Year- seasonal
- Attack duration
  - Seconds, minutes, hours, days
- Attack frequency
  - 24 hour distribution
  - Use of pain diaries
- Onset of present problem
  - Age at onset, associated events, trauma
- Severity
  - Verbal or visual analogue scales
- Quality
  - Verbal descriptions; stabbing, burning
  - Structured questionnaires: McGill
- Associated features or signs
  - Local, systemic
- Aggravating factors
  - Local: thermal, function
  - Systemic: dialysis, stress
- Alleviating factors
  - Endogenous; sleep
  - Exogenous; analgesics, massage
- Impact on daily function
  - Lost work days, marital relations, wakes
- Personal and Social History
  - Occupation, stress, function. Psychosocial evaluation
- Family History
  - Headache, facial pain, bereavement
- Medical status
  - Hypertension
- Drug History
  - Analgesic drug abuse

may be localized as in swelling, redness, sweating, tearing, rhinorrhea, and ptosis, or generalized such as nausea, photophobia and dizziness. There may be sensory changes associated with the pain complaint. Some patients may not be aware of a neurological deficit and we recommend a basic examination of the cranial nerves, as outlined in Table 1.3. If there are findings, the specific modes of sensory changes should be evaluated, as discussed in detail in Chapter 3, Measuring and Assessing Pain.

Drug history as pertains to the pain condition. Patients often forget the drugs and dosages they are taking, and should bring documentation with them on their first visit. The most reliable method is to request a physician's summary or a drug card; medical alert bracelets and hospital release notes are also valuable sources of information. It is imperative to record what drugs the patient has tried to alleviate pain. These may be over-the-counter (OTC) drugs or physician-prescribed. Exact dosage, schedule and duration for each drug trial will indicate whether the full therapeutic potential was exploited.

Listening to the 'language of pain'. Patients with similar pain conditions may describe their pain in very different terms (Zborowsky 1969). This may reflect differences in culture, education or the actual physical experience of pain, no doubt influenced by genetic factors. Patients most often describe their pain in the 'physical' dimension, for example, severity and quality. Thus, a patient with trigeminal neuralgia may relate that their pain is severe and electric, or sharp. Additionally some patients may choose terms that describe an 'emotional' dimension; the same patient with trigeminal neuralgia may add that their pain is unbearable to live with, frightening or depressing. The choice of words to describe pain is therefore important and offers insight into the complete experience that pain patients endure (see Chapters 3 and 4). Psychosocial assessment of pain patients is therefore important (see Chapter 4). The application of questionnaires typically used in such assessments is time consuming but may be invaluable in preparing a treatment plan and assessing prognosis.

3.2. The Physical Examination

The physical examination of a patient who complains of pain aims at identifying the source and cause of pain, i.e. the affected structure and the pathophysiological process. Routine physical examination builds upon the history to formulate a differential diagnosis and may require further special tests.

A routine physical examination of the head and neck should include observation, clinical examination (e.g. palpation) and detection of functional and sensory deviations from the normal. One should look for facial asymmetry, change in colour and deviation or limitation of mouth opening. We palpate cervical and submaxillary lymph nodes, parotid and submandibular salivary glands, masticatory and neck muscles and the TMJ to detect any abnormality in texture, mobility or tenderness. A routine, basic examination of the cranial nerves is also performed (Table 1.3). An intraoral examination seeks possible sources of pain, e.g. carious lesions, mucosal erosions or ulcerations, and includes examination modalities such as inspection, probing, palpation and percussion. We summarize physical findings on a standardized form (Box 1.2), but the clinician may devise his/her own form of examination according to personal preferences.

3.3. The Differential: Confirmatory Tests

In addition to the routine physical examination, several tests may be required to confirm or refute the suspected diagnosis. These may be as simple as the application of a cold stimulus to a tooth with suspected pulpitis or more elaborate sensory testing (see Chapter 3). Radiographs and other means of imaging are still by far the most useful ancillary tests. These include the simple, relatively cheap, 'bite-wing' or periapical dental radiographs

Box 1.4 Model of Pain Diary Employed in Clinical Setting. QOL=Quality of Life

Patient's name:
On a scale of 0 to 10, when: 0=No pain, and 10=Strongest pain possible, mark 4 times a day your pain for that period (AM=morning, Mid.=midday, PM=afternoon. Ni.=night, only if wakes).

Day and date	Pain intensity				Medication prescribed	Remarks	
	AM	Mid.	PM	Ni.		Side effects, escape drugs (No., type)	Effect on QOL
1							
2							
3							
4							
5							
6							
20							
21							
22							
23							
24							
25							
26							
27							
28							

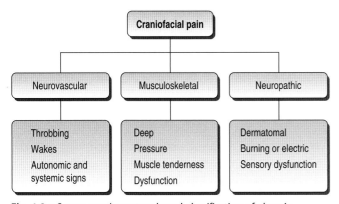

Fig. 1.2 • Symptomatic, system-based classification of chronic craniofacial pain.

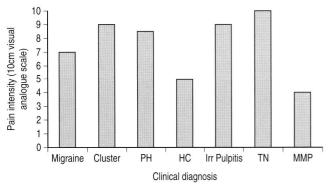

Fig. 1.3 • Mean pain severity in various craniofacial pain disorders. PH=paroxysmal hemicrania, HC=hemicrania continua, Irr Pulpitis= irreversible pulpitis, TN=trigeminal neuralgia, MMP=masticatory myofascial pain.

(Chapter 5) and the more sophisticated, neuroimaging techniques such as computerized tomography (CT) or magnetic resonance imaging (MRI).

The decision when to refer a patient with chronic orofacial pain for advanced neuroimaging is often complex, particularly under current financial constraints in healthcare systems. Most studies dealing with this issue relate specifically to headache or trigeminal neuralgia, but the guidelines may easily be adopted for orofacial pain in general (Frishberg *et al* 2000; Sandrini *et al* 2004).

Among patients with normal neurological examinations and headaches diagnosed as migraine or tension type, the prevalence of significant intracranial abnormalities on neuroimaging is approximately 0.2 and 0%, respectively (Frishberg *et al* 2000). Undiagnosable headaches have a higher prevalence of intracranial abnormalities but studies report varying, inconsistent figures ranging from 0 to 6.7% (Frishberg *et al* 2000). Positive neurological findings are intuitively suggestive of an intracranial abnormality; see also trigeminal neuralgia discussion in Chapter 11. However, the predictive value of an intracranial abnormality by a positive neurological exam is surprisingly low at around 3%; this is due to the very low initial probability of intracranial abnormalities. Patient complaints of neurological symptoms will significantly increase this risk (Frishberg *et al* 2000). The absence of findings on the neurological examination significantly decreases (but does not eliminate) the likelihood of finding a significant lesion on neuroimaging (Frishberg *et al* 2000). When considering neuroimaging the orofacial pain practitioner should

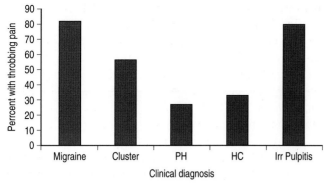

Fig. 1.4 • Percent of patients reporting a throbbing quality in various craniofacial pain disorders. PH=paroxysmal hemicrania, HC= hemicrania continua, Irr Pulpitis=irreversible pulpitis.

specifically request extracranial areas to be examined (jaws, submandibular space) as these are often excluded on routine imaging.

The indications for advanced neuroimaging are shown in Box 1.5. In individual cases with pronounced anxiety, imaging may be indicated to alleviate emotional distress. The number of studies comparing CT to MRI is limited but suggests that MRI may be more sensitive than CT for identifying clinically insignificant abnormalities. However, MRI may not be more sensitive for identifying clinically significant pathology relevant to the cause of headache (Frishberg *et al* 2000). Thus the choice of modality and the region to be scanned needs to be based on a differential diagnosis.

Table 1.3	Basic Cranial Nerve Examination	
Test	**Result**	**Pathway/Cranial Nerve**
Group A (Cranial nerves I, II, III, IV, VI and VIII)		
Shine a light into the patient's pupil (test both sides)	Tests the pupillary light reflex: Pupils should constrict bilaterally	Afferent is the optic nerve (I) and efferent the occulomotor (III)
Ask the patient to close his eyes; seal one nostril and smell coffee, tobacco or eugenol packed in unmarked containers	Positive identification of smell	Tests olfactory nerve function (II). Note that patients with colds or allergies may have a reduced ability
Ask the patient to seal one ear and whisper numbers contralaterally	Accurate repetition	Tests the vestibulocochlear nerve (VIII)
Ask the patient to follow your finger with his eyes in the following directions:	Accurate and smooth tracking of finger movements by both eyes simultaneously	Tests the occulomotor (III), trochlear (IV) and abducens (VI) nerves
Group B (Cranial nerves V, VII)		
Ask the patient to look laterally and up with their eyes: gently stimulate the cornea with a wisp of cotton wool	Tests the corneal reflex; causes immediate closure of the eyelids	Afferent is the trigeminal nerve and efferent the facial. Contact lenses will interfere
Ask the patient to identify, with eyes closed, sharp, blunt and thermal stimuli in the upper, middle and lower face	Accurate identification of stimuli and area tested	Sensory branches of the trigeminal (V) nerve
Ask the patient to clench teeth	Feel for symmetrical contraction of masticatory (e.g. masseter) muscles	Motor branch of the trigeminal (V) nerve
Ask patient to raise eyebrows, close their eyes, smile and whistle	Symmetrical movements, good muscle strength	Facial (VII) nerve function
Place sweet, salty, sour stimuli on tongue	Accurate identification	Chorda tympani branch of facial nerve
Group C (Cranial nerves IX, XI and XII)		
Ask patient to rotate head to both sides, then raise shoulders—all against mild manual resistance	Symmetrical movement. Good muscle strength	Accessory (XI) nerve
Ask the patient to say 'aah'	The uvula and soft palate should be raised symmetrically	Glossopharyngeal (IX) nerve
Ask the patient to perform tongue movements		Hypoglossal (XII) nerve

Clear Indication

- Unexplained abnormal neurological finding (e.g. numbness)

Possible Indication

- Headache worsened by Valsalva manoeuvre
- Headache causing awakening from sleep
- New headache in the older population
- Progressively worsening headache or rapidly increasing headache frequency

3.4. The Diagnosis

Routines in medicine are very effective, as they add confidence especially to the inexperienced, sometimes save time, and ensure a comprehensive gathering of clinical information. Thus, in principle, the diagnosis should follow the history, physical examination and ancillary tests. However, gathering information on its own does not make a diagnosis! What is one then supposed to do with all this information? As any experienced clinician will attest to, clinical information gathering is a back and forth process, mainly dictated by the diagnostic process and the possible differential diagnoses considered. Indeed, the experienced clinician often formulates initial diagnostic hypotheses very early on in the clinical setting. At a certain point, and usually quite early, the routine is departed from and these hypotheses are tested through the asking of specific questions. The difference is that while 'routine' questions expect an 'open' answer, such as 'Where do you feel your pain?', most 'hypothesis-generated questions' aim at a 'closed' yes or no answer. For example, 'Does bending your head aggravate pain?' in patients where sinusitis is suspected, or 'Does the tooth react painfully to a cold stimulus?' when a carious lesion in a vital tooth is suspected. If the answer, whether to an oral question or to a physical test, 'satisfies' the hypothesis the examiner usually proceeds with another hypothesis-generated question, but if the answer leads to a dead-end clinicians often return to the routine methodology. Ultimately, enough 'positive' pieces of information have been clustered together to confirm the hypothesis (diagnosis), and usually also some 'negative' pieces of information that enable one to refute other possible diagnoses.

Clustering of information is a very useful tool in the process of decision-making, as it reduces the number of fragments of information one deals with and facilitates the process. Over the years, we have developed a clustering system for diagnostic entities that is especially useful for the more difficult diagnostic process of *chronic* orofacial pain. This system divides chronic orofacial pain into three main symptomatic classes: musculoskeletal,

neurovascular and neuropathic (Benoliel et al 1994), detailed in Fig. 1.2, and Box 1.6. Examine these entities and the cluster of signs and symptoms relevant for each class of these diagnostic entities. After studying Box 1.6, we suggest one proceed to Table 1.4 for a description of the diagnostic process generated by hypotheses based on pain location, and to Table 1.5 when based on the temporal behaviour and characteristics of the pain. This system allows for proceeding from signs and symptoms, as presented by the patient, to the disease process hypothesized by the clinician ('Diagnostic hypothesis'). It is entirely legitimate, after considering a diagnosis, to keep testing it by gathering further information. Referring to points addressed in the column of 'Information critical for hypothesis testing' of Tables 1.4 and 1.5 further specific information is requested at all levels: history, physical examination and ancillary tests. The ability to start the diagnostic process from pain-location (Table 1.4) or from pain-characteristics (Table 1.5) allows for versatility of the interview method and for cross-checking one's hypothesis generation in more than one way.

This method for diagnosis of chronic orofacial pain, while presented at the introductory part of the book, is a recommended reference when reading subsequent chapters. It is especially useful for the chapters dealing with chronic orofacial pain of musculoskeletal, neurovascular or neuropathic origin.

4. The Pain Patient

The pain patient who is undiagnosed may be particularly worried that they have cancer or some other threatening disease. Prospective studies suggest a relationship between psychological distress and pain, which may operate both ways; see Chapter 4 (Magni *et al* 1994; Hotopf *et al* 1998). A high level of psychological distress is often a predictor of the onset of future pain or the development of chronic pain. Conversely, ongoing orofacial pain is often associated with psychological distress (Macfarlane *et al* 2002b). Research shows that patients with chronic craniofacial pain suffer from psychological distress, increased depression, impaired social performance and decreased quality of life (see Chapters 7, 9–11). Thus, chronic orofacial pain patients develop maladaptive or illness behaviour patterns (Macfarlane *et al* 2002b) that are important factors affecting their management and prognosis.

5. The Confounders: Patient Variability, Impact on Diagnosis and Therapy

Patients differ from each other in many respects that influence diagnostic considerations, for example, responses to

Box 1.6 Typical Clusters of Signs and Symptoms in the Main Chronic Orofacial Pain Entities

1. Musculoskeletal Orofacial Pain (MOP)

TMJ (temporomandibular joint pain)

- ☐ Pain fairly localized to TMJ area
- ☐ Click/crepitation of TMJ
- ☐ Deviation of mouth opening toward affected joint
- ☐ TMJ painful on palpation
- ☐ Pain on function (biting on contralateral side to affected TMJ)

MMP (masticatory myofascial pain)

- ☐ Pain, mostly unilateral, at angle of mandible and front of ear, diffuse
- ☐ Masticatory muscle tenderness on palpation, mostly on affected side
- ☐ Jaw dysfunction (limited opening, tiredness on chewing)
- ☐ Pain on function (such as: yawning, chewing, talking)

TTH (tension-type headache)

- ☐ Pain, bilateral, at temples and occipital areas
- ☐ Pain pressing and annoying
- ☐ Periodic or chronic
- ☐ Anorexia
- ☐ Nausea

2. Neurovascular Craniofacial Pain (NCP)

Migraine

- ☐ Strong, unilateral headache
- ☐ Pain is throbbing
- ☐ Periodic (day or two, couple of times a month)
- ☐ Occasionally wakes from sleep toward morning
- ☐ Photophobia/phonophobia
- ☐ Nausea and vomiting
- ☐ Tearing, occasional
- ☐ Patient seeks rest in a dark quiet place

CHA (cluster headache)

- ☐ Periorbital unilateral very strong, throbbing pain
- ☐ Clusters of active periods of pain (6-10 weeks, mostly once a year)
- ☐ At active period 1-2 attacks/24 hours, clockwise regularity
- ☐ Typical attack 45-60 minutes duration
- ☐ Wakes from sleep (REM locked?)
- ☐ Tearing, one eye on affected side
- ☐ Rhinorrhea, one nostril on affected side
- ☐ Redness, ptosis and miosis of eye on affected side possible
- ☐ Patient paces around restlessly

CPH (chronic paroxysmal hemicrania)

- ☐ Periorbital and temporal, unilateral strong pain
- ☐ Short (minutes) paroxysmal pain attacks
- ☐ Occasionally wakes from sleep

- ☐ Tearing, cojunctival injection, one eye on affected side
- ☐ Rhinorrhea, one nostril on affected side
- ☐ Head movement may trigger pain

SUNCT (short lasting unilateral, neuralgiform, headache attacks with conjunctival injection and tearing)

- ☐ Periorbital unilateral severe pain
- ☐ Paroxysmal short (seconds) attacks
- ☐ Pain precipitated by touch of eyebrow
- ☐ Conjunctival injection, tearing

NVOP (neurovascular orofacial pain)

- ☐ Mid-face, peri- and intra-oral pain
- ☐ Spontaneous or evoked (mostly by cold food ingestion)
- ☐ Occasional swelling or redness of cheek
- ☐ Wakes from sleep
- ☐ Nausea
- ☐ Tearing, one eye on affected side, possible
- ☐ Mostly periodic but may be chronic

HC (hemicrania continua)

- ☐ Unilateral, moderate-intensity, headache with no side shifts
- ☐ Chronic (>3 months), daily non-remitting
- ☐ Rarely wakes from sleep
- ☐ Mild tearing, one eye on affected side
- ☐ Mild rhinorrhea, one nostril on affected side
- ☐ Occasionally, eye redness, ptosis and miosis on affected side,

3. Neuropathic Orofacial Pain (NOP)

Trigeminal neuralgia (TN)

- ☐ Unilateral pain trigeminal nerve area (mostly 2nd and 3rd divisions)
- ☐ Paroxysmal electric-like very short (seconds) strong pain
- ☐ Pain attack accompanied by facial tic
- ☐ Triggered by light touch, vibration, and other non-painful stimuli
- ☐ After triggering there is a refractory period
- ☐ No sensory deficit

Traumatic neuropathies (CRPS-I/II)

- ☐ Pain location associated with history of trauma
- ☐ Pain continuous, mostly burning quality
- ☐ Allodynia
- ☐ Oedema/redness
- ☐ Trophic changes (mostly in CRPS/II)
- ☐ Sensory deficit (in CRPS/II)
- ☐ Dysaesthesia (in CRPS/II)

TMJ = temporomandibular joint; REM = rapid eye movement; CRPS = complex regional pain syndrome.

Table 1.4	Diagnostic Process and Hypothesis Generation Based on Pain Location	
Location (Unilateral)	Diagnostic Hypothesis	Information Critical for Hypothesis Testing
Frontotemporal*	Migraine Hemicrania continua	Pain attack duration Patterns of periodicity Photo- and/or phonophobia Nausea
Orbital and periorbital	Cluster headache Paroxysmal hemicrania SUNCT	Pain attack duration Attacks/day Periodicity Tearing, rhinorrhea SUNCT trigged by touch
Preauricular, angle of mandible	TMJ pain Masticatory muscle pain	Aggravated by chewing Mouth opening dysfunction TMJ tenderness, click Masticatory muscle tenderness
Mid-face, perioral or intraoral	Trigeminal neuralgia NVOP	Attack duration Triggered by touch, vibration Evoked by cold/hot foods Tearing, rhinorrhea

*If pain is bilateral, consider tension-type headache (TTH).
SUNCT=short lasting unilateral, neuralgiform headache attacks with conjunctival injection and tearing; TMJ=temporomandibular joint; NVOP=neurovascular orofacial pain.

Table 1.5	Diagnostic Process and Hypothesis Generation Based on Temporal Pain Behaviour and Characteristics	
Temporal Pain Behaviour and Characteristics	Diagnostic Hypothesis	Information Critical for Hypothesis Testing
Short, paroxysmal	Trigeminal neuralgia Paroxysmal hemicrania SUNCT	Pain location Duration of pain attack Triggering/evoking stimuli Autonomic signs Wakes from sleep
Periodic, throbbing	Migraine Cluster headache NVOP	Pain location Duration of pain attack Periodicity Autonomic signs Nausea
Continuous, pressing	TTH TMJ MMP Hemicrania continua CRPS-I/II	Pain location, Laterality Aggravates by chewing Dysfunctional mouth opening TMJ tenderness, Click Masticatory muscle tenderness History of trauma Sensory abnormality

SUNCT=short lasting unilateral, neuralgiform headache attacks with conjunctival injection and tearing; NVOP=neurovascular orofacial pain; TTH=tension-type headache; TMJ=temporomandibular joint; MMP=masticatory muscle pain; CRPS=complex regional pain syndrome (types I or II).

pain medications, attitudes to healthcare and behavioural responses to chronic pain. Below we discuss the effects of three important factors: genetics, gender and culture and ethnicity.

5.1. Genetics

The sequencing of the human genome has elucidated the presence of 30,000-40,000 human genes. Some of these genes and protein end-products will emerge as new therapeutic targets for chronic pain. For some pain syndromes, we have information on genetic polymorphisms that may affect disease occurrence; this area is covered in the clinical chapters (7, 9–11). Information concerning genetically controlled drug toxicity and common adverse drug reactions will be available on an individual basis. Genetically governed interindividual differences are also found in the drug-transport proteins and drug targets (receptors), altering the pharmacokinetics and

pharmacodynamics of a variety of drugs. For example, the analgesic potency of morphine is partly dictated by variations in the expression of mu-opioid receptors. Polymorphisms in this receptor lead to interindividual differences in responses to pain and its relief by opioid drugs (Uhl et al 1999). Pain modulation is impaired in certain ethnic groups and it is postulated that some of this effect may be related to increased stress (Mechlin et al 2005). It becomes clear that genetic considerations will become integral to the diagnostic and therapeutic process of chronic pain.

5.2. Gender

There have been extensive reports on the effects of gender on the epidemiology of pain syndromes and on pain thresholds. Women suffer significantly more from migraines, tension-type headaches, facial pains, fibromyalgia and TMDs (Jensen et al 1993; Rasmussen 1995;

Rauhala *et al* 2000; Breslau and Rasmussen 2001; Huang *et al* 2002; Yunus, 2002). In general, females do not seek treatment for orofacial pain significantly more than men (Macfarlane *et al* 2003). However, in temporomandibular disorders females usually demand more care than men (Epker and Gatchel 2000), probably related to more severe symptoms (Levitt and McKinney 1994). Both hormone replacement therapy and use of oral contraceptives have been associated with increased risk of TMD (LeResche *et al* 1997; Dao *et al* 1998); see Chapter 7. Under experimental conditions, women consistently demonstrate a lowered pain threshold, often affected by the stage of the menstrual cycle and by exogenous hormones such as oral contraceptives (Fillingim *et al* 1998; Fillingim and Ness 2000). Injection of capsaicin into the forehead induced trigeminal sensitization and evoked gender-specific sensory and vasomotor responses, with menstruating females generally showing the strongest manifestations (Gazerani *et al* 2005). Post-extraction and experimental pain in women responds better to opioid therapy than that in men (Gear *et al* 1999; Fillingim 2002). However, males and females may differ in their response to nonsteroidal anti-inflammatory drugs (NSAIDs), and females enjoy less analgesia with ibuprofen than males (Walker and Carmody 1998). Others found no gender-based differences using ibuprofen nor in the level of induced placebo analgesia after tooth extraction (Averbuch and Katzper 2001, 2002).

The practical applications of gender differences are still unclear. However, menstrual-related changes in pain sensitivity associated with increased analgesic use, epidemiological data concerning pain syndromes in women and pharmacological traits particular to each gender are areas in which the continued accumulation of knowledge will aid the pain physician.

5.3. Culture and Ethnicity

The role of ethnicity in the individual's reaction to pain was highlighted almost forty years ago in the now classical book *People in Pain* (Zborowsky 1969). The book deals with the attitudes and reaction to pain in three American ethnic groups and points to striking differences. More recent research examines racial and ethnic variability affecting the pain experience (Morris 2001; Lasch 2002;).

The terms 'culture', 'ethnicity' and 'race' are often used interchangeably, most probably because of the difficulty in accurately defining them. Because of massive population migration, intermarriage and genetic polymorphisms, populations such as Africans, Whites and Asians are more genetically heterogeneous within than across groups. Indeed, anthropologists and biologists are increasingly defining race as a social construct and not a scientific category (Morris 2001). This is not to say that genetically distinct physiological or medical traits in 'ethnic' populations (e.g. Tay-Sachs or drug metabolism such as glucose-6-phosphate dehydrogenase enzyme deficiency) do not exist, but these traits cannot solely define ethnicity.

Cultural and social factors are the foundation for the expression and management of pain (Lasch 2002). These factors affect our patients' experience of pain, behavioural responses, seeking of healthcare and adherence to treatment (Hobara 2005). In a multiracial environment we must understand these factors and attempt to positively modify the way we practise pain medicine. Examples that highlight the influence of culture and beliefs on the experience and interpretation of pain include the reliance of some ethnic groups on religion to cope with pain (Morris 2001; Lasch 2002) and differences in the use of local anaesthetic for dental treatment (Moore *et al* 1998a,b). Pain sensitivity, secondary hyperalgesic area and pressure pain thresholds following capsaicin injection to the forehead were assessed in which South Indians showed significantly greater pain responses than Caucasians (Gazerani and Arendt-Nielsen 2005). Ethnic differences in pain tolerance reflect traits in the affective dimension of pain; these differences are not innate but learned and even modified at later stages by the environment (Morris 2001).

However, it is becoming increasingly important to appreciate cultural factors that influence healthcare workers. Although no difference has been observed between ethnic groups in the amounts of self-administered analgesia for acute pain, significant differences were shown to occur between the amount of analgesia prescribed to these subgroups (Ng *et al* 1996). Ethnocultural background may influence a clinician's assessment of pain intensity in patients (Sheiner *et al* 1999), and minorities may be at risk for inadequate pain control (Lasch 2002). Therefore, one must be aware of the cultural factors that affect the way patients respond to pain and its management, as well as understand the way the 'ethnicity' of clinicians and patients may influence healthcare delivery.

6. The Aims: Treatment and Follow-up

The initial aim of the diagnostic process is to initiate the patient on a treatment plan; the ultimate, but elusive, aim is the eradication of pain. This may involve multiple modalities that ideally aim to eradicate pain. Patients with acute pain are usually alarmed and made anxious by this sudden, mostly unexpected, change in their state of well being, and need a lot of reassurance. An accurate diagnosis, empathic explanation and effective treatment are important in reassuring patients and obtaining their confidence. Treatment of acute pain often includes physical intervention, e.g. tooth pulp extirpation, and the use of analgesics (see Chapters 5, 6 and 15). Dentists do this almost every day and the vast majority of patients enjoy rapid and complete relief from acute dental pain within a short time.

Chronic pain, as its name implies, is long-standing and is often associated with comorbidities such as negative changes in function, drug abuse, psychosocial dysfunction and depression (see Chapter 4 and also 7, 9–11). Consequently the aims of therapy in chronic or recurrent pain cannot be limited to the alleviation of pain but must include the restoration of quality of life and function, and the prevention or elimination of drug abuse. Chronic orofacial pain is difficult to eradicate, particularly certain syndromes such as traumatic neuropathies, which is why we refer to the 'management' of chronic orofacial pain rather than its 'treatment'. It is important to explain to the patient the goals of pain management, often defined as >50% reductions in pain intensity or frequency, which are often way below the patient's initial expectations. Furthermore, results may not be obtained as quickly as patients would wish; multiple drug trials for months at a time, prolonged physiotherapy and psychological interventions are often needed before attaining a reasonable, 'successful', result.

6.1. Success

So how do we define success? As much as pain is an individual experience, a 'successful outcome' is often an individual, highly personalized result. Some patients with a reduction of more than 50% in pain intensity following permanent ingestion of psychotropic drugs may be dissatisfied, unhappy and incapable of maintaining normal employment. On the other hand, a patient may be able to function normally following less than 50% reduction in pain intensity obtained with physiotherapy and cognitive behavioural therapy (see Chapters 4, 7). Just as we have come to appreciate that pain is a complex and individual experience, therapeutic outcome needs to assess a broader spectrum including factors such as restoration of function and psychosocial status. In a highly simplified paradigm, we essentially need to balance the patient's expectations with the physician's possibilities. A more realistic model appreciates that the patient's expectations are a complex result of a painful experience within a context of cultural and ethnic influences, current employment, views on health and disease and other variables.

6.2. Follow-up

The use of pain diaries is very useful for follow-up, assessing treatment results, and often for confirming diagnosis. To ensure compliance, a diary is kept as simple as possible (Box 1.4), but can be modified to meet individual needs. The patient records pain intensity and its effect on quality of life on a numerical scale from 0 to 10, at different times of the day (including night if the pain wakes from sleep). The diary also records dosages of the prescribed drugs, escape drugs if utilized and adverse pharmacological effects. The diary is sufficient for 28 days and makes it possible to adjust treatment according to pain response and side effects. Patients' reaction to the utilization of the pain diary is usually very positive; they feel their pain symptoms are taken seriously, and are reassured by the attention given to their response to therapy.

In addition to the above, the pain diary is essential in controlling drug abuse. Chronic pain patients often abuse many drugs, some prescribed and some obtained OTC. Often drugs prescribed in the past are still taken and added to those currently used; unless specifically instructed, patients often 'forget' to stop previous medications. The recording of 'escape drugs' in the diary (usually analgesics, utilized to control breakthrough pain), in addition to the prescribed medications, facilitates the detection of drug abuse. Drug consumption in response to breakthrough pain is a learned response that may lead to dependence. By following the pattern and amount of escape drug used, the physician can advise the patient on adequate scheduling and help break the habit of taking additional medications. This is achieved by shifting the patient from 'on demand' to 'per schedule' consumption of the escape drug, and gradually decreasing the amount consumed. As a rule, for chronic pain it is always advisable to prescribe medications per schedule rather than per demand, as the latter usually leads to more drug abuse and dependence (Stimmel 1983).

6.3. Bottom Line

While we aim to eradicate or alleviate all pain, we are a long way from optimal patient care. Some of the best drugs will offer substantial relief to some of the patients, but certainly not all patients will be pain-free despite the treatment (see clinical chapters and Chapter 16). For many patients, and particularly those who do not respond well to therapy, means for better coping with agony and despair must be offered. We can help the patient to increase adaptive skills in order to minimize pain-related stress and avoid unnecessary illness behaviour by means of psychological pain management, such as cognitive behavioural therapy (CBT). This approach, discussed in detail in Chapter 4 on the psychological aspects of chronic orofacial pain, offers an effective mode for improving coping skills. Of special concern are also patients with trauma-related pain, who many times suffer from post-traumatic stress disorder (PTSD) and need early psychological intervention (see Chapter 13).

7. The Set-up: A Pain Clinic

Pain is one of the prime reasons for seeking medical attention. In most instances of orofacial pain, the patient's main route is to look for help at the dental clinic (see above), or see the family physician. In most cases, especially those with acute pain, patient management and treatment result are easily attained. However, when things get complicated and as the orofacial region is anatomically dense the orofacial pain clinic becomes a necessity. The pain clinic and the physicians who run it approach chronic pain as a disease and offer expertise on the pathophysiology of pain, pain medication for both acute and chronic pain and alternative treatment options; see Chapters 4, 12, 15–17. An additional strength of the pain clinic is its ability to utilize a multidisciplinary team approach that involves other professionals, e.g. psychologists, physiotherapists. The concept of the pain clinic is not new and has developed over the years from a centre offering management alternatives for pre-diagnosed patients (e.g. intrathecal injections, regional blocks, surgical interventions) to a centre that diagnoses, manages and follows up patients in pain.

The orofacial pain clinic is therefore involved in the diagnostic process and management of craniofacial pain. Although we rely heavily on pharmacotherapy, we perform other modalities as appropriate, such as muscle trigger-point injection, arthrocentesis of the TMJ, acupuncture, hypnotherapy, night guards and physiotherapy. We often consult with our colleagues, especially from neurosurgery, neurology and otolaryngology, and refer patients for psychiatric evaluation and for CBT. This intimate relation with other members of the medical community has become a two-way channel for patient referral, communication, and the constant enrichment of knowledge.

References

Averbuch M, Katzper M (2002) A search for sex differences in response to analgesia. *Arch Intern Med* **160**(22):3424–3428.

Benoliel R, Sharav Y (2006) Accurate diagnosis of facial pain. *Cephalalgia* **26**(7):902; author reply 903.

Benoliel R, Eliav E, Elishoov H, *et al* (1994) Diagnosis and treatment of persistent pain after trauma to the head and neck. *J Oral Maxillofac Surg* **52**(11):1138–1147; discussion 1147–1148.

Benoliel R, Elishoov H, Sharav Y (1997) Orofacial pain with vascular-type features. *Oral Surg Oral Med Oral Pathol Oral Radiol Endod* **84**(5):506–512.

Breslau N, Rasmussen BK (2001) The impact of migraine: Epidemiology, risk factors, and co-morbidities. *Neurology* **56**(6 Suppl 1):S4–S12.

Brousseau M, Manzini C, Thie N, *et al* (2003) Understanding and managing the interaction between sleep and pain: an update for the dentist. *J Can Dent Assoc* **69**(7):437–442.

Czerninsky R, Benoliel R, Sharav Y (1999) Odontalgia in vascular orofacial pain. *J Orofac Pain* **13**(3):196–200.

Dao TT, Knight K, Ton-That V (1998) Modulation of myofascial pain by the reproductive hormones: a preliminary report. *J Prosthet Dent* **79**(6):663–670.

Dworkin SF, LeResche L (1992) Research diagnostic criteria for temporomandibular disorders: review, criteria, examinations and specifications, critique. *J Craniomandib Disord* **6**(4):301–355.

Epker J, Gatchel RJ (2000) Prediction of treatment-seeking behavior in acute TMD patients: practical application in clinical settings. *J Orofac Pain* **14**(4): 303–309.

Fillingim RB (2002) Sex differences in analgesic responses: evidence from experimental pain models. *Eur J Anaesthesiol Suppl* **26**:16–24.

Fillingim RB, Ness TJ (2000) Sex-related hormonal influences on pain and analgesic responses. *Neurosci Biobehav Rev* **24**(4): 485–501.

Fillingim RB, Maixner W, Kincaid S, *et al* (1998) Sex differences in temporal summation but not sensory-discriminative processing of thermal pain. *Pain* **75**(1):121–127.

Frishberg BM, Rosenberg JH, Matchar DB, *et al* (2000) *Evidence-Based Guidelines in the Primary Care Setting: Neuroimaging in Patients with Nonacute Headache*. American Academy of Neurology. Available at: http://www.aan.com/professionals/practice/pdfs/gl0088.pdf.

Gazerani P, Arendt-Nielsen L (2005) The impact of ethnic differences in response to capsaicin-induced trigeminal sensitization. *Pain* **117**(1–2): 223–229.

Gazerani P, Andersen OK, Arendt-Nielsen L (2005) A human experimental capsaicin model for trigeminal sensitization. Gender-specific differences. *Pain* **118**(1–2):155–163.

Gear RW, Miaskowski C, Gordon NC, *et al* (1999) The kappa opioid nalbuphine produces gender- and dose-dependent analgesia and antianalgesia in patients with postoperative pain. *Pain* **83**(2):339–345.

Goulet JP, Lavigne GJ, Lund JP (1995) Jaw pain prevalence among French-speaking Canadians in Quebec and related symptoms of temporomandibular disorders. *J Dent Res* **74** (11):1738–1744.

Harris CD (2005) Neurophysiology of sleep and wakefulness. *Respir Care Clin N Am* **11**(4):567–586.

Hirshkowitz M (2004) Normal human sleep: an overview. *Med Clin North Am* **88**(3):551–565, vii.

Hobara M (2005) Beliefs about appropriate pain behavior: cross-cultural and sex differences between Japanese and Euro-Americans. *Eur J Pain* **9**(4):389–393.

Hotopf M, Mayou R, Wadsworth M, *et al* (1998) Temporal relationships between physical symptoms and psychiatric disorder. Results from a national birth cohort. *Br J Psychiatry* **173**:255–261.

Huang GJ, LeResche L, Critchlow CW, *et al* (2002) Risk factors for diagnostic subgroups of painful temporomandibular disorders (TMD). *J Dent Res* **81**(4):284–288.

Iadarola JM, Caudle RM (1997) Good pain, bad pain. *Science* **278** (5336):239–240.

Jensen R, Rasmussen BK, Pedersen B, *et al* (1993) Prevalence of oromandibular dysfunction in a general population. *J Orofac Pain* **7**(2):175–182.

Kelman L, Rains JC (2005) Headache and sleep: examination of sleep patterns and complaints in a large clinical sample of migraineurs. *Headache* **45**(7): 904–910.

Lasch KE (2002) *Culture and Pain*. Pain, Clinical Updates; X(5). Available at: http://www.iasp-pain.org

Lavigne GJ, Goulet JP, Zuconni M, *et al* (1999) Sleep disorders and the dental patient: an overview. *Oral Surg Oral Med Oral Pathol Oral Radiol Endod* **88**(3):257–272.

LeResche L, Saunders K, Von Korff MR, *et al* (1997) Use of exogenous hormones and risk of temporomandibular disorder pain. *Pain* **69**(1–2):153–160.

Levitt SR, McKinney MW (1994) Validating the TMJ scale in a national sample of 10,000 patients: demographic and epidemiologic characteristics. *J Orofac Pain* **8**(1):25–35.

Macfarlane TV, Blinkhorn AS, Davies RM, *et al* (2002a) Oro-facial pain in the community: prevalence and associated impact. *Community Dent Oral Epidemiol* **30**(1):52–60.

Macfarlane TV, Kincey J, Worthington HV (2002b) The association between psychological factors and oro-facial pain: a community-based study. *Eur J Pain* **6**(6):427–434.

Macfarlane TV, Blinkhorn AS, Davies RM, *et al* (2003) Factors associated with health care seeking behaviour for orofacial pain in the general population. *Community Dent Health* **20** (1):20–26.

McMillan AS, Wong MC, Zheng J, *et al* (2006) Prevalence of orofacial pain and treatment seeking in Hong Kong Chinese. *J Orofac Pain* **20**(3):218–225.

Magni G, Moreschi C, Rigatti-Luchini S, *et al* (1994) Prospective study on the relationship between depressive symptoms and chronic musculoskeletal pain. *Pain* **56**(3):289–297.

Mechlin MB, Maixner W, Light KC, *et al* (2005) African Americans show alterations in endogenous pain regulatory mechanisms and reduced pain tolerance to experimental pain procedures. *Psychosom Med* **67**(6):948–956.

Merskey H, Bogduk N (1994) *Classification of Chronic Pain: Descriptions of Chronic Pain Syndromes and Definition of Pain Terms*, 2nd edn. Seattle: IASP Press.

Moldofsky H (2001a) Sleep and pain. *Sleep Med Rev* **5**(5):385–396.

Moldofsky HK (2001b) Disordered sleep in fibromyalgia and related myofascial facial pain conditions. *Dent Clin North Am* **45**(4):701–713.

Moore R, Brodsgaard I, Mao TK, *et al* (1998a) Acute pain and use of local anesthesia: tooth drilling and childbirth labor pain beliefs among Anglo-Americans, Chinese, and Scandinavians. *Anesth Prog* **45**(1):29–37.

Moore R, Brodsgaard I, Mao TK, *et al* (1998b) Perceived need for local anesthesia in tooth drilling among Anglo-Americans, Chinese, and Scandinavians. *Anesth Prog* **45**(1):22–28.

Morris DB (2001) *Ethnicity and Pain.* Pain, Clinical Updates 2001; IX(4). Available at: http://www.iasp-pain.org

Ng B, Dimsdale JE, Rollnik JD, *et al* (1996) The effect of ethnicity on prescriptions for patient-controlled analgesia for post-operative pain. *Pain* **66**(1):9–12.

Ng KF, Tsui SL, Chan WS (2002) Prevalence of common chronic pain in Hong Kong adults. *Clin J Pain* **18**(5):275–281.

Nicholson B, Verma S (2004) Comorbidities in chronic neuropathic pain. Pain Med **5**(Suppl 1):S9–S27.

Okeson JP(1996). *Orofacial Pain: Guidelines for Assessment, Classification, and Management.* American Academy of Orofacial Pain. Illinois: Quintessence Publishing.

Olesen J, Bousser M-G, Diener HC, *et al* (2004) The International Classification of Headache Disorders, 2nd edition. *Cephalalgia* **24**(Suppl 1):24–150.

Rains JC, Poceta JS (2005) Sleep-related headache syndromes. *Semin Neurol* **25**(1):69–80.

Rasmussen BK (1995) Epidemiology of headache. *Cephalalgia* **15** (1):45–68.

Rauhala K, Oikarinen KS, Jarvelin MR, *et al* (2000) Facial pain and temporomandibular disorders: an epidemiological study of the Northern Finland 1966 Birth Cohort. *Cranio* **18**(1):40–46.

Riley JL, 3rd, Gilbert GH, Heft MW (1998) Orofacial pain symptom prevalence: selective sex differences in the elderly? *Pain* **76**(1-2):97–104.

Sabatowski R, Galvez R, Cherry DA, *et al* (2004) Pregabalin reduces pain and improves sleep and mood disturbances in patients with post-herpetic neuralgia: results of a randomised, placebo-controlled clinical trial. *Pain* **109**(1–2):26–35.

Sandrini G, Friberg L, Janig W, *et al* (2004) Neurophysiological tests and neuroimaging procedures in non-acute headache: guidelines and recommendations. *Eur J Neurol* **11**(4):217–224.

Sharav Y (2005) Orofacial pain: how much is it a local phenomenon? *J Am Dent Assoc* **136**(4):432, 434, 436.

Sharav Y, Benoliel R (2001) Primary vascular-type craniofacial pain. *Compend Contin Educ Dent* **22**(2):119–122, 124–126, 128 *passim*; quiz 132.

Sharav Y, Leviner E, Tzukert A, *et al* (1984) The spatial distribution, intensity and unpleasantness of acute dental pain. *Pain* **20**(4):363–370.

Sheiner EK, Sheiner E, Shoham-Vardi I, *et al* (1999) Ethnic differences influence care giver's estimates of pain during labour. *Pain* **81**(3):299–305.

Stimmel B (1983) *Pain, Analgesia and Addiction: The Pharmacologic Treatment of Pain.* New York: Raven Press.

Uhl GR, Sora I, Wang Z (1999) The mu opiate receptor as a candidate gene for pain: polymorphisms, variations in expression, nociception, and opiate responses. *Proc Natl Acad Sci USA* **96**(14):7752–7755.

Vgontzas AN, Chrousos GP (2002) Sleep, the hypothalamic-pituitary-adrenal axis, and cytokines: multiple interactions and disturbances in sleep disorders. *Endocrinol Metab Clin North Am* **31**(1):15–36.

Walker JS, Carmody JJ (1998) Experimental pain in healthy human subjects: gender differences in nociception and in response to ibuprofen. *Anesth Analg* **86**(6):1257–1262.

Yunus MB (2002) Gender differences in fibromyalgia and other related syndromes. *J Gend Specif Med* **5**(2):42–47.

Zborowsky M (1969) *People in Pain.* San Francisco: Jossey-Bass.

Zebenholzer K, Wober C, Vigl M, *et al* (2005) Facial pain in a neurological tertiary care centre—evaluation of the International Classification of Headache Disorders. *Cephalalgia* **25**(9):689–699.

Zebenholzer K, Wober C, Vigl M, *et al* (2006) Facial pain and the second edition of the International Classification of Headache Disorders. *Headache* **46**(2): 259–263.

Zelman DC, Brandenburg NA, Gore M (2006) Sleep impairment in patients with painful diabetic peripheral neuropathy. *Clin J Pain* **22**(8):681–685.

CHAPTER 2

Anatomy and neurophysiology of orofacial pain

Michael Tal and Marshall Devor

1. Introduction

When it comes to pain, dentists take a bad rap. 'Going to the dentist' universally conjures up fears of painful procedures, the whirring angst of the high-speed drill, huge syringes and blood-curdling extractions. Nothing could be more unfair; dentists are angels of pain relief. The patient who enters a dental clinic with a mind-gouging toothache is almost certain to leave within an hour with the problem resolved, the pain gone. And not only gone, but gone permanently, with very little likelihood of pain recurrence. This happy ending is most unlikely if you visit a rheumatologist with a painful hip, or an orthopaedist with an aching back. On the other hand, some painful conditions in the trigeminal region are much more difficult to treat than dental caries. Consideration of the anatomy and physiology of craniofacial innervation, with comparison to innervation at segmental levels, can provide useful insights into what works, what doesn't and why.

1.1. Pain in the Orofacial and Cranial Region

All tissues of the body receive sensory innervation, with the sole exception of the brain parenchyma. Although the fundamental patterns of innervation and of information processing are similar throughout the body, the orofacial and cranial region has certain peculiarities that motivate special focus on this region with respect to pain. Most strikingly, the head is functionally unique, mounted as it is on a narrow stalk (the neck), subject to continuous accelerations in all three planes, and containing the vestibule to the digestive system and the lungs, the special sensory organs and, most important, the brain. The head is also subject to a variety of chronic pain syndromes that do not have obvious parallels in other parts of the body: headache, toothache and trigeminal neuralgia, for example. It is by no means clear why these conditions do not occur in spinal structures. In this chapter we review the anatomy and physiology of the pain system that serves the orofacial and cranial region, and consider the features that set it apart from other somatic tissues.

1.2. Normal (Nociceptive), Inflammatory and Neuropathic Pain

1.2.1. Basic Pain Types

Normally, pain is felt when signals originating in thinly myelinated (Aδ) and/or unmyelinated (C) nociceptive afferents reach a conscious brain. Its purpose is protective. Examples are burning your tongue or biting your lip. The sensation felt (pain) matches the stimulus (noxious). This is *normal* (or *nociceptive*) pain.

Minor tissue injuries, burns, abrasions and infections often cause ongoing pain and tenderness (hypersensibility). This is *inflammatory* pain. Current pain nomenclature divides tenderness into two aspects: pain in response to a normally painless stimulus is *allodynia*. In allodynia, the sensation felt in the inflamed tissue (pain) no longer matches the stimulus (non-noxious). Excessive pain in response to a stimulus expected to be painful is *hyperalgesia* (Merskey and Bogduk 1994). Classically the allodynia and hyperalgesia caused by everyday injuries have been explained by a putative increase in the responsiveness of nociceptor endings (*peripheral sensitization*) resulting from chemical inflammatory mediators released in the injured tissue. The resulting sensitized nociceptors respond at substantially reduced threshold, to lukewarm water for example, resulting in *heat allodynia* (i.e. pain to a normally non-painful warm stimulus). Some C fibres do not respond to any applied stimulus under normal conditions, but begin to respond during inflammation. These are called *silent* or *sleeping* nociceptors (Schmidt *et al* 1995).

Peripheral sensitization may well account for thermal allodynia. There is also good evidence that sensitization of normal and silent nociceptors to mechanical forces contributes to pain on movement and weight-bearing in joints and in other deep tissues where significant mechanical forces are brought to bear. However, it has become increasingly clear that this is *not* the correct explanation of tactile allodynia in which light touch to irritated tender skin and mucous membranes is felt as painful. The reduction in the response threshold of nociceptors to tactile stimuli is much smaller than that to heat. Afferent nociceptors in inflamed skin do not generally respond to light brushing of tender skin even though this brushing is painful (Schmelz *et al* 1996; Banik and Brennan 2004). *Tactile allodynia* in the skin has another cause (see below).

A third type of pain, *neuropathic*, results from injury or disease of nerves or central nervous system (CNS) structures. This type of pain resembles tissue inflammation in the sense that spontaneous pain and hypersensibility are usually present. However, it differs from inflammatory pain as the injury/disease is in neural tissue. This distinction is not without problems. Pain due to inflammation in a major nerve trunk (*neuritis*) is generally considered neuropathic (Eliav *et al* 1999). On the other hand, all peripheral tissues are innervated, so minor trauma to skin, muscle, joint, etc., also injures nerve fibres, or at least changes their local chemical milieu. And yet it would be odd to list painful abrasions or cutaneous infections as examples of neuropathic pain. Nomenclature aside, from the point of view of mechanism, there turns out to be considerable overlap between neuropathic and inflammatory pain processes. Indeed, at segmental levels, and even more so in the craniofacial area, we often do not know whether a particular chronic pain diagnosis is nociceptive, inflammatory or neuropathic.

Normal and inflammatory pain are adaptive design features of the nervous system. They constitute an alarm bell. Temporary hyper-responsiveness to stimuli in inflammatory pain provides warning, and protects against further damage by reducing use of the body part and by suppressing activity in general. Neuropathic pain, in contrast, reflects abnormal (pathophysiologic) functioning of a damaged pain system. It is maladaptive, the equivalent of a defective alarm system that produces false alarms.

1.2.2. Tactile Allodynia and Central Sensitization

There is now strong evidence that tenderness to the touch (tactile allodynia) following both inflammation and frank nerve injury results from abnormal signal amplification in the CNS rather than from sensitized nociceptors. The process is called *central sensitization*, and it results from a variety of injury-evoked pathophysiological changes (see below). In the presence of central sensitization peripheral input entering the CNS along non-nociceptive, thickly myelinated, Aβ touch afferents evokes pain (Campbell *et al* 1988; Gracely *et al* 1992; Torebjork *et al* 1992). Since mechanical rather than thermal hypersensibility is the most common cause of suffering and disability in chronic

pain patients, pain signalled by Aβ afferents is as important as pain signalled by nociceptors. *Aβ pain* constitutes a revolution in our understanding of both inflammatory and neuropathic pain.

1.2.3. The Paradox of Neuropathic Pain

Neuropathic pain in the craniofacial area, as elsewhere, is a significant problem for both theoretical understanding and clinical management. It is fundamentally paradoxical. Just as cutting a telephone wire leaves the line dead, cutting axons should deaden sensation. Sure enough, complete denervation of a body part does result in numbness, the hallmark *negative* symptom of neuropathy. Yet nerve trauma and disease are also frequently associated with *positive* symptoms and signs, some resembling inflammation and others unique. These include:

(a) spontaneous paraesthesias (e.g. *pins-and-needles*), dysaesthesias (unpleasant paraesthesias) and frank pain;
(b) allodynic and hyperalgesic response to stimuli in the partially denervated regions;
(c) pain evoked by deep palpation and by movement of the neck, jaw, etc.; and
(d) electric shock-like paroxysms and *hyperpathia*.

These pathophysiological pain states are discussed below.

2. Sensory and Motor Innervation of Craniofacial Structures

2.1. Sensory Neurons

Somatovisceral sensation is due to innervation by primary sensory neurons (*primary afferents*). These neurons reside in the dorsal root ganglia (DRGs) for spinal structures, and in cranial root ganglia for the head except for the back of the scalp, which is innervated by sensory cells in the upper cervical DRGs. The bodies of sensory cells have a distinctive *pseudounipolar* structure unlike any other cell in the nervous system. With rare exceptions (notably MesV, the mesencephalic nucleus of the trigeminal nerve, see below) the sensory ganglia are located in a bony cavern between adjacent vertebrae or at the base of the skull, and have two axonal processes (Fig. 2.1). One process travels from the cell body through a peripheral nerve, usually containing motor and sensory axons, and terminates in one or more sensory endings in innervated tissue. The other runs from the cell body, through the dorsal root or cranial nerve root, and ends in a cluster of pre-synaptic terminals within the CNS. Sensory neurons also reside in parasympathetic and enteric ganglia (Janig 2006). These ganglia are cell clusters intrinsic to certain tissues, notably the alimentary canal, and can be thought of as remnants of a primitive, distributed nervous system capable of carrying out complex functions,

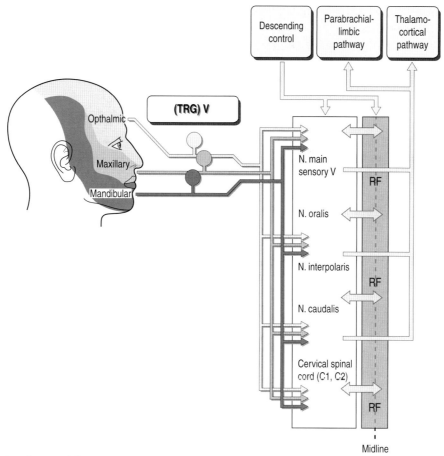

Fig. 2.1 • Major neuronal pathways of the trigeminal system. Primary sensory neurons of the trigeminal ganglion (TRG), and their peripheral distributions to the V1, V2 and V3 territories, are shown on the left. Note that sensory ganglia of the facial (VII), glossopharyngeal (IX) and vagus (X) nerves also innervate craniofacial structures, as do the spinal C1 and C2 dorsal root ganglia. TRG afferents end in the main sensory V nucleus, and in the spinal trigeminal complex. Second order neurons of these nuclei provide ascending pathways, mostly crossed, to the reticular formation (RF, greyshading) a variety of brainstem and diencephalic structures, especially the thalamic relay nuclei. The latter nuclei project to the cerebral cortex. Descending pathways modulate the flow of ascending trigeminal sensory signals.

such as peristalsis, independent of the brain. Our sensory experience of the gut and other visceral organs, however, is thought to be due exclusively to pseudounipolar neurons of the DRGs and cranial nerve ganglia. It is unlikely that signals that originate in sensory neurons in the parasympathetic or enteric ganglia reach consciousness. Parasympathetic ganglia reside in, and serve, some craniofacial structures, but there are no enteric-type ganglia in the head. The most rostral ones are in the myenteric plexus of the upper oesophagus.

2.2. Peculiarities of Craniofacial Sensory Innervation

There are several anatomical and functional features of primary afferent neurons of the trigeminal (and other cranial nerve) ganglia that distinguish them from neurons of the spinal DRGs, although the functional significance of these differences is not necessarily obvious. These include:

2.2.1. Fibre Types

The ratio of myelinated (A-) to non-myelinated (C-) afferent fibres is higher in trigeminal nerve tributaries

than in spinal nerves. Cranial nerves have relatively few C fibres (Darian-Smith 1966; Young and King 1973). Related to this, many of the thermoreceptors that innervate the orofacial area have thinly myelinated Aδ fibres while in other parts of the body most thermoreceptors are C fibres. The tooth pulp chamber is also known to have a high proportion of A-fibre nociceptors compared to the more frequent C-fibre nociceptors at spinal level (Jyväsjärvi and Kniffki 1989; Mengel et al 1996). This yields a higher mean conduction velocity for trigeminal versus spinal nociceptive signalling, which is in any event faster because of the shorter propagation distances in the head. The reasons for this emphasis on speed are not clear.

Hoffmann and Matthews (1990) reported that peripheral nerves in the head also contain fewer sympathetic efferent axons than somatic peripheral nerves, and argued that this may bear a relationship to the relative infrequency of sympathetically maintained pain states (SMP) in the trigeminal region. The hallmark of SMP is pain relief following sympathetic block or sympatholysis. Interestingly, trigeminal cutaneous and intracerebral blood vessels receive parasympathetic as well as sympathetic innervation (Kaji et al 1991; Uddman et al 1999).

At segmental levels parasympathetic innervation of blood vessels is uncommon if it exists at all.

2.2.2. Teeth

The teeth are unique structures with no homologue at spinal levels. A tooth is an open-ended vital, innervated, calcified box (dentin and cementum) filled with soft neural tissue (pulp chamber), and coated orally with a relatively non-vital hard tissue that is not innervated (enamel). There is a clear resemblance to the ends of skeletal long bones with the non-innervated (synovial) cartilage being homologous to dental enamel (Fig. 2.2).

2.2.3. MesV

The trigeminal mesencephalic nucleus (MesV), located at the mesopontine junction, is a unique sensory structure. It contains cell bodies of primary afferent proprioceptors, Ia afferents, that innervate the jaw-closing muscles (masseter, temporalis and medial pterygoid) and the periodontium. It is, in essence, a cranial nerve ganglion *displaced* into the brain, the only example of this architecture in the CNS. The axons of muscle and periodontal afferents of MesV neurons travel in the motor rather than the sensory root of the trigeminal nerve. The functional significance of this anomaly is unclear, although there is a hint of special neural processing in the fact that, unlike DRGs and normal cranial nerve ganglia, MesV neurons receive synaptic input. Another hint is that while at spinal levels opposing extensor and flexor muscle blocks are roughly equal in size, in the orofacial motor system there is asymmetry. Jaw-closing muscles, the flexors, are massive and powerful with rich muscle spindle and Golgi tendon organ innervation. The jaw-opening muscles, the extensors, are small and delicate and lack muscle spindles and Golgi tendon organs (Lennartsson 1980).

2.2.4. Embryonic Origin

The largest of the cranial nerve ganglia, the trigeminal ganglion (TRG) is in essence constructed by fusion of three ganglia associated with the ophthalmic, maxillary and mandibular branches of the trigeminal complex. All DRG neurons at spinal levels originate in the embryonic neural crest. The TRG, in contrast, contains many neurons of ectodermal (placodal) origin as well as neurons of neural crest origin (Le Douarin and Kalcheim 1999).

2.3. Innervation of the Head

2.3.1. Overview

The cranial nerves that support pain sensation are *mixed nerves*, meaning that they also contain somatic and autonomic motor axons. This should not matter much as, normally, axons that share a nerve trunk are functionally independent. However, in the event of nerve injury adjacent axons may interact and this may contribute to pain pathophysiology. A suspected example of this is SMP (see below).

Somatic and visceral sensory innervation. Innervation of the orofacial region is provided mainly by the trigeminal nerve (cranial nerve V), and partly by the glossopharyngeal (IX) and vagus (X) nerves with a very minor contribution from the facial nerve (VII). The back of the scalp is innervated primarily by dorsal roots of the C1 and C2 spinal segments (Fig. 2.3). With the exception of MesV, the relevant primary sensory neurons are all located in the corresponding cranial nerve ganglia or DRGs. The *special* senses, smell, vision, taste, hearing and the vestibular sense, are served by cranial nerves I, II, VII and VIII. The trigeminal nerve (V) is by far the most important cranial nerve for pain.

Voluntary motor innervation (including somatic and branchial divisions). External ocular muscles are innervated

Fig. 2.2 • The structural analogy between teeth and epiphysial bone ends may provide useful insights into pain mechanisms in calcified tissues in general. As illustrated in this schematic diagram, tooth enamel is analogous to articular hyaline cartilage (note that neither is innervated), dentine is analogous to subchondral bone, the tooth pulp is analogous to bone marrow, and the external soft tissues of the tooth (gingiva and periodontal ligament) are analogous to synovial soft tissue and periosteum of the joint. There are also important differences between tooth and bone innervation.

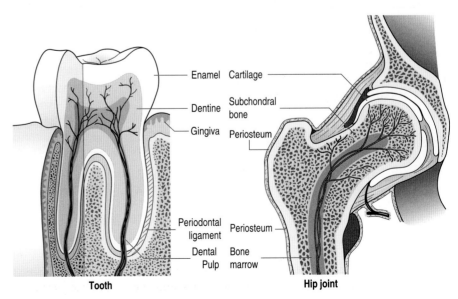

Enamel — Cartilage
Dentine — Subchondral bone
Gingiva — Periosteum
Periodontal ligament — Periosteum
Dental Pulp — Bone marrow

Tooth   **Hip joint**

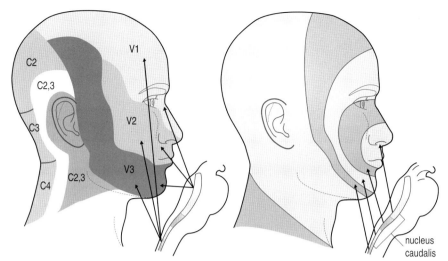

Fig. 2.3 • Craniofacial input to the trigeminal nuclear complex forms a somatotopic map continuous with that of the spinal dorsal horn, and similarly organized (drawing on the left). In addition, there appears to be a separate mapped representation of the ipsilateral intraoral and facial structures onto laminae I and II of nucleus caudalis and the upper cervical dorsal horn. This representation takes the form of concentric semicircular rings (drawing on the right). The nose and lips (snout) map rostrally in nucleus caudalis while the jaw, forehead and scalp map caudally.

by the oculomotor (III), trochlear (IV) and abducens nerves (VI). The facial *muscles of expression* are innervated by the facial nerve (VII). The muscles of mastication are served mostly by the motor branch of the trigeminal nerve (Vm). The muscles that control swallowing and the larynx are served by the glossopharyngeal (IX) and the vagus nerves (X). The spinal accessory nerve (XI) innervates certain muscles of the neck and shoulder, the hypoglossal nerve (XII) supplies motor innervation to the muscles of the tongue, and the C1 and C2 ventral roots supply muscles underlying the scalp.

Autonomic motor innervation. The entire sympathetic supply to smooth muscles and glands of the head above the neck, including cranial vasculature, is from motoneurons of the superior cervical sympathetic ganglion. These are driven, in turn, by preganglionic sympathetic neurons of the upper part of the spinal intermediolateral column. Parasympathetic ganglia are located within or near the cranial structures that they innervate (*juxtamural*), and they are driven by preganglionic motoneurons that reside in the brainstem parasympathetic motor nuclei. The axons of the preganglionic motoneurons reach their target juxtamural ganglia via the oculomotor (III), facial (VII), glossopharyngeal (IX) and vagus (X) cranial nerves. The motoneurons of the parasympathetic ganglia, in turn, have short axons which innervate nearby smooth muscle and glands, in the trigeminal distribution also including blood vessels (Kaji *et al* 1991; Ramien *et al* 2004).

2.3.2. The Trigeminal Nerve

The trigeminal nerve (V) is the largest of the cranial nerves, named because it branches into three major peripheral divisions, the ophthalmic (V1), the maxillary (V2) and the mandibular (V3) nerves. These *map* the face from forehead to jaw. Their sensory axons innervate most tissues of the head except for the back of the skull, the angle of the mandible and parts of the ear and throat. All three divisions contribute sensory fibres to the meninges and the

intracranial blood vessels and venous sinuses via a small nerve branch, equivalent to the spinal dorsal ramus, which leaves the nerve just distal to the TRG. The brain parenchyma, including the retina, does not receive any nociceptive innervation.

Except for MesV, the primary sensory neurons of all three divisions reside in the TRG, also termed Gasserian or semilunar ganglion. Although merged within a single perineurial/dural capsule, the three divisions of this *fused* ganglion are preserved; cells of V1, V2 and V3 do not intermingle much in the TRG. The topographic layout of the TRG is largely preserved as axons leave the ganglion and pass into the trigeminal root on their way to the brain. This permits the neurosurgeon to target trigeminal pain sources regionally by selective fibre transaction in the trigeminal root (see Chapter 12). This facility is not available for dorsal roots at spinal levels. Trigeminal motor fibres originate in pontine trigeminal motor nuclei. They exit the brain as a coherent bundle in the trigeminal root, bypass the TRG and then follow mandibular nerve (V3) tributaries into the masseter, temporalis, pterygoid and digastric (anterior belly) muscles, and some small muscles in the soft palate and middle ear.

The ophthalmic division (V1). This branch is the smallest of the three trigeminal nerve tributaries. After entering the orbit through the superior orbital fissure, the ophthalmic nerve splits into the frontal, nasociliary and lacrimal nerves. These supply the upper eyelid, forehead and scalp, the sphenoid, ethmoid and nasal sinus cavities, the orbital contents and the upper part of the nose.

The maxillary division (V2). This branch exits the cranium through the foramen rotundum and enters the pterygopalatine fossa. Preganglionic secretomotor fibres that exit the brain in the facial nerve (VII) join V2 en route to the parasympathetic sphenopalatine ganglion (also called the pterygopalatine ganglion). This large ganglion is an important target for pain control, not so much because of its autonomic role, but because of its location. *Sphenopalatine ganglion blocks* also block the adjacent maxillary nerve trunk, and it is for this reason that they provide at least temporary relief in sphenopalatine neuralgia, certain persistent headaches and migraine, herpes zoster pain of the face and some atypical facial pains (Klein *et al* 2001; Yarnitsky *et al* 2003). The maxillary nerve provides innervation of facial bones and then continues anteriorly to enter the orbit through the inferior orbital fissure as the infraorbital nerve. This nerve provides postganglionic parasympathetic innervation to the lacrimal and salivatory glands, and to the mucosal glands of the maxilla (the hard and soft palate, gums, maxillary sinuses). It also provides sensory innervation to teeth of the upper jaw and to skin of the middle part of the face including the lower part of the nose (Fig. 2.3).

The mandibular division (V3). This branch is the largest of the trigeminal nerves and the only one that carries voluntary motor fibres. It exits the cranium through the foramen ovale and divides into four tributaries in the infratemporal fossa: the auriculotemporal, inferior alveolar, lingual and buccal nerves. The auriculotemporal nerve provides sensory innervation to skin of the temporal region, including the ear lobe, and to the temporomandibular joint (TMJ). It also carries postganglionic parasympathetic motor axons from the otic ganglion that serve the parotid gland. The inferior alveolar nerve enters the mandibular canal and supplies the teeth of the lower jaw. Its mental nerve branch emerges through the mental foramen to supply the skin of the cheek, the mucous membrane of the lower lip and the vestibular gingiva of the mandibular teeth from the foramen anteriorly to the midline. The lingual nerve innervates the anterior two thirds of the tongue, the floor of the oral cavity and the lingual periodontium. The buccal nerve (named also *long buccal* to distinguish it from the motor buccal branch of VII) innervates the mucous membrane, vestibular gingiva and the gums posterior to the mental foramen. The chorda tympani nerve, a branch of the facial nerve (VII), joins the lingual nerve in the infratemporal fossa carrying taste fibres from the anterior two-thirds of the tongue, and parasympathetic supply to the submandibular and sublingual salivary glands.

2.4. Pain and Specific Craniofacial Structures

2.4.1. Skin

The skin of the face and scalp, including its innervation, is fundamentally the same as the skin in other parts of the body. It is served by a variety of heavily myelinated low-threshold mechanoreceptive afferents (Aβ fibres), thinly myelinated afferents including Aδ nociceptors, and unmyelinated C fibres, many of which are nociceptors. It is now recognized that there are many cutaneous C fibres in the limbs that respond to light touch. Their role in sensation is not yet clear (Olausson *et al* 2002). It has not been determined

yet whether these *C tactile* afferents also occur in the trigeminal system. Among the C nociceptors a substantial fraction are silent and cannot be activated by any natural stimulus except when sensitized by inflammation. Many non-human mammals have giant motile facial hairs, *vibrissae*, with follicles richly innervated by both nociceptors and low-threshold Aβ afferents which are sensitive to the direction and dynamics of vibrissal bending. The vibrissae are actively whisked back and forth and, like fingertips, provide the animal with essential detailed touch information.

2.4.2. Intranasal and Intraoral Mucosa

The surface of the nasal and oral cavities, including the cranial air sinuses, is covered with a mucous-secreting epithelial membrane, and a special keratinized mucosa on the dorsal surface of the tongue. This tissue is served by the same families of trigeminal primary afferent neurons as serve the skin, including a rich contribution by C polymodal nociceptors. Absence of the tough, poorly penetrable external corium layer of skin, however, provides for much easier access of mechanical, chemical and thermal stimuli to sensory receptor endings in mucosal tissues. It also permits enhanced access to drugs such as local anaesthetics, and a route of delivery of drugs to capillary beds and the circulatory system. The oral cavity is richly invested with receptors for touch and cold sensation, but many areas have little sensitivity to heat. This is why the anterior part of the hard palate is prone to burns; there is no feeling there that food items are too hot (Junge 1998). Ongoing pain in conditions such as burning mouth disorder is very likely due to abnormal activity of intraoral thermal afferents. Inflammation is not obvious in burning mouth disorder. This has led to the hypothesis that the abnormal neural activity underlying this type of pain may be neuropathic in origin (Yilmaz *et al* 2007) (see Chapter 11).

2.4.2.1. Nasal Cavity and Smell
The olfactory epithelium, on the upper nasal turbinate bones, has the same trigeminal innervation as all other nasal and oral mucosas. The intense burning sensation that follows sniffing of irritating substances such as ammonia or spicy horseradish is thought to be due to the activation of trigeminal C-fibre chemo-nociceptors, not olfactory receptors. Likewise, the sneezing reflex is mediated by trigeminal afferent input. Trigeminal chemo-nociception must be distinguished from olfactory chemo-sensation. The latter is based on an entirely different physiology and functional architecture, and a different cranial nerve, the olfactory nerve (I) (and in non-human mammals also the vomeronasal nerve). The sensory cell bodies of trigeminal nerve chemo-nociceptors are pseudounipolar neurons located in the TRG, with entry into the CNS in the brainstem trigeminal complex. Olfactory receptor neurons do not reside in a ganglion, but rather within the nasal olfactory epithelium itself. They are ciliated bipolar neurons with axons that enter the brain along the olfactory nerve (I) with their first synapse in the olfactory bulbs.

2.4.2.2. Oral Cavity, the Tongue, Taste and Flavour

The same distinction must be made between chemo-nociception in the oral cavity and the sense of taste. Taste chemoreceptors are specialized non-neural transduction cells within the taste buds of the tongue and pharynx. The taste receptor cells activate axonal endings of myelinated visceral primary afferents of the chorda tympani nerve, whose cell bodies reside in the geniculate ganglion of the facial nerve (VII). They do not belong to the trigeminal nerve (V), and are not normally associated with pain in the oral cavity. Pain sensation in the oral cavity, including on the tongue, is due to trigeminal nerve (V) primary afferent nociceptors whose cell bodies reside in the TRG.

Tastants are molecules that activate taste chemoreceptors, and give rise to the five basic taste modalities: sweet, sour, salty, bitter and umami (the taste of monosodium glutamate (MSG)). Olfactants are the much larger family of molecules that activate olfactory receptor neurons and give rise to a sensation of smell. Olfactants can access the olfactory epithelium via the nostrils and also from the oral cavity via the pharynx. The flavour of food is due at least as much to olfactory stimulation via these two routes as it is to taste buds on the tongue. The *taste* of piquant food items such as hot peppers (which contain capsaicin) is due to neither taste nor olfactory receptors, but to trigeminal sensory endings in the tongue, palate, gums, nasal cavity, etc. Trigeminal innervation is likewise responsible for all other somatosensory discrimination in the oral cavity, such as heat, cold and pinprick. Finally, low-threshold mechanoreceptors of the oral mucosa and tongue, together with periodontal and jaw muscle proprioceptors, provide a sense of the texture of food. These various sources of sensory input, taste, olfaction, oral mechanosensation and proprioception are integrated in the cerebral cortex to provide the final complex sensory experience that we associate with eating fine food.

Interestingly, there are occasional reports in which food items, not painful in themselves, are reported to trigger pain. The most common example is migraine, which is sometimes triggered by eating yellow cheese and chocolate, or by drinking coffee or red wine. It is not clear whether this is due to the taste/smell of these foods, or to some chemical absorbed into the circulation. Headache can also be triggered by drinking orange juice, or by eating pineapple, pickled onions or food items that contain MSG, tyramine or sucrose (see Chapter 9). There are also reports that various gustatory stimuli to the tongue, such as sweet, can induce sweating in the trigeminal nerve distribution. In some patients taste and smell induce paroxysmal pain attacks resembling trigeminal neuralgia (Sharav *et al* 1991; Helcer *et al* 1998; Goldstein *et al* 2004). The triggering mechanism is unknown.

2.4.2.3. Pharynx and Larynx

As noted, the absence in the oral mucosa of the skin's cornified outer layer permits easy access of stimulants (mechanical, thermal and chemical) to mucosal sensory receptors, and also easy access of applied drugs to the underlying vasculature. An interesting example of the former is the tingling, almost painful sensation in the back of the throat caused by drinking carbonated fizzy drinks. This sensation is due to the response of trigeminal acid-sensing chemo-nociceptors activated by carbonic acid in the drink (Simons *et al* 2000). The absence of a cornified layer also poses special problems for the prevention of viral and bacterial infection via the nasal and oral cavities. Protective enzymes are present in the saliva to help deal with this problem. Nonetheless, infection and irritation with consequent painful inflammation in this area is common.

The mucosa of the larynx, including the laryngeal surface of the epiglottis, the false and true vocal folds, and the arytenoid region, contain one of the most dense concentrations of sensory nerve endings in the human body (Mu and Sanders 2000; Uno *et al* 2004). This provides a sensory basis for coughing, gagging and other reflexes that protect the lungs. Even brief loss of these functions may lead to life-threatening conditions such as entry of food into the lungs, and to infections such as pneumonia. The internal superior and recurrent laryngeal nerves, branches of the vagus nerve (X), supply the sensory innervation to this area.

2.4.3. Cornea and Conjunctiva

Like skin and mucosa, the outer surface of the eye, the transparent cornea and the opaque white conjunctiva, has a specialized epithelial outer layer that is innervated by both sensitive mechanoreceptor and nociceptor endings. Both low- and high-threshold afferents contribute to the eye blink reflex. This defensive (protective) reflex is homologous to the flexion reflex at spinal levels, but unique in the body for being triggered also by weak stimuli such as dust particles and air puffs, and not just noxious stimuli. Tearing, another important protective reflex of the cornea–conjunctiva, is activated mainly by chemical irritation and results in parasympathetic activation of the main and accessory lacrimal glands (see also trigeminoparasympathetic reflex discussed in Chapter 10). Mechanical trauma (*scratched* cornea) and radiant heat injury provoke pain originating in the cornea. Interestingly, destruction of corneal innervation by radial keratectomy surgery causes persistent pain coupled with reduced response to stimuli, but only in about 25% of patients. This may be due to microneuromas, and hence fall into the category of neuropathic pain. Regeneration and recovery takes many months (Belmonte and Tervo 2006).

The iris also has nociceptive innervation, although the lens and retina do not. When surgeons lightly touch the iris in the absence of adequate local anaesthesia, patients report pain. Reflex hyperconstriction of the iris can evoke pain which is relieved by mydriatic agents. It is unlikely that pain can originate in the retina as laser tacking of a detached retina is not painful.

2.4.4. Muscles

Musculoskeletal pain, after excessive physical exercise for example, is a part of everyday living. Overuse of the masticatory (jaw) and other orofacial muscles is no exception. It has been suggested that the main cause of the deep tissue pain during exercise is reduced blood flow and reduced tissue oxygenation (see Chapter 7). This compromises the metabolic status of nociceptive sensory endings, and causes depolarization, firing and pain (Martens and Moeyersoons 1990). An additional potential mechanism is accumulation of various substances in the exercised muscle that excite muscle nociceptors and/or sensitize them, increasing responses to muscle contractions that are normally non-painful (Graven-Nielsen and Mense 2001; Graven-Nielsen *et al* 2003; Hoheisel *et al* 2004). In experimental studies involving intramuscular injection of algesic substances that might be present in exercised muscle, pain is induced. Candidate mediators include low pH (acidic) buffer, hypertonic saline, ATP, glutamate, potassium chloride, capsaicin, bradykinin, serotonin and L-ascorbic acid. It is not unlikely that under pathological conditions characterized by ongoing muscle pain and tenderness such as fibromyalgia and masticatory myofascial pain, algesic substances accumulate in abnormally high concentrations activating muscle nociceptors, and/or these nociceptors become abnormally sensitized (Graven-Nielsen and Mense 2001). Building on this idea it has been postulated that chronic tension-type headache may be due to abnormal and excessive activity of jaw, head and neck muscles. However, experimental support for this model is uncertain (Stohler *et al* 1996; see also Chapter 7).

2.4.5. Teeth and Bones

Teeth are a source of both pain and low-threshold mechanosensation. Like other hard tissues, they have two quite different types of nociceptive innervation (Fig. 2.2). One is extrinsic, the innervation of the periodontium and gingiva at the base of teeth, and the periosteum of bones. The second is the intrinsic (internal), nociceptive innervation associated with tooth pulp and bone marrow. Many pulpal afferents end in fine dentinal tubules in teeth, and in Haversian canals in porous bone (see also Chapter 5). The enamel of teeth, and the epiphysial cartilage of long bones, is not innervated. The intrinsic innervation of teeth and bones is not known to provide a conscious sensory experience in health. Rather, it reports on damage such as a broken tooth, dental caries or bone metastases. When people complain about *toothache*, the source of the pain may be extrinsic or intrinsic. The associated sensations as described in Chapter 5, however, are subtly different, providing the clinician a hint of the real source. There is also low-threshold touch and proprioceptive input from teeth, which originates in the periodontium and associated gingival soft tissues. This contributes to the fine control of mastication (see below). Like the fine hand flexor control required to pick up an egg without cracking the shell, the forces applied during jaw closure in mastication must be finely controlled to permit effective biting and chewing without breaking teeth.

Non-classical nociceptive intrinsic innervation. It is widely held that the only sensation that can be elicited by stimulation of the intrinsic (pulpal) innervation of teeth is pain (Byers 1984; Brannstrom 1992). However, noxious stimulation or peripheral sensitization by inflammatory mediators is not required to evoke tooth pain. Weak stimuli applied to healthy exposed dentin, such as by light touch and even air-puffs, evoke sharp tooth pain. This situation, pain evoked by weak stimuli in healthy individuals, appears to be unique to the tooth. A potential explanation derives from the unusual properties of tooth pulp afferents. Within the tooth pulp, sensory axon endings are of fine diameter, and conduct in the Aδ- and C-fibre range. But as they exit from the tooth many of these axons have the properties of large-diameter, fast-conducting Aβ fibres (Cadden *et al* 1983). Moreover, retrograde labelling shows that the cell soma of most pulpal afferents within the TRG are of medium and large diameter and express corresponding neurochemical markers (e.g. RT-97). Likewise, they are not depleted by neonatal capsaicin treatment like most small-diameter TRG neurons (Fried *et al* 1988). These are properties of low-threshold mechanosensitive afferents. Remarkably, however, many (although not all) of these large neurons terminate in the superficial layers of the trigeminal dorsal horn (Marfurt and Turner 1984), and many express peptides and neurotrophic receptors normally associated with C-fibre nociceptors. These include CGRP, ret (the GDNF receptor) and trkA, although not SP or IB4 (a marker of non-peptidergic nociceptors; Silverman and Kruger 1987; Fried *et al* 1989; Byers and Narhi 1999; Yang *et al* 2006). It is possible that by virtue of their Aβ characteristics the large-diameter tooth pulp afferents respond to weak stimuli, but by virtue of their peptide neurotransmitter content they activate pain-signalling neurons in the trigeminal brainstem, evoking pain. The tooth pulp also contains a small population of small-diameter afferents that have the characteristics typical of Aδ and C nociceptors.

The only exception to tooth pulp stimulation evoking pain seems to be the non-painful tingling sensation felt during electrical stimulation of the tooth using threshold currents. This is called *pre-pain* (McGrath *et al* 1983; Virtanen *et al* 1987). Apparently the tooth pulp also contains some Aβ axons that signal non-painful sensation. With large numbers of low-threshold nociceptors in the tooth pulp, it is hard to imagine in what natural circumstances such low-threshold touch afferents might be activated selectively. Numerous sympathetic efferents are also present in the tooth pulp. These presumably serve pulpal vasculature and perhaps dentine (Matthews 1970; Cadden *et al* 1983; Byers 1984; Dong *et al* 1985, 1993; Holland *et al* 1987; Jyväsjärvi *et al* 1988).

The sensory endings of intrapulpal afferents have an unusual anatomy. Many end within fine tubules in the dentin. Specifically, about 40% of these tubules contain free nerve endings that extend ~100 μm, and sometimes as far as 200 μm from the pulp, across the odontoblastic layer and into the dentin (Byers and Narhi 1999). But this still leaves them about 1–3 mm from the dentinoenamel junction. Given the considerable distance of the nerve endings from the outer layer of the dentin it is not clear how gentle dentinal stimulation activates these endings and causes pain. For chemical stimuli the gap is presumably crossed by diffusion and for thermal stimuli by conduction. For mechanical stimuli the popular *hydrodynamic theory* posits that stimuli to the dentin cause movement of fluid within the tubules. The fluid pressure then mechanically displaces the membrane of the nerve ending, depolarizing and activating it. Inflammation of dentinal endings may increase their sensitivity to applied stimuli, but it is clear that such sensitization is not required as healthy dentin exposed in dental procedures is sensitive. There is no good evidence of synapses or gap junctions between the nerve fibre endings and odontoblasts. For a comprehensive discussion of tooth innervation and function, see Byers and Narhi (1999).

Less is known about the intrinsic innervation of bones than of teeth. For example, aspiration of marrow from skeletal bone shafts and the pelvis is painful, as are intramedullary tumours in skeletal bones. This is in keeping with a sensory role for intrinsic innervation, as in teeth. Pursuing this analogy, we have suggested that erosion of epiphysial cartilage in osteoarthritis may result in pain due to direct application of weight-bearing forces to exposed, innervated, subchondral bone in the same way that mechanical force applied to exposed dentin, healthy or inflamed, is painful (Niv *et al* 2003). However, anecdotal reports from neurosurgeons indicate that in awake patients undergoing craniotomy, after the fascia and periosteum have been locally anaesthetized drilling through the marrow chamber of flat bones of the calvarium is not noticeably painful. Likewise, tumours within the mandibular bone tend not to be painful unless they breach the bone and press on nearby nerves or innervated tissues. Interestingly, certain chemotherapeutic agents, such as vincristine, are known to cause decalcifying lesions in bones of the jaw, while sparing skeletal bone. These observations suggest a fundamental difference in the sensory role of the intrinsic innervation of cranial versus skeletal bones, perhaps due to differences in embryonic origin.

Low-threshold extrinsic innervation. The periodontal apparatus, which serves as an interface between the tooth and its socket in the alveolar bone, supplies the CNS with mechanoreceptor signals about tooth loads for the neural control of jaw movements. When this information is not available, e.g. during dental anaesthesia, the control of forces that move the jaw is severely impaired. Low-threshold nerve fibres have been described in all four parts of the apparatus: the periodontal ligament, the adjacent gingiva, the cementum and the alveolar bone. Ruffini-like nerve endings are located among the collagen fibres in the periodontal ligament that anchor the root of the tooth to the jawbone (Byers 1985). The ligament also contains endings that appear to be proprioceptive although no clear encapsulated receptors have been found here (Biemesderfer

et al 1978; Byers *et al* 1989, 1999). In the gingiva, neural endings resembling Meissner and Ruffini corpuscles have been described at the papillary and subpapillary lamina, in addition to free nerve endings. These might provide information about tooth displacement (Johnsen and Trulsson 2003, 2005; Macefield 2005). It is uncertain whether the cementum is innervated, but nerve endings have been described in alveolar bone in human specimens (Abarca *et al* 2006). Beyond their role in the control of jaw movement, it is possible that low-threshold periodontal afferents play a role in pain. Specifically, in the presence of central sensitization, they could yield Aβ pain. This could account for sensitivity of healthy tissue (teeth and gingiva) neighbouring an inflamed, painful tooth.

2.4.6. Craniocervical Joints and Mastication

Temporomandibular joint. The TMJ, the articulation of the condylar process of the mandible in the glenoid fossa of the temporal bone, permits opening and closing of the jaw. The articular surfaces of these bones are covered with fibrous (non-cellular, non-vascular) cartilage and sealed with a synovial membrane. The capsule is covered externally by periosteum which extends over the mandible and the temporal bone. Proprioceptors of the TMJ provide sensory input about jaw position, and the force being applied by the masticatory muscles. The joint is also innervated by trigeminal nerve nociceptors as is the periarticular connective tissue (Hutchins *et al* 2000; Kyrkanides *et al* 2002; Ichikawa *et al* 2004; Oliveira *et al* 2005). The actual articular surfaces have been thought to lack nerve endings (Davidson *et al* 2003). However, new evidence suggests that the human articular disk, a unique layer of fibrous cartilage within the synovial space which separates the two articular surfaces of the mandible, does contain sensory nerve endings that are probably low-threshold proprioceptors (Asaki *et al* 2006). The relative paucity of low-threshold sensory endings in the TMJ contrasts with their widespread distribution in the associated muscles, tendons and periodontal ligaments. This has led to the suggestion that the sensory regulation of mastication is due primarily to these surrounding structures while the nociceptive innervation of the TMJ contributes to limiting excessive force application and the detection of injury (Capra 1987; Andoh *et al* 1988). The nociceptors no doubt also contribute to pain in disorders of the TMJ (Broton *et al* 1988). Despite the fact that it is not a weight-bearing joint like the knee or hip, the jaw-closing musculature is capable of generating substantial forces which are applied to the joint (Tanaka *et al* 2006). Painful disorders of the TMJ exact a considerable toll of suffering and disability; see Chapter 8.

Jaw-closing reflex. Stretch of the jaw closer muscle (masseter) activates Ia muscle spindle afferents. The result is reflex masseter contraction and jaw closing. This is a classic monosynaptic stretch (myotactic) reflex, common to many somatic joints. The cell bodies of the muscle spindle afferents are located in MesV, and they connect monosynaptically with the jaw closer motoneurons in the trigeminal motor nucleus. When the jaws close and the apposing teeth make contact, proprioceptors of the masseter are suddenly unloaded, and masseter contraction stops, preventing breakage of the teeth. The jaw-closing reflex also contributes to stabilization of the jaw, preventing it from bouncing during walking and running by maintaining a fixed open–closed jaw position (Lund *et al* 1984; Miles *et al* 2004). There is no evidence for a stretch reflex in the jaw opener muscles. This is consistent with the observation that the opener muscles lack muscle spindles and a Golgi tendon organ (Abbink *et al* 1998).

Jaw-opening reflex. This is a protective reflex that, combined with unloading of the jaw-closing reflex, prevents breakage of tooth cusps by excessive bite force, and protects soft oral tissues (gums, tongue) from being bitten. It is basically like the spinal flexor reflex. Forceful tooth occlusion activates nociceptive (*flexor reflex*) afferents in the periodontium and in soft tissue caught between the teeth, triggering reflex contraction of jaw opener muscles and inhibition of jaw closer muscles. This occurs within about 15 ms. As in limb flexion it is a disynaptic protective reflex, but unlike the limbs, it acts bilaterally.

Mastication. Early in the twentieth century Sherrington (1906) proposed that reciprocating activities of jaw-opening and jaw-closing reflexes might constitute the basic motor synergy of mastication. In this scheme, food stimuli to the lips or mouth initiate jaw-opening. The resulting stretch of the masseter triggers the jaw-closing response. This stretches opener muscles once again triggering jaw-opening, and so forth. Although this heuristic concept held for years, it has since been replaced in light of more recent neurophysiological evidence. Problems with the old model included the observation that lesioning the proprioceptors of MesV, and thus eliminating the jaw-closing reflex, did not totally abolish the masticatory rhythm (Goodwin and Luschei 1974). Likewise, paralysis of the jaw muscles did not eliminate rhythmic masticatory patterns in the brainstem or the motor nerves (Dellow and Lund 1971; Goldberg and Tal 1978; Goldberg and Chandler 1981). It is now known that the masticatory rhythm is produced by brainstem central pattern generator (CPG) circuitry, like running, flying and breathing (Camhi 1984). The masticatory CPG is located within the rostral medullary reticular formation (Chandler and Tal 1986; Nakamura and Katakura 1995).

Neck joints. Neck pain, though not as common as low back pain, is encountered frequently. It is considered one of the most common chronic pain conditions and a major problem in modern society (Manchikanti *et al* 2002). Nociceptive innervation of various structures in the cervical spine, including facets, intervertebral discs, muscles and ligaments is capable of causing neck pain and shoulder pain, but also headache (see Chapter 13). The same is true of neuropathy associated with injury to upper cervical DRGs, spinal roots and spinal nerves. Since the structures and innervation are spinal, neck pain is normally managed within the framework of orthopaedics despite the frequent referral of pain to the head.

2.4.7. Intracranial Structures (Brain, Dura, Blood Vessels)

The brain parenchyma is not innervated by sensory axons. For this reason insertion of intracranial probes and neurosurgical excisions can be carried out in awake patients without pain. However, two intracranial structures do have a sensory innervation, the meninges and the vasculature. The dura, including the sinuses and tentorium, is innervated primarily by Aδ and C nociceptors as documented by both the presence of histological markers such as substance P and calcitonin gene related peptide (CGRP), and by electrophysiological responses of afferent fibres to noxious stimuli. The density of innervation is highest near major dural blood vessels and sinuses. Opening the dura and cauterizing dural blood vessels in awake patients requires the use of local anaesthesia. In the presence of meningeal inflammation even modest mechanical stimulation of the dura can evoke pain. This is usually described as dull and poorly localized, consistent with the proposal that sensitized dural afferents contribute to headache pain, including migraine (Pietrobon and Striessnig 2003; Strassman *et al* 2004). Pain is said to be the only sensation evoked by stimulation of the intracranial meninges, regardless of whether the stimulus is electrical, mechanical, thermal or chemical (Ray and Wolff 1940; Penfield and Rasmussen 1955).

The larger intracranial blood vessels, arterial and venous, also have nociceptive Aδ- and C-fibre innervation based on immunolabelling. However, clamping or cauterizing such vessels in conscious patients is usually not accompanied by reports of pain. An exception is the rich vascular bed overlying the insular cortex and on the temporal operculum. Stimulation of blood vessels and arachnoid in conscious patients during open dissection of this region for the removal of tumours is a source of intense pain (Pereira *et al* 2005).

2.4.8. Pain Associated with Strong Stimulation of Special Sense Organs

Unpleasant sensations and frank pain can be evoked by irritating chemical stimulation of the tongue and the olfactory epithelium. Although some of these chemicals can activate taste buds and olfactory receptors, the result is taste and smell sensation. As noted earlier, evoked pain sensations are due to activation of trigeminal chemo-nociceptors rather than to impulses generated in taste or smell afferents. However, stimulation of the retina with intense *blinding* light is usually considered to be unpleasant if not frankly painful, and intense noise is sometimes described as painful, not just unpleasant on aesthetic grounds. Interestingly, these sensations are often enhanced during migraine and other neurovascular headaches (phonophobia, photophobia; see Chapters 9 and 10).

2.5. Autonomic Innervation of Trigeminal Structures

Sympathetic and parasympathetic efferents. The autonomic nervous system is a purely motor (efferent) system. It contains no sensory neurons. Nonetheless, sympathetic nerve fibres are thought to play an important indirect role in a number of painful conditions. They do this by regulating regional blood flow and temperature, and also by interacting directly with sensory nerve fibres, particularly in the event of nerve injury (sympathetically maintained pain (SMP), see 2.7.2.2). It is not known whether parasympathetic efferents also play a role in pain, although this prospect deserves consideration, particularly in light of the evidence for parasympathetic innervation of craniofacial vasculature noted below.

Sympathetic and parasympathetic nerve fibres end on and control smooth muscles and glands. In the orofacial area autonomic innervation controls salivation, lacrimation, mucosal secretion, vascular smooth muscle tone, intraocular smooth muscles, thermoregulation (vasomotor and pilomotor fibres) and sweating (sudomotor fibres). There is also evidence that sympathetic endings affect bone remodelling (Haug and Heyeraas 2006). In structures with parasympathetic innervation, such as the iris, control is through a balance between sympathetic and parasympathetic tone. In other structures only sympathetic innervation is present. In somatic blood vessels, for example, constriction and dilatation are served by different types of sympathetic efferents, vasoconstrictors and vasodilators (Janig 2006). However, recent evidence indicates that cutaneous and probably intracranial blood vessels in the head have parasympathetic innervation, a rarity at spinal levels (Kaji *et al* 1991; Ramien *et al* 2004). A role for this innervation in migraine has been proposed (Yarnitzky *et al* 2003). Moreover, these fibres begin to sprout following partial nerve injury, like sympathetic endings. Based on this observation it has been proposed that parasympathetic sprouting may contribute to trigeminal neuropathic pain (Ramien *et al* 2004; Grelik *et al* 2005).

The sympathetic innervation of the head originates in the most rostral intermediolateral horn cells, located in the upper thoracic and lower cervical segments of the spinal cord. Axons exit the cord via the segmental ventral roots, ascend in connectives of the sympathetic chain and end synaptically on neurons in the superior cervical sympathetic ganglion. Postganglionic axons of superior cervical sympathetic ganglion neurons ascend into the head as the superior cervical sympathetic nerve trunk, which parallels the carotid artery. They then distribute to their smooth muscle (e.g. vascular) and glandular end-targets.

The parasympathetic outflow to the orofacial area originates in parasympathetic brainstem nuclei associated with cranial nerves III, VII, IX and X, which constitutes the cranial part of the craniosacral parasympathetic outflow. Preganglionic parasympathetic fibres of the oculomotor nerve (III) originate in motoneurons in the midbrain Edinger-Westfal nucleus and end in the ciliary ganglion. The postganglionic axons innervate the iris (papillary sphincter) and ciliary muscles of the eye. Preganglionic parasympathetic fibres of the facial nerve (VII) originate in motoneurons of the upper medullary lacrimal and salivatory nuclei and end in ganglia associated with the lacrimal, submandibular and sublingual salivatory and nasal mucous glands. These ganglia send postganglionic axons into the glands. Preganglionic parasympathetic fibres of the glossopharyngeal nerve (IX) originate in the inferior salivatory nucleus and end in the otic ganglion. The postganglionic axons innervate the parotid salivatory gland. Preganglionic parasympathetic fibres of the vagus nerve (X) originate in the medullary dorsal motor nucleus of the vagus nerve. A minority serve structures in the neck, with the large majority leaving the head to supply thoracic and abdominal organs (Janig 2006). The cranial parasympathetic innervation supports numerous trigemino-parasympathetic reflexes such as tearing upon irritation of the cornea, salivation triggered by the taste of a good steak and mucous secretion in the presence of allergens (see Chapter 10).

CNS control. The limbic cortex (notably the insula), the hypothalamus and specific brainstem circuitry provide executive control for both the sympathetic and the parasympathetic compartments of the autonomic nervous system (Janig 2006). Since there are no preganglionic sympathetic motoneurons in the brain, all sympathetic commands are passed along descending tracts of the spinal cord and then pass back up into the head via the sympathetic chain. Most sympathetic and parasympathetic function is organized as spinal and brainstem reflexes that, in turn, are modulated by the forebrain structures noted. The iris is dually innervated, by sympathetic and parasympathetic efferents. Bright light induces pupillary constriction (myosis, parasympathetic); dim light induces pupillary dilatation (mydriasis, sympathetic). Both responses are driven via retinal projections to the upper brainstem. Sympathetic and parasympathetic outflow can also be initiated centrally as psychomotor events. For example, sadness on notification of the death of a loved one may initiate parasympathetically driven tearing, and sudden fear from a thunderclap sympathetic-driven vasoconstriction (paling).

2.6. Central Representation of Orofacial and Cranial Structures

2.6.1. Somatosensory Input to the Trigeminal Brainstem

Orofacial input to the brainstem trigeminal nuclear complex is in many ways analogous to input into the spinal cord from segmental DRGs. This is particularly so caudally where there is a continuous transition from the cervical spinal dorsal horn to the trigeminal nucleus caudalis. Further rostrally within the trigeminal nuclear complex it less resembles the organization of the spinal cord. The continuum of grey matter that receives primary afferent input from the TRG is designated, from caudal to rostral, the nucleus caudalis, nucleus interpolaris, nucleus oralis and the main sensory nucleus of the trigeminal complex (*main sensory V*) (Fig. 2.1). All of the nuclei caudal to main sensory V are sometimes collectively called the *spinal trigeminal complex*. Like DRG input at spinal levels, entering trigeminal root afferents bifurcate in an ascending and descending white matter tract overlying the grey matter of the trigeminal nuclei. But because entry is at the level of the pons, adjacent to nucleus oralis, the descending part of the trigeminal tract is much longer than the ascending part (O'Connor *et al* 1986; Li *et al* 1993a).

Fine diameter nociceptive afferents make up a particularly important component of the descending spinal trigeminal tract, which in this sense is the functional equivalent of Lissauer's tract at spinal levels. As these primary afferent axons run caudally they drop terminal arborizations into the underlying grey matter of the spinal trigeminal complex. Many continue caudally 2–3 segments into the cervical dorsal horn. The structure of the nucleus caudalis resembles that of the cervical dorsal horn, including its laminar distribution of second-order sensory neurons and superficial zone resembling the substantia gelatinosa. For this reason the caudal extent of the nucleus caudalis is often called the trigeminal medullary dorsal horn. Most large diameter fibres of the trigeminal root end synaptically in the grey matter near their level of entry, i.e. in the nucleus oralis, interpolaris and main sensory V. Functionally, therefore, this region more closely resembles the deeper layers of the dorsal horn.

As at spinal segmental levels, the synaptic action of primary afferents of all types is excitatory, and dependent upon glutamate as the primary neurotransmitter. Nociceptors, in addition, contain and release a large variety of peptide neuromodulators including substance P, CGRP, somatostatin and vasoactive intestinal polypeptide (VIP). Like the superficial spinal dorsal horn, cells in the superficial laminae of nucleus caudalis tend to respond preferentially to nociceptive input. Cells of deeper laminae respond to low-threshold touch input or a combination of nociceptive and touch input. The latter are wide dynamic range (WDR) neurons. Few nociceptive afferents ascend as far as main sensory V and hence cells in this nucleus respond almost exclusively to light tactile stimuli on the face and in the oral cavity. In this sense main sensory V corresponds to the dorsal column nuclei (nuclei gracilis and cuneatus), the spinal cord's medullary relay for light touch sensation.

Again resembling the spinal dorsal horn, somatosensory input from the orofacial region forms a topographic map-like representation in the trigeminal complex (Strassman and Vos 1993). Sensory fibres of the ophthalmic division (V_1) end ventrolaterally while fibres from the mandibular division (V_3) end dorsomedially. Thus, the ipsilateral face is represented along the length of the brainstem trigeminal complex, inverted (chin up and forehead down)

(Figs 2.3, 2.4). This arrangement is similar to the spinal topographic map where the proximal part of each dermatome (e.g. the shoulder) is represented ventrolaterally while the distal part (e.g. the finger tips) is represented dorsomedially. The intranasal and intraoral mucosas, and the tooth pulps, are individually represented in the map. Likewise, nociceptive input from cranial nerves VII, IX and X (pharynx and parts of the ear) also converges on nucleus caudalis, completing the topographic map of the head.

Nociceptive-specific (mostly in nucleus caudalis) and WDR cells (in all of the spinal trigeminal nuclei) are driven by noxious stimuli and presumably mediate the sensation of pain. This is despite the fact that nuclei interpolaris and oralis lack a structure resembling the substantia gelatinosa, and do not receive many direct nociceptive afferents from the TRG. In fact, most nociceptive input to these nuclei derives from the nucleus caudalis. That is, nucleus caudalis neurons receive direct primary afferent nociceptive input and then relay it to the interpolar and oral nuclei via second-order ascending fibres of the trigeminal complex (Dubner *et al* 1978; Chiang *et al* 2002). Lesions of nucleus caudalis suppress nociceptive responses of interpolar and oral neurons to noxious stimulation, including those of the mucosa and tooth pulp, although these responses are not abolished completely (Sessle 2000). Surgical transection of the descending tract of V (*trigeminal tractotomy*) can thus relieve pain in the orofacial region both by reducing descending nociceptive drive to the nucleus caudalis and by functionally blocking ascending relay fibres from nucleus caudalis to nuclei interpolaris and oralis. Unfortunately, the pain relief is rarely permanent (Sjoqvist 1950).

2.6.2. Ascending Trigeminal Pathways

Outputs of the trigeminal nuclear complex also follow the general organizational plan of the spinal cord, with certain differences. Trigeminal signals, light touch and nociceptive, ascend towards the thalamus and then the cortex following two families of trigeminothalamic pathways, a lateral 'neotrigeminothalamic pathway' and a medial 'paleo-trigeminothalamic pathway'. Many of these fibres drop collateral branches along their route in the brainstem reticular formation and in specific brainstem nuclei. The term 'trigeminobulbothalamic pathway' therefore best describes this system just as 'spino-bulbothalamic pathway' best describes fibres that ascend from the spinal cord towards the thalamus. The trigeminal complex also has thalamic projections that specialize in conveying detailed light touch signals, analogous to the dorsal column–medial lemniscus system. These fibres originate in the rostral parts of the complex, mostly in main sensory V. Finally, a variety of pathways convey trigeminal signals to the hypothalamus, the basal forebrain and limbic areas of the telencephalon including the amygdaloid complex. Together, these pathways subserve both the sensory-discriminative aspects of pain sensation from the face, and the motivational-emotional aspects (Beggs *et al* 2003; Dostrovsky and Craig 2006).

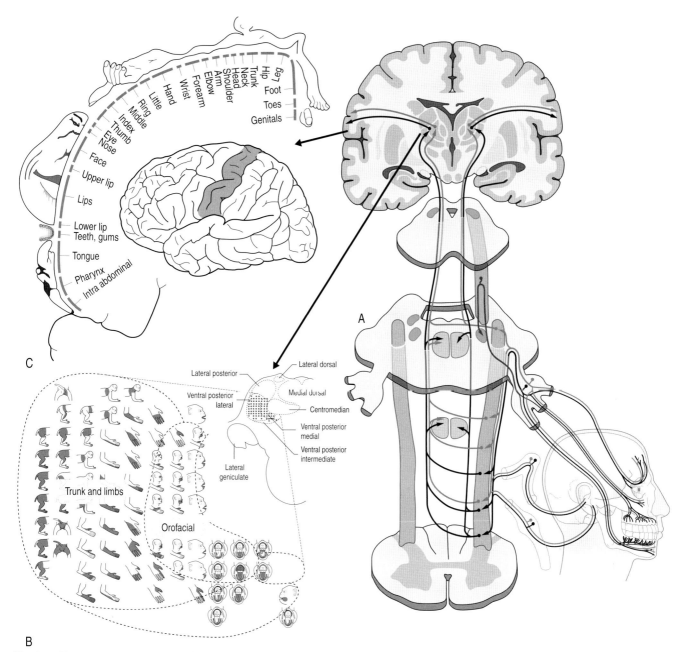

Fig. 2.4 • The somatotopic mapping of primary sensory input in the spinal trigeminal complex is reflected in somatotopic representations at higher way-stations in the trigeminal pathway (A). The somatotopic map of craniofacial and spinal-somatic structures in the ventrobasal complex (nuclei VPL and VPM) is shown in the lower left (B) (Mouncastle and Henneman 1952). The somatotopic map of craniofacial and spinal-somatic structures in the primary somatosensory cortex (S1) is shown in the upper left (C).

2.6.2.1. Trigemino-bulbothalamic Pathways

Most projection neurons of the trigeminal complex cross the midline near the level at which the neurons reside and contribute to the trigeminothalamic stream. Along the length of the medulla and pons this somewhat diffuse scattering of axons joins the more compact white matter of the ascending spinothalamic tract completing its map-like representation of the body surface: the contralateral hindlimb laterally, then the contralateral forelimb and trunk, and far medially the contralateral face.

Lateral and medial pathways to the thalamus. Like the spino-bulbothalamic tract, the trigemino-bulbothalamic projections contain axons of all neuronal types, nociceptive and low-threshold selective, as well as WDR. Not all of these ascending axons reach the thalamus, but those that

do terminate map-like in the contralateral nucleus ventralis posterior medialis (VPM), in the medial division of the somatosensory ventrobasal complex (VB). VPM, together with the dorsolaterally adjacent nucleus ventralis posterior lateralis (VPL), which maps the body below the neck, form the principal somatosensory relay to the somatosensory cortex. Inputs to VPM tend to come preferentially from trigeminal WDR and touch selective neurons, with fewer from nociceptive selective neurons of nucleus caudalis. A small part of the input to VPM comes from the ipsilateral trigeminal complex. A small region in the most medial part of VPM maps intraoral structures including the teeth (Kelly 1985; Krout *et al* 2002).

Many ascending axons of the trigeminal complex also contribute synaptic input to parts of the thalamus located medial to the VPL–VPM. Two such areas are of particular note: the posterior nuclear group of the thalamus (PO), just caudal to VPL–VPM, and the thalamic intralaminar nuclei, including the centromedial, parafascicular and paracentral nuclei. Inputs to these medial nuclei tend to come preferentially from WDR and nociceptive-selective neurons of the nucleus caudalis, bilaterally, resulting in receptive fields that are large and respond preferentially to noxious stimuli. However, they also receive light touch input from the more rostral trigeminal nuclei. Other medially located thalamic nuclei also receive input from the trigeminal complex including the mediodorsal nucleus (MD), the thalamic midline nuclei and the ventromedial thalamic area (Peschanski 1984; Carstens et al 1990; Williams et al 1994; Krout et al 2002; Craig 2004).

Some authors believe that pain sensation is due exclusively, or almost exclusively, to the nociceptive-selective neurons in lamina I of the spinal and trigeminal dorsal horn, with the numerous WDR neurons of deeper layers being largely irrelevant (Craig 2003). This view focuses blinkered interest on the connections of the lamina I neurons, ignoring nociceptive input to WDR neurons of lamina V and deeper spinal laminae. Two small thalamic subnuclei have been identified in monkeys and man that receive input preferentially from lamina I neurons, VMpo and MDvc. They have hence been promoted as specific relays for burning pain and itch. Lower mammals do not appear to have equivalent nuclei, leading to the speculation that they do not *feel* pain in the same way that we do (Craig 2003, 2004).

In addition to thalamic projections, ascending trigeminothalamic axons, crossed and uncrossed, drop collateral branches in a variety of brainstem structures caudal to the thalamus that lie along their trajectory. The most prominent of these are the medullary, pontine and mesencephalic reticular formation, the parabrachial complex and the deep layers of the superior colliculus. These connections can be thought of as the trigeminal equivalent of the spinobulbar (spinoreticular) pathways. They probably play a variety of sensory, autonomic and neuroendocrine roles in addition to conscious pain perception. For example, the somatosensory map in the deep superior colliculus participates in body orientation to somatosensory stimuli (Drager and Hubel 1975).

Trigeminolemniscal fibres. The rostral nuclei of the trigeminal complex, especially nucleus oralis and main sensory V, bear some resemblance to the dorsal column nuclei in the sense of receiving direct input from the TRG and containing cells that respond selectively to low-threshold tactile and proprioceptive stimuli, with small receptive fields and high spatial resolution. Axons of these neurons cross the midline as a part of trigeminothalamic tract, join the medial lemniscus and terminate mainly in the VPM. For this reason they are sometimes called *trigeminolemniscal* fibres. Although didactic, the concept of a dual pathway for light touch input, paralleling the spinal dorsal column–medial lemniscus system and the spinothalamic system, is a bit overstated. Ascending spinothalamic projections

of dorsal horn laminae III and IV neurons are just as good an analogy. Unlike the dorsal column nuclei, main sensory V is not displaced from the segments of afferent input, and its thalamic projections follow the general trajectory of the rest of the trigeminothalamic axons.

2.6.2.2. Thalamocortical Relations

Classical somatosensory cortex. Thalamocortical neurons of VPL and VPM, the *specific* somatosensory nuclei of the thalamus, project via the thalamocortical radiations to the ipsilateral postcentral gyrus. They end there topographically, mainly in the primary somatosensory cortex (S1), with synaptic terminations mostly in lamina IV. Axons of VPM neurons end in the face region of the S1 map, in the ventrolateral part of the postcentral gyrus. The body and feet end dorsomedially in this gyrus (Fig. 2.4). The S1 cortical area devoted to the head is disproportionately large in comparison to the representation of the rest of the body. Likewise, the representation of the mouth, perioral region and the tongue, and in animals the vibrissae of the snout (whiskers), is disproportionately large in comparison with the rest of the head. The size of these cortical representations reflects the density of innervation, and presumably the functional importance of these body parts, rather than their physical size. Some neurons of S1 respond to noxious inputs as well as to touch and vibration, although most are poor at encoding the intensity of noxious stimuli in terms of firing frequency. Nociceptive selective neurons appear to be rare, or absent in S1.

Thalamocortical neurons of VPL and VPM also project to a smaller, secondary somatosensory cortical area, ventral and posterior to S1. This area, S2, forms an additional complete body–head map. Both the lateral and the medial groups of thalamic nuclei project to both S1 and S2. However, the lateral nuclei (VPL, VPM) preferentially target S1, while the medial nuclei preferentially target S2 (Dostrovsky and Craig 2006). As a result tooth pain, for example, leads to localized, bilateral activation in both S1 and S2 (Jantsch et al 2005). The distinction between S1 and S2 is only the beginning of cortical differentiation. Especially in higher primates, including humans, S1 and S2 each contain numerous complete map representations of the contralateral body surface. Although the functional meaning of this is not entirely clear, the tendency of each to have somewhat different receptive field properties (e.g. skin vs. deep tissues, input from slow vs. rapidly adapting afferents) suggests that they specialize in processing specific types of sensory information. How this information is reassembled into a unified percept remains a mystery.

Neurons of PO and the intralaminar thalamic nuclei also project to S1 and S2. However, in addition, they terminate in a diffuse and widespread manner in much broader regions of the cerebral cortex. These relatively *nonspecific* projections are thought to contribute to generalized functions such as cortical arousal and wake–sleep states. However, they may also make a contribution to conscious pain sensation.

Pathways to limbic cortex and the cerebellum. The results of non-invasive functional imaging in humans subjected to noxious stimuli have brought to the fore somatosensory projection areas at a distance from the classical somatosensory cortices S1 and S2. A variety of non-S1/S2 cortical areas show *activations* in functional imaging (positron emission tomography (PET), functional magnetic resonance imaging (fMRI) and magnetoencephalography (MEG)). The areas with the most prominent and reliable responses are the anterior part of the cingulate cortex (ACC), parts of the prefrontal cortex and the insular cortex (Peyron *et al* 2000). These and several of the other non-classical cortical targets are noteworthy as being integral parts of the *limbic system*. The limbic system is a highly interconnected network of cortical and subcortical brain areas that together control the autonomic and neuroendocrine nervous systems, and are intimately related to motivational and emotional behaviours such as hunger, thirst, sex, nesting, fear and anger. This has led to the concept that these limbic cortical areas process the motivational-emotional aspects of pain, in contrast to the sensory-discriminative aspects which are processed by the classical somatosensory cortex (Rainville *et al* 1997; Peyron *et al* 2000; Johansen *et al* 2001; Strigo *et al* 2003). The limbic cortical areas activated by painful stimuli, including ACC and the insula, receive their somatosensory input mostly from the medial group of thalamic nuclei, notably MD, VM, PO and the intralaminar group. That means that they receive much of their trigeminal sensory information from nucleus caudalis, and tend to have large receptive fields with a prominent nociceptive component as well as a low-threshold component.

A final *surprise* that derives from functional imaging in humans is the consistent activations observed in the cerebellum during painful stimuli, and their correlation with felt pain intensity (Peyron *et al* 2000). It has been known for generations that the cerebellum receives heavy somatosensory input from the spinal cord and trigeminal complex, including nociceptive input. Some of this input is direct, via the spinocerebellar and trigeminocerebellar tracts, and some is indirect, relayed by the reticular formation (Ikeda 1979; Matsushita *et al* 1982). In the past, this input has been presumed to serve in the context of motor control, e.g. motor accommodation to unexpected noxious stimuli. In light of the new results, we need to take seriously the possibility that the cerebellum is also involved in pain perception.

2.6.2.3. Ascending Extrathalamic Trigeminal Pathways

The prevailing concept of the classical somatosensory cortex being 'the seat of pain perception' (despite evidence to the contrary, see below) delayed appreciation of ascending trigeminosensory pathways that bypass the thalamic VPL–VPM nuclei, or avoid the cortex altogether. The advent of sensitive neuroanatomical tracing methods and of non-invasive brain imaging in humans has focused more attention on alternative pain pathways. As noted,

the *affect* of pain sensation, how aversive it feels, is currently thought to be conveyed by non-VPL–VPM thalamo-cortical routes to the limbic cortex. In addition, however, there are somatosensory routes to the forebrain that do not pass through the thalamus. The three noted below are the most prominent. The functional role of these extra-thalamic pathways for trigeminal sensory processing is not well understood. Do they contribute to conscious pain discrimination and affect? Do they contribute to autonomic and neuroendocrine control? Do they play a role in arousal? Do they contribute to memory formation?

Parabrachial-amygdaloid pathway. There is a prominent projection from the trigeminal nuclear complex, particularly nucleus caudalis, to the ipsilateral lateral and Kolliker-Fuse divisions of the parabrachial complex. This region also receives visceral afferent input, including nociceptive input, from the vagus nerve (X), relayed through the nucleus of the solitary tract (NTS). From the parabrachial nucleus information passes to the central nucleus of the amygdala. This pathway may be important for fear and avoidance responses (Bernard and Besson 1990). The parabrachial nucleus also relays nociceptive information to the hypothalamus and basal forebrain.

Hypothalamus and basal forebrain. Direct projections from the trigeminal complex, both nucleus caudalis and the more rostral nuclei, have been traced into the hypothalamus and the basal forebrain (Ring and Ganchrow 1983; Carstens *et al* 1990; Iwata *et al* 1992; Zagon *et al* 1994; Li *et al* 1997; Malick and Burstein 1998; Malick *et al* 2000). These connections are presumed to play a role in the generation of autonomic and neuroendocrine responses, and to contribute to emotional and motivational states. Several of these target areas have direct projections to the cortex.

Septum, hippocampus and basal ganglia. Direct nociceptive projections from the trigeminal complex have also been traced into the preoptic area, the diagonal band nuclei, the septum, amygdala and orbitofrontal cortex (Burstein and Giesler 1989). These provide potential routes for nociceptive signals to access the hippocampal formation. Nociceptive responses have been recorded in neurons of the caudate putamen and the globus pallidus (Carelli and West 1991; Zagon *et al* 1994). A recent trans-synaptic tracer study has provided anatomical evidence of a nociceptive pathway from the spinal cord to the striatum (Braz *et al* 2005). An equivalent trigeminal pathway is very likely to exist. Together, these pathways imply a role for trigeminal nociceptive input to the subcortical forebrain in motor function, affect, learning and memory.

2.6.3. Trigeminal Pain Is Subject to Descending Control

The most important contribution of Melzack and Wall's 'gate control' theory of pain was the concept that pain sensation is subject to modulation, both by inputs from the periphery and by signals that derive from the brain itself. We have discussed pathways that *evoke* pain sensation. There is also a significant projection from the brainstem trigeminal complex to areas thought to *modulate* pain, notably the rostroventromedial medulla (RVM) and the periaqueductal grey (PAG). The PAG, via relays in the RVM and lateral medulla, suppresses the forward transmission of nociceptive signals within the trigeminal complex. This is done both by inhibiting the ability of primary afferent nociceptors to activate second-order pain-signalling neurons (presynaptic inhibition) and by postsynaptic inhibition of second-order neurons, at least partly through inhibitory interneurons (Li *et al* 1993b,c; Sessle 2000; Ren and Dubner 2002).

The fact that trigeminal nociceptive signals can activate PAG-induced pain inhibition means that a feedback loop is in place. Pain inhibits pain. The PAG is also activated by circulating opiates, both endogenous (endorphins) and those administered therapeutically. The resulting pre- and postsynaptic inhibition in the spinal trigeminal complex, and in the spinal cord, is believed to be the primary analgesic mechanism of morphine and other analgesic opiates. Only at high opiate concentrations is there also direct inhibition of trigeminal pain-signalling neurons. Some forms of context-related analgesia (e.g. the 'placebo effect') are suppressed by pharmacological block of mu-opiate receptors. This suggests that complex processes such as anticipation, expectation, conditioning and belief, processes that undoubtedly play out in the cerebral cortex, may generate pain inhibition by opioid (enkephalinergic) activation of the PAG. Recently it has become clear that activity in some neurons of the rostromedial medulla (and elsewhere) facilitates pain transmission, rather than inhibiting it. Cerebral modulation of trigeminal pain is a two-way process (Ren and Dubner 2002).

2.6.4. Cerebral Representation of Pain

Pain, by definition, is a sensory and emotional event experienced by a conscious brain. There has never been much doubt that the pathways leading to pain perception end in the cerebral cortex. However, closer consideration of this dogma leaves some perplexing questions.

Microelectrode recordings in animals, and noninvasive functional imaging in humans, show excitations in many brain areas following pain-provoking stimulation of the skin and internal organs (Peyron *et al* 2000). As noted earlier, these include structures long known as key parts of the somatosensory system (e.g. VPL–VPM, and S1 and S2 cortex), *novel* areas of limbic cortex (e.g. ACC and the insula), as well as subcortical areas not classically thought of as somatosensory processors (e.g. the cerebellum and the corpus striatum). Noxious stimulation of different organs, skin versus viscera for example, reveals different if overlapping patterns of cortical activation, appropriate to the different *feels* evoked. Moreover, some cortical activations, particularly in ACC, track reported pain unpleasantness and not the intensity of the applied stimulus when the

two are dissociated by manipulations such as placebo and hypnotic suggestion (Rainville *et al* 1997; Strigo *et al* 2003).

All of these observations are as expected of a cortical pain analyser. However, other observations are not as expected. The most important is that direct electrical stimulation of the cortical convexity, including areas activated by painful stimuli, almost never evokes a report of pain in awake patients (Penfield and Rasmussen 1955; Libet 1973). Stimulation of cortical areas associated with vision, hearing, smell and (non-painful) touch readily arouse the appropriate percepts. It may be argued that the structures relevant for pain sensation are buried in the mid-sagittal (ACC) or Sylvian sulci (insula) and are hard to access by surface stimulation. However, it is very rare for epileptic seizures to include auras that are painful even though the underlying cortical discharge frequently includes, indeed often favours, the buried limbic cortices. A recent report of pain evoked in a small number of epileptic patients by depth electrodes on the insular cortex is an exception (Ostrowsky *et al* 2002). However, it has been shown that direct stimulation of the meninges and blood vessels that overlie the insular cortex evokes pain sensation (Pereira *et al* 2005). These vessels have rich nociceptive innervation from the TRG. Thus, the claim that pain is evoked by insular cortex stimulation using depth electrodes may be confounded by stimulation of local non-neural tissue.

Another retort sometimes given is that pain is complex and multiply represented in the cortex such that unlike vision, hearing, smell and touch, to evoke pain by cortical stimulation requires simultaneous activation at numerous locations. However, epileptic seizures often activate widespread areas simultaneously, and as noted, they are rarely painful. One might argue that the widespread activity must be precisely patterned. However, if this were the case, then disruption of this complex pattern, as is expected to occur in the presence of brain lesions, ought to eliminate pain sensation. In fact, focal lesions in areas active during pain, and even massive cortical lesions, do not produce analgesia. On the contrary, cortical strokes are often followed by chronic neuropathic post-stroke pain (Boivie *et al* 1989; see also Chapter 11). Lesions in cortical areas thought to subserve vision, hearing, smell and touch do not behave in this way. Patients with lesions in the primary visual cortex, for example, are perceptually blind, although they may have some residual visually guided function. It is unjustified to rule out the possibility that the neural computations that generate pain experience play out subcortically rather than in the cerebral cortex. Note that in contrast to the cortex, pain is readily evoked by focal (microelectrode) stimulation in areas of the thalamus and brainstem (Dostrovsky 2000).

2.7. Pathophysiology and Neural Plasticity in the Orofacial Area

Normal (nociceptive) pain and associated nocifensive reflexes such as tearing, blinking, sneezing and reflex withdrawal (including the jaw-opening reflex) are designed to minimize tissue damage. Likewise, associated ascending pain signals and hypersensibility help to protect from further damage and permit learning of avoidance strategies. However, there are a variety of chronic orofacial pain states that do not appear to have adaptive value. Specific pain diagnoses of this sort include myofascial pain, headaches, trigeminal and other cranial nerve neuralgias, burning mouth disorder and atypical facial pain. These and related conditions, which constitute a major burden for patient and therapist alike, will be discussed in considerable detail in later chapters in this volume. Here we consider pathophysiological processes thought to underlie these problematic chronic pain syndromes (also see Chapter 11).

2.7.1. What Needs Explaining?

Sensory dysfunction in chronic orofacial pain states. Abnormalities of sensation in chronic orofacial diagnoses include two categories of *positive* phenomena: (1) spontaneous paraesthesias, dysaesthesias and pain, and (2) abnormal sensation and pain evoked by natural stimuli. Evoked pain may include bizarre distortions of sensation in space and time that come under the umbrella heading of *hyperpathia*.

In addition to these positive sensory abnormalities there may also be *negative* changes. These too fall into the categories of spontaneous and evoked. Nerve block using local anaesthetics or injury of a nerve reduces or eliminates the ability to evoke sensation by stimuli applied distally. However, the complete elimination of spontaneous sensation is much more difficult to achieve. For example, local anaesthetic block of the mandibular nerve eliminates sensation of stimuli applied to the lip, but it does not erase feelings of the existence of the lip, leaving the impression that there is a hole in the face. Rather, such nerve blocks lead to a sensation of *numbness*, described by most people as the sensation of a tingling and swollen lip. A swollen lip and absence of a lip are two qualitatively different sensations; a quick look in the mirror is enough to confirm that the lip itself is not in fact swollen. The dental patient's sensation of a 'swollen lip' is actually phantom limb sensation. Likewise, when all nerves of a limb are blocked, subjects report feeling a (non-painful) phantom limb (Melzack and Bromage 1973) rather than absence of the limb. Lesions of the parietal cortex sometimes lead to true erasure of the limb from the patient's perceptual body schema: denial by the patient that the limb belongs to him. We are not aware of this phenomenon occurring in the head or parts of the head.

Spontaneous (ongoing) pain. Spontaneous (ongoing) pain is present at rest when no (intentional) stimulus is applied. Whether the pain is truly stimulus-independent, or actually associated with occult stimuli related to blood chemistry, growths, autonomic nervous system activity, hormones or other internal physiological factors is often unknown. It is a bad habit to refer to ongoing pain simply as 'pain'.

Stimulus-evoked pain. Alterations of evoked sensation include pain by stimuli that are normally painless (allodynia) as well as exaggerated pain from normally painful stimuli (hyperalgesia). Amplified sensation may affect the skin, oral or nasal mucosa, vasculature, meninges, etc. Pain may also be evoked by jaw movement and flexion of the neck, or by focal pressure to deep tissue *tender* or *trigger* points in muscle, tendons and joints. There are many potential causes of tissue tenderness, but they all ultimately boil down to the question of neural signals generated by the stimulus. For example, exaggerated sensation may be due to *trivial* peripheral factors such as altered viscoelastic or thermal conductive properties of the tissue intervening between the stimulus and the nociceptive nerve endings. The same stimulus would then activate a large afferent pain signal. Still in the periphery, nociceptive sensory endings may be sensitized by inflammation or due to neuropathology. An example of the latter is the development of local hypersensitivity at a site where a small nerve branch has been pinched as it crossed a fascial plane (microneuroma). Finally, augmented pain sensation may be due to changes in CNS signal processing. In general, when the source of pain is not at the surface, it is inherently difficult to analyze the root cause and even whether the problem is nociceptive, inflammatory or neuropathic. This uncertainty is common in craniofacial pain syndromes.

Altered sensory quality. The words that people with chronic pain use to describe their sensory experience can be informative, particularly in the case of chronic pain associated with neural damage and disease. Some words are generic, and common to nociceptive, inflammatory and neuropathic pain. But some are characteristic of neuropathy in general, or even of particular neuropathic pain syndromes (Bouhassira *et al* 2005). For example, spontaneous burning pain occurs in postherpetic neuralgia (PHN), a neuropathic pain condition, but it also occurs after an acute burn, an example of normal nociceptive pain. However, patients with nerve injuries often describe spontaneous and evoked shooting pains and electric shock-like paroxysms, sensations uncommon except in neuropathy. The closest (presumably) nociceptive equivalent occurs when the radial nerve is percussed against bone at the elbow ('hitting your funny-bone'). Another abnormal sensation specific to neuropathy is *hyperpathia*, a constellation of pain descriptors that do not occur normally or in inflamed tissue. In hyperpathia, sensation shows odd temporal and spatial convergence. A gentle tap on the back of the hand may feel dull, as if felt through a boxing glove. But with repeated tapping, say once or twice a second for 10–20 seconds, the sensation 'winds up', becoming stronger and stronger until it reaches a painful crescendo. Hyperpathic sensations also spread in space; localized touch may trigger a stinging sensation that spreads up the arm (Kugelberg and Lindblom 1959; Noordenbos 1959; Gottrup *et al* 2003). There are several chronic pain conditions specific to the craniofacial area that have distinctive sensory characteristics. These include trigeminal neuralgia and migraine.

Phantom limb pain and anaesthesia dolorosa ('deafferentation pain'). Special mention needs to be made of neuropathic sensations experienced in parts of the body that no longer exist or that are completely numb due to major nerve injury, traumatic or surgical (Wynn-Parry 1980; Nikolajsen and Jensen 2001). The body part continues to be felt as a *phantom*, and is painful some of the time in most patients, and most of the time in some patients. In the trigeminal region phantom ear and nose are occasionally reported after amputation, and pain is often described in anaesthetic areas following major nerve or cranial root injury (anaesthesia dolorosa; Benoliel *et al* 2005). Anaesthesia dolorosa may also be a complication of tumours and therapeutic transection of major trigeminal nerve tributaries, the TRG or the trigeminal root, procedures carried out in an attempt to control pain in trigeminal neuralgia (White and Sweet 1969). Phantom limb pain has been claimed to occur following extraction of teeth (Marbach and Raphael 2000), but this pain is probably better understood as an example of more typical traumatic neuropathic pains. Many patients with neuropathic pain, including phantoms and anaesthesia dolorosa, report exacerbating factors such as emotional upset or cold weather, and that temporary relief may be provided by massage, warming, etc. Distortions in body schema reported by amputees with phantom limbs (e.g. telescoping) are not common in the orofacial region. However, upper limb amputees sometimes report that stimuli on the face are felt in (i.e. referred to) the phantom arm. Pain that follows nerve injury, distal to the sensory ganglion, is often mistakenly referred to as 'deafferentation pain'. This is an unfortunate term as it implies a specific pain mechanism, loss of afferent input. In fact, as explained below, far from eliminating afferent input, nerve injury may actually generate such input, ectopically. Deafferentation pain should be reserved for cases in which there has been nerve root injury central to the ganglion, or removal of the ganglion itself. 'Peripheral neuropathic pain' is the appropriate term for pain due to orofacial peripheral nerve injury. Incorrect use of the diagnostic term deafferentation pain may actually distract from the true pain mechanism and delay effective treatment. It is essential to realize that pain following neural injury peripheral and central to the trigeminal ganglion is likely to have different causes.

2.7.2. Trigeminal Neuropathic Pain

2.7.2.1. Precipitating Events and Variability

Any type of neural damage or disease, physical, chemical or metabolic, that has the effect of inducing pathology in a peripheral nerve (neuropathy), sensory or autonomic ganglion (ganglionopathy) or cranial nerve/dorsal root (radiculopathy) may precipitate peripheral neuropathic pain. Typical precipitating events are trauma (frequently iatrogenic), infection, inflammation, tumours, metabolic abnormalities, malnutrition, ischaemia, vascular abnormalities, neurotoxins (including chemotherapeutic agents), radiation, inherited mutations and autoimmune attack. If damage occurs suddenly 'injury discharge' may cause acute pain sensation. But in general, peripheral neuropathic pain results from secondary pathophysiological changes that develop over time in the peripheral (PNS) and central nervous system.

There are two basic forms of pathological change, dys- or demyelination and various degrees of axonopathy. Disruption of the ability of peripheral axons to conduct nerve impulses causes negative sensory abnormalities such as hypoaesthesia and anaesthesia. It is more challenging to understand positive sensory symptoms and signs such as pain, and why they are common in some diagnoses and not in others. A related challenge is to understand the notorious variability in pain from patient to patient even when the precipitating neuropathy is essentially identical. Environmental and psychosocial factors play a role. However, there is accumulating evidence for the existence of genetic polymorphisms that affect susceptibility to pain given a fixed neural pathology. Such 'pain susceptibility genes' must be distinguished from 'disease susceptibility genes', mutations that predispose to acquiring particular types of nerve pathology that may be painful (Mogil 2004). The fact that the link between pathological changes in nerve and sensory symptoms is non-trivial suggests that objective indicators of neuropathology must be interpreted with caution. There may be significant neural dysfunction without obvious pathology, and there may be significant pathology without obvious motor or sensory abnormalities. In general, electrophysiological parameters used in the limbs, such as nerve conduction studies, are not available in the orofacial region because of short conduction distances. Histological methods such as nerve and skin-punch biopsies have not been applied much to trigeminal structures, and are unlikely to be acceptable in exposed areas of the face. However, there are many circumstances in which these methods might provide useful information.

2.7.2.2. Neuropathic Pain Mechanisms

The paradox of neuropathic pain, amplified sensation following disruption of conduction pathways, is rooted in the misconception that nerves are like copper telephone cables. True, primary afferents convey electrical signals from the periphery to the CNS, but the analogy does not go much beyond that. Axons are not wires but live, protoplasmic extensions of specialized cells. The biology of these cells needs to be taken seriously (Devor 2006a,b). How do they respond to demyelination and axonopathy, and how do they interact with their PNS and CNS neighbours?

Spontaneous firing and pain in neuropathy. When a peripheral nerve is damaged, the severed or demyelinated axons can no longer pass impulses efficiently from periphery to centre. This is the cause of negative sensory symptoms such as numbness, and also negative motor symptoms such as weakness (e.g. Bell's palsy). However, severed or demyelinated axons may also undergo changes in their functional properties (their *phenotype*) that cause positive symptoms. The most important of these is the emergence of electrical hyperexcitability and the consequent generation of abnormal impulse discharge at ectopic locations in the neuron (Burchiel and Wyler 1978; Bongenhielm and Robinson 1996, 1998; Devor 2006a). For the most part, nerve injury does not cause the death of sensory cell bodies in the TRG, or loss of afferent connections in the trigeminal brainstem. Ectopically generated impulses are therefore conducted into the CNS where they evoke paraesthesias, dysaesthesias and pain. In addition, abnormal discharge in injured neurons, perhaps together with abnormal discharge in nearby uninjured neurons (Gracely *et al* 1992; Tsuboi *et al* 2004) may trigger central sensitization, amplifying the sensory effects of both the abnormal spontaneous discharge and signals evoked in normal residual afferents by natural stimulation. In this way, both injured and nearby non-injured sensory neurons contribute to neuropathic pain sensation.

It is expected that the sensation evoked by spontaneous (and evoked) ectopic discharge can be related to the type of afferent involved. For example, thermal sensibility to heat and cold stimuli is normally due to the activation of specific thermosensitive C and $A\delta$ afferents. It is thus likely that spontaneous burning pain, a common symptom in patients with peripheral neuropathy (e.g. burning mouth disorder or post herpetic neuralgia, Chapter 11), is due to activity in peripheral thermal nociceptors and/or CNS pathways normally involved in heat sensation. The key difference is that due to the pathology these pathways are now active at normal body temperature.

Neural response to injury and ectopic discharge. The cascade of events that leads to spontaneous ectopic discharge and spontaneous pain in severed (and perhaps also in demyelinated) afferents begins with blockade of the normal flow of neurotrophic signalling molecules between the periphery and the sensory cell body. This triggers a change in the quantity of various of the proteins synthesized (*expressed*) by the cell body and exported to both peripheral and central axon endings (Boucher and McMahon 2001). Some proteins start to be expressed in excess (*upregulation* of gene expression) while the synthesis of others is reduced (*downregulation*; Costigan *et al* 2002; Xiao *et al* 2002). Upregulation of Na^+ channel types combined with downregulation of K^+ channel types is probably the immediate cause of hyperexcitability (Kocsis and Devor 2000; Waxman 2002; Devor 2006a). Disrupted delivery (*trafficking*) of transported molecules, notably the accumulation of Na^+ channels at sites of axonal injury including zones of demyelination, also contributes to hyperexcitability (Devor *et al* 1989; Waxman 2002; Devor 2006a). The biophysical process whereby changes in the density of specific ion channels lead to membrane

resonance, repetitive firing capability and ectopic discharge is rapidly coming into focus (Amir *et al* 2002; Devor 2006a).

Evoked pain. Gentle percussion over sites of nerve injury, areas of entrapment, tumour infiltration, neuromas, etc., typically evokes an intense stabbing or electric shock-like sensation. This pain, the 'Tinel sign', is thought to be due to the development of ectopic neuropathic mechanosensitivity at these sites. In the event of injuries that leave the nerve in-continuity a second Tinel may be evoked further distally, at the farthest position reached by regenerating axon sprouts. Pain may also occur on tapping along the trajectory of an injured nerve. This activates freely outgrowing sprouts or sprouts that have become trapped along the course of the nerve. Pain evoked by jaw opening sometimes has this paroxysmal neuropathic quality, suggesting that traction on a mandibular nerve branch might activate local ectopic mechanosensitive trigger sites. Likewise, pain evoked by tapping a tooth, or by deep palpation at tender spots, may be due to this mechanism. For example, ectopic mechanosensitivity of injured axon ends may account for teeth that are tender to percussion for years following root canal therapy despite no radiological or clinical evidence of periapical pathology (see Chapter 11). Destruction of the tooth pulp, or tooth extraction, leaves a neuroma at the base of the tooth.

Ectopic mechanosensitivity is also a feature of spinal roots locally demyelinated by stenosis in the spinal canal, entrapped in the constricted space of root foraminae (e.g. in the neck), or damaged by continuous percussion by an arterial loop. The latter is thought to underlie pain in trigeminal neuralgia (see below and Chapter 11). Interestingly, momentary mechanical probing of ectopic pacemaker sites frequently evokes discharge that long outlasts the stimulus itself. Such *afterdischarge* is the likely explanation of aftersensations, trigger-points and triggered pain paroxysms that may be evoked by pressure applied at nerve loci which have been injured (Devor *et al* 2002; Gottrup *et al* 2003).

Exacerbating factors. Both spontaneous and pressure-evoked pains may be exacerbated by a variety of additional factors that tend to depolarize and excite sensory axons and neuronal somata that have become hyperexcitable due to injury or disease. Notable among these are ectopic responses to circulating catecholamines, and noradrenaline released from nearby postganglionic sympathetic axons. This 'sympathetic–sensory coupling' may account for painful flare-ups at times of emotional upset. Injured sympathetic axon ends sprout and proliferate in the skin and other peripheral tissue, and at nerve injury sites and neuromas. In addition, intact sympathetic endings associated with blood vessels may sprout within sensory ganglia and engulf neuronal cell bodies, causing excitation and pain (McLachlan *et al* 1993; Shinder *et al* 1999; Grelik *et al* 2005). However, there is some debate as to whether sympathetic sprouting indeed occurs in the cranial TRG as it does in sensory ganglia at spinal levels (Davis *et al* 1994; Bongenhielm *et al* 1999; Benoliel *et al* 2001). Sympathetic–sensory coupling may be an important substrate for sympathetically maintained chronic pain states (Harden *et al* 2001).

Afferent response to local and circulating inflammatory mediators is a second example of ectopic chemosensitivity. Proinflammatory cytokines such as IL-1 and IL-6 are candidate mediators of the generalized aching feeling associated with many disease states. Abnormal discharge may also arise from temperature changes, ischaemia, hypoxia, hypoglycaemia and other conditions capable of locally depolarizing afferent neurons at sites at which they have developed local resonance and ectopic pacemaker capability (Devor 2006a). It is important to recall that whereas sensory endings of specialized nociceptive neurons may be sensitive to these chemical and physical stimuli in the intact nervous system, nerve trunks and sensory ganglia do not normally respond to them. The key change in neuropathic pain is not the appearance of excitatory physical and chemical stimuli, but rather the emergence of abnormal sensitivity to these stimuli.

Allodynia and 'Aβ pain'. Pain in response to light touch of the skin, tactile allodynia, is a common symptom in neuropathy. The simplest explanation is reduced response threshold in nociceptive afferents, the classic 'excitable nociceptor hypothesis'. However, there is precious little evidence that fibres that were originally nociceptors ever come to respond to the very weak tactile stimuli that typically evoke allodynia in neuropathy, or even in inflamed tissues (Banik and Brennan, 2004; Tsuboi *et al* 2004; Shim *et al* 2005). Rather, tactile allodynia appears to be a sensory response to impulse activity in low-threshold mechanosensitive Aβ afferents. This touch signal is abnormally *amplified* in the CNS by one or a combination of CNS changes triggered by nerve injury that are collectively called central sensitization. Aβ afferents normally signal touch and vibration sense, but in neuropathy (and inflammation) they can evoke 'Aβ pain' (Woolf 1983; Campbell *et al* 1988; Torebjork *et al* 1992). A proposed example is tenderness of the scalp during migraine. Aβ afferents activated by touching skin or brushing hair are amplified centrally and rendered painful (Burstein *et al* 2000). The discovery that tactile allodynia is primarily or exclusively signalled by low-threshold mechanoreceptive afferents overturns the classical dogma that all pain is due to Aδ and C nociceptors.

It is relatively easy to recognize Aβ pain when it occurs in the skin; light touch is painful. However, it is likely that low-threshold afferent innervation of deep structures can also induce Aβ pain in the event of pathology. Thus, pain evoked by deep palpation or jaw movements may not always be due to sensitized deep nociceptors. Low-threshold mechanoreceptor activation in the presence of central sensitization is a possible alternative. It is even possible that proprioceptive input contributes in this way to muscle ache. We must assume that central sensitization also causes *ectopic* spontaneous activity in Aβ fibres to be felt

as painful, and likewise for Aβ fibre activity evoked at ectopic sites by mechanical and other applied stimuli. Central sensitization also amplifies afferent input of nociceptors, rendering painful stimuli more painful than normal (hyperalgesia).

Hyperpathia. Hyperpathic sensory peculiarities and their underlying causes have attracted relatively little attention, particularly in the trigeminal region. Pathophysiological behaviour of injured sensory neurons, however, coupled with central sensitization, echo the bizarre symptoms of hyperpathia and are probably responsible for them (Devor 2006a). For example, repeated stimulation may result in an incremental build-up of discharge in axotomized DRG and (hence) in postsynaptic spinal neurons, recalling *windup* of sensation in hyperpathia. It has also been demonstrated that injured sensory neurons communicate with one another through ephaptic (electrical) coupling, and through a novel non-synaptic, neurotransmitter-mediated mechanism called axonal and DRG 'cross excitation' (Amir and Devor 1996). Neuron-to-neuron crosstalk of this sort could account both for windup and for hyperpathic spread of sensation from the site of stimulation. This form of crosstalk is also thought to underlie paroxysmal pains in trigeminal neuralgia (the 'Ignition Hypothesis'; Devor *et al* 2002, see Chapter 11).

2.8. The Relation of PNS Injury to Central Sensitization

The term central sensitization deserves special comment. The phenomenon was first described in experiments in which nociceptors were activated by tissue injury or electrical stimulation (Woolf 1983). This caused transiently enhanced response of dorsal horn neurons to touch stimuli, and tactile allodynia in awake animals. Some authors continue to limit use of the term to functional changes that are dependent on nociceptive afferent activity and which reverse rapidly when the impulse activity is blocked (Gracely *et al* 1992; Torebjork *et al* 1992; Ji *et al* 2003). The best documented mechanism of this sort involves the recruitment of N-methyl D-aspartate (NMDA)-type glutamate receptors on postsynaptic nociceptive and WDR neurons in lamina I, II and V and deeper neurons of the dorsal horn (Willis 1992), which have both nociceptive and low-threshold input. These receptors are inactive at normal resting potential due to $Mg2+$ block of their central ion pore. Depolarization due to afferent nociceptor activity displaces the $Mg2+$ block and enables enhanced response of NMDA receptors to glutamate released from afferents, most notably large-diameter Aβ touch afferents (hence Aβ pain). Essentially, the effectiveness of the low-threshold input is enhanced in central sensitization; the same weak stimulus drives the neurons at higher rates, resulting in pain.

However, many other potential central sensitizing mechanisms have been revealed since (Devor 2006c). This has led to a broader definition of central sensitization that encompasses all of the central changes that tend to increase spinal gain (amplification) whether or not they are labile, and whether or not they are closely linked to impulse traffic in afferent nociceptors. Such changes include altered expression and release of neuromodulatory peptides from primary afferent terminals (e.g. downregulation of the inhibitory neuropeptide galanin); spinal disinhibition by selective loss of inhibitory interneurons containing GABA, glycine, taurine and/or endogenous opiates; altered gene expression and consequent hyperexcitability of intrinsic spinal neurons; denervation supersensitivity; sprouting of low-threshold afferent terminals into the superficial dorsal horn; release by *activated* microglia and astocytes of proinflammatory compounds; upregulation of postsynaptic transcription factors and other transmembrane signalling molecules (e.g. pERK, CREB); suppression of brainstem descending inhibition and augmentation of brainstem descending facilitation.

All of these changes can apparently be triggered by nerve injury (and some by peripheral inflammation), although in most instances little is known about the relation of the injury to the central change. The three fundamental possibilities are depolarization due to impulse traffic per se, the action of neuroactive substances released within the spinal cord by impulse traffic, and trophic interactions between primary afferents and postsynaptic neurons in the dorsal horn that may or may not be directly related to impulse traffic (Devor 2006b). Interestingly, there is evidence that in the presence of chronic inflammation or neuropathy, Aβ afferents begin to synthesize and release the very peptides, e.g. SP and CGRP, that are normally present only in nociceptors and are thought to trigger central sensitization when released in the CNS (Molander *et al* 1994; Noguchi *et al* 1995; Neumann *et al* 1996; Weissner *et al* 2006). Through this mechanism Aβ afferents may acquire the ability not only to signal pain, but also to trigger and maintain central sensitization.

2.9. Pain Mechanisms and Craniofacial Pain Diagnoses

In this chapter we have considered the variety of physiological and pathophysiological mechanisms that underlie pain in the craniofacial area. In some conditions precipitating factors, signs, symptoms and response to treatment are strongly suggestive of a particular pain mechanism. In others, causes of pain may be ambiguous or multiple. As a prelude to the comprehensive discussion of specific pain diagnoses presented in the following chapters, we will close by considering the relation of a selection of these diagnoses to the pain mechanisms just discussed.

2.9.1. Nociceptive (Normal) Pain

The hallmark of nociceptive pain is a response appropriate in terms of intensity and quality to the stimulus applied. Pain in response to an acute trauma or burn, pinprick, sniffing of a strong irritant chemical, accidental biting of the lip or a grain of sand on the cornea are all examples of normal pain. Spontaneous pain in the absence of a defined stimulus or pain in response to a non-noxious stimulus is not normal. They indicate an inflammatory or a neuropathic process.

2.9.2. Inflammatory Pain

Inflammation is a near-universal response to tissue injury or disease, and it is usually signalled by the clinical quadruple response of heat, reddening, swelling and pain ('calor, rubor, tumor, dolor'), and the expression of a variety of cellular markers. However, inflammation is not always accompanied by pain, and its presence with pain does not necessarily exclude neuropathy, or even normal nociception, as the most relevant pain mechanism. Simple inflammatory pain due to peripheral sensitization of nociceptors is the likely mechanism when there is pain on pressure, and abnormal sensitivity to heat or cold. Examples include painful cutaneous or mucosal ulcerations, or periapical disease. Spontaneous burning pain may be present, indicating that heat-sensitized nociceptors are firing at normal body temperature. When there is tenderness to light touch or other weak mechanical stimuli, swallowing in the presence of a sore throat or tonsillitis for example, a different mechanism is indicated. Specifically, such tenderness might be due to central sensitization of low-threshold mechanoreceptor input. That is, it might reflect Aβ pain.

Interestingly, there may be an inflammatory response without spontaneous pain or even noticeable tenderness in conditions with intact epithelium/mucosa (e.g. candidiasis and non-erosive lichen planus; see Chapter 5), and even in the presence of open ulcers. Examples of the latter are facial leishmaniasis, a parasitic infection common in the underdeveloped world, chronic periodontal disease and some chronic periapical radiolucencies. It is not clear why ulceration from leishmaniasis infection is basically painless while ulceration from herpes zoster infection, for example, is typically intensely painful. Research on inflammation with respect to pain has typically stressed the large variety of mediator substances present ('inflammatory soup'). Little attention has been given to the possibility that different lesions may be characterized by different mediators, only some of which induce sensitization and pain.

Even if an inflammatory lesion does not generate pain-provoking mediators, it may nonetheless cause intense pain if present in an enclosed space. Pressure build-up within the tooth pulp chamber in pulpitis, or periapical abscess, may be enough to activate normal nociceptive endings even if they have not been mechanosensitized by inflammatory mediators. Release of the pressure under these conditions causes instant pain relief even though the mediator substances are still present. This is an example of normal (nociceptive) pain caused secondarily by inflammation. Painful osteomyelitis due to infection in the mandibular bone marrow may have a similar source, as may tumours within the medullary bone canal such as in multiple myeloma. Elevated intracranial pressure can cause headache, likely by activating mechano-nociceptors in the meninges, particularly the dura, and perhaps blood vessels. This effect is no doubt exacerbated when the nociceptive endings are sensitized by inflammatory mediators as in meningitis. A leading hypothesis holds that ongoing activity of meningeal endings sensitized by an as-yet unknown mechanism is the primary pain source in migraine. This activity also triggers and maintains central sensitization, amplifying the pain and rendering Aβ input from intra- and extracranial sources (e.g. skin and hair afferents) painful (Burstein *et al* 2000; see Chapter 9).

2.9.3. Neuropathic Pain

Trigeminal neuralgia (tic doloreux), and to a lesser extent the other cranial nerve neuralgias, are the most recognizable neuropathic pains of the head. Nothing quite like trigeminal neuralgia, with its intense recurring lightning pains, occurs at spinal levels. It is widely held that trigeminal neuralgia results from a demyelinating lesion in the trigeminal root, or less frequently in the descending trigeminal tract where the demyelination is thought to be due to microvascular compression, tumour or multiple sclerosis (see Chapter 11). The distinctive characteristics of this condition can be explained in terms of known pathophysiological properties of injured sensory axons (Devor *et al* 2002). However, it is not clear why these symptoms rarely take such dramatic form at spinal levels.

A neuropathic condition much more common than trigeminal neuralgia is herpes zoster, and postherpetic neuralgia. Well known also at spinal levels, pain is likely due to ectopic hyperexcitability of virus-infected TRG and DRG neurons. Interestingly, another common source of neuropathic pain in the limbs and trunk, diabetic neuropathy, has only minimal effects in the head. This is probably because metabolically compromised sensory neurons of the TRG are nonetheless able to support their distal axon ends given the short length of the axons and the rich blood supply typical of the head and neck. These factors also appear to protect cranial innervation from a variety of inherited dying-back neuropathies which affect the limbs but rarely the head.

Like segmental nerves, cranial nerves are subject to neuropathy due to focal injury. Trauma to trigeminal nerve tributaries, e.g. due to mandibular fracture, nerve compression and iatrogenic causes, frequently generates neuropathic pain as do tumours and local infections. Trigeminal neuropathic pain, where the lesion is distal to the TRG, must be distinguished from trigeminal neuralgia in which the lesion is proximal to the TRG. A major mystery is why destruction of dental nerves by tooth extraction and root canal treatment so rarely causes

neuroma pain; see Chapter 11. Perhaps these neurons are less likely than others to develop ectopic excitability (Tal and Devor 1992). Another possible explanation is enhanced retrograde degeneration of the cell body due to the proximity of the lesion to the ganglion. If many of the TRG neurons that innervate the pulp chamber of a particular tooth die back, then they will not be present to generate ectopic firing and to cause neuroma pain. Loss of these neurons, however, would result in only minor brainstem deafferentation, and would therefore not be expected to trigger deafferentation pain and anaesthesia dolorosa.

When inflammation affects sensory endings in innervated tissue, causing pain, the pain is inflammatory. However, inflammation sometimes occurs along the course of a nerve trunk, in the presence of infection, for example, or in the early stages of malignancy. Resulting injury (e.g. demyelination) may induce ectopic firing in the injured axons, resulting in neuropathic pain (Eliav *et al* 1999, 2001; Benoliel *et al* 2002). Neuropathic changes secondary to trauma, compression and in-continuity inflammation may be important causes of atypical odontalgia, referred pain and altered sensation in rhinosinusitis (Benoliel *et al* 2006) and other atypical facial pain syndromes.

2.9.4. Pain Mechanisms and Pain Management

A satisfactory answer to the 'hard problem' of *how* neural activity gives rise to conscious perception remains as far off as it ever was. But it does. Pain management is normally empirical. We learn diagnoses and for each the treatments that may be effective. But the ability to go beyond routine, to solve problems that are atypical, can be greatly facilitated by an understanding of the underlying pain process. The key question to ask is 'Where are the neural impulses coming from that are causing this patient's pain?'

Acknowledgements

We thank Kaj Fried, Rami Burstein, Margaret Byers and the volume editors for helpful comments on the manuscript. The authors' research on trigeminal pain mechanisms is supported, among other sources, by the Hebrew University Center for Research on Pain.

References

Abarca M, Steenberghe D, Malevez C, *et al* (2006) The neurophysiology of osseointegrated oral implants. A clinically underestimated aspect. *J Oral Rehabil* **33**:161–169.
Abbink JH, van der Bilt A, Bosman F, *et al* (1998) A comparison of jaw-opener and jaw-closer muscle activity in humans to overcome an external force counteracting jaw movement. *Exp Brain Res* **118**:269–278.
Amir R, Devor M (1996) Axonal cross-excitation in nerve-end neuromas: comparison of A- and C-fibers. *J Neurophysiol* **68**:1160–1166.

Amir R, Liu C-N, Kocsis JD, *et al* (2002) Oscillatory mechanism in primary sensory neurones. *Brain* **125**:421–435.

Andoh S, Uemura (Sumi) M, Kawagishi S, *et al* (1988) An HRP study of primary afferent and postganglionic sympathetic neurones which innervate the temporomandibular joint in the cat. *Japan J Oral Biol* **30**:772–785.

Asaki S, Sekikawa M, Kim YT (2006) Sensory innervation of temporomandibular joint disk. *J Orthop Surg (Hong Kong)* **14**:3–8.

Banik RK, Brennan TJ (2004) Spontaneous discharge and increased heat sensitivity of rat C-fiber nociceptors are present in vitro after plantar incision. *Pain* **112**:204–213.

Beggs J, Jordan S, Ericson AC, *et al* (2003) Synaptology of trigemino- and spinothalamic lamina I terminations in the posterior ventral medial nucleus of the macaque. *J Comp Neurol* **459**:334–354.

Belmonte C, Tervo TT, (2006) Pain in and around the eye. In: McMahon SL, Koltzenburg M (eds) *Wall and Melzack's Textbook of Pain*, 5th edn. London: Churchill Livingstone, pp 887–901.

Benoliel R, Eliav E, Tal M (2001) No sympathetic nerve sprouting in rat trigeminal ganglion following painful and non-painful infraorbital nerve neuropathy. *Neurosci Lett* **297**:151–154.

Benoliel R, Wilensky A, Tal M, *et al* (2002) Application of a pro-inflammatory agent to the orbital portion of the rat infraorbital nerve induces changes indicative of ongoing trigeminal pain. *Pain* **99**:567–578.

Benoliel R, Birenboim R, Regev E, *et al* (2005) Neurosensory changes in the infraorbital nerve following zygomatic fractures. *Oral Surg* **99**:657–665.

Benoliel R, Quek S, Biron A, *et al* (2006) Trigeminal neurosensory changes following acute and chronic paranasal sinusitis. *Quint Int* **37**:437–443.

Bernard JF, Besson JM (1990) The spino (trigemino) pontoamygdaloid pathway: electrophysiological evidence for an involvement in pain processes. *J Neurophysiol* **63**:473–490.

Biemesderfer BL, Munger DL, Dubner R (1978) The pilo-Ruffini complex: a non-sinus hair and associated slowly-adapting mechanoreceptor in primate facial skin. *Brain Res* **142**:197–222.

Boivie J, Leijon G, Johansson I (1989) Central post-stroke pain - a study of the mechanisms through analyses of the sensory abnormalities. *Pain* **37**:173–185.

Bongenhielm U, Robinson PP (1996) Spontaneous and mechanically evoked afferent activity originating from myelinated fibres in ferret inferior alveolar nerve neuromas. *Pain* **67**:399–406.

Bongenhielm U, Robinson PP (1998) Afferent activity from myelinated inferior alveolar nerve fibers in ferrets after constriction or section and regeneration. *Pain* **74**:123–132.

Bongenhielm U, Boissonade FM, Westermark A, *et al* (1999) Sympathetic nerve sprouting fails to occur in the trigeminal ganglion after peripheral nerve injury in the rat. *Pain* **82**:283–288.

Boucher TJ, McMahon SB (2001) Neurotrophic factors and neuropathic pain. *Curr Opin Pharmacol* **1**:66–72.

Bouhassira D, Attal N, Alchaar H, *et al* (2005) Comparison of pain syndromes associated with nervous or somatic lesions and development of a new neuropathic pain diagnostic questionnaire (DN4). *Pain* **114**:29–36.

Brannstrom M (1992) Etiology of dentin hypersensitivity. *Proc Finn Dent Soc* **88**:7–13.

Braz JM, Nassar MA, Wood JN, *et al* (2005) Parallel 'pain' pathways arise from subpopulations of primary afferent nociceptor. *Neuron* **47**:787–793.

Broton JG, Hu JW, Sessle BJ (1988) Effects of temporomandibular joint stimulation on nociceptive and nonnociceptive neurons of the cat's trigeminal subnucleus caudalis (medullary dorsal horn). *J Neurophysiol* **59**:1575–1589.

Burchiel KJ, Wyler AR (1978) Ectopic action potential generation in peripheral trigeminal axons. *Exp Neurol* **62**:269–281.

Burstein R, Giesler GJ Jr (1989) Retrograde labeling of neurons in the spinal cord that project directly to nucleus accumbens or the septal nuclei in the rat. *Brain Res* **497**:149–154.

Burstein R, Potrebic S (1993) Retrograde labeling of neurons in the spinal cord that project directly to the amygdala or the orbital cortex in the rat. *J Comp Neurol* **335**:469–485.

Burstein R, Yarnitsky D, Goor-Aryeh I, *et al* (2000) An association between migraine and cutaneous allodynia. *Ann Neurol* **47**:614–624.

Byers MR (1984) Dental sensory receptors. *Int Rev Neurobiol* **25**:39–94.

Byers MR (1985) Sensory innervation of periodontal ligament of rat molar consists of unencapsulated Ruffini-like mechanoreceptors and free nerve endings. *J Comp Neurol* **231**:500–518.

Byers MR, Dong WK (1989) Comparison of trigeminal receptor location and structure in the periodontal ligament of different types of teeth from the rat, cat, and monkey. *J Comp Neurol* **279**:117–127.

Byers MR, Narhi MV (1999) Dental injury models: experimental tools for understanding neuroinflammatory interactions and polymodal nociceptor functions. *Crit Rev Oral Biol Med* **10**: 4–39.

Cadden SW, Lisney SJ, Matthews B (1983) Thresholds to electrical stimulation of nerves in cat canine tooth-pulp with A beta-, A delta- and C-fibre conduction velocities. *Brain Res* **261**:31–41.

Camhi JM (1984) *Neuroethology*. Sunderland MA: Sinauer, pp 289–329.

Campbell JN, Raja SN, Meyer RA, *et al* (1988) Myelinated afferents signal the hyperalgesia associated with nerve injury. *Pain* **32**:89–94.

Capra NF (1987) Localization and central projections of primary afferent neurons that innervate the temporomandibular joint in cats. *Somatosens Res* **4**:201–213.

Carelli RM, West MO (1991) Representation of the body by single neurons in the dorsolateral striatum of the awake, unrestrained rat. *J Comp Neurol* **309**:231–249.

Carstens E, Leah J, Lechner J, *et al* (1990) Demonstration of extensive brainstem projections to medial and lateral thalamus and hypothalamus in the rat. *Neuroscience* **35**:609–626.

Chandler SH, Tal M (1986) The effects of brain stem transections on the neuronal networks responsible for rhythmical jaw muscle activity in the guinea pig. *J Neurosci* **6**:1831–1842.

Chiang CY, Hu B, Hu JW, *et al* (2002) Central sensitization of nociceptive neurons in trigeminal subnucleus oralis depends on integrity of subnucleus caudalis. *J Neurophysiol* **88**:256–264.

Costigan M, Befort K, Karchewski L, *et al* (2002) Replicate high-density rat genome oligonucleotide microarrays reveal hundreds of regulated genes in the dorsal root ganglion after peripheral nerve injury. *BMC Neurosci* **3**:16–28.

Craig AD (2003) A new view of pain as a homeostatic emotion. *Trends Neurosci* **26**:303–307.

Craig AD (2004) Distribution of trigeminothalamic and spinothalamic lamina I terminations in the macaque monkey. *J Comp Neurol* **477**:119–148.

Darian-Smith I (1966) Neural mechanisms of facial sensation. *Int Rev Neurobiol* **9**:301–395.

Davidson JA, Metzinger SE, Tufaro AP, *et al* (2003) Clinical implications of the innervation of the temporomandibular joint. *J Craniofac Surg* 235–239.

Davis BM, Albers KM, Seroogy KB, *et al* (1994) Overexpression of nerve growth factor in transgenic mice induces novel sympathetic projections to primary sensory neurons. *J Comp Neurol* **349**:464–474.

Dellow PG, Lund JP (1971) Evidence for central timing of rhythmical mastication. *J Physiol* **215**:1–13.

Devor M (2006a) Response of nerves to injury in relation to neuropathic pain. In: McMahon SL, Koltzenburg M (eds) *Wall and Melzack's Textbook of Pain*, 5th edn. London: Churchill Livingstone, pp 905–927.

Devor M (2006b) Peripheral nerve generators of neuropathic pain. In: Campbell JN, Basbaum AI, Dray A, *et al* (eds) *Emerging Strategies for the Treatment of Neuropathic Pain*. Seattle: IASP Press, pp 37–68.

Devor M (2006c) Central changes after nerve injury. In: Willis W, Schmidt R (eds) *Encyclopedia of Pain*. Berlin: Springer-Verlag.

Devor M, Keller CH, Deerinck T, *et al* (1989) Na$^+$ channel accumulation on axolemma of afferents in nerve end neuromas in Apteronotus. *Neurosci Lett* **102**:149–154.

Devor M, Amir R, Rappaport ZH (2002) Pathophysiology of trigeminal neuralgia: the ignition hypothesis. *Clin J Pain* **18**:4–13.

Dong WK, Chudler EH, Martin RF (1985) Physiological properties of intradental mechanoreceptors. *Brain Res* **334**:389–394.

Dong WK, Shiwaku T, Kawakami Y, *et al* (1993) Static and dynamic responses of periodontal ligament mechanoreceptors and intradental mechanoreceptors. *J Neurophysiol* **69**:1567–1582.

Dostrovsky JO (2000) Role of thalamus in pain. *Prog Brain Res* **129**:245–257.

Dostrovsky JO, Craig AD (2006) Ascending projection systems. In: McMahon SL, Koltzenburg M (eds) *Wall and Melzack's Textbook of Pain*, 5th edn. London: Churchill Livingstone, pp 187–203.

Drager UC, Hubel DH (1975) Physiology of visual cells in mouse superior colliculus and correlation with somatosensory and auditory input. *Nature* **253**:203–204.

Dubner R, Sessle BJ, Storey AT (eds) (1978) *The Neural Basis of Oral and Facial Function*. New York: Plenum Press, pp 26–36.

Eliav E, Herzberg U, Ruda MA, *et al* (1999) Neuropathic pain from an experimental neuritis of the rat sciatic nerve. *Pain* **83**:169–182.

Eliav E, Benoliel R, Tal M (2001) Inflammation with no axonal damage of the rat saphenous nerve trunk induces ectopic discharge and mechanosensitivity in myelinated axons. *Neurosci Lett* **311**:49–52.

Fried K, Aldskogius H, Hildebrand C (1988) Proportion of unmyelinated axons in rat molar and incisor tooth pulps following neonatal capsaicin treatment and/or sympathectomy. *Brain Res* **463**:118–123.

Fried K, Arvidsson J, Robertson B, *et al* (1989) Combined retrograde tracing and enzyme/immunohistochemistry of trigeminal ganglion cell bodies innervating tooth pulps in the rat. *Neuroscience* **33**:101–109.

Goldberg LJ, Chandler SH (1981) Evidence for pattern generator control of the effects of spindle afferent input during rhythmical jaw movements. *Can J Physiol Pharmacol* **59**:707–712.

Goldberg LJ, Tal M (1978) Intracellular recording in trigeminal motoneurons of the anesthetized guinea pig during rhythmic jaw movements. *Exp Neurol* **58**:102–110.

Goldstein DS, Pechnik S, Moak J, *et al* (2004) Painful sweating. *Neurology* **63**:1471–1475.

Goodwin GM, Luschei ES (1974) Effects of destroying spindle afferents from jaw muscles on mastication in monkeys. *J Neurophysiol* **37**:967–981.

Gottrup H, Kristensen AD, Bach FW, *et al* (2003) Aftersensations in experimental and clinical hypersensitivity. *Pain* 103:57–64.

Gracely R, Lynch S, Bennett GJ (1992) Painful neuropathy: altered central processing, maintained dynamically by peripheral input. *Pain* **51**:175–194.

Graven-Nielsen T, Mense S (2001) The peripheral apparatus of muscle pain: evidence from animal and human studies. *Clin J Pain* **17**:2–10.

Graven-Nielsen T, Jansson Y, Segerdahl M, *et al* (2003) Experimental pain by ischaemic contractions compared with pain by intramuscular infusions of adenosine and hypertonic saline. *Eur J Pain* **7**:93–102.

Grelik C, Bennett GJ, Ribeiro-da-Silva A (2005) Autonomic fibre sprouting and changes in nociceptive sensory innervation in the rat lower lip skin following chronic constriction injury. *Eur J Neurosci* **21**:2475–2487.

Harden RN, Baron R, Janig W (2001) *Complex Regional Pain Syndrome*, Progress in Pain Research and Management, vol. 22. Seattle: IASP Press.

Haug SR, Heyeraas KJ (2006) Modulation of dental inflammation by the sympathetic nervous system. *J Dent Res* **85**:488–495.

Helcer M, Schnarch A, Benoliel R, *et al* (1998) Trigeminal neuralgic-type pain and vascular-type headache due to gustatory stimulus. *Headache* **38**:129–131.

Hoffmann KD, Matthews MA (1990) Comparison of sympathetic neurons in orofacial and upper extremity nerves: implications for causalgia. *J Oral Maxillofac Surg* **48**:720–726.

Hoheisel U, Reinohl J, Unger T, *et al* (2004) Acidic pH and capsaicin activate mechanosensitive group IV muscle receptors in the rat. *Pain* **110**:149–157.

Holland GR, Matthews B, Robinson PP (1987) An electrophysiological and morphological study of the innervation and reinnervation of cat dentine. *J Physiol* **386**:31–43.

Hutchins B, Spears R, Hinton RJ, *et al* (2000) Calcitonin gene-related peptide and substance P immunoreactivity in rat trigeminal ganglia and brainstem following adjuvant-induced inflammation of the temporomandibular joint. *Arch Oral Biol* **45**:335–345.

Ichikawa H, Fukunaga T, Jin HW, *et al* (2004) VR1-, VRL-1- and P2X3 receptor-immunoreactive innervation of the rat temporomandibular joint. *Brain Res* **1008**:131–136.

Ikeda M (1979) Projections from the spinal and the principal sensory nuclei of the trigeminal nerve to the cerebellar cortex in the cat, as studied by retrograde transport of horseradish peroxidase. *J Comp Neurol* **184**:567–585.

Iwata K, Kenshalo DR Jr, Dubner R, *et al* (1992) Diencephalic projections from the superficial and deep laminae of the medullary dorsal horn in the rat. *J Comp Neurol* **321**:404–420.

Janig W (2006) *Integrative Action of the Autonomic Nervous System: Neurobiology of Homeostasis*. Cambridge: Cambridge University Press.

Jantsch HH, Kemppainen P, Ringler R, *et al* (2005) Cortical representation of experimental tooth pain in humans. *Pain* **118**:390–399.

Ji RR, Kohno T, Moore KA, *et al* (2003) Central sensitization and LTP: do pain and memory share similar mechanisms? *Trends Neurosci* **26**:696–705.

Johansen JP, Fields HL, Manning BH (2001) The affective component of pain in rodents: direct evidence for a contribution of the anterior cingulate cortex. *Proc Natl Acad Sci USA* **98**:8077–8082.

Johnsen SE, Trulsson M (2003) Receptive field properties of human periodontal afferents responding to loading of premolar and molar teeth. *J Neurophysiol* **89**:1478–1487.

Johnsen SE, Trulsson M (2005) Encoding of amplitude and rate of tooth loads by human periodontal afferents from premolar and molar teeth. *J Neurophysiol* **93**:1889–1897.

Junge D (1998) *Oral Sensorimotor Function*. St. Louis, MO: Medico Dental Media International.

Jyväsjärvi E, Kniffki KD (1989) Afferent C fibre innervation of cat tooth pulp: confirmation by electrophysiological methods. *J Physiol* **411**:663–675.

Kaji A, Maeda T, Watanabe S (1991) Parasympathetic innervation of cutaneous blood vessels examined by retrograde tracing in the rat lower lip. *J Auton Nerv Syst* **32**:153–158.

Kelly JP (1985) Trigeminal system. In: Kandel E, Schwartz JH (eds) *Principles of Neural Science*, 2nd edn. Norwalk, CT: Appleton and Lange, pp 562–570.

Klein RN, Burk DT, Chase PF (2001) Anatomically and physiologically based guidelines for use of the sphenopalatine ganglion block versus the stellate ganglion block to reduce atypical facial pain. *Cranio* **19**:48–55.

Kocsis JD, Devor M (2000) Altered excitability of large-diameter cutaneous afferents following nerve injury: consequences for chronic pain. In: Devor M, Rowbotham M, Wiesenfeld-Hallin Z (eds) *Proceedings of the 9th World Congress on Pain*, Progress in Pain Research and Management, vol. 17. Seattle: IASP Press, pp 119–136.

Krout KE, Belzer RE, Loewy AD (2002) Brainstem projections to midline and intralaminar thalamic nuclei of the rat. *J Comp Neurol* **448**:53–101.

Kugelberg E, Lindblom U (1959) The mechanism of the pain in trigeminal neuralgia. *J Neurol Neurosurg Psychiatry* **22**:36–43.

Kyrkanides S, Tallents RH, Macher DJ, *et al* (2002) Temporo-mandibular joint nociception: effects of capsaicin on substance P-like immunoreactivity in the rabbit brain stem. *J Orofac Pain* **16**:229–236.

Le Douarin NM, Kalcheim C (1999) *The Neural Crest*. Cambridge: Cambridge University Press, p 163.

Lennartsson B (1980) Number and distribution of muscle spindles in the masticatory muscles of the rat. *J Anat* **130**:279–288.

Li YQ, Kaneko T, Shigemoto R, *et al* (1997) Distribution of trigeminohypothalamic and spinohypothalamic tract neurons displaying substance P receptor-like immunoreactivity in the rat. *J Comp Neurol* **378**:508–521.

Li YQ, Takada M, Ohishi H, *et al* (1993a) Collateral projections of trigeminal ganglion neurons to both the principal sensory trigeminal and the spinal trigeminal nuclei in the rat. *Exp Brain Res* **93**:205–212.

Li YQ, Takada M, Shigenaga Y, *et al* (1993b) Collateral projections of single neurons in the nucleus raphe magnus to both the sensory trigeminal nuclei and spinal cord in the rat. *Brain Res* **602**:331–335.

Li YQ, Takada M, Mizuno N (1993c) Collateral projections of single neurons in the periaqueductal gray and dorsal raphe nucleus to both the trigeminal sensory complex and spinal cord in the rat. *Neurosci Lett* **153**:153–156.

Libet B (1973) Electrical stimulation of cortex in human subjects, and conscious sensory aspects. In: Iggo A (ed) *Handbook of Sensory Physiology*, vol II. Berlin: Springer-Verlag, pp 743–790.

Lund JP, Drew T, Rossignol S (1984) A study of jaw reflexes of the awake cat during mastication and locomotion. *Brain Behav Evol* **25**:146–156.

Macefield VG (2005) Physiological characteristics of low-threshold mechanoreceptors in joints, muscle and skin in human subjects. *Clin Exp Pharmacol Physiol* **32**:135–144.

McGrath PA, Gracely RH, Dubner R (1983) Non-pain and pain sensation induced by tooth pulp stimulation. *Pain* **15**:377–388.

McLachlan E, Janig W, Devor M, *et al* (1993) Peripheral nerve injury triggers noradrenergic sprouting within dorsal root ganglia. *Nature* **363**:543–546.

Malick A, Burstein R (1998) Cells of origin of the trigeminohypothalamic tract in the rat. *J Comp Neurol* **400**:125–144.

Malick A, Strassman RM, Burstein R (2000) Trigeminohypothalamic and reticulohypothalamic tract neurons in the upper cervical spinal cord and caudal medulla of the rat. *J Neurophysiol* **84**:2078–2112.

Manchikanti L, Singh V, Rivera J, *et al* (2002) Prevalence of cervical facet joint pain in chronic neck pain. *Pain Physician* **5**:243–249.

Marbach JJ, Raphael KG (2000) Phantom tooth pain: a new look at an old dilemma. *Pain Med* **1**:68–77.

Marfurt CF, Turner DF (1984) The central projections of tooth pulp afferent neurons in the rat as determined by the transganglionic transport of horseradish peroxidase. *J Comp Neurol* **223**:535–547.

Martens MA, Moeyersoons JP (1990) Acute and recurrent effort-related compartment syndrome in sports. *Sports Med* **1**:62–68.

Matsushita M, Ikeda M, Okado N (1982) The cells of origin of the trigeminothalamic, trigeminospinal and trigeminocerebellar projections in the cat. *Neuroscience* **7**:1439–1454.

Matthews B (1970) Nerve impulses recorded from dentine in the cat. *Arch Oral Biol* **15**:523–530.

Melzack R, Bromage PR (1973) Experimental phantom limbs. *Exp Neurol* **39**:261–269.

Mengel MK, Jyväsjärvi E, Kniffki KD (1996) Evidence for slowly conducting afferent fibres innervating both tooth pulp and periodontal ligament in the cat. *Pain* **65**(2-3):181–188.

Merskey H, Bogduk N (eds) (1994) *Classification of Chronic Pain. Descriptions of Chronic Pain Syndromes and Definitions of Pain Terms*. Seattle: IASP Press.

Miles TS, Flavel SC, Nordstrom MA (2004) Control of human mandibular position during locomotion. *J Physiol* **554**:216–226.

Mogil JS (ed) (2004) *The Genetics of Pain*, Progress in Pain Research and Management, vol. 28. Seattle: IASP Press.

Molander C, Hongpaisan J, Persson JK (1994) Distribution of c-fos expressing dorsal horn neurons after electrical stimulation of low threshold sensory fibers in the chronically injured sciatic nerve. *Brain Res* **64**:74–82.

Mountcastle VB, Henneman E (1952) The representation of tactile sensibility in the thalamus of the monkey. *J Comp Neurol* **97**:409–439.

Mu L, Sanders I (2000) Sensory nerve supply of the human oro- and laryngopharynx: a preliminary study. *Anat Rec* **258**:406–420.

Nakamura Y, Katakura N (1995) Generation of masticatory rhythm in the brainstem *Neurosci Res* **23**:1–19.

Neumann S, Doubell TP, Leslie TA, *et al* (1996) Inflammatory pain hypersensitivity mediated by phenotypic switch in myelinated primary sensory neurons. *Nature* **384**:360–364.

Nikolajsen L, Jensen TS (2001) Phantom limb pain. *Br J Anesth* **87**:107–116.

Niv D, Gofeld M, Devor M (2003) Causes of pain in degenerative bone and joint disease: a lesson from vertebroplasty. *Pain* **105**:387–392.

Noguchi K, Kawai Y, Fukuoka T, *et al* (1995) Substance P induced by peripheral nerve injury in primary afferent sensory neurons and its effect on dorsal column nucleus neurons. *J Neurosci* **15**:7633–7643.

Noordenbos W (1959) *Pain*. Amsterdam: Elsevier.

O'Connor TP, van der Kooy D (1986) Pattern of intracranial and extracranial projections of trigeminal ganglion cells. *J Neurosci* **6**:2200–2207.

Olausson H, Lamarre Y, Backlund H, *et al* (2002) Unmyelinated tactile afferents signal touch and project to insular cortex. *Nat Neurosci* **5**:900–904.

Oliveira MC, Parada CA, Veiga MC, *et al* (2005) Evidence for the involvement of endogenous ATP and P2X receptors in TMJ pain. *Eur J Pain* **9**:87–93.

Ostrowsky K, Magnin M, Ryvlin P, *et al* (2002) Representation of pain and somatic sensation in the human insula: a study of responses to direct electrical cortical stimulation. *Cereb Cortex* **12**:376–385.

Penfield W, Rasmussen T (1955) *The Cerebral Cortex of Man*. New York: MacMillan.

Pereira LC, Modesto AM, Sugai R, *et al* (2005) Pain sensitive cerebral areas and intracranial structures revealed at fully awake craniotomies for primary intracranial tumor resection. Abstracts IASP 11th World Congress on Pain. Seattle: IASP Press.

Peschanski M (1984) Trigeminal afferents to the diencephalon in the rat. *Neuroscience* **12**:465–487.

Peyron R, Laurent B, Garcia-Larrea L (2000) Functional imaging of brain responses to pain: A review and meta-analysis. *Neurophysiol Clin* 263–288.

Pietrobon D, Striessnig J (2003) Neurobiology of migraine. *Nat Rev Neurosci* **4**:386–398.

Rainville P, Duncan GH, Price DD, *et al* (1997) Pain affect encoded in human anterior cingulate but not somatosensory cortex. *Science* **277**:968–971.

Ramien M, Ruocco I, Cuello AC, *et al* (2004) Parasympathetic nerve fibers invade the upper dermis following sensory denervation of the rat lower lip skin. *J Comp Neurol* **469**:83–95.

Ray BS, Wolff HG (1940) Experimental studies on headache. Pain sensitive structures of the head and their significance in headache. *Arch Surg* **41**:813–856.

Ren K, Dubner R (2002) Descending modulation in persistent pain: an update. *Pain* **100**:1–6.

Ring G, Ganchrow D (1983) Projections of nucleus caudalis and spinal cord to brainstem and diencephalon in the hedgehog (*Erinaceus europaeus* and *Paraechinus aethiopicus*): a degeneration study. *J Comp Neurol* **216**:132–151.

Schmelz M, Schmidt R, Ringkamp M, *et al* (1996) Limitation of sensitization to injured parts of receptive fields in human skin C-nociceptors. *Exp Brain Res* **109**:141–147.

Schmidt R, Schmelz M, Forster C, *et al* (1995) Novel classes of responsive and unresponsive C nociceptors in human skin. *J Neurosci* **15**:333–341.

Sessle BJ (2000) Acute and chronic craniofacial pain: brain stem mechanisms of nociceptive transmission and neuroplasticity, and their clinical correlates. *Crit Rev Oral Biol Med* **11**:57–91.

Sharav Y, Benoliel R, Shnarch A, *et al* (1991) Idiopathic trigeminal pain associated with gustatory stimuli. *Pain* **44**:171–174.

Sherrington CS (1906) *The Integrative Action of the Nervous System.* Yale University Press: New Haven.

Shim B, Kim DW, Kim BH, *et al* (2005) Mechanical and heat sensitization of cutaneous nociceptors in rats with experimental peripheral neuropathy. *Neuroscience* **132**:193–201.

Shinder V, Govrin-Lippmann R, Cohen S, *et al* (1999) Structural basis of sympathetic-sensory coupling in rat and human dorsal root ganglia following peripheral nerve injury. *J Neurocytol* **28**:743–761.

Silverman JD, Kruger L (1987) An interpretation of dental innervation based upon the pattern of calcitonin gene-related peptide (CGRP)-immunoreactive thin sensory axons. *Somatosens Res* **5**:157–175.

Simons C, Dessirier J-M, Carstens M, *et al* (2000) The tingling sensation of carbonated drinks is mediated by a carbonic anhydrase-dependent excitation of trigeminal nociceptive neurons. In: Devor M, Rowbotham MC, Wiesenfeld-Hallin Z (eds) *Proceedings of the 9th World Congress on Pain Progress in Pain Research and Management*, vol 16. Seattle: IASP Press, pp 225–232.

Sjoqvist O (1950) Surgery of cords and pain routes in medulla and brain stem. *Rev Neurol (Paris)* **83**:38–40.

Stohler CS, Zhang X, Lund JP (1996) The effect of experimental jaw muscle pain on postural muscle activity. *Pain* **66**:215–221.

Strassman AM, Vos BP (1993) Somatotopic and laminar organization of fos-like immunoreactivity in the medullary and upper cervical dorsal horn induced by noxious facial stimulation in the rat. *J Comp Neurol* **331**:495–516.

Strassman AM, Weissner W, Williams M, *et al* (2004) Axon diameters and intradural trajectories of the dural innervation in the rat. *J Comp Neurol* **473**:364–376.

Strigo IA, Duncan GH, Boivin M, *et al* (2003) Differentiation of visceral and cutaneous pain in the human brain. *J Neurophysiol* **89**:3294–3303.

Tal M, Devor M (1992) Ectopic discharge in injured nerves: comparison of trigeminal and somatic afferents. *Brain Res* **579**:148–151.

Tanaka E, Yamano E, Dalla-Bona DA, *et al* (2006) Dynamic compressive properties of the mandibular condylar cartilage. *J Dent Res* **85**:571–575.

Torebjork H, Lundberg L, LaMotte RH (1992) Central changes in processing of mechanoreceptive input in capsaicin-induced secondary hyperalgesia in humans. *J Physiol* **448**:765–780.

Tsuboi Y, Takeda M, Tanimoto T, *et al* (2004) Alteration of the second branch of the trigeminal nerve activity following inferior alveolar nerve transection in rats. *Pain* **111**:323–334.

Uddman R, Tajti J, Moller S, *et al* (1999) Neuronal messengers and peptide receptors in the human sphenopalatine and otic ganglia. *Brain Res* **826**:193–199.

Uno T, Koike S, Bamba H, *et al* (2004) Capsaicin receptor expression in rat laryngeal innervation. *Ann Otol Rhinol Laryngol* **113**:356–358.

Virtanen ASJ, Huopaniemi T, Narhi MVO, *et al* (1987) The effect of temporal parameters on subjective sensations evoked by electrical tooth stimulation. *Pain* **30**:361–371.

Waxman SG (ed.) (2002) *Sodium Channels and Neuronal Hyperexcitability*, Novartis Foundation. Symposia. West Sussex: Wiley.

Weissner W, Winterson BJ, Stuart-Tilley A, *et al* (2006) Time course of substance P expression in dorsal root ganglia following complete spinal nerve transection. *J Comp Neurol* **497**:78–87.

White J, Sweet W (1969) *Pain and the Neurosurgeon*. Springfield, IL: Thomas, pp 123–256.

Williams MN, Zahm DS, Jacquin MF (1994) Differential foci and synaptic organization of the principal and spinal trigeminal projections to the thalamus in the rat. *Eur J Neurosci* **6**:429–453.

Willis W (ed.) (1992) *Hyperalgesia and Allodynia*. New York: Raven Press, pp 173–385.

Woolf CJ (1983) Evidence for a central component of postinjury pain hypersensitivity. *Nature* **306**:686–688.

Wynn-Parry CB (1980) Pain in avulsion lesions of the brachial plexus. *Pain* **9**:41–53.

Xiao HS, Huang QH, Zhang FX, *et al* (2002) Identification of gene expression profile of dorsal root ganglion in the rat peripheral axotomy model of neuropathic pain. *Proc Natl Acad Sci USA* **99**:8360–8365.

Yang H, Bernanke JM, Naftel JP (2006) Immunocytochemical evidence that most sensory neurons of the rat molar pulp express receptors for both glial cell line-derived neurotrophic factor and nerve growth factor. *Arch Oral Biol* **51**:69–78.

Yarnitsky D, Goor-Aryeh I, Bajwa ZH, *et al* (2003) Possible parasympathetic contributions to peripheral and central sensitization during migraine. *Headache* **43**:704–714.

Yilmaz Z, Renton T, Yiangou Y, *et al* (2007) Burning mouth syndrome as a trigeminal small fibre neuropathy: increased heat and capsaicin receptor TRPV1 in nerve fibres correlates with pain score. *J Clin Neurosci* **14**:864–871.

Young RF, King RB (1973) Fiber spectrum of the trigeminal sensory root of the baboon determined by electron microscopy. *J Neurosurg* **38**:65–72.

Zagon A, Totterdell S, Jones RS (1994) Direct projections from the ventrolateral medulla oblongata to the limbic forebrain: anterograde and retrograde tract-tracing studies in the rat. *J Comp Neurol* **340**:445–468.

CHAPTER 3

Measuring and assessing pain

Eli Eliav and Richard H Gracely

1. Introduction

Pain measurement is an essential element in any medical assessment, including diagnosis, monitoring of disease progress and evaluation of treatment effectiveness. Unfortunately there is no one common or easy method of pain measurement. Since pain is a personal and private experience that cannot be seen or felt by others, the methods that must be used for pain assessment include indirect, self report, physiological and behavioural methods. The target of these pain assessments should be multidimensional; pain is both a somatic sensation and an emotional state that evokes behaviours that minimize bodily harm and promote healing (Wall 1979). In this chapter we review current techniques employed in the assessment of pain.

Pain experience and intensity may vary among different populations and are affected by a broad range of factors. Emotional states may have divergent effects on the pain experience; fear can reduce pain, whereas anxiety may have enhancing effects. Particularly in chronic conditions anxiety and stress can aggravate pain (see also Chapter 4). The duration of pain is an important variable in pain assessment; long-lasting or frequent pain episodes can induce processes in the central nervous system that extend the normal duration of pain secondary to injury (see post-traumatic neuropathy, Chapter 11). The character of pain onset will also substantially affect the experience; pain that develops gradually may be quite different from pain that develops abruptly. Pain can occur at different periods of the day and it may be invalid to compare intensity of pain upon awakening to pain occurring during the day or during function. Moreover major variations in pain intensity can also occur during the day, the week (weekend headaches) and the month (menstrually related headaches). Pain localization may affect the pain experience. Similar pathological processes in different sites can produce different pain experiences. For example, pain induced by inflammation within a tooth pulp (pulpitis) or in the hip joint cannot be compared to inflammatory-related temporomandibular joint pain (capsulitis or osteoarthritis) despite the common mechanism (inflammatory process).

The word *pain* embraces many conditions and qualities. Pain can be throbbing, burning, aching, diffuse, tingling, stabbing, cramping and pressing. Some qualities are more specific to certain conditions. For example, migraine has a throbbing quality, while myofascial pain is pressing and dull. Electrical shock-like pain has been frequently associated with trigeminal neuralgia, whereas other neuropathic conditions are characterized by burning pain. However, it is not clear whether clinicians and patients use the same terms to describe the same sensations.

Pain intensity and frequency are probably the most important features measured to assess a patient's well being. However, pain quality, onset, duration, localization and other additional factors that modify the condition (alleviating or aggravating), occurrence of pain elsewhere in the body, and associated psychosocial problems must also be assessed.

Accurate measurement of the pain experience can be performed only with the assistance of several tools and methods. Drawing the painful area on a body map and a pain diary may provide necessary information for the pain location, duration, frequency and modifying factors. These methods should be standardized and used consistently with each patient. In the chapters on the major clinical pain syndromes (7–11, 13) there are extensive examples of the use of pain diaries, drawings and mapping of pain to aid in diagnosis and follow-up.

2. Methods for Pain Assessment

2.1. Pain Scales

2.1.1. Visual Analogue Scale

The visual analogue scale (VAS) is the most frequently used method to assess pain intensity. The scale is usually a horizontal (Joyce *et al* 1975; Huskisson *et al* 1983) or

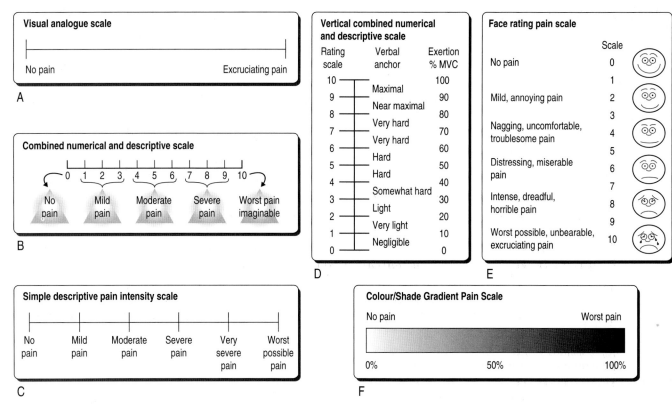

Fig. 3.1 • Scales commonly employed to assess pain severity. The choice of which scale to adopt is dictated by the setting (e.g. clinic, research project) and by the study population (e.g. children, adults); see text. (A) Simple visual analogue scale. (B) Combined numerical and descriptive pain scale. (C) Descriptive pain scale. (D) Combined numerical and descriptive vertical pain scale, MVC=maximal voluntary contraction. (E) Face rating pain scale. (F) Colour gradient pain scale.

vertical 10-cm line (Sriwatanakul *et al* 1983) labelled at each end by descriptors such as 'no pain' and 'worse pain ever' (Fig. 3.1). The patient marks the line to indicate pain severity and it is simply quantified by measuring the distance in centimetres from 0 (no pain) to the patient's marked rating. This method has been validated in a number of studies (Price and Dubner 1977; Belanger *et al* 1989; Choiniere *et al* 1989; Rosier *et al* 2002), but was found to be insufficient in others (Yarnitsky and Sprecher 1994). However this is a simple method to use in the clinical situation and also aids in monitoring treatment efficacy. A popular variation of the VAS that was designed for children or for patients who do not have the verbal skills to describe their symptoms is the Faces Pain Rating Scale (Fig. 3.1) (Bieri *et al* 1990; Wong and Baker 2001). This scale is comprised of a series of faces with different expressions. The facial expressions vary in a continuum from a happy face for 'no pain' to a very sad face for intense pain and often a written description accompanies each face. The patient is asked to choose the face that best describes their pain.

2.1.2. Numerical and Verbal Rating Scales

In the numerical rating scale, patients are asked to rate their pain on a scale from 0 to 10 or 0 to 100, in which 0 is no pain and the other end of the scale represents the worst possible pain (Jensen *et al* 1987). Alternatively, verbal descriptive scales incorporate specific words

organized to express the increasing and progressive intensity of pain. A category scale is a simple form of verbal scale and in clinical trials is usually composed of four pain descriptions such as none, mild, moderate or severe. Simple category scales can be used for rough comparisons or in addition to other pain scales and the number of categories can be increased to achieve greater resolution. Hybrid scales combine verbal scales with graphic rating or with numerical scales; the descriptors are placed in appropriate locations on the analogue scale (Naliboff *et al* 1997; Sternberg *et al* 2001). Nominal verbal scales include a list of qualitative descriptive words such as burning, cramping or pricking. This scale supplements pain intensity scales with additional clinically useful information.

There is no simple guide to the choice of pain scale. Numerical, visual and verbal scales have been validated in numerous studies and the choice must be specifically established considering the individual patient or research project in question. For example, it has been shown that elderly patients make fewer mistakes with verbal scales than with a VAS (Gagliese and Melzack 1997; Herr *et al* 2004). Using a numerical or verbal scale eliminates the task of marking a line, and therefore may be useful for patients with motor disability.

Visual analogue scales have been integrated in computerized systems that can calculate and measure pain over time (Gracely 1990; Graven-Nielsen *et al* 1997). The addition of the time element to the assessment of intensity can provide important information concerning pain pattern over time, prolonged stimulus-evoked pain sensations and spontaneous or specific factors that aggravate pain intensity. Computerized systems can also assess pain for longer periods of time using personal electronic devices. This method has been validated in pain-free patients and shown to be sensitive in a clinical trial (Jamison *et al* 2002; Gendreau *et al* 2003).

Most visual analogue, numerical or verbal pain scales rate pain as a unidimensional experience. More sophisticated questionnaires that address the multidimensional experience that pain induces have been developed.

2.2. Pain Questionnaires

2.2.1. The McGill Pain Questionnaire

The McGill Pain Questionnaire (MPQ) (Melzack 1975) is the most frequently used questionnaire for the multidimensional assessment of pain. The MPQ assesses three separate components of the pain experience: the sensory intensity, the emotional impact and the cognitive evaluation of pain. Patients are presented with 78 adjectives in 20 groups, and are instructed to select one from each group for the particular groups that most closely match their own pain experience. An overall score for each major dimension is obtained from the sum of either weighted scores or the ranks of the chosen word within the group.

Following translation of the MPQ to many languages it has been shown that people from different ethnic and educational backgrounds use similar adjectives to describe the same pain conditions (Gaston-Johansson *et al* 1990). In certain specific pain disorders characterized with typical adjectives, the questionnaire may also assist in diagnosis (Dubuisson and Melzack 1976; Melzack *et al* 1986). Moreover, the MPQ has been found to be sensitive to pain interventions, and therefore can evaluate treatment efficacy (Burchiel *et al* 1996; Nikolajsen *et al* 1996; Tesfaye *et al* 1996). In the orofacial pain region, the MPQ has been validated in trigeminal neuralgia, atypical odontalgia, tooth ache and Burning Mouth Syndrome (Grushka and Sessle 1984; Melzack *et al* 1986). A short form (MPQ-SF) that consists of 15 selected adjectives that patients score on a four-point scale and a VAS used for measurement of pain intensity is available (Fig. 3.2) (Gronblad *et al* 1990; Harden *et al* 1991; McGuire *et al* 1993; Gagliese and Melzack 1997).

Other multidimensional questionnaires have found common psychological patterns for patients in pain, regardless of aetiology, location, treatment or the medical or dental diagnosis (Turk and Rudy 1987, 1988, 1990).

2.2.2. The Research Diagnostic Criteria

The Research Diagnostic Criteria for Temporomandibular Disorders (RDC-TMD) is an example of a multidimensional questionnaire designed for TMDs (see Chapters 7

and 8) that was developed by Dworkin, LeResche and colleagues (Dworkin and LeResche 1992). This classification and assessment system includes two axes: Axis I comprises clinical and physical examination items and Axis II consists of pain-related and psychosocial disability ratings. The RDC-TMD can be used for diagnostic evaluation of TMDs and for pain and disability assessment, making it a useful tool for both clinical and research purposes. A multicentre study confirmed the reliability of the RDC-TMD for the most common TMD diagnoses (John *et al* 2005), and a validated questionnaire is available in various languages (go to: http://www.rdc-tmdinternational.org/). However, the RDC-TMD criteria are designed for joint- and muscle-related orofacial pains only. Other diagnostic criteria and tools such as those outlined by the American Academy of Orofacial Pain (Okeson 1996), the International Headache Society (Olesen *et al* 2004) and the International Association for the Study of Pain (Merskey and Bogduk 1994) must be employed for the diagnosis and assessment of neuropathic (Chapters 11 and 13) and neurovascular (Chapters 9 and 10) orofacial pain conditions.

2.3. Spontaneous and Behavioural Responses

Single or multidimensional pain scales are not useful for patients with language deficits or for children of preverbal age and in these cases pain assessment relies on observation. Facial expressions related to pain may serve as a limited tool for pain evaluation in infants or disabled patients (LeResche and Dworkin 1984; Carroll and Russell 1996). At present this is not a validated method; however, experienced clinicians can gather valuable information about a patient's pain experience from their facial expressions. In addition, observations of altered orofacial functions such as avoidance or altered biting or chewing patterns can signify the presence of orofacial pain (see Chapters 7 and 8).

2.4. Physiological Measurements

Autonomic responses such as heart rate, blood pressure, skin conductivity, pupil size or hormone release intensify during painful conditions (Drummond 1995a,b). Unfortunately these signs tend to diminish (habituate) over time. In addition, autonomic responses are not specific to pain, but are influenced by other factors such as startle response, anger or fear. Specific autonomic signs are common in neurovascular headaches particularly the trigeminal autonomic cephalgias (Chapter 10). Autonomic signs are also observed in complex regional pain syndrome (CRPS), which is, however, considered to be rare in the orofacial region (Chapter 11). In these specific syndromes physiological measurements as indicators of pain severity are complex and best avoided.

Fig. 3.2 • McGill Pain Questionnaire Short Form (MPQ-SF). The questionnaire includes a visual analogue scale, a map to define location and a short list of descriptive terms; see text.

Short form McGill pain questionnaire and pain diagram

(Reproduced with permission of author © Dr. Ron Melzack, for publication and distribution)

Date: _____

Name: _____

Check the column to indicate the level of your pain for each word, or leave blank if it does not apply to you.

	Mild	Moderate	Severe
1. Throbbing	____	____	____
2. Shooting	____	____	____
3. Stabbing	____	____	____
4. Sharp	____	____	____
5. Cramping	____	____	____
6. Gnawing	____	____	____
7. Hot-burning	____	____	____
8. Aching	____	____	____
9. Heavy	____	____	____
10. Tender	____	____	____
11. Splitting	____	____	____
12. Tiring-Exhausting	____	____	____
13. Sickening	____	____	____
14. Fearful	____	____	____
15. Cruel-Punishing	____	____	____

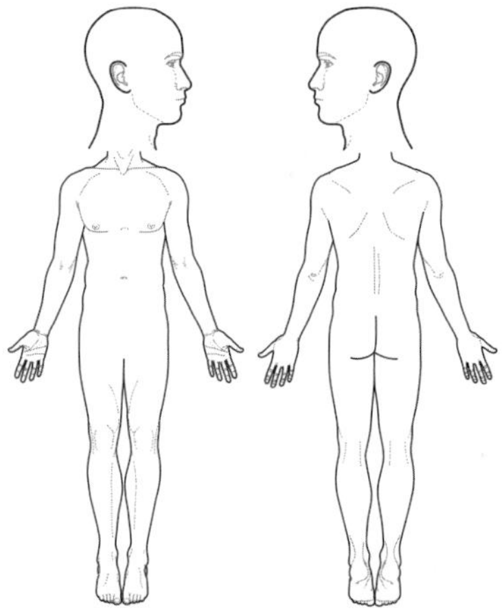

Mark or comment on the above figure where your have your pain or problems

Indicate on this line how bad your pain is — at the left end of line means no pain at all, at right end means worst pain possible

No pain _____ Worst possible pain

S	/33	A	/12	VAS	/10

2.5. Electromyography

This method measures action potentials from muscles as an indication of muscle activity. However, the correlation between muscle activity and orofacial pain conditions is debatable; this is extensively discussed in Chapter 7 (Glaros *et al* 1997; Gramling *et al* 1997; Liu *et al* 1999). Orofacial pain conditions can alter trigeminal reflex activities, suggesting a connection between the nociceptive pathways and trigeminal reflexes (Tal and Goldberg 1981; Tal *et al* 1981; Tal 1984; Tal and Sharav 1985; Sharav and Tal 1995). However, this extensively studied method has never been validated as a clinical tool for pain assessment.

2.6. Microneurography

Neurophysiological recording from peripheral nerve fibres in animal studies provides valuable information on neuronal function and pain mechanisms. A similar method has been developed for use in humans to explore the characteristics of nociceptors, mainly different populations of C fibres (Weidner *et al* 2000, 2002, 2003), and this method has been employed to assess function in the trigeminal system (Jaaskelainen *et al* 2005). Microneurography is an excellent research tool that directly evaluates primary afferent function. However, the invasive nature of the method and significant requirements for subject compliance limit its clinical utility.

2.7. Imaging

Standard imaging techniques are very useful for diagnosis but not for pain assessment. There is no correlation between the extent of a lesion or tissue damage established by imaging and the magnitude of pain severity.

Functional magnetic resonance imaging (fMRI) and positron emission tomography (PET) are used in research laboratories to assess brain activity associated with pain. These studies and earlier EEG studies mapped the areas in the brain that appear to be involved in pain perception (Coghill *et al* 2001; Bentley *et al* 2003; Frot and Mauguiere

2003). Recent findings suggest the presence of brain-augmented pain processing in patients suffering from fibromyalgia (Gracely *et al* 2003). However, these promising techniques are not clinically applicable to pain measurement as yet. Similar to most other pain studies using brain imaging methods, the studies average group data to investigate pain processing mechanisms. Therefore these studies have not examined the ability of these methods to provide clinically useful information about single subjects, and their possible utility in clinical decision-making.

3. Quantitative Sensory Testing

The term quantitative sensory testing (QST) embraces several methods used to quantify sensory nerve function. QST utilizes noninvasive assessment and quantification of sensory nerve function in patients with suspected neurological damage or disease. The common concepts in QST methods are that the assessment of normal and non-normal responses to various stimuli provides information about the functioning of the peripheral and central nervous system and that these responses can be quantified by the amount of physical stimuli required to evoke specific levels of sensory perception. External stimuli are usually mechanical, thermal or electrical. The response to gross external stimuli has been part of the formal neurological evaluation since the late nineteenth century. The concept is still valid and years of research and development of new tools have improved the benefit gained from such tests.

The establishment of normal QST ranges is complicated by numerous variables including probe or electrode size, stimulus frequency, site, rate of change, clinical environment, gender, age and ethnicity. Data from one assessment system cannot be easily transferred or compared to another. This variance can be reduced to some extent by routinely using the same methods and devices. For localized unilateral pathologies, expressing thresholds as the ratio between the ipsilateral (affected) and the contralateral (unaffected, control) sides improves consistency (Kemler *et al* 2000). Bilateral pathologies may be compared to adjacent dermatomes (see Case 3.1).

3.1. QST Methods

In general, QST methods can be divided into two broad classes. The first is based on a fixed set of stimuli and requires a response indicating the magnitude of the sensation evoked by each stimulus. This class is used for suprathreshold pain sensations. The response intensity can be measured with VAS, numerical or verbal scales as described earlier. In the second class the response is fixed and the stimulus varies; this is usually used to measure pain or sensory thresholds. These methods have been referred to as response-dependent and stimulus-

---

Case 3.1 Bilateral Mental Neuropathy, 45-year-old Female

This rare case of bilateral mental numbness following insertion of dental implants demonstrates the use of quantitative sensory testing in the orofacial pain clinic.

Present complaint

Bilateral numbness in the mental nerve territory. The area of paraesthesia on the right side is larger and accompanied by an intermittent mild burning sensation.

History of present complaint

Five days ago the patient underwent insertion of lower dental implants bilaterally (3 on the left side and 4 on the right). Immediately following resolution of the local anaesthesia the right side felt 'different', a sensation that developed into numbness within 24 hours. Two days following the procedure, left-side mental paraesthesia and numbness developed. For the last 24 hours the right-side paraesthesia is accompanied by a mild burning sensation.

Examination

Excluding the mental nerve territories, head and neck examination was unremarkable. Quantitative sensory testing employing electrical and thermal stimuli was performed in the mental and infraorbital nerve dermatomes respectively. Testing revealed that relative to the infraorbital dermatomes the mental dermatomes expressed elevated heat and electrical detection thresholds in the right side and a reduced electrical detection threshold in the left side (Fig. 3.3).

Relevant medical history

None.

Diagnosis

The history and findings indicated right-side nerve damage and left-side perineural inflammation. A computerized tomographic scan (Fig. 3.4) clearly showed impingement of a right implant in the inferior alveolar (mandibular) canal.

Treatment

60 mg of prednisone was initiated immediately; the dose was reduced by 10 mg each subsequent day for 5 days. Three days later the aberrant sensation on the left side disappeared while that on the right only improved slightly. A few days later the misplaced implant on the right side was surgically removed. Right-side pain was dramatically improved within three weeks, while sensory function returned only after 3 months. Compare this case to that described in Chapter 11 where removal of the implants resulted in no change in pain or sensory disturbance. It is possible that in Case 3.1 the amount of nerve damage was less than that inflicted in the case depicted in Figs.11.9A–C.

Conclusions

The left-side numbness was the result of perineural inflammation while the right-side aberrant sensation was related to direct nerve damage. Early intervention and the radiographic identification of an intact left inferior dental canal were good prognostic factors for the neural recovery of the left side. Compare this case to that presented in Chapter 11; removal of implants in that case did not improve symptoms.

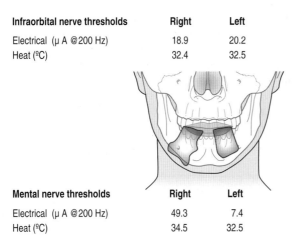

Infraorbital nerve thresholds	Right	Left
Electrical (μA @200 Hz)	18.9	20.2
Heat (ºC)	32.4	32.5

Mental nerve thresholds	Right	Left
Electrical (μA @200 Hz)	49.3	7.4
Heat (ºC)	34.5	32.5

Fig. 3.3 • Location of pain and sensory dysfunction for Case 3.1. Bilateral mental paraesthesia (grey areas) 3 days following insertion of dental implants. Sensory testing was performed with electrical and thermal stimuli. The right side demonstrated elevated heat and electrical detection thresholds, indicating nerve damage. The left side demonstrated normal heat detection threshold and reduced electrical detection threshold, indicating neuritis (inflammation).

dependent, respectively, and may be further classified on the basis of the type of data collected (modality employed, units, test, etc.).

In both classes the test accuracy is largely dependent on the patient's response, which can be biased either by delayed responses or by a range of expectations. These biases are controlled to some extent by more time-consuming psychophysical methods that deliver numerous stimuli, but are less controlled in typical fast assessments performed in a clinical setting. In many cases the features, such as hyperalgesia, are quite evident and appropriately assessed by the fast methods. Cases of more subtle sensory abnormalities may require the more extensive procedures.

The stimulus-dependent methods express results in terms of physical units of stimulus intensity, which avoids the use of subjective scaling units and provides a convenient measure for comparison between individuals and within individuals over time. Two main stimulus-dependent protocols are used: method of limits and method of levels.

In the 'method of limits' the subject is required to indicate detection of an increasing stimulus, or the disappearance of a decreasing stimulus. In pain studies, this method is

usually modified to present only ascending series to avoid excessively painful stimulation at the beginning of a descending series. This modification tends to be less accurate, mainly due to the fact that the method is sensitive to the patient's reaction time and errors of anticipation (Dyck et al 1990; Yarnitsky and Sprecher 1994). Yet, this is a simple fast method that can be very useful in situations in which the expected abnormalities are obvious, or as a means of determining the range of stimuli for further tests.

In the 'method of levels', a specific stimulus intensity is delivered and the subject signals whether the stimulus is detected or is painful. In adaptive methods such as the staircase procedure, the response is used to modify the intensity of future stimulation to track a specific subjective level such as pain threshold of 'moderate pain' (Gracely and Kwilosz 1988; Gracely et al 1988). Usually this method requires longer examination times; however, the method is more accurate and reliable.

Additional QST tests assess the subject's ability to discriminate in space rather than by sensory intensity. The 'two-point discrimination test' assesses the differentiation between two mechanical punctuate stimuli placed at variable distances on the skin. The recorded variable is the distance between stimuli while the stimulus intensity is fixed. This test has been used to evaluate nerve repair after surgery (Mackinnon and Dellon 1985). The two-point discrimination values on the face, lips (5 mm) and fingers (2–3 mm) are lower (more sensitive) than those on the back (39 mm) or abdomen (30 mm).

A QST examination must usually assess sensitivity at a number of locations. At the very least the painful, neighbouring and contralateral sites should be systematically mapped for pain and detection thresholds (Case 3.1). Sensory alterations beyond the primary site may indicate systemic disease or centrally mediated conditions, requiring further tests. Case 3.1 is interesting in that it demonstrates the diagnostic and therapeutic applicability of QST techniques in a patient complaining of bilateral numbness in the area of the mental nerve.

3.2. Levels of Sensation

An increasing stimulus can be described by three simple levels of sensation: detection threshold, pain threshold and pain tolerance. The threshold value describes the

Fig. 3.4 • Computerized tomography (CT) of the mandible in Case 3.1. The CT demonstrates the inserted implants and the proximity of the most distal implant on the right side to the inferior alveolar canal. Inset is a section through this area confirming the implant had penetrated the canal.

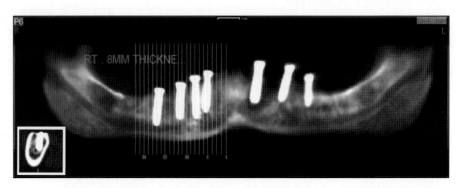

transition between the presence and qualities of sensation; in simple terms these describe the lowest stimulus level that is detected, produces pain or is unbearably painful. More complete descriptions include a level of probability. For example, the detection threshold can be described as a level that is sensed 50 or 75% of the time. Pain tolerance is defined as the highest stimulus level that a subject will willingly tolerate for stimuli with controllable magnitudes, or in the case of stimuli that are uncontrolled such as tourniquet ischaemia, the length of time the stimulus is endured. This latter class of stimuli is rarely used in QST but is often used in studies examining the recruitment of endogenous inhibitory controls in response to pain (Maixner *et al* 1995). In the presence of pathological states both the pain and detection thresholds can be either reduced or elevated.

3.3. Modalities and Nerve Fibres

Specific QST modalities selectively activate different sensory nerve fibres that fall into four major groups. Aα fibres are characterized by a thick coat of myelin (12–22 μm diameter, conduction velocity 70–120 m/sec) and conduct stimuli from neuromuscular spindles and Golgi tendon organs. Aβ fibres have a slightly thinner myelin coat (6–12 μm diameter, conduction velocity 35–70 m/sec) and mediate touch and vibratory sensations. Aβ fibres are preferentially activated by pulsed electrical stimuli at the threshold for detection.

Nociceptive and thermal stimuli are transmitted by thinner fibres. Aδ fibres possess a thin myelinated sheath (1–5 μm diameter, conduction velocity 4–30 m/sec) and are activated mainly by cold stimuli, fast onset mechanical stimuli, radiant (including laser) heat and punctuate mechanical stimulation such as a sharp pin. C fibres are unmyelinated (0.3–1.5 μm diameter, conduction velocity 0.4–2 m/sec) and comprise 60–90% of the cutaneous nerve fibres activated by heat stimuli. The polymodal nociceptors are an important subclass of C fibres that respond to chemical, mechanical and thermal nociceptive stimuli.

The most commonly used stimulus modalities for QST are mechanical, thermal, electrical and chemical. Each stimulus modality has unique characteristics and clinical relevance.

3.3.1. Mechanical Stimuli

Mechanical stimuli evoke sensations of prickle, vibration, pressure or touch. The tools used to evoke mechanical sensations include calibrated von Frey (or Semmes Weinstein) monofilaments for punctuate stimulation or electronic devices for quantitative punctate or vibration stimulation. A blunt needle (e.g. safety pin) or dental explorer can be used to test for sharp pain or a pricking sensation (pinprick). Pressure algometers provide quantitative values of blunt pressure sensitivity used mainly to assess the pressure pain threshold. A cotton swab can assess light touch over a larger area and, along with other stimuli such as an artist's brush or gauze, provide a moving stimulus that is particularly effective for the demonstration of dynamic mechanical allodynia.

Mechanical stimuli are translated to neural activity by several types of receptors. These receptors can be classified as either fast adapting or slowly adapting, which are defined by the rate of decline in neural activity during stimulation. Fast-adapting receptors are comprised of Meissner corpuscles, hair receptors and Pacinian corpuscles. Slowly adapting receptors are comprised of Merckel cell–neurite complexes, touch pads and Ruffini endings. Proprioception is mediated by muscle spindles located in muscle and by Golgi tendon organs which attach the muscles to bone and joint capsules and contain a group of endings similar in structure to the tactile receptors. Sensations evoked by vibration and light mechanical stimuli are conducted via the large Aβ myelinated nerve fibres described earlier.

Altered response to vibration has been found in diabetic neuropathy (Guy *et al* 1985) (not as severe and not as common as the altered response to heat) and in toxic and chemotherapy-related neuropathies (Chaudhry *et al* 1994). Uremic neuropathy and chronic inflammatory demyelinating polyradiculoneuropathies predominantly affect large myelinated fibres (Nielson 1974; Tegner and Lindholm 1985; Krajewski *et al* 2000). Allodynia to pressure has been observed over an inflamed joint; however, long-term arthritic conditions (>5 years) have been associated with hyposensitivity to light touch (Leffler *et al* 2002).

In orofacial evaluations, practitioners assess mechanical allodynia by tapping a tooth for the diagnosis of periapical, periodontal or other dental pathologies (Chapter 5). Prolonged hyperalgesia to cold stimuli on the tooth crown is pathognomonic of irreversible pulpitis. Elevated mechanical detection thresholds have been observed in an experimental model of muscular orofacial pain (Stohler *et al* 2001) and elevated vibrotactile threshold has been observed on the cheek skin in TMD patients (Hollins *et al* 1996). Increased sensitivity (allodynia) has been evaluated in the gingivae of patients diagnosed with atypical odontalgia (List *et al* 2006) and hyperalgesia (reduced pain threshold) was found up to 30 days following third molar extraction (Juhl *et al* 2006). Reduced detection thresholds to both electrical and mechanical stimuli have been demonstrated in the lingual and mental dermatomes 2 days following simple third molar extractions, normalizing to baseline levels 8 days following the procedure (Eliav and Gracely 1998). Muscle and generalized hypersensitivity is also consistently found in patients with fibromyalgia (Giesecke *et al* 2003; Gracely *et al* 2003; Petzke *et al* 2003).

3.3.2. Thermal Stimuli

Thermoreceptors are histologically described as having free, non-specialized nerve endings. In general, thermoreceptors are divided into low- and high-threshold receptors. The low-threshold receptors are activated by temperatures between 15 and 45 °C, which are usually not painful and the brief stimulus durations usually used for assessment do not damage tissue. The high-threshold receptors respond mainly to temperatures higher than 45 °C and lower than 15 °C. Warm sensation is conducted mostly via the slowly conducting unmyelinated C fibres, while the thinly myelinated Aδ fibres largely mediate cold sensation and are also responsible for the sensation of pricking heat pain.

The receptor channels involved in thermal sensation are the Vanilloid receptor subtype 1 (VR1) activated by temperatures above 41 °C, the Vanilloid receptor-like type 1 (VRL-1) activated by temperatures above 50 °C and the cold menthol receptor type 1 (CMR1) activated by a temperature range of 7–28 °C. Interestingly, these receptors are activated by chemical compounds such as capsaicin (the active component in hot chili pepper) that reduce the channel-opening temperature significantly in VR1 and VRL-1 receptors, while menthol-related compounds increase the sensitivity to cold via CMR1 receptors.

For both cold and warm sensations, the range of temperatures between 29 and 37 °C is an adaptation zone. Application of an experimental stimulus or natural object within this temperature zone to skin or mucosa is initially felt as warm or cold, but becomes neutral within minutes. This phenomenon of thermal adaptation must be considered while assessing the detection threshold; continuous or prolonged application may lead to erroneous values.

The temperatures that individuals report as painful vary, although temperatures above 45 °C and below 15 °C are generally considered to be painful. It is important to note that temperatures above 50 °C and below 0 °C can cause significant tissue damage. Thermal stimuli can be applied by heated objects, water, coolant sprays or more modern devices based on electrical, radiant or laser heat, while thermal stimuli based on the Peltier principle or circulating fluids can be used for both heat and cold stimulation.

Stimulus assessment can be affected by the skin temperature. Under normal conditions the face skin temperature is slightly elevated compared to the rest of the body (33–34 °C vs. 30–33 °C) (Verdugo et al 2004) and the temperature of the mucosa and tongue is higher still (34–35 °C and 36–37 °C, respectively) (Green and Gelhard 1987). Heat stimuli applied within the oral cavity are affected by mucosal thickness and the presence and quantity of saliva. In the dental office simple cold and heat sensory tests are commonly used to assess tooth pathology as described earlier (see also Chapter 5). Prolonged and intense thermally evoked pain suggests pulpitis, while a lack of response may indicate a non vital tooth.

Thermal tests provide information about the function of unmyelinated (C) and the thinly myelinated (Aδ) fibres. Heat stimuli can provide a fast initial Aδ response but either slow onset rates or repeated stimulation of the same location evokes C-fibre mediated sensations (Gracely

unpublished observations). Aδ fibres are also tested by cold stimulation. Altered thermal pain and detection thresholds have been reported in diabetic neuropathy (Report and recommendations of the San Antonio conference on diabetic neuropathy 1988; Dyck et al 1990; Navarro and Kennedy 1991), post herpetic neuralgia (Rowbotham and Fields 1996), fibromyalgia (Lautenbacher and Rollman 1997; Geisser et al 2003; Petzke et al 2003), chronic pelvic pain syndrome (Lee et al 2001) and small fibre sensory polyneuropathy (Holland et al 1998).

In the orofacial area, the results of studies applying thermal stimuli to assess patients with burning mouth syndrome (BMS) have been less conclusive (see Chapter 11). Thermal detection thresholds were similar in BMS patients and healthy volunteers, but thermal pain tolerance was significantly lower in BMS patients (Grushka et al 1987; Lamey 1996; Lamey et al 1996). Studies in patients with trigeminal neuralgia (Chapter 11) have found increased thresholds to warm and cold that are resolved after neurosurgical decompression of the trigeminal nerve root (Bowsher et al 1997; Miles et al 1997). The thermal detection threshold has been found to be elevated in patients suffering from chronic sinusitis or following acute facial trauma (Benoliel et al 2005, 2006).

3.3.3. Chemical Stimulation

As stated earlier, chemical compounds such as capsaicin and menthol can alter the performance of thermal receptors. Capsaicin, bee venom and mustard oil are used to induce experimental, dermal, mucosal (nasal gastric), muscular or tooth pain (Kobal 1985; Foster and Weston 1986; Coghill et al 1998; Sang et al 1998; Khalili et al 2001). Intramuscular infusion of hypertonic saline is used to induce experimental muscular orofacial pain as discussed in Chapter 7 (Svensson et al 2000; Stohler et al 2001).

The pain induced by chemical compounds may be specific but there is poor control of stimulus magnitude and resultant pain sensations, and minimal if any application for clinical pain assessment. Various chemical compounds are useful for the evaluation of taste and smell, and in dental practice pain induced by sweet compounds can be an important sign of exposed dentine and deep caries.

3.3.4. Electrical Stimulation

Electrical nerve stimulation evokes a non-natural sensation that is used extensively for sensory testing, sometimes with conflicting and inconsistent results (Hagberg et al 1990; Vecchiet et al 1991; Bendtsen et al 1997). However, electrical stimulation provides unique and useful properties for sensory assessment. Unlike other methods that naturally stimulate nerve receptors, electrical stimuli bypass the receptor to stimulate the primary afferent axon. As a result, primary neurons activated by electrical stimulation do not show the same temporal profile regarding 'sensitization, suppression or fatigue'.

In addition, at the threshold for detection, electrical stimuli exclusively activate the thickly myelinated fibres (Aβ). Thus, a comparison of the detection threshold to both mechanical and electrical stimuli can provide a differential method that isolates receptor and post-receptor processes in Aβ fibres. Changes in both thresholds or in only electrical detection threshold indicate a post-receptor process, while isolated changes in mechanical stimulation indicate a receptor process.

As previously stated, interpatient variability is a common problem in QST particularly with electrical sensory assessment. This inconsistency can be reduced by expressing the electrical detection thresholds as the ratio between the pathological and the contralateral control side (Kemler *et al* 2000). A study assessing sensory changes in diabetic neuropathy patients showed that electrical perception threshold to high-frequency stimulus (2000 Hz) correlates best with vibratory thresholds (large myelinated fibres) and the low-frequency stimulus (5 Hz) correlated with thresholds to the sensation of warm (Masson *et al* 1989).

In dentistry, electrical stimulation is used to assess tooth vitality; however, stimulus or response intensity does not correlate with tooth pathology. Electrical stimulation is used to assess taste and chorda tympani nerve function (Yamada and Tomita 1989; Murphy *et al* 1995). Chorda tympani nerve elevated taste threshold has been found in BMS patients (Eliav *et al* 2007). Electrical detection threshold is reduced (hypersensitivity) in joint-related TMDs (Eliav *et al* 2003), in early oral malignancy (Eliav *et al* 2002), in the first days following third molar extraction (Eliav and Gracely 1998) and in patients suffering from acute sinusitis (Benoliel *et al* 2006). Elevated threshold (hyposensitivity) is found in muscle-related TMD (Eliav *et al* 2003), chronic sinusitis and the delayed phase following facial trauma (Benoliel *et al* 2005).

In the presence of mechanical allodynia, the ratio between the electrical pain and detection threshold of less than 2.0 may indicate altered central nervous system processing of Aβ fibre input (Sang *et al* 2003). Such a result may be a sign of altered central pain modulation and central sensitization.

3.4. Clinical Relevance of QST

QST is an accepted tool for the assessment of diabetic neuropathies (Shy *et al* 2003) and other sensory abnormalities (Eliav *et al* 2004). However, although it is an important tool, currently QST cannot be used alone to diagnose neuropathies (Shy *et al* 2003). The results of thermal and electrical QST offer insight as to the pathological processes in the peripheral nerves (Case 3.1 and Table 3.1).

Mechanical nerve damage or total nerve transection is characterized by myelinated and unmyelinated nerve fibre hyposensitivity that clinically can be translated to elevated detection thresholds to heat, electrical and mechanical stimulation (Dao and Mellor 1998). Partial damage may be followed by either hypo- or hypersensitivity accompanied by ongoing neuropathic pain

Table 3.1	Interpretation of Quantitative Sensory Testing	
	Stimulus	
	Heat Stimulus	**Electrical Stimulus (High Frequency)**
Condition	Assessment of detection threshold of C, unmyelinated nerve fibres	Assessment of detection thresholds in Aβ myelinated nerve fibres
Inflammation (perineural, neuritis)	Unaffected	Hypersensitivity (reduced detection threshold)
Malignancy (malignant neuritis)	*Early stage:* Unaffected	*Early stage:* Hypersensitivity (reduced detection threshold)
	Late stage: Hyposensitivity (elevated, detection threshold)	*Late stage:* Hyposensitivity (elevated, detection threshold)
Nerve damage	Hyposensitivity (elevated, detection threshold)	*Late stage:* Hyposensitivity (elevated, detection threshold)*

*Hypersensitivity is rarely observed at a very early stage (reduced detection threshold).

(Benoliel *et al* 2001, 2002, 2005). In contrast to the neuropathic process of mechanical nerve damage, other specific nociceptive processes may provide a different, identifiable sensory signature. For example, early perineural inflammation produces short-lasting large myelinated nerve fibre hypersensitivity that clinically is revealed by reduced detection to electrical and mechanical stimuli. This increased sensitivity has been demonstrated in clinical and animal spinal nerve models (Eliav and Gracely 1998; Eliav *et al* 1999, 2001, 2002; Chacur *et al* 2001; Gazda *et al* 2001) and reproduced in a model of inflammatory trigeminal nerve neuropathy (Benoliel *et al* 2002).

QST can add a further dimension to pain evaluation. For example, allodynia is defined as pain due to stimulus which normally does not evoke pain. By employing QST the practitioner can distinguish between several allodynic conditions. By definition the pain threshold is reduced in all allodynia cases; however, the detection threshold and pain tolerance can decrease, increase or remain unchanged. Measurements such as the interval between detection and pain thresholds, and detection to pain ratio can be useful in these conditions. These features have been shown to have clinical significance in the assessment of centrally mediated pain conditions (Sang *et al* 2003).

Hyperalgesia is defined as an increased response to stimulus which is normally painful. Pain intensity can be measured with one of the tools described previously (as mentioned earlier the most commonly used tool is the VAS). However, similar to allodynia, there are several types of hyperalgesic conditions. Heat hyperalgesia, for example, is related to thin unmyelinated nerve fibres while tactile hyperalgesia may suggest involvement of myelinated fibres (see Chapter 11). Moreover, in addition to varying intensity any stimulus applied can vary both in frequency and in rate of change (increasing or decreasing rate).

The use of QST in the trigeminal system or other orofacial areas requires further research before being used in routine clinical practice; however, the field is sufficiently developed to aid diagnosis and the evaluation of treatment.

References

Report and recommendations of the San Antonio conference on diabetic neuropathy. Consensus statement. *Diabetes* 1988;**37**(7):1000–1004.

Belanger E, Melzack R, Lauzon P (1989) Pain of first-trimester abortion: a study of psychosocial and medical predictors. *Pain* **36**(3):339–350.

Bendtsen L, Jensen RA, Olesen J (1997) [Decreased pain threshold and tolerance in patients with chronic tension headache]. *Ugeskr Laeger* **159**(29):4521–4525.

Benoliel R, Eliav E, Iadarola MJ (2001) Neuropeptide Y in trigeminal ganglion following chronic constriction injury of the rat infraorbital nerve: is there correlation to somatosensory parameters? *Pain* **91**(1-2):111–121.

Benoliel R, Wilensky A, Tal M, *et al* (2002) Application of a pro-inflammatory agent to the orbital portion of the rat infraorbital nerve induces changes indicative of ongoing trigeminal pain. *Pain* **99**(3):567–578.

Benoliel R, Birenboim R, Regev E, *et al* (2005) Neurosensory changes in the infraorbital nerve following zygomatic fractures. *Oral Surg Oral Med Oral Pathol Oral Radiol Endod* **99**(6):657–665.

Benoliel R, Biron A, Quek SY, *et al* (2006) Trigeminal neurosensory changes following acute and chronic paranasal sinusitis. *Quintessence Int* **37**(6):437–443.

Bentley DE, Derbyshire SW, Youell PD, *et al* (2003) Caudal cingulate cortex involvement in pain processing: an inter-individual laser evoked potential source localisation study using realistic head models. *Pain* **102**(3):265–271.

Bieri D, Reeve RA, Champion GD, *et al* (1990) The Faces Pain Scale for the self-assessment of the severity of pain experienced by children: development, initial validation, and preliminary investigation for ratio scale properties. *Pain* **41**(2):139–150.

Bowsher D, Miles JB, Haggett CE, *et al* (1997) Trigeminal neuralgia: a quantitative sensory perception threshold study in patients who had not undergone previous invasive procedures. *J Neurosurg* **86**(2):190–192.

Burchiel KJ, Anderson VC, Brown FD, *et al* (1996) Prospective, multicenter study of spinal cord stimulation for relief of chronic back and extremity pain. *Spine* **21**(23):2786–2794.

Carroll JM, Russell JA (1996) Do facial expressions signal specific emotions? Judging emotion from the face in context. *J Pers Soc Psychol* **70**(2):205–218.

Chacur M, Milligan ED, Gazda LS, *et al* (2001) A new model of sciatic inflammatory neuritis (SIN): induction of unilateral and bilateral mechanical allodynia following acute unilateral peri-sciatic immune activation in rats. *Pain* **94**(3):231–244.

Chaudhry V, Rowinsky EK, Sartorius SE, *et al* (1994) Peripheral neuropathy from taxol and cisplatin combination chemotherapy: clinical and electrophysiological studies. *Ann Neurol* **35**(3):304–311.

Choiniere M, Melzack R, Rondeau J, *et al* (1989) The pain of burns: characteristics and correlates. *J Trauma* **29**(11):1531–1539.

Coghill RC, Sang CN, Berman KF, *et al* (1998) Global cerebral blood flow decreases during pain. *J Cereb Blood Flow Metab* **18**(2):141–147.

Coghill RC, Gilron I, Iadarola MJ (2001) Hemispheric lateralization of somatosensory processing. *J Neurophysiol* **85**(6):2602–2612.

Dao TT, Mellor A (1998) Sensory disturbances associated with implant surgery. *Int J Prosthodont* **11**(5):462–469.

Drummond PD (1995a) Lacrimation and cutaneous vasodilatation in the face induced by painful stimulation of the nasal ala and upper lip. *J Auton Nerv Syst* **51**(2):109–116.

Drummond PD (1995b) Noradrenaline increases hyperalgesia to heat in skin sensitized by capsaicin. *Pain* **60**(3):311–315.

Dubuisson D, Melzack R (1976) Classification of clinical pain descriptions by multiple group discriminant analysis. *Exp Neurol* **51**(2):480–487.

Dworkin SF, LeResche L (1992) Research diagnostic criteria for temporomandibular disorders: review, criteria, examinations and specifications, critique. *J Craniomandib Disord* **6**(4):301–355.

Dyck PJ, Karnes JL, Gillen DA, *et al* (1990) Comparison of algorithms of testing for use in automated evaluation of sensation. *Neurology* **40**(10):1607–1613.

Eliav E, Gracely RH (1998) Sensory changes in the territory of the lingual and inferior alveolar nerves following lower third molar extraction. *Pain* **77**(2):191–199.

Eliav E, Herzberg U, Ruda MA, *et al* (1999) Neuropathic pain from an experimental neuritis of the rat sciatic nerve. *Pain* **83**(2):169–182.

Eliav E, Benoliel R, Tal M (2001) Inflammation with no axonal damage of the rat saphenous nerve trunk induces ectopic discharge and mechanosensitivity in myelinated axons. *Neurosci Lett* **311**(1):49–52.

Eliav E, Teich S, Benoliel R, *et al* (2002) Large myelinated nerve fiber hypersensitivity in oral malignancy. *Oral Surg Oral Med Oral Pathol Oral Radiol Endod* **94**(1):45–50.

Eliav E, Teich S, Nitzan D, *et al* (2003) Facial arthralgia and myalgia: can they be differentiated by trigeminal sensory assessment? *Pain* **104**(3):481–490.

Eliav E, Gracely RH, Nahlieli O, *et al* (2004) Quantitative sensory testing in trigeminal nerve damage assessment. *J Orofac Pain* **18**(4):339–344.

Eliav E, Gracely RH, Nahlieli O, *et al* (2007) Evidence for chorda tympani dysfunction in burning mouth syndrome patients. *J Am Dent Assoc* **138**(5):628–633.

Foster RW, Weston KM (1986) Chemical irritant algesia assessed using the human blister base. *Pain* **25**(2):269–278.

Frot M, Mauguiere F (2003) Dual representation of pain in the operculo-insular cortex in humans. *Brain* **126**(Pt 2):438–450.

Gagliese L, Melzack R (1997) Chronic pain in elderly people. *Pain* **70**(1):3–14.

Gaston-Johansson F, Albert M, Fagan E, *et al* (1990) Similarities in pain descriptions of four different ethnic-culture groups. *J Pain Symptom Manage* **5**(2):94–100.

Gazda LS, Milligan ED, Hansen MK, *et al* (2001) Sciatic inflammatory neuritis (SIN): behavioral allodynia is paralleled by peri-sciatic proinflammatory cytokine and superoxide production. *J Peripher Nerv Syst* **6**(3):111–129.

Geisser ME, Casey KL, Brucksch CB, *et al* (2003) Perception of noxious and innocuous heat stimulation among healthy women and women with fibromyalgia: association with mood, somatic focus, and catastrophizing. *Pain* **102**(3):243–250.

Gendreau M, Hufford MR, Stone AA (2003) Measuring clinical pain in chronic widespread pain: selected methodological issues. *Best Pract Res Clin Rheumatol* **17**(4):575–592.

Giesecke T, Williams DA, Harris RE, *et al* (2003) Subgrouping of fibromyalgia patients on the basis of pressure-pain thresholds and psychological factors. *Arthritis Rheum* **48**(10):2916–2922.

Glaros AG, Glass EG, Brockman D (1997) Electromyographic data from TMD patients with myofascial pain and from matched control subjects: evidence for statistical, not clinical, significance. *J Orofac Pain* **11**(2):125–129.

Gracely RH (1990) Measuring pain in the clinic. *Anesth Prog* **37** (2–3):88–92.

Gracely RH, Kwilosz DM (1988) The Descriptor Differential Scale: applying psychophysical principles to clinical pain assessment. *Pain* **35**(3):279–288.

Gracely RH, Lota L, Walter DJ, *et al* (1988) A multiple random staircase method of psychophysical pain assessment. *Pain* **32**(1):55–63.

Gracely RH, Grant MA, Giesecke T (2003) Evoked pain measures in fibromyalgia. *Best Pract Res Clin Rheumatol* **17**(4):593–609.

Gramling SE, Grayson RL, Sullivan TN, *et al* (1997) Schedule-induced masseter EMG in facial pain subjects vs. no-pain controls. *Physiol Behav* **61**(2):301–309.

Graven-Nielsen T, McArdle A, *et al* (1997) In vivo model of muscle pain: quantification of intramuscular chemical, electrical, and pressure changes associated with saline-induced muscle pain in humans. *Pain* **69**(1–2): 137–143.

Green BG, Gelhard B (1987) Perception of temperature on oral and facial skin. *Somatosens Res* **4**(3):191–200.

Gronblad M, Lukinmaa A, Konttinen YT (1990) Chronic low-back pain: intercorrelation of repeated measures for pain and disability. *Scand J Rehabil Med* **22**(2):73–77.

Grushka M, Sessle BJ (1984) Applicability of the McGill Pain Questionnaire to the differentiation of 'toothache' pain. *Pain* **19**(1):49–57.

Grushka M, Sessle BJ, Howley TP (1987) Psychophysical assessment of tactile, pain and thermal sensory functions in burning mouth syndrome. *Pain* **28**(2):169–184.

Guy RJ, Clark CA, Malcolm PN, *et al* (1985) Evaluation of thermal and vibration sensation in diabetic neuropathy. *Diabetologia* **28**(3):131–137.

Hagberg C, Hellsing G, Hagberg M (1990) Perception of cutaneous electrical stimulation in patients with craniomandibular disorders. *J Craniomandib Disord* **4**(2):120–125.

Harden RN, Carter TD, Gilman CS, *et al* (1991) Ketorolac in acute headache management. *Headache* **31**(7):463–464.

Herr KA, Spratt K, Mobily PR, *et al* (2004) Pain intensity assessment in older adults: use of experimental pain to compare psychometric properties and usability of selected pain scales with younger adults. *Clin J Pain* **20**(4):207–219.

Holland NR, Crawford TO, Hauer P, *et al* (1998) Small-fiber sensory neuropathies: clinical course and neuropathology of idiopathic cases. *Ann Neurol* **44**(1):47–59.

Hollins M, Sigurdsson A, Fillingim L, *et al* (1996) Vibrotactile threshold is elevated in temporomandibular disorders. *Pain* **67**(1):89–96.

Huskisson EC, Sturrock RD, Tugwell P (1983) Measurement of patient outcome. *Br J Rheumatol* **22**(3 Suppl):86–89.

Jaaskelainen SK, Teerijoki-Oksa T, Forssell H (2005) Neurophysiologic and quantitative sensory testing in the diagnosis of trigeminal neuropathy and neuropathic pain. *Pain* **117**(3):349–357.

Jamison RN, Gracely RH, Raymond SA, *et al* (2002) Comparative study of electronic vs. paper VAS ratings: a randomized, crossover trial using healthy volunteers. *Pain* **99**(1–2):341–347.

Jensen MP, Karoly P, Huger R (1987) The development and preliminary validation of an instrument to assess patients' attitudes toward pain. *J Psychosom Res* **31**(3):393–400.

John MT, Dworkin SF, Mancl LA (2005) Reliability of clinical temporomandibular disorder diagnoses. *Pain* **118**(1–2):61–69.

Joyce CR, Zutshi DW, Hrubes V, *et al* (1975) Comparison of fixed interval and visual analogue scales for rating chronic pain. *Eur J Clin Pharmacol* **8**(6):415–420.

Juhl GI, Svensson P, Norholt SE, *et al* (2006) Long-lasting mechanical sensitization following third molar surgery. *J Orofac Pain* **20**(1):59–73.

Kemler MA, Schouten HJ, Gracely RH (2000) Diagnosing sensory abnormalities with either normal values or values from contralateral skin: comparison of two approaches in complex regional pain syndrome I. *Anesthesiology* **93**(3):718–727.

Khalili N, Wendelschafer-Crabb G, Kennedy WR, *et al* (2001) Influence of thermode size for detecting heat pain dysfunction in a capsaicin model of epidermal nerve fiber loss. *Pain* **91** (3):241–250.

Kobal G (1985) Pain-related electrical potentials of the human nasal mucosa elicited by chemical stimulation. *Pain* **22**(2): 151–163.

Krajewski KM, Lewis RA, Fuerst DR, *et al* (2000) Neurological dysfunction and axonal degeneration in Charcot-Marie-Tooth disease type 1A. *Brain* **123** (Pt 7):1516–1527.

Lamey PJ (1996) Burning mouth syndrome. *Dermatol Clin* **14**(2): 339–354.

Lamey PJ, Hobson RS, Orchardson R (1996) Perception of stimulus size in patients with burning mouth syndrome. *J Oral Pathol Med* **25**(8):420–423.

Lautenbacher S, Rollman GB (1997) Possible deficiencies of pain modulation in fibromyalgia. *Clin J Pain* **13**(3):189–196.

Lee JC, Yang CC, Kromm BG, *et al* (2001) Neurophysiologic testing in chronic pelvic pain syndrome: a pilot study. *Urology* **58**(2):246–250.

Leffler AS, Hansson P, Kosek E (2002) Somatosensory perception in a remote pain-free area and function of diffuse noxious inhibitory controls (DNIC) in patients suffering from long-term trapezius myalgia. *Eur J Pain* **6**(2):149–159.

LeResche L, Dworkin SF (1984) Facial expression accompanying pain. *Soc Sci Med* **19**(12):1325–1330.

List T, Leijon G, Helkimo M, *et al* (2006) Effect of local anesthesia on atypical odontalgia – A randomized controlled trial. *Pain* **122**(3):306–314.

Liu ZJ, Yamagata K, Kasahara Y, *et al* (1999) Electromyographic examination of jaw muscles in relation to symptoms and occlusion of patients with temporomandibular joint disorders. *J Oral Rehabil* **26**(1):33–47.

McGuire DB, Altomonte V, Peterson DE, *et al* (1993) Patterns of mucositis and pain in patients receiving preparative chemotherapy and bone marrow transplantation. *Oncol Nurs Forum* **20**(10):1493–1502.

Mackinnon SE, Dellon AL (1985) Two-point discrimination tester. *J Hand Surg [Am]* **10**(6 Pt 1):906–907.

Maixner W, Fillingim R, Booker D, *et al* (1995) Sensitivity of patients with painful temporomandibular disorders to experimentally evoked pain. *Pain* **63**(3):341–351.

Masson EA, Veves A, Fernando D, *et al* (1989) Current perception thresholds: a new, quick, and reproducible method for the assessment of peripheral neuropathy in diabetes mellitus. *Diabetologia* **32**(10):724–728.

Melzack R (1975) The McGill Pain Questionnaire: major properties and scoring methods. *Pain* **1**(3):277–299.

Melzack R, Terrence C, Fromm G, *et al* (1986) Trigeminal neuralgia and atypical facial pain: use of the McGill Pain Questionnaire for discrimination and diagnosis. *Pain* **27**(3):297–302.

Merskey H, Bogduk N (1994) *Classification of Chronic Pain: Descriptions of Chronic Pain Syndromes and Definition of Pain Terms*. Seattle: IASP Press.

Miles JB, Eldridge PR, Haggett CE, *et al* (1997) Sensory effects of microvascular decompression in trigeminal neuralgia. *J Neurosurg* **86**(2):193–196.

Murphy C, Quinonez C, Nordin S (1995) Reliability and validity of electrogustometry and its application to young and elderly persons. *Chem Senses* **20**(5):499–503.

Naliboff BD, Munakata J, Fullerton S, *et al* (1997) Evidence for two distinct perceptual alterations in irritable bowel syndrome. *Gut* **41**(4):505–512.

Navarro X, Kennedy WR (1991) Evaluation of thermal and pain sensitivity in type I diabetic patients. *J Neurol Neurosurg Psychiatry* **54**(1):60–64.

Nielson VK (1974) The peripheral nerve function in chronic renal failure. A survey. *Acta Med Scand Suppl* **573**:1–32.

Nikolajsen L, Hansen CL, Nielsen J, *et al* (1996) The effect of ketamine on phantom pain: a central neuropathic disorder maintained by peripheral input. *Pain* **67**(1):69–77.

Okeson JP (1996) *Orofacial Pain: Guidelines for Assessment, Classification, and Management.* The American Academy of Orofacial Pain. Illinois: Quintessence Publishing.

Olesen J, Bousser M-G, Diener HC, *et al* (2004) The International Classification of Headache Disorders, 2nd edition. *Cephalalgia* **24**(suppl 1):24–150.

Petzke F, Clauw DJ, Ambrose K, *et al* (2003) Increased pain sensitivity in fibromyalgia: effects of stimulus type and mode of presentation. *Pain* **105**(3):403–413.

Price DD, Dubner R (1977) Mechanisms of first and second pain in the peripheral and central nervous systems. *J Invest Dermatol* **69**(1):167–171.

Rosier EM, Iadarola MJ, Coghill RC (2002) Reproducibility of pain measurement and pain perception. *Pain* **98**(1–2):205–216.

Rowbotham MC, Fields HL (1996) The relationship of pain, allodynia and thermal sensation in post-herpetic neuralgia. *Brain* **119**(Pt 2):347–354.

Sang CN, Hostetter MP, Gracely RH, *et al* (1998) AMPA/kainate antagonist LY293558 reduces capsaicin-evoked hyperalgesia but not pain in normal skin in humans. *Anesthesiology* **89**(5):1060–1067.

Sang CN, Max MB, Gracely RH (2003) Stability and reliability of detection thresholds for human A-Beta and A-delta sensory afferents determined by cutaneous electrical stimulation. *J Pain Symptom Manage* **25**(1):64–73.

Sharav Y, Tal M (1995) Hypnotic analgesia and reflex activity. *Pain* **63**(3):391–392.

Shy ME, Frohman EM, So YT, *et al* (2003) Quantitative sensory testing: report of the Therapeutics and Technology Assessment Subcommittee of the American Academy of Neurology. *Neurology* **60**(6):898–904.

Sriwatanakul K, Kelvie W, Lasagna L, *et al* (1983) Studies with different types of visual analog scales for measurement of pain. *Clin Pharmacol Ther* **34**(2):234–239.

Sternberg WF, Bokat C, Kass L, *et al* (2001) Sex-dependent components of the analgesia produced by athletic competition. *J Pain* **2**(1):65–74.

Stohler CS, Kowalski CJ, Lund JP (2001) Muscle pain inhibits cutaneous touch perception. *Pain* **92**(3):327–333.

Svensson P, Miles TS, Graven-Nielsen T, *et al* (2000) Modulation of stretch-evoked reflexes in single motor units in human masseter muscle by experimental pain. *Exp Brain Res* **132**(1):65–71.

Tal M (1984) The threshold for eliciting the jaw opening reflex in rats is not increased by neonatal capsaicin. *Behav Brain Res* **13**(2):197–200.

Tal M, Goldberg LJ (1981) Masticatory muscle activity during rhythmic jaw movements in the anaesthetized guinea-pig. *Arch Oral Biol* **26**(10):803–807.

Tal M, Sharav Y (1985) Development of sensory and reflex responses to tooth-pulp stimulation in children. *Arch Oral Biol* **30**(6):467–470.

Tal M, Sharav Y, Devor M (1981) Modulation of the jaw-opening reflex by peripheral electrical stimulation. *Exp Neurol* **74**(3):907–919.

Tegner R, Lindholm B (1985) Vibratory perception threshold compared with nerve conduction velocity in the evaluation of uremic neuropathy. *Acta Neurol Scand* **71**(4):284–289.

Tesfaye S, Watt J, Benbow SJ, *et al* (1996) Electrical spinal-cord stimulation for painful diabetic peripheral neuropathy. *Lancet* **348**(9043):1698–1701.

Turk DC, Rudy TE (1987) Towards a comprehensive assessment of chronic pain patients. *Behav Res Ther* **25**(4):237–249.

Turk DC, Rudy TE (1988) Toward an empirically derived taxonomy of chronic pain patients: integration of psychological assessment data. *J Consult Clin Psychol* **56**(2):233–238.

Turk DC, Rudy TE (1990) The robustness of an empirically derived taxonomy of chronic pain patients. *Pain* **43**(1):27–35.

Vecchiet L, Giamberardino MA, Saggini R (1991) Myofascial pain syndromes: clinical and pathophysiological aspects. *Clin J Pain* **7**(Suppl 1):S16–S22.

Verdugo RJ, Bell LA, Campero M, *et al* (2004) Spectrum of cutaneous hyperalgesias/allodynias in neuropathic pain patients. *Acta Neurol Scand* **110**(6):368–376.

Wall PD (1979) On the relation of injury to pain. The John J. Bonica lecture. *Pain* **6**(3):253–264.

Weidner C, Schmidt R, Schmelz M, *et al* (2000) Time course of post-excitatory effects separates afferent human C fibre classes. *J Physiol* **527**(Pt 1):185–191.

Weidner C, Schmelz M, Schmidt R, *et al* (2002) Neural signal processing: the underestimated contribution of peripheral human C-fibers. *J Neurosci* **22**(15):6704–6712.

Weidner C, Schmidt R, Schmelz M, *et al* (2003) Action potential conduction in the terminal arborisation of nociceptive C-fibre afferents. *J Physiol* **547**(Pt 3):931–940.

Wong DL, Baker CM (2001) Smiling faces as anchor for pain intensity scales. *Pain* **89**(2–3):295–300.

Yamada Y, Tomita H (1989) Influences on taste in the area of chorda tympani nerve after transtympanic injection of local anesthetic (4% lidocaine). *Auris Nasus Larynx* **16**(Suppl 1):S41–S46.

Yarnitsky D, Sprecher E (1994) Thermal testing: normative data and repeatability for various test algorithms. *J Neurol Sci* **125**(1):39–45.

CHAPTER 4

Psychological aspects of chronic orofacial pain

Karen G Raphael and Donald S Ciccone

1. Introduction

It has been estimated that as many as 12% of cases seen in dental practices have pain that cannot be ascribed to a known physiological cause (Horowitz *et al* 1991). When organic factors appear insufficient to explain a complaint of pain, it may be tempting to assume that psychiatric and psychological factors must be involved. The goals of this chapter are, first, to review the evidence for this common assumption and, second, to introduce the reader to selected methods that have proven effective in managing psychological complications when present. In the first part of the chapter we address the potentially separate effects of psychological factors on pain onset and aetiology and on pain course. Models of how psychological factors can impact orofacial pain will also be reviewed and evaluated. In the second part we present a theoretical framework for psychological intervention, describe psychological methods shown to be effective in randomized controlled trials and conclude with a discussion of psychological screening and referral.

2. Comorbidity of Psychiatric and Chronic Orofacial Pain Conditions

Multiple reviews have noted that patients with various types of orofacial pain appear to be at risk of psychiatric disorder and psychological symptoms. In particular, migraineurs (see Chapter 9) may have increased risk of depression, anxiety and panic attacks (Breslau *et al* 1994a; Stewart *et al* 1994; Low and Merikangas 2003; Patel *et al* 2004; Scher *et al* 2005). Burning mouth syndrome (Chapter 11) appears to be comorbid with personality disorders (Maina *et al* 2005) and depression and anxiety disorders

(Bogetto *et al* 1998). Patients with temporomandibular disorders (TMD; Chapters 7 and 8) have an increased risk of depression (Gallagher *et al* 1991; Korszun *et al* 1996), particularly when the masticatory muscles rather than joint are involved (Kight *et al* 1999; Auerbach *et al* 2001; Huang *et al* 2002; Yap *et al* 2002). A diverse group of orofacial pain patients (Sherman *et al* 2005) and TMD patients in particular (De Leeuw *et al* 2005a) are reported to have elevated rates of post-traumatic stress disorder (PTSD). These patterns reflect, in part, the fact that psychiatric disorders and psychological symptoms are common among pain patients in general, not solely among orofacial pain patients. In fact, it has been argued that psychiatric comorbidity, especially depression, is more marked among a diverse group of patients with chronic pain conditions than among those with serious medical conditions such as cardiac disease or cancer (Banks and Kerns 1996).

Thus, it is likely that a large subset of patients presenting for orofacial treatment will have a comorbid psychiatric disorder. Establishing comorbidity between orofacial pain and psychiatric disorders does not provide an understanding of the nature of the conditions or the mechanisms through which they are linked. Indeed, their comorbidity provokes important questions about the relation of psychiatric disorders or subthreshold psychological symptoms to the aetiology and course of orofacial pain.

3. Psychological Factors and Orofacial Pain: An Overview of Explanatory Models

The cause of certain orofacial pain conditions is controversial or elusive. The danger for the orofacial pain specialist is in assuming that 'medically unexplained' orofacial pain is therefore 'psychologically explained'. The contribution of psychological factors to symptom presentation must be distinguished from their role as primary cause.

3.1. The Psychogenic Model

A purely psychological or 'psychogenic' model of orofacial pain, in which the patient presents symptoms in the absence of demonstrable pathology, derives in part from a half-century-old view of 'psychogenic pain' (Engel 1951, 1959) that has roots in psychoanalytic theory. In one of George Engel's early works (Engel 1951), 'atypical facial neuralgia' was posed as a model hysterical conversion syndrome. Engel notes that several of Sigmund Freud's monographs from the late nineteenth and early twentieth centuries describe facial neuralgias 'which proved to be hysterical' (p 376). The model of purely psychological orofacial pain continued to gain advocates in the 1960s and 1970s (Lascelles 1966; Lefer 1966; Moulton 1966; Lesse 1974), and concepts of atypical facial pain such as 'masked depression' were introduced (Lesse 1974; Violon 1980; Lehmann and Buchholz 1986). One publication even proposed that atypical facial pain can develop as 'a defense against psychosis' (Delaney 1976).

Moving into more recent approaches to the purely psychological model, the bible for classification of psychiatric disorder, the *Diagnostic and Statistical Manual of Mental Disorders IV* (DSM-IV) (American Psychiatric Association 1994), includes a classification of somatoform disorder labelled 'pain disorder' (or pain disorder associated with psychological factors in DSM-IV-TR; 'text revision'). A subtype of pain disorder is postulated to exist in which, in the absence of a general medical condition, psychological factors are viewed as the primary cause of onset, severity, exacerbation or pain maintenance. Similar is the ICD-10 (*International Classification of Diseases* (ICD) 10th revision, version for 2007. URL; http://www.who.int/classifications/apps/icd/icd10online/, accessed 12/2007) classification of 'persistent somatoform pain disorder' representing persistent and distressing pain that cannot be fully attributed to a physical cause and that occurs in the presence of psychological issues which are presumed to be causative. The International Headache Society's *International Classification of Headache Disorders*, second edition (ICHD-2), includes a classification for 'headache attributed to psychiatric disorder' but considers it to be a rare occurrence, with specific instances included in an appendix 'to encourage further research into this area' (Olesen *et al* 2004, p 121). Thus, standard diagnostic systems for pain and disease allow for the possibility of pain due primarily to psychological factors. A more recent trend is to retreat from the potential stigmatization (Marbach *et al* 1990; Werner and Malterud 2003) of a purely psychological or psychogenic pain model by invoking the euphemism of 'medically unexplained' pain (Marbach 1999; Smythe 2005).

Aside from the theoretical support offered from a psychoanalytic perspective, the concept of psychogenic pain is supported by several sources of data. The first is the striking comorbidity of several orofacial pain disorders with psychiatric disorders, as described earlier in this chapter. Second, the efficacy of tricyclic antidepressants in the treatment of orofacial pain may be viewed as support for a psychological aetiology. However, compelling evidence indicates that their mechanism of pain relief is independent of their antidepressant effect (Feinmann *et al* 1984; Sharav *et al* 1987; Cohen and Abdi 2001).

Many of the orofacial pain conditions sometimes considered to have primary psychological causes show an epidemiological preponderance in women. The striking preponderance of women with TMD (Dworkin *et al* 1990; LeResche 1997; Marbach *et al* 1997), burning mouth syndrome (Tammiala-Salonen *et al* 1993; Bergdahl and Bergdahl 1999), tension-type headache (Russell 2005) and migraine (Patel *et al* 2004; Lipton and Bigal 2005) parallels the preponderance of women with anxiety disorders (Regier *et al* 1990; Kessler *et al* 1994) and mood disorders (Kessler *et al* 1994; Weissman *et al* 1996), especially depression with somatic features such as pain (Silverstein 1999, 2002). Clinicians may tend to view women as having more psychosomatic illness, more emotional lability and more symptoms due to emotional factors (Unruh 1996).

Adding to the belief that orofacial pain can be due primarily to psychological factors, over and above comorbidity with specific psychiatric disorders, is that some chronic orofacial pain patients may present with distinct cognitive styles and personality characteristics. Clinicians who note the presence of such dysfunctional personality characteristics in their orofacial pain patients may be further encouraged to assume that pain is primarily due to psychological factors. For example, TMD patients may show affective inhibition and somatosensory amplification (Speculand *et al* 1981; Raphael *et al* 2000). One large study of patients with burning mouth syndrome (BMS) found that they had elevated rates of psychiatrically assessed personality disorder (Maina *et al* 2005), and another (Al Quran 2004) showed that BMS patients had higher scores than controls on scales of neuroticism but lower scores on measures such as openness and extraversion.

Refutation of the concept of psychogenic pain comes from several sources. First, while a female preponderance is common to several psychiatric conditions and several orofacial pain disorders, there are numerous other disorders with a high female-to-male ratio for which no psychological risk factors have been firmly identified. These include, among many others, dermatologic conditions (Robinson 2006), sexually transmitted diseases (Madkan *et al* 2006) and autoimmune diseases (Lockshin 2002). Tertiary factors that link orofacial pain and psychiatric disorder and are associated with female sex, such as oestrogenic hormones, may eventually be identified (LeResche *et al* 1997; Dao *et al* 1998; Macfarlane *et al* 2002). Second, elevated rates of psychiatric disorder in treatment-seeking patients may reflect the fact that psychiatric comorbidity increases the probability of an individual seeking treatment for any disorder (Galbaud du Fort *et al* 1993); whether these psychiatric comorbidities would indeed be detected in more representative community samples of individuals with various orofacial pain conditions has yet to be examined. Additionally, psychiatric comorbidity may well develop as a consequence of the stress of living with chronic pain. Indeed, one family study supported this explanation for masticatory muscle pain, in finding that patients with depression themselves had low rates of depression in their families, indicating that their depression was likely reactive to the stress of living with chronic orofacial pain (Dohrenwend *et al* 1999). Although the implications of this pattern of familial aggregation was not interpreted as reflecting reactive depression in pain patients, a similar observation was made decades earlier regarding the absence of family history of depression in atypical facial pain patients with depression themselves (Lascelles 1966).

Patient follow-up studies also provide evidence that psychological symptoms can develop in reaction to the stress of living with orofacial pain. A study of patients undergoing arthroscopy for TM joint pain (Dahlstrom *et al* 2000) found that some psychosocial variables did improve at a 3-month postoperative visit: specifically, a 'dysfunctional index' from the Multidimensional Pain Inventory (MPI) (Kerns *et al* 1985) consisting of high pain, high life interference, high affective distress and low perceived life control. Similarly, a five-year outcome study of TMD patients (Ohrbach and Dworkin 1998) found that those with high levels of psychological distress whose pain improved also showed improvement in psychological distress, suggesting that at least part of the distress for some TMD patients represents a reaction to their pain. The stigma of living with chronic orofacial pain (Marbach *et al* 1990) could induce a psychologically defensive response style (Raphael *et al* 2000). Indeed, patients' self-reports suggest that dysfunctional personality characteristics were not evident prior to the onset of orofacial pain, but manifested later (Vickers and Boocock 2005).

As described by Feinmann and Newton-John (2004: 361):

Failure to identify the cause of pain or to effect [sic] a cure is then interpreted as a sign that either the examination or test used was faulty (in this case, the test is often repeated many times)...or that the clinician was less than capable (so a different one is sought, often many times). As the patient becomes increasingly frustrated and despondent with the inability of the medical system to cure him or her, there may also be a change in the attitudes of the treating professionals toward the patient. The persistence of pain over time despite the application of multiple tests and multiple treatment approaches is interpreted as a sign of an underlying psychopathology, which only causes the patient further distress.

The major logical fallacy for the purely psychological model of orofacial pain is that it assumes that failure to find a biological marker for a particular orofacial pain condition implies that psychological factors must be primary. However, pain researchers increasingly recognize that the association between observable tissue damage or other identifiable pathological process and the presence or extent of pain is weak at best (Melzack and Wall 1996). Multiple factors, including genetic susceptibility to pain and neuronal plasticity, can at least partially explain the continuation of pain beyond localized healing and the lack of correlation between injury and pain.

3.2. Psychosocial Stress as the Link between Orofacial Pain and Psychological Symptoms

Another model would suggest that the link between orofacial pain and psychological factors may also be due to their shared association with psychosocial stress. In theory, stress might seem to be important in the genesis of orofacial pain, as experimental stress can modulate jaw reflexes (Lobbezoo *et al* 2002). Nevertheless, while stress may be associated with pain modulation and impaired coping, muscle hyperactivity is no longer considered a risk factor for muscle pain (see Chapter 7).

We differentiate here between psychosocial stress due to major life events (e.g. death of a loved one), hassles (e.g. more common, daily, small events such as a fight with a spouse) and chronic environmental burdens (e.g. financial problems, chronic medical illness), and the harmful consequences of stress, i.e. distress (Selye 1974). This distinction is important, because research often fails to differentiate the two. Thus, orofacial pain patients may have elevated levels of distress, but this does not necessarily mean that they were exposed to high levels of specific psychosocial sources of stress, over and above the stressful experience of living with pain.

3.2.1. Psychosocial Stress and TMDs

The role of psychosocial stress has been particularly implicated for TMDs. In shifting from earlier mechanistic theories of TMD aetiology (Costen 1934), the psychophysiological model of masticatory muscle pain aetiology was first proposed by Laszlo Schwartz in the 1950s (Schwartz 1956; Marbach 1991) and expanded later by Daniel Laskin (Laskin 1969). It focused on the muscle rather than the joint as a primary source of pain and integrated psychosocial factors as a cause. The foundation of the psychophysiological model of TMDs is that psychosocial stress initiates a distress response or *tension* in an individual, causing dysfunctional oral habits such as tooth grinding and clenching. These oral habits are presumed to promote muscle contraction and hyperactivity and subsequent facial pain (see Chapter 7 for further discussion).

This model has been widely adopted by members of the dental community. A 1993 survey in the Seattle, Washington, area (Le Resche *et al* 1993) found that stress was identified as a major factor by 92% of general dentists and specialists, as well as 85% of 'TMD experts' who were selected for their extensive contributions to the peer-reviewed literature on TMDs. Supporting these endorsements are research studies that find TMD patients, especially those with a myogenous disorder, to have an increased likelihood of reporting selective types of major life stressors (Speculand *et al* 1984; Marbach *et al* 1988) but not necessarily hassles (Wright *et al* 1991). An uncontrolled study (De Leeuw *et al* 2005b) also suggested that TMD patients have high exposure to traumatic stress, but lack of a control group makes interpretation of these findings difficult. What is particularly clear is that subjective distress, often mislabelled as *stress*, is elevated in TMD patients (Marbach *et al* 1988; Beaton *et al* 1991; Macfarlane *et al* 2001; Ferrando *et al* 2004; Glaros 2005; Pallegama *et al* 2005), but, as discussed earlier, this may be a consequence of living with pain rather than represent a reaction to other psychosocial stressors. Chronic pain is a powerful stressor.

Thus, compared to the widespread belief in the role of stress as a major factor in TMDs, the body of evidence for psychosocial stress in TMD onset is relatively limited. Retrospective reports of frequent stressful life events in TMD patients must be viewed with some degree of scepticism, given the unreliability of self-reported life event exposure even over periods as short as six months (Raphael *et al* 1991). Moreover, there is a possibility that high levels of distress in TMD patients may bias recall of prior life events in mood-congruent ways (Raphael and Cloitre 1994).

3.2.2. Psychosocial Stress and Other Orofacial Pain Conditions

While the role of psychosocial stress has been most often implicated for TMDs, research has also examined its role in other orofacial pain conditions. For example, although BMS patients were more likely to report psychological symptoms, psychiatric hospitalization and outpatient psychological treatment than non-pain controls, they did not report more recent life events (Eli *et al* 1994). The support for major life stress in BMS is confined to an uncontrolled study of 18 BMS patients who frequently reported acute stressors prior to pain onset (Hakeberg *et al* 2003). A similar uncontrolled study points to stress as a migraine precipitant; see Chapter 9 for a discussion on migraine triggers (Deniz *et al* 2004). A larger study (Zivadinov *et al* 2003) suggests that, although stress is mentioned as a common precipitant for both migraine and tension-type headache, it is cited more often among migraineurs. In contrast, patients with *typical* and *atypical* trigeminal neuralgia rarely implicate psychological factors as precipitants (Rasmussen 1991).

Although neither BMS nor trigeminal neuralgia has been clearly linked to psychosocial stress, headache may have some relationship. The 1985 Nuprin Pain Report (Sternbach 1986) found that self-reported stress and daily hassles were more often reported by a community sample of individuals who experienced at least one headache in the prior year. Although major life events do not appear to be associated with diverse types of headache (Martin and Theunissen 1993), 'perceived stress', a possible indicator of distress or daily hassles, has been associated with it. The role of major life events in headache was also discounted in another study, which still found daily hassles to be elevated in chronic headache patients, particularly among those with tension-type or mixed headache rather than migraine (De Benedittis and Lorenzetti 1992). Another study (Fernandez and Sheffield 1996) reported no relation between headache frequency and major life events, but a modest relationship between headache frequency and daily hassles. A small relationship has been detected between more frequent headache and major life events in several large-sample studies (Passchier *et al* 1991; Fernandez and Sheffield 1996; Reynolds and Hovanitz 2000), with the relationship restricted to younger individuals. Thus, while there may be some relationship between headache and psychosocial stress, most likely centred on daily hassles and headache frequency, its role in BMS and trigeminal neuralgia is not supported.

3.3. Psychosocial Characteristics as Risk Factors for Pain Onset

Distinct from the reductionistic and deterministic model of psychosocial characteristics as a primary *cause* of orofacial pain is the more integrative model of psychosocial characteristics as risk factors for pain onset, considered as part of a constellation of other factors affecting pain onset. A classic example is provided by Von Korff *et al* (1993), who examined depression as a risk factor for onset of five common pain symptoms, including TMD pain, when studying a large sample of adults at baseline and 3-year follow-up. They found that depression severity and chronicity increased the risk of new onset of severe headache and chest pain, but the relationship between baseline depression and later TMD pain onset was not significant. Nevertheless, the nonsignificant trend was in the predicted direction, in which new onset rates for TMD pain were 6% for those with normal scores on a depression symptom index but 12% for those with severe depressive symptoms or more chronic symptoms. In contrast, new onset of severe headache was significantly associated with more severe and more chronic depressive symptoms. New onset probabilities for severe headache were 3% for those with normal scores on a depression index but over 9% for those with severe depressive symptoms.

Most recently, results from a prospective cohort study of initially TMD-free young women were reported (Slade *et al* 2007). Depression, perceived stress and mood were associated with baseline pain sensitivity and were predictive of a two- to threefold increase in risk of TMD symptoms at 3-year follow-up. Interestingly, the effect of these psychological factors on TMD symptom onset was independent of variation in the gene encoding catechol-O-methyl-transferase (COMT), which was separately associated with increased risk of TMD onset (see Chapter 7).

To our knowledge, no studies of risk factors for onset of orofacial pain conditions other than TMDs have been conducted. Nevertheless, the available data suggest that psychological factors may be among the constellation of factors that increase risk of onset of TMDs. Consideration of psychological and psychosocial factors as one of many factors increasing risk of pain is consistent with a general biopsychosocial model of orofacial pain. As summarized by Sherman and Turk (2001:423):

The model presumes physical pathology, or at least physical changes in muscle, joints, and nerves that generate pain signals, but also presumes that psychological and social processes interact with pathology to result in overt expression of pain such as functional impairment, disability, and distress.

Although a variety of specifications of the biopsychosocial model of orofacial pain exist (e.g. Dworkin and Massoth 1994; Andrasik *et al* 2005; Suvinen *et al* 2005), it has been argued that, despite the important heuristic value of these models, they tend to be neglected because they fail to specify testable hypotheses (Dworkin *et al* 1999). A specific form of the biopsychosocial model, labelled the 'vulnerability-diathesis-stress' model (Dworkin *et al* 1999) proposes an interaction between a physiological predisposition (i.e. a diathesis from genetic vulnerability, or acquired vulnerability from prior exposures such as disease or injury) and psychosocial stress leading to development of a pain disorder. According to this view, psychosocial stress is pathogenic only for constitutionally susceptible individuals. Recent advances in psychiatric research support the interaction of gene and environment. For example, psychosocial stress affects risk of developing depression (Caspi *et al* 2003) or psychosis (van Os *et al* 2003) particularly for those with genetic or familial vulnerability.

Attempts to test a stress vulnerability model in pain disorders in general and orofacial pain specifically are limited to date, despite the heuristic appeal of the model. An example is provided by Janke *et al* (2004), who found that depression was a risk factor for the development of tension-type headaches during and after a laboratory stress task, at least among those with a history of prior tension-type headaches. A series of studies on TMD pain (Yemm 1971a,b; Mercuri *et al* 1979; Kapel *et al* 1989; Flor *et al* 1991; Nicholson *et al* 2000) suggests that TMD patients have an increased risk of reacting to experimental stressors with increased EMG activity. While these stress reactivity studies have sometimes been interpreted to suggest that those with chronic TMD have a specific vulnerability to stress, whether such patterns were evident prior to the establishment of a pain disorder is unknown. In fact, numerous studies contradict the role of muscle hyperactivity in pain onset (see Chapter 7).

3.4. Psychosocial Characteristics as Risk Factors for Course and Outcome for Orofacial Pain

Although our review of the literature suggests that the concept of psychogenic orofacial pain is misguided, limited available data support the idea that psychosocial factors can influence the risk of onset of at least some orofacial pain conditions. Where psychological and psychosocial factors become more prominent is in explaining the course of and disability associated with pain conditions. For example, why do some patients who have a TMD experience it as a minor inconvenience, while others with the same disorder become disabled? Why do some have symptoms for only a couple of weeks, while others have a lifelong pattern of facial pain exacerbations and remissions?

3.4.1. Psychosocial Characteristics as Risk Factors for TMD Outcome

Once again, the bulk of the research literature on the role of psychological factors in the course of chronic orofacial pain focuses on TMDs. One study examined the relation between clinical and psychological variables and 5-year outcome for individuals with TMDs (Ohrbach and Dworkin 1998). It found that changes in depression and anxiety over the 5 years were not consistently related to degree of improvement in pain intensity, but that baseline depression and anxiety tended to be highest in the group whose symptoms were considered to be worse at 5-year follow-up. Notably, changes in physical measures were not consistently related to changes in pain at follow-up, suggesting 'at best only an indirect relationship between TMD pain report and clinical status for both the physical and psychological domains' (p 322). Mixed findings were also reported by Rammelsberg and colleagues (Rammelsberg *et al* 2003). They found that those myofascial TMD patients whose symptoms were remitted at 5-year follow-up were more likely than those with persistent or recurrent pain to be depressed at baseline. However, patients whose pain remitted at follow-up were the only group of subjects whose depression also significantly decreased at follow-up. The authors interpret this finding as suggesting that baseline depression was actually caused by their baseline pain severity. Another study (Garofalo *et al* 1998) examined physical and psychological variables that determined whether acute TMD pain was considered to be chronic at 6-month follow up. Although higher levels of both depression and nonspecific physical symptoms at baseline predicted chronic pain status at 6 months, neither factor was significant in a multivariate model that controlled for type of TMD (with myogenous TMD most likely to be chronic) or characteristic pain intensity at baseline. A similar study (Riley *et al* 2001) found that TMD patient satisfaction with improvement and subjective pain relief at 8 months following initial evaluation for treatment was predicted by initial symptoms of anxiety but not depression. They also found that patients who engaged in pretreatment use of cognitive coping strategies, including distancing from pain, coping self-statements and ignoring pain, had more satisfactory status at follow-up. These findings also suggest the potential utility of cognitive behaviour therapy (see 4.2.2) in TMD patients.

Other studies have found baseline psychological factors to predict pain severity at a later point. Auerbach and colleagues (Auerbach *et al* 2001) reported that TMD pain severity at a variable follow-up period was associated with baseline depression severity. Similarly, Epker and colleagues (Epker *et al* 1999) found that TMD patients who continued to have TMD pain at 6-month follow-up differed from those whose pain remitted by having more baseline depression. In a related publication (Wright *et al* 2004), patients who were classified on a prior algorithm as at high risk of progressing from acute to chronic TMD pain (Epker *et al* 1999) were further characterized as having elevated scores on self-report measures of depression and coping, as well as interview-based measures of major psychiatric disorder and personality disorders. A study by Fricton and Olsen (1996) found that various factors associated with depression, including low self-esteem and feeling worried, were associated with post-treatment symptom improvement among chronic TMD patients.

In contrast to studies supporting some role of psychological factors as predictors of TMD course, one study (Suvinen *et al* 1997) found that none of the baseline psychological measures examined, including affective disturbance and anxiety, predicted rapid versus slow response to conservative treatment of TMD. In another study, baseline depressive symptoms showed a nonsignificant trend towards prediction of treatment response, following 6 months of conservative treatment for TMDs (Grossi *et al* 2001). Negative findings were also reported by Steed (1998), who found that a general scale assessing anxiety, depression and frustration and another assessing chronic and recent stress were elevated among TMD patients at initial symptoms, but neither scale related to symptoms at time of 'maximum medical improvement', as judged by the treating clinician. Of course, the subjectivity in determining the time of maximum medical improvement creates interpretive problems. A well-cited paper by Rudy and colleagues (Rudy *et al* 1995) concludes that

'dysfunctional' TMD patients with the highest degree of psychological distress showed greater improvement in pain than other TMD patients receiving conservative, standardized treatment, but a careful review of their findings suggests that this pattern was found for only a self-report measure of pain symptoms but not muscle pain on palpation.

Review of the relatively large body of literature on psychological factors in the course of TMDs leads to the conclusion that results are mixed. Differences in defining successful outcome, assessing psychological symptoms and sample size are among the factors likely to explain this inconsistent pattern. Regardless of the explanation, psychological factors have not been able to consistently forecast the outcome of treatment or the clinical course of TMD symptoms. Nevertheless, psychological treatment studies of TMD have yielded promising results (see below), suggesting that such factors may yet prove to be clinically significant.

3.4.2. Psychosocial Characteristics as Risk Factors for Outcome in Other Orofacial Pain Disorders

The smaller body of literature on psychological factors as predictors of course of other orofacial pain conditions is also inconsistent. For example, in a mixed group of *psychogenic* facial pain patients (Feinmann *et al* 1984), treatment outcome at 12 months was predicted by a history of an adverse major life event prior to pain onset. In a later 4-year follow-up (Feinmann 1993) of the same group of patients (later labelled by the author as having 'chronic idiopathic facial pain') presence of a baseline psychiatric diagnosis did not predict pain status at 4-year follow-up. Finally, in an 8-year follow-up of juvenile-onset migraine or tension-type headache (Guidetti *et al* 1998), presence of baseline psychiatric comorbidity predicted a worse outcome.

3.5. Shared Pathogenesis for Psychiatric Disorders and Orofacial Pain

Finally, another model of the relation between psychiatric conditions (or less severe psychological symptoms) and orofacial pain is that they have a shared pathogenesis. This model has been suggested as explaining the general pain–depression relationship (Bair *et al* 2003), the general pain–PTSD relationship (Asmundson *et al* 2002) and, more specifically, the orofacial pain–depression relationship (Korszun 2002). For example, at the neurobiological level, neurotransmitters such as serotonin and norepinephrine have been implicated in both pain modulation and psychiatric disorders (Ward *et al* 1982; Stahl and Briley 2004). Stress vulnerability may be implicated in both depression and facial pain, probably involving dysregulation of the hypothalamic-pituitary-adrenal (HPA) axis (Korszun 2002). At a psychological level, vulnerability to negative affectivity or dysphoric states (Kirmayer *et al* 1994; Von Korff and Simon 1996) may link psychological symptoms with somatic symptoms, including orofacial pain. It has also been proposed (Krueger *et al* 2004) that chronic pain is linked to psychiatric disorders such as depression and anxiety through a specific tendency of certain individuals to express distress inwards ('internalizing disorders') rather than outwards through antisocial behaviour, substance abuse and impulsivity ('externalizing disorders').

For fibromyalgia, a condition that is itself comorbid with myofascial TMD (Plesh *et al* 1996; Aaron *et al* 2000), several studies have established that fibromyalgia and depression share familially mediated risk factors (Arnold *et al* 2004; Raphael *et al* 2004). Specifically, these studies established that having a family member with fibromyalgia places an individual at increased risk for depression, and having a family member with depression places an individual at increased risk for fibromyalgia. A shared vulnerability explanation has been proposed specifically for migraine and depression (Breslau *et al* 1994a, 2003), with evidence of bidirectional influences, so that depressed individuals have an increased risk of migraine and individuals with migraine have an increased risk of developing depression. Additional studies suggest that the bidirectional relationship applies to migraine but not other severe headaches (Breslau *et al* 2000).

3.6. Psychological Factors and Illness Behaviour

Despite a long history of speculation, the evidence for psychosocial factors as a primary cause of orofacial pain is weak. On the other hand, consistent with a biopsychosocial perspective on chronic orofacial pain, psychosocial factors may trigger an episode of pain in susceptible individuals, may cause pain exacerbation and may lead to a more chronic course of pain. However, on these last points, the literature is inconsistent. One possible conclusion is that psychological factors have small and inconsistent effects on orofacial pain symptoms. However, inconsistent prediction from psychological factors does not mean primary prediction from physical factors: as Ohrbach and Dworkin (1998) have shown, prediction of 5-year outcome of TMD pain from either physical or psychological measures is weak.

To understand the juncture at which psychological factors become critical, it is first necessary to distinguish between disease and illness (see Fig. 4.1). Disease refers to the objective evidence of a pathological state. In the case of chronic pain syndromes, including but not limited to orofacial pain, externally verifiable evidence of an underlying pathological state causing and maintaining the pain may often be lacking or only tentatively present. Illness refers to patients' beliefs and views of their ill health and is inferred from symptom reports and behaviour. The traditional biomedical model views

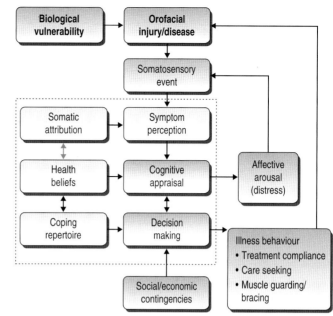

Fig. 4.1 • A cognitive-behavioural model of affective arousal and illness behaviour in patients with chronic orofacial pain.

psychological factors as a secondary factor, influencing the transition from disease and illness to clinical outcome; it assumes that biological processes are sufficient to cause both disease and illness. In contrast, the biopsychosocial model (Drossman 1998) views psychological factors as contributing to the expression of disease and illness. While psychological factors are again viewed as affecting ultimate clinical outcome, they are viewed as having the potential to exert influences on illness and disease, even at a biological level.

Empirical data clearly support the importance of psychological and psychosocial factors as affecting illness behaviour. Although we focus here on the sparse literature examining these factors for orofacial pain patients specifically, there exists a much broader literature on the relation between psychosocial factors and adjustment to diverse pain conditions (Keefe *et al* 2004). Particularly relevant is the concept of catastrophizing (see also below). Pain-related catastrophizing is characterized by an extreme focus on pain, exaggeration of the threat associated with the pain and feelings of helplessness related to the control of pain. While catastrophizing has been related to pain severity in diverse conditions, even during dental hygiene treatment (Sullivan and Neish 1998), it may be particularly relevant as a predictor of illness behaviour following the onset of orofacial pain. For example, Turner and colleagues (Turner *et al* 2005) reported that catastrophizing was associated with pain severity, activity interference and number of healthcare visits among TMD patients.

The nature of the specific psychosocial factors predicting healthcare seeking may differ, depending on the specific orofacial pain diagnosis. One study (Epker and Gatchel 2000) reported that affective distress predicted treatment-seeking behaviour for those with a myofascial TMD, but treatment-seeking for patients with TM joint conditions was better predicted by other factors such as psychological introversion.

Despite the small body of literature specifically examining illness behaviour in orofacial pain, it cannot be overemphasized that the broader body of literature on psychological factors in all type of chronic pain is relevant. Samuel Dworkin (1994: 862) has written:

> TMD is primarily a chronic pain condition sharing many important features with other common chronic pain conditions. Such a perspective places TMD within the same biopsychosocial model currently used to study and manage all illness, including common chronic pain conditions.

While these issues have been relatively more often explored for TMDs, the application of a biopsychosocial model for the understanding and treatment of all orofacial pain conditions is strongly advocated.

Despite our cautious interpretation of the literature, which suggests that psychological factors do not cause orofacial pain or may not reliably predict the outcome of traditional orofacial pain therapy, we nevertheless assert that psychological factors are likely to be important in clinical practice. This belief stems from the fact that orofacial pain is clearly associated with increased risk of psychiatric disorder, as well as increased likelihood of subthreshold psychological symptoms (see above). When present, these factors can amplify or distort the perception of pain and thus compromise the accuracy of symptom reporting. In the behavioural realm, psychological factors can undermine motivation to comply with therapeutic instruction and impede efforts to correct maladaptive illness behaviour. Psychological factors may not be an issue for many (or even most) patients with orofacial pain but, when present, they may threaten the outcome of an otherwise effective treatment. Moreover, the presence of psychiatric disorder, or even psychological distress in the absence of full-fledged disorder, may be sufficient to significantly diminish quality of life. Therefore, it merits clinical attention from the orofacial pain practitioner. In the section that follows, we examine selected psychological methods used to treat such patients and argue for the value of routine psychological screening.

4. Psychological Management of Chronic Orofacial Pain

Patients with orofacial pain are confronted with the prospect of living indefinitely with an ailment that does not respond to therapy. While psychosocial factors may or may not *cause* orofacial pain, they largely determine the impact of illness on emotional and behavioural

functioning. Depending on the patient's repertoire of coping skills, he or she may respond adaptively by minimizing pain-related stress and avoiding unnecessary illness behaviour that may exacerbate pain. Alternatively, the patient may respond maladaptively by exaggerating or catastrophizing pain, thereby increasing emotional distress and the likelihood of pain-related restrictions in physical activity (Turner *et al* 2001). The emotional and behavioural consequences of orofacial pain, whether adaptive or maladaptive, are not dictated by pathophysiology alone but by the patient's beliefs about his or her illness (in accord with the biopsychosocial model). The goals of psychological treatment are thus to identify maladaptive cognitive and behavioural responses and provide remedial training as necessary to reduce pain-related distress and minimize interference with daily functioning.

Before discussing psychological techniques used to achieve these aims, it will be helpful to provide an overview of the human information processing system. The theoretical orientation selected for this purpose is called the cognitive-relational model (Lazarus 1991). In the next section we use a slightly abridged version of this model to explain how changes in cognition lead to corresponding changes in pain-related affect and coping behaviour. It should be acknowledged, however, that important components of the theory have yet to undergo scientific testing. Nevertheless, the model provides a framework for our discussion of psychological intervention and is widely accepted among pain clinicians. Our goal will be to familiarize the non-specialist with a treatment approach that has produced promising results in patients with chronic orofacial pain (Dworkin *et al* 2002; Turner *et al* 2006) and, at the same time, has been widely used to treat psychiatric disorders in the general population (Beck 2005). Specifically, we will introduce the reader to cognitive psychotherapy (Beck 1976; Ellis 1994), followed by a brief discussion of adjunctive techniques including biofeedback and relaxation training (Crider *et al* 2005). Finally, we describe screening procedures that permit dental practitioners to identify patients most likely to profit from mental health services and provide a rationale for referral that may facilitate communication with reluctant patients.

4.1. Cognitive-Behavioural Theory of Illness Behaviour

The core assumption of the cognitive model is that humans do not respond directly to a stimulus event but rather to a cognitive interpretation of that event (Ellis 1962). Our emotional and behavioural responses to orofacial pain, for example, depend on whether we perceive it as a threat or simply a temporary inconvenience. According to the cognitive model, threat perception triggers a response from the sympathetic nervous system as well as action tendencies that govern overt responses in the form of illness behaviour. It is not within the scope of this discussion to examine the assumptions underlying a cognitive-relational theory of human behaviour (Lazarus 1991). Nevertheless, it may be useful to illustrate the central role of cognition in regulating emotional and behavioural responses to pain. An early demonstration of this role was provided by Beecher (1956), who interviewed soldiers about wounds they had received in battle. He was struck by the fact that some of the soldiers expressed an 'optimistic, even cheerful, state of mind' despite having sustained an objectively painful injury. This emotional reaction to pain was explained by the fact that serious injury required relocation to the relative safety of a field hospital. He concluded that the personal significance of an injury and not its objective severity was primarily responsible for the ensuing emotional response. It may, therefore, be important to understand what the patient thinks about orofacial pain if our goal is to mitigate its effects on emotional and physical functioning.

Figure 4.1 provides an overview of human information processing showing that sensory events, including pain, are subject to routine cognitive appraisal. A fundamental tenet of the model is that virtually all transactions with the environment are subject to cognitive interpretation and evaluation. Persistent face pain, for example, may be perceived as a symptom of disease or, alternatively, as an uncomfortable but benign sensation. The interpretation of somatosensory information is made in accordance with pre-existing knowledge about causes of facial pain and the likelihood of disease (among other factors). After deciding how to categorize this event, the individual is faced with the task of evaluating its personal significance. If pain sensation is judged to be a threat (labelled *unbearable* or *awful*) a corresponding affective response is mobilized and the individual is biologically prepared for 'flight or fight'. Unfortunately, in the case of chronic pain, such a response is unnecessary, since it fails to warn of impending danger, and is potentially maladaptive. Advantages and disadvantages of various behavioural options may be weighed as the individual decides how to cope with the problem at hand. Behavioural options are selected from an existing repertoire of skills and reflect efficacy expectations or beliefs about personal coping ability.

The presence of social and economic disincentives in the environment may further influence the choice of coping options. The patient may know, for example, that expressions of pain and suffering are met with increased social support or that treatment seeking enables him or her to avoid social (or work) obligations (Ciccone *et al* 1999). The consequences of faulty cognitive appraisal and ineffective coping may exacerbate pain, compromise the outcome of dental therapy and lead to emotional and behavioural problems requiring mental health intervention.

In sum, the model portrayed in Fig. 4.1 conveys a dynamic process in which pain-related affect and coping behaviour interact with orofacial pain symptoms. The processes of interpretation and evaluation are iterative

and subject to modification as new information or experiences are acquired. The model does not imply that cognitive processing entails conscious reflection and/or deliberation. In fact, automaticity is more likely the norm as thinking habits and perceptual bias become overlearned. To efficiently interpret the meaning of a rapidly changing environment, humans may necessarily rely on a set of perceptual rules and unconscious assumptions that can be deployed quickly and effortlessly (Glaser and Kihlstrom 2005).

4.2. Psychological Management of Chronic Orofacial Pain

Even though the dental practitioner may never conduct psychotherapy, he or she may wish to integrate dental treatment within a comprehensive plan that includes a mental health component. This is sufficient justification for the non-specialist to consider the methods used to treat pain-related psychological dysfunction. Before describing these methods, however, it is useful to distinguish between the goals of psychotherapy and those of the orofacial pain specialist. While the dentist is appropriately focused on symptom reduction or even alleviation, the psychotherapist is focused on ameliorating stress, minimizing dysfunctional illness behaviour, and treating comorbid psychiatric disorder, when present. Although some patients have reported a reduction in pain following psychological treatment (Morishige *et al* 2006; Turner *et al* 2006), we believe the primary justification for referral should be to reduce emotional distress and/or minimize pain-related impairment. It is worth noting that the goal(s) of psychological treatment remain the same, whether the distress developed in response to chronic pain or existed prior to onset. In either case, psychological dysfunction undermines quality of life and may compromise the outcome of dental therapy (Turner *et al* 2001; Dworkin *et al* 2002). The most popular psychological treatment for patients with chronic orofacial pain and the one we describe in this chapter is called cognitive behavioural therapy or CBT. Other psychological techniques, such as psychodynamic therapy, may also be appropriate and effective but, as yet, have not been tested in rigorous clinical trials.

4.2.1. Evidence-Based Psychological Treatment

Controlled trials of CBT for patients with chronic orofacial pain have yielded promising results. Unfortunately, almost all of these clinical trials have focused on TMD to the exclusion of other, less prevalent, orofacial pain conditions. Nevertheless, we believe that the results of these studies generalize beyond the treatment of TMD. This is likely since CBT is known to be effective in patients with chronic pain regardless of pain location and irrespective of whether pain is explained or unexplained (Morley *et al* 1999; Sharpe *et al* 2001; McCracken and Turk 2002; Turk 2003). The most recent trial involving TMD was reported by Turner et al (2006), who compared four sessions of CBT administered over 8 weeks to a usual care control group that received an equivalent amount of therapist attention but no active psychological treatment. The CBT group received the same usual care supplemented by instruction in cognitive coping and relaxation training. When the groups were assessed 12 months later, Turner *et al* found that CBT-treated patients reported a significant reduction in jaw pain and improved masticatory function compared to control patients. An earlier study by the same group compared six sessions of CBT plus conservative care to conservative care only for TMD patients 'who demonstrated poor psychosocial adaptation' (Dworkin *et al* 2002). When assessed 4 months after enrolment, patients in the CBT group reported significantly less pain and improved ability to control self-rated TMD symptoms. Similar results have also been reported by Gardea *et al* (2001), who administered twelve sessions of CBT to patients with TMD. When compared to a no-treatment control group one year later, CBT-treated patients reported significant reductions in pain severity and pain-related disability, as well as improved mandibular function. Finally, Turk *et al* (1996) compared two treatment protocols for TMD; one included CBT while the other provided 'nondirective, supportive counseling'. The group that received CBT 'demonstrated significantly greater reductions in pain, depression, and medication use'. In addition, only the CBT group showed 'continued improvements . . . on pain associated with muscle palpation, self-reported pain severity, depression, and use of medications.' Similar results have been reported for other orofacial pain disorders including chronic tension-type headache (McCrory *et al* 2001) and migraine without aura (Goslin *et al* 1999). While the preceding clinical trials provide a strong evidence base from which to recommend CBT for patients with chronic orofacial pain, it is perhaps more impressive to consider the larger body of evidence showing that CBT is effective for the most common forms of psychiatric disorder (Butler *et al* 2006) including depression (Scott 2001) and generalized anxiety disorder (Durham *et al* 1994; Linden *et al* 2005). Since our primary justification for psychological referral is to treat emotional distress and behavioural dysfunction rather than pain sensation, we submit that this larger body of evidence is equally relevant to our choice of treatment modality. At present, the consensus appears to favour CBT as the preferred mode of psychological intervention for patients with chronic pain.

In the next section we provide a brief introduction to cognitive therapy, a core component of CBT, originally developed by Albert Ellis (1955, 1962) and Aaron Beck (1976). Afterwards, we describe the use of biofeedback and related relaxation training for achieving improved self-control over dysfunctional muscle activity in patients with myofascial TMD (Crider *et al* 2005) and reducing autonomic hyperarousal in patients with tension-type or migraine headache (Goslin *et al* 1999; McCrory *et al* 2001).

4.2.2. Cognitive Therapy

As suggested by the model in Fig. 4.1, the goal of cognitive therapy is to produce a philosophical shift in the way patients think about negative events or, more specifically, the way they think about orofacial pain. The process of achieving cognitive change, sometimes called 'cognitive restructuring', has been described in detail by Walen *et al* (1992) among others. The limited goal of this section is to provide an overview of this treatment using the ABC framework originally proposed by Albert Ellis (1962, 1994). The three components of the model are designated as follows: 'A' is an antecedent event such as chronic pain; 'B' is a belief or belief system giving rise to a subjective interpretation of the event; and 'C' denotes the emotional and/or behavioural consequence of the event. After a stimulus is detected at A, we immediately interpret its personal significance or meaning at B which, in turn, elicits an emotional response as well as an illness behaviour at C. For purposes of this discussion, the cognitive process used to construct a mental representation of the stimulus is called an 'inference'. This type of activity occurs whenever we recognize a stimulus as functionally equivalent to one encountered in the past. Using prior knowledge to infer the meaning of new events allows us to unconsciously access properties or attributes of stimuli that were not directly observed or perceived (Hommel *et al* 2001). At least two types of inference are required to interpret the significance of events in our environment (Walen *et al* 1992). The first is descriptive and serves to identify or categorize the event in question. For example, hearing a loud noise may be perceived as a car backfiring or as a gunshot. After categorizing the event (inferring the source of the noise) we are left with the task of appraising its significance. The same event may be appraised as threatening or irrelevant, depending on prior knowledge of similar auditory events and expectations of coping ability. If we are standing next to a window and perceive gunshots coming from the street, we might decide to seek cover in anticipation of danger. On the other hand, if we perceive car noises instead of gunshots, we may not react at all. Identical stimuli can thus give rise to vastly different emotional and behavioural responses, depending on their cognitive interpretation. Despite the central role of cognition in regulating human behaviour, the inference process is notoriously fallible. Humans often rely on faulty logic ('jumping to conclusions') as they strive to decipher the personal significance of their changing environment. This leads to the second assumption underlying cognitive therapy, namely that faulty inference and mistaken appraisal are responsible for eliciting maladaptive emotion and self-defeating illness behaviour. In cognitive therapy, the goal is to dispute these 'thinking mistakes' and replace them with beliefs that are logical or more consistent with empirical observation. Persistent depression, anxiety and anger are said to be 'unhealthy' emotions and thus products of irrational belief whereas sadness, concern and annoyance are 'healthy' emotions and products of rational belief.

One of the most common of all thinking mistakes and the frequent subject of therapeutic intervention is called catastrophizing. As the name implies, this refers to the mistaken belief that difficult or unpleasant events are literally unbearable or catastrophic. Patients with chronic orofacial pain, for example, often use melodramatic language to describe their symptoms as 'devastating' or 'awful'. This type of exaggerated appraisal, according to cognitive theory, elicits an intense affective and behavioural response out of proportion to the sensory event. By definition, chronic pain is unpleasant but not 'unbearable' since patients actually bear or tolerate the sensation for months or even years. An alternative (rational) belief might be substituted as follows 'My problem is exceptionally painful at times but it is hardly unbearable or more than I can stand.' Another common thinking error occurs when patients insist that they must or 'should' have what they desire. For example, a cure for chronic pain is highly advantageous and thus preferable but hardly necessary. When patients confuse what they need with what they prefer (by demanding a cure), they unwittingly increase their emotional discomfort. Demanding pain relief may also lead to dysfunctional coping by motivating patients to go 'doctor shopping' or engage in excessive medical visitation. These emotional and behavioural consequences are maladaptive since they compromise quality of life and, in certain circumstances, exacerbate pain severity.

The process by which a therapist challenges and hopefully modifies the patient's irrational belief is called cognitive disputing. This is achieved by asking patients to explain or defend their logical fallacies or unproven assumptions. Typical examples of disputing include 'Where is the evidence that it would be awful?' or 'Why do things have to be the way you want them to be?' As noted earlier, the aim is not to correct grammatical or linguistic errors but to produce profound changes in the way patients evaluate the consequences of a negative life event. In the case of patients who catastrophize, for example, the therapist explains that chronic pain, unlike acute pain, does not signal the onset of physical injury (or tissue damage). The patient is advised that habitual use of a word such as 'unbearable' to describe pain sensation is understandable but likely to prove self-defeating. Cognitive therapists believe that catastrophic thought causes self-inflicted stress, which they refer to as 'emotional pain'. This is above and beyond the 'physical pain' caused by an orofacial pain disorder. In the language of the therapeutic 'cover story', the catastrophizing patient is said to be confronted with 'two types of pain' instead of one. According to the cognitive model, catastrophizing is a form of evaluative inference or misappraisal leading to an unnecessary flight or fight response. Once the patient expresses a willingness to correct this thinking habit, the therapist may begin disputing by asking for proof that the pain is actually unbearable as opposed to

extremely uncomfortable. Therapeutic benefits are contingent upon the patient believing and not simply understanding that pain exacerbations are tolerable despite being unpleasant. The shift from irrational to rational thought is accomplished gradually through repeated disputation during the session and frequent practice outside the clinic in the form of weekly 'homework assignments'. For example, the patient might be encouraged to resist the natural temptation to label an exacerbation as 'awful' and instead substitute the rational belief that 'pain is bad at times but all the evidence shows that I can certainly stand it.'

Aside from catastrophic appraisal, there are other common thinking *mistakes* that may compromise psychological adjustment. For example, patients have been known to engage in any or all of the following:

Demandingness	'My life should not be so difficult or uncomfortable.' 'You should be more understanding.' 'Doctors should be able to control my pain.'
Fortune telling	'Since I have been unable to function at work or home for a long time, I'll never be able to function again.' 'I'll never be able to enjoy myself again now that I have this pain problem.'
Self-downing	'Since I can't do the things I used to, I'm less of a person and not as good as other people.' 'I have to please others and when I don't (or can't) that proves I'm inadequate or worthless.'
All or none	'If I can't enjoy all of the activities I used to then I can't enjoy anything.' 'In order for treatment to be successful I have to be completely better and not just partly better.'

The cognitive therapist has an extensive repertoire of philosophical and empirical disputing strategies available to address each of these erroneous beliefs. It is beyond the scope of this chapter, however, to describe these strategies in more detail. The interested reader is referred to comprehensive manuals prepared by Walen *et al* (1992) and Beck *et al* (1979). Whilst the vast majority of pain practitioners will not practise psychotherapy, it is possible to collaborate with the psychotherapist by reinforcing a rational acceptance of chronic pain and offering a realistic appraisal of pain severity. In particular, it may be useful for the practitioner to refrain from catastrophic or absolutistic language when describing pain symptoms or past treatment failures (e.g. 'I know the pain can be unbearable at times'; 'There has to be a solution for your problem'). The practitioner may also wish to shift the focus of treatment away from pain *alleviation* in favour of pain *management* and restoration of functional capacity. This allows the patient to expect waxing and waning of symptoms without a promise of symptom remission. Despite the presence of pain and physical restrictions, the patient can be encouraged to maintain an adequate activity level, avoid excessive rest, correct defective posture and poor body mechanics and, when physically possible, resume domestic and work-related chores.

4.2.3. Adjunctive Modalities: Biofeedback and Relaxation Training

The aim of biofeedback training is to provide patients with information or *feedback* about physiological activity for the purpose of bringing that activity under voluntary control. The biofeedback device usually includes a sensor that detects and records information about bodily functions (such as skin temperature, blood pressure or muscle tension) and an electronic amplifier that converts this information into an auditory or visual display that can be monitored by the patient in real time. In most clinical applications, the device allows patients to access physiological events that may otherwise go unnoticed or that lie outside the boundaries of human proprioception. The assumption is that, with the aid of biofeedback, patients may be able to bring physiological activity under voluntary (cognitive) control. One of the first clinical demonstrations of this technique was reported by Budzynski and Stoyva (1969), who trained patients with tension headache to lower muscle activity using surface electromyographic (sEMG) feedback.

A number of studies have evaluated the clinical efficacy of sEMG training for patients with myofascial TMD (Crider *et al* 2005). The usual aim of this training is to reduce hypertonicity and/or hyperactivity of the masseter and anterior temporalis muscles. Training may target elevated tension in the muscle at rest or, more realistically, provide patients with an opportunity to reduce hyperactivity during or after a routine motor task (e.g. chewing). Aside from *re-educating* the muscles of mastication, biofeedback may also be used to facilitate generalized relaxation (Gardea *et al* 2001). In this case, the biofeedback device provides information about one or more parameters of the autonomic nervous system, such as skin temperature or electrodermal activity. By providing access to hand temperature during thermal biofeedback, for example, patients may acquire a hand warming response and thereby reduce sympathetically mediated arousal. At present, there is insufficient evidence to show that specialized sEMG biofeedback to correct abnormal muscle function in the face is any more or less effective than biofeedback-assisted relaxation to lower physiological arousal. A direct comparison of relaxation training with and without biofeedback for patients with myofascial TMD found that both were effective, producing improvement in 70 and 71% of patients, respectively (Brooke and Stenn 1983). Reduced arousal was apparently sufficient to reduce TMD symptoms without explicit sEMG training. These findings strongly suggest

that reduced tension in the masseter muscle may not be necessary to achieve a good clinical outcome and are consistent with a large body of literature (see above and Chapter 7) critiquing the role of muscle hyperactivity in pain.

While the underlying mechanism may not be known, the efficacy of biofeedback for myofascial TMD is less in doubt. Crider *et al* (2005) identified six randomized controlled trials and, of these, five yielded significant 'evidence for the efficacy of biofeedback-based treatments of TMD compared to appropriate control conditions'. The clinical utility of biofeedback when used alongside (or instead) of other conservative modalities, such as physical rehabilitation or oral splint therapy, has not been established. Finally, we should emphasize that the preceding trials were limited to patients who reported pain upon palpation of masticatory muscles and cannot be generalized to patients with TMD pain primarily related to joint problems.

While biofeedback has played a limited role in the treatment of myofascial TMD, it has been widely accepted as a front-line therapy for patients with tension-type or migraine headache. Behavioural treatments for headache have been recognized by, among others, the American Medical Association (1983), the National Institutes of Health (Anonymous 1996) and the World Health Organization (Holroyd and Penzien 1993). A meta-analysis by Goslin *et al* (1999) examined the efficacy of behavioural therapy, including biofeedback, for migraine without aura. Biofeedback alone or in combination with CBT and relaxation training produced dramatic (32–49%) reductions in migraine activity compared to untreated controls (5%). Thermal and EMG modalities were equally effective but neither was superior to relaxation training without biofeedback. A similar meta-analysis of behavioural treatments for tension-type headache reached similar conclusions (McCrory *et al* 2001). Relatively few studies have compared the efficacy of biofeedback or other behavioural modalities to pharmacotherapy, but the few that have suggest they are equally efficacious. Holroyd *et al* (2001), for example, compared tricyclic antidepressant therapy with 'stress management' for tension-type headache. The latter included instruction in cognitive coping and relaxation but no biofeedback. When delivered alone, medication and stress management produced 'clinically significant' improvement in headache activity for 35 and 38% of patients, respectively. When delivered together in a combined treatment group, they produced improvement in 64% of patients.

As noted earlier, the theoretical rationale used to justify biofeedback for patients with myofascial TMD has been called into question. Similar doubts have been raised about the mechanism underlying thermal biofeedback for migraine (Mullinix *et al* 1978) and about the mechanism underlying EMG biofeedback for tension-type headache (Andrasik and Holroyd 1980). In an effort to test the muscle tension hypothesis, Holroyd *et al* (1984) trained one group of patients to decrease muscle tension (as per the hypothesis) while training another to produce an increase. This was achieved by altering the feedback contingency so that decreased EMG activity was fed back as increased and vice versa. All patients were led to believe that training would lead to decreased muscle tension. At the same time, Holroyd *et al* manipulated outcome expectations by informing one group that they were 'highly successful' while informing others that they were only 'moderately successful'. Headache activity improved regardless of whether participants were trained to increase or decrease muscle tension. Moreover, those with the best outcomes were those led to believe they were highly successful at the biofeedback task. Whereas changes in muscle tension could not account for observed reductions in headache activity, the investigators showed that changes in cognition, specifically in self-efficacy beliefs, were correlated with clinical outcomes. This study does not rule out the muscle tension hypothesis but it does raise questions about whether other factors, such as cognitive expectations, might be more important determinants of headache activity. It remains to be seen whether other psychological treatments, aside from biofeedback, can effect similar changes in self-efficacy leading to similar improvements in headache symptoms.

4.3. Screening Patients for Psychiatric Disorder or Psychological Dysfunction

Although the orofacial pain specialist may play a supportive role, psychological intervention is ideally provided by a mental health clinician (psychologist or psychiatrist) with specialized training in behavioural medicine and chronic pain. In this section we address two fundamental issues facing the orofacial pain practitioner: (1) When should I request a psychological evaluation or consultation? and (2) How do I explain the referral to my patient?.

Given the prevalence of psychiatric disorders in this population (see above) and the possibility that subclinical psychological dysfunction can undermine even the most appropriate intervention, we and others (McCreary *et al* 1992; Dworkin *et al* 2002) believe that routine psychological screening of orofacial pain patients is justified. The decision to screen, however, is not without consequences, since the pain practitioner incurs a professional obligation to refer once he or she becomes aware that a patient is suffering from psychological dysfunction. It is therefore advisable to identify low-cost or subsidized mental health services in the community, before deciding whether to implement screening procedures. Once the decision is made to proceed, it is advisable to screen all patients who receive a diagnosis of chronic orofacial pain without exception, rather than limiting the assessment to those suspected of psychological involvement. This

allows the orofacial pain clinician to inform patients that screening is routine and not reserved for *special* cases. In addition, the detection of psychiatric disorder or psychological dysfunction can be subtle and medical practitioners are notoriously poor at this task (Cassano and Fava 2002).

4.3.1. Screening Instruments

Patients at risk of psychiatric disorder or suffering from psychological distress may be identified by one or more screening questionnaires administered at initial assessment. One of the most comprehensive instruments available for this purpose is the Patient Health Questionnaire (PHQ). Originally intended for primary care settings, the PHQ is self-administered and provides algorithmic diagnoses based on DSM-IV criteria for eight psychiatric disorders: major depression; other depressive disorder; panic; other anxiety disorder; binge eating; bulimia nervosa; somatoform disorder; alcohol use or dependence. Patients are instructed to code each symptom based on how often it bothered them over the preceding two weeks: 'not at all', 'several days', 'more than half the days', or 'nearly every day'. Aside from a psychiatric diagnosis, these ratings also yield a continuous measure of syndrome severity. The section on symptom reporting contains 15 ailments that account for over 90% of physical complaints reported by outpatients in primary care (Kroenke *et al* 1990). Patients rate each of these symptoms as 'not bothered', 'bothered a little', or 'bothered a lot'. Spitzer and colleagues (Spitzer *et al* 1999, 2000) conducted two separate validity studies involving 6000 adults attending primary care and obstetrics-gynaecology clinics, respectively. Both found adequate levels of agreement between PHQ diagnoses and those derived from clinical interviews by independent mental health clinicians. According to Spitzer *et al* (1999) most completed questionnaires (85%) could be reviewed by a physician in under three minutes. The PHQ is currently available as a free download for clinical (noncommercial) purposes at http://www.pdhealth.mil/guidelines/downloads/appendix2.pdf.

A Spanish language version has also been developed and is equally well validated (Diez-Quevedo *et al* 2001).

The PHQ is sufficiently sensitive to identify most cases of psychiatric disorder and/or psychological dysfunction. It does not, however, explicitly screen for PTSD, which may be prevalent in patients with orofacial pain (see above). One recent study estimates that as many as 23% of these patients may screen positive for this disorder (Sherman *et al* 2005). This is potentially important for the pain practitioner since PTSD is known to be associated with increased pain and is highly treatable in the acute stage (Foa *et al* 2000). Left undetected, it may compromise the efficacy of otherwise appropriate therapy. Fortunately, a brief screening instrument developed by Weathers *et al* (1993) is available with known diagnostic sensitivity and specificity (91 and 72%, respectively)

(Prins *et al* 2003). It consists of four items that are answered either Yes or No:

In your lifetime, have you ever had any experience that was so frightening, horrible, or upsetting that, in the past month, you... (Circle Y for Yes or N for No)

1. *Had nightmares about it or thought about it when you did not want to?*
2. *Tried hard not to think about it or went out of your way to avoid situations that reminded you of it?*
3. *Were constantly on guard, watchful, or easily startled?*
4. *Felt numb or detached from others, activities, or your surroundings?*

Patients with two or more 'Yes' responses are at risk of PTSD and should be referred for psychological evaluation, if not already under the care of a mental health provider.

4.3.2. Referral to a Mental Health Provider

Before making a mental health referral, the pain practitioner may wish to offer the patient a rationale for combining mental health services with existing physical and pharmacological approaches. One approach is to suggest that there are 'two types of pain', one of physical or biological origin (even if unknown) and the other of emotional origin. The reader is advised that this 'cover story' is not intended to suggest an actual dualism. Instead, the goal is to introduce the subject of coping by drawing a distinction between physical versus emotional problems. While patients often have little or no control over pain sensation (the physical problem), they have (or can acquire) control over their emotional distress (the emotional problem). The unfortunate choice often confronting the patient with chronic orofacial pain is either to (1) make a difficult situation more unpleasant by disturbing him/herself about it or (2) make the best of a difficult situation by minimizing emotional distress. The pain practitioner may wish to explain this dilemma and, at the same time, refer the patient to a mental health provider by paraphrasing the following narrative:

Chronic or long lasting pain, like the kind you have, sometimes forces people to make changes in the way they live. Sometimes you have to cut back on activities at home or at work and sometimes you even have to give up activities you enjoy. When this happens, it's normal for most of us to get upset or feel stressed out. The problem is that the added stress can actually aggravate the pain problem, making it worse than it already is. When this happens we wind up with two problems for the price of one. In order for us to manage the pain in the most effective way possible, it is important for you to learn how to live with this problem without getting yourself overly stressed or upset. This

means you have to develop an unusual coping ability that most people never have to think about. But when you have chronic pain it's something you have to take seriously. That's why I want you to see a colleague of mine who specializes in helping patients with {TMD; headache; etc}. He/she can help you minimize your pain-related stress and give us the best chance possible for a good treatment outcome. How do you feel about this suggestion? Do you have any questions about what I'm saying?

In summary, when referring the patient to a mental health provider, the pain practitioner ideally treats the pain as 'real' (not of psychogenic origin) while shifting the emphasis of treatment away from symptom alleviation and towards the restoration of function and the acquisition of enhanced coping ability.

5. Conclusions

We have shown that psychiatric disorders as well as sub-threshold symptoms of distress are prevalent in patients with chronic orofacial pain. Left untreated, these psychological factors may undermine quality of life, despite appropriate conservative or surgical intervention. Our critical review of the literature strongly refutes a psychogenic explanation, but there is evidence showing that psychological factors can affect the course of orofacial pain symptoms. While not present in all cases, these factors play an important role for some patients and deserve the attention of the orofacial pain practitioner. The preceding evidence-based review of psychological methods and suggestions for routine psychological screening may assist the non-specialist in identifying patients likely to profit from a collaborative care or interdisciplinary approach that includes mental health consultation.

References

Aaron LA, Burke MM, Buchwald D (2000) Overlapping conditions among patients with chronic fatigue syndrome, fibromyalgia, and temporomandibular disorder. *Arch Intern Med* **160**(2):221–227.

Al Quran FA (2004) Psychological profile in burning mouth syndrome. *Oral Surg Oral Med Oral Pathol Oral Radiol Endodont* **97**(3):339–344.

American Psychiatric Association (1994) *Diagnostic and Statistical Manual of Mental Disorders*, 4th edn. Washington, DC: American Psychiatric Association.

Andrasik F, Holroyd KA (1980) A test of specific and nonspecific effects in the biofeedback treatment of tension headache. *J Consult Clin Psychol* **48**(5):575–586.

Andrasik F, Flor H, Turk DC (2005) An expanded view of psychological aspects in head pain: the biopsychosocial model. *Neurol Sci* **26**(2):S87–S91.

Anonymous (1996) Integration of behavioural and relaxation approaches into the treatment of chronic pain and insomnia. NIH Technology and Assessment Panel on Integration of Behavioural and Relaxation Approaches into the Treatment of Chronic Pain and Insomnia. *JAMA* **267**(4):313–318, July 24–31.

Arnold LM, Hudson JI, Hess EV, *et al* (2004) Family study of fibromyalgia. *Arthritis Rheum* **50**(3):944–952.

Asmundson GJ, Coons MJ, Taylor S, *et al* (2002) PTSD and the experience of pain: research and clinical implications of shared vulnerability and mutual maintenance models. *Can J Psychiatry* **47**(10):930–937.

Auerbach SM, Laskin DM, Frantsve LM, *et al* (2001) Depression, pain, exposure to stressful life events, and long-term outcomes in temporomandibular disorder patients. *J Oral Maxillofac Surg* **59**(6):628–633.

Bair MJ, Robinson RL, Katon W, *et al* (2003) Depression and pain comorbidity: a literature review. *Arch Intern Med* **163**(20):2433–2445.

Banks SM, Kerns RD (1996) Explaining high rates of depression in chronic pain: a diathesis-stress framework. *Psychol Bull* **119**:95–110.

Beaton RD, Egan KJ, Nakagawa-Kogan H, *et al* (1991) Self-reported symptoms of stress with temporomandibular disorders: comparisons to healthy men and women. *J Prosthet Dent* **65**(2):289–293.

Beck AT (1976) *Cognitive Therapy and the Emotional Disorders*. New York: International Universities Press.

Beck AT (2005) The current state of cognitive therapy: a 40-year retrospective. *Arch Gen Psychiatry* **62**(9):953–959.

Beck AT, Rush AJ, Shaw BF, *et al* (1979) *Cognitive Therapy of Depression*. New York: Guilford Press.

Beecher HK (1956) Relationship of significance of wound to the pain experienced. *JAMA* **161**:1609.

Bergdahl M, Bergdahl J (1999) Burning mouth syndrome: prevalence and associated factors. *J Oral Pathol Med* **28**(8):350–354.

Bogetto F, Maina G, Ferro G, *et al* (1998) Psychiatric comorbidity in patients with burning mouth syndrome. *Psychosom Med* **60**(3):378–385.

Breslau N, Merikangas K, Bowden CL (1994a) Comorbidity of migraine and major affective disorders. *Neurology* **44**(10 Suppl 7).

Breslau N, Davis GC, Schultz LR, *et al* (1994b) Joint 1994 Wolff Award Presentation. Migraine and major depression: a longitudinal study. *Headache* **34**(7):387–393.

Breslau N, Schultz LR, Stewart WF, *et al* (2000) Headache and major depression: is the association specific to migraine? *Neurology* **54**(2):308–313.

Breslau N, Lipton RB, Stewart WF, *et al* (2003) Comorbidity of migraine and depression: investigating potential etiology and prognosis. *Neurology* **60**(8):1308–1312.

Brooke RI, Stenn PG (1983) Myofascial pain dysfunction syndrome–how effective is biofeedback-assisted relaxation training? *Adv Pain Res Ther* **5**:809–812.

Budzynski TH, Stoyva JM (1969) An instrument for producing deep muscle relaxation by means of analog information feedback. *J Appl Behav Analysis* **2**(4):231–237.

Butler AC, Chapman JE, Forman EM, *et al* (2006) The empirical status of cognitive-behavioral therapy: a review of meta-analyses. *Clin Psychol Rev* **26**(1):17–31.

Caspi A, Sugden K, Moffitt TE, *et al* (2003) Influence of life stress on depression: moderation by a polymorphism in the 5-HTT gene. *Science* **301**(5631):386–389.

Cassano P, Fava M (2002) Depression and public health: an overview. *J Psychosom Res* **53**(4):849–857.

Ciccone DS, Just N, Bandilla EB (1999) A comparison of economic and social reward in patients with chronic nonmalignant back pain. *Psychosom Med* **61**(4):552–563.

Cohen SP, Abdi S (2001) New developments in the use of tricyclic antidepressants for the management of pain. *Curr Opin Anaesthesiol* **14**:505–511.

Costen J (1934) A syndrome of ear and sinus symptoms dependent upon disturbed function of the temporomandibular joint. *Ann Otol* **43**:1–15.

Crider A, Glaros AG, Gevirtz RN (2005) Efficacy of biofeedback-based treatments for temporomandibular disorders. *Appl Psychophysiol Biofeed* **30**(4):333–345.

Dahlstrom L, Widmark G, Carlsson SG (2000) Changes in function and in pain-related and cognitive-behavioral variables after arthroscopy of temporomandibular joints. *Eur J Oral Sci* **108**(1):14–21.

Dao TT, Knight K, Ton-That V (1998) Modulation of myofascial pain by the reproductive hormones: a preliminary report. *J Prosthet Dent* **79**(6):663–670.

De Benedittis G, Lorenzetti A (1992) The role of stressful life events in the persistence of primary headache: major events vs. daily hassles. *Pain* **51**(1):35–42.

Delaney JF (1976) Atypical facial pain as a defense against psychosis. *Amer J Psychiatry* **133**(10):1151–1154.

De Leeuw R, Bertoli E, Schmidt JE, *et al* (2005a) Prevalence of post-traumatic stress disorder symptoms in orofacial pain patients. *Oral Surg Oral Med Oral Pathol Oral Radiol Endodont* **99**(5):558–568.

De Leeuw R, Bertoli E, Schmidt JE, *et al* (2005b) Prevalence of traumatic stressors in patients with temporomandibular disorders. *J Oral Maxillofac Surg* **63**(1):42–50.

Deniz O, Aygul R, Koczk N, *et al* (2004) Precipitating factors of migraine attacks in patients with migraine with and without aura. *The Pain Clinic* **16**:451–456.

Diez-Quevedo C, Rangil T, Sanchez-Planell L, *et al* (2001) Validation and utility of the patient health questionnaire in diagnosing mental disorders in 1003 general hospital Spanish inpatients. *Psychosom Med* **63**(4):679–686.

Dohrenwend BP, Raphael KG, Marbach JJ, *et al* (1999) Why is depression comorbid with chronic myofascial face pain? A family study test of alternative hypotheses. *Pain* **83**(2):183–192.

Drossman DA (1998) Presidential address: Gastrointestinal illness and the biopsychosocial model. *Psychosom Med* **60**(3):258–267.

Durham RC, Murphy T, Allan T, *et al* (1994) Cognitive therapy, analytic psychotherapy and anxiety management training for generalised anxiety disorder. *Br J Psychiatry* **165**(3):315–323.

Dworkin RH, Hetzel RD, Banks SM (1999) Toward a model of the pathogenesis of chronic pain. *Sem Clin Neuropsychiatry* **4**(3):176–185.

Dworkin SF (1994) Perspectives on the interaction of biological, psychological and social factors in TMD. *J Amer Dent Assoc* **125**(7):856–863.

Dworkin SF, Massoth DL (1994) Temporomandibular disorders and chronic pain: disease or illness? *J Prosthet Dent* **72**(1):29–38.

Dworkin SF, Huggins KH, LeResche L, *et al* (1990) Epidemiology of signs and symptoms in temporomandibular disorders: clinical signs in cases and controls. *J Amer Dent Assoc* **120**(3):273–281.

Dworkin SF, Turner JA, Mancl L, *et al* (2002) A randomized clinical trial of a tailored comprehensive care treatment program for temporomandibular disorders. *J Orofac Pain* **16**(4):259–276.

Eli I, Kleinhauz M, Baht R, *et al* (1994) Antecedents of burning mouth syndrome (glossodynia)–recent life events vs. psychopathologic aspects. *J Dent Res* **73**(2):567–572.

Ellis A (1955) New approaches to psychotherapy techniques. *J Clin Psychol* **11**(3):207–260.

Ellis A (1962) *Reason and Emotion in Psychotherapy*. Secaucus NJ: Citadel Press.

Ellis A (1994) *Reason and Emotion in Psychotherapy*, rev. and updated. New York: Birch Lane Press.

Engel GL (1951) Primary atypical facial neuralgia: an hysterical conversion symptom. *Psychosom Med* **13**:375–396.

Engel GL (1959) 'Psychogenic' pain and the pain-prone patient. *Am J Med* **26**:899–918.

Epker J, Gatchel RJ (2000) Prediction of treatment-seeking behavior in acute TMD patients: practical application in clinical settings. *J Orofac Pain* **14**(4):303–309.

Epker J, Gatchel RJ, Ellis E 3rd (1999) A model for predicting chronic TMD: practical application in clinical settings. *J Amer Dent Assoc* **130**(10):1470–1475.

Feinmann C (1993) The long-term outcome of facial pain treatment. *J Psychosom Res* **37**(4):381–387.

Feinmann C, Newton-John T (2004) Psychiatric and psychological management considerations associated with nerve damage and neuropathic trigeminal pain. *J Orofac Pain* **18**(4):360–365.

Feinmann C, Harris M, Cawley R (1984) Psychogenic facial pain: presentation and treatment. *Br Med J (Clin Res Ed)* **288** (6415):436–438.

Fernandez E, Sheffield J (1996) Relative contributions of life events versus daily hassles to the frequency and intensity of headaches. *Headache* **36**(10):595–602.

Ferrando M, Andreu Y, Galdon MJ, et al (2004) Psychological variables and temporomandibular disorders: distress, coping, and personality. *Oral Surg Oral Med Oral Pathol Oral Radiol Endodont* **98**(2):153–160.

Flor H, Birbaumer N, Schulte W, et al (1991) Stress-related electromyographic responses in patients with chronic temporomandibular pain. *Pain* **46**(2):145–152.

Foa EB, Keane TM, Friedman MJ (2000) Effective treatments for PTSD: practice guidelines from the International Society for Traumatic Stress Studies. Guilford Press.

Fricton JR, Olsen T (1996) Predictors of outcome for treatment of temporomandibular disorders. *J Orofac Pain* **10**(1):54–65.

Galbaud du Fort G, Newman SC, Bland RC (1993) Psychiatric comorbidity and treatment seeking. Sources of selection bias in the study of clinical populations. *J Nerv Ment Dis* **181** (8):467–474.

Gallagher RM, Marbach JJ, Raphael KG, et al (1991) Is major depression comorbid with temporomandibular pain and dysfunction syndrome? A pilot study. *Clin J Pain* **7** (3):219–225.

Gardea MA, Gatchel RJ, Mishra KD (2001) Long-term efficacy of biobehavioral treatment of temporomandibular disorders. *J Behav Med* **24**(4):341–359.

Garofalo JP, Gatchel RJ, Wesley AL, et al (1998) Predicting chronicity in acute temporomandibular joint disorders using the research diagnostic criteria. *J Amer Dent Assoc* **129** (4):438–447.

Glaros AG (2005) The role of parafunctions, emotions and stress in predicting facial pain. *J Am Dent Assoc* **136**:451–458.

Glaser J, Kihlstrom JF (2005) Compensatory automaticity: unconscious volition is not an oxymoron. In: Hassin RR, Uleman JS, Bargh JA (eds) *The New Unconscious*. New York: Oxford University Press.

Goslin RE, Gray RN, McCrory DC, et al (1999) Behavioral and physical treatments for migraine headache. Technical review 2.2: Agency for Health Care Policy and Research.

Grossi ML, Goldberg MB, Locker D, et al (2001) Reduced neuropsychologic measures as predictors of treatment outcome in patients with temporomandibular disorders. *J Orofac Pain* **15**(4):329–339.

Guidetti V, Galli F, Fabrizi P, et al (1998) Headache and psychiatric comorbidity: clinical aspects and outcome in an 8-year follow-up study. *Cephalalgia* **18**(7):455–462.

Hakeberg M, Hallberg LR, Berggren U (2003) Burning mouth syndrome: experiences from the perspective of female patients. *Eur J Oral Sci* **111**(4):305–311.

Holroyd KA, Penzien DB (1993) *Self-Management of Recurrent Headache*. Geneva, Switzerland: World Health Organization.

Holroyd KA, Penzien DB, Hursey KG, et al (1984). Change mechanisms in EMG biofeedback training: cognitive changes underlying improvements in tension headache. *J Consult Clin Psychol* **52**(6):1039–1053.

Holroyd KA, O'Donnell FJ, Stensland M, et al (2001) Management of chronic tension-type headache with tricyclic antidepressant medication, stress management therapy, and their combination: a randomized controlled trial. *JAMA* **285**(17):2208–2215.

Hommel B, Musseler J, Aschersleben G, et al (2001) The Theory of Event Coding (TEC): a framework for perception and action planning. *Behav Brain Sci* **24**(5):849–878.

Horowitz LG, Kehoe L, Jacobe E (1991) Multidisciplinary patient care in preventive dentistry: idiopathic dental pain reconsidered. *Clin Prevent Dent* **13**(6):23–29.

Huang GJ, LeResche L, Critchlow CW, et al (2002) Risk factors for diagnostic subgroups of painful temporomandibular disorders (TMD). *J Dent Res* **81**(4):284–288.

Janke EA, Holroyd KA, Romanek K (2004) Depression increases onset of tension-type headache following laboratory stress. *Pain* **111**(3):230–238.

Kapel L, Glaros AG, McGlynn FD (1989) Psychophysiological responses to stress in patients with myofascial pain-dysfunction syndrome. *J Behav Med* **12**(4):397–406.

Keefe FJ, Rumble ME, Scipio CD, et al (2004) Psychological aspects of persistent pain: current state of the science. *J Pain* **5**(4):195–211.

Kerns RD, Turk DC, Rudy TE (1985) The West Haven-Yale Multidimensional Pain Inventory (WHYMPI). *Pain* **23**(4): 345–356.

Kessler RC, McGonagle KA, Zhao S, et al (1994) Lifetime and 12-month prevalence of DSM-III-R psychiatric disorders in the United States. Results from the National Comorbidity Survey. *Arch Gen Psychiatry* **51**(1):8–19.

Kight M, Gatchel RJ, Wesley L (1999) Temporomandibular disorders: evidence for significant overlap with psychopathology. *Health Psychol* **18**(2):177–182.

Kirmayer LJ, Robbins JM, Paris J (1994) Somatoform disorders: personality and the social matrix of somatic distress. *J Abnorm Psychol* **103**(1):125–136.

Korszun A (2002) Facial pain, depression and stress - connections and directions. *J Oral Pathol Med* **31**(10):615–619.

Korszun A, Hinderstein B, Wong M (1996) Comorbidity of depression with chronic facial pain and temporomandibular disorders. *Oral Surg Oral Med Oral Pathol Oral Radiol Endod* **82**(5):496–500.

Kroenke K, Arrington ME, Mangelsdorff AD (1990) The prevalence of symptoms in medical outpatients and the adequacy of therapy. *Arch Intern Med* **150**(8):1685–1689.

Krueger RF, Tackett JL, Markon KE (2004) Structural models of comorbidity among common mental disorders: connections to chronic pain. *Adv Psychosom Med* **25**:63–77.

Lascelles RG (1966) Atypical facial pain and depression. *Br J Psychiatry* **112**(488):651–659.

Laskin DM (1969) Etiology of the pain-dysfunction syndrome. *J Amer Dent Assoc* **79**:147–153.

Lazarus RS (1991) *Emotion and Adaptation*. New York: Oxford University Press.

Lefer L (1966) A psychoanalytic view of a dental phenomenon: psychosomatics of the temporomandibular joint pain dysfunction syndrome. *Contemp Psychoanal* **2**(2):135–150.

Lehmann HJ, Buchholz G (1986) [Atypical facial neuralgia or depressive facial pain. Diagnostic aspects of a well-demarcated form of masked depression]. [German]. *Fortschr Neurol-Psychiatr* **54**(5):154–157.

LeResche L (1997) Epidemiology of temporomandibular disorders: implications for the investigation of etiologic factors. *Crit Rev Oral Biol Med* **8**(3):291–305.

Le Resche L, Truelove EL, Dworkin SF (1993) Temporomandibular disorders: a survey of dentists' knowledge and beliefs. *J Am Dent Assoc* **124**(5):90–94, 97–106.

LeResche L, Saunders K, Von Korff MR, et al (1997) Use of exogenous hormones and risk of temporomandibular disorder pain. *Pain* **69**(1–2):153–160.

Lesse S (1974) Atypical facial pain of psychogenic origin: a masked depression syndrome. In: Lesse S (ed.) *Masked Depression*. New York: Jason Aronson, pp 302–317.

Linden M, Zubraegel D, Baer T, et al (2005) Efficacy of cognitive behaviour therapy in generalized anxiety disorders. Results of a controlled clinical trial (Berlin CBT-GAD Study). *Psychother Psychosom* **74**(1):36–42.

Lipton RB, Bigal ME (2005) The epidemiology of migraine. *Am J Medicine* **118**(Supp 1):3S–10S.

Lobbezoo F, Trulsson M, Jacobs R, et al (2002) Topical review: modulation of trigeminal sensory input in humans: mechanisms and clinical implications. *J Orofac Pain* **16**(1):9–21.

Lockshin MD (2002) Sex ratio and rheumatic disease: excerpts from an Institute of Medicine report. *Lupus* **11**(10):662–666.

Low NC, Merikangas KR (2003) The comorbidity of migraine. *CNS Spectrums* **8**(6):433–434.

McCracken LM, Turk DC (2002) Behavioral and cognitive-behavioral treatment for chronic pain: outcome, predictors of outcome, and treatment process. *Spine* **27**(22):2564–2573.

McCreary CP, Clark GT, Oakley ME, *et al* (1992) Predicting response to treatment for temporomandibular disorders. *J Craniomandib Disord* **6**(3):161–169.

McCrory DC, Penzien DB, Hasselblad V, *et al* (2001) *Evidence Report: Behavioral and Physical Treatments for Tension-Type and Cervicogenic Headache.* Des Moines, IA: Foundation for Chiropractic Education and Research.

Macfarlane TV, Gray RJM, Kincey J, *et al* (2001) Factors associated with the temporomandibular disorder, pain dysfunction syndrome (PDS): Manchester case-control study. *Oral Diseases* **7**(6):321–330.

Macfarlane TV, Blinkhorn AS, Davies RM, *et al* (2002). Association between female hormonal factors and oro-facial pain: study in the community. *Pain* **97**(1–2):5–10.

Madkan VK, Giancola AA, Sra KK, *et al* (2006) Sex differences in the transmission, prevention, and disease manifestations of sexually transmitted diseases. *Arch Dermatol* **142**:365–370.

Maina G, Albert U, Gandolfo S, *et al* (2005) Personality disorders in patients with burning mouth syndrome. *J Personal Disord* **19**(1):84–93.

Marbach JJ (1991) Laszlo Schwartz and the origins of clinical research in TMJ disorders. *NY State Dent J* **57**(2):38–41.

Marbach JJ (1999) Medically unexplained chronic orofacial pain. Temporomandibular pain and dysfunction syndrome, orofacial phantom pain, burning mouth syndrome, and trigeminal neuralgia. *Med Clin North Am* **83**(3):691–710.

Marbach JJ, Lennon MC, Dohrenwend BP (1988) Candidate risk factors for temporomandibular pain and dysfunction syndrome: psychosocial, health behavior, physical illness and injury. *Pain* **34**(2):139–151.

Marbach JJ, Lennon MC, Link BG, *et al* (1990) Losing face: sources of stigma as perceived by chronic facial pain patients. *J Behav Med* **13**(6):583–604.

Marbach JJ, Ballard GT, Frankel MR, *et al* (1997) Patterns of TMJ surgery: evidence of sex differences. *J Amer Dent Assoc* **128** (5):609–614.

Martin PR, Theunissen C (1993) The role of life event stress, coping and social support in chronic headaches. *Headache* **33**(6):301–306.

Melzack R, Wall PD (1996) *The Challenge of Pain*, 2nd updated edn. Harmondsworth: Penguin Global.

Mercuri LG, Olson RE, Laskin DM (1979) The specificity of response to experimental stress in patients with myofascial pain dysfunction syndrome. *J Dent Res* **58**(9):1866–1871.

Morishige E, Ishigaki S, Yatani H, *et al* (2006) Clinical effectiveness of cognitive behavior therapy in the management of TMD. *Int J Prosthodont* **19**(1):31–33.

Morley S, Eccleston C, Williams A (1999) Systematic review and meta-analysis of randomized controlled trials of cognitive behaviour therapy and behaviour therapy for chronic pain in adults, excluding headache. *Pain* **80**(1–2):1–13.

Moulton RE (1966) Emotional factors in non-organic temporomandibular joint pain. *Dent Clin North Amer* 609–620.

Mullinix JM, Norton BJ, Hack S, *et al* (1978) Skin temperature biofeedback and migraine. *Headache* **17**(6):242–244.

Nicholson RA, Townsend DR, Gramling SE (2000) Influence of a scheduled-waiting task on EMG reactivity and oral habits among facial pain patients and no-pain controls. *Applied Psychophysiol Biofeed* **25**(4):203–219.

Ohrbach R, Dworkin SF (1998) Five-year outcomes in TMD: relationship of changes in pain to changes in physical and psychological variables. *Pain* **74**(2–3):315–326.

Olesen J, Bousser M-G, Diener HC, *et al* (2004) The International Classification of Headache Disorders, 2nd edn. *Cephalalgia* **24**(Suppl 1):24–150.

Pallegama RW, Ranasinghe AW, Weerasinghe VS, *et al* (2005) Anxiety and personality traits in patients with muscle related temporomandibular disorders. *J Oral Rehabil* **32**(10):701–707.

Passchier J, Schouten J, van der Donk J, van Romunde LK (1991) The association of frequent headaches with personality and life events. *Headache* **31**(2):116–121.

Patel NV, Bigal ME, Kolodner KB, *et al* (2004) Prevalence and impact of migraine and probable migraine in a health plan. *Neurology* **63**(8):1432–1438.

Plesh O, Wolfe F, Lane N (1996) The relationship between fibromyalgia and temporomandibular disorders: prevalence and symptom severity. *J Rheumatol* **23**(11): 1948–1952.

Prins A, Ouimette P, Kimerling R, *et al* (2003) The primary care PTSD screen (PC-PTSD): development and operating characteristics. *Primary Care Psychiatry* **9**(1):9–14.

Rammelsberg P, LeResche L, Dworkin S, Mancl L (2003) Longitudinal outcome of temporomandibular disorders: a 5-year epidemiologic study of muscle disorders defined by research diagnostic criteria for temporomandibular disorders. *J Orofac Pain* **17**(1):9–20.

Raphael KG, Cloitre M (1994) Does mood-congruence or causal search govern recall bias? A test of life event recall. *J Clin Epidemiol* **47**(5):555–564.

Raphael KG, Cloitre M, Dohrenwend BP (1991) Problems of recall and misclassification with checklist methods of measuring stressful life events. *Health Psychol* **10**(1):62–74.

Raphael KG, Marbach JJ, Gallagher RM (2000) Somatosensory amplification and affective inhibition are elevated in myofascial face pain. *Pain Med* **1**(3):247–253.

Raphael KG, Janal MN, Nayak S, *et al* (2004) Familial aggregation of depression in fibromyalgia: a community-based test of alternate hypotheses. *Pain* **110**(449–460).

Rasmussen P (1991) Facial pain. IV. A prospective study of 1052 patients with a view of: precipitating factors, associated symptoms, objective psychiatric and neurological symptoms. *Acta Neurochirurgica* **108**(3–4):100–109.

Regier DA, Narrow WE, Rae DS (1990) The epidemiology of anxiety disorders: the Epidemiologic Catchment Area (ECA) experience. *J Psychiatr Res* **2**:3–14.

Reynolds DJ, Hovanitz CA (2000) Life event stress and headache frequency revisited. *Headache* **40**(2):111–118.

Riley JL 3rd, Myers CD, Robinson ME, Bulcourf B, Gremillion HA (2001) Factors predicting orofacial pain patient satisfaction with improvement. *J Orofac Pain* **15**(1):29–35.

Robinson JK (2006) Anatomical and hormonal influences on women's dermatologic health. *JAMA* **295**(12): 1443–1445.

Rudy TE, Turk DC, Kubinski JA, Zaki HS (1995) Differential treatment responses of TMD patients as a function of psychological characteristics. *Pain* **61**(1):103–112.

Russell MB (2005) Tension-type headache in 40-year-olds: a Danish population-based sample of 4000. *J Headache Pain* **6**(6):441–447.

Scher AI, Bigal ME, Lipton RB (2005) Comorbidity of migraine. *Curr Opin Neurol* **18**(3):305–310.

Schwartz LL (1956) A temporomandibular joint pain-dysfunction syndrome. *J Chronic Dis* **3**:284–293.

Scott J (2001) Cognitive therapy for depression. *Br Med Bull* **57**:101–113.

Selye H (1974) *Stress without Distress*. Philadelphia: Lippincott.

Sharav Y, Singer E, Schmidt E, Dionne RA, Dubner R (1987) The analgesic effect of amitriptyline on chronic facial pain. *Pain* **31**(2):199–209.

Sharpe L, Sensky T, Timberlake N, Ryan B, Brewin CR, Allard S (2001) A blind, randomized, controlled trial of cognitive-behavioural intervention for patients with recent onset rheumatoid arthritis: preventing psychological and physical morbidity. *Pain* **89**(2–3):275–283.

Sherman JJ, Turk DC (2001) Nonpharmacologic approaches to the management of myofascial temporomandibular disorders. *Curr Pain Headache Rep* **5**(5):421–431.

Sherman JJ, Carlson CR, Wilson JF, Okeson JP, McCubbin JA (2005) Post-traumatic stress disorder among patients with orofacial pain. *J Orofac Pain* **19**(4):309–317.

Silverstein B (1999) Gender difference in the prevalence of clinical depression: the role played by depression associated with somatic symptoms. *Amer J Psychiatry* **156**(3):480–482.

Silverstein B (2002) Gender differences in the prevalence of somatic versus pure depression: a replication. *Amer J Psychiatry* **159**(6):1051–1052.

Slade GD, Diatchenko K, Bhalang K, *et al* (2007) Influence of psychological factors on risk of TMD. *J Dent Res* **86**:1120–1125.

Smythe HA (2005) Temporomandibular joint disorder and other medically unexplained symptoms in rheumatoid arthritis, osteoarthritis, and fibromyalgia.[Comment]. *J Rheumatol* **32**(12):2288–2290.

Speculand B, Goss AN, Spence ND, Pilowsky I (1981) Intractable facial pain and illness behaviour. *Pain* **11**(2):213–219.

Speculand B, Hughes AO, Goss AN (1984) Role of recent stressful life events experience in the onset of TMJ dysfunction pain. *Community Dent Oral Epidemiol* **12**(3):197–202.

Spitzer RL, Kroenke K, Williams JB (1999) Validation and utility of a self-report version of PRIME-MD: the PHQ primary care study. Primary Care Evaluation of Mental Disorders. Patient Health Questionnaire. *JAMA* **282**(18):1737–1744.

Spitzer RL, Williams JB, Kroenke K, *et al* (2000) Validity and utility of the PRIME-MD patient health questionnaire in assessment of 3000 obstetric-gynecologic patients: the PRIME-MD Patient Health Questionnaire Obstetrics-Gynecology Study. *Am J Obstet Gynecol* **183**(3):759–769.

Stahl S, Briley M (2004) Understanding pain in depression. *Hum Psychopharmacol* **19**(1):S9–S13.

Steed PA (1998) TMD treatment outcomes: a statistical assessment of the effects of psychological variables. *Cranio* **16**(3):138–142.

Sternbach RA (1986) Pain and 'hassles' in the United States: findings of the Nuprin pain report. *Pain* **27**(1):69–80.

Stewart W, Breslau N, Keck PE Jr (1994) Comorbidity of migraine and panic disorder. *Neurology* **44**(10 Suppl 7).

Sullivan MJ, Neish NR (1998) Catastrophizing, anxiety and pain during dental hygiene treatment. *Community Dent Oral Epidemiol* **26**(5):344–349.

Suvinen TI, Hanes KR, Reade PC (1997) Outcome of therapy in the conservative management of temporomandibular pain dysfunction disorder. *J Oral Rehabil* **24**(10):718–724.

Suvinen TI, Reade PC, Kemppainen P, *et al* (2005) Review of aetiological concepts of temporomandibular pain disorders: towards a biopsychosocial model for integration of physical disorder factors with psychological and psychosocial illness impact factors. *Eur J Pain* **9**(6):613–633.

Tammiala-Salonen T, Hiidenkari T, Parvinen T (1993) Burning mouth in a Finnish adult population. *Community Dent Oral Epidemiol* **21**(2):67–71.

Turk DC (2003) Cognitive-behavioral approach to the treatment of chronic pain patients. *Reg Anesth Pain Med* **28**(6):573–579.

Turk DC, Rudy TE, Kubinski JA, *et al* (1996) Dysfunctional patients with temporomandibular disorders: evaluating the efficacy of a tailored treatment protocol. *J Consult Clin Psychol* **64**(1):139–146.

Turner JA, Dworkin SF, Mancl L, *et al* (2001) The roles of beliefs, catastrophizing, and coping in the functioning of patients with temporomandibular disorders. *Pain* **92**(1-2):41–51.

Turner JA, Brister H, Huggins K, *et al* (2005) Catastrophizing is associated with clinical examination findings, activity interference, and health care use among patients with temporomandibular disorders. *J Orofac Pain* **19**(4):291–300.

Turner JA, Mancl L, Aaron LA (2006) Short- and long-term efficacy of brief cognitive-behavioral therapy for patients with chronic temporomandibular disorder pain: a randomized, controlled trial. *Pain* **121**(3):181–194.

Unruh AM (1996) Gender variations in clinical pain experience. *Pain* **65**(2-3):123–167.

van Os J, Hanssen M, Bak M, Bijl RV, Vollebergh W (2003) Do urbanicity and familial liability coparticipate in causing psychosis?. *Amer J Psychiatry* **160**(3):477–482.

Vickers ER, Boocock H (2005) Chronic orofacial pain is associated with psychological morbidity and negative personality changes: a comparison to the general population. *Aust Dent J* **50**(1):21–30.

Violon A (1980) The onset of facial pain. A psychological study. *Psychotherapy & Psychosomatics* **34**(1):11–16.

Von Korff M, Simon G (1996) The relationship between pain and depression. *Br J Psychiatry Suppl* **30**:101–108.

Von Korff M, Le Resche L, Dworkin SF (1993) First onset of common pain symptoms: a prospective study of depression as a risk factor. *Pain* **55**(2):251–258.

Walen SR, DiGiuseppe R, Dryden W (1992) *A Practitioner's Guide to Rational-Emotive Therapy*, 2nd edn. New York: Oxford University Press.

Ward NG, Bloom VL, Dworkin S, *et al* (1982) Psychobiological markers in coexisting pain and depression: toward a unified theory. *J Clin Psychiatry* **43**(8 Pt 2):32–41.

Weathers FW, Litz BT, Herman DS, Huska JA, Keane TM (1993) The PTSD Checklist (PCL): reliability, validity, and diagnostic utility. Annual Conference of the International Society for Traumatic Stress Studies, October 25, San Antonio, TX.

Weissman MM, Bland RC, Canino GJ, *et al* (1996) Cross-national epidemiology of major depression and bipolar disorder. *JAMA* **276**(4):293–299.

Werner A, Malterud K (2003) It is hard work behaving as a credible patient: encounters between women with chronic pain and their doctors. *Social Science & Medicine* **57**(8):1409–1419.

Wright AR, Gatchel RJ, Wildenstein L, *et al* (2004) Biopsychosocial differences between high-risk and low-risk patients with acute TMD-related pain. *J Amer Dent Assoc* **135**(4):474–483.

Wright J, Deary IJ, Geissler PR (1991) Depression, hassles and somatic symptoms in mandibular dysfunction syndrome patients. *J Dent* **19**(6):352–356.

Yap AU, Tan KB, Chua EK, Tan HH (2002) Depression and somatization in patients with temporomandibular disorders. *J Prosthet Dent* **88**(5):479–484.

Yemm R (1971a) A comparison of the electrical activity of masseter and temporal muscles of human subjects during experimental stress.*Arch Oral Biol* **16**(3):269–273.

Yemm R (1971b) Comparison of the activity of left and right masseter muscles of normal individuals and patients with mandibular dysfunction during experimental stress. *J Dent Res* **50**(5):1320–1323.

Zivadinov R, Willheim K, Sepic-Grahovac D, *et al* (2003) Migraine and tension-type headache in Croatia: a population-based survey of precipitating factors. *Cephalalgia* **23**(5):336–343.

CHAPTER 5

Acute orofacial pain

Yair Sharav and Rafael Benoliel

1. Introduction

Acute orofacial pain is primarily associated with the teeth and their supporting structures (the periodontium). Most frequently, dental pain is due to dental caries, although a broken filling or tooth-abrasion may also cause dental sensitivity. Other oral pains are periodontal or gingival in origin. Acute dental and periodontal pain is frequently rated as moderate to severe in intensity or from 60 to 100 on a 100-mm visual analogue scale (Sharav *et al* 1984). Pain is conceived of as deep and unpleasant. In about 60% of cases pain is not localized but spreads into remote areas of the head and face. There is considerable overlap in pain referral patterns for maxillary and mandibular sources, and the source of pain cannot be predicted from the pain location. Consequently, maps of facial pain spread patterns are of no use in the diagnosis of the source of dental pain. Pain spread is positively correlated with pain intensity and stronger pain tends to spread more (Fig. 5.1). Pain spread is also not dependent on the tissue affected by the pathological process, e.g. dental or periodontal structures (Sharav *et al* 1984). The nociceptive mechanisms responsible for this pain spread are of central origin, resulting from interactions between primary nociceptive afferents and trigeminothalamic neurons. Factors which may be important for the extensive pain spread patterns in the facial area include convergence of primary afferents from different areas on common dorsal horn neurons, the large receptive fields of the wide dynamic range (WDR) neurons and the somatotopic organization (Sessle 2005). As pain intensity increases, neurons whose receptive field centre lies within the source of pain would increase their activity, activating a larger receptive field, and also activating somatotopically adjacent neurons.

Caries and symptom progression. Initially, when the carious lesion is located in the superficial layer of the dentine, the tooth is sensitive to various stimuli such as change in temperature and sweet substances, but pain is not spontaneous and does not occur without an external stimulation. As the lesion penetrates deeper into the tooth the pain produced by these stimuli becomes stronger and lasts longer. Eventually, when the carious lesion approaches the tooth pulp, a strong, spontaneous, paroxysmal pain that is usually intermittent in nature develops. If microorganisms and products of tissue disintegration invade the area around the root apex, the tooth becomes very sensitive to chewing, touch and percussion. Usually at that stage the paroxysmal, intermittent pain acquires a continuous boring nature and the tooth is no longer sensitive to changes in temperature. The development of symptoms therefore follows the progression of pathology and the dental structures involved: initially dentine, followed by pulp and ultimately the periodontal tissues (Fig. 5.2). In clinical practice the demarcation between these various stages is sometimes indistinct; for example, the tooth may be sensitive simultaneously to temperature changes and to chewing.

Pain arising from the oral mucosa may be localized and associated with a detectable erosive or ulcerative lesion or of a diffuse nature resulting from widespread irritation of the oral mucosa. However, pain descriptors on their own are not usually sufficient as a diagnostic

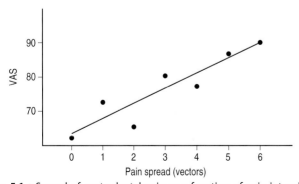

Fig. 5.1 • Spread of acute dental pain as a function of pain intensity. Pain intensity is described on a 0–100 mm visual analogue scale (VAS). Pain spread denotes the number of locations on the face that the pain has spread to. It is clear that pain spread is a function of pain intensity. (Based on data from Sharav *et al* 1984.)

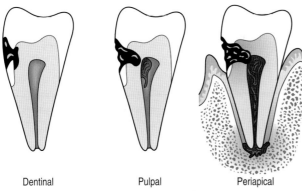

Dentinal   Pulpal   Periapical

Fig. 5.2 • Acute dental pain presented at three progressive consecutive stages of caries penetration. Dentinal pain is associated with caries penetrating into the dentine. Pulpal pain is associated with deep caries penetration approaching the dental pulp. Periapical pain occurs when the inflammatory process invades into the periapical area.

Table 5.1	Anamnestic Details of Dental and Periodontal Pain			
Pain Origin	**Localization**	**Character**	**Intensity**	**Aggravated by**
Dental				
Dentinal	Poor	Evoked, does not outlast stimulus	Mild to moderate	Hot, cold, sweet, or sour foods
Pulpal	Very poor	Spontaneous, paroxysmal, intermittent	Moderate to severe	Hot, cold, sometimes chewing
Periodontal				
Periapical or lateral	Good	Continues for hours, deep, boring	Moderate to severe	Chewing

Table 5.2	Physical and Radiographic Signs of Dental and Periodontal Pain		
Pain Origin	**Associated Signs**	**Diagnostic Findings**	**Radiology**
Dental			
Dentinal	Caries, exposed dentine, defective restorations	Sensitive to cold application, pain moderate, no overshoot	Proximal caries, defective restorations
Pulpal	Deep caries, extensive restorations	Strong pain to cold application with overshoot, may be tender to percussion	Deep caries or restorations, pulp exposure
Periodontal			
Periapical	Periapical tenderness, redness and swelling. Vertical tooth mobility.	Very tender to percussion, non-vital tooth-pulp	Usually no periapical changes at acute stage
Lateral	Periodontal tenderness, redness and swelling. Tooth mobility.	Tender to percussion, deep pocket on probing	Alveolar bone resorption

tool, and orofacial diseases must be validated by other diagnostic procedures such as physical examination and radiographs. The anamnestic details of dental and periodontal pain are described in Table 5.1 and the physical and radiographic signs in Table 5.2.

Epidemiology. Epidemiological data on dental pain are sparse and of poor quality and its reported prevalence in community dwelling adults ranges from 12 to 40%, depending on the description of dental pain used (Locker and Grushka 1987; Lipton *et al* 1993; Pau *et al* 2003).

2. Dental Pain

2.1. Dentinal Pain

Symptoms. The pain originating in dentine is described as a sharp, deep sensation usually evoked by an external stimulus and subsides within a few seconds. Hot, cold,

sweet, sour and sometimes salty foods and drinks are usually among the external stimuli that may produce pain. Extreme changes in temperature (e.g. hot soup followed by ice cream) may cause pain in intact, non-affected teeth but this is usually mild and transient. In most cases, however, tooth pain evoked by external stimuli such as cold food indicates allodynia, and some pathological state of the tooth should be suspected. Pain is poorly localized, often only to an approximate area within two or three teeth adjacent to the affected tooth. Frequently, the patient is unable to distinguish whether the pain originates from the lower or the upper jaw. However, patients rarely make localization errors across the midline, and posterior teeth are more difficult to localize than anterior ones (Friend and Glenwright 1968). A wide two-point discrimination threshold exists when teeth are electrically stimulated; patients are therefore unable to precisely localize which teeth are being stimulated (Van Hassel and Harrington 1969).

Physical and radiographic signs. The most common processes associated with dentine pain are early dental caries, defective restorations and areas of exposed dentine, e.g. abrasion or erosion of the enamel, and exposed roots due to gingival recession or periodontal therapy (Chabanski and Gillam 1997; von Troil *et al* 2002). Most frequently these can be found and identified by means of direct observation and examination with a sharp dental probe. Duplication of pain produced by controlled application of cold or hot stimuli to various teeth in the suspected area is useful in identifying the affected tooth. Areas of exposed dentine, e.g. abrasion and erosion of the enamel, or roots exposed due to gingival recession, are scratched with a sharp dental probe in order to evoke pain and locate the source of pain. Not all areas of exposed dentine are sensitive and therefore these are not necessarily a source of pain.

The *bite-wing* dental radiograph (Fig. 5.3A) is a very useful diagnostic aid in these cases, especially when the caries lesion is situated on a proximal tooth surface not easily visualized by direct observation and not accessible to probing. The *periapical* dental radiograph is useful for assessing processes affecting the tooth root (Fig. 5.3B).

2.1.1. The Cracked Tooth Syndrome

Symptoms. In addition to the symptoms typical for dentinal pain, the patient may also complain of a sharp pain, elicited by biting, that resolves immediately after pressure on the teeth ceases. Localization of the source of pain is not precise, although the affected area can often be limited to two or three adjacent teeth. The patient usually also complains of pain and discomfort associated with cold and hot stimuli in the area. These complaints indicate that there may be a crack in the dentine, the so-called 'cracked tooth syndrome' (Cameron 1976; Goose 1981). These incompletely fractured teeth may be associated with long-lasting diffuse orofacial pain and are difficult to diagnose (Brynjulfsen *et al* 2002).

Physical and radiographic signs. The main diagnostic challenge is localizing the affected tooth, especially as the crack is not readily detected and radiographs are not helpful. Localization of the affected tooth can be achieved by causing the crack to widen, and thus duplicate the pain. This can be achieved by the following techniques:

1. Percussion or pressure on the cusps of the suspected teeth at different angles (Fig. 5.4A).
2. Asking the patient to bite on individual cusps using a fine wooden stick or a predesigned bite stick (these are available commercially).
3. Probing firmly around margins of fillings and in suspected fissures (Fig. 5.4B).

Possible additional diagnoses, with signs and symptoms resembling the cracked tooth syndrome, may include occlusal abrasion resulting in exposed dentine or a cracked filling. However, these can be readily detected visually and with the aid of a sharp explorer. A similar but distinct entity, a vertical root fracture, may produce similar symptomatology and is discussed under periodontal pain.

2.1.2. Treatment of Dentinal Pain

Dentinal pain due to caries is best treated by removal of the carious lesion and restoring the tooth. Sensitivity usually disappears within a day or two, although when the carious lesion is deep the tooth may remain sensitive to cold stimulation for a week or two. Treatment of the cracked tooth depends on the state of the tooth (existing restorations, periodontal condition) and the extent of the fracture.

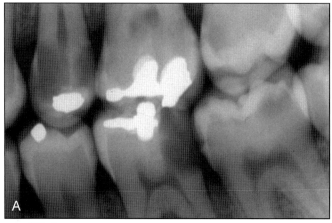

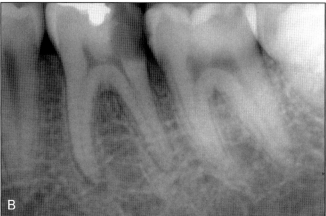

Fig. 5.3 • (A) Bite-wing radiograph of left side demonstrates multiple locations with deep caries, especially teeth 25 and 36. (B) Periapical radiograph of #36 demonstrates deep caries and widening of periodontal ligament and periapical radiolucency (especially at mesial root).

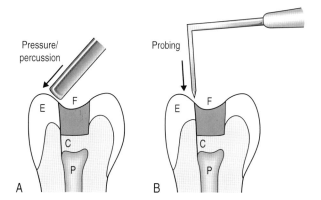

Fig. 5.4 • Detecting a crack in dentine (A) by oblique percussion or pressure on one cusp, or (B) by firm probing between filling and tooth with a sharp explorer, in order to *widen* the crack. This will activate dentinal and/or pulpal nociceptive mechanisms. E=enamel, F=filling, P=pulp chamber, C=crack.

Existing restorations associated with tooth fractures may be replaced with adhesive restorative materials; these may be successful but are associated with postoperative sensitivity (Opdam and Roeters 2003). Often removal of an existing restoration allows the localization and extent of the fracture to be identified. Isolated fractures of single cusps may be treated by their removal and subsequent tooth restoration. In some cases crowning the tooth is inevitable but root canal treatment is usually not indicated.

Hypersensitive (exposed) dentine, acidic foods and beverages will enhance dentinal sensitivity. These can be treated by interventions that reduce dentinal tubule permeability or reduce sensitivity of dentinal neurons. Desensitizing toothpastes with ingredients such as stannous fluoride or potassium nitrate will improve symptoms for most cases (Miller *et al* 1994; Poulsen *et al* 2001; Brookfield *et al* 2003). Fluid flow can be reduced by a variety of physical and chemical agents that induce a smear layer or block the tubules. Tubule-blocking agents include resins, glass ionomer cements and bonding agents; strontium chloride or acetate; aluminium, potassium or ferric oxalates; silica or calcium-containing materials; and protein precipitants (Hargreaves and Seltzer 2002; Brookfield *et al* 2003). The use of CO_2 and Nd:YAG lasers for cervical hypersensitivity was also found to be effective, with no recorded damage to the tooth pulp (Lan and Liu 1996; Zhang *et al* 1998; Kimura *et al* 2000). Good oral hygiene is essential in reducing the sensitivity of dentine exposed at the root surface.

2.2. Pulpal Pain

Symptoms. Pain associated with pulp disease is spontaneous, strong, often throbbing and exacerbated by changes in temperature, sweet foods and pressure on the carious lesion. When pain is evoked it outlasts the stimulus (unlike stimulus-induced dentinal pain) and can be excruciating for many minutes (Table 5.1). Similarly to dentinal pain, localization is poor and seems to be even poorer when pain becomes more intense (Mumford 1982). Pain tends to radiate or refer to the ear, temple and cheek but there are no definitive pain radiation patterns, and there is a considerable overlap in pain reference locations of maxillary and mandibular teeth (Sharav *et al* 1984; Falace *et al* 1996). Pain, however, does not usually cross the midline. Patients may describe pain in different ways and a continuous dull ache can be periodically exacerbated (by stimulation or spontaneously) for short (minutes) or long (hours) periods (Cohen 1996).

Pain may increase and throb when the patient lies down, and in many instances wakes the patient from sleep (Sharav *et al* 1984). Pain originating from the pulp is frequently not continuous and abates spontaneously; the precise explanation for such abatement is unclear (Seltzer 1978). This episodic, sharp, paroxysmal, non-localized pain may lead to the misdiagnosis of other conditions that mimic pain of pulp origin (e.g. cluster headache, trigeminal neuralgia; see Chapters 10 and 11).

Although pain is the most common symptom of a diseased pulp, no correlation exists between specific pain characteristics and the histopathological status of the pulp (Seltzer *et al* 1963; Tyldesley and Mumford 1970). Furthermore, despite the fact that pain associated with pulpitis is severe there are many instances when a tooth can progress to pulpal necrosis without pain. Thus, approximately 40% of 2202 teeth treated endodontically had no history of spontaneous pain or of prolonged pain to thermal stimulation (Michaelson and Holland 2002).

Physical and radiographic signs. The initial aim of the diagnostic process is to identify the affected tooth and then to assess the state of the tooth pulp in order to determine treatment. Localization of the affected tooth is achieved through the same methods detailed in the previous section on dentinal pain (Table 5.2). The application of heat or cold to the teeth should be done very carefully because these can cause excruciating pain. The application of a cold stimulus is commonly used to diagnose pulpal conditions. Application of ethyl chloride on a pledget of cotton wool usually induces a short, mildly painful response from intact teeth. In reversible pulpitis pain response is increased (hyperalgesia) and outlasts the stimulus, usually by less than 10 seconds. In irreversible pulpitis application of ethyl chloride results in excruciating pain that outlasts the stimulus for well beyond 10 seconds. Percussion aids in localizing the affected tooth as about 80% of teeth with painful pulpitis are tender to percussion. Non-vital pulps do not react to cold application. In teeth with secondary dentine a stronger cold stimulus may be needed to elicit a reaction (e.g. propane/butane), but this is not recommended for use in cases where irreversible pulpitis is suspected as it induces extremely strong pain. Pulp vitality may also be assessed with electrical pulp testers. The state of the pulp cannot be judged from one single symptom and should be based on the combination of several signs and symptoms (Cohen 1996).

Treatment. Depending on the diagnosis, treatment may aim at conserving the pulp, extirpating it or extracting the tooth. Pulpal pain normally disappears immediately after treatment. Systemic penicillin administration has clearly no effect on pain amelioration or prognosis of irreversible pulpitis (Nagle *et al* 2000). Clinical evidence indicates that when pain is severe, or there is a previous history of pain in the affected tooth, the tooth is in the irreversible category and treatment dictates endodontic therapy or extraction. On the other hand when pain is mild or moderate with no previous history of pain, which indicates normal pulpal vitality, and there is no pain to percussion, the pulp is in the reversible category, and the tooth pulp should be preserved by caries removal and indirect pulp capping (Bender 2000). Irreversible pulpitis may occur following prosthetic tooth preparation or after conservative restoration of carious teeth. In these cases the restoration or temporary prosthesis should be checked and repaired if needed and the pain managed with analgesic drugs. A recent study indicates that spontaneous pain,

Table 5.3	Clinical Characteristics That Help to Decide Whether the Tooth-Pulp Should Be Preserved (Reversible) or Extirpated (Irreversible) in Cases of Painful Pulpitis		
Characteristics	**Reversible**	**Irreversible**	
Pain intensity	Mild	Severe	
History of spontaneous pain	No	Yes	
Pain duration	Short	Prolonged, recurrent	
Temperature sensitivity	Mild, short-lasting	Strong, overshoot	
Percussion	Usually not tender	Tender	
Caries removal	Usually no exposure	Very often clear pulp exposure	
X-rays	Early caries or shallow restoration, recent tooth preparation	Deep caries, or restoration with no secondary dentine	

Case 5.1 Acute Pulpitis, a 22-year-old Female

Primary complaint

Suffers for the past 2 days from strong, paroxysmal pain in the lower left jaw. Pain radiates to the ear, and wakes the patient from sleep.

Findings

The bite-wing radiograph (Fig. 5.3A) exhibits more than one deep carious location, and therefore imposes difficulty in locating the source of this spontaneous pain. The source of pain is detected by means of the physical examination. A periapical radiograph of #36 (Fig. 5.3B) demonstrates periapical radiolucency. Note that periapical radiolucency and tenderness to percussion coexist with strong pain to cold stimulation.

Diagnosis and treatment

The diagnosis was irreversible pulpitis. The tooth pulp was extirpated, with subsequent complete pain relief.

Comment

The history and type of pain indicate the diagnosis of acute pulpitis. While the type of pain was typical for acute pulpitis, locating the affected tooth was somewhat problematic due to more than one possible source. The source of the acute, spontaneous, severe pain was evident from the signs of the physical examination. Although both #25 and #36 responded with strong pain to cold application, only #36 exhibited overshoot and tenderness to percussion. It should be noted that periapical radiolucency and tenderness to percussion coexisted with strong pain to cold stimulation.

with a history of previous pain, and prolonged pain on cold stimuli were significantly more frequent in patients with chronic (irreversible) pulpitis (Cisneros-Cabello and Segura-Egea 2005). One should be aware, however, that these indications are under debate and some controversies exist (Bergenholtz and Spangberg 2004). The clinical characteristics that dictate treatment indications for teeth with painful pulpitis are summarized in Table 5.3.

Case 5.1 demonstrates a patient with irreversible pulpitis.

2.3. Mechanisms of Dental Pain

The mechanisms of dentinal sensitivity and pain have been extensively reviewed (Brannstrom 1962; Anderson et al 1970; Olgart 1985; Byers and Narhi 1999). Morphologically, nerve fibres may penetrate into the dentine approximately as far as halfway along the odontoblastic process but certainly do not reach the dento-enamel junction (Fig. 5.5) (Byers and Kish 1976; Byers and Narhi 1999). Furthermore, the concept that the odontoblast has a role as a sensory receptor of the dentine has not been substantiated (Byers et al 1982). While there is some evidence for gap junctions between nerves and odontoblasts (Ushiyama 1989) it is not conclusive (Matthews and Sessle 2000). Experimental pain may be induced by applying various stimuli to exposed dentine, i.e. drying by application of absorbent paper or a stream of air, mechanical stimulation (e.g. cutting, scratching, probing) and changes in osmotic pressure, pH or temperature. However, the application of well-established algesic substances, such as potassium chloride, acetylcholine, 5-hydroxytryptamine (5-HT), bradykinin and histamine, to exposed dentine does not evoke pain (Anderson and Naylor 1962; Brannstrom 1962). All

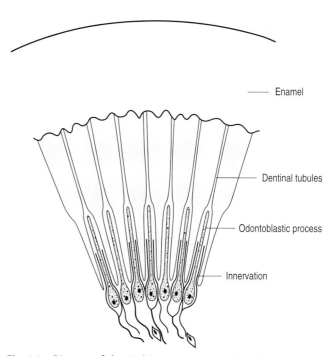

Fig. 5.5 • Diagram of dentinal innervation. Note that the intratubular odontoblastic process penetrates only about half of the dentinal tubule. Also, not all dentinal tubules are innervated. The percentage of innervated tubules decreases from the tip of the crown towards the root (Byers et al 1999).

Enamel / Dentinal tubules / Odontoblastic process / Innervation these substances can produce pain, however, when placed on a skin blister base (Armstrong *et al* 1953). The limited distribution of nerve fibres in dentine and the fact that neuroactive chemicals fail to stimulate or anaesthetize dentine led to the proposal of the hydrodynamic mechanism by Brannstrom (1963). According to Brannstrom's hypothesis the movement of extracellular fluid that fills the dentinal tubules will distort the pain-sensitive nervous structure in the pulp and predentinal area and activate mechanoreceptors to produce pain. The smear layer left by drilling must be removed to allow this shift in tubule fluid (Ahlquist *et al* 1994). Several other theories have been proposed such as the so-called neural theory and odontoblast transduction theory, but most of the evidence up to now supports the hydrodynamic theory (Matthews and Sessle 2000). It seems that the dentinal tubules act as passive hydraulic links between the site of stimulation and nerve endings sensitive to pressure at the pulpal end in the underlying pulp. The pressure-sensitive neurons are A fibres and are much more sensitive to outward than inward flow through the dentinal tubules (Narhi *et al* 1992). Fibres with conduction velocities in the C-fibre range do not appear to be pressure sensitive (Andrew and Matthews 2000). It is suspected that, unlike pulpal C fibres, A fibres are relatively insensitive to inflammatory mediators (Olgart 1985). On the other hand it was found that leukotriene B4 (LTB4) can sensitize pulpal Aδ fibres and may be a long-lasting hyperalgesic factor, which may contribute to pain of pulpal origin (Madison *et al* 1992). Pulpal C nociceptors seem, however, to have a predominant role in transmitting pain from inflamed pulp tissue (Hargreaves and Seltzer 2002). Additionally, specific tooth-pulp stimuli (particularly electric stimulation) may evoke sensations other than pain (Sessle *et al* 1979). Mediation of non-pain sensations by a distinct population of afferents was suggested by the results of stimuli that induce temporal summation (McGrath *et al* 1983). Based upon temporal and spatial summation experiments nonpainful, *pre-pain* and painful sensations from electrical tooth-pulp stimulation seem to be evoked by the same A-fibre populations (Brown *et al* 1985; Virtanen *et al* 1987). A more recent review points to the fact that many of the myelinated fibres in the pulp are of the Aβ type, and may be responsible for the pre-pain sensation evoked by electrical stimulation, thus supporting the hypothesis of two distinct populations of afferents (Narhi *et al* 1992).

Pain mechanisms underlying pulpal pain are related to inflammation and include a host of mediators found in the pulp, such as cholinergic and adrenergic neurotransmitters, prostaglandins and cyclic adenosine monophosphate (cAMP) (Byers and Narhi 2002; Hargreaves and Seltzer 2002). Some substances, such as prostaglandins (particularly PGE2), serotonin and bradykinin contribute to tooth-pulp nerve excitability, and PGE2 enhances bradykinin-evoked calcitonin gene-related peptide (CGRP) release in bovine dental pulp (Goodis *et al* 2000). Bradykinin released during inflammation may contribute to the

initiation of neurogenic inflammation in dental pulp, and may regulate pulpal response to injury or inflammation. Recently, it was demonstrated that the expression of substance P (SP), a neuropeptide with a major role in nociception, significantly increases with caries progression. Of clinical significance was the fact that this increase in SP was significantly greater in carious specimens that were painful than in carious asymptomatic specimens (Rodd and Boissonade 2000). SP causes vasodilatation by acting directly on smooth muscle cells and indirectly by stimulating histamine release from mast cells. Additionally SP increases microvascular permeability, oedema formation and subsequent plasma protein extravasation, which underlie its powerful proinflammatory properties (Lundy and Linden 2004). The characteristic oedema formation mediated by SP has been shown to be modulated by nitric oxide (Hughes *et al* 1990). Other factors to be considered are lowered oxygen tension and impaired microcirculation associated with increased intrapulpal pressure. The latter should be considered, taking into account the unique features of the pulp that is rigidly encased within dentine (Trowbridge and Kim 1996).

Neurophysiological and neurochemical central nervous system reactions occur as a result of the local inflammatory changes in the dental pulp, some of which have been recorded in trigeminal nuclei. These responses include significant changes in mechanoreceptive fields, altered response properties of brainstem neurons in the trigeminal nucleus and neuroplastic changes involving *N*-methyl D-aspartate (NMDA) receptor mechanisms (Chiang *et al* 1998; Hu *et al* 1990; Chattipakorn *et al* 2002; Sessle, 2005).

Erupted human teeth with incomplete root formation are often insensitive to electric tooth-pulp stimulation (Tal and Sharav 1985). This cannot be explained by the absence of innervation, as nerve fibres are already present at the time of eruption (Avery 1971). It was also demonstrated that masseteric reflex activity could be evoked in the absence of sensation when teeth with incomplete roots were electrically stimulated in children (Tal and Sharav 1985). These findings suggest that segmental reflex connections appear to be established before the cortical sensory projections are functional (Tal and Sharav 1985).

2.4. Differential Diagnosis of Odontalgia

Diagnosis of toothache is challenging because teeth often refer pain to other teeth as well as to other craniofacial locations (Sharav *et al* 1984). Other craniofacial pain disorders may refer to teeth and be expressed as toothache including pretrigeminal neuralgia, neurovascular orofacial pain or atypical pains associated with gustatory stimuli (Chapters 9 and 11) (Mitchell 1980; Fromm *et al* 1990; Sharav *et al* 1991; Helcer *et al* 1998; Sharav 2005). In this respect neurovascular orofacial pain is of great diagnostic importance and is discussed in Chapter 9 (Benoliel *et al* 1997;

Czerninsky *et al* 1999). Other conditions mimicking odontalgia may refer from the maxillary sinus or the ear; see Chapter 6. Pain may also be referred from more remote structures such as the carotid artery or from the heart, and mimic the symptoms of a toothache; Chapter 13 (Tzukert *et al* 1981; Roz *et al* 2005). Of particular importance is pain referred to the oral cavity associated with intracranial tumours; see Chapter 11 (Aiken 1981; Bullitt *et al* 1986).

3. Periodontal Pain

The periodontal tissues include the alveolar bone, the periodontal ligament and the gingivae. A major feature of periodontal disease is that it is usually painless. This is due to the fact that periodontal inflammation is chronic in nature, a fact also true for asymptomatic periapical rarifying osteitis lesions often detected on routine dental radiographs. The lack of pain may be partially explained by the lack of CGRP in gingival crevicular fluid (Lundy *et al* 1999, 2000). On the other hand, periodontal pain is usually experienced in response to localized acute inflammation. Pain originating in the structures surrounding the teeth is easily localized; the affected teeth are very tender on chewing and are readily localized by percussion. Periodontal pain usually results from an acute inflammatory process of the gingivae, the periodontal ligament and alveolar bone due to bacterial or viral infection. Aetiologically, three clinical conditions are possible:

1. Acute periapical inflammation as a result of pulp infection and pulp necrosis;
2. Acute periodontal infection associated with deep pocket formation that may result in a lateral periodontal abscess; and
3. Acute gingival bacterial or viral inflammation.

Although pain characteristics, ability to localize and pain-producing situations are similar in acute periapical and lateral periodontal abscess (Table 5.1), the physical and radiographic signs differ (Table 5.2). Treatment modalities are based on the aetiology of each condition and are therefore entirely different.

3.1. Acute Periapical Periodontitis

Symptoms. Pain associated with acute periapical inflammation is spontaneous, moderate to severe in intensity and long-lasting (hours). Pain is exacerbated by biting on the affected tooth and, in more advanced cases, even by closing the mouth and bringing the tooth into contact with the opposing teeth. In these cases, the tooth feels extruded and is very sensitive to touch. Frequently the patient reports symptoms of pulpal pain that preceded pain from the periapical area. The latter, although of a more continuous nature, is usually better tolerated than the paroxysmal and excruciating pulpal pain.

Localization of pain originating from the periapical area is usually precise and the patient is able to indicate the affected tooth. In this respect periodontal pain differs from the poorly localized dentinal and pulpal pain. The improved ability to localize the source of pain may be attributed to the proprioceptive and mechanoreceptive sensibility of the periodontium that is lacking in the pulp (Griffin and Harris 1974; van Steenberghe 1979). However, although localization of the affected tooth is usually precise, in approximately half the cases the pain is diffuse and spreads into the jaw on the affected side of the face (Sharav *et al* 1984).

Physical and radiographic signs. The affected tooth is readily located by means of gentle tooth percussion and the periapical vestibular area may be tender to palpation. The pulp of the affected tooth is non-vital; i.e. it does not respond to thermal changes or to electrical pulp stimulation. However, as mentioned earlier, in clinical practice pulpitis may not be sharply distinguished from acute periapical periodontitis, and pulpal as well as periapical involvement could occur at the same time. In these cases it is thought that algesic substances, both endogenous from pulp tissue damage or neurogenic inflammation and exogenous from bacterial toxins, invade the periapical area despite the fact that the pulp has not completely degenerated and can still react to stimuli such as temperature changes (Lundy and Linden 2004).

In more severe, purulent cases, swelling of the face associated with cellulitis is sometimes present (Fig. 5.6A) and can be associated with fever and malaise. The affected tooth may be extruded and mobile, both vertically and horizontally. Usually, when facial swelling appears, pain diminishes in intensity probably due to rupture of the local periosteum and the decrease in tissue pressure caused by pus accumulation. The diagnosis of these advanced cases is referred to as dentoalveolar abscess.

Case 5.2 is a patient with periapical periodontitis that developed into a dentoalveolar abscess.

Radiographs are of limited use in the diagnosis of acute periapical periodontitis as no periapical radiographic changes are detected in the early stages. If a radiographic periapical rarefying osteitis is noticed in a tooth that is sensitive to touch and percussion, the condition is then classified as re-acutization of chronic periapical periodontitis (as in Case 5.2). Many times, however, such a rarefying osteitis lesion is present in an otherwise asymptomatic situation. Furthermore, there is a lack of correlation between the radiographic picture and the microbiology or histology of the periapical lesion (Block *et al* 1976; Langeland *et al* 1977).

Pathophysiology. The recent discovery of a new class of protease-activated receptors (PARs) has shed light on enzyme-mediated sensory nerve activation, and especially on the important role of PAR-2 in disease states associated with inflammation (Vergnolle *et al* 1999). PAR-2 is co-expressed with SP and CGRP on sensory nerves, where it is involved in neurogenic inflammation and may also have a role in nociception (Steinhoff *et al* 2000). In fact, SP-immunoreactive nerve fibres have been

Case 5.2 Periapical Periodontitis with Acute Dentoalveolar Abscess, a 20-year-old Male

Primary complaint

Strong continuous pain on left side of face for the past 3 days; tooth #25 very sensitive to chewing. Swelling of left side of face developed rapidly since yesterday with marked relief in pain intensity.

Findings

The left side of the face is swollen (Fig. 5.6A). Tooth #25 is sensitive to percussion, does not respond to cold application and is slightly mobile; no periodontal pockets can be detected. A periapical radiograph (Fig.5.6B) demonstrates a deep disto-occlusal cavity in tooth #25 with a temporary filling, and a periapical radiolucency with concentric condensing osteitis.

Past history

Three months ago patient complained of discomfort on chewing, a sensitivity to cold foods on the left side of his mouth. A temporary filling of tooth #25 was performed. At first the tooth was very sensitive to cold foods, but then became comfortable until 3 days ago, when the strong pain started.

Comment

This is a *classic* case that starts with discomfort and pain due to caries, associated with dentinal allodynia and food impaction. Pulp irritation develops subsequent to cavity-preparation and placing of the temporary filling, which eventually leads to pulp necrosis. A periapical lesion develops asymptomatically and some 3 months later an acute exacerbation with strong pain occurs due to acute periapical periodontitis.

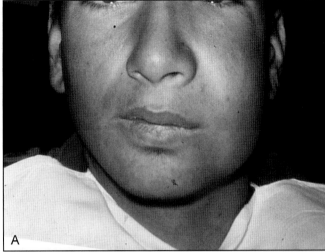
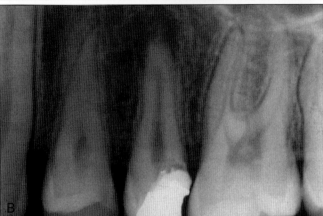

Fig. 5.6 • (A) Acute swelling of the left side of the face (cellulitis) due to acute dentoalveolar abscess of tooth #25. Note swelling of left cheek, left lower eyelid *closing* the eye, and the disappearance of the left nasolabial fold due to swelling. Also the left nostril and left upper lip are swollen (Case 5.2). (B) Periapical radiograph that demonstrates a deep disto-occlusal cavity in tooth #25 with a temporary filling, and a periapical radiolucency with concentric condensing osteitis (Case 5.2).

found in the vicinity of tryptase-positive mast cells (tryptase constitutes the major protein released during mast cell degranulation) in human periapical granulomas (Kabashima *et al* 2002). Of special interest is the fact that the gingival crevicular fluid around teeth with acute pain of pulpal origin demonstrated increased levels of SP and neurokinin-A compared with healthy teeth, and these levels decreased significantly 1 week after pulpectomy (Awawdeh *et al* 2002). Further evidence that pulpal pain can induce neurogenic inflammatory reactions is obtained from experimental painful tooth stimulation that induces a local elevation in metalloproteinase-8, a major tissue-destructive protease in gingival crevicular fluid that is lacking in the pulp (Avellan *et al* 2005).

Treatment. While the pain originates from the periodontal periapical tissues, the source of insult and infection usually lies within the pulp chamber and the root canal. The primary aim of treatment is to eliminate this source. The pulp chamber is opened and the root canal cleansed and dressed in accordance with current endodontic practice. There is no difference in postoperative pain between a calcium-hydroxide or a corticosteroid-antibiotic root canal dressing after biomechanical

preparation of teeth with acute apical periodontitis (Fava 1998). Patients with localized periapical pain or swelling generally recover quickly with local treatment, and there is no demonstrable benefit from penicillin supplementation (Fouad *et al* 1996). Furthermore, amoxicillin plus clavulanic acid was not more effective than penicillin in these cases (Lewis *et al* 1993). The conclusions from a systematic review were that an apical abscess should be drained through a pulpectomy or incision and drainage, and antibiotics are of no additional benefit (Matthews *et al* 2003). However, if cellulitis, fever and malaise are present, systemic administration of antibiotics is recommended. Antibiotics should also be prescribed in addition to abscess drainage and tooth debridement in immunocompromised patients. Various antibiotics at standard doses (amoxicillin, clindamycin or erythromycin stearate) were prescribed to 759 patients with acute dentoalveolar abscesses associated with swelling and pyrexia (>38.5°C) after initial abscess drainage or extraction (Martin *et al* 1997). It was found that in most patients 2–3 days of antibiotics was sufficient. However, the lack of a control group without antibiotics limits the conclusions from this study. Grinding the tooth to prevent contact with the opposing teeth helps to relieve pain. Grinding should be performed carefully, keeping in mind the eventual treatment plan. Teeth that are to be restored with a plastic restoration should be carefully ground with the aid of articulating paper. In contrast, teeth that are to be crowned may be more liberally ground.

3.2. Lateral Periodontal Abscess

Symptoms. Pain characteristics of a lateral periodontal abscess are very similar to those of acute periapical periodontitis (Tables 5.1 and 5.2). The pain is continuous, moderate to severe in intensity and well localized and is exacerbated by biting on the affected tooth.

Physical and radiographic signs. During examination swelling and redness of the gingiva may be noticed, usually located more coronally than in acute periapical lesions. The swelling is tender to palpation and the affected tooth is sensitive to percussion and may be mobile and slightly extruded; in more severe cases, cellulitis, fever and malaise may occur. A deep periodontal pocket is usually located around the tooth (Fig. 5.7A); once probed, pus exudation may occur with occasional pain relief. Frequently, probing is quite painful and has been correlated to the degree of the inflammatory process (Heft *et al* 1991). The anterior region is extremely sensitive; probing of the gums in healthy subjects is twice as painful in the area of the maxillary incisors than in that of the molar teeth (Heins *et al* 1998). The tooth pulp is usually vital; i.e. it reacts normally to temperature changes and electrical stimulation. The pulp may occasionally be slightly hyperalgesic in these cases and sometimes pulpitis and pulpal pain may develop due to retrograde infection from a deep periodontal pocket (see the section on perio-endo lesions below). It was shown in a sample of 29 patients (Herrera *et al* 2000a) that more than 75% of the abscesses demonstrated oedema, redness and swelling, and 90% of the patients reported pain. Bleeding occurred in all abscesses, while suppuration on sampling was detected in 66%. Mean associated pocket depth was 7.28 mm, and 79% of teeth presented some degree of mobility. Cervical lymphadenopathy was seen in 10% of patients, while elevated leucocyte counts were observed in 32%.

Abscess formation usually results from a blockage of drainage from a deep periodontal pocket, and is frequently associated with a deep infrabony pocket and teeth with root furcation involvement. A deep infrabony pocket is therefore usually present on the radiograph (Fig. 5.7B). Acute periodontal abscesses may also be associated with dental implants (Ibbott *et al* 1993).

Pathophysiology. High prevalences of putative periodontal pathogens including *Fusobacterium nucleatum, Peptostreptococcus micros, Porphyromonas gingivalis, Prevotella intermedia* and *Bacteroides forsythus* were found in periodontal abscesses (Herrera et al 2000a).

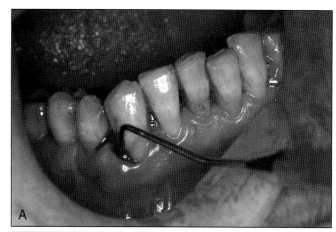

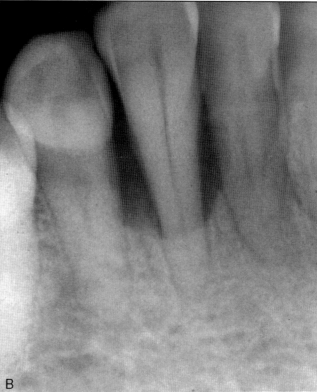

Fig. 5.7 • (A) Lateral periodontal abscess associated with pain, swelling and a 10-mm periodontal pocket. (B) Infrabony periodontal pocket.

Significant differences in the levels of prostaglandin E2 (PGE2) and LTB4 were found between patients with and without periodontitis. The PGE2 and LTB4 levels correlated with clinical parameters and reduced markedly after phase-1 of periodontal treatment (Tsai *et al* 1998). It is interesting that the levels of PGE2 correlated with the severity of the periodontal status, and the levels of LTB4 correlated with gingival inflammation.

Treatment. Gentle irrigation and curettage of the pocket should be performed. A vertical incision for drainage is recommended when the abscess is fluctuant but cannot be adequately approached through the pocket. Acute lateral periodontal abscess causes rapid alveolar bone destruction (Fig. 5.7B), hence the need for early and prompt intervention. If necessary, selective grinding of the tooth should be performed to avoid contact with the opposing teeth, reduce pain and restore tooth stability. When cellulitis, fever and malaise are present, systemic antibiotic administration may be recommended. As in periapical periodontitis, the need for antibiotic supplementation, in addition to local treatment, is unclear (Herrera *et al* 2000b). Pain usually subsides within 24 hours of treatment.

3.2.1. Interrelationships between Pulpal and Periodontal Diseases: 'Perio-endo' Lesions (Fig. 5.8)

Deep periodontal pockets can sometimes involve accessory canals (in the furcation or laterally) and extensive lesions can reach the root apex of the tooth and cause retrograde pulp inflammation (Fig. 5.8B). The major initial symptom is sensitivity to temperature changes, a situation that may progress to irreversible pulpitis and periapical periodontitis. A second possibility is that of an apical abscess which exudates through a periodontal pocket (Fig. 5.8A). In this case pain can be minimal due to the release of pressure through the pocket, or sometimes an exacerbation into an acute dentoalveolar abscess may occur. Finally, the co-occurrence of symptomatic active periodontal disease together with independent endodontic pathology is a possibility and is termed a *true* combined lesion.

Treatment. Treatment for all these situations is initially endodontic, followed by conventional periodontal treatment. The prognosis of endodontic lesions causing periodontal symptomatology is better than that in periodontally initiated or in combined lesions.

3.2.2. Vertical Root Fracture

A fracture of the tooth that involves most of the root will induce pain on biting. Root fractures are more common in endodontically treated teeth that have been restored with a post and core. Pain on biting in such cases is therefore of periodontal origin. Initially there may be no clinical or radiographic signs. An isolated periodontal pocket in the area of the fracture is often found. Disease progression usually leads to a typical radiographic picture of a lengthwise rarefying osteitis. If left untreated infection and abscess formation may occur. Currently, the only treatment option for vertical root fractures is extraction.

3.3. Gingival Pain

Gingival pain may occur as a result of mechanical irritation such as food impaction, acute inflammation associated with a partially erupted tooth (pericoronitis) or an acute bacterial or viral infection.

3.3.1. Food Impaction

Symptoms. Food impaction, as the name implies, is a situation when food is forced during meals in between two teeth and presses on the gums. The patient complains of a localized pain that develops between two teeth after meals, especially when food is fibrous (e.g. meat, celery). The pain is associated with a feeling of pressure and discomfort that is annoying and sometimes severe (Sharav *et al* 1984). The patient may report that pain gradually diminishes until evoked again at the next meal, or the pain may be relieved immediately by removing the food impacted between the teeth with a tooth pick or dental floss.

Physical and radiographic signs. Upon examination, a faulty contact between two adjacent teeth is noticed so that food is usually trapped between these teeth; the gingival papilla is tender to touch and bleeds easily. The two adjacent teeth are usually sensitive to percussion. Food impaction should be treated promptly as it may cause cervical caries and interdental alveolar bone resorption (Jernberg *et al* 1983).

Treatment. The cause of the faulty contact between the teeth is often a carious lesion, and restoring the tooth will

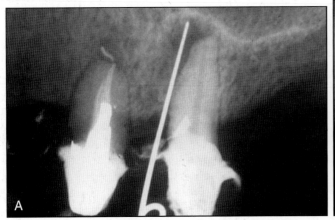
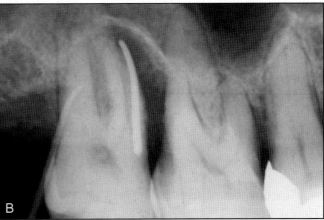

Fig. 5.8 • The two radiographs demonstrate the following. (A) Endo-perio lesion: a silver point was inserted into the pocket and a well-demarcated periapical radiolucent lesion was also demonstrated. The tooth pulp was non-vital and could be approached by drilling through the temporary acrylic crown without using any local anaesthesia. (B) Perio-endo lesion: the mesial pocket is demonstrated with a gutta percha point, and approaches the apex of the mesiobuccal root of the upper second molar. In this case the tooth pulp was vital and the patient complained of strong pain to hot and cold foods, and sometimes of strong spontaneous pain that lasted for 10–15 minutes.

eliminate pain. In some cases though the contacts are tight food impaction may occur, and creating anatomical escape grooves adjacent to the marginal ridge may eliminate food impaction (Newell *et al* 2002).

3.3.2. Pericoronitis

Acute pericoronal infections are common in teeth that are incompletely erupted and are partially covered by a flap or operculum of gingival tissue.

Symptoms. Pain, which may be severe, is usually located at the distal end of the arch of teeth in the lower jaw. Pain is spontaneous and may be exacerbated by closing the mouth. In more severe cases, pain is aggravated by swallowing and results in limited mouth opening.

Physical and radiographic signs. Upon examination, the operculum is acutely inflamed (red, oedematous) and frequently an indentation of the opposing tooth can be seen on the swollen gingival flap. Occasionally there is fever, malaise and restricted mouth opening.

Pathophysiology. A study of 2151 patients with pericoronitis found that the peak age of occurrence was from 21 to 25 years, and the most frequent predisposing factors were upper respiratory infection (38%) and stress (22%) (Newell *et al* 2002). Bacteriologic studies in 37 cases of pericoronitis indicated that spirochetes (55%) and fusiform bacteria (84%) are extremely common. In addition to obligate anaerobic bacteria, a predominantly facultative anaerobic microflora was cultured: *Streptococcus milleri* (78% of samples), *Stomatococcus mucilaginosus* (71%) and *Rothia dentocariosa* (57%). It was concluded that *S. milleri*, well-known for its ability to cause suppurative infections, is most likely involved in the pathogenesis of acute severe pericoronitis of the lower third molar (Peltroche-Llacsahuanga *et al* 2000). The lack of a normal control limits the conclusion from this study. In a recent study 10 patients with pericoronitis and 10 healthy controls were investigated for the presence of tumour necrosis factor-α (TNF-α) (Beklen *et al* 2005). Expectedly, TNF receptors (TNF-R1 and TNF-R2) were found in macrophage- and fibroblast-like cells, vascular endothelial cells in post-capillary venules and basal epithelial cells in pericoronitis, but were only weakly expressed in controls. It was concluded that the potent proinflammatory cytokine, TNF-α, plays a role in the pain and inflammation associated with pericoronitis (Beklen *et al* 2005).

Treatment. Irrigation of debris between the operculum and the affected tooth with saline or antibacterial agent (e.g. chlorhexidine 0.5%) should be performed. Trauma can be eliminated by grinding or extracting the opposing tooth. Systemic antibiotic administration is recommended when limited mouth opening occurs or the patient is febrile. Microbiological cultures were obtained from 26 patients with pericoronitis; 9 out of 26 samples contained β-lactamase-producing strains (Sixou *et al* 2003). The infection in pericoronitis is multimicrobial, predominantly caused by β-lactamase-producing anaerobic microorganisms, and

first-line treatment suggested is amoxicillin with clavulanic acid (Gutierrez-Perez 2004; Bresco-Salinas *et al* 2006).

3.3.3. Acute Necrotizing Ulcerative Gingivitis

Symptoms. This is an ulcerative gingival disease characterized by pain, bleeding and papillary necrosis (Bermejo-Fenoll and Sanchez-Perez 2004). Soreness and pain are characteristically felt at the margin of the gums. Pain is intensified by eating and tooth brushing; these activities are usually accompanied by gingival bleeding. In the early stages some patients may complain of a feeling of tightness around the teeth. A metallic taste is sometimes experienced and usually there is a foetid odor from the mouth. Pain is fairly well localized to the affected areas, but in cases with widespread lesions pain is experienced throughout the mouth. Fever and malaise are sometimes present.

Physical and radiographic signs. Necrosis and ulceration are present on the marginal gingiva with different degrees of gingival papillary destruction. An adherent greyish slough represents the so-called pseudo-membrane present in the acute stage (Fig. 5.9). Acute herpetic infection of the gums (herpetic gingivostomatitis) can sometimes resemble acute necrotizing ulcerative gingivitis (ANUG), but the clinical appearance and associated signs and symptoms are different. The papillary necrosis typical of ANUG (Fig. 5.9) is absent in the herpetic infection, while herpetic lesions create a typically 'punched-out' appearance located at the gingival margin.

Relatively little is known about the epidemiology of ANUG in normal adolescent populations. Most studies have comprised special target groups, such as military recruits, HIV patients or severely malnourished subjects (Jimenez *et al* 2005). In patients ($n = 101$) with HIV infection or AIDS, ANUG was found in about 28% (Bendick *et al* 2002). On the other hand, in 9203 students aged 12–21 years in Santiago, Chile, the estimated prevalence of

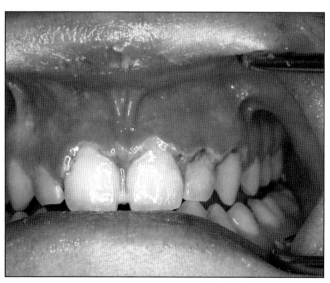

Fig. 5.9 • Acute necrotizing ulcerative gingivitis (ANUG). Note destruction of gingival papilla and pseudo-membrane at the marginal border.

ANUG was 6.7% (Lopez *et al* 2002). Of 19 944 patients examined at a periodontal clinic in Cape Town, South Africa, less than 0.5% were found to have ANUG, and the study demonstrated significant seasonal variation in the occurrence of the disease (Arendorf *et al* 2001).

Pathophysiology. ANUG is considered to be an acute opportunistic gingival infection caused by bacterial plaque. It appears more frequently in undernourished children and young adults as well as in patients with immunodeficiency. Its pathogenesis involves factors related to the oral microbiology and its invasive ability as well as factors associated with the host, including capillary and immunological disorders.

Treatment. Treatment includes swabbing and gentle irrigation of the ulcerative lesions, preferably with chlorhexidine or an oxidizing agent (hydrogen peroxide), and scaling and cleaning the teeth. Systemic antibiotics are recommended especially when fever and malaise are present (Brook 2003).

4. Mucosal Pain

Pain originating from the oral mucosa can be either localized or of a more generalized diffuse nature. Localized pain is usually associated with a detectable erosive or ulcerative lesion whilst diffuse pain may be associated with a widespread infection, a systemic disease or other unknown factors. The localized pain associated with a detectable lesion results from physical, chemical or thermal trauma, viral infection or lesions of unknown origin. Pain is usually mild to moderate but when there is irritation, mechanically or by sour, spicy or hot foods, may become quite severe and last for some minutes.

Detailed descriptions of the various lesions of the oral mucosa are beyond the scope of this chapter and only the most common lesions, recurrent aphthous stomatitis and acute herpetic gingivostomatitis, are briefly discussed.

4.1. Localized Mucosal Pain

4.1.1. Aphthous Lesions

Recurrent aphthous ulcers represent a very common but poorly understood mucosal disorder. They occur in men and women of all ages, races and geographic regions. It is estimated that at least 1 in 5 individuals has at least once been afflicted with aphthous ulcers. The condition is classified as minor, major and herpetiform on the basis of ulcer size and number.

Local trauma, stress, food intake, drugs, hormonal changes and vitamin and trace element deficiencies may precipitate attacks. Local and systemic conditions and genetic, immunological and microbial factors all may play a role in the pathogenesis of recurrent aphthous ulceration (RAU). No principal cause has been discovered but an autoimmune pathophysiology is suspected. Since the aetiology is unknown, diagnosis is entirely based on history and clinical criteria and no laboratory procedures exist to confirm the diagnosis (Natah *et al* 2004).

Recurrent aphthous stomatitis is characterized by a prodromal burning sensation from 2 to 48 hours before an ulcer appears. Although small in diameter (0.3–1.0 cm) this lesion may be quite painful and induces a painful regional lymphadenopathy. In the mild form, healing occurs within 10 days and pain is usually mild to moderate in severity. In the more severe forms (major aphthous ulcers), deep ulcers occur which may be confluent, are extremely painful and interfere with speech and eating. Such lesions may last for months, heal slowly and leave scars.

Treatment is mostly symptomatic, including the application of a topical protective emollient for the mild form and the use of topical corticosteroids and tetracycline to decrease healing time for the more severe form (Ylikontiola *et al* 1997; Lo Muzio *et al* 2001). Recently, cyanoacrylate has been used as an effective tissue adhesive for steroids and tetracycline (Ylikontiola *et al* 1997; Kutcher *et al* 2001). The use of diclofenac, a topical nonsteroidal anti-inflammatory drug (NSAID), was also found effective (Saxen *et al* 1997).

4.1.2. Acute Herpetic Gingivostomatitis

Oral infections caused by herpes simplex type 1 are widespread, even among otherwise healthy people. While most of these herpetic infections are mildly symptomatic, young children are at risk for developing extensive oropharyngeal vesicular eruptions when first infected with the virus. This initial outbreak is known as primary herpetic gingivostomatitis. There has been a general trend for the mean age of patients with acute herpetic stomatitis to increase and currently the majority of cases (>50%) suffer the first attack during their third decade (Main 1989; Chauvin and Ajar 2002). Diagnosis can be performed clinically and confirmed by laboratory tests. Although this is a self-limiting disease, symptoms may persist for 2 weeks, causing significant mouth discomfort, fever, lymphadenopathy and difficulty eating and drinking. The incidence of oral herpes simplex infection is particularly high in immunocompromised patients, and occurs in up to 50% of hospitalized patients with acute leukaemia (Greenberg *et al* 1987). Proper diagnosis and treatment are essential, particularly in elderly and immunocompromised patients. Cytology (Tzanck testing) may serve as a useful adjunct in diagnosis, but rapid and highly specific detection of human herpes simplex type-1 in saliva is possible by in vitro amplification using the polymerase chain reaction (Robinson *et al* 1992).

Treatment. Some young children may require hospitalization for management of dehydration and pain control (Blevins 2003). A soft bland diet preceded by a local anaesthetic mouth rinse is recommended. Oral hygiene may be maintained by rinsing with a mild bicarbonate or saline solution or a non-alcoholic solution of 0.2% chlorhexidine. Antiviral agents such as acyclovir and famciclovir should be considered part of early management of primary herpetic gingivostomatitis. Providing supportive care and educating parents about transmission of the virus are important (Chauvin and Ajar 2002; Blevins 2003).

4.2. Diffuse Mucosal Pain

When generalized diffuse pain is felt in the oral mucosa, it usually has a burning nature and may be accompanied by a dysgeusia, predominantly of a bitter metallic quality. This pain may result from a direct insult to the tissues due to bacterial, viral or fungal infection, which can be identified by the characteristic appearance of the oral mucosa. Diagnosis is aided by microbiological and other laboratory examinations. In cases of chronic fungal infection (candidiasis), possible underlying aetiological factors such as prolonged broad spectrum antibiotic therapy, immunodeficiencies and other debilitating factors should be investigated (Terai and Shimahara 2005). Radiation therapy to the head and neck region may result in acute mucositis with severe generalized mucosal pain (Kolbinson et al 1988). Decreased salivary flow is a late sequela of radiation therapy that may result in chronic pain and discomfort of the oral mucosa. Burning sensation of the oral mucosa, particularly the tongue, may result from systemic diseases, such as chronic iron-deficiency anaemia, and may be associated with atrophic glossitis (Terai and Shimahara 2005). This is usually associated with observable atrophic changes of the tongue, in particular absence of filiform and fungiform papillae. Atrophic glossitis and burning mouth sensations have also been associated with *Helicobacter pylori* colonization of tongue mucosa, and nutritional deficiency (Drinka et al 1993; Bohmer and Mowe 2000; Gall-Troselj et al 2001).

A large proportion of patients, mostly women between the ages of 50 and 70 years, complain of a burning sensation in the mouth and the tongue, with no observable changes in the oral mucosa and with no detectable underlying systemic changes. This group of patients is usually diagnosed as having burning mouth syndrome (BMS) or burning mouth disorder (BMD), discussed in Chapter 11.

5. Pain from Salivary Glands

Pain from the salivary glands is usually associated with salivary gland duct blockage. Pain from salivary glands is localized to the affected gland, and is of moderate to severe intensity. The salivary gland is swollen and very tender to palpation. Salivary flow from affected glands is reduced and sometimes completely abolished. Pain is intensified by increased saliva production, such as when starting meals, and pain can be induced by applying an acidic stimulant (citric acid is the standard stimulant) to the tongue. Many cases of salivary gland blockage are associated with ascending bacterial infection of the gland. Pus may be secreted from the salivary duct when the gland is infected, and pain may be associated with fever and malaise.

Blockage of the salivary duct may be caused by a calcified calculus, often identifiable on a radiograph, or it may be blocked by a radiolucent mucin plug formation. Ultrasound or sialography can aid in diagnosis (Haring 1991; Murray et al 1996).

In children the most common causes of pain from salivary glands are mumps and acute recurrent parotitis. Recurrent parotitis of childhood is a rare condition of unknown aetiology, probably immunologically mediated. The major clinical features that distinguish it from other causes of parotid swelling are the lack of pus and recurrent episodes. A clinical diagnosis can often be confirmed by ultrasound (Leerdam et al 2005). Recently a new method, combining a salivary intraductal endoscopic technique, was introduced for diagnosis and treatment of these cases (Nahlieli et al 2004).

Treatment. When blockage is diagnosed, surgical or endoscopic approaches are indicated to remove the blockage (Nahlieli et al 2003). In the acute bacterial infection stage antibiotic therapy is recommended. No antibiotics are recommended for mumps or recurrent parotitis (Leerdam et al 2005).

References

Ahlquist M, Franzen O, Coffey J, et al (1994) Dental pain evoked by hydrostatic pressures applied to exposed dentin in man: a test of the hydrodynamic theory of dentin sensitivity. *J Endod* **20**(3):130–134.

Aiken A (1981) Facial pain — toothache or tumour?. *Int J Oral Surg* **10**(Suppl 1):187–190.

Anderson DJ, Naylor MN (1962) Chemical excitants of pain in human dentine and dental pulp. *Arch Oral Biol* **7**:413–415.

Anderson DJ, Hannam AG, Mathews B (1970) Sensory mechanisms in mammalian teeth and their supporting structures. *Physiol Rev* **50**(2):171–195.

Andrew D, Matthews B (2000) Displacement of the contents of dentinal tubules and sensory transduction in intradental nerves of the cat. *J Physiol* **529**(Pt 3):791–802.

Arendorf TM, Bredekamp B, Cloete CA, et al (2001) Seasonal variation of acute necrotising ulcerative gingivitis in South Africans. *Oral Dis* **7**(3):150–154.

Armstrong D, Dry RM, Keele CA, et al (1953) Observations on chemical excitants of cutaneous pain in man. *J Physiol* **120**(3):326–351.

Avellan NL, Sorsa T, Tervahartiala T, et al (2005) Painful tooth stimulation elevates matrix metalloproteinase-8 levels locally in human gingival crevicular fluid. *J Dent Res* **84**(4):335–339.

Avery JK (1971) Structural elements of the young normal human pulp. *Oral Surg Oral Med Oral Pathol* **32**(1):113–125.

Awawdeh LA, Lundy FT, Linden GJ, et al (2002) Quantitative analysis of substance P, neurokinin A and calcitonin gene-related peptide in gingival crevicular fluid associated with painful human teeth. *Eur J Oral Sci* **110**(3):185–191.

Beklen A, Laine M, Venta I, et al (2005) Role of TNF-alpha and its receptors in pericoronitis. *J Dent Res* **84**(12):1178–1182.

Bender IB (2000) Reversible and irreversible painful pulpitides: diagnosis and treatment. *Aust Endod J* **26**(1):10–14.

Bendick C, Scheifele C, Reichart PA (2002) Oral manifestations in 101 Cambodians with HIV and AIDS. *J Oral Pathol Med* **31**(1):1–4.

Benoliel R, Elishoov H, Sharav Y (1997) Orofacial pain with vascular-type features. *Oral Surg Oral Med Oral Pathol Oral Radiol Endod* **84**(5):506–512.

Bergenholtz G, Spangberg L (2004) Controversies in endodontics. *Crit Rev Oral Biol Med* **15**(2):99–114.

Bermejo-Fenoll A, Sanchez-Perez A (2004) Necrotising periodontal diseases. *Med Oral Patol Oral Cir Bucal* **9**(Suppl):114–119; 108–114.

Blevins JY (2003) Primary herpetic gingivostomatitis in young children. *Pediatr Nurs* **29**(3):199–202.

Block RM, Bushell A, Rodrigues H, et al (1976) A histopathologic, histobacteriologic, and radiographic study of periapical endodontic surgical specimens. *Oral Surg Oral Med Oral Pathol* **42**(5):656–678.

Bohmer T, Mowe M (2000) The association between atrophic glossitis and protein-calorie malnutrition in old age. *Age Ageing* **29**(1):47–50.

Brannstrom M (1962) The elicitation of pain in human dentine and pulp by chemical stimuli. *Arch Oral Biol* **7**:59–62.

Brannstrom M (1963) Dentin sensitivity and aspiration of odontoblasts. *J Am Dent Assoc* **66**:366–370.

Bresco-Salinas M, Costa-Riu N, Berini-Aytes L, et al (2006) Antibiotic susceptibility of the bacteria causing odontogenic infections. *Med Oral Patol Oral Cir Bucal* **11**(1):E70–75.

Brook I (2003) Microbiology and management of periodontal infections. *Gen Dent* **51**(5):424–428.

Brookfield JR, Addy M, Alexander DC, et al (2003) Consensus-based recommendations for the diagnosis and management of dentin hypersensitivity. *J Can Dent Assoc* **69**(4):221–226.

Brown AC, Beeler WJ, Kloka AC, et al (1985) Spatial summation of pre-pain and pain in human teeth. *Pain* **21**(1):1–16.

Brynjulfsen A, Fristad I, Grevstad T, et al (2002) Incompletely fractured teeth associated with diffuse longstanding orofacial pain: diagnosis and treatment outcome. *Int Endod J* **35**(5):461–466.

Bullitt E, Tew JM, Boyd J (1986) Intracranial tumors in patients with facial pain. *J Neurosurg* **64**(6):865–871.

Byers MR, Kish SJ (1976) Delineation of somatic nerve endings in rat teeth by radioautography of axon-transported protein. *J Dent Res* **55**(3):419–425.

Byers MR, Narhi MV (1999) Dental injury models: experimental tools for understanding neuroinflammatory interactions and polymodal nociceptor functions. *Crit Rev Oral Biol Med* **10**(1):4–39.

Byers MR, Narhi MVO (2002) Nerve supply of the pulpodentin complex and response to injury. In: Hargreaves KM, Goodies HE (eds) *Seltzer and Bender's Dental Pulp*. Chicago: Quintessence, pp 151–179.

Byers MR, Neuhaus SJ, Gehrig JD (1982) Dental sensory receptor structure in human teeth. *Pain* **13**(3):221–235.

Cameron CE (1976) The cracked tooth syndrome: additional findings. *J Am Dent Assoc* **93**(5):971–975.

Chabanski MB, Gillam DG (1997) Aetiology, prevalence and clinical features of cervical dentine sensitivity. *J Oral Rehabil* **24**(1):15–19.

Chattipakorn SC, Sigurdsson A, Light AR, et al (2002) Trigeminal c-Fos expression and behavioral responses to pulpal inflammation in ferrets. *Pain* **99**(1–2):61–69.

Chauvin PJ, Ajar AH (2002) Acute herpetic gingivostomatitis in adults: a review of 13 cases, including diagnosis and management. *J Can Dent Assoc* **68**(4): 247–251.

Chiang CY, Park SJ, Kwan CL, et al (1998) NMDA receptor mechanisms contribute to neuroplasticity induced in caudalis nociceptive neurons by tooth pulp stimulation. *J Neurophysiol* **80**(5):2621–2631.

Cisneros-Cabello R, Segura-Egea JJ (2005) Relationship of patient complaints and signs to histopathologic diagnosis of pulpal condition. *Aust Endod J* **31**(1):24–27.

Cohen S (1996) Endodontic diagnosis. In: Cohen S, Burnse RC (eds) *Pathways of the Pulp*. St. Louis: CV Mosby.

Czerninsky R, Benoliel R, Sharav Y (1999) Odontalgia in vascular orofacial pain. *J Orofac Pain* **13**(3):196–200.

Drinka PJ, Langer EH, Voeks SK, et al (1993) Nutritional correlates of atrophic glossitis: possible role of vitamin E in papillary atrophy. *J Am Coll Nutr* **12**(1):14–20.

Falace DA, Reid K, Rayens MK (1996) The influence of deep (odontogenic) pain intensity, quality, and duration on the incidence and characteristics of referred orofacial pain. *J Orofac Pain* **10**(3):232–239.

Fava LR (1998) Acute apical periodontitis: incidence of post-operative pain using two different root canal dressings. *Int Endod J* **31**(5):343–347.

Fouad AF, Rivera EM, Walton RE (1996) Penicillin as a supplement in resolving the localized acute apical abscess. *Oral Surg Oral Med Oral Pathol Oral Radiol Endod* **81**(5):590–595.

Friend LA, Glenwright HD (1968) An experimental investigation into the localization of pain from the dental pulp. *Oral Surg Oral Med Oral Pathol* **25**(5):765–774.

Fromm GH, Graff-Radford SB, Terrence CF, et al (1990) Pre-trigeminal neuralgia. *Neurology* **40**(10):1493–1495.

Gall-Troselj K, Mravak-Stipetic M, Jurak I, et al (2001) Helicobacter pylori colonization of tongue mucosa–increased incidence in atrophic glossitis and burning mouth syndrome (BMS). *J Oral Pathol Med* **30**(9):560–563.

Goodis HE, Bowles WR, Hargreaves KM (2000) Prostaglandin E2 enhances bradykinin-evoked iCGRP release in bovine dental pulp. *J Dent Res* **79**(8):1604–1607.

Goose DH (1981) Cracked tooth syndrome. *Br Dent J* **150**(5):224–225.

Greenberg MS, Cohen SG, Boosz B, et al (1987) Oral herpes simplex infections in patients with leukemia. *J Am Dent Assoc* **114**(4):483–486.

Griffin CJ, Harris R (1974) Innervation of human periodontium. I. Classification of periodontal receptors. *Aust Dent J* **19**(1):51–56.

Gutierrez-Perez JL (2004) Third molar infections. *Med Oral Patol Oral Cir Bucal* **9**(Suppl):122–125; 120–122.

Hargreaves KM, Seltzer SIE (2002) Pharmacologic control of dental pain. In: Hargreaves KM, Goodies HE (eds) *Seltzer and Bender's Dental Pulp*. Chicago: Quintessence, pp 205–225.

Haring JI (1991) Diagnosing salivary stones. *J Am Dent Assoc* **122**(5):75–76.

Heft MW, Perelmuter SH, Cooper BY, et al (1991) Relationship between gingival inflammation and painfulness of periodontal probing. *J Clin Periodontol* **18**(3):213–215.

Heins PJ, Karpinia KA, Maruniak JW, et al (1998) Pain threshold values during periodontal probing: assessment of maxillary incisor and molar sites. *J Periodontol* **69**(7):812–818.

Helcer M, Schnarch A, Benoliel R, et al (1998) Trigeminal neuralgic-type pain and vascular-type headache due to gustatory stimulus. *Headache* **38**(2):129–131.

Herrera D, Roldan S, Gonzalez I, et al (2000a) The periodontal abscess (I). Clinical and microbiological findings. *J Clin Periodontol* **27**(6):387–394.

Herrera D, Roldan S, Sanz M (2000b) The periodontal abscess: a review. *J Clin Periodontol* **27**(6):377–386.

Hu JW, Sharav Y, Sessle BJ (1990) Effects of one- or two-stage deafferentation of mandibular and maxillary tooth pulps on the functional properties of trigeminal brainstem neurons. *Brain Res* **516**(2):271–279.

Hughes SR, Williams TJ, Brain SD (1990) Evidence that endogenous nitric oxide modulates oedema formation induced by substance P. *Eur J Pharmacol* **191**(3):481–484.

Ibbott CG, Kovach RJ, Carlson-Mann LD (1993) Acute periodontal abscess associated with an immediate implant site in the maintenance phase: a case report. *Int J Oral Maxillofac Implants* **8**(6):699–702.

Jernberg GR, Bakdash MB, Keenan KM (1983) Relationship between proximal tooth open contacts and periodontal disease. *J Periodontol* **54**(9):529–533.

Jimenez LM, Duque FL, Baer PN, *et al* (2005) Necrotizing ulcerative periodontal diseases in children and young adults in Medellin, Colombia, 1965–2000. *J Int Acad Periodontol* **7**(2):55–63.

Kabashima H, Nagata K, Maeda K, *et al* (2002) Involvement of substance P, mast cells, TNF-alpha and ICAM-1 in the infiltration of inflammatory cells in human periapical granulomas. *J Oral Pathol Med* **31**(3):175–180.

Kimura Y, Wilder-Smith P, Yonaga K, *et al* (2000) Treatment of dentine hypersensitivity by lasers: a review. *J Clin Periodontol* **27**(10):715–721.

Kolbinson DA, Schubert MM, Flournoy N, *et al* (1988) Early oral changes following bone marrow transplantation. *Oral Surg Oral Med Oral Pathol* **66**(1):130–138.

Kutcher MJ, Ludlow JB, Samuelson AD, *et al* (2001) Evaluation of a bioadhesive device for the management of aphthous ulcers. *J Am Dent Assoc* **132**(3):368–376.

Lan WH, Liu HC (1996) Treatment of dentin hypersensitivity by Nd:YAG laser. *J Clin Laser Med Surg* **14**(2):89–92.

Langeland K, Block RM, Grossman LI (1977) A histopathologic and histobacteriologic study of 35 periapical endodontic surgical specimens. *J Endod* **3**(1):8–23.

Leerdam CM, Martin HC, Isaacs D (2005) Recurrent parotitis of childhood. *J Paediatr Child Health* **41**(12):631–634.

Lewis MA, Carmichael F, MacFarlane TW, *et al* (1993) A randomised trial of co-amoxiclav (Augmentin) versus penicillin V in the treatment of acute dentoalveolar abscess. *Br Dent J* **175**(5):169–174.

Lipton JA, Ship JA, Larach-Robinson D (1993) Estimated prevalence and distribution of reported orofacial pain in the United States. *J Am Dent Assoc* **124**(10):115–121.

Lo Muzio L, della Valle A, Mignogna MD, *et al* (2001) The treatment of oral aphthous ulceration or erosive lichen planus with topical clobetasol propionate in three preparations: a clinical and pilot study on 54 patients. *J Oral Pathol Med* **30**(10):611–617.

Locker D, Grushka M (1987) Prevalence of oral and facial pain and discomfort: preliminary results of a mail survey. *Community Dent Oral Epidemiol* **15**(3):169–172.

Lopez R, Fernandez O, Jara G, *et al* (2002) Epidemiology of necrotizing ulcerative gingival lesions in adolescents. *J Periodontal Res* **37**(6):439–444.

Lundy FT, Linden GJ (2004) Neuropeptides and neurogenic mechanisms in oral and periodontal inflammation. *Crit Rev Oral Biol Med* **15**(2):82–98.

Lundy FT, Shaw C, McKinnell J, *et al* (1999) Calcitonin gene-related peptide in gingival crevicular fluid in periodontal health and disease. *J Clin Periodontol* **26**(4):212–216.

Lundy FT, Salmon AL, Lamey PJ, *et al* (2000) Carboxypeptidase-mediated metabolism of calcitonin gene-related peptide in human gingival crevicular fluid–a role in periodontal inflammation? *J Clin Periodontol* **27**(7):499–505.

McGrath PA, Gracely RH, Dubner R, *et al* (1983) Non-pain and pain sensations evoked by tooth pulp stimulation. *Pain* **15**(4): 377–388.

Madison S, Whitsel EA, Suarez-Roca H, *et al* (1992) Sensitizing effects of leukotriene B4 on intradental primary afferents. *Pain* **49**(1):99–104.

Main DM (1989) Acute herpetic stomatitis: referrals to Leeds Dental Hospital 1978-1987. *Br Dent J* **166**(1):14–16.

Martin MV, Longman LP, Hill JB, *et al* (1997) Acute dentoalveolar infections: an investigation of the duration of antibiotic therapy. *Br Dent J* **183**(4):135–137.

Matthews B, Sessle BJ (2000) Peripheral mechanisms of orofacial pain. In: Lund JP, Lavigne GJ, Dubner R, *et al* (eds) *Orofacial pain from Basic Science to Clinical Management*. Chicago: Quintessence, pp 37–46.

Matthews DC, Sutherland S, Basrani B (2003) Emergency management of acute apical abscesses in the permanent dentition: a systematic review of the literature. *J Can Dent Assoc* **69**(10):660.

Michaelson PL, Holland GR (2002) Is pulpitis painful? *Int Endod J* **35**(10):829–832.

Miller S, Truong T, Heu R, *et al* (1994) Recent advances in stannous fluoride technology: antibacterial efficacy and mechanism of action towards hypersensitivity. *Int Dent J* **44**(1 Suppl 1):83–98.

Mitchell RJ (1980) Variations in blood group frequencies in a single population: the Isle of Man. *Hum Biol* **52**(3):499–506.

Mumford JM (1982) *Orofacial Pain*, 3rd edn. Edinburgh: Churchill Livingstone.

Murray ME, Buckenham TM, Joseph AE (1996) The role of ultrasound in screening patients referred for sialography: a possible protocol. *Clin Otolaryngol Allied Sci* **21**(1):21–23.

Nagle D, Reader A, Beck M, *et al* (2000) Effect of systemic penicillin on pain in untreated irreversible pulpitis. *Oral Surg Oral Med Oral Pathol Oral Radiol Endod* **90**(5):636–640.

Nahlieli O, Shacham R, Bar T, *et al* (2003) Endoscopic mechanical retrieval of sialoliths. *Oral Surg Oral Med Oral Pathol Oral Radiol Endod* **95**(4):396–402.

Nahlieli O, Shacham R, Shlesinger M, *et al* (2004) Juvenile recurrent parotitis: a new method of diagnosis and treatment. *Pediatrics* **114**(1):9–12.

Narhi M, Jyväsjärvi E, Virtanen A, *et al* (1992) Role of intradental A- and C-type nerve fibres in dental pain mechanisms. *Proc Finn Dent Soc* **88**(Suppl 1):507–516.

Natah SS, Konttinen YT, Enattah NS, *et al* (2004) Recurrent aphthous ulcers today: a review of the growing knowledge. *Int J Oral Maxillofac Surg* **33**(3):221–234.

Newell DH, John V, Kim SJ (2002) A technique of occlusal adjustment for food impaction in the presence of tight proximal contacts. *Oper Dent* **27**(1):95–100.

Olgart LM (1985) The role of local factors in dentin and pulp in intradental pain mechanisms. *J Dent Res* 64 Spec No:572–578.

Opdam NJ, Roeters JM (2003) The effectiveness of bonded composite restorations in the treatment of painful, cracked teeth: six-month clinical evaluation. *Oper Dent* **28**(4):327–333.

Pau AK, Croucher R, Marcenes W (2003) Prevalence estimates and associated factors for dental pain: a review. *Oral Health Prev Dent* **1**(3):209–220.

Peltroche-Llacsahuanga H, Reichhart E, Schmitt W, *et al* (2000) Investigation of infectious organisms causing pericoronitis of the mandibular third molar. *J Oral Maxillofac Surg* **58**(6):611–616.

Poulsen S, Errboe M, Hovgaard O, *et al* (2001) Potassium nitrate toothpaste for dentine hypersensitivity. *Cochrane Database Syst Rev* (2):CD001476.

Robinson PA, High AS, Hume WJ (1992) Rapid detection of human herpes simplex virus type 1 in saliva. *Arch Oral Biol* **37**(10):797–806.

Rodd HD, Boissonade FM (2000) Substance P expression in human tooth pulp in relation to caries and pain experience. *Eur J Oral Sci* **108**(6):467–474.

Roz TM, Schiffman LE, Schlossberg S (2005) Spontaneous dissection of the internal carotid artery manifesting as pain in an endodontically treated molar. *J Am Dent Assoc* **136**(11): 1556–1559.

Saxen MA, Ambrosius WT, Rehemtula al KF, *et al* (1997) Sustained relief of oral aphthous ulcer pain from topical diclofenac in hyaluronan: a randomized, double-blind clinical trial. *Oral Surg Oral Med Oral Pathol Oral Radiol Endod* **84**(4):356–361.

Seltzer S (1978) *Pain Control in Dentistry – Diagnosis and Management*. Philadelphia: JB Lippincott.

Seltzer S, Bender IB, Ziontz M (1963) The dynamics of pulp inflammation: correlations between diagnostic data and actual histologic findings in the pulp. *Oral Surg Oral Med Oral Pathol* **16**:969–977.

Sessle BJ (2005) Peripheral and central mechanisms of orofacial pain and their clinical correlates. *Minerva Anestesiol* **71**(4): 117–136.

Sessle BJ, Bradley RM, Dubner R, *et al* (1979) Dental neuroscience. *New Dent* **10**(4):32–38.

Sharav Y (2005) Orofacial pain: how much is it a local phenomenon? *J Am Dent Assoc* **136**(4):432, 434, 436.

Sharav Y, Leviner E, Tzukert A, *et al* (1984) The spatial distribution, intensity and unpleasantness of acute dental pain. *Pain* **20**(4):363–370.

Sharav Y, Benoliel R, Schnarch A, *et al* (1991) Idiopathic trigeminal pain associated with gustatory stimuli. *Pain* **44**(2):171–174.

Sixou JL, Magaud C, Jolivet-Gougeon A, *et al* (2003) Microbiology of mandibular third molar pericoronitis: incidence of beta-lactamase-producing bacteria. *Oral Surg Oral Med Oral Pathol Oral Radiol Endod* **95**(6):655–659.

Steinhoff M, Vergnolle N, Young SH, *et al* (2000) Agonists of proteinase-activated receptor 2 induce inflammation by a neurogenic mechanism. *Nat Med* **6**(2):151–158.

Tal M, Sharav Y (1985) Development of sensory and reflex responses to tooth-pulp stimulation in children. *Arch Oral Biol* **30**(6):467–470.

Terai H, Shimahara M (2005) Atrophic tongue associated with Candida. *J Oral Pathol Med* **34**(7):397–400.

Trowbridge H, Kim S (1996) Pulp development structure and function. In: Cohen S, Burnse RC (eds) *Pathways of the Pulp*, 7th edn. St Louis: CV Mosby.

Tsai CC, Hong YC, Chen CC, *et al* (1998) Measurement of prostaglandin E2 and leukotriene B4 in the gingival crevicular fluid. *J Dent* **26**(2):97–103.

Tyldesley WR, Mumford JM (1970) Dental pain and the histological condition of the pulp. *Dent Pract Dent Rec* **20**(10):333–336.

Tzukert A, Hasin Y, Sharav Y (1981) Orofacial pain of cardiac origin. *Oral Surg Oral Med Oral Pathol* **51**(5):484–486.

Ushiyama J (1989) Gap junctions between odontoblasts revealed by transjunctional flux of fluorescent tracers. *Cell Tissue Res* **258**(3):611–616.

Van Hassel HJ, Harrington GW (1969) Localization of pulpal sensation. *Oral Surg Oral Med Oral Pathol* **28**(5):753–760.

van Steenberghe D (1979) The structure and function of periodontal innervation. A review of the literature. *J Periodontal Res* **14**(3):185–203.

Vergnolle N, Hollenberg MD, Sharkey KA, *et al* (1999) Characterization of the inflammatory response to proteinase-activated receptor-2 (PAR2)-activating peptides in the rat paw. *Br J Pharmacol* **127**(5):1083–1090.

Virtanen AS, Huopaniemi T, Narhi MV, *et al* (1987) The effect of temporal parameters on subjective sensations evoked by electrical tooth stimulation. *Pain* **30**(3):361–371.

von Troil B, Needleman I, Sanz M(2002) A systematic review of the prevalence of root sensitivity following periodontal therapy. *J Clin Periodontol* **29**(Suppl 3): 173–177; discussion 195-196.

Ylikontiola L, Sorsa T, Hayrinen-Immonen R, *et al* (1997) Doxymycine-cyanoacrylate treatment of recurrent aphthous ulcers. *Oral Surg Oral Med Oral Pathol Oral Radiol Endod* **83**(3):329–333.

Zhang C, Matsumoto K, Kimura Y, *et al* (1998) Effects of CO2 laser in treatment of cervical dentinal hypersensitivity. *J Endod* **24**(9):595–597.

CHAPTER 6

Otolaryngological aspects of orofacial pain

Menachem Gross and Ron Eliashar

1. Introduction

Orofacial pain is a relatively common complaint in both general medical and dental practice. Otolaryngologists are often involved when primary disorders of the ear, nose and throat, or head and neck are the source of pain. This chapter deals with the differential diagnosis of common painful disorders affecting the ears, sinonasal and facial area and the throat (see Tables 6.1, 6.2, 6.3).

2. Ear Pain

Earache or otalgia is quite common among both children and adults. It can vary from mild pain to an excruciating severe, dull, aching, or lancinating pain. Otalgia may be associated with sensations such as a sense of fullness in the ear, burning, throbbing, tenderness or itching. The exact incidence of otalgia is not known. Adults tend to suffer from fewer ear problems and less otalgia than children. Children are mostly affected, since acute otitis media (which is the most common cause of otalgia) occurs mainly in young people (Murtagh 1991).

Otalgia may be caused by several different medical conditions. Detailed history and physical examination with directed studies as indicated can clarify the source of the pain. Based on the resultant findings, the disease is classified as primary or secondary (referred) otalgia (Tables 6.1, 6.2).

Primary otalgia is due to a disease in the ear itself (a direct cause of earache) and the most serious problems are usually caused by infection. The areas most commonly involved in causing pain, or becoming infected, are the external ear and the middle ear. Pain in the external ear radiates most often to the vertex and to the temple, but may sometimes spread towards other areas of the head. Often patients cannot differentiate between pain originating in the inner ear and pain whose source is in the external or middle ear (Harvey 1992).

Secondary or referred otalgia (Table 6.2) is pain which stems from another region or location in the body and radiates to the ear (an indirect cause of earache). Because of the nature of the ear's sensory innervation a wide variety of disorders can produce referred otalgia. Branches of the trigeminal, facial, glossopharyngeal and vagus cranial nerves all participate, as well as the lesser occipital and the great auricular cervical nerve roots. The ear thus shares its sensory innervation with other head and neck structures, including the face, eyes, jaws, teeth, pharynx and larynx.

The incidence of referred otalgia increases with age. Up to 50% of cases suffering from otalgia are caused by referred pain from non-ear-related problems, whereas the other half are due to dental disorders (Yanagisawa and Kveton 1992). Diseased molars are the most common dental cause of secondary otalgia and cause severe unremitting pain which often worsens when cold fluids enter the oral cavity (see Chapter 5).

Muscular pain originating in the muscles, tendons or fascia of the head or neck such as myofascial pain and tension-type headache (Chapter 7) can also produce ear pain. The pain is constant, dull and aching and usually with no throbbing quality (Wazen 1989). Movement of the jaw or the head worsens the pain. Prolonged clenching the teeth, abnormal jaw movements and dental disease may cause a type of muscle spasm known as protective muscle splinting (Chapter 7).

Pharyngeal and laryngeal diseases cause referred otalgia via the glossopharyngeal nerve (Yanagisawa and Kveton 1992). Associated symptoms may include dysphagia, throat pain and breathing difficulty. Following recent tonsillectomy, patients virtually always complain of postoperative otalgia (Wazen 1989).

Persistent earache with a normal ear examination increases the suspicion of carcinoma, especially when associated with haemoptysis, weight loss, tooth pain or difficulty in swallowing (Thaller and DeSilva 1987). Otalgia is one of the earliest symptoms of carcinoma of the pyriform sinus, although neoplasia-producing otalgia may also be located in the larynx, oesophagus,

Table 6.1	Causes of Primary Otalgia	
Classification	**Condition**	**Comments for Entities Not Covered in This Chapter**
Auricular disorders	Auricular cellulitis	
	Auricular trauma	Injury to the ear may cause hyperaemia, abrasions, lacerations and auricular haematoma in cases of blunt trauma. The haematoma should be drained to relieve pain and to prevent abscess formation and auricular deformity such as 'cauliflower ear'.
	Relapsing polychondritis	
Disorders of the external ear	Impacted cerumen	Wax may obstruct the ear canal and may cause pain, itching and temporary hearing loss. Wax is removed by irrigation or by rolling it with a blunt curette or loop.
	Foreign object in the external ear	Insertion of foreign bodies such as beads, erasers and beans, is often by children. Foreign body should be removed by raking it out with a blunt hook.
	Furuncle of the external ear canal	
	Otitis externa	
	Necrotizing otitis externa	
	Ramsay Hunt syndrome (herpes zoster oticus)	
Disorders of the middle ear	Otitis media	
	Myringitis bullosa	
	Traumatic tympanic membrane rupture	The tympanic membrane may be perforated by objects placed in the external canal, by sudden overpressure, such as an explosion, a slap or diving, or by sudden negative pressure. This results in sudden severe pain followed by bleeding from the ear. Spontaneous closure of the perforation is usual. Persistent perforation is an indication for myringoplasty.
	Eustachian tube dysfunction	
	Barotrauma	

nasopharynx, lungs, tonsils or tongue (Wazen 1989; Harvey 1992; Nestor and Ngo 1994; Morgan *et al* 1995). Amundson (1990) stresses that unilateral ear pain in an adult who is a heavy smoker or a heavy drinker is probably caused by cancer until ruled out.

2.1. Common Diseases Causing Primary Otalgia

2.1.1. Auricular Cellulitis

Auricular cellulitis is a diffuse, spreading, acute infection of the auricular skin or subcutaneous structures, characterized by hyperaemia and oedema with no cellular necrosis or suppuration. The most common pathogen is *Streptococcus pyogenes* (Group-A, β-hemolytic streptococcus). *Staphylococcus aureus* occasionally causes superficial auricular cellulitis, which is less extensive than that of streptococcal origin. The infective process involves the entire auricle including the auricular lobule. The infection can occur spontaneously or following acute external otitis, chronic auricular dermatitis or trauma (such as auricular piercing). Primary treatment includes parenteral antibiotic therapy such as oxacillin or cefazolin.

2.1.2. Relapsing Polychondritis

Relapsing polychondritis (RP) is an episodic inflammatory condition of the cartilaginous and non-cartilaginous tissues that causes progressive destruction of the head and neck cartilages, predominantly those of the ear, nose and laryngotracheobronchial tree (Gergely *et al* 2004). Other affected structures may include the eye, the cardiovascular system, small and large peripheral joints and the middle and inner ear (Lucente *et al* 1995; Staats *et al* 2002; Gergely *et al* 2004). The aetiology is unknown; however, the pathogenesis is most likely autoimmune (Gergely *et al* 2004). Signs and symptoms of RP of the auricle include auricular cellulitis, typically with a sudden onset of unilateral or bilateral auricular pain, tenderness, swelling and redness, with sparing of the lobules. The pain and redness usually disappear within 2–4 weeks but may recur. A definitive diagnosis of RP is made by biopsy of the affected cartilaginous tissue that demonstrates infiltration of the cartilage and perichondrial tissues with neutrophils and lymphocytes and loss of cartilaginous matrix. Mild cases may respond to symptomatic treatment with aspirin, indomethacin or other nonsteroidal anti-inflammatory drugs (NSAIDs). Severe cases are initially treated with systemic corticosteroids with tapering of the dose in accordance with the clinical response. In very severe cases addition of an immunosuppressive agent such as cyclophosphamide is required.

Table 6.2 Causes of Secondary Otalgia

Classification	Condition	Comment
Dental problems	Infant teething Pain of eruption Impacted third molars (wisdom teeth) Dental infections in the upper back teeth Fractured tooth Dry socket following dental extraction Gingivitis and other periodontal disease	See Chapter 5
Infections	Upper respiratory tract infection	An acute usually viral infection of the respiratory tract with inflammation in the nose, throat, larynx and trachea. It is associated with watery nasal secretions, sore throat, cough and referred otalgia through glossopharyngeal nerve.
	Sinusitis	See section on facial pain in this chapter
	Infection of the throat: tonsillitis, pharyngitis, peritonsillar abscess	Covered under throat pain in this chapter
	Laryngitis	Acute viral inflammation of the larynx is associated with unnatural change of voice, throat pain and referred otalgia via the vagus nerve
	Salivary gland infection	See Chapter 5
Diseases of the joints and muscles of the lower jaw	Masticatory muscles disorders Temporomandibular joint (TMJ) dysfunction	See Chapter 7 See Chapter 8
Head and neck muscle spasms		See Chapter 7
The removal of tonsils	Post-tonsillectomy pain	Following tonsillectomy patients have throat pain and may feel a referred pain in one or both ears via the glossopharyngeal nerve. This pain vanishes within a few weeks.
Cervical spine problems		See Chapter 13
Inflammation of the blood vessels in the temple: temporal arteritis		See Chapter 13
Neuralgic disorders	Trigeminal neuralgia Glossopharyngeal neuralgia	See Chapter 11
	Arnold's nerve cough syndrome	Reflex cough, caused by chronic irritation of auricular branch of vagus (X) nerve. It is associated with attack of suboccipital stabbing or burning pain and auricular pain.
Cancer of the head or neck		See Chapters 13 and 14

2.1.3. Furuncle of the External Ear Canal

Furuncle of the external ear canal is an acute, tender, perifollicular inflammatory nodule resulting from infection by *S. aureus*. The initial nodule evolves into a pustule with central necrosis, which later discharges a sanguineous purulent exudate. A furuncle causes localized pain within the external auditory meatus, which is intensified by local pressure. Treatment includes surgical drainage of the furuncle, systemic antibiotic therapy with oxacillin or cefazolin.

2.1.4. Acute Otitis Externa

Acute otitis externa (AOE) is an infective condition involving the external ear canal usually caused by a Gram-negative rod such as *Pseudomonas aeruginosa* or *Escherichia coli*; however, *S. aureus* or, rarely, a fungus may also be causative agents (Sander 2001). Often this infection is predisposed by moisture in the external ear canal such as in warm-moist climates or after bathing. Injury caused by attempts to clean or scratch an itching ear as in patients suffering from contact dermatitis (from

Table 6.3 Differential Diagnosis of Facial Pain: Otolaryngologist's Viewpoint

Classification	Entity	Comment for Entities Not Covered in This Chapter
Sinonasal pain	Rhinosinusitis	
	Mucosal contact point headache	
	Intranasal tumour	Nasal obstruction and local nasal pain may occur as the intranasal tumour enlarges, especially if it invades nerves.
	Granulomatous diseases of the nose	Wegener's granulomatosis and sarcoidosis may affect the nasal cavity causing congestion, nasal secretions and local pain due to destructive lesions of soft tissue cartilage, and bone.
Midfacial segment pain		
Atypical facial pain	(recently renamed as persistent idiopathic facial pain)	See also Chapter 11
Scuba diving causing pain	Sinus pain Tension-type headache or muscle pain Carbon dioxide toxicity Decompression sickness headache	
Neuralgias	Trigeminal Sphenopalatine	See Chapter 11
Primary headaches	Tension headache Migraine Cluster headache Chronic paroxysmal hemicrania	See Chapter 7 See Chapter 9 See Chapter 10 See Chapter 10

earrings or earphones), allergic dermatitis or seborrheic dermatitis is another common cause (Hirsch 1992). A variant of AOE is 'swimmer's ear', a condition caused by a combination of external ear canal trauma and humidity during the swimming season (Agius *et al* 1992). Signs and symptoms of AOE include mild to severe otalgia associated with purulent discharge from the external ear canal. Auricular movement or pressure on the tragus intensifies the pain. The otalgia can become extreme as the canal swells and becomes

blocked. Appropriate treatment includes topical application of a combination of antibiotic and corticosteroid eardrops, instilled directly into the ear canal. Irrigation of the ear canal with either hydrogen peroxide or 70% alcohol can temporarily stop the pain and itching.

2.1.5. Necrotizing Otitis Externa

Necrotizing external otitis (NEO) is an infection which starts as an external otitis caused by *P. aeruginosa* and progresses into an osteomyelitis of the temporal bone (Sander 2001). This disease commonly occurs in elderly diabetic patients and occasionally in immunocompromised patients (Handzel and Halperin 2003). The disease spreads outside the external ear canal through the fissures of Santorini which are two slits located at the anterior cartilaginous external canal wall and the osseo-cartilaginous junction into the skull base. It is characterized by persistent severe otalgia, purulent otorrhea and granulation tissue in the external ear canal (Handzel and Halperin 2003). Pre-auricular and temporomandibular joint pain intensified by opening the mouth or by chewing may be present. Severe headache in the temporal or occipital areas may accompany the earache. The severity of the pain can give a clue to the diagnosis. In severe cases, facial nerve involvement may occur, indicating an invasive infection. Other cranial nerve palsies, such as IX, X, XI and XII, may also occur. Imaging evaluation by computed tomography (CT) usually demonstrates soft tissue infiltration and bone destruction (Guy *et al* 1991). Technetium[99] bone-scan is usually positive and is highly sensitive to NEO. Treatment includes good control of the diabetes and prolonged therapy with an anti-pseudomonal antibiotic such as ciprofloxacin for at least 6 weeks in addition to local therapy for the otitis externa. Surgical debridement through a mastoidectomy approach is occasionally required to control the spread of the infection.

2.1.6. Ramsay Hunt Syndrome (Herpes Zoster Oticus)

Ramsay Hunt Syndrome (RHS), also called herpes zoster oticus, is a herpes virus-3 infection (varicella-zoster virus infection which causes chickenpox and shingles) of the geniculate ganglion (facial nerve ganglion) (Kuhweide *et al* 2002). The virus spreads from the geniculate ganglion to the facial nerve and to the adjacent vestibulocochlear (XIII) nerve (Kuhweide *et al* 2002). The syndrome consists of unilateral facial paralysis, severe ear pain on the same side as the infection, tinnitus, vertigo and herpetic blistering rash or vesicles on the pinna, external canal and sometimes the roof of the mouth, in the distribution of the sensory branches of the facial nerve. Other cranial nerves may be involved and some degree of meningeal inflammation may occur (Ko *et al* 2000). RHS is usually more painful than Bell's palsy. It is rare in healthy people and occurs more commonly in people with a weakened immune system, such as the elderly (Burke *et al* 1982). Diagnosis of RHS is based on the clinical symptoms and signs. Prompt treatment with corticosteroids and antiviral medications such as acyclovir and famciclovir reduces the symptoms and improves recovery (Morrow 2000; Kinishi *et al* 2001). Overall, chances of recovery are better if treatment is started within 3 days of the onset of symptoms. Certain degrees of hearing loss or facial paralysis may become permanent (Morrow 2000). Recovery may be complicated if the nerve grows back to the wrong areas (synkinesis); this may cause inappropriate responses, such as tearing when laughing or chewing (crocodile's tears). Some may start blinking when talking or eating.

2.1.7. Acute Otitis Media

Acute otitis media (AOM) is an infection of the middle ear cavity. AOM occurs most frequently in infants and children, particularly between the ages of 3 months and 3 years, although it can occur at any age. AOM usually follows or accompanies an upper respiratory infection (URI) or a reduced immune response with no special reason. AOM is the second most common childhood disease after URI. The first complaint is usually persistent, severe otalgia, which is often caused by an accumulation of fluid and pressure behind the tympanic membrane (TM). Other symptoms include hearing loss, fever, chills, irritability and a feeling of fullness and pressure in the affected ear. Spontaneous drainage of pus or a clear or bloody fluid from the middle ear is common, and may indicate perforation of the TM. An otoscopic examination reveals abnormal findings of the TM, including an erythematous and bulging TM, middle ear effusion, non-distinct anatomical middle ear landmarks, displaced or absent TM light reflex and decreased TM mobility on pneumatic otoscopy. The most common bacterial pathogen in AOM is *Streptococcus pneumoniae*, followed by *Haemophilus influenzae* and *Moraxella catarrhalis*. These three organisms are responsible for more than 95% of all AOM cases with a bacterial aetiology. The most important factors in the pathogenesis of a middle ear infection are eustachian tube dysfunction and direct extension of infectious processes from the nasopharynx into the middle ear cleft. AOM is treated with painkillers and systemic antibiotics such as oral amoxicillin. Topical analgesics such as tetracaine applied by eardrops and nasal decongestants such as xylometazoline can be helpful. Antibiotic therapy relieves the symptoms, hastens resolution of the infection and reduces the chance for developing complications (such as mastoiditis or meningitis). Myringotomy (small incision of the TM) should be considered in cases of a bulging TM or a persistent earache.

2.1.8. Myringitis Bullosa

Myringitis bullosa (MB) is an inflammatory infection of the TM caused by a viral or a bacterial infection. *Mycoplasma pneumoniae* and *S. pneumoniae* are the most common bacteria responsible for MB. The disease is characterized by very painful vesicles on the tympanic membrane that may be full with a serous or haemorrhagic fluid. An upper respiratory tract infection can precede the ear manifestations. Pain is severe, starts suddenly, persists for 24–72 hours and is due to the TM blisters, which appear between the richly innervated outer epithelium and the middle fibrous layers of the TM (Woo *et al* 1992; Marais and Dale 1997). Bullae involving the TM may also extend towards portions of the external auditory canal immediately adjacent to the TM. Objective cochlear and vestibular involvement manifested by sensorineural or mixed-type hearing loss and vertigo have been reported in patients suffering from MB (Eliashar *et al* 2004). Treatment includes analgetic and antibiotic therapy such as azithromycin which is efficacious against the major known pathogens causing MB.

2.1.9. Eustachian Tube Dysfunction

The middle ear is connected to the nasopharynx by the eustachian tube (ET). The ET enables normal fluids to drain from the middle ear, and has an important role in equalizing the pressure in the middle ear when atmospheric pressure of ambient air shifts. Acute obstruction of the ET, mainly in cases of URI, may cause otalgia. This is especially common in small children, whose ET is naturally shorter and more horizontal. ET obstruction also occurs when there is an increase of postnasal drainage (PND) or allergy (Derebery and Berliner 1997; Grimmer and Poe 2005). As the PND drains posteriorly into the nasopharynx around the opening of the ET, it gets irritated and swollen and eventually becomes blocked on one or both sides. When this happens, surrounding tissue absorbs the air in the affected tube, creating a vacuum, which causes the differences in pressure to pull the tympanic membrane inward, the result being a sensation of fullness and pain. Hearing can be slightly impaired and the ears can feel blocked or stuffed. To improve ET function, topical vasoconstrictors such as xylometazoline may be instilled into each nasal cavity.

2.1.10. Barotrauma

Barotitis media (BM), also known as 'aerotitis', represents damage to the middle ear and tympanic membrane due to ambient pressure changes. When a sudden increase in the ambient pressure occurs, air must move from the nasopharynx into the middle ear in order to maintain equilibrium on both sides of the TM. In cases of eustachian tube dysfunction, the pressure in the middle ear is below the ambient pressure, and the relative negative pressure in the middle ear results in retraction of the TM and transudation of blood from vessels. Very severe and sudden pressure differences may rupture the TM, causing bleeding in the middle ear with severe earache and conductive hearing loss. A perilymphatic fistula through the oval or round windows can occur, causing sensorineural hearing loss and vertigo. Baro-trauma commonly occurs with altitude changes, such as in descent of an airplane, deep sea diving, scuba diving or driving in the mountains (Mirza and Richardson 2005). Otalgia is the most common complaint of scuba divers and is experienced at some point by almost every diver (Clenney and Lassen 1996). Some divers call it the 'ear squeeze'. A person with an acute URI or allergic rhinitis should be advised to abstain from diving. Topical application of a nasal vasoconstrictor such as xylometazoline before any activity associated with descent and pressure changes can prevent barotrauma.

3. Facial Pain

Facial and sinus pain complaints are commonly encountered by physicians. Facial pain is usually referred to otolaryngology, dental, and neurologic clinics, and often needs a multidisciplinary evaluation. Facial pain is located in the area below the eyebrows or the supraorbital rims, extending along the course of one or more trigeminal dermatomes. Headaches are located in the forehead and temporal regions. Facial pain may be due to either local disease of any one of the major facial structures or a condition affecting their innervation. The latter can occur anywhere between the posterior cranial fossa and the distal ends of the trigeminal nerve. The prevalence of facial pain of paranasal sinus origin has probably been overestimated. Patients' expectations are often tempered by their own prior diagnosis of 'sinusitis' guided by their knowledge of the location of the sinuses, or by their primary-care physician. However, many of these patients are found to have no evidence of sinonasal disease and there is an increasing awareness among general physicians and otolaryngologists that neurological causes are responsible for most of the suffering experienced by patients with facial pain or headache. The 'gold standard' in establishing a sinonasal aetiology is a diagnosis made after a personal history, a careful physical examination, imaging studies, response to medical and surgical treatment and an extended follow-up period. Patients who undergo normal nasal endoscopy or CT scan are often found to suffer from a range of neurological causes (West and Jones 2001). When the ostia of the sinuses are found to be patent and the mucosa healthy, the probability that a sinonasal disease or an anatomic variation is the cause of pain is eliminated (West and Jones 2001).

3.1. Common Diseases Causing Facial Pain

3.1.1. Sinonasal Disorders Causing Pain: The Neurobiology of Primary Sinonasal Pain

The trigeminal nerve is the main facial sensory supply. The ophthalmic (V1) and maxillary (V2) divisions of the trigeminal nerve provide sensation to the mucosa of the sinonasal cavity. These nerve branches terminate as extensive uncovered nerve terminal endings next to the basal cells of the nasal epithelium (Baraniuk 2001). Nasal pain is mediated by Aδ fibres—the fast-responding, primarily mechanoreceptive pain fibres—and by C fibres—the slower, unmyelinated fibres associated with a duller pain from mechanothermal and chemosensory stimulation (Baraniuk 2001). Recent theories of sinonasal pain from 'contact points' or pressure from sinus inflammation are based upon substance P (SP) release from trigeminal sensory neurons located in the nasal mucosa (Stammberger and Wolf 1988; Chow 1994; Clerico 1995; Clerico et al 1997). This may be accompanied by the release of various other neuropeptides such as calcitonin gene-related peptide (CGRP) and vasoactive intestinal peptide (VIP), which appear to be involved in the inflammatory cascade (Baraniuk 2001). The local stimulation of the trigeminal fibres leads to both a painful orthodromic and an antidromic response, typified by vasodilatation and hypersecretion (Stammberger and Wolf 1988; Baraniuk 2001). Despite this frequently cited mechanism for contact point sinonasal pain, it is poorly documented and highly controversial (Abu-Bakra and Jones 2001a,b; Jones 2004).

3.1.2. Rhinosinusitis

Rhinosinusitis is a group of disorders characterized by inflammation of the mucosa of the nose and paranasal sinuses. The term 'rhinosinusitis' is used instead of 'sinusitis' due to the fact that sinusitis is almost always accompanied by concurrent nasal airway inflammation, and in many cases, sinusitis is preceded by rhinitis. Rhinosinusitis is a leading healthcare problem which may affect up to 14% of the adult population and costs more than $2 billion in direct medical costs (Anand et al 1997). Rhinosinusitis is increasing in prevalence and incidence and has been estimated to affect approximately 31 million patients in the United States each year (International Rhinosinusitis Advisory Board 1997).

A common presenting symptom of acute rhinosinusitis is facial pain or headache. The pain is usually accompanied by other symptoms such as nasal congestion, anterior and posterior purulent nasal drainage and hyposmia or anosmia. The pain is a subjective complaint; however, tenderness on percussion is a function of spinal cord pain processing (hyperalgesia). People with acute rhinosinusitis have a significantly lower pain and sensory detection threshold in their sinus regions when compared to a healthy control group (Meltzer et al 2004; Benoliel et al 2006). Sinus pain caused by inflammation induced by infection (bacterial or viral) or allergic rhinosinusitis occurs when exudate blocks the sinus ostium and exerts pressure which stimulates local trigeminal nerve fibres. The local release of proinflammatory and proalgesic mediators is an early mechanism (this is probably as important as the pressure).

The development of rhinosinusitis depends on a variety of environmental and host factors and is considered to be a disease with multifactorial causes. Host factors include genetic or congenital conditions (e.g. cystic fibrosis, immotile cilia syndrome), allergic rhinitis, sinonasal anatomic abnormalities and systemic diseases. Environmental factors include infectious agents, trauma, noxious chemicals and iatrogenic causes.

There are two principal systems of classification and diagnostic criteria relating headaches and sinus disease: the working definitions for acute rhinosinusitis (ARS), subacute rhinosinusitis (SRS) and chronic rhinosinusitis (CRS) recommended by the American Academy of Otolaryngology-Head and Neck Surgery (AAO-HNS), and the International Headache Society (IHS) criteria (Lanza and Kennedy 1997; Benninger *et al* 2003; Meltzer *et al* 2004; Olesen *et al* 2004). As expected the IHS classification relates to diseases that may induce facial pain or headache whilst the AAO-HNS classification is concerned primarily with the disease process itself.

The different types of rhinosinusitis can be diagnosed clinically in most patients based on the history and physical examination. Physical examination includes otoscopy, anterior rhinoscopy, percussion over the areas of the paranasal sinuses and oropharyngeal and neck examination. Nasal endoscopy and imaging evaluation are not required for an initial diagnosis of any form of rhinosinusitis. However, these modalities may be very helpful in definitive diagnosis of rhinosinusitis. Patients with recurrent or complicated sinus disease may require imaging. Computerized tomography is superior to radiography because the latter are imprecise at determining the extent of the disease and the patency of the sinus ostium (Lanza and Kennedy 1997; Sinus and Allergy Health Partnership 2004). CT scanning of the sinonasal region has two major roles in rhinosinusitis:

1. To define the anatomy of the sinuses before surgery; and
2. To aid in the diagnosis and management of CRS or recurrent rhinosinusitis.

3.1.3. Acute Rhinosinusitis

Acute rhinosinusitis is an inflammatory condition involving the paranasal sinuses and the lining of the nasal passages, where the symptoms and signs last up to 4 weeks (Lanza and Kennedy 1997) (see Tables 6.4, 6.5). The symptoms resolve completely, and after the disease has been treated, antibiotics are no longer required.

The most common cause of ARS is a community-acquired viral infection leading to a self-limiting period of upper respiratory symptoms, such as nasal discharge, nasal congestion and coughing (Meltzer *et al* 2004). Human rhinovirus is the most common cause of viral ARS. Other viruses include coronavirus, influenza A and B virus,

Table 6.4	Clinical Criteria for the Diagnosis of Acute Rhinosinusitis (ARS)	
	Criteria	**Comments**
Major factors:	Purulent anterior nasal discharge Purulent-discoloured posterior nasal drainage Nasal obstruction or blockage Facial pain/pressure/ congestion/fullness Hyposmia or anosmia Fever	A diagnosis of rhinosinusitis is possible if: (a) 2 or more major symptoms or (b) 1 major symptom and 2 or more minor symptoms are present.
Minor factors:	Headache Ear pain/pressure/ fullness Halitosis Dental pain Cough Fever (all non-acute) Fatigue	Nasal purulence in itself is a strong indicator of an accurate diagnosis. Headache/facial pain or pressure as sole symptoms is not indicative of ARS. Similarly fever as a sole symptom is not indicative of ARS.

Table 6.5	The IHS Criteria for the Diagnosis of Headache/Facial Pain due to Rhinosinusitis	
	Diagnostic Criteria	**Comment**
A	Frontal headache accompanied by pain in one or more regions of the face, ears or teeth and fulfilling criteria C and D	
B	Clinical, nasal endoscopy, computerized tomography and/or magnetic resonance imaging, and/or laboratory evidence of acute or acute-on-chronic rhinosinusitis	Clinical evidence includes purulent nasal discharge, nasal obstruction, hyposmia or anosmia and/ or fever
C	Headache and facial pain develop simultaneously with onset or acute exacerbation of rhinosinusitis	
D	Headache and/or facial pain resolve within 7 days after remission or successful treatment of acute or acute-on-chronic rhinosinusitis	Chronic sinusitis is not validated as a cause of headache or facial pain unless there is re-acutization.

parainfluenza virus, respiratory syncytial virus and adenovirus. Occasionally, a secondary bacterial infection of the paranasal sinuses occurs and requires specific antimicrobial therapy (Meltzer *et al* 2004). Allergic rhinitis, nasal polyposis, foreign body in the nasal cavity, trauma, dental infection and other factors leading to inflammation of the nose and paranasal sinuses can also predispose individuals to develop ARS.

Commonly isolated bacteria in patients with ARS include *S. pneumonia*, non-typeable *H. influenzae* and *M. catarrhalis* (Sinus and Allergy Health Partnership 2004). *Streptococcus pneumonia* and non-typeable *H. influenzae* account for more than 75% of bacterial isolates (Meltzer *et al* 2004). Other streptococcal species, anaerobic bacteria and *S. aureus* are responsible for a small percentage of cases. Nosocomial rhinosinusitis often occurs in patients who require extended periods of intensive care, which involve prolonged nasotracheal intubation or a nasogastric tube. Isolates from hospitalized patients usually contain Gram-negative enterics such as *P. aeruginosa*, *Klebsiella pneumoniae*, *Enterobacter* spp., *Proteus mirabilis*, *Serratia marcescens*, and coagulase-negative *S. aureus* (Meltzer *et al* 2004).

The diagnosis of ARS focuses on clinical history and physical examination with radiographic diagnosis playing a supportive role (Sinus and Allergy Health Partnership 2004). The clinical diagnostic criteria for ARS as defined by the Task Force on Rhinosinusitis of the AAO-HNS include major and minor symptoms or signs, with a disease duration of less than 4 weeks (Table 6.4). According to this classification, facial pain or pressure is regarded as a major symptom, whereas headache is considered to be a minor symptom (Lanza and Kennedy 1997; Meltzer *et al* 2004). This classification was designed to be used by both primary care physicians and specialists. A diagnosis of rhinosinusitis is possible if two or more major symptoms or one major symptom and two or more minor symptoms are present. However, nasal purulence is a strong indicator of an accurate diagnosis. Facial pain or pressure alone does not constitute a suggestive history in the absence of another major nasal symptom or sign. Fever in itself does not constitute a strongly suggestive history in the absence of another major nasal symptom or sign. The IHS diagnostic criteria for sinusitis-related headache reiterate the requirement of clinical findings of acute sinusitis, along with a reversible 'sinus headache'; see Table 6.5 (Olesen *et al* 2004).

ARS has four basic clinical courses: resolution, development of adverse sequelae, development of a symptomatic CRS and development of a silent CRS.

In the immunocompetent person living in the general community, ARS is typically believed to be induced by viruses and does not require antibiotics for the first 10–14 days. Symptomatic relief may be obtained by the use of topical application of a nasal decongestant such as xylometazoline and oral acetaminophen. The presence of severe headache or facial pain, high fever, and brain, eye or lung complications indicate secondary bacterial infection and antibiotics are indicated (Meltzer *et al* 2004).

In cases where no complications occur but the symptoms and signs persist for more than 10–14 days, bacteria are presumed to predominate and the patient can benefit from initiating antibiotic therapy as described below (Meltzer *et al* 2004).

Expert recommendation is divided about the appropriate therapy for ARS and ranges from symptomatic treatment alone (Snow *et al* 2001) to a prolonged course of antibiotic therapy effective against β-lactamase-producing organisms (Winther and Gwaltney 1990). Primary care and specialty physicians demonstrate variability in treatment approaches (Piccirillo *et al* 2001). No benefit for antibiotic therapy has been demonstrated for the treatment of ARS diagnosed by clinical criteria alone (Stalman *et al* 1997) and one study showed no overall benefit for seven days of penicillin V compared to placebo (Hansen *et al* 2000). However, there are indications that early antibiotics are of benefit for patients with the most severe maxillofacial pain symptoms at baseline (Williams *et al* 2003). Success rates for amoxicillin, trimethoprim-sulfamethoxazole or erythromycin compared to newer, broader spectrum antibiotics are similar (Piccirillo *et al* 2001). Therefore, current data do not support the use of newer, more expensive, non-penicillin antibiotics for first-line empiric therapy (Williams *et al* 2003). Among the newer, wider-spectrum antibiotics efficacy was similar but amoxicillin-clavulanate had significantly more adverse effects than cephalosporins (Williams *et al* 2003). Therefore, differences in adverse effects and costs should be considered when choosing a second-line antimicrobial therapy. Based on a meta-analysis, ARS should be treated with amoxicillin 500 mg three times daily for 10 days (Williams *et al* 2003). For penicillin-allergic patients, several cephalosporins and macrolides have been shown to be equivalent to amoxicillin (Williams *et al* 2003). Based on limited data, there is no convincing evidence that adjuvant treatment such as topical nasal decongestants or nasal corticosteroids improve clinical outcomes.

3.1.3.1. Acute Maxillary Rhinosinusitis

Acute maxillary rhinosinusitis is the most common affliction of all paranasal sinuses and the most common sinus disease causing facial pain (Fig. 6.1). The pain is usually

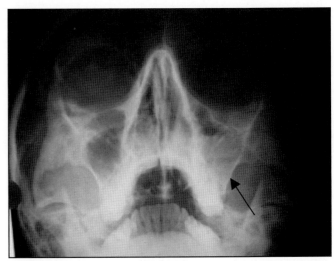

Fig. 6.1 • Plain film demonstrating left acute maxillary rhinosinusitis with air-fluid level in the left maxillary sinus (arrow).

related to the affected maxillary antrum, but is often referred to the upper teeth (whose roots are intimately related to the floor of the maxillary sinus, see Fig. 6.3) or to the forehead. Purulent nasal discharge in the middle nasal meatus and sensitivity to percussion over the cheek or teeth confirm the diagnosis.

3.1.3.2. Sinonasal Toothache

Diseases in the maxillary sinus mucosa may refer pain to the upper teeth. The pain is usually felt in several teeth as dull, aching or throbbing. Occasionally, the pain is associated with pressure below the eyes. It increases when bending the head, applying pressure over the sinuses, coughing or sneezing. Tests performed on the teeth, such as applying ice, chewing and percussion, may increase pain from a sinonasal origin. A history of URI, nasal congestion or other sinus problem is suspicious of a sinus toothache. Thorough dental examination (clinical and radiographic) excludes a primary dental cause.

3.1.3.3. Acute Ethmoiditis

Acute ethmoiditis causes pain at the root of the nose or behind the eye. Seldom does ethmoiditis occur as an isolated infection. More often it is part of an acute pansinusitis involving the maxillary and frontal sinuses as well. Purulent anterior and posterior nasal discharge and tenderness over the inner canthus of the eye are characteristic. The pain may spread laterally into the orbit or radiate to the temporal region. Occasionally, an orbital complication (such as periorbital cellulitis or abscess) may occur due to spreading of the infection into the orbit through the thin lamina papyracea.

3.1.3.4. Acute Frontal Rhinosinusitis

Acute suppurative frontal rhinosinusitis is not very common, apparently because of the vertical nature of the frontal sinus and its natural advantage of a dependent drainage through the nasofrontal duct (Fig. 6.2). Thus, the common forehead pain is seldom due to an underlying frontal rhinosinusitis.

The characteristic pain is over the affected sinus and often along the upper orbital rim. The pain may radiate to the vertex and behind the eye. Tenderness is usually felt in the frontal sinus or along its floor. When frontal sinusitis is complicated by osteomyelitis of the frontal bone, the pain is prominent, diffuse and intense, often worsening at night keeping the patient awake.

3.1.3.5. Acute Sphenoiditis

Acute sphenoiditis is rare and is characterized by a wide variety of types and distributions of pain. These include severe occipital headache, retro-orbital dull and aching pain and a stabbing pain at the vertex. Definitive diagnosis is by CT scan.

3.1.3.6. Subacute Rhinosinusitis

Subacute rhinosinusitis represents a continuum of the natural progression of ARS which has not resolved. SRS is diagnosed after 4 weeks duration of symptoms or signs

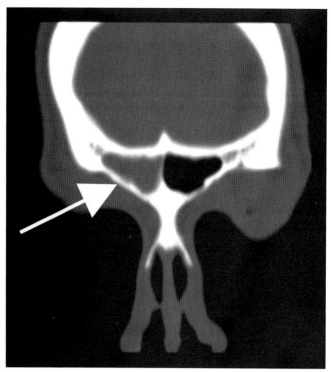

Fig. 6.2 • Coronal CT scan demonstrating right acute frontal rhinosinusitis with opacification of the right frontal sinus (arrow).

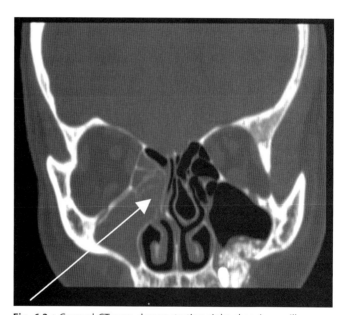

Fig. 6.3 • Coronal CT scan demonstrating right chronic maxillary rhinosinusitis with complete opacification of the right maxillary sinus and obstruction of the sinus ostium (arrow).

of rhinosinusitis, and lasts up to 12 weeks (Lanza and Kennedy 1997).

3.1.4. Chronic Rhinosinusitis

Chronic rhinosinusitis is divided into two major categories, including CRS with nasal polyposis (CRSwNP) and CRS with no nasal polyposis. The clinical diagnostic criteria suggested by the AAO-HNS for CRS include major and minor symptoms or signs, with disease duration of 12 weeks or more; see Table 6.6 (Lanza and Kennedy 1997; Meltzer *et al* 2004).

Symptoms of CRS are generally the same as those of ARS. However, they are usually milder and include only one symptom such as postnasal drip, headache, nasal obstruction or facial pain. CRS has not been defined as a cause of headache or facial pain according to the IHS diagnostic criteria, unless relapsing into an acute stage (Olesen *et al* 2004). The most recent otolaryngologic literature regarding CRS includes 'facial pain and pressure' as a major factor in CRS, with 'headache' as a minor factor, but suggests that facial pain and pressure or headache alone are not suggestive of CRS in the absence of other major nasal symptoms or signs (Lanza 2004). Other causes of headache or facial pain should be considered in the differential diagnosis of such cases.

Bacterial infection as a causative factor in patients with CRS is controversial, but is regarded as a relatively important factor. A comparatively new hypothesis regarding the pathogenesis of CRS is related to colonization of the sinonasal mucosa with microorganisms such as superantigen-producing *S. aureus*, colonizing fungi, or biofilms, and the host response to their presence (Meltzer *et al* 2004). A recent study has shown increased sensory thresholds in the skin over sinuses diagnosed with CRS, suggesting some form of peripheral nerve damage (Benoliel *et al* 2006).

CRS has four basic clinical courses: resolution, persistence, development of adverse sequelae and progression to generalized airway reactivity.

CRS is predominantly a medical condition where surgery can relieve symptoms and sometimes bring about a reversal in the course of the disease.

Table 6.6	Clinical Criteria for the Diagnosis of Chronic Rhinosinusitis (CRS)	
	Criteria	**Comments**
Major factors	Nasal obstruction Facial congestion Facial pain/pressure/fullness Nasal discharge (anterior/posterior purulent discharge) Loss of smell	Symptoms of CRS are milder than in the acute form. CRS may present with only one symptom such as postnasal drip, headache/facial pain or nasal obstruction.
Minor factors	Fatigue Headache Ear pain/pressure Cough Halitosis Dental pain Fever	Note, however, that according to the IHS CRS has not been validated as a cause of headache/facial pain.

3.1.4.1. Chronic Maxillary Rhinosinusitis

The most characteristic symptom of this condition is persistent purulent rhinorrhea with localization of pus in the middle meatus (Fig. 6.3). CRS in the maxillary sinus seldom gives rise to facial pain or headache, except during an episode of acute exacerbation or with progression towards maxillary pyocele or maxillary osteomyelitis.

3.1.4.2. Chronic Frontal Rhinosinusitis

Pain is seldom a symptom of CRS of the frontal sinus. This condition is usually part of chronic pansinusitis which involves the ethmoid and maxillary sinuses, the most common symptom being chronic purulent nasal discharge.

3.1.5. Mucosal Contact Point Pain

Stammberger and Wolf (1988) postulated that variations in the anatomy of the nasal cavity result in mucus stasis, infection and ultimately facial pain (Stammberger and Wolf 1988). They also stated that mucosal contact points could result in the release of substance P, a recognized neuropeptide and transmitter in nociceptive fibres. Other authors have adopted this concept to explain how pain might be induced by anatomical variants such as a concha bullosa (a pneumatized middle turbinate) or a pneumatized superior turbinate touching the septum (Morgenstein and Krieger 1980; Blaugrund 1989; Goldsmith *et al* 1993; Clerico and Fieldman 1994; Clerico 1996). According to the IHS, the assumptions related to certain otolaryngologic conditions often considered to induce headaches have not been sufficiently validated. These include deviation of the nasal septum, hypertrophy of turbinates and atrophy of sinus membranes. However, mucosal contact point pain is defined in the IHS appendix; see Table 6.7 (Olesen *et al* 2004).

3.2. Midfacial Segment Pain

Midfacial segment pain (MSP) may have all the same pain characteristics as tension headache, but affects the face and may involve the nasion, under the bridge of the nose, either side of the nose, the periorbital region, the retroorbital region or across the cheeks (Jones 2004). The forehead is often affected as well. It is described as a dull ache, a feeling of pressure or tightness. Some patients may feel that their nose is blocked although they have no nasal airway obstruction. The forehead and occipital region are affected simultaneously in approximately 60% of patients (Jones 2004). There are no consistent exacerbating or relieving factors. The pain can be chronic or episodic, and the skin and soft tissues over the forehead or cheek may be sensitive. Nasal endoscopy and CT scan of the paranasal sinuses are normal. MSP is the commonest cause of non-rhinologic facial pain seen in otolaryngological practice.

The aetiology of MSP is uncertain and may be myofascial or neurovascular in origin. However, Olesen's theory,

Table 6.7	Proposed IHS Diagnostic Criteria for Mucosal Contact Point Headache

Criteria	Comments
A Intermittent pain localized to the periorbital and medial canthal or temporozygomatic regions and fulfilling criteria C and D.	This is a new addition to the IHS appendix and is not completely validated.
B Clinical, endoscopic and/or CT imaging evidence of mucosal contact points without acute rhinosinusitis.	
C Evidence that the pain can be attributed to mucosal contact based on at least one of the following: 1. The pain corresponds to gravitational changes in mucosal congestion as the patient moves between upright and recumbent postures. 2. Abolition of pain within 5 minutes after diagnostic topical application of local anaesthesia to the middle turbinate using placebo or other controls.	Abolition as defined in criteria C2 means complete pain relief with a visual analogue score of 0.
D Pain resolves within 7 days, and does not recur, after surgical removal of mucosal contact points.	

which integrates the effects of myofascial afferents, the activation of peripheral nociceptors and their convergence on the caudal nucleus of the trigeminal nerve, along with qualitative changes in the central nervous system, provides one of the best models (Olesen 1991; Jensen and Olesen 2000). The treatment of choice in this condition is amitriptyline for a period of 6 months (Jones 2004).

3.3. Atypical Facial Pain (Persistent Idiopathic Facial Pain)

Atypical facial pain (AFP) is characterized by deep, achy, ill-defined, pulling or crushing pain, involving diffuse areas of the face in the territory of the trigeminal nerve. This term has recently been changed by the IHS to persistent idiopathic facial pain; see also Chapter 11. The pain fluctuates in intensity and severity. Occasionally, patients use terms such as 'sharp' or 'knifelike' to describe the pain. The pain often worsens at night, and can be aggravated by activity. Sometimes pain is

continuous. In the majority of cases, only one side of the face is affected, but pain on both sides is also possible. The pain may move from one part of the face to another, and may be accompanied by complaints such as 'mucus moving' in the sinuses (Jones 2004). Interestingly, the pain often crosses the recognized neurological dermatomes. AFP is more common in women over the age of 40.

In some AFP cases the symptoms may initially appear similar to trigeminal neuralgia, but they progress towards an AFP pattern. Whereas trigeminal neuralgia is characterized by quick episodes of jabbing or lancinating pain, AFP attacks always last longer than a few seconds, usually minutes or hours (see Chapters 11 and 13). Moreover, no trigger points on the face are detected in AFP. Many patients suffering from AFP show a significant psychological disturbance or a history of depression, and are unable to function normally as a result of the pains (Jones 2004). AFP usually has no specific cause. However, injury of any peripheral or proximal branch of the trigeminal nerve due to facial trauma or skull base fracture can produce this disorder. This possibility is extensively discussed in Chapter 13.

Medical treatment of AFP is often difficult and less satisfactory than treatment of trigeminal neuralgia. The treatment of choice is amitriptyline for a period of 6 months (see Chapters 11 and 16). Conventional analgesic drugs, including opioids, can also be effective with selected individuals, often accompanied by a comprehensive pain management programme.

3.4. Scuba Diving Facial Pain

Diving pain has spoiled the diving vacation of many scuba divers. Several causes have been associated with pain and diving.

Sinus pain. Sinus barotraumas, also known as 'sinus squeeze', is due to failure to equalize pressure during descent. Pressurized air cannot be forced into the sinuses. The air within the sinus contracts and causes the walls of the sinus to bleed. This is accompanied by intense, sharp pain. Common causes of sinus barotraumas include allergic rhinitis, vasomotor rhinitis, nasal deformity, nasal polyposis, acute URI and chronic irritation (such as smoking, diesel fumes, chemicals and prolonged use of decongestant nasal drops). Symptoms include pain in the area of the affected sinus or in the upper teeth (when the maxillary sinus is involved) and nose bleeding. The frontal sinuses are the most frequently affected, because the nasofrontal duct draining the frontal sinus is longer and more tortuous. A 'reverse squeeze' occurs during ascent, when air in the sinus expands without any ability to escape and is extremely painful. The situation is self-limiting, because air is gradually absorbed into the tissues lining the sinuses. When a sinus squeeze occurs, a slow ascent to the surface that generally alleviates most of the pain is recommended. Because the sinus may be filled with blood, the patient is at high risk of developing consequent sinusitis. Antibiotic therapy along with oral and nasal topical decongestants to promote drainage is recommended. Persistence of severe pain with no signs of acute rhinosinusitis may be treated by a short course of steroids. Diving is not recommended for patients with URI.

Tension-type headache. Symptoms of a tension-type headache include headache and pain in the nape (see Chapter 7). Tension headaches may be caused by muscle strain due to anxiety and muscular rigidity. To prevent the development of muscle strain, and consequently a tension headache, divers must learn to adopt a proper posture and relax in the water.

Carbon dioxide toxicity. A dull throbbing headache after diving is usually caused by carbon dioxide toxicity. This type of pain is common in divers and is caused by an accumulation of carbon dioxide in the body. Hypoventilation usually happens when a scuba diver does not inhale long deep breaths from the air tank, or not often enough. The best therapy for this type of headache is slow, deep breaths in order to reduce the carbon dioxide retention. Carbon dioxide-induced headaches do not respond well to pain relievers.

Decompression sickness headache. Headaches can be a symptom of decompression sickness (DCS). DCS is caused by the formation of bubbles when dissolved nitrogen is discharged from the tissues on ascent. Associated symptoms include joint pain and swelling, skin rash, itching, dizziness, nausea, vomiting, tinnitus (ringing inside the ears) and extreme exhaustion. A scuba diver is at a higher risk of DCS when he does not decompress after a long or deep dive, before surfacing, or when he ascends too quickly or makes a panic ascent.

3.5. Sphenopalatine Neuralgia

Sphenopalatine neuralgia (SPN) also known as 'Sluder's neuralgia' is characterized by a unilateral headache behind the eyes with pain in the upper jaw or soft palate (Sluder 1910, 1913; Ahamed and Jones 2003). Pain in the back of the nose, teeth, temple, occiput or neck may also occur. The pain is associated with sinonasal congestion, swelling of the nasal mucous membranes, tearing and redness of the face (Ahamed and Jones 2003). SPN is more common in women, with the ratio being 2:1. SPN should be distinguished from a cluster headache, although both are characterized by similar symptoms. However, SPN pain lasts longer and is associated with inflamed nasal mucosa on the involved side. SPN is evidently caused by an irritation of the sphenopalatine ganglion from intranasal infection, deformity or scarring. A topical decongestant may occasionally alleviate the nasal symptoms. Ganglion blocks (either by intranasal application or by direct injection) are effective for controlling the pain (Puig *et al* 1998; Day 1999).

3.6. Migraine and Sinus Headache

The IHS classification system lists operational diagnostic criteria for migraine as shown in Chapter 9 (Olesen *et al* 2004). Migraine is a common cause of headache or facial pain. Despite the high prevalence of migraine, over 50% of migraineurs remain undiagnosed by their physicians (Lipton *et al* 2001). Recent publications have stated that 'sinus' headache patients, at least those with no obvious signs of infection, have a 58–88% incidence of a migraine-type headache (Perry *et al* 2004; Schreiber *et al* 2004). Migraine can cause similar symptoms to rhinosinusitis, such as facial pain, nasal congestion and rhinorrhea. This form of migraine has been termed 'facial migraine' and is discussed further in Chapter 9.

A certain proportion of the patients attending an ENT clinic suffer from some facial pain resulting from migraine. In some clinical studies, 90% of self- or physician-diagnosed sinus headaches met the criteria of IHS migraine-type headache and were treated satisfactorily by anti-migraine treatments (Cady and Schreiber 2004). A recent prospective evaluation of 100 sequential patients who complained of sinus headaches demonstrated that 86% of patients had migraine or 'probable migraine', and only 3% had actual ARS-related headaches (Mudgil *et al* 2002).

The reason for the high rate of sinus headache patients misdiagnosed by their physicians is related to the pathophysiology of migraine and to the nature of nasal pain. The neurovascular theory of migraine implicates the nervous system as being the initiator of the process, and the blood vessel involvement occurring as a consequence of the neuronal process. This migraine model identifies the starting point in the central nervous system followed by a sensitization of the peripheral neurons of the trigeminal nerve, including those which supply sensation to the meninges. When the peripheral early phase is not treated in time, central sensitization at the level of the caudal nucleus of the trigeminal nerve occurs, with concomitant repetitive firing of the involved neurons, and pain in the distribution of the ophthalmic (V1) and/or maxillary branch (V2) of the trigeminal nerve. These nerves also provide sensation to the mucosa of the sinonasal cavity and are involved in the neurobiology of primary sinonasal pain. The early sensitization phase is accompanied by cutaneous allodynia (pain induced by stimulation which is normally non-painful) in the majority of patients (80%), and often occurs in the distribution of V1 and V2 (Cady and Schreiber 2004). This may include stimulation of the nose, such as while breathing cold air. A migraine attack may include secondary nasal symptoms, which are probably mediated by stimulation of the parasympathetic nervous system via the superior salivatory nucleus of the facial nerve (VII); this reflex activation is extensively discussed in Chapters 9 and 10. A report on patients with sinus headaches which fulfil the migraine criteria demonstrated that 84% reported sinus pressure,

82% sinus pain, 63% nasal congestion, 40% rhinorrhea, 38% watery eyes and 27% 'itchy' nose (Schreiber *et al* 2004). Occasionally, sinonasal disease or nasal allergy can play a role in triggering migraine which may respond to nasal steroids or to leukotriene antagonists (Cady and Schreiber 2004). The appearance of 'neurogenic rhinitis' along with a sinus headache in patients with migraine is often misunderstood and contributes to misdiagnosis.

The duration of a sinus headache and sinus symptoms is important for differentiating ARS from a migraine attack. In contrast to ARS, a migraine headache typically resolves within 72 hours. Bacterial ARS pain typically worsens after 5–7 days and is usually associated with hyposmia or anosmia, fever, cough, maxillary dental pain and ear fullness or pressure. The diagnostic features of facial migraine are primarily based on the patient's history and on the features reminiscent of typical migraine headaches as defined by the IHS (see Chapter 9).

4. Throat Pain

Throat pain or a sore throat is a common symptom. It is described as pain, discomfort or raw feeling of the throat, especially when swallowing. The vast majority of sore throats are caused by viral infections of the pharynx or tonsils. Many people experience a mild sore throat at the beginning of a common cold. The differential diagnosis of sore throat also includes various diseases of the oropharynx.

4.1. Acute Pharyngitis

Acute pharyngitis (AP) is an infection of the pharynx, which may involve the tonsils. AP may be a part of a generalized URI, or it may be a specific localized infection inside the pharynx. The most common cause of AP is a viral infection, but it can also be caused by a bacterial infection, such as group A *Streptococcus*, *M. pneumoniae* and *Chlamydia pneumoniae*. The viruses causing viral pharyngitis are highly contagious and tend to spread quickly, especially during the winter season. Throat symptoms include soreness, scratchiness or irritation. Associated symptoms include fever and discomfort with swallowing or odynophagia. Fever is more prominent in young children than in adults. Most viral pharyngitis cases are accompanied by a flu or cold, along with a stuffy runny nose, sneezing and generalized aches such as arthralgia and muscle pain. Nonproductive cough and hoarseness may also be present. Oedema and erythema of the pharyngeal walls are the typical findings on physical examination. Pharyngeal exudation occurs infrequently and is generally less effusive than in patients suffering from bacterial pharyngitis.

The most common viruses causing viral pharyngitis are rhinovirus and adenovirus. Other less common viruses include Epstein-Barr virus (EBV), herpes simplex virus (HSV), influenza virus, parainfluenza virus, coronavirus, coxsackievirus, echovirus, respiratory syncytial virus (RSV) and cytomegalovirus (CMV).

Rhinovirus. Rhinovirus, which is responsible for the common cold, is one of the most common causes of viral pharyngitis. The virus does not invade the pharyngeal mucosa but causes oedema and hyperaemia of the mucous membranes, and increases the secretory activity of the mucous glands. Bradykinin and lysyl-bradykinin are generated in the nasal mucous membranes and stimulate pain nerve endings.

Adenoviral pharyngitis. Adenoviral pharyngitis is common among young children and military recruits. The most common adenovirus types causing pharyngitis are adenovirus types 1–3 and 5, which directly invade the pharyngeal mucosa. Specific symptoms include fever, sore throat (more intense than that of the common cold) and conjunctivitis.

EBV pharyngitis. EBV pharyngitis is usually associated with infectious mononucleosis (IM).

Oedema and hyperaemia of the pharyngeal mucosa and uvula with enlargement of the tonsils are characteristic signs. Approximately 50% of patients with IM have greywhite thick patches of exudates distributed over the tonsils and pharyngeal walls, thus mimicking a streptococcal pharyngitis. Palatal petechiae associated with IM tend to be confined to the soft palate. An inflammatory exudate and nasopharyngeal lymphoid hyperplasia (adenoiditis) may also develop. Body temperature is usually high and may reach up to 104°F/40°C. Generalized lymphadenopathy is common in IM and is usually prominent in the anterior and posterior cervical triangles. Splenomegaly and hepatomegaly are present in approximately 50% and 10–15% of patients respectively. Patients suffering from IM who are treated with ampicillin may develop a diffuse, pruritic maculopapular eruption.

Herpetic pharyngitis. Herpetic pharyngitis is caused by herpes simplex virus types 1 and 2. This infection is commonly observed in children and young adults. HSV may cause gingivitis or stomatitis. A sore throat with associated gingivostomatitis is the typical presenting symptom. Other associated symptoms include fever, odynophagia, myalgia and malaise.

Enteroviral pharyngitis. Enteroviral pharyngitis is usually caused by coxsackievirus or echovirus. Enteroviral lesions in the oropharyngeal mucosa are usually a result of secondary infection of the endothelial cells in small mucosal vessels, occurring during viraemia. Coxsackievirus infection is common in the late summer and early fall and may cause the pathologies described below.

Herpangina. Herpangina is usually caused by group-A coxsackieviruses and tends to occur in epidemics, most commonly in infants and children. It is characterized by multiple, small (1–2 mm), greyish papulovesicular lesions on the tonsils, tonsillar pillars, uvula or soft palate. The lesions may occasionally grow up to 4 mm or have an erythematous ring as large as 10 mm. The vesicles become shallow ulcers in about 3 days and heal after a few days. The pharynx is usually not involved.

Associated symptoms include a sudden onset of fever with a sore throat, headache, anorexia and frequently pain in the neck, abdomen and extremities.

Acute lymphonodular pharyngitis. Acute lymphonodular pharyngitis is caused by coxsackievirus A10 and is characterized by a distribution of oral and pharyngeal lesions similar to those seen in herpangina. However, the lesions are protruding, whitish to yellowish nodules, and do not evolve into vesicles or ulcers. They remain papular and become greyish-white and nodular, secondary to infiltration by lymphocytes.

Hand-foot-and-mouth disease. Hand-foot-and-mouth disease is usually caused by coxsackievirus A16 and is characterized by 4–8 mm ulcers on the tongue, buccal mucosa and occasionally the tonsillar pillars. Vesicular exanthems develop on the hands and feet and in infants occasionally in the diaper area.

Differentiating viral from bacterial pharyngitis solely on the basis of physical examination is not easy. In viral pharyngitis the total white blood cell count may initially be slightly high, followed by a decrease to fewer than 5000 cells after 4–7 days of illness in around 50% of the cases. Atypical lymphocytosis is frequently associated with viral pharyngitis. In IM pharyngitis, the peripheral blood smear reveals relative and absolute lymphocytosis, with more than 10% atypical lymphocytes. Liver function test results are abnormal in 90% of IM cases. A mononucleosis spot test (Monospot) is usually positive and allows rapid screening for heterophile antibodies. IgM antibody to EBV capsid antigen and antibody to early antigen are useful for diagnosing an acute infection, particularly in heterophile negative cases. Rapid streptococcal antigen test and bacterial culture of a throat swab are negative. Leukopenia and proteinuria may be seen in influenza virus pharyngitis.

Treatment of viral pharyngitis includes bed rest, saltwater gargling and fluid intake. Analgesics and antipyretics are used to relieve pain and fever.

4.2. Acute Tonsillitis

Acute tonsillitis is inflammation of the palatine tonsils, usually due to group A β-hemolytic streptococcus (GABHS), or less commonly to a viral infection. Acute tonsillitis caused by *Streptococcus* species usually occurs in children aged 5–15 years. Approximately 10–20% of sore throats in adults are caused by streptococcal infection. Fever, chills, sore throat, foul breath, dysphagia, odynophagia and tenderness in the angle of the jaw characterize acute tonsillitis. The pain is frequently referred to the ears. Physical examination reveals hyperaemic and swollen palatine tonsils, uvula, tongue base and pharyngeal walls, with irregular, thin, nonconfluent patches of white exudates on the tonsils, forming the typical appearance of follicular tonsillitis. Submandibular lymph nodes are often enlarged and tender. Leukocytosis with an increased neutrophil count (shift to the left) is commonly

present in bacterial infections. Mere reliance on clinical criteria, such as the presence of follicular exudate, erythema, fever and lymphadenopathy, is not an accurate means for distinguishing streptococcal from viral tonsillitis. Throat culture is the gold standard for detecting GABHS tonsillitis with a sensitivity of 80–95%. Rapid antigen detection test (RADT) detects the presence of GABHS cell wall carbohydrate from swabbed material and is considered less sensitive than throat cultures. However, RADT has a high specificity and produces results in significantly less time than a throat culture.

Chronic tonsillitis. Chronic tonsillitis is characterized by chronic sore throat, halitosis, recurrent tonsillitis and persistent tender cervical lymph nodes. A polymicrobial bacterial population is observed in most cases, with α- and β-hemolytic streptococcal species, *S. aureus*, *H. influenzae* and *Bacteroides* species identified.

Complications of GABHS tonsillitis are classified into suppurative and nonsuppurative. The nonsuppurative complications include scarlet fever, acute rheumatic fever and post-streptococcal glomerulonephritis. Suppurative complications include peritonsillar, parapharyngeal and retropharyngeal cellulites and/or abscess.

Treatment of acute streptococcal tonsillitis includes adequate hydration and caloric intake. Analgesics and antipyretics are used to relieve pain and fever. GABHS infection obligates antibiotic therapy. Antibiotic therapy is directed towards:

1. Prevention of acute rheumatic fever;
2. Prevention of suppurative complications;
3. Abatement of clinical symptoms and signs; and
4. Reduction in transmission of GABHS to close contacts.

Penicillin is the treatment of choice in streptococcal tonsillitis.

4.3. Peritonsillar Cellulitis and Abscess

Peritonsillar infection, also known as 'Quincy's angina', is an infection located between the tonsil and the superior pharyngeal constrictor muscle. The most common pathogen causing peritonsillar cellulitis/abscess is GABHS. Anaerobic *Bacteroides* can also cause this type of infection. Presenting symptoms include severe throat pain, especially on swallowing, fever, drooling, foul breath, trismus, hot potato voice and unilateral referred otalgia. Limited mouth opening (trismus) is always present in varying severity. The tonsil and uvula are displaced medially by the peritonsillar infection. The soft palate and the anterior pillar are swollen and hyperaemic. Unilateral enlarged and tender submandibular lymph nodes are present. Peritonsillar cellulitis without pus formation usually responds to intravenous penicillin therapy. Drainage along with intravenous penicillin is required in peritonsillar abscess. Peritonsillar abscess tends to recur and tonsillectomy is usually indicated.

4.4. Lingual Tonsillitis

Lingual tonsillitis is an infection of the lymphatic tissue located in the base of the tongue. Most patients with lingual tonsillitis have already had palatine tonsillectomy. Lingual tonsillitis presents with fever, sore throat, glossal pain, dysphagia, muffled voice and pain at the level of the hyoid bone during swallowing. Lingual tonsillitis is visible only by means of a laryngeal mirror or fibre-optic examination. The base of the tongue is enlarged and oedematous and covered by exudates. The pharynx may appear normal or mildly hyperaemic. The anterior neck may be tender at the level of the hyoid bone, and cervical and submandibular adenopathy may be observed. Treatment includes intravenous penicillin.

4.5. Parapharyngeal Space Infection

The parapharyngeal space (PPS) (i.e. lateral pharyngeal space, pharyngomaxillary space, pterygomaxillary space, pterygopharyngeal space) occupies an inverted pyramidal area lateral to the superior constrictor muscles, and bounded by multiple components of the fascial system. The styloid process divides the PPS into an anterior or prestyloid compartment and a neurovascular or post-styloid compartment.

Parapharyngeal space infections (PPSI) may follow an infection in the pharynx, tonsils, adenoids, teeth, parotid gland, peritonsillar area, submandibular space, retropharyngeal space, Bezold abscess (mastoid abscess on the inner aspect of the mastoid tip along the digastric ridge) and adjacent lymph nodes. Despite the multitude of well-defined potential sources, in nearly half of the cases, the aetiology cannot be defined. Signs and symptoms of PPSI differ depending on whether the prestyloid or post-styloid compartment is involved. Anterior PPSI is characterized by pain in the angle of the jaw, preauricular area, ear and adjacent upper neck. Rotating the head and neck to the contralateral side intensifies the pain. Other symptoms include dysphagia, odynophagia, drooling, trismus (due to medial pterygoid muscle irritation), fever, chills and malaise. Oedema and medial displacement or bulging of the lateral pharyngeal wall and tonsil are hallmarks of PPSI. Swelling, induration and tenderness at the angle of the mandible are also commonly observed. Dyspnea and other symptoms of airway obstruction may occur in severe cases.

Posterior PPSI is not associated with trismus or tonsillar displacement and may have no localizing signs on examination. Despite this, the patients appear to be toxic with parotid space swelling. Involvement of the neurovascular structures may lead to complications such as cranial neuropathies, Horner's syndrome, septic internal jugular thrombosis and carotid artery rupture.

CT scan of the neck (with contrast medium) facilitates the diagnosis and assessment of the extent of PPSI. A recent manuscript redefines PPSI into two different disorders that are clinically and therapeutically relevant (Sichel et al 2006):

1. Parapharyngeal lymphadenitis—infection located in the posterior part of the PPS with no invasion into the parapharyngeal fat and with no extensions into other cervical spaces except the adjacent retropharyngeal space. This condition is relatively benign, and intravenous antibiotics and nonsurgical treatment are recommended.
2. Parapharyngeal abscess—infection in the anterior part of the PPS involving the parapharyngeal fat. May also be termed deep neck abscess. Diffusion into the mediastinum and other severe complications are frequent. Early diagnosis, aggressive intravenous antibiotics and urgent surgical drainage are recommended.

4.6. Retropharyngeal Space Infection

The retropharyngeal space (RPS) lies between the visceral division of the middle layer of the deep cervical fascia behind the pharyngeal constrictors and the alar division of the deep layer of the deep cervical fascia posteriorly. Retropharyngeal space infection (RPSI) may follow infection in the nasopharynx, oropharynx, sinonasal region and rarely mastoiditis. RPSI may also occur directly after a traumatic perforation of the posterior pharyngeal wall or oesophagus, or indirectly, from the parapharyngeal space. Most RPSIs in children are secondary to URI, whereas trauma or foreign bodies cause most RPSIs in adults. Retropharyngeal lymph nodes tend to regress by the age of 5, causing infection in this area to be much more common in children than in adults. RPSI may drain into the prevertebral space and through this space into the chest, thus causing mediastinitis. Symptoms of RPSI include sore throat, dysphagia, stiff neck, fever and rarely posterior neck and shoulder pain aggravated by swallowing. Examination reveals anterior displacement or bulging of one or both sides of the posterior pharyngeal wall due to involvement of lymph nodes, which are distributed lateral to the midline fascial raphe. Lateral neck radiograph (demonstrating widening of the retropharyngeal space) and CT scan with contrast of the neck facilitate diagnosis and assessment of the extent of RPSI. Early diagnosis is important and treatment with aggressive intravenous antibiotics is mandatory. Transoral incision and drainage is recommended in cases with abscess formation.

4.7. Ludwig's Angina

Ludwig's angina is a potentially life-threatening, rapidly expanding and spreading, gangrenous cellulitis of the submandibular space. Swelling of this region can compromise the airway. Most Ludwig's angina infections are odontogenic, usually from the second or third mandibular molar. Other causes include peritonsillar or parapharyngeal abscesses, mandibular fracture, oral lacerations or piercing, and rarely submandibular sialadenitis. Predisposing factors include dental caries, recent dental treatment, systemic illnesses (such as diabetes mellitus), malnutrition, alcoholism, compromised immune system (such as AIDS) and organ transplantation. The term 'Ludwig's angina' is reserved for infections meeting the following five criteria:

1. A cellulitic process (not an abscess) of the submandibular space;
2. Involvement of only the submandibular space, although this might be bilateral and spread into secondary spaces;
3. The finding of gangrene with foul serosanguineous fluid on incision, but no frank purulence;
4. Involvement of the fascia, muscle and connective tissue, with sparing of the glandular tissue; and
5. Direct spread of infection rather than spread by lymphatics.

The most common microbes involved are usually *Streptococcus* species and oral anaerobic bacteria. Symptoms include painful neck swelling, tooth pain, dysphagia, odynophagia, dyspnea, fever and malaise. Ludwig's angina is characterized by a brawny induration of the mouth floor and suprahyoid region (bilaterally), with elevation or protrusion of the tongue, thus potentially obstructing the airway. Other signs include a tender, firm swelling in the submental and anterior neck without fluctuance, tachypnea, stridor, trismus, muffled or 'hot potato' voice and drooling. The white blood cell count is high with a 'shift to the left'. Airway management is the primary therapeutic concern. Airway control by endotracheal intubation is mandatory. Therapy includes intravenous broad-spectrum antibiotics and occasionally drainage of the swelling through a cervical incision with placement of drains. Dental treatment may be needed to treat the initiating tooth infection. Complications such as sepsis and descending necrotizing mediastinitis may occur through the retropharyngeal space and carotid sheath.

References

Abu-Bakra M, Jones NS (2001a) Does stimulation of nasal mucosa cause referred pain to the face? *Clin Otolaryngol Allied Sci* **26**(5):430–432.

Abu-Bakra M, Jones NS (2001b) Prevalence of nasal mucosal contact points in patients with facial pain compared with patients without facial pain. *J Laryngol Otol* **115**(8):629–632.

Agius AM, Pickles JM, Burch KL (1992) A prospective study of otitis externa. *Clin Otolaryngol Allied Sci* **17**(2):150–154.

Ahamed SH, Jones NS (2003) What is Sluder's neuralgia? *J Laryngol Otol* **117**(6):437–443.

Amundson LH (1990) Disorders of the external ear. *Prim Care* **17**(2):213–231.

Anand VK, Osguthorpe JD, Rice D (1997) Surgical management of adult rhinosinusitis. *Otolaryngol Head Neck Surg* **117**(3 Pt 2): S50–S52.

Baraniuk JN (2001) Neurogenic mechanisms in rhinosinusitis. *Curr Allergy Asthma Rep* **1**(3):252–261.

Benninger MS, Ferguson BJ, Hadley JA, *et al* (2003) Adult chronic rhinosinusitis: definitions, diagnosis, epidemiology, and pathophysiology. *Otolaryngol Head Neck Surg* **129**(3 Suppl): S1–S32.

Benoliel R, Quek S, Biron A, *et al* (2006) Trigeminal neurosensory changes following acute and chronic paranasal sinusitis. *Quint Int* **37**(6):437–443.

Blaugrund SM (1989) Nasal obstruction. The nasal septum and concha bullosa. *Otolaryngol Clin North Am* **22**(2):291–306.

Burke BL, Steele RW, Beard OW, *et al* (1982). Immune responses to varicella-zoster in the aged. *Arch Intern Med* **142**(2):291–293.

Cady RK, Schreiber CP (2004) Sinus headache: a clinical conundrum. *Otolaryngol Clin North Am* **37**(2):267–288.

Chow JM (1994) Rhinologic headaches. *Otolaryngol Head Neck Surg* **111**(3 Pt 1):211–218.

Clenney TL, Lassen LF (1996) Recreational scuba diving injuries. *Am Fam Physician* **53**(5):1761–1774.

Clerico DM (1995) Sinus headaches reconsidered: referred cephalgia of rhinologic origin masquerading as refractory primary headaches. *Headache* **35**(4):185–192.

Clerico DM (1996) Pneumatized superior turbinate as a cause of referred migraine headache. *Laryngoscope* **106**(7):874–879.

Clerico DM, Fieldman R (1994) Referred headache of rhinogenic origin in the absence of sinusitis. *Headache* **34**(4):226–229.

Clerico DM, Evan K, Montgomery L, *et al* (1997) Endoscopic sinonasal surgery in the management of primary headaches. *Rhinology* **35**(3):98–102.

Day M (1999) Sphenopalatine ganglion analgesia. *Curr Rev Pain* **3**(5):342–347.

Derebery MJ, Berliner KI (1997) Allergic eustachian tube dysfunction: diagnosis and treatment. *Am J Otol* **18**(2):160–165.

Eliashar R, Gross M, Saah D, *et al* (2004) Vestibular involvement in myringitis bullosa. *Acta Otolaryngol* **124**(3):249–252.

Gergely P Jr, Poor G (2004) Relapsing polychondritis. *Best Pract Res Clin Rheumatol* **18**(5):723–738.

Goldsmith AJ, Zahtz GD, Stegnjajic A, *et al* (1993) Middle turbinate headache syndrome. *Am J Rhinology* **7**:17–23.

Grimmer JF, Poe DS (2005) Update on eustachian tube dysfunction and the patulous eustachian tube. *Curr Opin Otolaryngol Head Neck Surg* **13**(5):277–282.

Guy RL, Wylie E, Tonge KA (1991) Computed tomography in malignant external otitis. *Clin Radiol* **43**(3):166–170.

Handzel O, Halperin D (2003) Necrotizing (malignant) external otitis. *Am Fam Physician* **68**(2):309–312.

Hansen JG, Schmidt H, Grinsted P (2000) Randomised, double blind, placebo controlled trial of penicillin V in the treatment of acute maxillary sinusitis in adults in general practice. *Scand J Prim Health Care* **18**(1):44–47.

Harvey H (1992) Diagnosing referred otalgia: The ten Ts. *J Cranio Pract* **10**(4):333–334.

Hirsch BE (1992) Infection of the external ear. *Am J Otolaryngol* **13**(3):145–155.

International Rhinosinusitis Advisory Board (1997) Infectious rhinosinusitis in adults: classification, etiology and management. *Ear Nose Throat J* **76**(12 Suppl):1–22.

Jensen R, Olesen J (2000) Tension-type headache: an update on mechanisms and treatment. *Curr Opin Neurol* **13**(3):285–289.

Jones NS (2004) Midfacial segment pain: implications for rhinitis and sinusitis. *Curr Allergy Asthma Rep* **4**(3):187–192.

Kinishi M, Amatsu M, Mohri M, *et al* (2001) Acyclovir improves recovery rate of facial nerve palsy in Ramsay Hunt syndrome. *Auris Nasus Larynx* **28**(3): 223–226.

Ko JY, Sheen TS, Hsu MM (2000) Herpes zoster oticus treated with acyclovir and prednisolone: clinical manifestations and analysis of prognostic factors. *Clin Otolaryngol Allied Sci* **25**(2):139–142.

Kuhweide R, Van de Steene V, Vlaminck S, *et al* (2002) Ramsay Hunt syndrome: pathophysiology of cochleovestibular symptoms. *J Laryngol Otol* **116**(10): 844–848.

Lanza DC (2004) Diagnosis of chronic rhinosinusitis. *Ann Otol Rhinol Laryngol* **193**(Suppl):10–14.

Lanza DC, Kennedy DW (1997) Adult rhinosinusitis defined. *Otolaryngol Head Neck Surg* **117**(3 Pt 2):S1–S7.

Lipton RB, Stewart WF, Diamond S, *et al* (2001) Prevalence and burden of migraine in the United States: data from the American Migraine Study II. *Headache* **41**(7):646–657.

Lucente FE, Lawson W, Novick NL (1995) *The External Ear*. Philadelphia: WB Saunders.

Marais J, Dale BAB (1997) Bullous myringitis: a review. *Clin Otolaryngol* **22**(6):497–499.

Meltzer EO, Hamilos DL, Hadley JA, *et al* (2004) Rhinosinusitis: Establishing definitions for clinical research and patient care. *Otolaryngol Head Neck Surg* **131**(6 Suppl):S1–62.

Mirza S, Richardson H (2005) Otic barotrauma from air travel. *J Laryngol Otol* **119**(5):366–370.

Morgan NJ, Skipper JJ, Allen GM (1995) Referred otalgia: An old lesson. *Br J Oral Maxillofac Surg* **33**(5):332–333.

Morgenstein KM, Krieger MK (1980) Experiences in middle turbinectomy. *Laryngoscope* **90**(10 Pt 1):1596–1603.

Morrow MJ (2000) Bell's palsy and herpes zoster oticus. *Curr Treat Options Neurol* **2**(5):407–416.

Mudgil SP, Wise SW, Hopper KD, *et al* (2002) Correlation between presumed sinusitis-induced pain and paranasal sinus computed tomographic findings. *Ann Allergy Asthma Immunol* **88**(2):223–226.

Murtagh J (1991) The painful ear. *Aust Fam Physician* **20**(12): 1779–1783.

Nestor JJ, Ngo LK (1994) Incidence of facial pain caused by lung cancer. *Otolaryngol Head Neck Surg* **111**(1):155–156.

Olesen J (1991) Clinical and pathophysiological observations in migraine and tension-type headache explained by integration of vascular, supraspinal and myofascial inputs. *Pain* **46**(2): 125–132.

Olesen J, Bousser MG, Diener HC, *et al* (2004) The International Classification of Headache Disorders, 2nd Edition. *Cephalalgia* **24**(Suppl 1):1–160.

Perry BF, Login IS, Kountakis SE (2004) Nonrhinologic headache in a tertiary rhinology practice. *Otolaryngol Head Neck Surg* **130** (4):449–452.

Piccirillo JF, Mager DE, Frisse ME, *et al* (2001) Impact of first-line vs second-line antibiotics for the treatment of acute uncomplicated sinusitis. *JAMA* **286**(15):1849–1856.

Puig CM, Driscoll CL, Kern EB (1998) Sluder's sphenopalatine ganglion neuralgia–treatment with 88% phenol. *Am J Rhinol* **12** (2):113–118.

Sander R (2001) Otitis externa: a practical guide to treatment and prevention. *Am Fam Physician* **63**:927–936, 941–942.

Schreiber CP, Hutchinson S, Webster CJ, *et al* (2004) Prevalence of migraine in patients with a history of self-reported or physician-diagnosed 'sinus' headache. *Arch Intern Med* **164** (16):1769–1772.

Sichel JY, Attal P, Hocwald E, *et al* (2006) Redefining parapharyngeal space infections. *Ann Otol Rhinol Laryngol* **115** (2):117–123.

Sinus and Allergy Health Partnership (2004) Antimicrobial treatment guidelines for acute bacterial rhinosinusitis. *Otolaryngol Head Neck Surg* **130**(1):S1–S50.

Sluder G (1910) The syndrome of sphenopalatine ganglion neurosis. *New York Med J* **140**:868–878.

Sluder G (1913) Etiology, diagnosis, prognosis and treatment of sphenopalatine neuralgia. *J Am Med Assoc* **61**:1202–1206.

Snow V, Mottur-Pilson C, Hickner JM (2001) Principles of appropriate antibiotic use for acute sinusitis in adults. *Ann Intern Med* **134**(6):495–497.

Staats BA, Utz JP, Michet CJ Jr (2002) Relapsing polychondritis. *Semin Respir Crit Care Med* **23**(2):145–154.

Stalman W, van Essen GA, van der Graaf Y, *et al* (1997) Maxillary sinusitis in adults: an evaluation of placebo-controlled double-blind trials. *Fam Pract* **14**(2):124–129.

Stammberger H, Wolf G (1988) Headaches and sinus disease: the endoscopic approach. *Ann Otol Rhinol Laryngol Suppl* **134**:3–23.

Thaller SR, DeSilva A (1987) Otalgia with a normal ear. *Am Fam Physician* **36**(4):129–136.

Wazen JJ (1989) Referred otalgia. *Otolaryngol Clin N Am* **22** (6):1205–1215.

West B, Jones NS (2001) Endoscopy-negative, computed tomography-negative facial pain in a nasal clinic. *Laryngoscope* **111**(4 Pt 1):581–586.

Williams JW Jr, Aguilar C, Cornell J, *et al* (2003) Antibiotics for acute maxillary sinusitis. *Cochrane Database Syst Rev* (2): CD000243.

Winther B, Gwaltney JM Jr (1990) Therapeutic approach to sinusitis: antiinfectious therapy as the baseline of management. *Otolaryngol Head Neck Surg* **103**(5 Pt 2):876–878; discussion 878–879.

Woo JKS, Van Hasselt CA, Gluckman PGC (1992) Myringitis bullosa haemorrhagica: clinical course influenced by tympanosclerosis. *J Laryngol Otol* **106**(2):162–163.

Yanagisawa K, Kveton JF (1992) Referred otalgia. *Am J Otolaryngol* **13**(6):323–327.

CHAPTER 7

Masticatory myofascial pain, and tension-type and chronic daily headache

Rafael Benoliel and Yair Sharav

1. Introduction and Classification

This chapter focuses on masticatory muscle myofascial pain (MMP) and tension-type headaches (TTH) and examines their relationships to each other and to fibromyalgia (FM). We review the chronic daily headaches (CDH) as a group and specifically chronic tension-type headache and new daily persistent headache. Other CDHs such as chronic migraine (Chapter 9), chronic trigeminal autonomic cephalgias including hemicrania continua (Chapter 10) and medication overuse headache (Chapter 13) are covered in designated chapters. MMP is one of the entities found within a diagnostic umbrella termed temporomandibular disorders (TMD); a classification that includes ailments of the temporomandibular joints (TMJ) and masticatory muscles (Dworkin and LeResche 1992; Okeson 1996). TMJ disorders are reviewed in Chapter 8.

The International Headache Society (IHS) clearly defines TMJ pain but relates to MMP only as a possible initiating factor in TTH (Olesen *et al* 2004). For TMDs the IHS classification is therefore limiting, and orofacial pain specialists have tended to use two widely accepted systems that clearly subclassify TMDs into TMJ and masticatory muscle disorders: the Research Diagnostic Criteria for Temporomandibular Disorders (RDC-TMD) and the definitions of the American Academy of Orofacial Pain (AAOP) (Dworkin and LeResche 1992; Okeson 1996). These two classification systems are very similar but are distinguished by the meticulous inclusion criteria of muscle sites and the separation of MMP into with or without limitation of opening in the RDC-TMD system (Table 7.1). The RDC-TMD system has been extensively tested and translated into various languages so that it has wide universal acceptance. In addition to the physical diagnosis (Axis I) the RDC-TMD system assesses psychological, behavioural and psychosocial factors (Axis II); forms may be downloaded from http://www.rdc-tmdinternational.org/. Axis II parameters are further discussed below and in Chapter 4. Research on TMDs should therefore employ the RDC-TMD criteria although for routine clinical use the AAOP criteria are preferred by some clinicians. AAOP criteria may be augmented by psychosocial assessment employing accepted techniques (see later and Chapter 4).

TMDs are amongst the most common orofacial pain syndromes in the general population (Lipton *et al* 1993). TTH is the most common primary headache (Lyngberg *et al* 2005a) with referral of pain to the orofacial region suspected in some cases. Orofacial pain specialists are therefore regularly required to diagnose and manage these patients.

1.1. Clinical Approach

A thorough pain history must be recorded including specific questions on masticatory dysfunction. Pain location should be augmented by drawings that outline the extent and referral pattern of pain (see Fig. 7.1A, Case 7.1).

A routine head and neck examination must be performed including cranial nerve assessment. Specifically the interincisal mouth opening should be recorded in millimetres (mm) and any deviation or accompanying pain adequately described. In all musculoskeletal patients it is imperative to carefully palpate the regional muscles (masticatory/pericranial, cervical) and TMJ to locate tender areas or trigger points. Muscle trigger points refer pain and are distinct from muscle tenderness which reflects a generalized sensitivity over the affected muscle. The patient's reaction and assessment of resultant pain or tenderness should be recorded. Particularly in MMP the

Table 7.1	Diagnostic Criteria for Masticatory Muscle Myofascial Pain

Myofascial Pain (AAOP[a])	Myofascial Pain Without/With* Limited Opening (RDC-TMD[b])
	Axis I: Physical findings

– Regional dull, aching pain:
  • Aggravated by mandibular function.
	– Complaint of pain of muscle origin:
	  • In jaw, temples, face, preauricular or auricular at rest or during function.

– Hyperirritable sites or trigger points:
  • Frequently found within a taut band of muscle tissue or fascia
  • Provocation of these trigger points alters the pain complaint and reveals a pattern of referral *>50% reduction of pain is inducible by muscle stretch preceded by trigger point treatment with: Vapocoolant spray, or Local anaesthetic injection.
– Signs and symptoms that may accompany pain:
  • Sensation of muscle stiffness;
  • Sensation of acute malocclusion, not clinically verified;
  • Ear symptoms, tinnitus, vertigo, toothache, tension-type headache;
  • Decreased mouth opening; passive stretching increases opening by >4 mm; Soft end feel
  • Hyperalgesia in the region of referred pain.
	– Pain associated with localized areas of tenderness to palpation in muscle.
	– Pain on palpation in ≥3 sites of the following sites and at least one of which is ipsilateral to the pain complaint (right/left muscles count for separate sites):
	  • R/L temporalis: posterior, middle, anterior, tendon (8 sites);
	  • R/L masseter: origin, body, insertion (6 sites);
	  • R/L posterior mandibular region (2 sites);
	  • R/L submandibular region (2 sites);
	  • R/L lateral pterygoid region (2 sites).
	– Myofascial pain as above accompanied by:
	  • Stiffness of muscles;
	  • *Pain-free unassisted mandibular opening of <40 mm;
	  • *With assistance an increase of ≥5 mm in mandibular opening.

	Axis II: Psychosocial comorbidity[c]

– No psychosocial assessment required.	– Pain intensity and pain-related disability:
	  • Graded chronic pain scale;
	  • Jaw disability checklist.
	– Depression and somatization:
	  • Symptom Checklist for Depression and Somatization (SCL-90).

Adapted from Okeson (1996) and Dworkin and LeResche (1992).
[a] American Academy of Orofacial Pain.
[b] Research Diagnostic Criteria for Temporomandibular Disorders.
[c] Other validated measures may be used; see text and Chapter 4.

examination is crucial in diagnosis; it is therefore essential to develop a reliable technique whereby even and consistent pressure is applied across all patients (Dworkin *et al* 1990a). Clinical signs are difficult to measure with consistency and interrater reliability for some signs of MMP is not good, so close conformity with accepted classification criteria and thorough self-calibration is essential (John *et al* 2005). Examiner calibration rather than professional experience seems to be the most important factor for reliable measurement of TMD symptoms (Leher *et al* 2005). It is advisable to practise pressure application on weight scales using the fingers or thumbs and aiming at a pressure of about 4 kg (8.8 lbs). We usually begin by applying pressure on unaffected regions (e.g. forehead, shoulder) so as to allow the patient to familiarize himself with the technique. Patient response is recorded for each muscle or joint and graded from 0 to 3; where 0 is no pain, 1 is mild, 2 is moderate and 3 is severe (Fumal and Schoenen 2005). Ratings may then be summated to give a total tenderness score. MMP and fibromyalgia patients consistently display more

tenderness and more involved muscles than controls (Dworkin *et al* 1990a), but the findings in TTH are inconsistent and vary between patients (Olesen *et al* 2004; Ashina *et al* 2005). Radiation of pain or referral to particular sites is not a constant feature. Most masticatory muscles are examined extraorally except for the lateral pterygoid, which is approached from the upper retromolar region. The temporalis muscle has an insertion to the coronoid process that may be palpated intraorally. Patients should be questioned on other body pains and these areas examined if need be.

In the general population clicking or popping joints are very common and may occur during opening and/or closing; these may often be an isolated symptom requiring no treatment. The interincisal opening at each 'click' and associated deviation in mouth opening should be recorded. At times joint sounds may be pathognomonic of underlying disease; for example, crepitation (feels and sounds like sand, or walking on snow) commonly occurs in degenerative joint disease. Since the TMJs are connected by the mandible, joint sounds are often

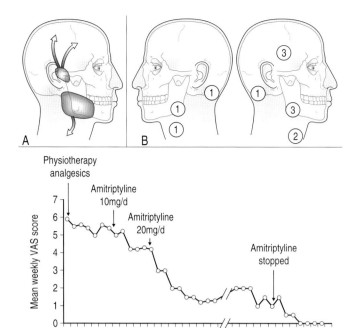

Fig. 7.1 • (A) Pain location in Case 7.1. (B) Muscle tenderness in Case 7.1; tenderness is graded from 1 to 3 (mild to severe). The ipsilateral masseter and temporal muscles were the most tender (scored 3). The contralateral masseter muscle was also mildly tender. Additionally the suboccipital and sternocleidomastoid muscles were mild to moderately tender bilaterally. (C) Case 7.1's pain diary.

transduced to the opposite side and careful examination is required. Lateral and protrusive movements of the jaw should be examined and irregularities or concomitant pain recorded. Joint pain should also be examined and recorded under ipsilateral and contralateral loading (biting a bite stick).

Intraoral examination should rule out dental pathology and assess the occlusion for gross problems and/or recent changes that may have been caused by a TMD. The dentition and periodontal tissues should be assessed for possible pathology.

2. Temporomandibular Disorders

2.1. Study Design and Reliability

Depending on specific subdiagnosis, the cardinal features of TMDs include muscle and/or joint pain, joint sounds and masticatory dysfunction. Many studies have therefore focused on the prevalence of these TMD signs and symptoms without us knowing their clinical significance. Moreover, because studies address a number of symptoms, conclusions as to the behaviour of any one sign or symptom should be arrived at with care. Other studies have reported on samples of patients seeking treatment or on convenience samples that are misrepresentative of the population. A major problem has been the use of diverse inclusion and exclusion criteria by different groups. This is reflected in the diverse terminology used

in the literature: mandibular dysfunction, craniomandibular disorders. We have substituted these terms with TMD throughout this chapter. The universal use of accepted research criteria will no doubt increase our understanding of the processes involved, the epidemiology and our diagnostic skills in TMDs. The use of the term TMD is widespread; however, research on epidemiology, treatment response, natural history and genetic factors must clearly differentiate between the diagnostic subgroups.

When examining the literature it is important to assess the study design, statistical power and the presence of confounding variables. For example studies of pain and bruxism very often ignore confounding parameters such as anxiety and therefore the results may be misrepresentative. It is important to ascertain what parameters the study assessed: patient report or physical findings of signs and symptoms by examination. There are usually more physical findings than the patient is aware of (LeResche 1997). The physical assessment of patients in TMD studies requires standardization of methods, reliability data and interrater calibration (Dworkin *et al* 1990b). The double-blind placebo-controlled trial is the gold standard for therapeutic interventions but may be problematic in some physical therapy modalities. Comparative studies of different interventions are needed to identify the more efficacious treatments. Evidence-based therapies in TMDs are rare and expert opinion or personal preference often replace a sound scientific approach. Whilst clinical experience and individual judgement are important in the assessment and treatment of patients, the incorporation of evidence-based principles is essential.

2.2. Epidemiology

Temporomandibular disorders are recognized as the most common chronic orofacial pain condition with no significant differences found between racial groups (Dworkin *et al* 1990a; Yap *et al* 2003). As previously defined TMD refers to a group of pain conditions and dysfunctions and not all epidemiological studies have used the same classification or differentiated between muscle and joint disorders (LeResche *et al* 1991). Indeed, inclusion criteria employed in studies prior to modern classifications encompassed a number of disorders into one entity. This questions the current validity of much of the epidemiologic research performed before criteria and diagnoses were standardized (Dworkin and LeResche 1992; Okeson 1996).

2.2.1. Signs and Symptoms versus Treatment Need

Studies reveal that 6–93% of the general population have or report signs and symptoms of TMD (Locker and Slade 1988; De Kanter *et al* 1993). There is great disparity between study results with prevalences of common signs such as clicking joints ranging from 6 to 48%, suggesting

Case 7.1 Masticatory Myofascial Pain, 27-year-old Female

Married, 2 children. Employed as a senior secretary in a law firm for the past 6 years.

Present complaint

Pain on the right side of the face particularly around the angle of the mandible and the preauricular region (Fig. 7.1A). The pain was constant and recently pain severity had become worse; graded around 6 on a 10-cm visual analogue scale (VAS). Pain severity fluctuated throughout the day and was worse in the afternoon or following chewing or yawning. Other than mild neck discomfort the patient reported no generalized symptoms. The patient had no record of absenteeism from work and reported that she slept well. Pain had occasionally referred to the teeth but her dentist had not detected pathology. Descriptors for pain quality were pressure, dull and annoying.

History of present complaint

Present for the past 4 months but previous to that had occurred and remitted for some months.

Physical examination

Extraoral examination revealed regional muscle tenderness (Fig. 7.1B) bilaterally but was more pronounced in the ipsilateral masseter and temporalis muscles. Interincisal mouth opening was 34 mm and accompanied by pain. Examiner-assisted opening was 39 mm with severe pain. No TMJ sounds were detected and the joints were not tender. Cranial nerve examination was normal.

Intraoral examination and full mouth radiographs revealed no dental problems.

Relevant medical history

Diagnosed with hypothyroidism 4 years previously and treated with 100 µg thyroxine daily.

Diagnosis

Masticatory muscle myofascial pain (MMP).

Diagnostic and treatment considerations

Conservative treatment options were discussed with the patient. It was decided to initiate therapy with analgesics (ibuprofen 400 mg three times daily for 10 days) and physiotherapy for the jaw and neck muscles (see text). The patient was also referred to her family physician to check on her thyroid status. Over the next 6 weeks the patient reported no significant improvement and began to complain of disturbed sleep and increased neck discomfort (Fig. 7.1C); thyroid hormone and thyroid-stimulating hormone levels were normal. Amitriptyline (10 mg at bedtime) was therefore initiated together with continuing physiotherapy. Based on response and side effects the dose was increased to 20 mg at bedtime and over a period of 15 weeks the pain severity decreased to a mean VAS of 1. The patient reported increasingly longer periods during the day when she was pain free. On examination the masticatory muscles were not significantly tender and unassisted, pain-free mouth opening was 41 mm. The patient was then lost to follow-up for about 12 weeks and subsequently returned and requested that the amitriptyline be withdrawn. She also commented that during intensive work at her desk pain was aggravated. The amitriptyline was withdrawn and the patient was instructed to continue physiotherapy and obtain advice regarding ergonomics in her immediate work environment. Over the next 4–5 weeks the patient reported no significant pain and was discharged.

---

that the methodology and definitions account for the observed variability.

Moreover data are lacking on the significance of these highly prevalent signs and symptoms. We cannot reliably predict which signs and symptoms will deteriorate and therefore justify early treatment. Clinical judgment alone is relied upon to decide which signs and symptoms will be treated but clinical judgment varies and in the absence of clear criteria this alone cannot be relied upon. Based on available data clear indications for treatment are pain and/or significant dysfunction.

The data should therefore reflect the severe cases (pain and/or dysfunction) that need treatment. For example, although signs or symptoms of dysfunction are extremely common, only 3–11% are assessed as needing treatment (Solberg et al 1979; Magnusson et al 2000). TMD-related facial pain has been found to occur in 4–12% of the population (Goulet et al 1995; Macfarlane et al 2002; Nilsson et al 2005) and severe symptoms are reported by 10% of subjects

(LeResche 1997). These figures are compatible with the data on the percentage of individuals who seek treatment (1.4–7%) (De Kanter et al 1993; Goulet et al 1995). Masticatory muscle and TMJ tenderness were found in 15 and 5%, respectively, of a large population examined (Gesch et al 2004a) but are self-reported by about 4 and 6–8%, respectively, suggesting that muscular tenderness is less bothersome to patients (Kamisaka et al 2000; Katz and Heft 2002). Longitudinal studies suggest that symptoms of TMD fluctuate considerably, particularly in MMP patients, and progression to severe pain and dysfunction of the masticatory system is rare (Raphael and Marbach 1992; Magnusson et al 2000). MMP has been clearly shown to be a chronic or fluctuating pain condition; over 5 years 31% of patients suffered continuous MMP, 36% experienced recurrent pain and 33% remitted (Rammelsberg et al 2003). Clinical experience confirms that there is extreme symptom fluctuation with new symptoms appearing as often as old ones disappear. Significant predictors of persistence were high baseline pain frequency, painful palpation sites and other body sites with pain (Rammelsberg *et al* 2003).

2.2.2. Age Distribution of TMDs

Signs and symptoms of TMD have been found in all age groups, peaking in 20–40 year olds (Tallents *et al* 1991; Levitt and McKinney 1994). Signs of TMD have been described in children and adolescents (List *et al* 1999) but are usually mild (Thilander *et al* 2002). In a group of adolescents treatment need was assessed at 7% (List *et al* 1999; Wahlund 2003). TMDs may also occur in edentulous patients (Dervis 2004). Accumulated evidence suggests that *symptoms* in the elderly may be lower than in the general population but some studies show a slight elevation in the prevalence of some *signs* in this age group (Dworkin *et al* 1990a; Levitt and McKinney 1994). These signs usually include asymptomatic joint sounds and limited mouth opening (Schmitter *et al* 2005). In a longitudinal study on elderly patients signs and symptoms of TMD tended to decrease over the follow-up period (Osterberg *et al* 1992). These data suggest that TMDs are not progressive and most symptoms resolve with increasing age.

2.2.3. Gender

There is a female preponderance of TMD signs and symptoms especially of muscular origin (LeResche 1997; Magnusson *et al* 2000). Most studies also report that the vast majority of patients (up to 80%) who seek treatment are females (LeResche 1997; White *et al* 2001; Anastassaki and Magnusson 2004). Back pain, headache and TMD-related pain were found to increase significantly with increasing pubertal development in girls (LeResche *et al* 2005a). Additionally women TMD patients generally have more severe physical and psychological symptoms than do men (Levitt and McKinney 1994). TMD pain and related symptoms appear to improve over the course of pregnancy but this is not paralleled by improvements in psychological distress (LeResche *et al* 2005b). This is most likely associated with the dramatic hormonal changes occurring during pregnancy. Indeed, TMD pain in women is highest at times of lowest oestrogen and may also be related to periods of rapid oestrogen change (LeResche *et al* 2003). These gender effects are examined further in the section on TMD pathophysiology below.

2.3. Personal and Societal Impact of TMDs

Although progression to severe TMD-related pain and dysfunction is rare the personal and societal impact of TMDs is significant. TMD patients significantly request sick leave more often, visit a physician more frequently and utilize more physical therapy services than controls (Kuttila *et al* 1997). It has been estimated that disabling

TMDs cause about 18 lost workdays annually for every 100 working adults in the United States (Dworkin and LeResche 1993). During the early 1990s it was calculated that approximately 3.6 million acrylic splints are constructed yearly in the USA to treat TMDs and bruxism, accounting for an annual expenditure of US$990 million (not adjusted for inflation): 3% of the total US dental healthcare expenditure (Pierce *et al* 1995). TMD subjects use significantly more healthcare services than controls with about 50% more mean costs in drug utilization, outpatient visits and specialist services (White *et al* 2001). Most of the increased costs were accounted for by about 10% of TMD subjects, probably the most severely affected (White *et al* 2001).

3. Masticatory Myofascial Pain

3.1. Clinical Features

The masticatory muscles involved in jaw closure include the masseter, temporalis and medial pterygoids. The lateral pterygoids are involved in opening and protrusive movements and in articular disc/condylar stabilization whilst the digastric muscles assist in mouth opening. Other pericranial and cervical muscles are concomitantly involved or provide support and stability during mastication, speech and swallowing. MMP is characterized primarily by pain and tenderness from the jaw-closing muscles. The specialized function of the masticatory muscles, the presence of bilateral joints with occluding teeth and their important roles in chewing produce specific clinical features such as significant masticatory dysfunction. In addition the intimate anatomical relations produce complex and overlapping referral patterns.

At present the diagnosis of MMP is based on the history and clinical examination of the patient; Table 7.1 lists clinical criteria for diagnosis (Dworkin and LeResche 1992; Okeson 1996). No classification system is perfect and clinical diagnosis needs to rely on more than just a list of criteria. For example, most clinicians would be comfortable with diagnosing a patient as MMP in the presence of chronic orofacial pain and dysfunction and only two painful muscle sites; the RDC-TMD criteria require ≥3 tender muscle sites.

Location and quality. MMP is characterized by regional, unilateral pain. Patients typically localize the pain to areas around the ear, the angle/body of the mandible and the temporal region (Fig. 7.2). Referral patterns include intraoral, auriculotemporal, supraorbital and maxillary areas depending on the muscles involved and the intensity of the pain (Fricton *et al* 1985; Simons *et al* 1999; Wright 2000; Svensson and Graven-Nielsen 2001). At times the pain refers diffusely throughout one side of the face, compounding diagnosis (Wright 2000). Although MMP is typically a unilateral pain syndrome it may also occur bilaterally particularly when associated

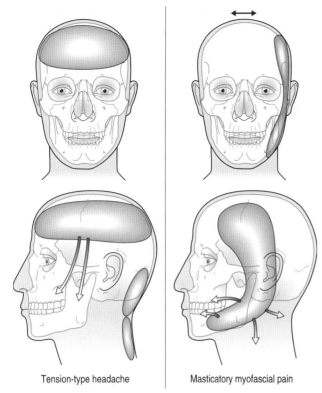

Tension-type headache | Masticatory myofascial pain

Fig. 7.2 • Typical pain location in tension-type headache and in masticatory myofascial pain.

with generalized disorders such as fibromyalgia (Rhodus *et al* 2003). Pain quality is dull, heavy, tender or aching and rarely throbbing (Kino *et al* 2005). Emotive descriptors such as tiring and troublesome are often reported by MMP patients (Kino *et al* 2005). Pain severity may fluctuate during the day but is usually about 3–5 on a 10-cm visual analogue scale, and varies considerably across patients (van Grootel *et al* 2005; Kino *et al* 2005).

Temporal pattern. Some patients experience the most intense pain in the morning (21%) or late afternoon (79%) and others have no fixed pattern; fortunately the pain rarely wakes (van Grootel *et al* 2005). Pain-free days may be reported and on a painful day average pain duration is about 5.5 hours (van Grootel *et al* 2005). Typically MMP is characterized by chronicity with reported onset months to several years previously (Rammelsberg *et al* 2003; Kino *et al* 2005). The temporal pain pattern varies considerably between patients.

Triggers. Pain may be aggravated during jaw function with transient spikes of pain occurring spontaneously (Fricton *et al* 1985; Okeson 1996); indeed pain on function may be the patient's primary complaint.

Associated signs. In addition to pain there may be deviation of the mandible on opening, fullness of the ear, dizziness and soreness of the neck (Sharav *et al* 1978; Blasberg and Chalmers 1989). Dizziness has been associated with pain in the sternocleidomastoid muscle and ear stuffiness with spasm of the medial pterygoid (Sharav *et al* 1978). Some patients may report tinnitus that is correlated with the number of tender muscles (Camparis *et al* 2005).

Tinnitus often improves with treatment together with other TMD signs and symptoms (Wright and Bifano 1997).

Physical findings. Examination usually reveals limited mouth opening (less than 40 mm, interincisal) with a soft-end feel. The presence of limited mouth opening in an MMP patient may also indicate TMJ pathology that may be clinically difficult to diagnose (Schmitter *et al* 2004). Tenderness to palpation is usually present in ipsilateral masticatory muscles and is a distinguishing feature of MMP patients (Dworkin *et al* 1990a). The masseter is the muscle most commonly involved (> 60%); the medial pterygoid and temporalis muscles are tender in about 40–50% of cases, commonly unilaterally (Sharav *et al* 1978). The sternocleidomastoid, trapezius and suboccipital muscles are usually tender in 30–45% of patients, very often bilaterally (Sharav *et al* 1978).

Typically there are localized tender sites and trigger points in muscle, tendon or fascia (Fricton *et al* 1985; McMillan and Blasberg 1994; Okeson 1996). A hypersensitive bundle or nodule of muscle fibre of harder than normal consistency is the physical finding most often associated with a trigger point. Trigger points may be associated with a twitch response when stimulated. Additionally trigger point palpation may also provoke a characteristic pattern of regional referred pain and/or autonomic symptoms (Dao *et al* 1994a; Okeson 1996; Simons *et al* 1999). Areas of referred pain may include perioral and intraoral (teeth) structures and depend on the muscles involved and the intensity of pain (Stohler *et al* 2001; Svensson *et al* 2003a). Referral to the teeth may be prominent and may often cause misdiagnosis as dental pathology. Referral of pain from trigger points in the deep part of the masseter muscle includes the TMJ and ear, causing possible misdiagnosis with intra-articular or ear disorders (see Chapters 6 and 8). Trigger points may be active (induce clinical symptoms) or latent, in which case they only induce pain on stimulation. It is suggested that muscle overload may activate latent trigger points (Gerwin *et al* 2004; Simons 2004). In our experience tender points are far more common in MMP patients than are trigger points; the RDC-TMD criteria relate to this by expanding its definition to include tender points. Indeed as discussed later, the presence or absence of trigger points seems unnecessary in the diagnosis of chronic musculoskeletal conditions such as fibromyalgia, myofascial pain and probably MMP (Wolfe *et al* 1992).

3.2. Differential Diagnosis

MMP needs to be differentiated from other conditions that may affect the masticatory muscles. Inflammation of a muscle or myositis secondary to infection or trauma is commonly seen in dental practice. Myositis is usually associated with a pertinent history or significant clinical findings such as muscle or regional swelling, redness and dental or periodontal infection. The affected muscles are tender, located in the vicinity of the inflammation and accompanied by limitation of mouth opening. Myositis may precede or be associated with a painful contraction or myospasm in the regional muscles that is of acute onset. Treatment of these involves the effective eradication of the initiating cause and analgesics in accordance with pain intensity (Chapters 5 and 15). Active physiotherapy aids in restoring normal mouth opening. Local muscle pain may occur some 24–48 hours after acute overuse of the masticatory muscles: delayed-onset muscle soreness similar to that observed in other body muscles following exercise. Treatment should be tailored to reported symptomatology and usually includes analgesics and physiotherapy.

Pain referral to intraoral structures has often caused serious misdiagnosis and unwarranted dental treatment; this can be easily avoided by careful clinical and radiographic examination. The differentiation from painful TMJ disorders may also be complex due to overlapping symptomatology; regional pain, pain-referral patterns and pain evoked by mandibular movement are common to both MMP and TMJ disorders (see Chapter 8). Careful clinical assessment and follow-up is essential. The clinician must be alert to the possible contribution of systemic comorbidities. Hypothyroidism, statin use, connective tissue disease and acquired immunodeficiency syndrome may cause a diffuse myalgia and need investigating in relevant situations.

The occurrence of regional primary or metastatic tumours may induce TMD-like symptomatology and should be excluded. Although relatively rare the continuing reports in the literature suggest that such misdiagnosis is possible (Mostafapour and Futran 2000; Treasure 2002). Warning signs include pain of sudden onset or acute worsening of existing pain, focal neurological findings, a lack of response to therapy and atypical distribution or characteristics of the pain. Particularly, patients with a history of previous malignancy are at risk and should be referred for relevant imaging studies (see Fig. 7.3).

3.3. Additional Diagnostic Tools

The doubtful role of muscle hyperactivity in the pathophysiology of MMP as discussed below suggests that

the use of EMG measurements is not useful in patient diagnosis and management (Baba *et al* 2001). Moreover surface EMG recordings are often contaminated by the muscles of facial expression. Pressure algometers attempt to accurately assess pressure pain thresholds but are affected by rate of application, gender and site (Baba *et al* 2001). Neurophysiological methods and quantitative sensory testing (QST) are excellent tools for assessing trigeminal somatosensory function and the contribution of the central nervous system (CNS) in orofacial pain conditions, making them useful for research (see Chapter 3). QST techniques measure pain and sensory thresholds to electrical, mechanical and thermal stimuli and are able to distinguish TMJ from MMP cases but are time-consuming (Eliav *et al* 2003).

3.4. Pathophysiology

Aetiologic theory of TMDs, much of it based on deep-rooted historical concepts reviewed below, is clouded by controversy. Current evidence supports that the induction of myofascial pain involves the interplay between a peripheral nociceptive source in muscle, a faulty CNS component (sensitization) and decreased coping ability (Mense 2003). In MMP patients specifically it is widely accepted that a complex interaction of variable intrinsic and extrinsic factors act to induce craniofacial pain and dysfunction. The clinical presentation and symptoms of MMP resemble muscular pain disorders elsewhere in the body. Similarly it is thought that the pathophysiology of MMP may share mechanisms with entities such as regional myofascial pain, tension-type headache and fibromyalgia.

3.4.1. Historical Perspective of TMD Concepts

The first description of a TMD-like entity emphasized the aetiologic importance of tooth loss. This established the concept that regional musculoskeletal pain was invariably associated with the dental occlusion and other anatomical factors such as skeletal relationships. The resultant structural and mechanistic concepts of TMD aetiology remain unproven but widely publicized. In view of such concepts dentists have treated TMDs whilst other

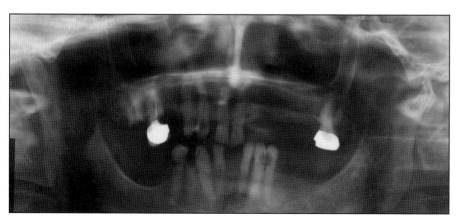

Fig. 7.3 • Metastatic lesion to left condyle mimicking a temporomandibular disorder. The condylar anatomy is distorted and a pathological fracture is present. The patient had a previous adenocarcinoma of the breast.

medical specialties have cared for additional chronic musculoskeletal craniofacial pains such as TTH. This has unfortunately resulted in a separation of MMP from other chronic regional pain syndromes, such as TTH, regional myofascial pains or FM. However, data expressing common ground between TTH and MMP are available, suggesting that we need to re-examine the present nosological separation.

Historically the diagnosis of pain associated with TMDs has been approached under more than a dozen names including the temporomandibular joint dysfunction syndrome and the myofascial pain dysfunction (MPD) syndrome, reflecting the confusion surrounding its aetiology and often its therapy. Research in the late 1950s attempted to shift attention from the TMJ to the muscles of mastication. Early studies also emphasized the contribution of psychological factors to TMDs, leading to the psychophysiological theory. Psychological components as contributing factors in TMDs were demonstrated by extensive work on large patient populations and it was hypothesized that parafunctional activities to relieve psychological stress led to muscle fatigue, spasm and pain; see Chapter 4. Recent research has shown that MMP patients consistently suffer higher levels of distress than those with articular TMDs (Ferrando et al 2004; Galdón et al 2006). However, some TMD patients suffer from complex psychosocial disorders and the role of such influences as initiating factors remains unclear, particularly in TMJ-related TMDs (Suvinen et al 2005a).

Early theories offered 'one cause one disease' hypotheses but accumulating data indicating a more complex TMD aetiology disproved these. New theories combining stress and occlusal disharmonies were subsequently proposed but the focus remained on occlusal adjustment as preferred therapy. The most popular current concepts are the multifactorial (Okeson 1996; Woda and Pionchon 1999) and biopsychosocial (Dworkin and Burgess 1987) theories. Both of these concepts propose a complex interaction between environmental, emotional, behavioural and physical factors in the aetiology of TMDs. However, specific risk factors involved may or may not be active in any given case and therefore do not answer the question of why the individual patient develops a TMD. Thus whilst these concepts are helpful at a population or group level they may be limited when faced with the individual patient.

Some aetiological factors have received wide acceptance. A proportion of acute TMD patients report a clear association with trauma. In chronic cases the initiation of pain is also often associated with a history of trauma but whether this is the aetiology, a cofactor or a trigger in the process is unclear. Importantly, however, the psychological status and psychosocial functioning of the patient have emerged as central in determining the establishment of chronic muscular pain and its treatment response (Suvinen et al 2005b).

In the following section we overview current thinking on possible factors that may be active in the initiation and maintenance of chronic muscle pain. It will become clear to the reader that there is evidence for the involvement of multiple mechanisms at the level of the muscles, the peripheral nervous system (PNS) and the central nervous system but that the net result is at present inconclusive. In our view the complex and heterogeneous clinical phenotype of muscle pain (tension-type headache, myofascial pain, fibromyalgia) probably involves different parameters (PNS versus CNS) maybe at different levels of activity. For example, fibromyalgia may mainly be an expression of CNS dysfunction whilst myofascial pain may involve peripheral mechanisms that may over time initiate central changes.

3.4.2. Muscle Pain

The sensation of muscle pain is usually the result of activation of polymodal muscle nociceptors; groups III and IV, functionally and anatomically equivalent to Aδ and C fibres, respectively. These fibres have a high stimulation threshold and, under normal conditions, are therefore not activated to physiologic movement or normal muscle stretch. However, muscle nociceptors may be sensitized by peripherally released neuropeptides that increase their response to suprathreshold stimuli and may induce long-term changes in the central nervous system, such as central sensitization (Mense 2003). Damage to individual muscle cells releases sufficient intracellular adenosine triphosphate to activate purinergic receptors and induce pain.

However, there are subgroups of patients with muscle pain such as in fibromyalgia where pain may not be dependent on any peripheral input. Indeed as discussed below pain can occur secondary to a dysfunctional descending antinociceptive system or overactive descending facilitatory system, or due to a loss of central inhibitory neurons (see also Chapter 11).

3.4.3. Nervous System Alterations in TMD Patients

There have been numerous studies documenting neurophysiological characteristics of TMD patients. Unfortunately many of these did not differentiate between muscular and joint-based aetiologies so that their usefulness is extremely limited. Moreover, most of these studies have been inconclusive and have largely been replaced by quantitative sensory testing and functional studies of the sensory system.

QST studies frequently reveal abnormal somatosensory processing in TMD patients. Large myelinated fibre hypersensitivity was shown in the skin overlying TMJs in patients with clinical pain and TMJ pathology (Eliav et al 2003). However, patients with MMP demonstrated superficial (skin) large myelinated nerve fibre hyposensitivity

(Eliav *et al* 2003). Similarly, MMP patients show higher detection, discomfort and pain thresholds (decreased sensitivity) to stimuli applied to the skin over the masseter muscle (Hagberg *et al* 1990). Within the patient group, those with the greatest spontaneous pain had the lowest threshold values. Tonic muscular pain has been shown to induce an elevation of detection threshold to graded monofilaments both in the affected and in the contralateral side, suggesting involvement of central mechanisms (Stohler *et al* 2001). Impaired vibrotactile function and discrimination from the skin overlying muscles in MMP patients has been shown (Hollins and Sigurdsson 1998).

In contrast, lowered pressure-pain thresholds in deep tissues have been consistently reported in MMP patients, suggesting peripheral sensitization of muscle nociceptors (Hedenberg-Magnusson *et al* 1997; Maixner *et al* 1998; Svensson *et al* 2001). What exactly activates the peripheral muscle nociceptor and induces muscle hyperalgesia is unclear. Stimuli may include peripheral chemical or mechanical agents and trigger point activity (see below) in addition to reactive or even primary central mechanisms that may lead, for example, to neurogenic inflammation (Svensson and Graven-Nielsen 2001). Experimental inflammatory conditions of the TMJ and pericranial muscles lead to changes classically associated with central sensitization which can be reversed with central delivery of *N*-methyl-D-aspartate (NMDA) antagonists (Sessle 1999). These findings implicate central neuroplasticity in initiating and maintaining chronic muscle pain.

Altered pain regulation is suggested by findings of significantly more prevalent generalized body pain (e.g. fibromyalgia and back pain) and headache in TMD patients (John *et al* 2003). In support of this theory, TMD patients exhibit lower pain thresholds, greater temporal summation of mechanically and thermally evoked pain, stronger aftersensations and multisite hyperalgesia (Maixner *et al* 1998; Sarlani *et al* 2004). These indicate generalized hyperexcitability of the central nervous system and generalized upregulation of nociceptive processing (decreased inhibition or increased facilitation) and have been suggested as important pathophysiologic mechanisms (Sarlani *et al* 2004). In support of this hypothesis, pain from TMDs was not attenuated after peripheral noxious stimuli (ischaemic tourniquet test), which would normally activate noxious inhibitory modulation, suggesting differential or faulty recruitment of inhibitory controls (Maixner *et al* 1995). The response of MMP patients to experimental ischaemic pain was subsequently shown to also depend on depression and somatization scores (Sherman *et al* 2004). This suggests a complex interaction between psychosocial and biological variables in TMD patients.

Patients with TMD show enhanced C-fibre-mediated temporal summation to thermal stimuli applied to either the face or the forearm compared to control subjects and have impaired ability to discriminate stimulus frequency (Maixner *et al* 1998). These findings further suggest a component of central hyperexcitability which contributes to the enhanced pain sensitivity observed in TMD patients. In clinical studies about two-thirds of facial pain patients report widespread pain outside the craniocervical region (Turp *et al* 1998). However, no generalized hypersensitivity in MMP patients has been shown in other experiments (Carlson *et al* 1998). Thus although some cases of MMP have multisite hyperalgesia, others do not—a situation reflected in clinical experience. This may suggest two clinical and possibly therapeutic subtypes of MMP: with or without extracranial muscle involvement. Alternatively multisite hyperalgesia may be a graded, time-dependent phenomenon (Svensson and Graven-Nielsen 2001), and indeed experimental studies show that somatosensory sensitivity develops in the presence of experimental jaw muscle pain (Svensson *et al* 1998a).

3.4.4. Trigger Points, Muscle Hypoperfusion and Muscle Pain

Myofascial pain syndrome whether in the facial area, head or other body parts is often characterized by the presence of trigger points (Gerwin *et al* 2004; Simons 2004). It is thought that muscular pain arises from trigger points and indeed in many MMP patients pressure on a trigger point will activate intense pain and induce referral to characteristic sites. The muscle around a trigger point (TrP) is usually hard and may be nodular or appear as a taut band. Data suggest that TrPs are found in the area of the neuromuscular junction at the motor endplate and that these are tonically active, resulting in localized contraction that together with adjacent active endplates contributes to the formation of the taut band or nodule (Gerwin *et al* 2004). The continuous electrophysiological activity of motor endplates is secondary to unchecked release of acetylcholine. Endplate activity or noise is significantly more common in myofascial pain patients than in controls. Continued contraction in the area of TrPs leads to localized hypoxia (hypoperfusion), lowered pH and the accumulation of proinflammatory mediators (Simons 2004; Shah *et al* 2005). Lowered pH increases the activity of peripheral receptors including the vanilloid receptor, further sensitizing muscle nociceptors (Mense 2003). This localized contraction in TrPs is not, however, associated with generalized muscle hyperactivity so this should not be confused with the hyperactivity theory discussed below. The appearance of active TrPs is thought to be related to muscle trauma particularly eccentric muscle lengthening during contraction (Gerwin *et al* 2004). However, experiments directed at inducing such damage have largely been inconclusive (see below).

It has been suggested that muscle hypoperfusion may be the primary factor in initiating muscle pain, possibly due to changes in sympathetic control (Maekawa *et al* 2002). Moreover the unchecked motor endplate activity described above develops sensitivity to sympathetic nervous system activity (Gerwin *et al* 2004). Similarly sensitized nociceptors may be activated by sympathetic activity. Thus, the sympathetic nervous system is capable of independently initiating all the features of myofascial pain (Maekawa *et al* 2002; Mense 2002). There is insufficient data at present to entirely endorse or refute this hypothesis.

3.4.5. Muscle Lesion and Trauma

It has been increasingly recognized that traumatic events in the craniofacial region lead to chronic TMD pain, similar to chronic post-traumatic headache. Trauma can be classified as macrotrauma (e.g. head injury) or microtrauma (e.g. dental treatment) (Huang *et al* 2002). Trauma history is present in significant numbers of patients with TMD (Pullinger and Seligman 1991; Huang *et al* 2002) and has been documented to cause regional myofascial pain (Benoliel *et al* 1994).

Indirect trauma as in hyperextension-flexion injury to the cervical complex (whiplash) has been implicated in the aetiology of TMDs (Klobas *et al* 2004). However, long-term follow-up of whiplash patients does not indicate an increased risk for chronic TMD (Barnsley *et al* 1994; Ferrari *et al* 1999; Kasch *et al* 2002). In summary there is insufficient substantial clinical data to support a causative role for whiplash in TMD (Kolbinson *et al* 1997).

Whether post-traumatic TMD patients suffer more severe symptoms or are more resistant to treatment is unclear (De Boever and Keersmaekers 1996; Kolbinson *et al* 1997; Steed and Wexler 2001). There are indications that early intervention with a conservative approach (physical therapy, tricyclics, nonsteroidal anti-inflammatory drugs (NSAIDs)) significantly improves prognosis of post-traumatic cases (Benoliel *et al* 1994).

3.4.6. Muscle Hyperactivity and Bruxism

For many years it was believed that abnormal patterns of muscle activity were crucial in the initiation and maintenance of chronic muscle pain. It was proposed that a painful muscle lesion led to tonic excitation of muscle afferents (hyperactivity) that led to muscle overwork, tiredness and spasm. This would in turn reactivate the muscle nociceptors establishing the 'vicious cycle' of pain spasm/hyperactivity pain, a process adopted as an aetiologic factor in TMDs. In the orofacial region bruxism was adopted as a specific aetiological factor particularly when associated with occlusal disharmony. These theories are discussed and critically analysed in the following sections (Lobbezoo and Lavigne 1997).

3.4.6.1. Bruxism

Bruxism may be defined as involuntary activity of the jaw musculature characterized by nonfunctional (unrelated to chewing or swallowing) clenching, grinding or gnashing of teeth and may occur whilst the patient is awake or asleep (sleep bruxism (SB)) (Kato *et al* 2003). Additionally bruxism may be a primary phenomenon or associated with neurologic, psychiatric, post-traumatic disorders or as a side effect of drugs, smoking or alcohol (Kato *et al* 2003; Winocur *et al* 2003; Ahlberg *et al* 2004). Primary SB is defined as a sleep disorder or parasomnia which is not an abnormality of the processes responsible for sleep and awake states per se but an undesirable physical phenomenon that occurs during sleep.

Bruxism is most common in children (7–38%) and tends to decline with age to about 5% in subjects aged 45–65 years but these figures are based largely on self-reported frequencies (Lavigne and Montplaisir 1994; Ohayon *et al* 2001; Granada and Hicks 2003; Cheifetz *et al* 2005).

It is important to appreciate that rhythmic masticatory muscle activity (RMMA) produces positive EMG findings that may occur with no tooth grinding (Lavigne *et al* 2001). RMMA is extremely common and occurs in 60% of healthy controls and may easily be mistaken for tooth grinding (Lavigne *et al* 1996). However, the number of RMMA episodes in bruxers is three times higher than in controls and is associated with tooth grinding in 33% of episodes (Lavigne *et al* 2001).

Sleep bruxism is considered an arousal phenomenon or a sleep parasomnia (Kato *et al* 2003; Lobbezoo *et al* 2006). SB occurs most often when the sleep stage is suddenly shifted to a lighter one; mostly during stage 1 or 2 of sleep, and rarely at the deep stages (3 and 4) (Dettmar *et al* 1987). SB is not observed during bursts of REM sleep, when the arousal threshold is quite high (Kato *et al* 2003). It appears therefore that light sleep or the lightening of sleep, either externally applied or internally originated, is important for the occurrence of bruxism (Bader and Lavigne 2000; Lavigne *et al* 2001).

The presence of stress secondary to normal work life has been associated with increased frequency of self-reported bruxism (Ahlberg *et al* 2004). A positive relationship was also found between increased urinary epinephrine and high levels of nocturnal masseter muscle activity, implying that sleep bruxism is stress-related (Clark *et al* 1980). Experimental stress in normal individuals increases masticatory muscle EMG activity, supporting the theory that stress induces muscular hyperactivity (Intrieri *et al* 1994). One study showed that stress produces a selective idiosyncratic muscular response at the site of pain in patients suffering from a chronic muscular pain condition such as back pain or MMP (Flor *et al* 1992). In summary the aetiology of sleep bruxism is currently thought to be related to changes in the central/autonomic nervous system that may be modulated by stress (Kato *et al* 2003).

Bruxism may cause muscle hypertrophy and severe damage to the dentition. The parafunctional forces applied during bruxism have also been suggested in the aetiology of dental implant failure, periodontal tissue damage and tooth fracture. Hypothetically the repetitive overloading of the TMJ and muscles by bruxing movements may cause tissue damage leading to TMDs. It is possible that muscle overload may initiate or reactivate trigger points (see above) in susceptible individuals. Additionally an association between bruxism and MMP that involves occlusal disharmonies that in turn induce muscle hyperactivity, joint overloading and pain has been proposed.

In order to be able to establish a cause and effect relationship between bruxism and MMP the evidence needs to be examined with several criteria as basic tenets: bias, chance and confounders are absent; the association is consistent; bruxism must precede MMP; some type of relation exists between the degree of bruxism and the severity of the MMP (i.e. a dose–response); and the association makes epidemiologic sense (Lobbezoo and Lavigne 1997). We will now examine whether occlusal discrepancies induce muscle hyperactivity and whether occlusal discrepancies or muscle hyperactivity can cause MMP.

3.4.6.2. Muscle Pain, Bruxism and Occlusal Derangement

A relation between bruxism and MMP is based on the vicious cycle theory where an occlusal interference is supposed to induce hyperactivity and spasm of the affected muscle, which in turn leads to ischaemia secondary to blood vessel compression. Ischaemic contractions are painful and activate muscle nociceptors; by this mechanism the vicious cycle is closed. Whilst the extent of the occlusal 'interference' may be minute it supposedly upsets proprioceptive feedback and triggers bruxism with spasm of masticatory muscles. These assumptions have been refuted by experiments demonstrating that artificial occlusal discrepancies tend to reduce bruxism rather than enhance it (Rugh et al 1984) and by the lack of correlation between oral parafunctions and pain intensity in TMD patients (van der Meulen et al 2006). Clinically no correlation has been found between bruxism and muscle tenderness (Pergamalian et al 2003).

Prerequisites for such an aetiology would be that MMP patients demonstrate persistently elevated activity of masticatory muscles at rest and show a consistent relation to malocclusion. Although EMG activity recorded from masticatory muscles in some patients is higher, later studies have shown that this activity fails to accurately define patients versus controls (Glaros et al 1997). Recent studies have avoided the issue of muscle hyperactivity but have examined the effects of acute artificial occlusal interferences on parameters such as facial pain, chewing ability and jaw fatigue instead (Le Bell et al 2006). There is no doubt in our minds that acute malocclusions will cause extreme discomfort. However, this experimental setup does not parallel the clinical situation in MMP patients where purported malocclusions occur slowly and are accompanied by skeletal growth and adaptation. Indeed the effects in these studies were most prominent on occlusal discomfort and chewing problems with TMD patients showing reduced adaptation (Le Bell et al 2006). Their results show that the TMD patients undergoing placebo intervention also had a tendency to develop mild symptoms, in some cases comparable to the non-TMD population with active interferences (Le Bell et al 2006). This would seem to indicate that TMD patients have less adaptive capabilities to both active and control interventions, but leaves the precise relationship between TMD pain and occlusion unanswered.

Several long-term follow-up studies have also shown no consistent pattern between occlusal variables and TMDs (Carlsson et al 2002). In patients awaiting full dentures no statistically significant correlations were found between signs and symptoms of TMD and occlusal errors or freeway space (Dervis 2004). Studies show no occlusal factors to be consistently associated with TMD onset and no malocclusion is able to accurately predict TMD incidence (Gesch et al 2004b; Pahkala and Qvarnstrom 2004). Taken together the data indicate that occlusal factors seem to be of minor if any importance in the aetiology of TMDs.

3.4.6.3. Bruxism and Orofacial Pain

Excessive bruxism with insufficient relaxation, as in jaw clenching, is thought to lead to muscle ischaemia and pain. In this context the most widespread belief is that MMP is induced by repetitive tooth clenching, grinding or abnormal posturing of the jaw. These habits are, however, extremely common and statistically have not been proven to induce MMP. Evidence for masticatory muscle hyperactivity in the aetiology of MMP is largely indirect, and relies mostly on experimental tooth clenching.

The theory that muscle hyperactivity can cause pain is based on accumulated data that prolonged and unaccustomed exercise is followed by transient local muscle soreness. Exercise-induced muscle soreness appears on the following day and, in the absence of repeated vigorous exercise, gradually disappears in one week. These exercises usually involve eccentric lengthening (isotonic) contractions of the involved muscle with subsequent injury suggested as the mechanism. Damage was found, however, to be less likely following isometric and shortening exercises, a situation most likely to occur in tooth clenching and tooth grinding. Histochemical and histological research on rodents has also supported the hypothesis that lengthening contractions produce more damage than shortening contractions (Armstrong et al 1983).

Additionally the vicious cycle theory predicted that MMP patients would demonstrate increased muscle activity both at rest and during contraction. However, it remains to be unequivocally proven that MMP patients do in fact show higher muscle activity than controls. Studies in TMD patients have shown that maintained muscular activity is an inconsistent finding; some show no differences (Carlson et al 1993), others small increases (Glaros et al 1997) and still others small decreases relative to controls (Intrieri et al 1994). The observed increases in activity are minimal and there is no evidence that this can lead to muscle pain (Svensson and Graven-Nielsen 2001). The specificity of increased EMG activity is questionable and open to contamination by the muscles of facial expression, which become active during pain (LeResche *et al* 1992).

Functional studies in TMD patients show that EMG activity in the jaw-closing muscles occurs when the patient attempts to open the mouth (Yemm 1979). During painful mastication EMG activity of jaw-closing muscles is decreased in the agonist phase and slightly increased in the antagonist phase (Turp *et al* 2002). Indeed activity in muscle nociceptors tends to induce inhibition of the alpha motoneuron pool during contraction (Lund and Stohler 1994). Furthermore, patients with MMP demonstrate shorter endurance at submaximal contractions (Clark *et al* 1984; Gay *et al* 1994) and a substantially reduced biting force compared to controls, which has been attributed to muscle pain and tenderness (Buchner *et al* 1992; Shiau *et al* 2003). In summary, these findings are likely to reflect a protective mechanism that avoids further tissue damage, and do not lend support to the hypothesis of increased muscle activity in MMP patients.

Whether MMP can occur secondary to experimental muscle contractions is also unclear. Studies demonstrating immediate post-contraction hyperaemia suggest that pain is secondary to contraction-induced ischaemia (Clark *et al* 1991). A prolonged increase in tissue fluid pressure following experimental tooth clenching in man and muscle oedema in MMP patients has been demonstrated, suggesting an inflammatory response (Christensen 1971; Ariji *et al* 2004).

Masticatory muscle pain has been studied experimentally using two general approaches. Exogenous models of pain involve the injection of algesic substances into muscle and are discussed later in this section. Endogenous models of experimental pain have been studied extensively and involve the persistent contraction or exercise of masticatory muscles (Svensson and Graven-Nielsen 2001). Sustained high-force jaw contractions, by tooth grinding as an isotonic exercise (Christensen 1971) and by tooth clenching as an isometric exercise (Christensen 1981), induce muscle pain in normal volunteers. Protrusive exercises induce soreness on the same day which lasts till evening; however, no delayed muscle soreness or jaw movement restriction was reported (Scott and Lundeen 1980). Indeed much of the work on endogenous models of experimental muscle pain has not reported on the presence of delayed muscle pain. Pain is difficult to induce following sustained isometric protrusive contractions and no significant post-experimental changes were found in maximum active pain-free opening, lateral excursion and jaw pain for up to 7 days following the experiment (Clark *et al* 1991). Patients with a diagnosis of MMP are characterized by unilateral muscle pain which has been rarely reproduced experimentally. Moreover replication of some of these studies did not consistently produce pain and no significant site specificity was found — even when the exercise was intended to cause such specificity (Bowley and Gale 1987). This may be due

to the extensive 'coactivation' of many muscles. Even in more recent experiments some subjects (25–30%) appeared to be very susceptible to developing muscle pain during or after stressful exercises, while other subjects did not; thus, there was a clear vulnerability factor apparent (Glaros and Burton 2004). There is further support for this susceptibility theory in experiments on muscle pain patients versus healthy controls. Jaw muscle pain patients are able to do only a fraction of the work performed by healthy subjects (Clark *et al* 1984), and a reduced endurance capacity was found in those with either active or past jaw muscle pain when compared to that in controls (Choy and Kydd 1988). Additional data indicate that muscles in TMD patients are a priori weaker than in controls and may predispose them to pain (Buchner *et al* 1992).

Obviously these intensive experimental exercises are not identical to the chronic parafunctional activities which occur in patients. For example, chronic low-level clenching induces muscle pain but again only in a subset of patients (Glaros *et al* 1998). It has also been found that self-reported clenching is more consistently associated with MMP than grinding although there was no cause and effect relationship established (Velly *et al* 2003). The reliability of self-reported bruxing habits is problematic; 85–90% of the population will report that at some time they have ground or clenched their teeth (Bader and Lavigne 2000). Many patients who self-report tooth grinding admit that this was first brought to their attention by their dentist (Marbach *et al* 1990). The reliability of clinician judgements of bruxism has been found to be extremely poor (Marbach *et al* 2003). Notwithstanding, self-reported clenching is frequently associated with MMP (Huang *et al* 2002; Johansson *et al* 2006). However, the directionality of a possible cause and effect remains unproven and additionally bruxism and MMP may be clinical manifestations of a shared neuropathology.

Whilst the models described have not totally elucidated the mechanisms underlying MMP they have consistently shown that pain following experimental muscle contraction is of short duration and self-limiting. Thus sustained or repeated abnormal loading of the masticatory apparatus as in these experiments is of a doubtful primary role in chronic MMP. The role of overloading in TMJ disorders is discussed in Chapter 8.

If muscle hyperactivity is clearly related to MMP, bruxers should report more muscle pain. Some preliminary results suggest that a majority of patients with bruxism have pain levels and sleep quality comparable with MMP patients (Lavigne *et al* 1991). Myalgia is reported in only 20–30% of bruxers and it unclear whether this is a myofascial pain or a form of post-exercise muscle soreness (PEMS) (Lavigne *et al* 1996; Bader and Lavigne 2000). Recent studies show that only gender, joint clicking and other non-painful TMD symptoms are significantly related to nocturnal EMG activity or bruxism (Ahlberg *et al* 2004; Baba *et al* 2005). Moreover 19.7% of MMP patients report peak pain in the morning whilst in bruxers this is 83.3%, suggesting that the latter may indeed be a form of PEMS (Lavigne *et al* 1996; Camparis and Siqueira 2006). Additionally the bruxers with morning pain have fewer tooth grinding episodes than those without (Bader and Lavigne 2000). This may be due to a protective mechanism that reduces muscle activity in the presence of pain. Alternatively the high bruxers with no pain may have undergone an adaptive process (Bader and Lavigne 2000). When bruxers with and without TMD were compared, no significant differences in bruxism levels or sleep patterns were present (Camparis *et al* 2006). In contrast a study on adult bruxers revealed frequent complaints of orofacial and bodily pain and 65% reported frequent headaches in the morning (Bader *et al* 1997). However, the patients in Bader *et al* (1997) reported more comorbid features such as anxiety and tension than those in Lavigne *et al*'s studies (e.g. Lavigne *et al* 1996).

In summary, available data do not support the traditional concept of myofascial pain induced or maintained by muscle hyperactivity (Lund *et al* 1991). Moreover examining the available data vis-à-vis the ideal criteria for establishing a cause and effect relationship casts serious doubts on the validity of the hypothesis that muscle hyperactivity leads to chronic MMP. Bias and confounders such as anxiety, EMG activity from the muscles of facial expression and the separation of RMMA from actual grinding or clenching are not consistently excluded or accounted for. Daytime and sleep bruxism may be different in their effects on the masticatory system but these have not been separated in studies. The association between bruxism and MMP is inconsistent; experimental models show a high degree of selectivity and no prolonged muscle pain. No dose–response is present as demonstrated by the facts that bruxers do not report extremely high levels of MMP and high-activity bruxers in fact complain less of morning muscle pain than do low-level bruxers. Finally the association makes little epidemiologic sense: TMDs are rare in children in whom bruxism is most common and TMD/MMP peaks in young adults when bruxism is shown to be decreasing in frequency. There is little evidence to support SB in the aetiology of MMP but the role of bruxing and clenching habits particularly in the daytime are as yet unclear (Lobbezoo *et al* 2006). Additionally we have little data on the ability of such bruxing habits to activate or initiate trigger points in masticatory muscles in a fashion similar to that suggested for myofascial pain in other regions (Simons 2004).

3.4.6.4. Does Orofacial Pain Lead to Muscle Hyperactivity?
Experimental muscle pain models induced by external stimuli are referred to as exogenous. These external stimuli include the injection of algesic substances that induce reliable models of muscle pain and include hypertonic saline (Graven-Nielsen *et al* 1998), neuropeptides such as serotonin or bradykinin (Babenko *et al* 1999) and capsaicin (Marchettini *et al* 1996). These models have shed light onto the referral patterns, pain quality, neuropharmacology and sensorimotor mechanisms underlying MMP.

An experiment on humans examined the effect of unilateral tonic muscle pain on EMG activity in the masseter and temporal muscles bilaterally (Stohler *et al* 1996). Muscle pain was induced by the infusion of hypertonic saline into the masseter muscle unilaterally and resulted in increased activity in all muscles. However, asking the patients to imagine pain of similar intensity (sham pain) also increased muscle activity to similar levels. The muscles of facial expression were also activated in reaction to both real and sham pain so that they were responsible for the increases in EMG activity (Stohler *et al* 1996). These findings have been confirmed in further studies and overall there is little experimental evidence to support jaw muscle pain as a long-term inducer of increased muscle activity (Svensson and Graven-Nielsen 2001; Ro *et al* 2002). Moreover orofacial pain tends to reduce bite force in both humans and animals (High *et al* 1988; Benoliel *et al* 2002) and blocking pain restores forceful contractions (High *et al* 1988).

Based on the above, the vicious cycle theory is untenable and an alternative model is needed to explain motor changes in patients with muscle pain and disorders.

3.4.7. The Pain Adaptation Model

The pain adaptation model is based on data from chronic musculoskeletal pain conditions (including that of TMDs) and proposes that the observed changes in motor function are secondary to chronic pain and mediated at the spinal level (Lund *et al* 1991). Changes in masticatory muscle function, secondary to experimental muscle pain as described earlier, support this model and confirm clinical complaints of dysfunction in muscular TMD patients (Svensson and Graven-Nielsen 2001). Injection of hypertonic saline into the jaw muscles induces pain with a significant reduction in jaw movements and in EMG activity during the agonist phase accompanied by a small increase in antagonist muscle activity (Graven-Nielsen *et al* 1997; Svensson *et al* 1998b). The pain adaptation model suggested that pain will induce inhibition of alpha motoneurons during jaw closing and facilitate these during antagonist (opening) activity (Lund *et al* 1991). This model therefore accurately fits the currently available data.

If muscle dysfunction is not the cause of pain but rather part of the spectrum of a 'pain-adaptation' response then some of the parafunctions including some of the bruxing habits can no longer be considered as a primary aetiological mechanism of pain in MMP (Lund *et al* 1991). However, the precise association between bruxism and MMP remains unclear at this stage.

3.4.8. The Temporomandibular Joint and Masticatory Myofascial Pain

Theoretically, trauma or noxious stimulation of TMJ tissues can produce a sustained excitation of masticatory muscles that may serve to protect the masticatory system from potentially damaging movements and stimuli (Sessle and Hu 1991). Clinically, the frequent comorbidity of arthralgia and myalgia (Huang *et al* 2002) has led to such hypotheses linking their aetiologies, but these have not been proven (Schiffman *et al* 1992). Such comorbidity may reflect sensitization and referral patterns mediated by primary afferents in the TMJ and muscles of mastication co-synapsing on dorsal horn neurons (convergence). Moreover experimental injection of algesic chemicals into the TMJ resulted in sustained reflex increase in EMG activity of jaw-opening muscles; excitatory effects were also seen in jaw-closing muscles but were generally weaker (Broton and Sessle 1988). While such effects may be related to clinically based concepts of myofascial dysfunction (e.g. splinting, myospastic activity and trigger points), the weak effects in jaw-closing muscles and the stronger effects in antagonist muscles suggest associations more in keeping with protective, withdrawal-type reflexes (Sessle and Hu 1991). Based upon the present available data it seems that pain originating in the TMJ contributes minimally to the development of MMP.

3.4.9. Skeletal Morphological Features

The association between certain skeletal morphological features and the prevalence of TMD has been the focus of much controversy. Data presented in early reviews and in recent research indicate that the distribution of major occlusal categories in TMD patients does not differ significantly from the normal population (Greene and Marbach 1982) and that no single occlusal problem can accurately predict TMD onset (Egermark *et al* 2001; Mohlin *et al* 2004).

3.4.9.1. Orthodontics
The possibility that orthodontic treatment in any of its many forms may lead to the initiation or deterioration of TMDs is of great concern. Recent research suggests that orthodontics does not entail an increased risk to developing either signs or symptoms of TMD (Egermark *et al* 2001, 2005; Henrikson and Nilner 2003; Mohlin *et al* 2004). Moreover in meta-analyses no study indicating that traditional orthodontic treatment increased the prevalence of TMD was found (Kim *et al* 2002; How 2004). Some mild signs such as soft click or tenderness on palpation were occasionally reported but these are difficult to accurately assess and asymptomatic clicks are considered physiological. The occlusion and the TMJ are important factors in successful orthodontic treatment and stability; once again the question remains as to the connection between these and TMDs. Evidence suggests that there is very little if any scientific evidence to support this connection.

3.4.10. Psychosocial Correlates

Chronic pain, from whatever source, is in many patients associated with psychological distress and psychosocial disturbances. These levels of distress may significantly impact on patient compliance and treatment outcomes. Although a minority of TMD patients will manifest significant psychological distress and psychosocial disturbances, the level of distress often predicts treatment demand and outcome (Epker and Gatchel 2000; Raphael *et al* 2000a). Indeed patients with chronic pain who finally do attend for treatment usually have more severe pain, distress and a poorer prognosis. Thus although psychosocial factors are not seen as aetiological factors in TMDs they have an important role in treatment response and transition to chronicity.

Currently psychosocial factors are considered important variables in chronic MMP; see Chapter 4. Patients with MMP are frequently found to suffer from other stress-related disorders such as migraine, backache, nervous stomach and gastrointestinal ulcers (Turp *et al* 1997; Korszun *et al* 1998; Aaron and Buchwald 2003). Elevated urinary concentrations of catecholamines and 17-hydroxy steroids in these patients suggest higher stress levels (Vanderas *et al* 2001).

Several methods for measuring the emotional results of stress or the intensity of environmental stress have been designed. These methods are employed as secondary endpoints in the assessment of outcomes in the treatment of chronic pain. The methodologies have recently been reviewed, and the Beck Depression Inventory (BDI) and the Profile of Mood States questionnaire are recommended for the assessment of treatment outcomes and for research in chronic pain (Dworkin *et al* 2005). For TMDs the RDC-TMD criteria have been extensively applied. Depression, as assessed by the BDI, and lack of sleep have been found to be significantly increased in TMD patients (Selaimen *et al* 2006). Cognitive coping abilities in response to injury and pain are also thought important in TMDs. Two aspects of coping emerge as therapeutically relevant in TMDs: control or adjustment in response to pain and the recruitment of maladaptive coping strategies such as catastrophizing in an attempt to control pain (Suvinen *et al* 2005b). A positive response to TMD treatment has been correlated to increased coping abilities (Schnurr *et al* 1991).

Studies suggest that stress-related disorders may underlie or contribute to the development of TMD chronicity and may therefore be viewed as perpetuating rather than initiating factors (Garofalo *et al* 1998; Epker *et al* 1999). Indeed TMD patients with increased self-efficacy measures suffered lower levels of pain, disability or psychological distress and reported greater use of an active, adaptive pain-coping strategy (Brister *et al* 2006). These findings form the basis for biobehavioural interventions described in Chapter 4.

3.4.11. Genes, Culture, Gender and Susceptibility

Genetic influences on TMD development have recently been shown (Diatchenko *et al* 2005). The study examined the effects of catecholamine-*O*-methyltransferase (COMT) on pain perception and found that the COMT genotype is highly associated with human pain perception. More relevant, the authors demonstrated an association between a genetic polymorphism that impacts risk for developing MMP; possession of a protective haplotype reduced the risk by a factor of 2.3 (Diatchenko *et al* 2005). The cultural and possibly genetic effects of chronic TMD pain on patient behaviour have also been recently highlighted (Reiter *et al* 2006). Despite no differences in the physical parameters of RDC-TMD diagnosis (Axis I) there were significant differences between two distinct ethnic populations in their psychosocial response (Axis II). However, a study on female MMP patients and their first-degree relatives revealed no evidence that there is any familial aggregation (Raphael *et al* 1999).

3.4.11.1. Gender and TMDs

The effects of gender on the epidemiology of pain syndromes and on pain thresholds have been extensively reported. Women suffer significantly more from migraines, tension-type headaches, fibromyalgia and TMDs. Under experimental conditions women consistently demonstrate a lowered pain threshold often affected by the stage of the menstrual cycle and by exogenous hormones such as oral contraceptives (Fillingim and Ness 2000). Both hormone replacement therapy and use of oral contraceptives have been associated with increased risk of TMD (LeResche *et al* 1997; Dao *et al* 1998) — although another report failed to confirm this association (Hatch *et al* 2001). In a study examining progression to chronicity in acute TMD patients, significant differences between men and women were observed (Phillips *et al* 2001). Overall more psychosocial distress was present in all patients progressing to chronicity but specifically women with a muscle disorder were extremely likely to become chronic pain sufferers. The pressure–pain thresholds of muscles in female MMP patients increased significantly by 16–42% in the follicular and luteal phases but remained low in the perimenstrual phase (Isselee *et al* 2002). The VAS pain ratings did not correspond with pressure–pain thresholds and could not predict the cycle phases so that the precise relationship between pain and the menstrual cycle was unclear.

There is evidence that oestrogen and nerve growth factor (NGF) may interact in the regulation of nociceptive processes. When NGF was systemically administered to healthy human subjects muscle pain particularly in the craniofacial region was observed but was more pronounced in women than in men (Petty *et al* 1994). Interactions between NGF and oestrogen have been shown (Gollapudi and Oblinger 1999) but the mechanisms involved in TMDs are unclear.

The injection of glutamate into the masseter muscle or the temporomandibular joint of the rat induced significantly greater muscle activity in female rats (Cairns *et al* 2002). Gonadectomy significantly reduced the magnitude of muscle activity in female rats following glutamate injection into the TMJ, a phenomenon partially reversible by the delivery of oestrogen (Cairns *et al* 2002). These studies clearly demonstrate that there are sex-related differences in glutamate-evoked jaw muscle activity that are female sex hormone dependent. Recent experimental studies have shown that ovarian steroids are able to regulate neuropeptides, particularly neuropeptide Y and galanin, in trigeminal ganglia (Puri *et al* 2005). These neuropeptides are involved in pain pathways and in neuronal reaction to injury.

The applications of gender differences in TMDs are unclear. In addition to gender-specific interactions between neuropeptides and hormones, the continued accumulation of knowledge pertaining to gender-related changes in pain sensitivity and analgesic use may elucidate further pathophysiological mechanisms.

3.4.12. Pathophysiology: Summary

It is clear that many factors may be active in the aetiology of TMDs in general and MMP in particular (Fig. 7.4). Host susceptibility plays a role in MMP at a number of levels. Some patients may be more prone than others to develop trigger points secondary to muscle injury — genetically influenced injury response. Other genetically influenced physical traits such as pain modulation and pharmacogenomics may then interact with psychological traits to determine disease onset and progression and indeed whether pain develops. Additionally environmental parameters such as ethnicity, culture and stress are essential variables in the patient's coping abilities and demand for treatment. The effects of gender are paramount and may be expressed via interactions between hormones and nociceptive pathways as well as environmental and cultural issues.

Any of the aetiologic agents discussed may contribute to MMP in one patient but not in another, who may require a single or a combination of aetiological factors to develop MMP. We are still unable, however, to accurately identify these factors in the individual patient so as to tailor a focused, mechanism-based treatment plan. Notwithstanding, available treatment options are able to offer adequate management for most MMP cases.

3.5. Treatment

Treatment of TMDs with a variety of conservative methods consistently results in high (75–90%) success rates (Dworkin *et al* 2002; De Laat *et al* 2003; Anastassaki and Magnusson 2004; Ekberg and Nilner 2004; Michelotti *et al* 2004). In general treatment is aimed at palliation and is based on clinical diagnosis; since the aetiology is unclear no treatment is curative. An interesting approach is to identify individual factors in specific patients and attempt to recognize their roles as possible predisposing, initiating and perpetuating factors (Okeson 1996).

Fig. 7.4 • Factors affecting the transition from acute to chronic temporomandibular disorder.

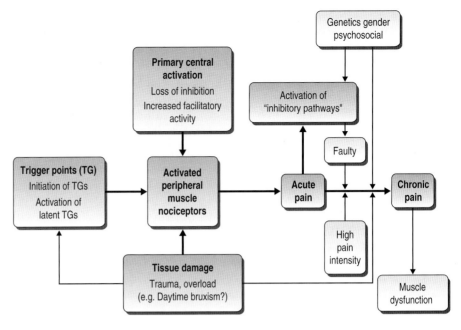

Individual factors may serve any or all of these roles in different patients.

Extensive research in the field of TMD therapy shows that there is no compelling data to support any intervention as capable of disease eradication or modification (Stohler and Zarb 1999). Moreover conservative therapies are consistently successful and are in no way inferior to more invasive or irreversible procedures such as surgery, occlusal adjustment or prosthetic rehabilitation (Anastassaki and Magnusson 2004). The data support a conservative approach to the management of TMDs. This is reinforced by findings that the natural history of MMP includes an extensive number of patients that will either substantially fluctuate or remit over time and rarely progress to severe pain (Magnusson *et al* 2000; Rammelsberg *et al* 2003). Patient's beliefs, medical status, type of employment and personal preference may often dictate the treatment plan; the patient should therefore be actively involved in the decision-making process.

Therapy for MMP falls into four categories: physical, pharmacological, psychological and trigger point injection and is often multidisciplinary (Sherman and Turk 2001; Benoliel *et al* 2003). Treatment of MMP very often combines conservative interventions and different centres have variable protocols depending on patients' signs and symptoms and personal preferences. Treatment duration is usually 4–6 months but in selected cases may be longer.

Most MMP patients seek treatment to alleviate pain; significant reduction or eradication of pain must then be one of the primary aims. However, treatment aims in chronic MMP patients are usually more complex and ambitious; these are summarized in Table 7.2. The assessment of treatment outcome should be based on accurate assessment of pain intensity and frequency (Chapter 3) and the evaluation of changes in psychosocial comorbidity (see Chapter 4).

Table 7.2	Treatment Aims in Masticatory Myofascial Pain
Aims	**Examples of Available Therapies**
Reduce pain	Simple analgesics, tricyclic antidepressant drugs, rest.
Restore function and range of motion	Physiotherapy. Reduce pain. Trigger injection. Vapocoolant.
Decrease aggravating or contributing factors	Identify specific variables acting in the individual patient and attempt to eradicate. These may include emotional and physical variables.
Increase bite comfort	Occlusal appliances.
Increase muscle strength	Physiotherapy. Restore function.
Reduce psychological distress	Empathy, information. Referral for counseling, cognitive behavioural therapy when needed.
Prevent drug abuse	Careful monitoring of drug use, efficient and prophylactic pain therapy.
Restore social functioning	Cooperation with family physician, family members. Referral for social and emotional help/counselling.

3.5.1. Chronicity in Myofascial Pain

The transition from acute to chronic MMP is dictated partly by response to initial treatment and is therefore discussed in this section. Attempts at designing models for predicting chronicity in TMD patients have revealed that high characteristic pain intensity and the presence of myofascial pain (versus TMJ disorders) were the most significant predictors of chronicity (Epker *et al* 1999). High pain intensity, high disability score, higher scores of emotional distress and being female with myofascial pain were predictors of chronicity (Garofalo *et al* 1998). Patients developing chronicity differed significantly in numerous biopsychosocial variables (e.g. they suffered from more current anxiety disorders, mood disorders and somatization disorders). TMD patients not responding to treatment were found to suffer from significantly higher rates of fatigue and sleep disturbances (Grossi *et al* 2001). It has been suggested that the development of chronicity involves neuroplastic changes in medullary dorsal horn, including functional and morphologic changes. At the same time endogenous factors, such as descending inhibition, are working to attenuate these changes and may vary in effect between patients. These findings are consistent with the theory that prolonged and intense nociceptive input is one of the initiating factors for chronicity with decreased biopsychosocial abilities, gender-related variables in pain modulation and generalized symptomatology possibly acting as perpetuating factors.

3.5.2. Physical and Combined Modalities

Most pain physicians with experience in the field of MMP will attest to the success of conservative physical therapy, including muscle exercise, thermal packs and oral splints. However, few, if any, of these therapies have been unequivocally proven in controlled trials. Often reassurance and education of the patient, combined with simple muscle exercises for masticatory and neck muscles, will result in pain alleviation and restored mandibular function (De Laat *et al* 2003; Michelotti *et al* 2004). Chewing exercises may be beneficial for some MMP patients but following vigorous exercises there may be increased pain (Dao *et al* 1994b; Gavish *et al* 2002). Based on accepted principles (Simons 2004), we use simple active stretch exercises performed by the patient: two minimal mouth openings followed by a gentle and slow maximal opening (stretch) without causing extreme pain. Wooden or plastic tongue spatulas may be used by the patient as a dynamic record of maximal opening attained. These exercises are performed three times every 1 or 2 hours. Patients with suboccipital and cervical muscle tenderness or chronic pain will benefit from the addition of active neck exercises. Rotation of the head and ear to shoulder movements with mild 'stretching' to each side (three times each) are similarly prescribed every 1–2 hours. Under normal conditions patients will rotate the head by about 70° whilst ear–shoulder movements are inherently more limited (40°).

Muscle tenderness may be also treated with vapocoolant sprays and concomitant stretching; 'spray and stretch' (Simons 2004). This usually induces immediate relief and is often employed as a diagnostic test (Table 7.1). Other techniques commonly used such as ultrasound and thermal packs have not been rigorously assessed. However, since these are conservative approaches individual patients who benefit from their use should be encouraged to continue. Transcutaneous electrical nerve stimulation (TENS) was not superior to placebo, although both induced improvement in pain and maximal opening in TMDs (Taylor *et al* 1987). Flat occlusal splints were shown to be superior to TENS in the treatment of TMJ-associated symptoms (Linde *et al* 1995). There is some evidence to support the use of low-level laser therapy in TMD patients particularly in MMP (Cetiner *et al* 2006). When combined with an exercise program laser therapy significantly improved symptoms more than in exercise alone (Kulekcioglu *et al* 2003). However, there was no advantage in adding laser therapy when pain intensity was specifically analysed (Kulekcioglu *et al* 2003).

A physical self-regulation (PSR) programme consisting of training in breathing, postural relaxation and proprioceptive re-education has been shown to be superior to conservative therapy (flat-plane intraoral appliance and self-care instructions) at 6-month follow-up (Carlson *et al* 2001). In a further study conservative treatment by specialists was compared with a structured self-care programme in TMD patients with minimal levels of psychosocial dysfunction (Dworkin *et al* 2002). The specialist treatments included splints, physiotherapy, analgesics, muscle relaxants and patient education (diet and parafunctional habits). There were no limitations on the combinations of treatments or on the number of visits. The self-care program incorporated cognitive behavioural therapy and self-care techniques such as relaxation. One year later both groups showed improvement in all clinical and self-report categories measured (Dworkin *et al* 2002). However, the patients in the self-care programme showed significantly decreased TMD pain, decreased pain-related interference in activity and reduced number of painful masticatory muscles, and required fewer visits. These studies indicate the importance of education and self-care in the management of TMDs.

3.5.3. Occlusal Adjustments and the Management of TMDs

There is no doubt in our minds that occlusion is of paramount importance in restorative and prosthetic dentistry. The question remains as to the relationship between TMDs and occlusion. The historical importance of occlusion in the aetiology of TMDs, although largely unproven, led to the extensive use of occlusal adjustment. It is true that occlusal adjustment may induce pain relief in some cases but the irreversible nature of this procedure is problematic. To date there is divergence of opinion concerning occlusal and skeletal factors in TMDs. A large number of general and specialist dentists still view occlusal factors as important in the pathophysiology and management of TMDs and many continue to equilibrate the occlusion as therapy for TMDs. Based on published research and clinical experience irreversible occlusal adjustment or rehabilitation for the treatment of TMDs is in our view contraindicated. Patients with prosthodontic needs will benefit from sound prosthodontic rehabilitation; that should not be confused with the treatment of TMDs. We summarize the available data but this is not to be misunderstood as in any way endorsing occlusal adjustment for TMD. To those who remain unconvinced we advise the use of reversible techniques such as splints.

Comparing occlusal adjustment with conservative care it was found that the clinical dysfunction score was significantly diminished only in the latter treatment group (Wenneberg et al 1988). A further study presented results of occlusal adjustment as significantly improving subjective symptoms in TMD patients (Vallon et al 1991). However, there was no significant change within or between groups with regard to frequency of headaches, the number of tender muscles, facial pain or pain on mandibular movements (Vallon et al 1991). When compared to counselling occlusal adjustment was beneficial but only in the short term and not across all symptoms (Vallon et al 1995). Occlusal adjustment aimed at removing presumed structural risks was significantly associated with a reduced incidence of TMD over a 4-year follow-up (Kirveskari et al 1998). However, the groups were relatively small (total $n = 127$) and there was no examiner calibration. Moreover mock adjustment removed no enamel at all and to test that the true occlusal equilibration was indeed the important factor the control groups should have had non-relevant occlusal areas 'adjusted'.

The sum results of the studies supporting adjustment presented above are equivocal. Factors not considered in these studies are the irreversible nature of occlusal adjustments and that these adjustments are not stable over time and tend to partially recur (Hellsing 1988). Moreover occlusal adjustment shows no advantage over any other conservative and reversible therapy. Large reviews and meta-analyses uniformly conclude that occlusal adjustment has no current evidence base to support its use (Forssell and Kalso 2004; Koh and Robinson 2004). It becomes apparent that occlusion plays a minor if any role in the aetiology and therefore the treatment of TMDs (McNamara 1997; De Boever et al 2000).

3.5.4. Occlusal Splints

Occlusal splints may be soft or hard and may be fabricated with full or partial tooth coverage. A recent example of a new type of partial coverage bite plate is the 'nociceptive trigeminal inhibition tension suppression system' (NTI) that has been advocated for the treatment of headache (Shankland 2002). Some splints are designed with the aim to reposition the mandible in a new maxillo-mandibular relation (repositioning splints). Soft appliances are probably as efficacious as hard splints in the management of MMP but are difficult to adjust and repair (Turp et al 2004). Repositioning appliances have been used extensively to treat internal derangements (ID) of the TMJ and aim to 'recapture' the disc (see Chapter 8). Whilst these appliances may successfully capture discs in ID with reduction in the short term, they fail to do so at all for ID without reduction or osteoarthritis (Eberhard et al 2002). Moreover long-term stability of successful treatment is usually not good and clicks or abnormal disc positions tend to recur (Lundh and Westesson 1989; Tallents et al 1990). Recent studies show that repositioning appliances have no significant benefit over stabilization appliances in the treatment of TMJ sounds (Tecco et al 2004). Additionally repositioning splints may induce irreversible occlusal changes and are therefore not recommended. In the management of TMJ disorders splints are sometimes constructed to reduce TMJ loading by providing occlusal contacts in the posterior region only (Nitzan 1994).

Flat occlusal splints (relaxation or stabilizing splints) are in widespread use and provide even occlusal contacts; these may be constructed for the upper or lower jaw. Stabilization splints are effective in the management of TMJ arthralgia; see Chapter 8 (Ekberg 1998). There seems to be no difference in effect between flat splints and splints designed to provide canine guidance on lateral excursions of the mandible (Conti et al 2006). We are reluctant to use partial coverage splints due to the inherent potential to cause permanent occlusal changes and the lack of evidence for any advantage over flat splints (Magnusson et al 2004; Al Quran and Kamal 2006). To avoid occlusal changes all patients with any appliance must be instructed not to wear it all the time. Additionally appliances must be regularly checked and repaired if need be. We have seen cases where the splint has fractured in the area of the last molars (the thinnest part) and has allowed the selective overeruption of these teeth, therefore causing an anterior open bite.

Meta-analyses consistently demonstrate benefit for oral splints in TMDs in general (Forssell and Kalso 2004). The most recent meta-analytic review concludes that 'stabilization splint therapy may be beneficial for reducing pain severity at rest and on palpation and depression when compared to no treatment' (Al-Ani et al 2005). There have been several studies investigating the efficacy of occlusal appliances in the treatment of MMP (Kuttila et al 2002; Ekberg and Nilner 2004; Wassell et al 2006). Most have resulted in improvement in both active and placebo arms (non-occluding splints) of the trial with only marginal superiority of the active splint (Turp et al 2004). Similar effects of non-occluding splints on TMJ pain and clicking have been observed (Conti et al 2006). The presence of widespread pain reduces the effectiveness of oral splints and suggests that these should be prescribed for patients with regional myofascial face pain only (Raphael and Marbach 2001). The number needed to treat (NNT) for occlusal appliances in the treatment of TMDs has been calculated (Forssell and Kalso 2004). NNT calculates the number of patients that need to be treated to obtain 1 patient with $\geq 50\%$ reduction of worst pain. For oral splints an NNT of 6 was obtained for TMJ pain and of 4.3 for MMP. The relatively good success rate and highly conservative nature of splints accounts for their extensive use (Pierce *et al* 1995). However, splints entail substantial costs in their manufacture and maintenance. A recent study suggests that splint therapy, both high-cost laboratory-processed or chairside thermoplastic splints, offers no significant advantage over conservative self-care strategies (Truelove *et al* 2006). The self-care strategies include jaw relaxation, reduction of parafunction, thermal packs, physiotherapy, stress reduction and the use of NSAIDs (Truelove *et al* 2006).

The exact mode of action of splints is unproven. Splints may reduce sleep bruxism (Clark *et al* 1979) but both control and placebo splints induce similar reductions in muscle activity (Dube *et al* 2004). However, after prolonged wear of splints bruxing movements tend to recur and this occurs despite the fact that symptoms such as pain remain improved (Sheikholeslam *et al* 1986; Chung *et al* 2000). The above data and the lack of evidence for the role of muscle hyperactivity in TMDs confirm that reduction of bruxism is not the mode of action of splints in the relief of TMD. Currently splints are considered to act through nonspecific mechanisms probably involving behaviour-modifying properties.

3.5.5. Pharmacological

3.5.5.1. Simple Analgesics
Nonsteroidal anti-inflammatory drugs are used extensively in the management of pain and disability associated with joint disease. Although the antiplatelet and gastrointestinal safety profile of selective cyclooxygenase (COX)-2 inhibitors is superior they still have potentially serious side effects on the renal and cardiovascular system; see Chapter 15. For the treatment of TMDs calculations of NNTs for drugs versus placebo reveal encouraging figures of 2.7–3.5 (Forssell and Kalso 2004). Based on current evidence ibuprofen (400 mg 3 times daily) or etodolac (1200 mg daily) are efficacious (see Chapter 15). Simple analgesics or combination analgesics (e.g. codeine and paracetamol) may also provide good analgesia and may be safer than NSAIDs. In myofascial pain patients, ibuprofen combined with diazepam is superior to ibuprofen (Singer *et al* 1987). However, the use of benzodiazepines as analgesics is of questionable value and antidepressants, muscle relaxants and anticonvulsant drugs are more efficacious.

3.5.5.2. Antidepressants, Benzodiazepines, Muscle Relaxants and Antiepileptic Drugs
Amitriptyline at low doses (10–30 mg/day) is superior to placebo (Sharav *et al* 1987) and has been consistently reported as beneficial for patients with craniofacial myofascial pain, including predominantly muscular TMDs (Plesh *et al* 2000) and post-traumatic myofascial pain (Benoliel *et al* 1994). The use of clonazepam, a long-acting benzodiazepine with anticonvulsant properties, has been

beneficial (Harkins *et al* 1991), but the muscle relaxant cyclobenzaprine has proven superior to clonazepam in a recent study (Herman *et al* 2002). More recently gabapentin, a novel antiepileptic drug, has been tested in a randomized double-blind fashion for the treatment of MMP (Kimos *et al* 2007). Gabapentin showed to be clinically and statistically superior to placebo in reducing reported pain, masticatory muscle hyperalgesia and the impact of MMP on daily functioning. Reduction in muscle tenderness was observed after 8 weeks but the effects on pain appeared only after 12 weeks of therapy at a mean dose of about 3400 mg per day (Kimos *et al* 2007). The NNT was calculated at 3.4 for gabapentin in the treatment of MMP. Involvement of the sympathetic nervous system is suspected in MMP, similar to that observed in fibromyalgia (see below). Recent findings of genetically based abnormalities in catecholamine pathophysiology in MMP (Diatchenko *et al* 2005) theoretically support the treatment of MMP with adrenergic blockers; no controlled trials have as yet been published. More quality drug trials in craniofacial myofascial- and arthralgic-pain patients are needed, and treatment remains somewhat empirical.

3.5.6. Biobehavioural Therapy

Pain is a subjective experience with important affective, cognitive, behavioural and sensory components; see Chapter 4. Like other chronic pain syndromes, MMP is a complex entity associated with changes in mood, behaviour and attitudes to life in addition to drug abuse and secondary psychological gains. Therefore outcomes including restoration of functional activity, eradication of drug abuse and dependency, and rehabilitation of residual emotional distress need to be addressed. Careful review of such parameters as lost workdays, sleep disturbance and general functioning provide valuable insight as to the emotional well being of the patient. Patients reporting a high degree of disability, psychological distress or drug or alcohol abuse may suffer from underlying psychosocial distress. Sleep disturbances are often part of emotional disorders and are intimately related to a number of chronic pain syndromes (Brousseau *et al* 2003). Although experienced clinicians may obtain much information from an interview it is generally accepted that this is insufficient for a reliable psychosocial assessment (Oakley *et al* 1989). The assessment of psychological distress in MMP patients may be performed with the RDC-TMD questionnaire or with established alternatives (Turner and Dworkin 2004; Dworkin *et al* 2005).

Cognitive behavioural therapy (CBT) is an option and aims at altering negative overt behaviour, thoughts or feelings in chronic-pain patients and diminishing distress and suffering (Chapter 4). Whether separately or combined with other pain treatments, CBT produced significantly decreased pain, emotional distress and disability and are of proven efficacy in TMD patients (Turner *et al* 2006).

Biofeedback aims to teach the patient to control behaviour that is possibly part of the pain aetiology; see Chapter 4 (Crider and Glaros 1999). The lack of evidence for muscle hyperactivity in the aetiology of muscular TMDs questions the validity of this method. Indeed some studies have shown that headache improves whether patients increase or decrease muscle activity (Borgeat et al 1985). However, biofeedback is efficacious in regulating muscle tension in TMD patients with good long-term results (Flor and Birbaumer 1993) and the limited data available support the efficacy of EMG biofeedback treatments for TMD (Crider and Glaros 1999). This may be particularly useful for TMJ disorders associated with overloading; see Chapter 8. Combination of biofeedback with CBT techniques significantly improves treatment outcomes versus CBT alone (Mishra et al 2000; Gardea et al 2001).

3.5.7. Trigger Point Injections and Needling

Injections of local anaesthetics into 'trigger points' induce pain relief that may be prolonged beyond the effect of the anaesthetic agent (Simons 2004). The technique for the head and neck muscles is simple and involves the location and immobilization of the trigger point followed by injection using a standard dental syringe and 27-gauge needle; other body areas may require thicker needles (Fig. 7.5). Introducing the needle into the trigger point may induce sharp pain, muscle twitching or an unpleasant sensation. Prior to injection the overlying skin should be cleansed with an approved antiseptic. Some suggest that the needle be inserted 1–2 cm away from the trigger point and then advanced at an acute angle of 30° to the skin into the trigger point proper. Once an initial injection is performed (about 0.2 mL) the needle may be withdrawn to the level of the subcutaneous tissue, then redirected superiorly, inferiorly, laterally and medially, repeating the needling and injection process in each direction. All injections should be preceded

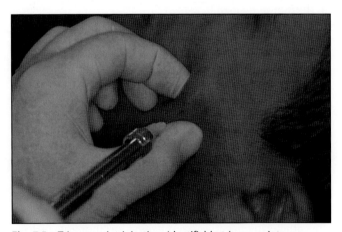

Fig. 7.5 • Trigger point injection. Identifiable trigger points are immobilized between two fingers and local anaesthetic solution is then injected. Injection should be performed at a number of points around the trigger. The needle should be retracted (but not withdrawn from the skin) and reinserted at each injection point. This technique combines the effects of local anaesthetic with the effects of 'needling'.

by aspiration to ensure that the needle is not in a blood vessel. Following injection the muscle should be gently mobilized. Stretch exercises and analgesics are prescribed postoperatively to ensure that mouth opening and muscle function remain improved. In myofascial pain patients, bupivacaine (0.5%) is equi-efficacious to botulinum toxin in the relief of pain and cost effectiveness would suggest the former's preferential use (Graboski et al 2005). We initially use mepivacaine (3%) to test patient response. If the results are encouraging and the patient needs further injections we may then employ bupivacaine (0.5%), although there are reports of bupivacaine-induced damage to muscle fibres. However, based on an extensive literature review direct (or 'dry') needling of myofascial trigger points appears to be an effective treatment, most likely because of the needle or placebo rather than the injection of either saline or active drug (Cummings and White 2001). Thus whether these needling therapies have efficacy beyond placebo is unclear. Dry needling of trigger points is very similar to some acupuncture techniques.

3.5.8. Complementary and Alternative Therapy

Patient interest in and demand for complementary or alternative medicine (CAM) is increasing; see Chapter 17. Approximately 20% of facial pain patients in a referral centre have attended a CAM specialist previously and up to 36% of TMD patients have reported treating their symptoms with CAM techniques (Chapter 17). The existing evidence supports the value of acupuncture for the management of idiopathic headaches and has shown promise in the management of TMDs (Chapter 17). However, well-planned studies need to assess the clinical value and cost-effectiveness of acupuncture and other CAM therapies for facial pain.

3.5.9. Treatment: Summary and Prognosis

Based on the review above the clinician may choose from a number of conservative therapeutic options that depend on the history, physical findings and comorbid signs in the individual patient (Fig. 7.6).

Chronicity of MMP is manifest by the increased need for long-term treatment of these patients (Wexler and McKinney 1999). However, prognosis in the majority of MMP patients is good and remission of pain and dysfunction is readily achieved for long periods.

4. Tension-Type Headaches

Tension-type headache is extremely common and most individuals will have experienced one in their lifetime (Rasmussen 1995). The IHS subclassifies TTH into episodic (infrequent and frequent), chronic and probable TTH; see Tables 7.3, 7.4. The individual attacks in these subentities have similar clinical features with some subtle differences; severity and the occurrence of mild nausea tend to increase

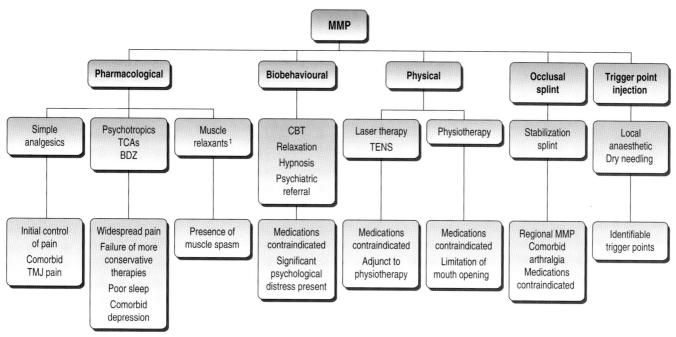

Fig. 7.6 • Treatment of masticatory myofascial pain (MMP). A wide variety of conservative treatment options are available. Choice is dictated by symptomatology, comorbid medical or psychological problems and physician or patient preference. (TCA, tricyclic antidepressants; BDZ, benzodiazepine; 1, muscle relaxants are recommended for short-term management).

Table 7.3	Diagnostic Criteria: Episodic Tension Type Headache (ETTH)	
Temporal Diagnostic Criteria Infrequent (I) ETTH		**Notes**
A	At least 10 episodes occurring <1 day per month on average (<12 days per year) and fulfilling criteria B–D.	TTH patients often present with clinical pericranial muscle tenderness. However, some cases do not and the role of muscle tenderness and hyperactivity is at present unclear. TTH has therefore been subclassified as with or without pericranial tenderness.
Temporal Diagnostic Criteria Frequent (F) ETTH		
A	At least 10 episodes occurring ≥1 but <15 days per month for at least 3 months (≥12 and <180 days per year) and fulfilling criteria B–D.	
Additional Diagnostic Criteria for Both IETTH & FETTH		**Notes**
B	Headache lasting from 30 minutes to 7 days.	
C	Headache has at least two of the following characteristics: 1. Bilateral location 2. Pressing/tightening (non-pulsating) quality 3. Mild or moderate intensity 4. Not aggravated by routine physical activity such as walking or climbing stairs.	Accumulating evidence suggests that some TTHs may be aggravated by exercise (see text).
D	Both of the following: 1. No nausea or vomiting (anorexia may occur) 2. No more than one of photophobia or phonophobia.	Mild migraines may be phenotypically similar to ETTH. Criteria D are very common in migraines.
E	Not attributed to another disorder.	Secondary headache has been excluded by history, examination and imaging if appropriate.

Based on Olesen *et al* (2004) with permission.

Table 7.4 Diagnostic Criteria: Chronic Tension-Type Headache[a]

	Diagnostic criteria	Notes
A	Headache occurring on ≥15 days per month on average for >3 months (≥180 days per year) and fulfilling criteria B–D	CTTH evolves from ETTH. Chronic headache starting de novo should be classified as NDPH[b]; see Table 7.5.
B	Headache lasts hours or may be continuous.	
C	Headache has at least 2 of the following: 1. Bilateral location 2. Pressing/tightening (non pulsating) quality 3. Mild or moderate intensity 4. Not aggravated by routine physical activity such as walking or climbing stairs.	
D	Both of the following: 1. No more than one of photophobia or phonophobia or mild nausea 2. Neither moderate or severe nausea nor vomiting.	These criteria may complicate differentiation with chronic migraine (Chapter 9) and cases may need careful follow-up (pain diaries) to accurately diagnose their headaches. CTTH is bilateral.
E	Not attributed to another disorder.	Secondary headaches have been ruled out. Medication overuse (MO) is common in chronic headache and may lead to MO headache; see text and Chapter 13.

Based on Olesen et al (2004) with permission.
[a] Based on the presence of muscle tenderness being subclassified as with or without pericranial muscle tenderness.
[b] New daily persistent headache.

with frequency. Pericranial muscle tenderness is an extremely common feature in TTH patients but since some patients do not demonstrate this feature the IHS subclassifies TTH as with or without pericranial tenderness.

4.1. Epidemiology and Genetics of Tension-Type Headache

TTH has a one-year prevalence in adults of over 80%, an incidence higher than migraine, and a lifetime prevalence of over 80% (Rasmussen 1995; Lyngberg et al 2005a). Population studies indicate that infrequent episodic TTH (IETTH) which occurs on average once per month is most common (48–59%) but does not usually require medical attention (Lyngberg et al 2005b; Russell 2005). One-year prevalence of frequent episodic TTH (FETTH) in the population is 18–43% and 10–25% report weekly headaches (Russell 2005; Jensen and Symon 2006).

The frequency and severity of TTH attacks are fundamental in estimating socioeconomic and personal impact. By definition patients with FETTH suffer more than one attack monthly but fewer than one headache every other day and this can have a significant impact on quality of life. Indeed FETTH patients report on average 3 missed days of work per month (Pryse-Phillips et al 1992). In one study 12% of TTH patients reported absence from work during the previous year because of headache (Stovner et al 2006). Considering the high prevalence of TTH this is a significant problem. TTH, in particular chronic TTH (CTTH), is thought to account for more than

10% of disease-related absenteeism in Denmark (Rasmussen et al 1992a). CTTH has a profound negative effect on the well being of patients with significantly reduced quality of life (Holroyd et al 2000).

The average onset age of TTH is 20–30 years with peak prevalence in the third to fifth decades (Lyngberg et al 2005b). However, up to 25% of school children report having TTH (Stovner et al 2006) and in the older population (>60 years) the prevalence is 20–30%. Post-adolescent females are only slightly more affected than males (ratio F:M=5:4) (Lyngberg et al 2005b; Jensen and Symon 2006).

Genetic studies reveal that first-degree relatives of CTTH sufferers are three times as likely to also suffer headaches relative to the population (Ostergaard et al 1997). This suggests that CTTH has important genetic factors. FETTH is significantly affected by environmental factors with evidence for only a minor genetic contribution (Ulrich et al 2004).

4.2. Episodic Tension-Type Headache

4.2.1. Clinical Features

Location. ETTH is almost exclusively bilateral (>90%) and is usually described as 'band-like' or 'cap-like' and affects, in order of frequency, the occipital, parietal, temporal or frontal areas (see Fig. 7.2) (Iversen et al 1990; Rasmussen et al 1991). Pain site may vary with intensity and between patients (Iversen et al 1990).

Quality and severity. Quality of pain is described by the vast majority of cases as pressure-like, dull or as a sensation of tightness (Iversen *et al* 1990). A throbbing character is rare in TTH, but has been reported in 14–20% of patients, particularly during more severe attacks (Iversen *et al* 1990; Inan *et al* 1994).

Pain of TTH is considered milder than migraine pain but the differences may not always be as striking as expected. Usually TTH is mild to moderate in intensity (Rasmussen *et al* 1991; Gobel *et al* 1994), but may become moderate to severe with an increase in headache frequency (Rasmussen 1996). This is in contrast to the pattern observed in migraine: an all or none phenomenon where pain severity is largely unaffected by headache frequency (Chapter 9).

Temporal pattern. The temporal features of individual ETTHs are extremely variable both within and between patients. TTH duration may range from 30 minutes to 7 days (Olesen *et al* 2004) with reported median duration ranging 4–13 hours (Pryse-Phillips *et al* 1992; Jensen 1996). The median frequency in the population ranges from one headache every 2 months to 2 headache days per month whilst in a clinic population it is expectedly higher at 6 days per month (Pryse-Phillips *et al* 1992; Gobel *et al* 1994). The IHS classification lists five diagnostic criteria for ETTH (listed A–E) with the first criterion (A) distinguishing, by temporal features, between infrequent and frequent ETTH (Table 7.3).

Long-term follow-up indicates that most (75%) ETTH patients continue to suffer episodic attacks but 25% report evolving into CTTH (Couch 2005; Jensen and Symon 2006). However, in another study 45% of patients with FETTH or CTTH experienced remission over a follow-up period of 12 years, suggesting that some TTH patients have a good long-term prognosis (Lyngberg *et al* 2005c). Negative prognostic factors for TTH included not being married, no physical activity and poor sleep (Lyngberg *et al* 2005c). ETTH is a chronic condition with an average duration prior to treatment of 9–12 years (Gobel *et al* 1994; Lyngberg *et al* 2005c).

Precipitating or aggravating factors. ETTH is commonly precipitated by a number of factors: stress, fatigue, disturbed meals, menstruation, alcohol and a lack of sleep (Spierings *et al* 2001; Karli *et al* 2005). These are similar to those reported by migraineurs (see Chapter 9).

TTH is usually not aggravated by physical activity (Iversen *et al* 1990). This has been considered a major differentiating factor from migraine where over 95% report aggravation by exercise (Rasmussen *et al* 1992b). However, there are reports that exercise may aggravate pain in 16–28% of TTH patients (Ulrich *et al* 1996; Koseoglu *et al* 2003).

Associated signs. A proportion of ETTH sufferers experience significant disability related to pain severity, frequency and accompanying features such as poor sleep (Lipton *et al* 2002). Sleep disturbances are common in TTH sufferers and fatigue is reported in up to 80% of cases. Lack of sleep is a common precipitant of TTH.

Accompanying symptoms are rare in the less frequent forms of TTH but mild to moderate anorexia is reported by 18% of cases (Rasmussen *et al* 1991). Occasional and mild photophobia (10%) or phonophobia (7%) has been observed (Iversen *et al* 1990; Rasmussen *et al* 1991).

Many patients will suffer both migraines and TTH that may further impact quality of life. Interestingly ETTH in migraine sufferers responds to sumatriptan, a migraine-specific drug, whilst in non-migraine patients it does not (Lipton *et al* 2000). This may suggest that mild migraines may phenotypically be very similar to ETTH (see Chapter 9).

4.3. Chronic Tension-Type Headache

CTTH is one of the subtypes of a more recent diagnostic family simply termed chronic daily headaches (CDH). The umbrella diagnosis of CDH is based on the daily or near daily occurrence of headaches.

4.3.1. Chronic Daily Headaches

The diagnosis of CDH is based on specific criteria that have been shown to accurately classify most cases (Silberstein *et al* 1996). Most importantly, CDHs are defined as occurring on at least 15 days per month and may be subdivided into two forms: primary or secondary (attributable to specific pathology). The most common secondary type of CDH is medication overuse headache (Chapter 13). Primary CDHs are mostly a continuation of their episodic counterparts and may be short or long-lasting (>4 hours per attack) and include chronic migraine (CM; Chapter 9), chronic trigeminal autonomic cephalgias including hemicrania continua (HC; Chapter 10), CTTH and new daily persistent headache (NDPH); the latter two entities are phenotypically similar and are described in this section. The diagnosis of NDPH is reserved for patients with daily headache with strictly no history of episodic migraine or ETTH. Since most patients with daily headache have a tendency to abuse analgesics (Bigal *et al* 2002) that themselves potentially induce headache, the primary CDHs must occur without drug abuse. The concept of CDH is clinically and epidemiologically useful but since it represents a family of entities with different therapeutic responses a specific diagnosis is essential for successful management.

The prevalence of CDH in the population, from children to the elderly, is about 2.5–5% and remains consistent across global studies (Hagen *et al* 2000; Lanteri-Minet *et al* 2003; Stovner *et al* 2006). CTTH has a global prevalence of 2–3% (Russell 2005; Jensen and Symon 2006) and chronic migraine has been estimated to occur in 1.3–2.5% of the population (Chapter 9). Therefore the vast majority of CDH patients in the population suffer from CTTH or CM. Chronic daily headache is very common in headache clinics. In one study 45% of 171 patients with a primary complaint of headache were diagnosed as suffering from

CDH; 62% of them had CM, 34% had CTTH, 2.6% had NDPH and 1.3% were diagnosed with HC (Deleu and Hanssens 1999). In paediatric headache clinics CDH may be rarer and account for about 5% of primary headaches (Raieli *et al* 2005). Most studies demonstrate that 25–38% of CDH patients are abusing analgesics (Castillo *et al* 1999; Wang *et al* 2000; Prencipe *et al* 2001). This would require persistence of symptoms following cessation of drug abuse prior to final diagnosis. Treatment of CDH depends on the specific diagnosis and is based on prophylactic regimens involving many classes of drugs (see Chapters 9, 10, 13 on the relevant disorders and Chapters 16 and 17 on the drugs commonly employed).

4.3.2. Clinical Features of Chronic Tension-Type Headache (Table 7.4)

Classically the patient with CTTH is middle-aged, female with a long headache history that began with episodic headaches 10–20 years previously and slowly increased in frequency (Bigal *et al* 2002; Solomon *et al* 1992; Scher *et al* 2003). The clinical features of CTTH are largely similar to those in FETTH with differences in accompanying features, treatment response and impact on quality of life.

Location and quality. In 80–98% of cases CTTH is bilateral and usually located in the frontal, temporal or frontotemporal regions (Rasmussen *et al* 1991; Solomon *et al* 1992; Bendtsen and Jensen 2004). Headaches limited to the occipital region have also been reported (Langemark *et al* 1988).

Pain quality is similar to that reported in ETTH and is mostly pressure-like and bilateral (Rasmussen *et al* 1991). Severity of CTTH in population and clinic studies reveal that the majority (78%) suffer moderate pain, some (14.8–16%) mild and very few (4–7.4%) severe (Rasmussen *et al* 1991; Manzoni *et al* 1995).

Temporal pattern. CTTH is characterized by a continuous or daily headache. Mean frequency obtained from patient diaries is 23–30 headache days per month (Jensen and Rasmussen 1996; Bendtsen and Jensen 2004).

Associated signs. Many CTTH patients demonstrate increased pericranial tenderness in regional muscles. This is more severe in trapezius, neck and sternocleidomastoid muscles but is also detectable in masseter and temporalis (Bendtsen *et al* 1996a). Headaches are often accompanied (32% of cases) by photo- or phonophobia (Langemark *et al* 1988). As reported for ETTH physical activity may worsen pain in a subgroup of CTTH patients (Rasmussen *et al* 1991; Manzoni *et al* 1995).

TTH sufferers report a lack of sufficient and of restorative sleep but this is a common finding in chronic pain patients and may also be related to depression (Palermo and Kiska 2005). Indeed as observed in other chronic pain conditions, depression and anxiety are common in CTTH patients (de Filippis *et al* 2005).

Photo- or phonophobia were reported by 17% of a population and 32% of a clinic-based study on CTTH patients

(Langemark *et al* 1988; Rasmussen *et al* 1991). Nausea was reported by 25% of CTTH patients in the population. CTTH may be diagnosed in cases with only one of photo-, phonophobia or mild nausea (Table 7.4; Olesen *et al* 2004).

4.3.3. Pathophysiology

Interrelationships between peripheral and central mechanisms probably underlie the initiation of TTHs but the exact aetiology is uncertain. It is interesting to note that the same aetiological factors are considered in TTH and in MMP, further suggesting common pathophysiology.

4.3.3.1. Pericranial Muscles as a Source of Pain

It is unclear whether the presence of pericranial muscle tenderness is the cause or the result of the headache. Moreover many patients with TTH present without pericranial myofascial tenderness.

Human experiments with intramuscular injection of algesic substances (usually hypertonic saline) induce pain and referral patterns characteristic of craniofacial myofascial syndromes. Injections into the sternocleidomastoid and trapezius muscles produce localized pain with referral to regions associated with TTH location (Jensen and Norup 1992; Simons *et al* 1999; Svensson *et al* 2003a; Schmidt-Hansen *et al* 2006). In contrast injection into the masseter, medial or lateral pterygoids refers pain to the teeth, angle of the mandible and temporomandibular joint and resembles the pain pattern observed in MMP (Svensson *et al* 2003a; Schmidt-Hansen *et al* 2006). Quality and intensity of resultant pain do not differ significantly between injection sites. This would suggest a prominent role for muscle nociceptors in the location and referral patterns of reported pain in TTH and MMP. Pain referral patterns also involve central convergence of peripheral afferents onto second-order neurons in subnucleus caudalis, central sensitization with expansion of receptive fields (Svensson *et al* 2003b) and activation of convergent thalamic neurons (Kawakita *et al* 1993).

4.3.3.2. Muscle Hyperactivity

Excessive contraction of muscles has been thought to play a major role in the pathophysiology of many myofascial disorders including TTH. Pericranial muscle activity in TTH patients has been shown to be variably normal or increased. Later studies have similarly been inconclusive but in summary there is no substantial evidence to support a causal relation between pericranial muscle hyperactivity and TTH. Some TTH patients do have increased muscle activity but this may be in line with the protective mechanisms proposed by the pain adaptation model (Lund *et al* 1991). Moreover contamination of EMG recordings by the muscles of facial expression is an important confounding variable.

Experimental chewing (concentric exercises) with or without temporal artery ischaemia induces a bilateral dull head pain (Gobel and Cordes 1990). TTH was induced by prolonged tooth clenching with muscle tenderness that preceded the onset of headache by several hours (Jensen and Olesen 1996). Prolonged experimental frontalis muscle contraction, however, failed to produce headaches in a group with relatively frequent TTH (Lacroix and Corbett 1990). Moreover a further study on TTH patients showed no significant differences in the induction of headache between active clenching and holding a toothpick between their lips as a control procedure (Neufeld *et al* 2000). Both groups, however, developed more headaches than in non-TTH patients under the same experimental conditions. This would suggest that abnormalities in central pain transmission or modulation alter the susceptibility of patients to develop headache and are more important than muscle strain induced, for example, by jaw clenching. Similar conclusions may be derived from an experiment testing headache onset following static contraction of the trapezius muscle; although more TTH patients developed headache than did controls there was no significant difference in headache development between the active and the placebo procedure (tibial muscle contraction) in patients or controls (Christensen *et al* 2005). Eccentric exercises are proposed to induce ultrastructural muscle damage and thus lead to pain. This has been postulated to involve abnormalities in muscle blood flow but experiments show this is normal in CTTH patients (Ashina 2004). During static contraction diminished flow was noted but was unassociated with ischaemia or inflammation (Ashina 2004). Headache has been produced following various experimental muscle exercises but is usually short lasting even following prolonged exercises (Arima *et al* 1999). Thus the role of pericranial muscle tenderness in TTH remains unclear; in TTH patients with muscle tenderness it has been suggested that the mechanisms involve persistent nociceptive input leading to central sensitization that is negatively affected by faulty central modulation. This hypothesis is very similar to that proposed for MMP but leaves the origin of the peripheral nociceptive activity unanswered.

4.3.3.3. Biopsychosocial Parameters

The complex relationships between chronic pain and psychosocial pathology have been increasingly investigated, including in the field of headache. Significant psychopathology is observed in a minority of headache patients in the population, although those with significant problems are more likely to seek treatment for their headaches (Lake *et al* 2005). For example, patients with recurrent headaches (e.g. TTH or migraines) exhibit significantly more psychiatric comorbidity (Breslau *et al* 2003). Significant psychopathology complicates headache management and is associated with a reduced prognosis. Individuals with recurrent TTH report more stressful events and judge them to have more impact on their lives (Wittrock and Myers 1998). TTH sufferers also seem to recruit different coping strategies for both stress and pain (Wittrock and Myers 1998). However, there is little evidence of differences in physiological responses to stressful events (Wittrock and Myers 1998). Coping abilities have not been extensively studied in TTH but catastrophizing may be more common in TTH sufferers. In summary the cause and effect relationship between TTH and psychosocial problems is unclear but may affect treatment outcome.

4.3.3.4. Peripheral and Central Neural Mechanisms

In both ETTH and CTTH there is a high proportion of patients with tenderness of the myofascial tissues (including tendons) that is present during and between attacks, suggesting peripheral sensitization (Lipchik *et al* 2000; Neufeld *et al* 2000). Interestingly muscle tenderness correlates with frequency and intensity of TTH and often the relief of TTH is accompanied by reduced muscle tenderness (Bendtsen and Jensen 2000). Once again the peripheral mechanism associated with these findings remains unclear.

However, it has been suggested that sensitivity in the pericranial muscles may be secondary to changes in the central nervous system. In a trial on the initiation of TTH by tooth clenching it was found that FETTH patients who did not develop headache developed increased pressure pain thresholds, suggesting that clenching activated their antinociceptive system (Jensen and Olesen 1996). Interestingly the patients that did develop headache had no change in pressure pain thresholds. This suggests that patients unable to recruit endogenous antinociceptive pathways are more likely to develop headache (Jensen and Olesen 1996). This lends support to the hypothesis that muscle tenderness may be secondary to central sensitization and/or faulty supraspinal inhibitory or facilitatory mechanisms (Pielsticker *et al* 2005). The presence of central sensitization in CTTH is supported by findings of increased sensitivity to pressure, electrical and thermal stimuli at craniofacial and general body sites (Langemark *et al* 1993; Bendtsen *et al* 1996a). In most studies, pain detection and tolerance thresholds are also reduced in CTTH patients (Langemark *et al* 1993; Bendtsen *et al* 1996a). In contrast ETTH patients, other than those with FETTH, demonstrate normal pain detection thresholds (Jensen *et al* 1993a; Jensen 1996). In CTTH there is a significant correlation between generalized sensitivity and pericranial tenderness (Bendtsen *et al* 1996a; Jensen *et al* 1998). Since CTTH is most often a progression from FETTH it is likely that central sensitization in CTTH patients is induced by prolonged nociceptive inputs from myofascial tissues (Bendtsen 2000). Impairment of endogenous supraspinal pain modulation systems following experimental pain has been shown in CTTH patients (Sandrini *et al* 2006). The evidence thus suggests that peripheral mechanisms play a major role in ETTHs, whilst central mechanisms such as faulty inhibitory mechanisms and central sensitization are prominent in CTTH.

4.4. Treatment of Tension-Type Headache

Patient education is essential; there are accessible websites that explain headaches and their treatment (e.g. http://www.achenet.org/). The dangers of analgesic drug abuse must be made clear to the patient and every effort made to control it. Many patients with frequent ETTH or CTTH suffer from impaired function and quality of life often accompanied by emotional distress and drug abuse that needs careful and professional attention.

4.4.1. Pharmacological

The pharmacological management of TTH may be subdivided into abortive (individually treat the acute attack) or prophylactic approaches depending on headache frequency, patient preference and other factors. Abortive approaches are largely pharmacologic whilst psychologic, physiotherapeutic and TMD-aimed treatments have all been employed in the prophylactic treatment of TTH with varying degrees of success. Abortive pharmacotherapy should not be employed in CTTH as the high headache frequency may lead to analgesic abuse and medication overuse headache (see Chapter 13).

As abortive therapy mild analgesics or NSAIDs have been consistently proven efficacious and are considered first choice. Mild headaches may respond favourably to 1 g of paracetamol or aspirin (Steiner et al 2003). Ibuprofen (200–400mg) is superior to paracetamol and aspirin with better and faster pain relief (Schachtel et al 1996). Low-dose diclofenac is comparable to 400mg of ibuprofen (Kubitzek et al 2003). The more rapidly absorbed naproxen formulation, naproxen sodium (375–550mg), is effective in TTH and the higher dose was superior to 1 g paracetamol (Prior et al 2002). Overall, however, onset of pain relief is delayed in most of these drugs (Mathew and Ashina 2006). Based on efficacy and safety profiles expert recommendations suggest 800 mg ibuprofen or 825 mg naproxen sodium as drugs of choice (Mathew and Ashina 2006). Combination analgesics are often employed but may offer small advantage over single drugs and increase the risk of medication overuse headache. However, caffeine at doses from 130–200 mg has been proven to increase the efficacy of ibuprofen and other mild analgesics in the treatment of TTH, but caffeine carries a high addiction profile and should be carefully monitored (Diamond and Freitag 2001). In patients with CTTH, or coexisting migraine and ETTH, triptans have induced significant pain relief (Brennum et al 1992; Cady et al 1997).

Tricyclic antidepressants have been extensively studied as prophylactic agents and are superior to serotonin selective agents in TTH (Bendtsen et al 1996b). Amitriptyline is consistently efficacious in prophylactically reducing frequency, duration and severity of CTTH (Tomkins et al 2001). Interpreting these results to clinical practice and patient expectations needs extreme care; often statistically significant reductions in headache duration (e.g. from 11 to 8 hours) may be of doubtful significance to the patient (Fumal and Schoenen 2005). Nevertheless amitriptyline and other tricyclic antidepressants are widely used for CTTH. Indeed amitriptyline is effective in CTTH but not in ETTH, suggesting different pathophysiologic mechanisms. Amitriptyline should be initiated at 10 mg daily taken just before bedtime (see Chapter 17) and then titrated according to response and side effects. Studies on CTTH patients show that a higher dose is often needed (75 mg) (Fumal and Schoenen 2005). Based on the high frequency of pericranial muscle tenderness in TTH, investigators have tried muscle relaxants, including the use of botulinum toxin (see Stillman 2002). Large trials are needed to confirm early reports of success.

4.4.2. Nonpharmacological Interventions

Commonly used behavioural interventions for TTH include relaxation training, biofeedback training and cognitive behavioural (stress-management) therapy (Holroyd 2002). These treatments attempt to influence the frequency and the severity of headaches and emphasize the prevention of headache episodes. Relaxation and electromyographic biofeedback therapies are effective mainly in ETTH, providing on average a 50% reduction in headache activity (Bogaards and ter Kuile 1994). However, in CTTH patients the combination of stress management with a tricyclic antidepressant (amitriptyline $\leq$100 mg/d, or nortriptyline $\leq$75 mg/d) was more likely to produce clinically significant reductions in headache index scores than each therapy alone or placebo (Holroyd et al 2001).

Physical or manual therapies are often integrated into the treatment plan of TTH sufferers. Physiotherapy is more effective than massage therapy or acupuncture for the treatment of TTH and appears to be most beneficial for patients with a high frequency of headache episodes. Chiropractic manipulation may be beneficial for TTH, but the evidence is weak. Data are lacking regarding the efficacy of these treatments in reducing headache frequency, intensity, duration and disability in many commonly encountered clinical situations. Many of the published case series and controlled studies are of low quality and there is very little rigorous evidence clearly supporting the use of these modalities (Fernandez-de-Las-Penas et al 2006).

4.4.3. Temporomandibular Disorder Therapies in the Treatment of TTH

The interpretation of the relevant literature is hampered by the overwhelming majority of studies (>95%) that are not randomized, controlled or blinded. Uncontrolled studies show a reduction in severity and frequency of headaches following occlusal splints, occlusal adjustments or physiotherapy (Magnusson and Carlsson 1983). With no placebo control and poor definition of headache types these studies are of limited applicability. The use of stabilization splints in headache patients with concurrent TMD resulted in a significant reduction in headache frequency and analgesic use relative to a group treated by a neurologist (Schokker *et al* 1990). This would seem to make sense in that comprehensive treatment planning to include all pain-related problems is more likely to produce beneficial results. Moreover the splint group was examined more often by the treating physician, which may have subconscious beneficial effects on treatment outcome. No significant effect of occlusal adjustment on headache frequency was observed (Vallon *et al* 1995). The use of a new type of bite plate, the nociceptive trigeminal inhibition tension suppression system, for the treatment of migraines and TTH has recently been proposed (Shankland 2002). The original studies were all open and have not been duplicated. Moreover the NTI provides occlusal contacts in the anterior region only and may, with overuse, cause permanent occlusal changes.

In summary, standard TMD therapies may help some TTH patients, particularly those with concomitant MMP. However, as previously stated irreversible destruction of tooth structure as in occlusal adjustment has in our view not enough evidence. In selected cases a trial with a flat occlusal splint may be justified.

5. New Daily Persistent Headache

This chronic headache appears with no history of previous TTH or migraine and has been previously termed chronic headache with acute onset. The headache as defined by the IHS must become chronic within three days of onset (Table 7.5) and this is the major differentiating feature in relation to CTTH; compare Tables 7.4 and 7.5 (Olesen *et al* 2004).

5.1. Clinical Features

Location. Pain is bilateral in most patients (62–87%) (Li and Rozen 2002; Takase *et al* 2004). Location involves the temporal region alone (20%) or in combination with other sites in 46% of patients. In one series retro-orbital pain was reported by 40% of patients (Li and Rozen 2002). Occipital areas are involved in 40–60% of cases and a minority will describe pain throughout the head (10–18%) (Li and Rozen 2002).

Quality and severity. Pressure (54%) and throbbing (10–55%) qualities are the individual descriptors most commonly reported (Li and Rozen 2002; Takase *et al* 2004). Pain quality is varied and many patients describe their pain with combinations of descriptors such as pressure or tightening (73%) (Takase *et al* 2004). Stabbing (45%), aching (43%), dull (37%) and tightness (36%) are also frequently employed. More rarely burning (23%) or searing (4%) pain is reported.

Most patients (66%) report headache severity as usually moderate (4–6 on a 10-cm VAS), some (21%), however, report persistently severe pain (>6 VAS rating) (Li and Rozen 2002). In a series of 30 NDPH cases from Japan all reported severe unbearable pain (Takase *et al* 2004). These cases excluded post-viral cases (see below) so the differences in pain severity may reflect a diagnostic subgroup or cultural differences (Takase *et al* 2004).

	Table 7.5	Diagnostic Criteria for New Daily Persistent Headache (NDPH)	
	Diagnostic Criteria		**Notes**
A	Headache for >3 months fulfilling criteria B–D.		
B	Headache is daily and unremitting from onset or from <3 days from onset.		If headache evolves from tension-type headache (TTH), diagnosis should be chronic TTH (CTTH)
C	Headache has at least 2 of the following: 1. Bilateral location 2. Pressing/tightening (non pulsating) quality 3. Mild or moderate intensity 4. Not aggravated by routine physical activity such as walking or climbing stairs.		Criteria C–E are identical to those for CTTH and may complicate differentiation (see text and Table 7.4). Criterion B is essential for accurate diagnosis.
D	Both of the following; 1. No more than one of photophobia or phonophobia or mild nausea 2. Neither moderate or severe nausea nor vomiting.		
E	Not attributed to another disorder.		Secondary headaches have been ruled out. Medication overuse (MO) is common in chronic headache and may lead to MO headache; see text and Chapter 13.

Based on Olesen *et al* (2004) with permission.

Temporal features. Many patients can accurately recall the exact date of headache onset with a subsequently rapid progression to chronic pain (<3 days) (Li and Rozen 2002). The vast majority will report headache that is present continuously but about one-fifth suffer from a daily headache lasting a number of hours (Li and Rozen 2002; Takase *et al* 2004).

Headache onset. A recent infection or flu-like illness is reported in 30% of cases (Li and Rozen 2002). Extracranial surgery (12%) and stressful life event (12–20%) are also common precipitators but in 46–80% there were no identifiable precipitating factors (Li and Rozen 2002; Takase *et al* 2004). One series excluded post-viral NDPH cases so that the contribution of viral infections to NDPH onset and phenotype remains unclear (Takase *et al* 2004).

Accompanying signs/symptoms. Associated symptoms may include nausea (33–68%) or vomiting (23%), phonophobia (68%), photophobia (3–66%), lightheadedness (55%), stiff neck (50%), blurred vision (43%) and vertigo (11%) (Li and Rozen 2002; Takase *et al* 2004). Aura-type symptoms have been observed in a small fraction of patients (Li and Rozen 2002).

Aggravating/relieving factors. Stress, physical exertion and bright light were reported as aggravating factors in 33–40% of cases (Li and Rozen 2002). Headache relief was obtained by lying down in two-thirds or by being in a dark room by almost one half of patients (Li and Rozen 2002). Massage relieved pain in about a quarter and sleep only in a minority of cases (9%) (Li and Rozen 2002).

5.2. Epidemiology

Based on available studies a female preponderance is apparent (Li and Rozen 2002; Takase *et al* 2004). Age of onset in women (second to third decades) occurs earlier than in men (fifth decade) (Li and Rozen 2002). As discussed previously chronic daily headaches have a prevalence of about 2.5–5% in the general population. In a Spanish population NDPH was found in 0.1% and formed only 2–6.7% of all the CDHs identified (Castillo *et al* 1999; Colas *et al* 2004). In specialist clinics the proportion of CDH cases diagnosed as NDPH increases to 11–14% (Bigal *et al* 2002; Koenig *et al* 2002).

5.3. Pathophysiology

Since about one-third of patients describe a viral illness prior to headache onset it has been hypothesized that NDPH has an infectious aetiology. In support, over 80% of NDPH patients had evidence of active Epstein-Barr virus (EBV) infection, which was significantly higher than in controls (Diaz-Mitoma *et al* 1987). Over 60% of NDPH patients were actively excreting EBV in the oropharynx. Past but not active EBV infection was found in 5 out of 7 patients tested in a later study (Li and Rozen 2002). Other viral infections such as recent herpes simplex virus infection and cytomegalovirus have also been identified

in NDPH patients (Meineri *et al* 2004). Moreover bacterial agents have also been associated with NDPH, but the highly frequent reports of fever (34.2%) and painful cervical lymphadenopathy (56.5%) not reported in other studies suggests that this may be a distinct subgroup (Santoni and Santoni-Williams 1993). In a paediatric population with NDPH 43% reported onset of their symptoms during an infection and positive EBV serology was detected in half of these. However, how a viral infection leads to NDPH is unclear. Some suggest that subclinical meningitis may be involved (Evans 2003), and in support new onset headache after meningitis is quite common (Neufeld *et al* 1999).

Minor head injuries (23%) and surgery were also common precipitators of headaches, suggesting post-traumatic mechanisms may also be involved (see Chapter 11). Stressful life events are also frequently reported in NDPH patients but how these cause the onset of headache is unclear.

5.4. Treatment

There seem to be two subgroups of NDPH (Olesen *et al* 2004): those refractory to treatment (Takase *et al* 2004) and those that have a benign progression and will improve with or without therapy. Complete resolution was reported in 86% of male patients and in 73% of female patients over a period of 2 years.

Anecdotal evidence suggests that the novel antiepileptic drugs such as gabapentin and topiramate may be useful in the prophylactic treatment of NDPH. When a stepped approach that began with muscle relaxants and progressed through TCAs, SSRIs and AEDs was employed, it was found that 30% graded the result as 'moderate' or 'very' improved, but only 2 cases were cured (Takase *et al* 2004). The drugs used that were moderately to very successful were TCAs in 33% of cases and AEDs or muscle relaxants in 22% of cases each (Takase *et al* 2004). However, gabapentin and topiramate were not tested.

5.5. Differential Diagnosis

NDPH is phenotypically similar to CTTH; however, onset of NDPH is independent of ETTH or migraine that increases in frequency and NDPH may be very refractory to treatment. A number of disorders may also give rise to NDPH-like headaches (Goadsby and Boes 2002; Evans 2003). Low cerebrospinal fluid (CSF) volume headache is commonly encountered after lumbar puncture and is characteristically relieved by bed rest. Patients with chronic CSF leaks may report a history of lumbar puncture or epidural injection or vigorous exercises that involve strong Valsalva manoeuvres (e.g. lifting heavy objects). Headache is absent on waking and worsens during the day; lying down rapidly improves pain. Magnetic resonance imaging with gadolinium enhancement will usually identify the leak. Raised CSF pressure may occur secondary to tumours and induces headache. Subarachnoid haemorrhage (SAH) may be present with a normal or near normal neurologic examination and cause headache of moderate to severe intensity. Onset of SAH headache may be instantaneous in about half or develop over about 5 minutes (Evans 2003). Benign thunderclap headache (BTH) is also of sudden onset, reaching maximum intensity within 30 seconds. The headache may last several hours, but a less severe headache may persist for weeks. Some consider BTH to be symptomatic of SAH, cervical artery dissection (Chapter 13) or cerebral venous thrombosis (Olesen et al 2004). These entities should therefore be excluded in patients suspected of secondary NDPH.

6. Headache, Myofascial Pains and Fibromyalgia

Masticatory muscle pain has been suggested to be a localized expression of a spectrum of myofascial disorders with many similarities between MMP, TTH and fibromyalgia; it is not unusual that these entities coexist in patients (Meyer 2002). Indeed the segregation of MMP from other myofascial pain disorders of a more generalized type such as FM has been questioned (Widmer 1991).

6.1. Headache and Masticatory Myofascial Pain

Headache has been reported to be more common in adult patients with TMDs than in those without (Ciancaglini and Radaelli 2001; Aaron and Buchwald 2003), but often these results are not replicated in other studies or age groups (Liljestrom et al 2001). There are great similarities, and possible overlap, between patients suffering from headache and MMP. Age distribution, female preponderance and contributing psychophysiological mechanisms are shared. Muscle tenderness is a frequent finding in migraine and TTH patients, the distribution of which may be distinctly similar to that in MMP patients. Thus, two of the fundamental symptoms of MMP, pain of daily occurrence and tenderness of muscles to palpation, fail to properly differentiate between headache and MMP patients.

Migraineurs suffer no more TMDs than controls with no change in this association with increasing frequency of migraine (Jensen et al 1993a). The rate of migraine in MMP patients does not differ from that in the general population, so that MMP and migraine patients seem separate groups (Watts et al 1986). Children with migraine and migraine-type headache groups were recently shown to have the highest incidence of more severe TMD signs (Liljestrom et al 2001; Liljestrom et al 2005). Migraine sufferers have been found to report significantly more clenching habits that may relate them to some forms of

muscle pains (Steele et al 1991). An association between migraine and MMP is not clearly apparent; pathophysiology and clinical presentation are distinctly different. The role that neurovascular mechanisms, such as neurogenic inflammation, play in MMP is not entirely clear. Vascular headache is REM 'locked' and some data point to an REM-locked destructive form of bruxism that may link certain forms of muscle pain with vascular mechanisms (Ware and Rugh 1988; Dodick et al 2003). Moreover recent associations between migraine and fibromyalgia suggest that a relation with MMP may yet become apparent (Marcus et al 2005).

Despite stated similarities most MMP patients have pain and muscle tenderness on palpation unilaterally (Sharav et al 1978) whilst TTH and FM are predominantly bilateral pain syndromes (Henriksson and Bengtsson 1991). MMP is thought of as an initiating or perpetuating factor in TTH (Olesen et al 2004). TMD patients report headaches significantly more frequently and of higher severity (Ciancaglini and Radaelli 2001) and specifically MMP patients report a significantly higher incidence of TTH than controls (John et al 2003). A minor relationship between TMDs and TTH frequency was observed in one study (Jensen et al 1993b). Many of these studies use differing inclusion criteria that make it difficult to compare results. There is limited evidence for masticatory muscle tenderness (equivalent to MMP?) in patients with TTH. However, there is considerable overlap in the tender muscles needed for the diagnosis of MMP and TTH and this may suggest that MMP and TTH share pathophysiological mechanisms and often coexist. There is therefore no convincing evidence for the role of TMDs in the initiation of TTH.

6.2. Fibromyalgia

Fibromyalgia is a common condition characterized by widespread pain and the presence of tender points (Yunus et al 2000). Specifically the diagnosis of FM relies primarily on the report of widespread musculoskeletal pain for at least 3 months (Wolfe et al 1990). Additionally there must be at least 11 points of tenderness out of the 18 anatomical sites defined by the American College of Rheumatology (Wolfe et al 1990). These sites must be examined with the application of 4 kg of pressure and are distributed bilaterally and in both upper and lower body segments. In some cases FM may occur with a comorbid disease such as hypothyroidism or a connective tissue disease and is then termed concomitant FM (Wolfe et al 1990). Since treatment of these comorbid disorders does not always eradicate concomitant FM the term secondary FM is to be avoided.

Much controversy still surrounds FM as a disease entity and how it should be classified (Crofford and Clauw 2002; Wolfe 2003). Moreover the boundaries between FM and regional myofascial pains, such as MMP, are at times poorly demarcated despite established criteria (Scudds *et al* 1989; Wolfe *et al* 1990). A major differentiating feature between FM and regional myofascial pain is the presence of trigger points and a palpable band of tight muscle in regional myofascial pain as opposed to multiple tender points in FM. For MMP, trigger points are not an integral part of the RDC-TMD criteria whilst the AAOP requires hyperirritable sites or trigger points within muscles. By definition trigger points, on palpation, refer pain to a distant site but this condition for trigger points has been suggested as unnecessary, and trigger points may be considered active or latent, further fogging the boundaries between regional myofascial pain and FM. Moreover only regional pain and tenderness have been validated in FM and regional myofascial pain; the presence of trigger points may be unnecessary (Wolfe *et al* 1992). The other basic difference is the chronic, widespread, systemic character of FM as opposed to the acute, localized nature of myofascial pains (Wolfe *et al* 1990). However, FM often begins as a localized pain disorder and later becomes widespread whilst persistent myofascial pains may involve multiple sites and cause systemic symptoms (Inanici *et al* 1999). Many of the 'perpetuating factors' in myofascial pains are termed 'modulating factors' of FM: physical activity, cold, stress and weather changes. Indeed it has been suggested that FM and regional myofascial pain represent an overlapping spectrum (Meyer 2002).

The point prevalence of fibromyalgia is about 2–2.9%; females (3.4–4.9%) are affected more than males (0.5–1.6%) (Wolfe *et al* 1995; White *et al* 1999). Most commonly FM occurs in females aged 40–60 years (Neumann and Buskila 2003) and its onset is often linked to a preceding viral infection, trauma or mental stress (Buskila 2001). FM may begin as a regional pain and in a prospective trial back pain predicted FM whereas tender points and pain in the neck did not. Self-assessed depression, long-lasting pain and the presence of >3 associated symptoms were significant predictors for progression (Forseth *et al* 1999).

Pain in FM is usually located in the lower back, neck, shoulder, arms, hands, hips, thighs, knees, legs and feet (Yunus *et al* 1981; Wolfe *et al* 1990). Complaints of joint pains may accompany FM and may be the prominent feature in some patients. In the vast majority (85%) of patients with FM, pain is accompanied by stiffness particularly in the morning. Both of FM's cardinal symptoms, pain and stiffness, are aggravated by cold or humid weather, anxiety or stress, inactivity and poor sleep. FM symptomatology is complex and affects multiple modalities; common complaints include fatigue (75–90%), a feeling of swelling or paraesthesia (50% each), vertigo (60%), non-restorative sleep (70%) and psychological symptoms (60%). Fatigue, usually expressed by patients as feeling 'drained', is correlated to pain and poor sleep (Yunus *et al* 1981; White *et al* 1999). Paraesthesias and swelling usually affect the extremities and need careful neurological examination. Vertigo or dizziness is considered to be central in origin and may be accompanied by phonophobia or tinnitus. Sleep disturbances are extremely common and include difficulties in falling asleep (increased sleep latency), waking up during the night (decreased sleep efficiency) and feeling tired in the morning (non-refreshing sleep). Poor sleep correlates with pain, psychological distress and fatigue (Moldofsky 2001, 2002). Anxiety, depression and stress are prevalent in FM patients and psychological distress correlates with disease severity (Yunus *et al* 1991). Rarer signs include Raynaud's phenomenon, Sjögren-like symptoms and cognitive dysfunction. In established FM cases long-term follow-up shows that there is usually no further deterioration in symptomatology (Wolfe *et al* 1997).

The pathophysiology of FM is unclear (Vierck 2006). There is evidence for dysautonomia with increased neural sympathetic activation and a lack of an adequate sympathetic response to stressor or cardiovascular challenges (Martinez-Lavin 2004). Additionally FM presents features of a neuropathic pain syndrome (paraesthesias, allodynia), augmented CNS processing of pain (sensitization) and a deficit of endogenous pain inhibition (Gracely *et al* 2002). The data suggest that FM may be a generalized form of sympathetically maintained neuropathic pain. Dysfunction of the hypothalamic-pituitary-adrenal axis is thought to partly underlie sleep disorders, some pain symptoms and autonomic nervous system imbalance (Demitrack and Crofford 1998; Drewes 1999; Vgontzas and Chrousos 2002; Sarzi-Puttini *et al* 2006).

Many pharmacological and non-pharmacological approaches have been used to treat FM. Treatment aims at controlling pain and associated signs and improving functional and psychological disability. Tricyclic or other antidepressants and AEDs are probably the most effective pharmacological agents (Rao and Clauw 2004). Combining these with aerobic exercise and cognitive behavioural therapy may increase efficacy (Rao and Clauw 2004).

6.3. Temporomandibular Disorders and Fibromyalgia

Early reports on MMP/FM comorbidity suggested that a connection may exist between these entities. FM, by definition, is characterized by widespread pain so it is not surprising that many FM patients have signs of MMP (Henriksson and Bengtsson 1991). Additionally, pain outside the craniofacial region is common amongst TMD patients (Hagberg 1991). Some patients with MMP (18%) have signs suggestive of FM and up to 75% of FM patients demonstrate comorbid MMP (Hedenberg-Magnusson *et al* 1997; Korszun *et al* 1998; Rhodus *et al* 2003). Female patients with widespread pain are at significantly increased risk of developing TMDs, suggesting that TMDs may be related, and in continuum, to generalized muscle disorders (John *et al* 2003). Indeed patients with FM, regional myofascial pain such as

MMP and chronic fatigue syndrome (CFS) share many clinical features including myalgia, fatigue and disturbed sleep, suggesting a common aetiology (Cimino *et al* 1998). Additionally patients with FM and TMD have significantly elevated prevalence rates of irritable bowel syndrome, sleep disturbances and concentration difficulties (Aaron *et al* 2000). Fatigued patients are four times more likely to suffer from TMD than non-fatigued twin controls. Thus fatigue and fatigue-related symptoms are common in TMD but are also frequently reported by all chronic pain patients and probably related to somatization and depression (de Leeuw *et al* 2005).

There are many cases of MMP where muscle tenderness affects many sites in the head and neck but trigger points may be hard to find. These patients often have tender points and characteristics associating them with FM, e.g. disturbed sleep, anxiety and general fatigue. When the symptoms of FM patients are compared with those of patients with MMP, no symptoms are specific to MMP, suggesting that such local 'syndromes' of myofascial pain should be compiled to form one entity. Focusing on the one region in which pain is greatest may account for a restricted diagnosis such as MMP, when in effect this disorder can be a local symptom of a more generalized condition (Widmer 1991). Findings of faulty pain processing in MMP patients would seem to support this contention (Fillingim *et al* 1998; Maixner *et al* 1998). However, not surprisingly TMD patients are distinguishable from FM patients by a high prevalence rate of masticatory muscle tenderness and a reduced prevalence of fatigue, muscle weakness, migratory arthralgias and burning or shooting muscle pains (Aaron *et al* 2000). FM patients may also demonstrate lower pain thresholds and lower tolerance levels to experimental facial pain than TMD patients, suggesting differential processing of external stimuli (Hedenberg-Magnusson *et al* 1997). The vast majority of FM patients (94%) reported local pain from the temporomandibular region: most frequently the temple, the TMJ and the neck (Hedenberg-Magnusson *et al* 1999). About half of the patients complained about difficulties in jaw movements and about three-quarters reported tiredness of the jaws. Generalized body pain had a significantly longer duration than the onset of TMD symptoms, suggesting that FM starts in other parts of the body and later extends to the masticatory system. In a large study jaw pain was found in 35.4% of FM patients and in about 19% each of osteoarthritis and rheumatoid arthritis patients (Wolfe *et al* 2005). Jaw pain is associated with disease severity and the presence of jaw pain in FM patients correlated with a significantly reduced quality of life relative to FM without jaw pain (Wolfe *et al* 2005).

Female patients ($n=162$) with a previous diagnosis of MMP were re-examined 7 years later to elicit a history of comorbid FM (Raphael *et al* 2000b). Thirty-eight patients (23.5%) had a positive history of FM, but showed no difference in presenting signs and symptoms relating to MMP.

However, patients with a positive history of FM reported more MMP symptoms accompanied by more severe pain and increased emotional distress. In conclusion increased chronicity was observed for MMP patients with comorbid FM that also seemed to be more resistant to occlusal splint treatment (Raphael and Marbach 2001).

The data suggest similarities between MMP and generalized muscle disorders. Although it is clear that in many cases MMP is a local pain syndrome with minimal complaints in other areas of the body many cases present with complaints suggestive of a generalized widespread disorder. It may well be that there are two distinct MMP subgroups (with and without FM/widespread pain) or that the MMP phenotype is part of a spectrum of a possible progression to FM. It remains unclear, however, which MMP cases progress to FM.

6.4. Headache and Fibromyalgia

Tension-type headaches are very frequently (<50%) observed in FM patients (Yunus *et al* 1981, 2000). Similarities have been observed in the distribution of muscle tender points between recurrent headache patients and FM patients (Okifuji *et al* 1999). In patients with concomitant CDH and FM there was significantly more insomnia and more incapacitating headaches than in headache patients without fibromyalgia (Peres *et al* 2000). Within CDH both migrainous and nonmigrainous headaches have been similarly associated with generalized muscle pains (Hagen *et al* 2002). The most significant headache parameter associated with muscle pain was headache frequency and not headache diagnosis. These findings may indicate that musculoskeletal pains and chronic headaches (irrespective of diagnosis) may share central sensitization as a common aetiologic factor (Hagen *et al* 2002). In this and further studies a highly significant correlation was found between headaches and muscle pain in the upper body area, which may suggest segmental effects (Blau and MacGregor 1994).

Recent data on central nervous system dysregulation and widespread allodynia in migraine (see Chapter 9) suggest that in some cases migraine may form part of more widespread pain disorders such as FM. Migraines occur frequently in FM patients (Hudson *et al* 1992). Conversely FM was found in 36% of transformed migraine patients and the comorbidity was predicted by concomitant depression and insomnia (Peres *et al* 2001). A recent study on 100 FM patients found that 76% had headaches, most of which began prior to onset of FM (Marcus *et al* 2005) and the most common headache diagnosis was migraine alone or in combination with TTH. Characteristics of FM patients with headache were not different to those without headache so that they are not a distinct subgroup. The data suggest that migraine may form part of the FM phenotype. Based on the data showing considerable overlap between migraine, MMP, FM and TTH, comorbidity in any given patient is highly likely.

Acknowledgements

We thank Dr Karen Raphael for her input in the preparation of this chapter.

We thank Dr Karen Raphael for her input in the preparation of this chapter.

References

Aaron LA, Buchwald D (2003) Chronic diffuse musculoskeletal pain, fibromyalgia and co-morbid unexplained clinical conditions. *Best Pract Res Clin Rheumatol* **17**(4):563–574.

Aaron LA, Burke MM, Buchwald D (2000) Overlapping conditions among patients with chronic fatigue syndrome, fibromyalgia, and temporomandibular disorder. *Arch Intern Med* **160**(2):221–227.

Ahlberg J, Savolainen A, Rantala M, et al (2004) Reported bruxism and biopsychosocial symptoms: a longitudinal study. *Community Dent Oral Epidemiol* **32**(4):307–311.

Al-Ani Z, Gray RJ, Davies SJ, et al (2005) Stabilization splint therapy for the treatment of temporomandibular myofascial pain: a systematic review. *J Dent Educ* **69**(11):1242–1250.

Al Quran FA, Kamal MS (2006) Anterior midline point stop device (AMPS) in the treatment of myogenous TMDs: comparison with the stabilization splint and control group. *Oral Surg Oral Med Oral Pathol Oral Radiol Endod* **101**(6):741–747.

Anastassaki A, Magnusson T (2004) Patients referred to a specialist clinic because of suspected temporomandibular disorders: a survey of 3194 patients in respect of diagnoses, treatments, and treatment outcome. *Acta Odontol Scand* **62**(4):183–192.

Ariji Y, Sakuma S, Izumi M, et al (2004) Ultrasonographic features of the masseter muscle in female patients with temporomandibular disorder associated with myofascial pain. *Oral Surg Oral Med Oral Pathol Oral Radiol Endod* **98**(3):337–341.

Arima T, Svensson P, Arendt-Nielsen L (1999) Experimental grinding in healthy subjects: a model for postexercise jaw muscle soreness? *J Orofac Pain* **13**(2):104–114.

Armstrong RB, Ogilvie RW, Schwane JA (1983) Eccentric exercise-induced injury to rat skeletal muscle. *J Appl Physiol* **54**(1):80–93.

Ashina M (2004) Neurobiology of chronic tension-type headache. *Cephalalgia* **24**(3):161–172.

Ashina S, Babenko L, Jensen R, et al (2005) Increased muscular and cutaneous pain sensitivity in cephalic region in patients with chronic tension-type headache. *Eur J Neurol* **12**(7):543–549.

Baba K, Tsukiyama Y, Yamazaki M, et al (2001) A review of temporomandibular disorder diagnostic techniques. *J Prosthet Dent* **86**(2):184–194.

Baba K, Haketa T, Sasaki Y, et al (2005) Association between masseter muscle activity levels recorded during sleep and signs and symptoms of temporomandibular disorders in healthy young adults. *J Orofac Pain* **19**(3):226–231.

Babenko VV, Graven-Nielsen T, Svensson P, et al (1999) Experimental human muscle pain induced by intramuscular injections of bradykinin, serotonin, and substance P. *Eur J Pain* **3**(2):93–102.

Bader G, Lavigne G (2000) Sleep bruxism; an overview of an oromandibular sleep movement disorder. Review article. *Sleep Med Rev* **4**(1):27–43.

Bader GG, Kampe T, Tagdae T, et al (1997) Descriptive physiological data on a sleep bruxism population. *Sleep* **20**(11):982–990.

Barnsley L, Lord S, Bogduk N (1994) Whiplash injury. *Pain* **58**(3):283–307.

Bendtsen L (2000) Central sensitization in tension-type headache–possible pathophysiological mechanisms. *Cephalalgia* **20**(5):486–508.

Bendtsen L, Jensen R (2000) Amitriptyline reduces myofascial tenderness in patients with chronic tension-type headache. *Cephalalgia* **20**(6):603–610.

Bendtsen L, Jensen R (2004) Mirtazapine is effective in the prophylactic treatment of chronic tension-type headache. *Neurology* **62**(10):1706–1711.

Bendtsen L, Jensen R, Olesen J (1996a) Decreased pain detection and tolerance thresholds in chronic tension-type headache. *Arch Neurol* **53**(4):373–376.

Bendtsen L, Jensen R, Olesen J (1996b) A non-selective (amitriptyline), but not a selective (citalopram), serotonin reuptake inhibitor is effective in the prophylactic treatment of chronic tension-type headache. *J Neurol Neurosurg Psychiatry* **61**(3):285–290.

Benoliel R, Eliav E, Elishoov H, et al (1994) Diagnosis and treatment of persistent pain after trauma to the head and neck. *J Oral Maxillofac Surg* **52**(11):1138–1147; discussion 1147–1148.

Benoliel R, Wilensky A, Tal M, et al (2002) Application of a pro-inflammatory agent to the orbital portion of the rat infraorbital nerve induces changes indicative of ongoing trigeminal pain. *Pain* **99**(3):567–578.

Benoliel R, Sharav Y, Tal M, et al (2003) Management of chronic orofacial pain: today and tomorrow. *Compend Contin Educ Dent* **24**(12):909–920, 922–924, 926–928 passim; quiz 932.

Bigal ME, Sheftell FD, Rapoport AM, et al (2002) Chronic daily headache in a tertiary care population: correlation between the International Headache Society diagnostic criteria and proposed revisions of criteria for chronic daily headache. *Cephalalgia* **22**(6):432–438.

Blasberg B, Chalmers A (1989) Temporomandibular pain and dysfunction syndrome associated with generalized musculoskeletal pain: a retrospective study. *J Rheumatol Suppl* **19**:87–90.

Blau JN, MacGregor EA (1994) Migraine and the neck. *Headache* **34**(2):88–90.

Bogaards MC, ter Kuile MM (1994) Treatment of recurrent tension headache: a meta-analytic review. *Clin J Pain* **10**(3):174–190.

Borgeat F, Elie R, Larouche LM (1985) Pain response to voluntary muscle tension increases and biofeedback efficacy in tension headache. *Headache* **25**(7):387–391.

Bowley JF, Gale EN (1987) Experimental masticatory muscle pain. *J Dent Res* **66**(12):1765–1769.

Brennum J, Kjeldsen M, Olesen J (1992) The 5-HT1-like agonist sumatriptan has a significant effect in chronic tension-type headache. *Cephalalgia* **12**(6):375–379.

Breslau N, Lipton RB, Stewart WF, et al (2003) Comorbidity of migraine and depression: investigating potential etiology and prognosis. *Neurology* **60**(8):1308–1312.

Brister H, Turner JA, Aaron LA, et al (2006) Self-efficacy is associated with pain, functioning, and coping in patients with chronic temporomandibular disorder pain. *J Orofac Pain* **20**(2):115–124.

Broton JG, Sessle BJ (1988) Reflex excitation of masticatory muscles induced by algesic chemicals applied to the temporomandibular joint of the cat. *Arch Oral Biol* **33**(10):741–747.

Brousseau M, Manzini C, Thie N, et al (2003) Understanding and managing the interaction between sleep and pain: an update for the dentist. *J Can Dent Assoc* **69**(7):437–442.

Buchner R, Van der Glas HW, Brouwers JE, et al (1992) Electromyographic parameters related to clenching level and jaw-jerk reflex in patients with a simple type of myogenous cranio-mandibular disorder. *J Oral Rehabil* **19**(5): 495–511.

Buskila D (2001) Fibromyalgia, chronic fatigue syndrome, and myofascial pain syndrome. *Curr Opin Rheumatol* **13**(2):117–127.

Cady RK, Gutterman D, Saiers JA, et al (1997) Responsiveness of non-IHS migraine and tension-type headache to sumatriptan. *Cephalalgia* **17**(5):588–590.

Cairns BE, Sim Y, Bereiter DA, et al (2002) Influence of sex on reflex jaw muscle activity evoked from the rat temporomandibular joint. *Brain Res* **957**(2):338–344.

Camparis CM, Siqueira JT (2006) Sleep bruxism: clinical aspects and characteristics in patients with and without chronic orofacial pain. *Oral Surg Oral Med Oral Pathol Oral Radiol Endod* **101**(2):188–193.

Camparis CM, Formigoni G, Teixeira MJ, et al (2005) Clinical evaluation of tinnitus in patients with sleep bruxism: prevalence and characteristics. J Oral Rehabil 32(11):808–814.

Camparis CM, Formigoni G, Teixeira MJ, et al (2006) Sleep bruxism and temporomandibular disorder: clinical and polysomnographic evaluation. Arch Oral Biol 51:721–728.

Carlson CR, Okeson JP, Falace DA, et al (1993) Comparison of psychologic and physiologic functioning between patients with masticatory muscle pain and matched controls. J Orofac Pain 7(1):15–22.

Carlson CR, Reid KI, Curran SL, et al (1998) Psychological and physiological parameters of masticatory muscle pain. Pain 76(3):297–307.

Carlson CR, Bertrand PM, Ehrlich AD, et al (2001) Physical self-regulation training for the management of temporomandibular disorders. J Orofac Pain 15(1):47–55.

Carlsson GE, Egermark I, Magnusson T (2002) Predictors of signs and symptoms of temporomandibular disorders: a 20-year follow-up study from childhood to adulthood. Acta Odontol Scand 60(3):180–185.

Castillo J, Munoz P, Guitera V, et al (1999) Epidemiology of chronic daily headache in the general population. Headache 39(3):190–196.

Cetiner S, Kahraman SA, Yucetas S (2006) Evaluation of low-level laser therapy in the treatment of temporomandibular disorders. Photomed Laser Surg 24(5):637–641.

Cheifetz AT, Osganian SK, Allred EN, et al (2005) Prevalence of bruxism and associated correlates in children as reported by parents. J Dent Child (Chic) 72(2):67–73.

Choy E, Kydd WL (1988) Bite force duration: a diagnostic procedure for mandibular dysfunction. J Prosthet Dent 60(3):365–368.

Christensen LV (1971) Facial pain and internal pressure of masseter muscle in experimental bruxism in man. Arch Oral Biol 16(9):1021–1031.

Christensen LV (1981) Progressive jaw muscle fatigue of experimental tooth clenching in man. J Oral Rehabil 8(5):413–420.

Christensen MB, Bendtsen L, Ashina M, et al (2005) Experimental induction of muscle tenderness and headache in tension-type headache patients. Cephalalgia 25(11):1061–1067.

Chung SC, Kim YK, Kim HS (2000) Prevalence and patterns of nocturnal bruxofacets on stabilization splints in temporomandibular disorder patients. Cranio 18(2):92–97.

Ciancaglini R, Radaelli G (2001) The relationship between headache and symptoms of temporomandibular disorder in the general population. J Dent 29(2):93–98.

Cimino R, Michelotti A, Stradi R, et al (1998) Comparison of clinical and psychologic features of fibromyalgia and masticatory myofascial pain. J Orofac Pain 12(1):35–41.

Clark GT, Beemsterboer PL, Solberg WK, et al (1979) Nocturnal electromyographic evaluation of myofascial pain dysfunction in patients undergoing occlusal splint therapy. J Am Dent Assoc 99(4):607–611.

Clark GT, Rugh JD, Handelman SL (1980) Nocturnal masseter muscle activity and urinary catecholamine levels in bruxers. J Dent Res 59(10):1571–1576.

Clark GT, Beemsterboer PL, Jacobson R (1984) The effect of sustained submaximal clenching on maximum bite force in myofascial pain dysfunction patients. J Oral Rehabil 11(4):387–391.

Clark GT, Adler RC, Lee JJ (1991) Jaw pain and tenderness levels during and after repeated sustained maximum voluntary protrusion. Pain 45(1):17–22.

Colas R, Munoz P, Temprano R, et al (2004) Chronic daily headache with analgesic overuse: epidemiology and impact on quality of life. Neurology 62(8):1338–1342.

Conti PC, dos Santos CN, Kogawa EM, et al (2006) The treatment of painful temporomandibular joint clicking with oral splints: a randomized clinical trial. J Am Dent Assoc 137(8):1108–1114.

Couch JR (2005) The long-term prognosis of tension-type headache. Curr Pain Headache Rep 9(6):436–441.

Crider AB, Glaros AG (1999) A meta-analysis of EMG biofeedback treatment of temporomandibular disorders. J Orofac Pain 13(1):29–37.

Crofford LJ, Clauw DJ (2002) Fibromyalgia: where are we a decade after the American College of Rheumatology classification criteria were developed? Arthritis Rheum 46(5):1136–1138.

Cummings TM, White AR (2001) Needling therapies in the management of myofascial trigger point pain: a systematic review. Arch Phys Med Rehabil 82(7):986–992.

Dao TT, Lavigne GJ, Charbonneau A, et al (1994a) The efficacy of oral splints in the treatment of myofascial pain of the jaw muscles: a controlled clinical trial. Pain 56(1):85–94.

Dao TT, Lund JP, Lavigne GJ (1994b) Pain responses to experimental chewing in myofascial pain patients. J Dent Res 73(6):1163–1167.

Dao TT, Knight K, Ton-That V (1998) Modulation of myofascial pain by the reproductive hormones: a preliminary report. J Prosthet Dent 79(6):663–670.

De Boever JA, Keersmaekers K (1996) Trauma in patients with temporomandibular disorders: frequency and treatment outcome. J Oral Rehabil 23(2):91–96.

De Boever JA, Carlsson GE, Klineberg IJ (2000) Need for occlusal therapy and prosthodontic treatment in the management of temporomandibular disorders. Part I. Occlusal interferences and occlusal adjustment. J Oral Rehabil 27(5):367–379.

de Filippis S, Salvatori E, Coloprisco G, et al (2005) Headache and mood disorders. J Headache Pain 6(4):250–253.

De Kanter RJ, Truin GJ, Burgersdijk RC, et al (1993) Prevalence in the Dutch adult population and a meta-analysis of signs and symptoms of temporomandibular disorder. J Dent Res 72(11):1509–1518.

De Laat A, Stappaerts K, Papy S (2003) Counseling and physical therapy as treatment for myofascial pain of the masticatory system. J Orofac Pain 17(1):42–49.

de Leeuw R, Studts JL, Carlson CR (2005) Fatigue and fatigue-related symptoms in an orofacial pain population. Oral Surg Oral Med Oral Pathol Oral Radiol Endod 99(2):168–174.

Deleu D, Hanssens Y (1999) Primary chronic daily headache: clinical and pharmacological aspects. A clinic-based study in Oman. Headache 39(6): 432–436.

Demitrack MA, Crofford LJ (1998) Evidence for and pathophysiologic implications of hypothalamic-pituitary-adrenal axis dysregulation in fibromyalgia and chronic fatigue syndrome. Ann N Y Acad Sci 840:684–697.

Dervis E (2004) Changes in temporomandibular disorders after treatment with new complete dentures. J Oral Rehabil 31(4): 320–326.

Dettmar DM, Shaw RM, Tilley AJ (1987) Tooth wear and bruxism: a sleep laboratory investigation. Aust Dent J 32(6):421–426.

Diamond S, Freitag FG (2001) The use of ibuprofen plus caffeine to treat tension-type headache. Curr Pain Headache Rep 5(5): 472–478.

Diatchenko L, Slade GD, Nackley AG, et al (2005) Genetic basis for individual variations in pain perception and the development of a chronic pain condition. Hum Mol Genet 14(1):135–143.

Diaz-Mitoma F, Vanast WJ, Tyrrell DL (1987) Increased frequency of Epstein-Barr virus excretion in patients with new daily persistent headaches. Lancet 1(8530):411–415.

Dodick DW, Eross EJ, Parish JM, et al (2003) Clinical, anatomical, and physiologic relationship between sleep and headache. Headache 43(3):282–292.

Drewes AM (1999) Pain and sleep disturbances with special reference to fibromyalgia and rheumatoid arthritis. Rheumatology (Oxford) 38(11):1035–1038.

Dube C, Rompre PH, Manzini C, et al (2004) Quantitative polygraphic controlled study on efficacy and safety of oral splint devices in tooth-grinding subjects. J Dent Res 83(5): 398–403.

Dworkin RH, Turk DC, Farrar JT, et al (2005) Core outcome measures for chronic pain clinical trials: IMMPACT recommendations. Pain 113(1-2):9–19.

Dworkin SF, Burgess JA (1987) Orofacial pain of psychogenic origin: current concepts and classification. J Am Dent Assoc 115(4):565–571.

Dworkin SF, LeResche L (1992) Research diagnostic criteria for temporomandibular disorders: review, criteria, examinations and specifications, critique. *J Craniomandib Disord* **6**(4):301–355.

Dworkin SF, LeResche L (1993) Temporomandibular disorder pain: epidemiologic data. *APS Bulletin* **12**(April/May).

Dworkin SF, Huggins KH, LeResche L, et al (1990a) Epidemiology of signs and symptoms in temporomandibular disorders: clinical signs in cases and controls. *J Am Dent Assoc* **120**(3): 273–281.

Dworkin SF, LeResche L, DeRouen T, et al (1990b) Assessing clinical signs of temporomandibular disorders: reliability of clinical examiners. *J Prosthet Dent* **63**(5):574–579.

Dworkin SF, Huggins KH, Wilson L, et al (2002) A randomized clinical trial using research diagnostic criteria for temporomandibular disorders-axis II to target clinic cases for a tailored self-care TMD treatment program. *J Orofac Pain* **16**(1):48–63.

Eberhard D, Bantleon HP, Steger W (2002) The efficacy of anterior repositioning splint therapy studied by magnetic resonance imaging. *Eur J Orthod* **24**(4):343–352.

Egermark I, Carlsson GE, Magnusson T (2001) A 20-year longitudinal study of subjective symptoms of temporomandibular disorders from childhood to adulthood. *Acta Odontol Scand* **59**(1):40–48.

Egermark I, Carlsson GE, Magnusson T (2005) A prospective long-term study of signs and symptoms of temporomandibular disorders in patients who received orthodontic treatment in childhood. *Angle Orthod* **75**(4):645–650.

Ekberg E (1998) Treatment of temporomandibular disorders of arthrogeneous origin. Controlled double-blind studies of a non-steroidal anti-inflammatory drug and a stabilisation appliance. *Swed Dent J Suppl* **131**:1–57.

Ekberg E, Nilner M (2004) Treatment outcome of appliance therapy in temporomandibular disorder patients with myofascial pain after 6 and 12 months. *Acta Odontol Scand* **62**(6):343–349.

Eliav E, Teich S, Nitzan D, et al (2003) Facial arthralgia and myalgia: can they be differentiated by trigeminal sensory assessment? *Pain* **104**(3):481–490.

Epker J, Gatchel RJ (2000) Coping profile differences in the biopsychosocial functioning of patients with temporomandibular disorder. *Psychosom Med* **62**(1):69–75.

Epker J, Gatchel RJ, Ellis E, 3rd (1999) A model for predicting chronic TMD: practical application in clinical settings. *J Am Dent Assoc* **130**(10):1470–1475.

Evans RW (2003) New daily persistent headache. *Curr Pain Headache Rep* **7**(4):303–307.

Fernandez-de-Las-Penas C, Alonso-Blanco C, Cuadrado ML, et al (2006) Are manual therapies effective in reducing pain from tension-type headache?: a systematic review. *Clin J Pain* **22**(3):278–285.

Ferrando M, Andreu Y, Galdon MJ, et al (2004) Psychological variables and temporomandibular disorders: distress, coping, and personality. *Oral Surg Oral Med Oral Pathol Oral Radiol Endod* **98**(2):153–160.

Ferrari R, Schrader H, Obelieniene D (1999) Prevalence of temporomandibular disorders associated with whiplash injury in Lithuania. *Oral Surg Oral Med Oral Pathol Oral Radiol Endod* **87**(6):653–657.

Fillingim RB, Ness TJ (2000) Sex-related hormonal influences on pain and analgesic responses. *Neurosci Biobehav Rev* **24**(4): 485–501.

Fillingim RB, Fillingim LA, Hollins M, et al (1998) Generalized vibrotactile allodynia in a patient with temporomandibular disorder. *Pain* **78**(1):75–78.

Flor H, Birbaumer N (1993) Comparison of the efficacy of electromyographic biofeedback, cognitive-behavioral therapy, and conservative medical interventions in the treatment of chronic musculoskeletal pain. *J Consult Clin Psychol* **61**(4):653–658.

Flor H, Birbaumer N, Schugens MM, et al (1992) Symptom-specific psychophysiological responses in chronic pain patients. *Psychophysiology* **29**(4):452–460.

Forseth KO, Husby G, Gran JT, et al (1999) Prognostic factors for the development of fibromyalgia in women with self-reported musculoskeletal pain. A prospective study. *J Rheumatol* **26**(11):2458–2467.

Forssell H, Kalso E (2004) Application of principles of evidence-based medicine to occlusal treatment for temporomandibular disorders: are there lessons to be learned? *J Orofac Pain* **18**(1): 9–22; discussion 23–32.

Fricton JR, Kroening R, Haley D, et al (1985) Myofascial pain syndrome of the head and neck: a review of clinical characteristics of 164 patients. *Oral Surg Oral Med Oral Pathol* **60**(6):615–623.

Fumal A, Schoenen J (2005) Chronic tension-type headache. In: Goadsby PJ, Silberstein SD, Dodick D (eds) *Chronic Daily Headache*. Hamilton: BC Decker, pp 57–64.

Galdón MJ, Durá E, Andreu Y, et al (2006) Multidimensional approach to the differences between muscular and articular temporomandibular patients: coping, distress, and pain characteristics. *Oral Surg Oral Med Oral Pathol* **102**(1):40–46.

Gardea MA, Gatchel RJ, Mishra KD (2001) Long-term efficacy of biobehavioral treatment of temporomandibular disorders. *J Behav Med* **24**(4):341–359.

Garofalo JP, Gatchel RJ, Wesley AL, et al (1998) Predicting chronicity in acute temporomandibular joint disorders using the research diagnostic criteria. *J Am Dent Assoc* **129**(4):438–447.

Gavish A, Winocur E, Menashe S, et al (2002) Experimental chewing in myofascial pain patients. *J Orofac Pain* **16**(1):22–28.

Gay T, Maton B, Rendell J, et al (1994) Characteristics of muscle fatigue in patients with myofascial pain-dysfunction syndrome. *Arch Oral Biol* **39**(10):847–852.

Gerwin RD, Dommerholt J, Shah JP (2004) An expansion of Simons' integrated hypothesis of trigger point formation. *Curr Pain Headache Rep* **8**(6):468–475.

Gesch D, Bernhardt O, Alte D, et al (2004a) Prevalence of signs and symptoms of temporomandibular disorders in an urban and rural German population: results of a population-based Study of Health in Pomerania. *Quintessence Int* **35**(2):143–150.

Gesch D, Bernhardt O, Kirbschus A (2004b) Association of malocclusion and functional occlusion with temporomandibular disorders (TMD) in adults: a systematic review of population-based studies. *Quintessence Int* **35**(3):211–221.

Glaros AG, Burton E (2004) Parafunctional clenching, pain, and effort in temporomandibular disorders. *J Behav Med* **27**(1): 91–100.

Glaros AG, Glass EG, Brockman D (1997) Electromyographic data from TMD patients with myofascial pain and from matched control subjects: evidence for statistical, not clinical, significance. *J Orofac Pain* **11**(2):125–129.

Glaros AG, Tabacchi KN, Glass EG (1998) Effect of parafunctional clenching on TMD pain. *J Orofac Pain* **12**(2):145–152.

Goadsby PJ, Boes C (2002) New daily persistent headache. *J Neurol Neurosurg Psychiatry* **72**(Suppl 2):ii6–ii9.

Gobel H, Cordes P (1990) Circadian variation of pain sensitivity in pericranial musculature. *Headache* **30**(7):418–422.

Gobel H, Petersen-Braun M, Soyka D (1994) The epidemiology of headache in Germany: a nationwide survey of a representative sample on the basis of the headache classification of the International Headache Society. *Cephalalgia* **14**(2):97–106.

Gollapudi L, Oblinger MM (1999) Estrogen and NGF synergistically protect terminally differentiated, ERalpha-transfected PC12 cells from apoptosis. *J Neurosci Res* **56**(5): 471–481.

Goulet JP, Lavigne GJ, Lund JP (1995) Jaw pain prevalence among French-speaking Canadians in Quebec and related symptoms of temporomandibular disorders. *J Dent Res* **74**(11):1738–1744.

Graboski CL, Gray DS, Burnham RS (2005) Botulinum toxin A versus bupivacaine trigger point injections for the treatment of myofascial pain syndrome: a randomised double blind crossover study. *Pain* **118**(1-2):170–175.

Gracely RH, Petzke F, Wolf JM, et al (2002) Functional magnetic resonance imaging evidence of augmented pain processing in fibromyalgia. *Arthritis Rheum* **46**(5):1333–1343.

Granada S, Hicks RA (2003) Changes in self-reported incidence of nocturnal bruxism in college students: 1966-2002. *Percept Mot Skills* **97**(3 Pt 1):777–778.

Graven-Nielsen T, Svensson P, Arendt-Nielsen L (1997) Effects of experimental muscle pain on muscle activity and co-ordination during static and dynamic motor function. *Electroencephalogr Clin Neurophysiol* **105**(2):156–164.

Graven-Nielsen T, Fenger-Gron LS, Svensson P, *et al* (1998) Quantification of deep and superficial sensibility in saline-induced muscle pain–a psychophysical study. *Somatosens Mot Res* **15**(1):46–53.

Greene CS, Marbach JJ (1982) Epidemiologic studies of mandibular dysfunction: a critical review. *J Prosthet Dent* **48**(2):184–190.

Grossi ML, Goldberg MB, Locker D, *et al* (2001) Reduced neuropsychologic measures as predictors of treatment outcome in patients with temporomandibular disorders. *J Orofac Pain* **15**(4):329–339.

Hagberg C (1991) General musculoskeletal complaints in a group of patients with craniomandibular disorders (CMD). A case control study. *Swed Dent J* **15**(4):179–185.

Hagberg C, Hellsing G, Hagberg M (1990) Perception of cutaneous electrical stimulation in patients with craniomandibular disorders. *J Craniomandib Disord* **4**(2):120–125.

Hagen K, Zwart JA, Vatten L, *et al* (2000) Prevalence of migraine and non-migrainous headache–head-HUNT, a large population-based study. *Cephalalgia* **20**(10):900–906.

Hagen K, Einarsen C, Zwart JA, *et al* (2002) The co-occurrence of headache and musculoskeletal symptoms amongst 51 050 adults in Norway. *Eur J Neurol* **9**(5):527–533.

Harkins S, Linford J, Cohen J, *et al* (1991) Administration of clonazepam in the treatment of TMD and associated myofascial pain: a double-blind pilot study. *J Craniomandib Disord* **5**(3):179–186.

Hatch JP, Rugh JD, Sakai S, *et al* (2001) Is use of exogenous estrogen associated with temporomandibular signs and symptoms? *J Am Dent Assoc* **132**(3):319–326.

Hedenberg-Magnusson B, Ernberg M, Kopp S (1997) Symptoms and signs of temporomandibular disorders in patients with fibromyalgia and local myalgia of the temporomandibular system. A comparative study. *Acta Odontol Scand* **55**(6):344–349.

Hedenberg-Magnusson B, Ernberg M, Kopp S (1999) Presence of orofacial pain and temporomandibular disorder in fibromyalgia. A study by questionnaire. *Swed Dent J* **23**(5-6):185–192.

Hellsing G (1988) Occlusal adjustment and occlusal stability. *J Prosthet Dent* **59**(6):696–702.

Henrikson T, Nilner M (2003) Temporomandibular disorders, occlusion and orthodontic treatment. *J Orthod* **30**(2):129–137; discussion 127.

Henriksson KG, Bengtsson A (1991) Fibromyalgia–a clinical entity? *Can J Physiol Pharmacol* **69**(5):672–677.

Herman CR, Schiffman EL, Look JO, *et al* (2002) The effectiveness of adding pharmacologic treatment with clonazepam or cyclobenzaprine to patient education and self-care for the treatment of jaw pain upon awakening: a randomized clinical trial. *J Orofac Pain* **16**(1):64–70.

High AS, Macgregor AJ, Tomlinson GE, *et al* (1988) A gnathodynamometer as an objective means of pain assessment following wisdom tooth removal. *Br J Oral Maxillofac Surg* **26**(4):284–291.

Hollins M, Sigurdsson A (1998) Vibrotactile amplitude and frequency discrimination in temporomandibular disorders. *Pain* **75**(1):59–67.

Holroyd KA (2002) Behavioral and psychologic aspects of the pathophysiology and management of tension-type headache. *Curr Pain Headache Rep* **6**(5):401–407.

Holroyd KA, Stensland M, Lipchik GL, *et al* (2000) Psychosocial correlates and impact of chronic tension-type headaches. *Headache* **40**(1):3–16.

Holroyd KA, O'Donnell FJ, Stensland M, *et al* (2001) Management of chronic tension-type headache with tricyclic antidepressant medication, stress management therapy, and their combination: a randomized controlled trial. *Jama* **285**(17):2208–2215.

How CK (2004) Orthodontic treatment has little to do with temporomandibular disorders. *Evid Based Dent* **5**(3):75.

Huang GJ, LeResche L, Critchlow CW, *et al* (2002) Risk factors for diagnostic subgroups of painful temporomandibular disorders (TMD). *J Dent Res* **81**(4):284–288.

Hudson JI, Goldenberg DL, Pope HG, Jr., *et al* (1992) Comorbidity of fibromyalgia with medical and psychiatric disorders. *Am J Med* **92**(4):363–367.

Inan LE, Tulunay FC, Guvener A, *et al* (1994) Characteristics of headache in migraine without aura and episodic tension-type headache in the Turkish population according to the IHS classification. *Cephalalgia* **14**(2):171–173.

Inanici F, Yunus MB, Aldag JC (1999) Clinical features and psychological factors in regional soft tissue pain: comparison with fibromyalgia syndrome. *J Musculoskelet Pain* **7**:293–301.

Intrieri RC, Jones GE, Alcorn JD (1994) Masseter muscle hyperactivity and myofascial pain dysfunction syndrome: a relationship under stress. *J Behav Med* **17**(5):479–500.

Isselee H, De Laat A, De Mot B, *et al* (2002) Pressure-pain threshold variation in temporomandibular disorder myalgia over the course of the menstrual cycle. *J Orofac Pain* **16**(2):105–117.

Iversen HK, Langemark M, Andersson PG, *et al* (1990) Clinical characteristics of migraine and episodic tension-type headache in relation to old and new diagnostic criteria. *Headache* **30**(8):514–519.

Jensen K, Norup M (1992) Experimental pain in human temporal muscle induced by hypertonic saline, potassium and acidity. *Cephalalgia* **12**(2):101–106.

Jensen R (1996) Mechanisms of spontaneous tension-type headaches: an analysis of tenderness, pain thresholds and EMG. *Pain* **64**(2):251–256.

Jensen R, Olesen J (1996) Initiating mechanisms of experimentally induced tension-type headache. *Cephalalgia* **16**(3):175–182; discussion 138–179.

Jensen R, Rasmussen BK (1996) Muscular disorders in tension-type headache. *Cephalalgia* **16**(2):97–103.

Jensen R, Symon D (2006) Epidemiology of tension-type headache. In: Olesen J, Goadsby PJ, Ramadan NM, *et al* (eds) *The Headaches*, 3rd edn. Philadelphia: Lippincott Williams & Wilkins, pp 621–624.

Jensen R, Rasmussen BK, Pedersen B, *et al* (1993a) Muscle tenderness and pressure pain thresholds in headache. A population study. *Pain* **52**(2):193–199.

Jensen R, Rasmussen BK, Lous I (1993b) Oromandibular dysfunctions and provocation of headache. In: Olesen J, Schoenen J (eds) *Tension-Type Headache: Classification, Mechanisms and Treatment*. New York: Raven Press, pp 210–223.

Jensen R, Bendtsen L, Olesen J (1998) Muscular factors are of importance in tension-type headache. *Headache* **38**(1):10–17.

Johansson A, Unell L, Carlsson GE, *et al* (2006) Risk factors associated with symptoms of temporomandibular disorders in a population of 50- and 60-year-old subjects. *J Oral Rehabil* **33**(7):473–481.

John MT, Miglioretti DL, LeResche L, *et al* (2003) Widespread pain as a risk factor for dysfunctional temporomandibular disorder pain. *Pain* **102**(3):257–263.

John MT, Dworkin SF, Mancl LA (2005) Reliability of clinical temporomandibular disorder diagnoses. *Pain* **118**(1-2):61–69.

Kamisaka M, Yatani H, Kuboki T, *et al* (2000) Four-year longitudinal course of TMD symptoms in an adult population and the estimation of risk factors in relation to symptoms. *J Orofac Pain* **14**(3):224–232.

Karli N, Zarifoglu M, Calisir N, *et al* (2005) Comparison of pre-headache phases and trigger factors of migraine and episodic tension-type headache: do they share similar clinical pathophysiology? *Cephalalgia* **25**(6):444–451.

Kasch H, Hjorth T, Svensson P, *et al* (2002) Temporomandibular disorders after whiplash injury: a controlled, prospective study. *J Orofac Pain* **16**(2):118–128.

Kato T, Thie NM, Huynh N, *et al* (2003) Topical review: sleep bruxism and the role of peripheral sensory influences. *J Orofac Pain* **17**(3):191–213.

Katz J, Heft M (2002) The epidemiology of self-reported TMJ sounds and pain in young adults in Israel. *J Public Health Dent* **62**(3):177–179.

Kawakita K, Dostrovsky JO, Tang JS, *et al* (1993) Responses of neurons in the rat thalamic nucleus submedius to cutaneous, muscle and visceral nociceptive stimuli. *Pain* **55**(3):327–338.

Kim MR, Graber TM, Viana MA (2002) Orthodontics and temporomandibular disorder: a meta-analysis. *Am J Orthod Dentofacial Orthop* **121**(5):438–446.

Kimos P, Biggs C, Mah J, *et al.* (2007) Analgesic action of gabapentin on chronic pain in the masticatory muscles: A randomized controlled trial. *Pain* **127**(1–2):151–160.

Kino K, Sugisaki M, Haketa T, *et al* (2005) The comparison between pains, difficulties in function, and associating factors of patients in subtypes of temporomandibular disorders. *J Oral Rehabil* **32**(5):315–325.

Kirveskari P, Jamsa T, Alanen P (1998) Occlusal adjustment and the incidence of demand for temporomandibular disorder treatment. *J Prosthet Dent* **79**(4):433–438.

Klobas L, Tegelberg A, Axelsson S (2004) Symptoms and signs of temporomandibular disorders in individuals with chronic whiplash-associated disorders. *Swed Dent J* **28**(1):29–36.

Koenig MA, Gladstein J, McCarter RJ, *et al* (2002) Chronic daily headache in children and adolescents presenting to tertiary headache clinics. *Headache* **42**(6):491–500.

Koh H, Robinson PG (2004) Occlusal adjustment for treating and preventing temporomandibular joint disorders. *J Oral Rehabil* **31**(4):287–292.

Kolbinson DA, Epstein JB, Senthilselvan A, *et al* (1997) A comparison of TMD patients with or without prior motor vehicle accident involvement: initial signs, symptoms, and diagnostic characteristics. *J Orofac Pain* **11**(3):206–214.

Korszun A, Papadopoulos E, Demitrack M, *et al* (1998) The relationship between temporomandibular disorders and stress-associated syndromes. *Oral Surg Oral Med Oral Pathol Oral Radiol Endod* **86**(4):416–420.

Koseoglu E, Nacar M, Talaslioglu A, *et al* (2003) Epidemiological and clinical characteristics of migraine and tension type headache in 1146 females in Kayseri, Turkey. *Cephalalgia* **23**(5):381–388.

Kubitzek F, Ziegler G, Gold MS, *et al* (2003) Low-dose diclofenac potassium in the treatment of episodic tension-type headache. *Eur J Pain* **7**(2):155–162.

Kulekcioglu S, Sivrioglu K, Ozcan O, *et al* (2003) Effectiveness of low-level laser therapy in temporomandibular disorder. *Scand J Rheumatol* **32**(2):114–118.

Kuttila M, Kuttila S, Le Bell Y, *et al* (1997) Association between TMD treatment need, sick leaves, and use of health care services for adults. *J Orofac Pain* **11**(3):242–248.

Kuttila M, Le Bell Y, Savolainen-Niemi E, *et al* (2002) Efficiency of occlusal appliance therapy in secondary otalgia and temporomandibular disorders. *Acta Odontol Scand* **60**(4):248–254.

Lacroix JM, Corbett L (1990) An experimental test of the muscle tension hypothesis of tension-type headache. *Int J Psychophysiol* **10**(1):47–51.

Lake AE 3rd, Rains JC, Penzien DB, *et al* (2005) Headache and psychiatric comorbidity: historical context, clinical implications, and research relevance. *Headache* **45**(5):493–506.

Langemark M, Olesen J, Poulsen DL, *et al* (1988) Clinical characterization of patients with chronic tension headache. *Headache* **28**(9):590–596.

Langemark M, Bach FW, Jensen TS, *et al* (1993) Decreased nociceptive flexion reflex threshold in chronic tension-type headache. *Arch Neurol* **50**(10):1061–1064.

Lanteri-Minet M, Auray JP, El Hasnaoui A, *et al* (2003) Prevalence and description of chronic daily headache in the general population in France. *Pain* **102**(1–2):143–149.

Lavigne GJ, Montplaisir JY (1994) Restless legs syndrome and sleep bruxism: prevalence and association among Canadians. *Sleep* **17**(8):739–743.

Lavigne GJ, Velly-Miguel AM, Montplaisir J (1991) Muscle pain, dyskinesia, and sleep. *Can J Physiol Pharmacol* **69**(5):678–682.

Lavigne GJ, Rompre PH, Montplaisir JY (1996) Sleep bruxism: validity of clinical research diagnostic criteria in a controlled polysomnographic study. *J Dent Res* **75**(1):546–552.

Lavigne GJ, Rompre PH, Poirier G, *et al* (2001) Rhythmic masticatory muscle activity during sleep in humans. *J Dent Res* **80**(2):443–448.

Le Bell Y, Niemi PM, Jamsa T, *et al* (2006) Subjective reactions to intervention with artificial interferences in subjects with and without a history of temporomandibular disorders. *Acta Odontol Scand* **64**(1):59–63.

Leher A, Graf K, PhoDuc JM, *et al* (2005) Is there a difference in the reliable measurement of temporomandibular disorder signs between experienced and inexperienced examiners? *J Orofac Pain* **19**(1):58–64.

LeResche L (1997) Epidemiology of temporomandibular disorders: implications for the investigation of etiologic factors. *Crit Rev Oral Biol Med* **8**(3):291–305.

LeResche L, Dworkin SF, Sommers EE, *et al* (1991) An epidemiologic evaluation of two diagnostic classification schemes for temporomandibular disorders. *J Prosthet Dent* **65**(1):131–137.

LeResche L, Dworkin SF, Wilson L, *et al* (1992) Effect of temporomandibular disorder pain duration on facial expressions and verbal report of pain. *Pain* **51**(3):289–295.

LeResche L, Saunders K, Von Korff MR, *et al* (1997) Use of exogenous hormones and risk of temporomandibular disorder pain. *Pain* **69**(1–2):153–160.

LeResche L, Mancl L, Sherman JJ, *et al* (2003) Changes in temporomandibular pain and other symptoms across the menstrual cycle. *Pain* **106**(3):253–261.

LeResche L, Mancl LA, Drangsholt MT, *et al* (2005a) Relationship of pain and symptoms to pubertal development in adolescents. *Pain* **118**(1–2):201–209.

LeResche L, Sherman JJ, Huggins K, *et al* (2005b) Musculoskeletal orofacial pain and other signs and symptoms of temporomandibular disorders during pregnancy: a prospective study. *J Orofac Pain* **19**(3):193–201.

Levitt SR, McKinney MW (1994) Validating the TMJ scale in a national sample of 10,000 patients: demographic and epidemiologic characteristics. *J Orofac Pain* **8**(1):25–35.

Li D, Rozen TD (2002) The clinical characteristics of new daily persistent headache. *Cephalalgia* **22**(1):66–69.

Liljestrom MR, Jamsa A, Le Bell Y, *et al* (2001) Signs and symptoms of temporomandibular disorders in children with different types of headache. *Acta Odontol Scand* **59**(6):413–417.

Liljestrom MR, Le Bell Y, Anttila P, *et al* (2005) Headache children with temporomandibular disorders have several types of pain and other symptoms. *Cephalalgia* **25**(11):1054–1060.

Linde C, Isacsson G, Jonsson BG (1995) Outcome of 6-week treatment with transcutaneous electric nerve stimulation compared with splint on symptomatic temporomandibular joint disk displacement without reduction. *Acta Odontol Scand* **53**(2):92–98.

Lipchik GL, Holroyd KA, O'Donnell FJ, *et al* (2000) Exteroceptive suppression periods and pericranial muscle tenderness in chronic tension-type headache: effects of psychopathology, chronicity and disability. *Cephalalgia* **20**(7):638–646.

Lipton JA, Ship JA, Larach-Robinson D (1993) Estimated prevalence and distribution of reported orofacial pain in the United States. *J Am Dent Assoc* **124**(10):115–121.

Lipton RB, Stewart WF, Cady R, *et al* (2000) Wolfe Award. Sumatriptan for the range of headaches in migraine sufferers: results of the Spectrum Study. *Headache* **40**(10):783–791.

Lipton RB, Cady RK, Stewart WF, *et al* (2002) Diagnostic lessons from the spectrum study. *Neurology* **58**(9 Suppl 6):S27–31.

List T, Wahlund K, Wenneberg B, *et al* (1999) TMD in children and adolescents: prevalence of pain, gender differences, and perceived treatment need. *J Orofac Pain* **13**(1):9–20.

Lobbezoo F, Lavigne GJ (1997) Do bruxism and temporomandibular disorders have a cause-and-effect relationship? *J Orofac Pain* **11**(1):15–23.

Lobbezoo F, van Selms MK, Naeije M (2006) Masticatory muscle pain and disordered jaw motor behaviour: Literature review over the past decade. *Arch Oral Biol* **51**(9):713–720.

Locker D, Slade G (1988) Prevalence of symptoms associated with temporomandibular disorders in a Canadian population. *Community Dent Oral Epidemiol* **16**(5):310–313.

Lund JP, Stohler CS (1994) Effects of pain on muscular activity in temporomandibular disorders and related conditions. In: Stohler CS, Carlson DS (eds) *Biological and Psychological Aspects of Orofacial Pain*. Ann Arbor, MI: University of Michigan, pp 74–91.

Lund JP, Donga R, Widmer CG, *et al* (1991) The pain-adaptation model: a discussion of the relationship between chronic musculoskeletal pain and motor activity. *Can J Physiol Pharmacol* **69**(5):683–694.

Lundh H, Westesson PL (1989) Long-term follow-up after occlusal treatment to correct abnormal temporomandibular joint disk position. *Oral Surg Oral Med Oral Pathol* **67**(1):2–10.

Lyngberg AC, Rasmussen BK, Jorgensen T, *et al* (2005a) Incidence of primary headache: a Danish epidemiologic follow-up study. *Am J Epidemiol* **161**(11):1066–1073.

Lyngberg AC, Rasmussen BK, Jorgensen T, *et al* (2005b) Has the prevalence of migraine and tension-type headache changed over a 12-year period? A Danish population survey. *Eur J Epidemiol* **20**(3):243–249.

Lyngberg AC, Rasmussen BK, Jorgensen T, *et al* (2005c) Prognosis of migraine and tension-type headache: a population-based follow-up study. *Neurology* **65**(4):580–585.

Macfarlane TV, Blinkhorn AS, Davies RM, *et al* (2002) Oro-facial pain in the community: prevalence and associated impact. *Community Dent Oral Epidemiol* **30**(1):52–60.

McMillan AS, Blasberg B (1994) Pain-pressure threshold in painful jaw muscles following trigger point injection. *J Orofac Pain* **8**(4):384–390.

McNamara JA Jr (1997) Orthodontic treatment and temporomandibular disorders. *Oral Surg Oral Med Oral Pathol Oral Radiol Endod* **83**(1):107–117.

Maekawa K, Clark GT, Kuboki T (2002) Intramuscular hypoperfusion, adrenergic receptors, and chronic muscle pain. *J Pain* **3**(4):251–260.

Magnusson T, Carlsson GE (1983) A 21/2-year follow-up of changes in headache and mandibular dysfunction after stomatognathic treatment. *J Prosthet Dent* **49**(3):398–402.

Magnusson T, Egermark I, Carlsson GE (2000) A longitudinal epidemiologic study of signs and symptoms of temporomandibular disorders from 15 to 35 years of age. *J Orofac Pain* **14**(4):310–319.

Magnusson T, Adiels AM, Nilsson HL, *et al* (2004) Treatment effect on signs and symptoms of temporomandibular disorders–comparison between stabilisation splint and a new type of splint (NTI). A pilot study. *Swed Dent J* **28**(1):11–20.

Maixner W, Fillingim R, Booker D, *et al* (1995) Sensitivity of patients with painful temporomandibular disorders to experimentally evoked pain. *Pain* **63**(3):341–351.

Maixner W, Fillingim R, Sigurdsson A, *et al* (1998) Sensitivity of patients with painful temporomandibular disorders to experimentally evoked pain: evidence for altered temporal summation of pain. *Pain* **76**(1-2):71–81.

Manzoni GC, Granella F, Sandrini G, *et al* (1995) Classification of chronic daily headache by International Headache Society criteria: limits and new proposals. *Cephalalgia* **15**(1):37–43.

Marbach JJ, Raphael KG, Dohrenwend BP, *et al* (1990) The validity of tooth grinding measures: etiology of pain dysfunction syndrome revisited. *J Am Dent Assoc* **120**(3):327–333.

Marbach JJ, Raphael KG, Janal MN, *et al* (2003) Reliability of clinician judgements of bruxism. *J Oral Rehabil* **30**(2):113–118.

Marchettini P, Simone DA, Caputi G, *et al* (1996) Pain from excitation of identified muscle nociceptors in humans. *Brain Res* **740**(1-2):109–116.

Marcus DA, Bernstein C, Rudy TE (2005) Fibromyalgia and headache: an epidemiological study supporting migraine as part of the fibromyalgia syndrome. *Clin Rheumatol* **24**(6):595–601.

Martinez-Lavin M (2004) Fibromyalgia as a sympathetically maintained pain syndrome. *Curr Pain Headache Rep* **8**(5):385–389.

Mathew NT, Ashina M (2006) Acute pharmacotherapy of tension-type headaches. In: Olesen J, Goadsby PJ, Ramadan NM, *et al.* (eds) *The Headaches*, 3rd edn. Philadelphia: Lippincott Williams & Wilkins, pp 727–733.

Meineri P, Torre E, Rota E, *et al* (2004) New daily persistent headache: clinical and serological characteristics in a retrospective study. *Neurol Sci* **25**(Suppl 3):S281–282.

Mense S (2002) Do we know enough to put forward a unifying hypothesis? *J Pain* **3**(4):264–267; discussion 270–261.

Mense S (2003) The pathogenesis of muscle pain. *Curr Pain Headache Rep* **7**(6):419–425.

Meyer HP (2002) Myofascial pain syndrome and its suggested role in the pathogenesis and treatment of fibromyalgia syndrome. *Curr Pain Headache Rep* **6**(4):274–283.

Michelotti A, Steenks MH, Farella M, *et al* (2004) The additional value of a home physical therapy regimen versus patient education only for the treatment of myofascial pain of the jaw muscles: short-term results of a randomized clinical trial. *J Orofac Pain* **18**(2):114–125.

Mishra KD, Gatchel RJ, Gardea MA (2000) The relative efficacy of three cognitive-behavioral treatment approaches to temporomandibular disorders. *J Behav Med* **23**(3):293–309.

Mohlin BO, Derweduwen K, Pilley R, *et al* (2004) Malocclusion and temporomandibular disorder: a comparison of adolescents with moderate to severe dysfunction with those without signs and symptoms of temporomandibular disorder and their further development to 30 years of age. *Angle Orthod* **74**(3):319–327.

Moldofsky H (2001) Sleep and pain. *Sleep Med Rev* **5**(5):385–396.

Moldofsky H (2002) Management of sleep disorders in fibromyalgia. *Rheum Dis Clin North Am* **28**(2):353–365.

Mostafapour SP, Futran ND (2000) Tumors and tumorous masses presenting as temporomandibular joint syndrome. *Otolaryngol Head Neck Surg* **123**(4):459–464.

Neufeld JD, Holroyd KA, Lipchik GL (2000) Dynamic assessment of abnormalities in central pain transmission and modulation in tension-type headache sufferers. *Headache* **40**(2):142–151.

Neufeld MY, Treves TA, Chistik V, *et al* (1999) Postmeningitis headache. *Headache* **39**(2):132–134.

Neumann L, Buskila D (2003) Epidemiology of fibromyalgia. *Curr Pain Headache Rep* **7**(5):362–368.

Nilsson IM, List T, Drangsholt M (2005) Prevalence of temporomandibular pain and subsequent dental treatment in Swedish adolescents. *J Orofac Pain* **19**(2):144–150.

Nitzan DW (1994) Intraarticular pressure in the functioning human temporomandibular joint and its alteration by uniform elevation of the occlusal plane. *J Oral Maxillofac Surg* **52**(7):671–679; discussion 679–680.

Oakley ME, McCreary CP, Flack VF, *et al* (1989) Dentists' ability to detect psychological problems in patients with temporomandibular disorders and chronic pain. *J Am Dent Assoc* **118**(6):727–730.

Ohayon MM, Li KK, Guilleminault C (2001) Risk factors for sleep bruxism in the general population. *Chest* **119**(1):53–61.

Okeson JP (1996) *Orofacial Pain: Guidelines for Assessment, Classification, and Management*. American Academy of Orofacial Pain. Chicago: Quintessence Publishing.

Okifuji A, Turk DC, Marcus DA (1999) Comparison of generalized and localized hyperalgesia in patients with recurrent headache and fibromyalgia. *Psychosom Med* **61**(6):771–780.

Olesen J, Bousser M-G, Diener HC, *et al* (2004) The International Classification of Headache Disorders, 2nd Edition. *Cephalalgia* **24** (suppl 1):24–150.

Osterberg T, Carlsson GE, Wedel A, *et al* (1992) A cross-sectional and longitudinal study of craniomandibular dysfunction in an elderly population. *J Craniomandib Disord* **6**(4):237–245.

Ostergaard S, Russell MB, Bendtsen L, *et al* (1997) Comparison of first degree relatives and spouses of people with chronic tension headache. *Bmj* **314**(7087):1092–1093.

Pahkala R, Qvarnstrom M (2004) Can temporomandibular dysfunction signs be predicted by early morphological or functional variables? *Eur J Orthod* **26**(4):367–373.

Palermo TM, Kiska R (2005) Subjective sleep disturbances in adolescents with chronic pain: relationship to daily functioning and quality of life. *J Pain* 6(3):201–207.

Peres MFP, Kaup A, Zukerman OE, *et al* (2000) Fibromyalgia and chronic daily headache. *Cephalalgia* 20(4):302–303.

Peres MF, Young WB, Kaup AO, *et al* (2001) Fibromyalgia is common in patients with transformed migraine. *Neurology* 57(7):1326–1328.

Pergamalian A, Rudy TE, Zaki HS, *et al* (2003) The association between wear facets, bruxism, and severity of facial pain in patients with temporomandibular disorders. *J Prosthet Dent* 90(2):194–200.

Petty BG, Cornblath DR, Adornato BT, *et al* (1994) The effect of systemically administered recombinant human nerve growth factor in healthy human subjects. *Ann Neurol* 36(2):244–246.

Phillips JM, Gatchel RJ, Wesley AL, *et al* (2001) Clinical implications of sex in acute temporomandibular disorders. *J Am Dent Assoc* 132(1):49–57.

Pielsticker A, Haag G, Zaudig M, *et al* (2005) Impairment of pain inhibition in chronic tension-type headache. *Pain* 118(1-2):215–223.

Pierce CJ, Weyant RJ, Block HM, *et al* (1995) Dental splint prescription patterns: a survey. *J Am Dent Assoc* 126(2):248–254.

Plesh O, Curtis D, Levine J, *et al* (2000) Amitriptyline treatment of chronic pain in patients with temporomandibular disorders. *J Oral Rehabil* 27(10):834–841.

Prencipe M, Casini AR, Ferretti C, *et al* (2001) Prevalence of headache in an elderly population: attack frequency, disability, and use of medication. *J Neurol Neurosurg Psychiatry* 70(3):377–381.

Prior MJ, Cooper KM, May LG, *et al* (2002) Efficacy and safety of acetaminophen and naproxen in the treatment of tension-type headache. A randomized, double-blind, placebo-controlled trial. *Cephalalgia* 22(9):740–748.

Pryse-Phillips W, Findlay H, Tugwell P, *et al* (1992) A Canadian population survey on the clinical, epidemiologic and societal impact of migraine and tension-type headache. *Can J Neurol Sci* 19(3):333–339.

Pullinger AG, Seligman DA (1991) Trauma history in diagnostic groups of temporomandibular disorders. *Oral Surg Oral Med Oral Pathol* 71(5):529–534.

Puri V, Cui L, Liverman CS, *et al* (2005) Ovarian steroids regulate neuropeptides in the trigeminal ganglion. *Neuropeptides* 39(4):409–417.

Raieli V, Eliseo M, Pandolfi E, *et al* (2005) Recurrent and chronic headaches in children below 6 years of age. *J Headache Pain* 6(3):135–142.

Rammelsberg P, LeResche L, Dworkin S, *et al* (2003) Longitudinal outcome of temporomandibular disorders: a 5-year epidemiologic study of muscle disorders defined by research diagnostic criteria for temporomandibular disorders. *J Orofac Pain* 17(1):9–20.

Rao SG, Clauw DJ (2004) The management of fibromyalgia. *Drugs Today (Barc)* 40(6):539–554.

Raphael KG, Marbach JJ (1992) A year of chronic TMPDS: evaluating patients' pain patterns. *J Am Dent Assoc* 123(11):53–58.

Raphael KG, Marbach JJ (2001) Widespread pain and the effectiveness of oral splints in myofascial face pain. *J Am Dent Assoc* 132(3):305–316.

Raphael KG, Marbach JJ, Gallagher RM, *et al* (1999) Myofascial TMD does not run in families. *Pain* 80(1-2):15–22.

Raphael KG, Marbach JJ, Gallagher RM (2000a) Somatosensory amplification and affective inhibition are elevated in myofascial face pain. *Pain Med* 1(3):247–253.

Raphael KG, Marbach JJ, Klausner J (2000b) Myofascial face pain. Clinical characteristics of those with regional vs. widespread pain. *J Am Dent Assoc* 131(2):161–171.

Rasmussen BK (1995) Epidemiology of headache. *Cephalalgia* 15(1):45–68.

Rasmussen BK (1996) Migraine and tension-type headache are separate disorders. *Cephalalgia* 16(4):217–220; discussion 223.

Rasmussen BK, Jensen R, Olesen J (1991) A population-based analysis of the diagnostic criteria of the International Headache Society. *Cephalalgia* 11(3):129–134.

Rasmussen BK, Jensen R, Olesen J (1992a) Impact of headache on sickness absence and utilisation of medical services: a Danish population study. *J Epidemiol Community Health* 46(4):443–446.

Rasmussen BK, Jensen R, Schroll M, *et al* (1992b) Interrelations between migraine and tension-type headache in the general population. *Arch Neurol* 49(9):914–918.

Reiter S, Eli I, Gavish A, *et al* (2006) Ethnic differences in temporomandibular disorders between Jewish and Arab populations in Israel according to RDC/TMD evaluation. *J Orofac Pain* 20(1):36–42.

Rhodus NL, Fricton J, Carlson P, *et al* (2003) Oral symptoms associated with fibromyalgia syndrome. *J Rheumatol* 30(8):1841–1845.

Ro JY, Svensson P, Capra N (2002) Effects of experimental muscle pain on electromyographic activity of masticatory muscles in the rat. *Muscle Nerve* 25(4):576–584.

Rugh JD, Barghi N, Drago CJ (1984) Experimental occlusal discrepancies and nocturnal bruxism. *J Prosthet Dent* 51(4):548–553.

Russell MB (2005) Tension-type headache in 40-year-olds: a Danish population-based sample of 4000. *J Headache Pain* 6(6):441–447.

Sandrini G, Rossi P, Milanov I, *et al* (2006) Abnormal modulatory influence of diffuse noxious inhibitory controls in migraine and chronic tension-type headache patients. *Cephalalgia* 26(7):782–789.

Santoni JR, Santoni-Williams CJ (1993) Headache and painful lymphadenopathy in extracranial or systemic infection: etiology of new daily persistent headaches. *Intern Med* 32(7):530–532.

Sarlani E, Grace EG, Reynolds MA, *et al* (2004) Evidence for up-regulated central nociceptive processing in patients with masticatory myofascial pain. *J Orofac Pain* 18(1):41–55.

Sarzi-Puttini P, Atzeni F, Diana A, *et al* (2006) Increased neural sympathetic activation in fibromyalgia syndrome. *Ann N Y Acad Sci* 1069:109–117.

Schachtel BP, Furey SA, Thoden WR (1996) Nonprescription ibuprofen and acetaminophen in the treatment of tension-type headache. *J Clin Pharmacol* 36(12):1120–1125.

Scher AI, Stewart WF, Ricci JA, *et al* (2003) Factors associated with the onset and remission of chronic daily headache in a population-based study. *Pain* 106(1-2):81–89.

Schiffman EL, Anderson GC, Fricton JR, *et al* (1992) The relationship between level of mandibular pain and dysfunction and stage of temporomandibular joint internal derangement. *J Dent Res* 71(11):1812–1815.

Schmidt-Hansen P, Svensson P, Jensen T, *et al* (2006) Patterns of experimentally induced pain in pericranial muscles. *Cephalalgia* 26(5):568–577.

Schmitter M, Kress B, Rammelsberg P (2004) Temporomandibular joint pathosis in patients with myofascial pain: a comparative analysis of magnetic resonance imaging and a clinical examination based on a specific set of criteria. *Oral Surg Oral Med Oral Pathol Oral Radiol Endod* 97(3):318–324.

Schmitter M, Rammelsberg P, Hassel A (2005) The prevalence of signs and symptoms of temporomandibular disorders in very old subjects. *J Oral Rehabil* 32(7):467–473.

Schnurr RF, Rollman GB, Brooke RI (1991) Are there psychologic predictors of treatment outcome in temporomandibular joint pain and dysfunction? *Oral Surg Oral Med Oral Pathol* 72(5):550–558.

Schokker RP, Hansson TL, Ansink BJ (1990) The result of treatment of the masticatory system of chronic headache patients. *J Craniomandib Disord* 4(2):126–130.

Scott DS, Lundeen TF (1980) Myofascial pain involving the masticatory muscles: an experimental model. *Pain* 8(2):207–215.

Scudds RA, Trachsel LC, Luckhurst BJ, *et al* (1989) A comparative study of pain, sleep quality and pain responsiveness in fibrositis and myofascial pain syndrome. *J Rheumatol Suppl* **19**:120–126.

Selaimen CM, Jeronymo JC, Brilhante DP, *et al* (2006) Sleep and depression as risk indicators for temporomandibular disorders in a cross-cultural perspective: a case-control study. *Int J Prosthodont* **19**(2):154–161.

Sessle BJ (1999) The neural basis of temporomandibular joint and masticatory muscle pain. *J Orofac Pain* **13**(4):238–245.

Sessle BJ, Hu JW (1991) Mechanisms of pain arising from articular tissues. *Can J Physiol Pharmacol* **69**(5):617–626.

Shah JP, Phillips TM, Danoff JV, *et al* (2005) An in vivo microanalytical technique for measuring the local biochemical milieu of human skeletal muscle. *J Appl Physiol* **99**(5):1977–1984.

Shankland WE (2002) Nociceptive trigeminal inhibition–tension suppression system: a method of preventing migraine and tension headaches. *Compend Contin Educ Dent* **23**(2):105–108, 110, 112-113; quiz 114.

Sharav Y, Tzukert A, Refaeli B (1978) Muscle pain index in relation to pain, dysfunction, and dizziness associated with the myofascial pain-dysfunction syndrome. *Oral Surg Oral Med Oral Pathol* **46**(6):742–747.

Sharav Y, Singer E, Schmidt E, *et al* (1987) The analgesic effect of amitriptyline on chronic facial pain. *Pain* **31**(2):199–209.

Sheikholeslam A, Holmgren K, Riise C (1986) A clinical and electromyographic study of the long-term effects of an occlusal splint on the temporal and masseter muscles in patients with functional disorders and nocturnal bruxism. *J Oral Rehabil* **13**(2):137–145.

Sherman JJ, Turk DC (2001) Nonpharmacologic approaches to the management of myofascial temporomandibular disorders. *Curr Pain Headache Rep* **5**(5): 421–431.

Sherman JJ, LeResche L, Huggins KH, *et al* (2004) The relationship of somatization and depression to experimental pain response in women with temporomandibular disorders. *Psychosom Med* **66**(6):852–860.

Shiau YY, Peng CC, Wen SC, *et al* (2003) The effects of masseter muscle pain on biting performance. *J Oral Rehabil* **30**(10): 978–984.

Silberstein SD, Lipton RB, Sliwinski M (1996) Classification of daily and near-daily headaches: field trial of revised IHS criteria. *Neurology* **47**(4):871–875.

Simons DG (2004) Review of enigmatic MTrPs as a common cause of enigmatic musculoskeletal pain and dysfunction. *J Electromyogr Kinesiol* **14**(1):95–107.

Simons DG, Travell JG, Simons LS (1999). Head and neck pain. In: Travell JG, Simons DG (eds) *Myofascial Pain and Dysfunction: The Trigger Point Manual*, 2nd edn. Baltimore: Williams and Wilkins, pp 237–483.

Singer E, Sharav Y, Dubner R, *et al* (1987) The efficacy of diazepam and ibuprofen in the treatment of chronic myofascial orofacial pain. *Pain* (Suppl 4):583.

Solberg WK, Woo MW, Houston JB (1979) Prevalence of mandibular dysfunction in young adults. *J Am Dent Assoc* **98**(1):25–34.

Solomon S, Lipton RB, Newman LC (1992) Clinical features of chronic daily headache. *Headache* **32**(7):325–329.

Spierings EL, Ranke AH, Honkoop PC (2001) Precipitating and aggravating factors of migraine versus tension-type headache. *Headache* **41**(6):554–558.

Steed PA, Wexler GB (2001) Temporomandibular disorders–traumatic etiology vs. nontraumatic etiology: a clinical and methodological inquiry into symptomatology and treatment outcomes. *Cranio* **19**(3):188–194.

Steele JG, Lamey PJ, Sharkey SW, *et al* (1991) Occlusal abnormalities, pericranial muscle and joint tenderness and tooth wear in a group of migraine patients. *J Oral Rehabil* **18**(5):453–458.

Steiner TJ, Lange R, Voelker M (2003) Aspirin in episodic tension-type headache: placebo-controlled dose-ranging comparison with paracetamol. *Cephalalgia* **23**(1):59–66.

Stillman MJ (2002) Pharmacotherapy of tension-type headaches. *Curr Pain Headache Rep* **6**(5):408–413.

Stohler CS, Zarb GA (1999) On the management of temporomandibular disorders: a plea for a low-tech, high-prudence therapeutic approach. *J Orofac Pain* **13**(4):255–261.

Stohler CS, Zhang X, Lund JP (1996) The effect of experimental jaw muscle pain on postural muscle activity. *Pain* **66**(2-3): 215–221.

Stohler CS, Kowalski CJ, Lund JP (2001) Muscle pain inhibits cutaneous touch perception. *Pain* **92**(3):327–333.

Stovner LJ, Zwart JA, Hagen K, *et al* (2006) Epidemiology of headache in Europe. *Eur J Neurol* **13**(4):333–345.

Suvinen TI, Reade PC, Hanes KR, *et al* (2005a) Temporomandibular disorder subtypes according to self-reported physical and psychosocial variables in female patients: a re-evaluation. *J Oral Rehabil* **32**(3):166–173.

Suvinen TI, Reade PC, Kemppainen P, *et al* (2005b) Review of aetiological concepts of temporomandibular pain disorders: towards a biopsychosocial model for integration of physical disorder factors with psychological and psychosocial illness impact factors. *Eur J Pain* **9**(6):613–633.

Svensson P, Graven-Nielsen T (2001) Craniofacial muscle pain: review of mechanisms and clinical manifestations. *J Orofac Pain* **15**(2):117–145.

Svensson P, Arendt-Nielsen L, Houe L (1998a) Muscle pain modulates mastication: an experimental study in humans. *J Orofac Pain* **12**(1):7–16.

Svensson P, Graven-Nielsen T, Arendt-Nielsen L (1998b) Mechanical hyperesthesia of human facial skin induced by tonic painful stimulation of jaw muscles. *Pain* **74**(1):93–100.

Svensson P, List T, Hector G (2001) Analysis of stimulus-evoked pain in patients with myofascial temporomandibular pain disorders. *Pain* **92**(3):399–409.

Svensson P, Bak J, Troest T (2003a) Spread and referral of experimental pain in different jaw muscles. *J Orofac Pain* **17**(3):214–223.

Svensson P, Cairns BE, Wang K, *et al* (2003b) Glutamate-evoked pain and mechanical allodynia in the human masseter muscle. *Pain* **101**(3):221–227.

Takase Y, Nakano M, Tatsumi C, *et al* (2004) Clinical features, effectiveness of drug-based treatment, and prognosis of new daily persistent headache (NDPH): 30 cases in Japan. *Cephalalgia* **24**(11):955–959.

Tallents RH, Katzberg RW, Macher DJ, *et al* (1990) Use of protrusive splint therapy in anterior disk displacement of the temporomandibular joint: a 1- to 3-year follow-up. *J Prosthet Dent* **63**(3):336–341.

Tallents RH, Catania J, Sommers E (1991) Temporomandibular joint findings in pediatric populations and young adults: a critical review. *Angle Orthod* **61**(1):7–16.

Taylor K, Newton RA, Personius WJ, *et al* (1987) Effects of interferential current stimulation for treatment of subjects with recurrent jaw pain. *Phys Ther* **67**(3):346–350.

Tecco S, Festa F, Salini V, *et al* (2004) Treatment of joint pain and joint noises associated with a recent TMJ internal derangement: a comparison of an anterior repositioning splint, a full-arch maxillary stabilization splint, and an untreated control group. *Cranio* **22**(3):209–219.

Thilander B, Rubio G, Pena L, *et al* (2002) Prevalence of temporomandibular dysfunction and its association with malocclusion in children and adolescents: an epidemiologic study related to specified stages of dental development. *Angle Orthod* **72**(2):146–154.

Tomkins GE, Jackson JL, O'Malley PG, *et al* (2001) Treatment of chronic headache with antidepressants: a meta-analysis. *Am J Med* **111**(1):54–63.

Treasure T (2002) External auditory canal carcinoma involving the temporomandibular joint: two cases presenting as temporomandibular disorders. *J Oral Maxillofac Surg* **60**(4): 465–469.

Truelove E, Huggins KH, Mancl L, *et al* (2006) The efficacy of traditional, low-cost and nonsplint therapies for temporomandibular disorder: a randomized controlled trial. *J Am Dent Assoc* **137**(8):1099–1107; quiz 1169.

Turner JA, Dworkin SF (2004) Screening for psychosocial risk factors in patients with chronic orofacial pain: recent advances. *J Am Dent Assoc* **135**(8):1119–1125; quiz 1164–1165.

Turner JA, Holtzman S, Mancl L (2007) Mediators, moderators, and predictors of therapeutic change in cognitive-behavioral therapy for chronic pain. *Pain* **127**:276–286.

Turp JC, Kowalski CJ, Stohler CS (1997) Temporomandibular disorders–pain outside the head and face is rarely acknowledged in the chief complaint. *J Prosthet Dent* **78**(6): 592–595.

Turp JC, Kowalski CJ, O'Leary N, *et al* (1998) Pain maps from facial pain patients indicate a broad pain geography. *J Dent Res* **77**(6):1465–1472.

Turp JC, Schindler HJ, Pritsch M, *et al* (2002) Antero-posterior activity changes in the superficial masseter muscle after exposure to experimental pain. *Eur J Oral Sci* **110**(2):83–91.

Turp JC, Komine F, Hugger A (2004) Efficacy of stabilization splints for the management of patients with masticatory muscle pain: a qualitative systematic review. *Clin Oral Investig* **8**(4):179–195.

Ulrich V, Russell MB, Jensen R, *et al* (1996) A comparison of tension-type headache in migraineurs and in non-migraineurs: a population-based study. *Pain* **67**(2-3):501–506.

Ulrich V, Gervil M, Olesen J (2004) The relative influence of environment and genes in episodic tension-type headache. *Neurology* **62**(11):2065–2069.

Vallon D, Ekberg EC, Nilner M, *et al* (1991) Short-term effect of occlusal adjustment on craniomandibular disorders including headaches. *Acta Odontol Scand* **49**(2):89–96.

Vallon D, Ekberg E, Nilner M, *et al* (1995) Occlusal adjustment in patients with craniomandibular disorders including headaches. A 3- and 6-month follow-up. *Acta Odontol Scand* **53**(1):55–59.

Vanderas AP, Menenakou M, Papagiannoulis L (2001) Emotional stress and craniomandibular dysfunction in children. *Cranio* **19**(2):123–129.

van der Meulen MJ, Lobbezoo F, Aartman IH, *et al* (2006) Self-reported oral parafunctions and pain intensity in temporomandibular disorder patients. *J Orofac Pain* **20**(1): 31–35.

van Grootel RJ, van der Glas HW, Buchner R, *et al* (2005) Patterns of pain variation related to myogenous temporomandibular disorders. *Clin J Pain* **21**(2):154–165.

Velly AM, Gornitsky M, Philippe P (2003) Contributing factors to chronic myofascial pain: a case-control study. *Pain* **104**(3): 491–499.

Vgontzas AN, Chrousos GP (2002) Sleep, the hypothalamic-pituitary-adrenal axis, and cytokines: multiple interactions and disturbances in sleep disorders. *Endocrinol Metab Clin North Am* **31**(1):15–36.

Vierck CJ Jr (2006) Mechanisms underlying development of spatially distributed chronic pain (fibromyalgia). *Pain* **124**(3):242–263.

Wahlund K (2003) Temporomandibular disorders in adolescents. Epidemiological and methodological studies and a randomized controlled trial. *Swed Dent J Suppl* (164):inside front cover, 2–64.

Wang SJ, Fuh JL, Lu SR, *et al* (2000) Chronic daily headache in Chinese elderly: prevalence, risk factors, and biannual follow-up. *Neurology* **54**(2):314–319.

Ware JC, Rugh JD (1988) Destructive bruxism: sleep stage relationship. *Sleep* **11**(2):172–181.

Wassell RW, Adams N, Kelly PJ (2006) The treatment of temporomandibular disorders with stabilizing splints in general dental practice: one-year follow-up. *J Am Dent Assoc* **137**(8):1089–1098; quiz 1168–1089.

Watts PG, Peet KM, Juniper RP (1986) Migraine and the temporomandibular joint: the final answer? *Br Dent J* **161**(5):170–173.

Wenneberg B, Nystrom T, Carlsson GE (1988) Occlusal equilibration and other stomatognathic treatment in patients with mandibular dysfunction and headache. *J Prosthet Dent* **59**(4):478–483.

Wexler GB, McKinney MW (1999) Temporomandibular treatment outcomes within five diagnostic categories. *Cranio* **17**(1):30–37.

White BA, Williams LA, Leben JR (2001) Health care utilization and cost among health maintenance organization members with temporomandibular disorders. *J Orofac Pain* **15**(2):158–169.

White KP, Speechley M, Harth M, *et al* (1999) The London Fibromyalgia Epidemiology Study: the prevalence of fibromyalgia syndrome in London, Ontario. *J Rheumatol* **26**(7):1570–1576.

Widmer CG (1991) Chronic muscle pain syndromes: an overview. *Can J Physiol Pharmacol* **69**(5):659–661.

Winocur E, Gavish A, Voikovitch M, *et al* (2003) Drugs and bruxism: a critical review. *J Orofac Pain* **17**(2):99–111.

Wittrock DA, Myers TC (1998) The comparison of individuals with recurrent tension-type headache and headache-free controls in physiological response, appraisal, and coping with stressors: a review of the literature. *Ann Behav Med* **20**(2): 118–134.

Woda A, Pionchon P (1999) A unified concept of idiopathic orofacial pain: clinical features. *J Orofac Pain* **13**(3):172–184; discussion 185-195.

Wolfe F (2003) Stop using the American College of Rheumatology criteria in the clinic. *J Rheumatol* **30**(8):1671–1672.

Wolfe F, Smythe HA, Yunus MB, *et al* (1990) The American College of Rheumatology 1990 Criteria for the Classification of Fibromyalgia. Report of the Multicenter Criteria Committee. *Arthritis Rheum* **33**(2):160–172.

Wolfe F, Simons DG, Fricton J, *et al* (1992) The fibromyalgia and myofascial pain syndromes: a preliminary study of tender points and trigger points in persons with fibromyalgia, myofascial pain syndrome and no disease. *J Rheumatol* **19**(6):944–951.

Wolfe F, Ross K, Anderson J, *et al* (1995) The prevalence and characteristics of fibromyalgia in the general population. *Arthritis Rheum* **38**(1):19–28.

Wolfe F, Anderson J, Harkness D, *et al* (1997) Health status and disease severity in fibromyalgia: results of a six-center longitudinal study. *Arthritis Rheum* **40**(9):1571–1579.

Wolfe F, Katz RS, Michaud K (2005) Jaw pain: its prevalence and meaning in patients with rheumatoid arthritis, osteoarthritis, and fibromyalgia. *J Rheumatol* **32**(12):2421–2428.

Wright EF (2000) Referred craniofacial pain patterns in patients with temporomandibular disorder. *J Am Dent Assoc* **131**(9):1307–1315.

Wright EF, Bifano SL (1997) The relationship between tinnitus and temporomandibular disorder (TMD) therapy. *Int Tinnitus J* **3**(1):55–61.

Yap AU, Dworkin SF, Chua EK, *et al* (2003) Prevalence of temporomandibular disorder subtypes, psychologic distress, and psychosocial dysfunction in Asian patients. *J Orofac Pain* **17**(1):21–28.

Yemm R (1979) Neurophysiological studies of temporo-mandibular joint dysfunction. In: Zarb GA, Carlsson GE (eds) *The Temporomandibular Joint*. Copenhagen: Munksgaard, pp 215–237.

Yunus M, Masi AT, Calabro JJ, *et al* (1981) Primary fibromyalgia (fibrositis): clinical study of 50 patients with matched normal controls. *Semin Arthritis Rheum* **11**(1):151–171.

Yunus MB, Ahles TA, Aldag JC, *et al* (1991) Relationship of clinical features with psychological status in primary fibromyalgia. *Arthritis Rheum* **34**(1):15–21.

Yunus MB, Inanici F, Aldag JC, *et al* (2000) Fibromyalgia in men: comparison of clinical features with women. *J Rheumatol* **27**(2):485–490.

CHAPTER 8

Pain and dysfunction of the temporomandibular joint

Dorrit Nitzan, Rafael Benoliel, Gary Heir and Franklin Dolwick

1. Introduction

Temporomandibular disorders (TMD) refer to various conditions affecting the temporomandibular joint (TMJ), masticatory muscles and contiguous tissue components. Two common types of painful TMD are encountered: myogenous or muscle-generated pain (see Chapter 7), and arthrogenous or joint-generated pain. As discussed in Chapter 7 and below, the use of the term TMD is problematic; it forcefully integrates what are probably distinct biological entities into one diagnostic family. The pooling of data from epidemiologic, clinical and therapeutic studies of 'TMD' is therefore misleading. An overview of the overall epidemiology and general characteristics of TMDs was presented in Chapter 7.

This chapter focuses on pain and dysfunction originating in the TMJ proper, particularly as a result of disc derangements or osteoarthritis. Other relatively rare joint-related entities that may present as TMJ pain are extremely important in differential diagnosis but are beyond the scope of this chapter; some have been partly covered in other chapters (Table 8.1).

When discussing TMJ disorders the term 'internal derangement' is often used as a diagnosis. However, internal derangement is a classification, not a diagnosis, and includes disc displacements (joint derangements) and degeneration of the TMJ (Stegenga 2001). Joint *derangement* refers to a disarranged condition, focusing on a disturbance in mechanical operation. For accurate diagnosis the structures and the mechanical problem must be defined; for example disc displacement with reduction. On the other hand, joint *degeneration* is

associated with disintegration or tissue damage to the joint constituents, as is the case in TMJ osteoarthritis.

Many patients report the onset of TMJ symptoms subsequent to trauma; others describe an insidious onset with no apparent cause. However, accumulating data suggest that many TMJ disorders may primarily be due to overuse or overloading of the system. We review current thinking on pathogenesis, diagnosis and treatment and discuss pain and dysfunction of the TMJ based upon the biomechanical and biochemical events underlying pain and joint dysfunction. Although knowledge of the aetiology of TMJ disorders is limited, the prognosis of most TMJ problems is good and many patients improve spontaneously in terms of both signs and symptoms. Our treatment approach should therefore be in line with this natural process. Adopting a conservative treatment with an aim to reduce joint loading and inflammation, encourage healing and repair and restore function consistently results in successful outcomes for most of our patients.

2. Classification

We employ the diagnostic criteria published by the American Academy of Orofacial Pain (AAOP) (Okeson 1996) and by Dworkin and LeResche (1992) (Research Diagnostic Criteria for Temporomandibular Disorders, RDC-TMD). The systems are very similar in approach and content and their merits are described in Chapter 7; the AAOP's criteria are intuitive and highly applicable in the clinical setting whilst the RDC-TMD are extremely detailed (in both the examination technique to be used

Table 8.1 Differential Diagnosis: Entities Not Covered in This Chapter That May Present With TMJ Pain

Mechanism		Structure/Entity	Comments	Chapter
Referred	*Regional*	• Dental	Referral area related to pain intensity	5
		• Ear	Very common	6
		• Muscular	Very common; pterygoids, masseter	7
		• Neurovascular	Hemicrania continua	9, 10
		• Neuropathic	Glossopharyngeal, nervus intermedius neuralgias	11
	Distant	• Cardiac	Usually left-sided, associated with exertion	13
Systemic	*Autoimmune*	• Rheumatoid	Patient's primary disorder has usually been diagnosed and requires specific TMJ-related management	14
		• Psoriasis		
		• SLE		
		• MCTD		
		• Ankylosing spondylitis		
		• Systemic sclerosis		
Infectious	*Primary*	• Bacterial	Usually staphylococcal	14
	Reactive	• Reiter's syndrome		
Tumour	*Benign*	• Usually bone or cartilage	Uncommon: new onset malocclusion, painless swelling	14
	Malignant	• Primary	Uncommon, usually chondrosarcoma. Painful mass.	
		• Metastatic	More common than primary; breast, lung, prostate	
		• Referred pain	Nasopharyngeal carcinoma	
		• Post-therapy	Surgery, radiotherapy	

TMJ, temporomandibular joint; SLE, systemic lupus erythematosus; MCTD, multiple connective tissue disease.

and the diagnostic criteria) and should be employed for TMD research. However, the RDC-TMD do not include polyarthritides or tumours that affect the TMJ and do not deal at all with orofacial pain; this limits their application for routine use in specialized or oral and maxillofacial surgery clinics. Additionally the AAOP system is built upon and integrated with the International Headache Society's (IHS) classification of head and face pain (Olesen *et al* 2004); see Chapter 1. The combined systems thus allow for extensive diagnostic options.

3. Patient Assessment

3.1. Interview and Clinical Examination

Patient interview and evaluation, leading to accurate diagnosis, are the keys to appropriate treatment; but bear in mind that each piece of information may be misleading. It is therefore crucial to evaluate each patient as if assembling a new puzzle. A conclusion can be drawn only when all pieces are collected and properly placed; missing pieces should be looked for and accordingly misleading pieces should be recognized and discarded (see Chapter 1, The Diagnostic Process).

Accurate history taking and thorough physical examination techniques are beyond the scope of this chapter.

Examination of the TMJ is rarely performed without a thorough head and neck examination including masticatory, neck and pericranial muscles. The complete examination of the head and neck musculature is essential to diagnose comorbid muscle problems (Chapter 7).

The basic examination techniques and anamnestic approach to orofacial pain patients have been reviewed in Chapters 1 and 7. We therefore present only aspects of the diagnostic process relevant to patients with TMJ problems. In our practice, patient evaluation includes a self-filled questionnaire detailing demographic information and a comprehensive history of the main complaints in the patient's own words. This includes initial symptoms, their characteristics, onset and duration, triggering, modifying or aggravating factors and the presence of oral habits (e.g. clenching). Pure TMJ pain (but not referred pain) is usually accompanied by complaints of dysfunction such as reduced chewing ability. Location and referral patterns should be described in words and marked by the patient on a diagram of the head and neck region. Patients with pain of intra-articular origin usually locate pain in the joint that may radiate to adjacent structures, especially the ear. Pain is increased upon forced opening and on biting and/or chewing on the contralateral side. Severity of pain at rest and during function as well as the extent of any dysfunction should be assessed by using visual analogue scales (VAS) and drawings; see Chapter 3.

In addition to quantifying an admittedly subjective experience VAS records enable the clinician to assess changes over time and treatment response in a more objective manner (see also use of pain diaries; Chapter 1). Admittedly there is some disagreement as to the use of questionnaires but we find them time-saving and extremely useful.

A thorough history and examination (see Chapter 7) are important to exclude primary dental pathology or secondary occlusal problems such as deviation of the dental midline, missing teeth, collapsed or open bites. The patient's previous treatments such as drug dosages and duration, physical exercises and the result these obtained should be recorded. The patient's adherence to these treatment protocols is important—often treatment is prescribed but not carefully followed and may lead to 'treatment failure'. General health problems and current or past medications are highly relevant to diagnosis and treatment planning (see drug interactions and contraindications in Chapters 15 and 16). Psychosocial factors are important modifiers of disease progression and treatment response (see Chapters 4 and 7) and a basic psychosocial history, with or without the aid of pre-prepared forms, may be useful. The RDC-TMD clinical examination protocol and techniques are highly recommended. They include careful observation, determination and recording of clinical signs and symptoms.

The clinical examination of the TMJ should begin by allowing the clinician to familiarize himself with the patient (behaviour, relative sensitivity) and the articular problem. Examination and interview should be performed facing the patient so that responses can be adequately assessed. Following the initial interview, we begin by palpating the lateral pole of the joint in the preauricular area and asking the patient to perform basic jaw movements; this also familiarizes the patient with the examination procedures to follow. The joint should be carefully palpated with uniform pressure from its lateral aspect and posteriorly via the external auditory meatus both in the open and closed positions. The degree of resultant pain and sensitivity may be recorded on a simple ordinal scale (0=no pain, 1=mild pain, 2=moderate pain and 3=very painful) or employing a 10-cm VAS scale.

The presence and characteristics of joint sounds (Box 8.1) should be recorded. This may be performed digitally or via stethoscopic auscultation; often sounds are present continuously during movement or at particular positions and these should be recorded. Maximal unassisted and assisted interincisal mouth opening should be accurately measured with a millimetre ruler; the presence and pattern of deviation if it exists should be recorded. For example, persistent deviation to one side is characteristic of ipsilateral osteoarthritis or disc derangement without reduction. Deviation during opening that corrects itself following a joint sound (the classical 'S'-shaped mouth opening) is characteristic of ipsilateral disc displacement with reduction. Pain produced on assisted opening, its severity and very importantly its location

---

Box 8.1 Defining Joint Sounds

Click
- A brief and distinct sound of limited duration occurring during mandibular movement.
- The sound is usually of a 'sharp' or 'popping' nature.
- Clicking noises may occur during opening or closing jaw movements; when they occur on both the click is termed 'reciprocal'.
- Reproducible clicks refer to sounds consistently present on clinical examination and not only as a patient complaint.

Crepitus
- A sound that is present continuously during jaw movement and is therefore not brief, like a click.
- Crepitus reflects the noise of bone grinding against bone or cartilage on cartilage, and sounds or feels like the grinding of stones or walking on snow or sand.
- RDC-TMD further subdivides crepitus into coarse or fine crepitus.
- Coarse crepitus is not muffled and quite prominent whilst fine crepitus is a more subtle grating sound often over a longer period of jaw movements.
- Fine crepitus may often be described as a rubbing or crackling sound on a rough surface.

RDC-TMD, Research Diagnostic Criteria Temporomandibular Disorders.

---

should be carefully noted (Figs 8.1A and 8.1B). Other characteristics associated with limitation in jaw movement should be recorded when present; anchored disc phenomenon is associated with a strictly limited mouth opening whilst other disorders may allow increased opening with manual assistance. Other jaw movements such as protrusion and lateral excursions should be accurately assessed and measured on a millimetre (mm) scale, and the exact location of resultant pain recorded. These measurements are reliable in differentiating TMJ patients versus controls (Dworkin and LeResche 1992; Dworkin *et al* 2002; Celic *et al* 2003). A joint-loading test performed by biting on a wooden stick on the canines and molars on both sides followed by asking the patient to point to the pain location and define its intensity is useful (Fig. 8.2A). Intra-articular inflammatory processes are characterized by pain or sensitivity when the patient bites contralaterally to the affected TMJ whilst muscle disorders usually result in pain ipsilateral to the loading (Fig. 8.2B).

3.2. Imaging

Imaging of the TMJ is a complementary modality to clinical examination and is used to confirm diagnosis, aid in treatment planning and assess disease progress. Certain modalities such as arthrography (radiography with contrast medium) have greatly contributed to our understanding of TMJ disorders and the high correlation between specific clinical signs and anatomic disc

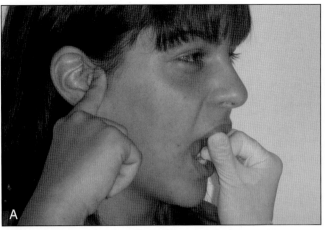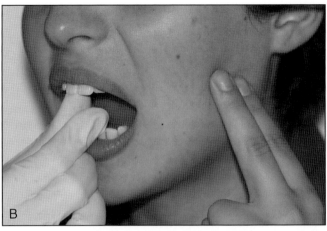

Fig. 8.1 • Forced or assisted opening. Assisted opening will often induce strong pain in the affected temporomandibular joint (A). In masticatory myofascial pain this is often localized over the masseter muscle (B). This examination also demonstrates the amount of opening that may be additionally gained by mild force; in muscle this may be substantial (5 mm or more), in disc displacement without reduction moderate (less than 4 mm) whilst in anchored disc phenomenon the limitation is 'hard' with no possibility of increase.

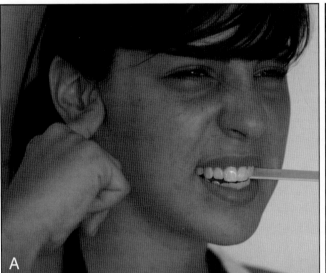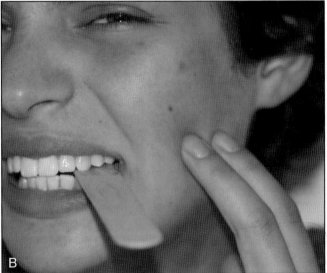

Fig. 8.2 • Loading test. In patients with painful intra-articular disorders or degeneration of the temporomandibular joints loading by clenching the teeth on a wooden stick or spatula induces pain located to the contralateral joint (A). In muscle disorders clenching usually induces ipsilateral pain over the masseter muscle (B).

derangements. The correlation was so high that arthrography is not needed today (Nitzan *et al* 1991a) and in any event has been replaced by magnetic resonance imaging (MRI). Indeed, clinical examination and the co-occurrence of certain signs may accurately predict the presence of some imaging abnormalities on MRI, such as effusion (Manfredini *et al* 2003). However, some clinical diagnoses do not always accurately predict the precise intra-articular disorder. Thus, the predictability of the clinical examination in disc displacement and TMJ osteoarthritis when compared to MRI or arthroscopy was 43–71% (Roberts *et al* 1991; Paesani *et al* 1992; Israel *et al* 1998). Following clinical assessment, imaging studies may be needed to complete the diagnostic process but careful patient selection is important.

For routine screening or evaluation, panoramic radiographs are adequate. For the basic evaluation of the TMJ, transpharyngeal and transcranial radiographs in the closed and open-mouth positions provide information on the hard tissue structures and range of movement (Brooks *et al* 1997). The decision to obtain other imaging modalities of the TMJ, such as computerized tomography (CT), MRI or bone scan should be deferred until the diagnostic process indicates a need for these. CT scanning provides the most complete three-dimensional reproduction of TMJ bone anatomy, but is not essential for diagnosis (see Fig. 8.3). CT is valuable in assessing the degree of joint degeneration or the possible presence of ankylosis, and essential mostly prior to open surgical intervention (Fig. 8.3). However, accurate information on all the soft tissue elements of the TMJ can only be obtained employing MRI. Indeed MRI may depict joint abnormalities not seen with any other imaging method and thus is the best method for making a thorough imaging assessment of the

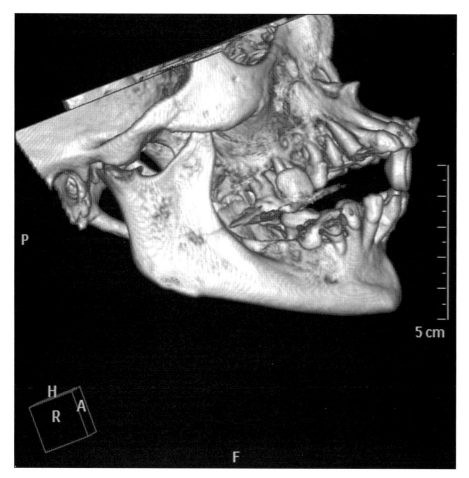

Fig. 8.3 • Three-dimensional (3D) computerized tomography. Reconstruction of images provides a 3D image that is especially useful for assessment of TMJ anatomy. In this case the right temporomandibular joint shows degenerative changes consistent with osteoarthritis and the presence of ankylosis.

TMJ, when this is indicated (Larheim 2005). When MRI is used, some disc displacements may be detected in asymptomatic individuals. Consecutive MRI images may be performed to create a dynamic representation of joint movement and this clearly shows the causes for limitation, such as anchored disc or disc displacements without reduction. Additionally, MRI is able to detect joint effusion and mandibular condyle marrow abnormalities (Takahashi *et al* 1999; Guler *et al* 2005). It is important to realize, however, that MRI as a sole modality is not sufficient for the diagnosis of TMJ pathologies and must be integrated with clinical and anamnestic findings (Emshoff *et al* 2003a; Widmalm *et al* 2006). Bone scanning (scintigraphy or radionuclide studies) offers information on the metabolic activity of bone, and can show increased activity in osteoarthritic joints, even in the absence of radiographic changes (Epstein *et al* 2002). Severe osteoarthritic joint degeneration associated with a negative bone scan indicates inactive disease, making scintigraphy an invaluable tool.

3.3. Other Special Tests

3.3.1. Joint Sounds

Diagnosis of many intra-articular disorders relies on the clinical detection and characterization of joint sounds;

different examiners may not agree on the presence and characteristics of these sounds (Dworkin *et al* 1990). Patient confirmation of digitally detected sounds improves the agreement between two independent examiners to about 90% (Goulet and Clark 1990). Techniques using vibration or sound sensors to characterize specific TMJ dysfunction conditions have been tested (Toolson and Sadowsky 1991; Ishigaki *et al* 1993). Unfortunately, these studies suffer from research design flaws that make their conclusions questionable (Baba *et al* 2001). Poor reproducibility of joint sounds can be best explained by the fact that joint sounds vary over time (Kononen *et al* 1996).

3.3.2. Laboratory Findings

Isolated TMJ disease will rarely be accompanied by changes in haematological, biochemical or autoimmune profiles. TMJ involvement in polyarthritides is, however, accompanied by a number of diagnostic and prognostic markers. Direct markers provide a measure of cellular response or changes in the affected tissues and are largely metabolic markers. One example is antigenic keratin sulphate (AgKS) found almost exclusively in articular cartilage. Tissue destruction releases these into body fluids, allowing them to be measured; in most patients with polyarticular osteoarthritis serum AgKS is high (Thonar *et al*

1985). Indirect markers have the ability to influence the metabolism of cells in the affected tissues and include proteolytic enzymes, growth factors and proinflammatory agents. Erythrocyte sedimentation rate and C-reactive protein are indirect systemic markers of inflammation. Inflammatory markers may also be assessed from synovial fluid as described in the pathophysiology section. Synovial fluid analysis is probably the most promising test in intra-articular disorders but is relatively more invasive than venipuncture.

Ultimately, the final diagnosis is based on the skilful integration and interpretation of the patient's complaint (pain, dysfunction), the history, the clinical examination and the radiographic and laboratory findings.

4. Diagnosis of TMJ Disorders

4.1. Historical Perspective

Till the late 1980s disorders of the TMJ and the muscles of mastication were pooled together under a variety of diagnostic terms such as temporomandibular dysfunction syndrome (TMPDS). However, it became clearly apparent in the 1980s that TMPDS included both muscular and joint-based problems that needed to be categorized separately (Eversole and Machado 1985). Concomitantly disc displacement was the postulated cause of joint pain, limited mandibular movement and joint sounds (Westesson and Rohlin 1984; Wilkes 1989; Milam and Schmitz 1995). Naturally at this point a variety of surgical interventions were developed to restore normal TMJ anatomy (disc displacements) and function that led to apparently successful outcomes. However, these procedures were based on limited awareness of the differential diagnosis and pathogenesis of TMJ pain and dysfunction. For example, patients with painless clicking joints but severe muscle pain underwent unwarranted surgical intervention. The result was severe joint and muscle pain accompanied by an inability to exercise the jaw, leading to further complications. Subsequently, many patients complained of recurring and severe signs and symptoms, leading to further, multiple surgical interventions. These repeated interventions sometimes resulted in such severe complications that a need and demand for joint replacements was created (Kent *et al* 1993; Dolwick and Dimitroulis 1994; Mercuri *et al* 1995). Thus, although TMJ pain and dysfunction as a clinical entity has been given much attention, efforts to explain the factor(s) underlying this phenomenon appeared only at a later stage (Haskin *et al* 1995; Zardeneta *et al* 1998).

4.2. Current Thinking

The reported results of therapeutic interventions aimed at disc displacements and data from recent research have stimulated a rethinking of the role played by disc displacement in TMJ complaints (Hall 1995). Disc displacement may be a physiological change (Scapino 1983), often diagnosed in normal individuals and not associated with joint pain (Kircos *et al* 1987a). Over one-third of joints in asymptomatic volunteers were found to have moderately or severely displaced discs (Katzberg *et al* 1996; Morrow *et al* 1996; Tallents *et al* 1996). Contralateral discs in asymptomatic joints of patients with unilateral TMJ problems were found to be displaced as often as the disc on the symptomatic side (Davant *et al* 1993). Conversely normal disc position is observed on imaging in about a quarter of clicking joints (Davant *et al* 1993). In addition, lavage of the upper joint compartment using arthroscopy (Sanders 1986; Nitzan *et al* 1990) or arthrocentesis (Nitzan *et al* 1997), neither of which change the disc position (Montgomery *et al* 1989; Moses and Poker 1989), were found to markedly improve function and alleviate pain. It has become clear that disc displacement is not always the underlying cause of clicking joints; see below. Thus, accurate diagnosis of the origin of pain and/or dysfunction is crucial prior to any treatment recommendations. Gradually, studies on the 'position of the disc' have shifted to the search for the intra-articular, bio-mechanical and biochemical events underlying joint pain and dysfunction (Nitzan and Dolwick 1991; Dolwick 1995).

5. The Temporomandibular Joint

Understanding the functional anatomy of the TMJ is essential for a thorough clinical examination, interpretation of findings and understanding the intricacies of the disorders that afflict this joint. The maintenance of a healthy and functional joint involves the interaction between its constituent tissues: bone, cartilage, synovium, capsule, disc, blood vessels and innervation. Since much of the articular cartilage is avascular, it is dependent on the synovial fluid for its nutrients, lubricating agents and metabolic homeostasis.

5.1. Anatomy and Function

The temporomandibular joint is a ginglymoarthrodial synovial joint, that is, a joint capable of hinge and sliding movements. It is encapsulated, bathed in synovial fluid, stress-bearing and capable of allowing opening, lateral and protrusive movement of the mandibular body. Condylar movements are protected from direct contact with the bony architecture of the fossa through an intricate system of fibrocartilage and synovial structures. The TMJ is unique, compared with other load-bearing joints, in anatomical, functional and genetic regulation (Luyten 1997).

There are two joint compartments separated by an inter-articular disc, and thus four articular surfaces. Joint rotation (hinge) occurs largely in the lower joint space whilst sliding (translation) occurs within the upper joint space. The articular surfaces, including the disc, are all fibrocartilage rather than chondrocartilage as in other joints.

Fibrocartilage is considered more resistant to tensile or shear forces associated with full-range mandibular movements. Articular cartilage is made up of collagen, proteoglycan and chondrocytes. A dense network of aggrecan (aggregating chondroitin sulphate proteoglycan) and collagen fibres provides the necessary biomechanical properties to cartilage (see below on loading). The TMJ is the only joint in the body with vascularized tissue within the capsular ligament. Jaw movements require active participation and perfect coordination between masticatory muscle bilaterally and both TMJs.

The articular disc is made up of dense fibrous connective tissue and divides the joint cavity into upper and lower joint spaces. The disc is shaped to match the condyle and fossa: concave inferiorly and convex superiorly. If sectioned anteroposteriorly the anterior portion (or anterior band) is thicker than its central portion (or intermediate zone). Posteriorly the articular disc is thickest (termed the posterior band). Both the posterior band and the intermediate zone thin laterally. Laterally and medially collateral ligaments attach the disc to the condylar head. It has been suggested that the disc imparts the TMJ with abilities to withstand impressive and prolonged compression, relative to joints without a disc (Tanaka *et al* 2004). It is significant, however, that patients who underwent meniscectomy presented excellent function 30 years later (Silver 1984; Eriksson and Westesson 1985; Tolvanen *et al* 1988; Takaku and Toyoda 1994).

During function the lateral and medial discal collateral ligaments, which attach the disc to the condyle, allow for rotational movement of the condyle on the inferior surface of the disc. The superior surface of the disc translates or slides along the posterior aspect of the articular eminence during full mouth opening. Limited lateral movements are also possible. During all movements of a normal TMJ the interarticular disc is always positioned between the fossa/eminence and condyle by the action of the superior lateral pterygoid muscle and the uppermost elastic properties of the posterior attachment known as the posterior, superior retrodiscal lamina of the retrodiscal tissue. Translation of the condyle occurs as a result of the action of the inferior lateral pterygoid muscle which protrudes the mandible, acting in concert with other mandibular depressors and the infra- and suprahyoid musculature. Movement of the disc is controlled during opening by the superior retrodiscal lamina which passively pulls the disc posteriorly as the condyle translates anteriorly. During closing, the superior lateral pterygoid muscle contracts eccentrically, stabilizing the disc against the distal slope of the articular eminence.

5.2. Load Distribution and Lubrication

The arrangement of the teeth, muscles and TMJ is similar to the arrangement of a class 3 lever and predicts that during clenching the TMJ is loaded by muscle activity. Experimental evidence demonstrates that forces acting on the TMJ are both compressive and tensile (Herring and Liu 2001; Sindelar and Herring 2005). The bone architecture of the condyle includes fine, vertically oriented bony trabeculae ideally suited for compressive loading. The articular eminence has thick cortices with the trabeculae oriented approximately transversely and suited for tensile and shearing forces (Herring and Liu 2001). The articular disc is also subjected to both compression and shearing (Sindelar and Herring 2005).

The normal articular surfaces are smooth and possess a high surface energy (Ghadially *et al* 1982; Bloebaum and Radley 1995; Hills 1996), thus requiring an efficient lubrication system. Indeed the smooth movements of the TMJ are possible as a result of sophisticated lubricating and shock-absorbing mechanisms. The synovial membrane, which lines the two layers of the joint capsule and the disc (except for the articulating surface), produces synovial fluid and supplies the nutritional needs of the joint (Dijkgraaf *et al* 1996). The lubricating abilities depend upon the synovial membrane and fluid, the disc and the articular cartilage. The latter are microporous, allowing permeability of the synovial fluid. The permeability and mechanical response of the joint are mutually dependent (de Bont *et al* 1985). It is important to understand that TMJ movements are responsible for the efficient generation of lubrication, blood supply, load absorption mechanism and normal mandibular growth.

The surface-active phospholipids protect the articular surfaces, and are highly effective as major boundary lubricants (Schwarz and Hills 1998; Hills 2000). The joint space is filled by the highly viscous synovial fluid (SF), containing hyaluronic acid (HA) and the glycoprotein lubricin (Swann *et al* 1981). HA is a polymer of D-glucuronic acid and D-N-acetylglucosamine, which is highly unstable and degrades under inflammatory conditions (Nitzan *et al* 2001). Lubricin is composed of ~44% protein, ~45% carbohydrates and ~11% surface-active phospholipids (Swann *et al* 1981), and is suggested to facilitate joint lubrication (Hills and Butler 1984; Schwarz and Hills 1998). Lubricin and proteolipid, which have been isolated from synovial fluid, seem to facilitate surface-active phospholipid deposition at articular surfaces (Schwarz and Hills 1998).

An electron-dense layer has been identified in the TMJ that maintains proper joint function and prevents adherence of the articular surfaces (Marchetti *et al* 1997). Osmiophilic layers with embedded vesicular structures have been demonstrated in the TMJ (Clark *et al* 1999). The dominant presence of phosphatidylcholine, a surface-active phospholipid, in rat TMJ was demonstrated in connection with hyaluronic acid and fibronectin (Rachamim *et al* 2001; Zea-Aragon *et al* 2005). Upon exposure to phospholipase A2 (PLA2) the osmiophilic droplet cluster in centrifuged SF degraded and the immunolabelling for phosphatidylcholine was clearly decreased (Zea-Aragon *et al* 2005). PLA2, part of the inflammatory process, is naturally secreted into the synovial fluid by the synoviocytes, chondrocytes and osteoblasts, and probably acts specifically on PLs. Addition of PLA2 to the SF, *in vitro*, significantly increases the measured friction (Hills and Monds 1998).

HA, although not itself a lubricant, forms a 'full fluid film' that keeps the articular surfaces apart and acts as a cushion, preventing generation of friction and thus has an indirect role in joint lubrication (Nitzan *et al* 2001). An *in vitro* study revealed that HA protects PL membranes (liposomes) from lysis by PLA2 by their mutual adherence (Nitzan *et al* 2001; Zea-Aragon *et al* 2005). The lubricating mechanism is therefore intricate and may be disturbed by disruption of any one of its elements; therapy by the specific injection of HA is thus of questionable value.

The normal subchondral bone contains (fatty) bone marrow and trabecular bone with many arterial terminal branches. Subchondral bone marrow accounts for more than 50% of the glucose, oxygen and water requirements of cartilage and is, therefore, important for cartilage metabolism (Imhof *et al* 2000). Additionally, shock absorption in synovial joints is shared by the articular cartilage and the subchondral bone; 1–3% of load forces are attenuated by cartilage while normal subchondral bone is able to attenuate about 30% of the loads (Imhof *et al* 2000). Thus, the subchondral bone has a role protecting articular cartilage from damage caused by excessive loading.

Various methods have been used to assess the amount of load generated in the TMJ. Forces of up to 17.7 kg have been recorded in Macaca monkeys and contact stress in human TMJs is similar to that in the hip and knee joints (Boyd *et al* 1990; Chen and Xu 1994). Intra-articular pressure indirectly measures load; it is negative under most conditions, and reaches high positive values in synovial joints only at the extremes of movement (Ward *et al* 1990). In weanling pigs, intra-articular pressure in the superior TMJ compartment was as high as 20 mmHg during masticatory movement (Ward *et al* 1990). In awake humans, intra-articular pressure in open mouth position is negative and becomes positive in clenched mouth position (Nitzan 1994). These fluctuating intra-articular pressures play a major role in governing joint nutrition, waste removal and condylar growth (Nitzan 1994).

5.3. Innervation

Studies have shown that the TMJ receives small diameter afferents (nociceptors), proprioceptors (including Ruffini, Pacinian), sympathetic and parasympathetic efferents (Dreessen *et al* 1990; Kido *et al* 1993, 1995, 2001; Uddman *et al* 1998; Haeuchi *et al* 1999). Surprisingly the articular proprioceptors become active only at extremes of jaw movement and it is postulated that muscle proprioceptors control routine jaw movements. Sensory innervation is largely from the mandibular branch of the trigeminal nerve via its auriculotemporal branch, although the masseteric and deep temporal branches also participate (Uddman *et al* 1998; Davidson *et al* 2003). Additionally there are fibres originating from the

upper cervical dorsal root ganglia (Uddman *et al* 1998); these may be important in patterns of pain referral. The intra-articular distribution pattern of these fibres is anatomically peripheral (i.e. present in the capsule and synovium) with the central parts of the articular disc, condylar head and fossa largely non-innervated. The periphery of the human articular disc is, however, sparsely innervated (Haeuchi *et al* 1999).

The sensation of pain requires the presence and activity of nociceptors but in normal circumstances most of the articular disc is avascular and largely non-innervated. Additionally the articular surfaces of the fossa, eminence and condyle are not innervated. Thus pain from within the joint is usually due to inflammation or injury of the capsule, the highly vascularized and innervated retrodiscal tissues or inflammation of the synovial tissues. The autonomic nervous system, particularly the sympathetic nervous system, is involved in the modulation of pain (see Chapters 2, 11).

5.3.1. Effects of Inflammation

Following inflammation clinical and experimental evidence suggests significant changes in the innervation pattern and neuronal characteristics of the TMJ. Following experimental TMJ arthritis in the rat, nerve sprouting into the central part of the articular disc has been shown to occur (Shinoda *et al* 2003). This was associated with behavioural changes, such as reduced food and water intake suggestive of pain. TMJ inflammation significantly increased numbers of heat-sensitive units and induced a lowered heat threshold (Takeuchi *et al* 2004). Mechanical thresholds also tended to be lower, suggesting that inflammation may sensitize nociceptors in the TMJ, and cause hyperalgesia and allodynia (Takeuchi *et al* 2004). There is also evidence for the establishment of central sensitization following TMJ inflammation. Expanded receptive fields, reduced thresholds to mechano stimulation and prolonged neuronal discharges have been documented following TMJ inflammation (Broton *et al* 1988; Sessle and Hu 1991; Iwata *et al* 1999; Lam *et al* 2005; Takeda *et al* 2005). The sympathetic nervous system has a significant pain-modulating capacity and this has been demonstrated in experimental arthritis of the TMJ (Rodrigues *et al* 2006).

Clinical correlates of these changes are difficult but have been documented. Inflammation of the TMJ is clinically characterized by a synovitis with increased vascularity and synovial hyperplasia usually accompanied by neuronal structures (Murakami *et al* 1991; Gynther *et al* 1994, 1998). Sensory thresholds of the skin overlying inflamed TMJs were significantly lower than in non-inflamed TMJs, indicating peripheral sensitization (Eliav *et al* 2003). These changes, and patient's pain ratings, were reversed by arthrocentesis, suggesting that inflammatory cytokines may have been responsible. Immunohistochemical analysis of articular discs from humans with disc displacements revealed more intense substance P (SP)-like reactivity than in control subjects (Yoshida *et al* 1999).

Taken together the evidence points to a dynamic response of the TMJ constituent tissues to inflammation and includes neuronal plasticity and neuroanatomical changes. Clinically this should be interpreted as indications for early, effective (but conservative) interventions in painful TMJ conditions. This may be valuable in the prevention of nerve sprouting and neuronal plasticity important in the establishment of chronic TMJ pain.

6. Pathophysiology of TMJ Disorders: General Factors

In the following section we examine the pathophysiological events associated with TMJ disorders under two major headings: intra-articular and extra-articular factors. These may be involved in various degrees in different pathologies; factors known to be specifically associated with particular diagnoses are further elaborated in individual sections.

6.1. Intra-articular Events

It is generally accepted that joint derangements involve a complex interaction between the tissues that make up the joint; these components may individually initiate disease but also interact to modify disease progression (Stegenga 2001; Martel-Pelletier *et al* 2006). There is debate regarding the initiating factor or event in joint derangements. Joint function remains normal as long as its adaptive capacity is not compromised (Boyd *et al* 1990; Stegenga *et al* 1991; Nitzan 1994; Milam and Schmitz 1995). Intrinsic and extrinsic overloading, immobilization and trauma are the major factors associated with joint derangement and disruption of its integrity (Stegenga *et al* 1991; Alexander 2004). Parafunction, such as clenching, is a good example of repetitive jaw motion associated with possibly high and unevenly distributed impact loading that may elicit marked damage to synovial joints such as the TMJ (Nitzan 1994). Overloading is capable of inducing direct and indirect cellular events, neuronal activation and the triggering of a cascade of molecular events that lead to the degradation of the joint constituents by a number of mechanisms. These events include the release of free radicals, neuropeptides, cytokines, proinflammatory agents, enzymes and growth factors (reviewed below). This leads to the establishment of conditions for joint derangement, degeneration and chronic pain. Immobilization may be caused by extra- or intra-articular factors (see 8.3). Excessive force, as in macrotrauma, leads to direct cellular and tissue damage with an additional massive release of intracellular contents. This type of injury with microbleeding may also be the source of redox active iron (Zardeneta *et al* 2000), which acts much in the same way as free radicals (see below).

6.1.1. Production of Free Radicals

Free radicals are highly unstable and reactive and will rapidly interact with surrounding molecules to initiate chemical reactions and/or induce tissue injury. Cells, such as synoviocytes, generate free radicals in response to excessive loading (Fukuoka *et al* 1993) and inflammatory cytokines (Kawai *et al* 2000). Free radicals may also be generated as a result of hypoxic-reperfusion cycles associated with overloading (Blake *et al* 1989; Merry *et al* 1991). Temporary hypoxia is a natural outcome of TMJ capillary bed compression occurring during loading (e.g. tooth clenching); re-oxygenation upon cessation of overloading may initiate a hypoxic-reperfusion cycle evoking non-enzymatic release of reactive oxygen species or ROS (i.e. superoxide and hydroxyl anions) (Blake *et al* 1989; Merry *et al* 1991). The highly reactive ROS may enter into rapid chemical reactions in various tissues or with important molecules in the synovial joint (Sheets *et al* 2006), that may lead to joint disease:

- Induction of neuropeptide release by sensory afferents (see below);
- Initiation of the formation of adhesions (Dijkgraaf *et al* 2003; Sheets *et al* 2006);
- Induction of inflammatory cytokines and activation of transcription of genes involved in the pathogenesis of joint disease (Fukuoka *et al* 1993);
- Inhibition of HA biosynthesis and initiation of its degradation, thus decreasing SF's viscosity (Merry *et al* 1991). ROS degradation of HA removes an essential protection mechanism. An *in vitro* study has shown that in the degraded form HA fails to protect continuity of the surface-active phospholipid layer (Dan *et al* 1996; Nitzan *et al* 2001). Thus, phospholipase-A2 secreted into the SF following any inflammatory event is able to extensively lyse surface-active phospholipids (Dan *et al* 1996; Nitzan *et al* 2001). This will reduce or eliminate the continuity of the boundary surfactant layer essential to the movement between articular surfaces. In the TMJ, uncovering of the articular surface is speculated to be an initiating factor in joint derangement such as disc displacement, or OA. PLA2 is also a key element in the production of fatty acid derivatives such as prostaglandins and leukotrienes; and
- Inhibition of the activity of proteolytic enzyme inhibitors by oxidation; e.g. tissue inhibitor of metalloproteases (TIMP) (Zardeneta *et al* 1998; Kanyama *et al* 2000; Shinoda and Takaku 2000), thus removing an important homeostatic mechanism.

6.1.2. Neuropeptides

Proinflammatory and nociceptive neuropeptides are released in the TMJ by nociceptive trigeminal nerve terminals found in the retrodiscal tissue and capsular ligaments. These include SP, calcitonin gene-related peptide (CGRP), neuropeptide Y (NPY) and vasoactive intestinal peptide (VIP) (Holmlund *et al* 1991; Appelgren *et al* 1995, 1998; Kopp 2001). SP and CGRP are released by sensory fibres, NPY by sympathetic fibres and VIP by parasympathetic fibres. Analysis of the synovial fluid of patients with TMJ disorders has shown elevated levels of CGRP (Sato *et al* 2004), SP (Henry and Wolford 2001), NPY and VIP (Alstergren *et al* 1995), providing further evidence that the human TMJ is innervated as described in rodent experiments (Haeuchi *et al* 1999). Neuropeptide release can be initiated by intra-articular mechanical and nociceptive stimuli as in overload; this effect is reversible by opioids. The primary effects (nociceptor activity, neurogenic inflammation) are followed by the appearance of various enzymes and cytokines that were linked by *in vitro* and *in vivo* studies to the biological activities leading to typical degenerative alterations (van der Kraan and van den Berg 2000; Pufe *et al* 2004a). It is important to appreciate that neuropeptides released by nerve terminals and the resultant neurogenic inflammation are normally essential elements of healing and repair and a disruption in this balance occurs in arthritis (Levine *et al* 2006).

6.1.3. Cytokines

Cytokines are small proteins released by cells that have specific effects on cell–cell communication or interaction, and cell behaviour. The cytokines include the interleukins (IL), lymphokines and cell signal molecules, such as tumour necrosis factor (TNF) and the interferons, which trigger inflammation. Among the cytokines reported in osteoarthritic joints are interleukin 1 (IL-1), interleukin 6 (IL-6) and TNF-α, which are associated with cartilage degradation (Rossomando *et al* 1992; Kopp 2001; Ogura *et al* 2002, 2005; Pufe *et al* 2004a). Some of these molecules are correlated with disease severity and may be used to predict therapeutic outcomes (Hamada *et al* 2006; Kaneyama *et al* 2007). Cytokines exert their effects via a number of mechanisms:

• Potent proinflammatory effects; accumulation of prostaglandins and other molecules; see below;
• IL-1 and TNF-α, which are known inducers of the synthesis and activation of metalloproteases by chondrocytes, possibly leading to increased tissue destruction;
• Stimulation of sensory nerve endings, inducing pain and the release of proinflammatory neuropeptides; and
• Generation of free radicals; see above.

6.1.4. Proinflammatory Agents

A number of molecules active in the inflammatory process (see Chapter 15) have been identified in disorders of the TMJ; some are closely related to clinical symptoms

and therapeutic response (Murakami *et al* 1998a; Alstergren and Kopp 2000; Kaneyama *et al* 2007). Significant correlations include levels of prostaglandin (PGE2) and pain on movement (Alstergren and Kopp 2000). PGE2 is involved in the pathogenesis of osteoarthritis and induces the production of cytokines, proteases and ROS.

6.1.5. Enzymes

These are released within the osteoarthritic joint by chondrocytes of the articular cartilage, by the lining cells of the synovial membrane and by the osteoblasts in subchondral bone. The enzymes are mainly metalloproteases, serine proteases, thiolproteases and aggrecanases; all are known for their collagen and proteoglycan lysis activity and have been detected in human TMJ disorders (Kanyama *et al* 2000; Yoshida *et al* 2006).

6.1.6. Bone Morphogenetic Proteins (BMP) and Growth Factors

Development of chondrocytes in articular cartilage is arrested prior to final maturation by growth factors, circumventing mineralization and apoptosis. The exact role these factors play in joint disease is unclear; they may be involved in attempts at repair (decompensation). On the other hand some growth factors have been shown to induce catabolic processes and activate proteases (Martel-Pelletier *et al* 2006). In osteoarthritic joints cartilage and osteophytes express growth factor genes, such as BMP-2 and –4, and VEGF, probably involved in allowing the cells to complete the maturation cycle (Martel-Pelletier *et al* 2006). Insulin growth factor (IGF-I), BMP-2 and transforming growth factor-β (TGF$_β$), which are related to matrix synthesis, have been identified in the synovial fluid of TMJ disorders (Gotz *et al* 2005; Matsumoto *et al* 2006). Once the exact mechanisms in osteoarthritis are elucidated, treatment of TMJ disorders will be improved (Detamore and Athanasiou 2005; Almarza and Athanasiou 2006).

6.1.7. Interactions and Progressive Damage

The continued presence of proinflammatory agents and neuropeptides will itself activate trigeminal fibres and further drive the production of neuropeptides—these interactions are schematically represented in Figure 8.4. As a result of the accumulation of free radicals, neuropeptides, cytokines and proteases there is damage to the lubrication system and the collagen structure of the cartilage, and an increased volume of proteoglycans. Damage to the lubrication system may lead to stickiness and increased friction of the disc and derangements (see below).

More rarely severe damage to the joint ensues. Cartilage swelling and softening occurs (chondromalacia) followed by the breakdown of cartilage by proteases (de Bont *et al* 1985) and release of proteoglycans into the synovial fluid (Israel *et al* 1997; Ratcliffe *et al* 1998). This

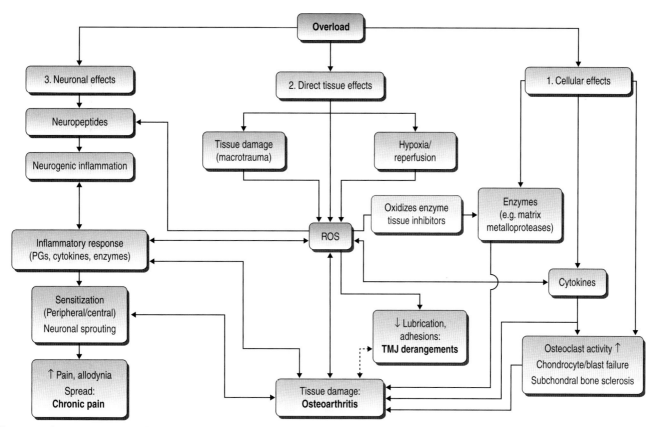

Fig. 8.4 • Schematic summary of events leading to pain and TMJ disorders (for details see text). Overload is considered to be a major factor in the initiation of articular tissue damage. It is important to appreciate that extra-articular factors, such as nutrition, atheromatous disease (hypoxia) or obesity, may predispose to joint disease; the overload may therefore be relative. Female gender is also a significant predisposing factor. Overload exerts its damaging effects via a number of mechanisms, including direct tissue, cellular and neuronal effects.

1. Cellular effects include the induction of cytokine and enzyme release from resident tissue cells. Released cytokines are proinflammatory and algesic molecules also known to induce the release of reactive oxygen species (ROS; see below). Cellular enzymes released are largely proteases that induce tissue damage. Mechanical overload also leads to increased activity of osteoclasts and chondrocyte/chondroblast failure, disturbing the TMJ's repair abilities and increasing tissue destruction.

2. Direct tissue effects are the result of damage (macrotrauma with massive tissue injury) and hypoxia reperfusion injury induced by repetitive capillary bed compression and release (e.g. clenching). Hypoxia reperfusion cycles result in the production of ROS that have multiple deleterious effects on joint function. ROS are able to induce direct tissue damage, they also induce the release of neuropeptides from afferent fibres, cytokines and enzymes from cells and the oxidation of tissue inhibitors of enzymatic proteases, thus increasing tissue destruction. The lubrication system is severely affected by ROS, leading to increased friction and the formation of adhesions. This may underlie the initiation of some TMJ derangements.

3. Neuronal effects are caused by mechanical activation of trigeminal afferents inducing peripheral release of neuropeptides and subsequent neurogenic inflammation. If unchecked, neurogenic inflammation induces an inflammatory response with classical proinflammatory agents (e.g. prostaglandins, PG) and induces the release of cytokines and tissue-damaging enzymes. Prolonged inflammation will result in neuronal changes (plasticity) including peripheral and central sensitization and neuronal sprouting into the central portion of the articular disc. These events are clinically represented as ongoing (spontaneous) pain, allodynia (pain on movement, touch) and spread of pain to adjacent structures (ear, temple, mandible).

results in weak cartilage that is unable to withstand loads and thus deforms. Signs of fibrocartilage disintegration include the appearance of vertical and horizontal splits and cartilage thinning (de Bont *et al* 1985; de Bont *et al* 1986). Moreover tissue loading results in chondroblast and chondrocyte failure and osteoclastic bone destruction, leading to impaired repair capacities and structural damage (Stegenga 2001). The role of altered bone physical properties is currently thought central to the onset of degenerative joint disease (see section 9.2.1).

Painful TMJs usually prevent the patient from performing mandibular movements. The above data stress the importance of maintaining joint movement (with minimal loading) so as to encourage elimination of damaging products and promote healing.

6.2. Extra-articular Factors

Recent evidence suggests that a number of extra-articular factors may significantly affect the initiation and progression of joint disease. These include nutrition, bone physiology, genetics and gender.

6.2.1. Nutrition

In general suppressed or abnormal synthesis related to insufficient or disturbed nutrition may manifest as degenerative disease. A direct connection between deficient nutrition and joint disorders in general (TMJ disorders included) is rare and has not been clearly established (Cimmino and Parodi 2005). However, recent research demonstrates that certain foods or nutritional supplements may offer protection from, or alleviate joint disorders (Ameye and Chee 2006). The anti-inflammatory effects of omega-3 fatty acids (see Chapter 17) are well established, and these supplements have been successfully applied in patients with rheumatoid arthritis (Goldberg and Katz 2007). There is also preliminary evidence for the beneficial effects of vitamins C and D in arthritic conditions (McAlindon 2006). Glucosamine with or without chondroitin sulphate is beneficial in arthritic conditions, but is of slow onset (Sarzi-Puttini *et al* 2005; Clegg *et al* 2006). Preliminary evidence suggests that these may be useful in TMJ disorders (Shankland 1998; Nguyen *et al* 2001; Thie *et al* 2001). Based on the above it is reasonable to predict that data demonstrating efficacy of these agents in TMJ disorders will continue to accumulate. Consequently these supplements will gradually be incorporated into the management of TMJ disorders.

6.2.2. Genetics

Genetic variations in the initiation and maintenance of chronic pain syndromes have been extensively studied (see Chapters 7, 9–11). The onset of masticatory muscle pain has been linked to variants (haplotype) of the gene encoding catecholamine-*O*-methyltransferase (COMT) (Diatchenko *et al* 2005). Mutations in genes encoding collagen have been associated with degenerative joint disease (Cimmino and Parodi 2005); however, no similar data are currently available for TMJ disorders but it seems reasonable that a genetic link will be established by future research.

6.2.3. Gender

Pain, dysfunction and clinical signs of TMJ osteoarthritis are more common in females than in males (Agerberg and Inkapool 1990; De Kanter *et al* 1993; Yap *et al* 2003). Although the reasons for this are unclear they are probably linked to the following findings:

- Recent evidence indicates that female hormones modulate the release of neuropeptides from trigeminal ganglion cells (Puri *et al* 2005).
- TMJ afferent activity following intra-articular glutamate injection (excitatory neurotransmitter) is greater in female than in male rats (Cairns *et al* 2001). Oestrogen increases the excitability of rat TMJ afferents and amplifies sensitization secondary to inflammation (Flake *et al* 2005, 2006). Experimental data suggest that testosterone may reduce TMJ damage by modifying the inflammatory response (Flake *et al* 2006).
- The central integration of pain signals originating from the TMJ region differs between male and female rats (Bereiter *et al* 2002) and varies over the oestrus cycle (Okamoto *et al* 2003). Pro-oestrus female rats

showed a higher level of central neuronal activation following TMJ inflammation than male rats (Bereiter *et al* 2002). Additionally morphine caused a greater dose-related reduction in nociceptive markers in males than in females.
- Various cell types within TMJs, including synoviocytes and neurons, express oestrogen receptors and their activation is thought to contribute to joint hypermobility, increased matrix metalloprotease activity and a decreased content of collagen and protein in the articular disc (Abubaker *et al* 1993, 1996).

Taken together the data suggest that females are more prone to tissue damage in the TMJ and that this damage expresses itself more severely. It also seems that females may be more resistant to pharmacologic treatment.

7. The Painful TMJ

Arthralgia is a term used in the RDC-TMD classification and is defined by the presence of sensitivity to pressure on the TMJ and joint pain on mandibular movements (Table 8.2): these signs usually indicate capsulitis. Many of the disorders and degenerative diseases of the TMJ are often painless. When pain is present it usually indicates an active inflammatory and/or a neuropathic process (see the section above on innervation). Because it is often difficult to accurately identify the underlying process we usually qualify our diagnoses as with or without pain. Similarly since many TMJ disorders present with or without dysfunction diagnoses should be similarly qualified. The following sections deal with individual clinical conditions: joint inflammation, derangements and joint degeneration. Within each section the clinical features are described, specific pathophysiological events highlighted and general treatment options outlined. Full descriptions of the individual treatment options can be found at the end of the chapter.

7.1. Capsulitis and Synovitis

The AAOP define capsulitis and synovitis together (Table 8.2). We will discuss these entities separately in an attempt to differentiate between the two conditions.

7.1.1. Capsulitis

Although there is little data concerning the clinical presentation of capsulitis, it is easily diagnosable. The patient complains of pain around the affected TMJ, particularly during function, and the joint is tender to pressure but not to loading. In pure capsulitis there are no joint sounds and no findings on plain radiography. However, capsulitis may accompany disc derangements.

Table 8.2 Diagnostic Criteria and Symptomatology of Capsulitis, Synovitis or Arthralgia

Parameters	AAOP[a]: Capsulitis, Synovitis[b]	RDC-TMD[c]: Arthralgia

Diagnostic signs	• Localized TMJ pain
	• Pain exacerbated by:
	  – Function
	  – Joint loading
	  – Palpation.
		• Pain on palpation of the joint on the lateral pole and/or via external auditory meatus
		• Complaint of:
		  – Pain over the joint;
		  – Pain on function; or
		  – Pain on assisted or unassisted mandibular movements
		• No coarse crepitus (see Box 8.1).

Findings or comments	• Pain may be present at rest. • Pain may cause limited range of movement. • Fluctuant swelling over affected TMJ may be found. • Ear pain may occur.	
Imaging	• A bright MRI (T2-weighted) signal may be detected if an effusion is present • No extensive osteoarthritic changes are detected.	• Not included
Authors' comments	• In our opinion synovitis is usually distinguishable from capsulitis by the presence of pain on joint loading with contralaterally applied occlusal force (load test); see text.	• Arthralgia is in our view a nonspecific term with specific criteria reminiscent of capsulitis; it has proven invaluable for research purposes. We recommend clinicians attempt to reach a clinical diagnosis that may have features of capsulitis, synovitis, etc. See text for further comments.

AAOP, American Academy of Orofacial Pain; RDC-TMD, Research Diagnostic Criteria Temporomandibular Disorders.
[a] Adapted from Okeson (1996).
[b] Clinically indistinguishable.
[c] Adapted from Dworkin and LeResche (1992).

Treatment should initially include analgesics or non-steroidal anti-inflammatory agents (NSAIDs; see Chapter 15), and physiotherapy to maintain joint mobility. Alternatively periarticular steroids have proven beneficial in our experience.

7.1.2. Synovitis

Characteristically TMJ synovitis causes spontaneous pain, local tenderness to palpation and evoked pain on mandibular movement. It is our opinion that pain on joint loading is a particular feature of synovitis not present in capsulitis. Rarely, fullness over the joint is detectable due to joint effusion, and may induce a sense of acute ipsilateral malocclusion. Joint effusion may be detectable with MRI. Synovitis may occur following external trauma to the joint (falls, blows, traffic accidents) or from joint overload such as repetitive and prolonged clenching. Treatment includes analgesics or NSAIDs, physiotherapy (with no loading) to maintain joint mobility and reduction of joint loading with an intraoral appliance (IOA; see below). In resistant cases arthrocentesis and/or intra-articular steroids have proven beneficial in our experience.

8. Derangements of the TMJ

In its broadest sense the term internal derangements of the TMJ includes all of the intra-articular disorders characterized by dysfunction based on localized anatomical faults (Stegenga 2001). Below we discuss derangements that are accompanied by significant dysfunction, including clicking joints, limited mouth opening and open lock.

8.1. The Clicking Joint

Clicking sounds from TMJs are very common and are reported in patients not seeking treatment: 8.9% in children (Keeling *et al* 1994) and 6–48% in larger population studies (Locker and Slade 1988; De Kanter *et al* 1993). Most often clicking joints are detected by the clinician in patients previously unaware they had joint sounds (Hardison and Okeson 1990), suggesting that clicking is not viewed by patients as a significant treatment-seeking symptom.

Although clicking is commonly considered the first sign of a TMJ derangement the clinical value of a clicking joint as a diagnosis is doubtful. Clicking sounds per se are of no prognostic value and are not an absolute indication for treatment; only 7% of patients with clicking joints progressed over 1–7.5 years to a bothersome problem (Randolph *et al* 1990). In a large study that followed up patients over a 20-year period, joint sounds rarely progressed to clinically significant problems (Magnusson *et al* 2000).

Persistent clicking is a condition characterized by joint sounds consistently occurring during function; usually at variable points during mandibular movement and usually asymptomatic. Clicking may not be a permanent feature of jaw movements and is referred to as intermittent clicking, a condition that is largely asymptomatic.

8.2. Persistent Click

The patient may present with clicking sounds upon mouth opening, closing or both. There is no limitation in mouth opening but when unilateral the mandible may deviate to the affected side on mouth opening. Clicking may be associated with mild to severe pain and sensitivity to palpation or on loading. These symptoms may cause limitation in function. Some patients may experience intermittent locking, where they are unable to open the jaw to their normal range, but this may be eliminated by active manipulation of the jaw. Joint noise may often be associated with, but is not caused by, muscle spasm.

Most often, persistent clicking is produced when an anteriorly displaced disc is reduced to its proper relationship with the condyle during mouth opening (Fig. 8.5). After reduction, the disc-condyle complex moves together as they slide down the posterior slope of the articular eminence, resulting in most cases in normal mouth opening. Upon closure of the mouth, the disc slips to its anteriorly displaced position and this is associated with a clicking sound during closure (Fig. 8.5). This pattern of joint clicking on opening and closing is referred to as a 'reciprocal click' and is pathognomonic of disc displacement with reduction; see below.

8.2.1. Disc Displacements

Disc displacement is defined as an abnormal anatomical relation between the condylar head and the articular disc when the teeth are in normal occlusion: in most cases the disc is anteriorly displaced. Disc displacements may be divided into two major categories: disc displacements with reduction (DDwR) and disc displacement without reduction (DDwoR) (see Fig. 8.5). Patients with DDwR or DDwoR account for about 9% of clinic patients, and may also be seen in conjunction with muscular disorders (8%) or together with osteoarthritis, joint pain and muscle disorders (12%) (Lobbezoo *et al* 2004). Disc displacements as diagnosed with the RDC-TMD criteria are relatively rare in the community—about 3%—and are more commonly seen with muscle disorders (8%) (Lobbezoo *et al* 2004).

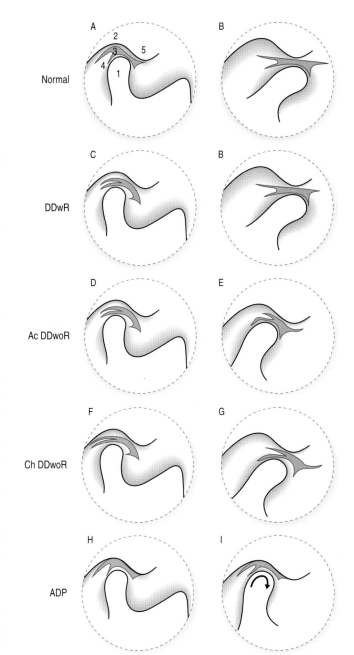

Fig. 8.5 • Schematic representation of condyle and articular disc movements in various disorders. In normal circumstances (A) the condyle (1) is located in the fossa (2) with the articular disc (3) located above and slightly anteriorly. The highly vascular and innervated retrodiscal tissues (4) do not articulate. (5) is the articular eminence. During opening (B) and closing, the disc and condyle are coordinated and move smoothly together. (C) In disc displacement with reduction (DDwR) the disc is anteriorly displaced. During opening the condyle meets the displaced disc, which causes a temporary obstacle to movement and thus deviation to the affected side. The condyle is able to reduce under the disc (opening click) and subsequently opening is undeviated and unlimited (B). On closing the condyle disc relation is again disturbed (closing click), leaving the disc displaced anteriorly. Disc displacement without reduction (DDwoR) may be (D) acute (Ac) or (F) chronic (Ch). (E) In Ac DDwoR the disc remains anteriorly displaced during opening movements, with limited mouth opening (35 mm or less). The repetitive forces during mouth opening eventually deform the disc structure and stretch the posterior attachment that has undergone adaptive changes to act as an articulating disc. Consequently mouth opening is far less limited (more than 35 mm) and may even approach normal values (G). In anchored disc phenomenon (ADP) the disc adheres to the fossa (H) and allows for rotatory movements only (I); thus mouth opening is severely limited (less than 30 mm). See text for further details.

8.2.2. Disc Displacement with Reduction (Table 8.3, Fig. 8.5)

Displacement of the articular disc is usually anteriorly or anteromedially (Prinz 1998a) but other rare displacements have been described (Westesson *et al* 1989; Huddleston Slater *et al* 2005). DDwR is characterized by a reproducible joint noise occurring during opening and closing mandibular movements (Okeson 1996). The click during opening occurs at about 20–25 mm interincisal opening; the click on closing invariably occurs at a smaller interincisal opening (15–20 mm) (Dworkin and LeResche 1992). Jaw movements on opening have a classical 'S' shape: initial deviation to the affected side and following a click returns to undeviated and unrestricted maximal opening.

Patients with DDwR are usually asymptomatic and may not even be aware of their joint sounds. TMJ sensitivity and pain may occur spontaneously or secondary to joint loading or other function. When present, pain is usually moderate but may occasionally be more severe (VAS scores of up to 7 on a 10-cm scale) (Conti *et al* 2006). When asked to protrude the jaw and then open, the click is usually eliminated (Dworkin and LeResche 1992).

8.2.2.1. Pathogenesis of Disc Displacement

Many aetiologic factors to explain the occurrence of disc displacement have been proposed. The suggestion that spasm of the superior head of the lateral pterygoid muscle is responsible for the displacement of the disc was rejected (Eriksson *et al* 1981; Mao *et al* 1992). Joint laxity might be a contributing factor but is not prevalent enough relative to the prevalence of disc displacement (Westling 1992). Trauma was thought to cause disc displacement; however, several studies have failed to confirm significant relationships between indirect trauma and disc displacement (Isacsson *et al* 1989; Katzberg *et al* 1996). For example, the prevalence of disc displacement in patients with and without history of whiplash is similar (Tasaki *et al* 1996).

Displacement of the disc seems to be caused by impairment of free articular movements caused by disruption of the lubrication system (Ogus 1981, 1987; Stegenga *et al* 1991; Nitzan 2001). It has been suggested that the lubrication system in the TMJ is relatively stable even with prolonged compression compared to other joints without disc (Tanaka *et al* 2004). Still, the adaptive capacity of the joint structures is often exceeded by prolonged overloading and the viscoelastic properties are affected, leading to increased shear stress in the disc which in turn leads to fatigue and damage. This is associated with generation of free radicals (Cai *et al* 2006) detrimental to the lubrication system (see Fig. 8.4) (Takahashi *et al* 1996; Nitzan *et al* 2002). It seems that as a result of repetitive disc hesitation the ligaments are gradually stretched (Ogus 1981). The disc adheres to the fossa, increasing disc mobility and finally inducing its displacement (Stegenga *et al* 1991; Nitzan 2001; Stegenga 2001) (Fig. 8.6). In support, TMJ arthrography in disc displacement with reduction demonstrates disfiguration of the lower compartment caused by the condyle sliding under the 'hesitating' disc and stretching the anterior wall of the capsule.

Accumulating data are driving research in the direction of the biological mechanisms of joint lubrication; thus disc mobility may be much more important than disc position (Benito *et al* 1998; Takatsuka *et al* 2005; Ohnuki *et al* 2006). Additional mechanisms potentially involved in disruption of disc mobility have been discussed earlier (see General Factors).

Table 8.3	Diagnostic Criteria and Symptomatology of Disc Displacement with Reduction (DDwR)	
Parameters	**AAOP**[a]	**RDC-TMD**[b]

Diagnostic signs	• Reproducible joint sounds on opening and closing movements of the mandible
	• Pain may be present
	  – Precipitated by joint movement
	• Deviation of mouth opening
	  – Coincides with opening click
	• Unrestricted maximal mouth opening
		• Reciprocal click on opening and closing[c]
		  – Click occurs on opening at an interincisal opening ≥5 mm than that on closing
		• May be accompanied by click on protrusion or lateral excursion[c]

Findings or comments	• Patients may report episodic and momentary impairment of jaw movement that may be resolved by mandibular movement or manipulation.	• The RDC-TMD criteria require that when DDwR is accompanied by pain a second diagnosis of joint pain or arthralgia (see Table 8.2) is made
Imaging	• Displaced disc that reduces on mouth opening • No extensive bone changes	• Not included

AAOP, American Academy of Orofacial Pain; RDC-TMD, Research Diagnostic Criteria Temporomandibular Disorders.
[a] Adapted from Okeson (1996).
[b] Adapted from Dworkin and LeResche (1992).
[c] Reproducible on two of three consecutive trials.

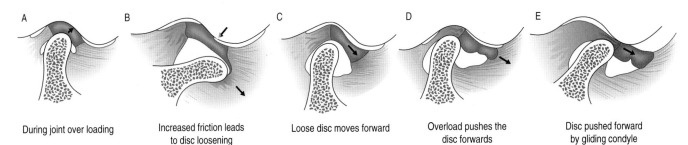

During joint over loading | Increased friction leads to disc loosening | Loose disc moves forward | Overload pushes the disc forwards | Disc pushed forward by gliding condyle

Fig. 8.6 • Pathophysiology of disc displacements. Displacement of the disc is thought to begin by the disruption of the lubrication system leading to increased friction during articular movements and subsequent tissue disruption.
In prolonged overloading the viscoelastic properties of the disc are damaged (A). Concomitant generation of free radicals disrupts the lubrication system, resulting in repetitive disc hesitation and gradual stretching of the ligaments. The disc adheres to the fossa (B), increasing disc mobility and finally inducing its displacement (C). The displaced disc is now repetitively pushed forwards, causing further displacement on clenching (E) with further displacement on opening and overloading of the posterior attachment (D); see text.

Data from Ogus (1981, 1987), Stegenga *et al* (1991), Takahashi *et al* (1996), Nitzan (2001) and Nitzan *et al* (2002).

8.2.3. Intermittent Clicking

Not all clicking joints have verifiable disc displacement and the question arises as to what causes clicking in these cases. Intermittent clicking may also be caused by disc hesitation or lagging as a result of 'stickiness' in the upper compartment following transient overloading or clenching (Prinz 1998b). The clicking noise is assumed to occur upon release of the disc or while the condyle moves against the lagging disc. Other possible mechanisms that may induce intermittent or persistent clicking include joint hypermobility (Johansson and Isberg 1991), enlargement of the lateral pole of the condyle (Griffin 1977), irregularities of the articular eminence (Pereira *et al* 1994a) and adhesions or intra-articular bodies (Bewyer 1989; Montgomery *et al* 1989).

8.2.4. Clicking Joint: Treatment Guidelines

The treatment of a clicking joint, including DDwR, is dictated primarily by the presence of pain or dysfunction. Reciprocal or intermittent click with no significant symptoms should not be treated. The majority of patients with DDwR do not progress to DDwoR (Sato *et al* 2003). Unfortunately, we currently have no means by which to predict which patients will deteriorate; see also discussion below on prognosis of disc displacements. In the presence of pain or dysfunction, therapy should begin with conservative options such as joint unloading (appliances, behavioural modification), physiotherapy and medication. This will improve pain but leaves clicking largely unaffected. When clicking is associated with severe joint pain with no response to non-surgical treatment, arthrocentesis may improve symptoms but clicking usually remains or recurs. Surgical arthroscopy, disc repositioning, condylotomy, discectomy or disc anchorage may be considered when an intolerable loud sound and/or pain resistant to conservative therapy persists. Each procedure should be enhanced by reducing joint loading and by physical therapy. Recurrence of clicking may and often occurs but is usually less annoying to the patient.

In cases where clicking is secondary to adhesions lavage of the upper compartment releases the disc and enables both the condyle and the disc to move simultaneously, preventing the clicking noise. Alternatively if clicking is caused by irregularities, anatomical changes or loose bodies an approach such as arthroscopy or surgery is recommended (Hall *et al* 2005; Smolka and Iizuka 2005; Gonzalez-Garcia *et al* 2006; Undt *et al* 2006; Dolwick 2007). Alleviation of symptoms is obtained regardless of the post-treatment disc position, which usually remains anteriorly displaced (Takatsuka *et al* 2005; Ohnuki *et al* 2006). It has therefore become evident that disc position may be relatively unimportant in TMJ disorders (Dolwick 1995).

8.3. Limited Mouth Opening

In general, the TMJ itself accounts for only a small proportion of disorders causing limitation. Most TMD disorders are muscular in origin (Lobbezoo *et al* 2004) and these account for most cases of limitation of mouth opening. TMJ disorders underlying limited mouth opening include disc displacement without reduction (Han *et al* 1999; Carvajal and Laskin 2000; Guler *et al* 2005) or closed lock (Emshoff *et al* 2000a,b; Reston and Turkelson 2003; Hamada *et al* 2006), anchored disc phenomenon (Nitzan 2003), fibrous ankylosis (McCain *et al* 1992) and osteoarthritis (Emshoff *et al* 2003b). Arthrocentesis seems efficient for these entities, other than for fibrous ankylosis (Montgomery *et al* 1989; Goudot *et al* 2000; Alpaslan and Alpaslan 2001; Guler *et al* 2005). However, it is important to realize that each of these is an independent disorder that requires an individually tailored approach based upon clear diagnostic criteria.

8.3.1. Disc Displacement without Reduction (Table 8.4, Fig. 8.5)

The basic alteration of disc position is the same as in DDwR only that in DDwoR the condyle is unable to

Table 8.4 Diagnostic Criteria and Symptomatology of Disc Displacement without Reduction (DDwoR)

Parameters	AAOP[a]: Acute	RDC-TMD[b]: With Limited Opening

Diagnostic signs	• Persistent marked limitation of mouth opening ≤35 mm
	• Deviation to the affected side on mouth opening
	• Markedly limited contralaterotrusion
		• History of limited mouth opening
		  – Unassisted opening ≤35 mm
		  – Passive stretch improves opening by ≤4 mm
		• Uncorrected deviation to the affected side on opening or contralateral excursion <7 mm
		• Absence of reciprocal click—other joint sounds allowable

Findings or comments	• Pain on forced mouth opening • History of clicking – Ceased when DDwoR began • Affected TMJ tender to palpation	• The RDC-TMD criteria require that when DDwoR is accompanied by pain a second diagnosis of arthralgia (joint pain, see Table 8.2) is made
Imaging	• Disc displaced that does not reduce on opening • No extensive osteoarthritic changes—mild to moderate changes allowable	• Not included
Authors' comments	• The current definition of acute DDwoR includes a subgroup of limited mouth opening caused by anchored disc phenomenon (ADP). The major factor that may finally differentiate is clinical response (mouth opening, pain) to arthrocentesis, which is dramatic in ADP and not so significant in DDwoR.	
Parameters	AAOP[a]: Chronic	RDC-TMD[b]: Without Limited Opening

Diagnostic signs	• History of sudden onset limited mouth opening that began >4 months ago	• History of limited mouth opening
		  – Unassisted opening >35 mm
		  – Passive stretch improves opening by ≥5 mm
		• Uncorrected deviation to the affected side on opening or contralateral excursion ≥7 mm
		• Absence of reciprocal click—other joint sounds allowable

Findings or comments	• If pain present, markedly less than in acute stage • History of clicking – Ceased when DDwoR began • Gradual resolution of mouth opening	
Imaging	• Disc displaced that does not reduce on opening • Moderate osteoarthritic changes allowable	• Evidence of non-reducing disc displacement on arthrography or MRI
Authors' comments	• The definition of limited mouth opening in our view includes an opening significantly less than the patient's original normal value	

AAOP, American Academy of Orofacial Pain; RDC-TMD, Research Diagnostic Criteria Temporomandibular Disorders; MRI, magnetic resonance imaging; TMJ, temporomandibular joint.
[a] Adapted from Okeson (1996).
[b] Adapted from Dworkin and LeResche (1992).

reduce onto the disc during opening. Accumulated data have shown that DDwoR may occur with or without clinically significant limited mouth opening (Dworkin and LeResche 1992); the AAOP refer to these as acute or chronic DDwoR, respectively, in the belief that adaptive changes that restore normal range of mouth opening in DDwoR occur over time (Okeson 1996). We define clinically significant limited mouth opening as less than 40 mm interincisal or when the patient subjectively reports

discomfort/dysfunction associated with an opening that is less than their usual maximal opening.

Early on, disc displacement without reduction is characterized by limited mouth opening (usually 25–35 mm) that usually develops gradually. A history of clicking is obligatory to make this diagnosis (Okeson 1996). Mouth opening is associated with deviation to the affected side and lateral excursion to the contralateral side is markedly limited. Assisted mouth opening is painful but usually results in an increase of about 4mm or less. The affected joint may be symptomatic, with localized pain occurring spontaneously or on jaw movements and loading. Pain over the affected TMJ is usually moderate with VAS scores of about 6, but may be more severe particularly in patients seeking treatment. Patients often complain of chewing problems and reduced masticatory efficiency (Peroz and Tai 2002). There is usually pain on palpation of the affected joint, and on loading (see Fig. 8.2). Pain is also due to stretching and overloading of the yet unadapted and highly innervated retrodiscal tissue. In the absence of problematic limitation of opening or pain, this disorder might remain unnoticed by the affected individual. Plain open-mouth or CT radiographs of the TMJ invariably demonstrate some condylar sliding, however limited. In arthrography and MRI, the disc is located in front of the condyle in both closed- and open-mouth positions.

Over time pain may be markedly reduced (VAS scores 1–2) and maximal opening may approach normal values (Choi *et al* 1994; Sato *et al* 1997, 1999). This stage is termed 'chronic DDwoR' by the AAOP (Okeson 1996) and 'DDwoR without limited opening' by the RDC-TMD (Dworkin and LeResche 1992).

8.3.1.1. Pathogenesis of Disc Displacement Without Reduction

The pathogenesis of DDwoR is thought to involve processes similar to those discussed earlier; see general pathophysiological processes (Fig. 8.4) and particular processes associated with DDwR (Fig. 8.6).

8.3.2. Prognosis of Disc Displacements

Some studies have suggested that disc displacements will naturally progress to osteoarthritis (Rasmussen 1981; de Leeuw *et al* 1994). However, osteoarthritis can afflict TMJs with or without discs (Eriksson and Westesson 1985; Takaku and Toyoda 1994; Tolvanen *et al* 1988), and may appear prior to signs of disc displacement (de Bont *et al* 1986; Pereira *et al* 1994b), suggesting that these disorders may be independent. Degenerative changes in the condyle are related to female gender, joint immobilization, increased load, atheromatous disease, increased age and a reduced dental arch length and less-to-disc position (Luder *et al* 1993; Luder 2002; Alexander 2004). Most prospective studies have shown that the vast majority of patients with symptomatic DDwoR either remain static or improve spontaneously (Lundh *et al* 1992; Sato *et al* 1997; Kurita *et al* 1998). The reduction in symptoms and restoration of function in DDwoR probably reflects adaptive intracapsular changes that include an increase in dense connective tissue, decreased vascularity and decreased innervation (Isberg and Isacsson 1986; Kurita *et al* 1989). These changes are also present in elderly individuals, irrespective of disc position, so they may be both adaptive and age-related events (Scapino 1991; Luder *et al* 1993; Pereira *et al* 1996). The end result is that the retrodiscal tissues are modified and able to act as a functional disc.

More recently disc mobility and not disc position has emerged as highly important in the prognosis of TMJ disorders (Benito *et al* 1998). This is interesting in that it links the lack of adequate joint lubrication to the development of advanced TMJ disorders.

8.3.3. Treatment of Disc Displacement Without Reduction

In early (acute) DDwoR patients with pain, conservative management may improve symptoms but mouth opening usually remains limited. Arthrocentesis will improve symptoms and marginally increase mouth opening; since arthrocentesis does not alter disc position this is to be expected. Arthrocentesis should be accompanied by conservative options such as joint unloading, appliances, behavioural modification, physiotherapy and analgesic or anti-inflammatory medication. This supportive mode of treatment encourages adaptation of the posterior attachment to act as a disc (Scapino 1991).

The decision to treat chronic DDwoR (or with no limited mouth opening) depends largely on the assessment of functional capabilities as described by the patient and the presence of pain. If treatment is offered it should include conservative options with or without arthrocentesis. Surgical options are considered for patients who remain with pain and significant dysfunction despite conservative management.

8.4. Anchored Disc Phenomenon (ADP) (Fig. 8.5, Case 8.1)

Anchored disc phenomenon is characterized by sudden severe and persistent limited mouth opening, ranging from 10 to 30mm (considerably lower than in disc displacement without reduction), with deviation towards the affected side of the mandibular midline on opening. The movement towards the contralateral side is limited and often painful. On protrusion, the mandible deviates towards the ipsilateral side. History of clicking is *not* obligatory (see DDwoR), but may be present in up to 70% of cases. There is usually no pain in the TMJ upon loading. Forced mouth opening evokes pain in the affected joint and is characterized by an inability to increase maximal opening; the limitation in ADP feels 'hard' relative to that in DDwoR. In long-lasting ADP, the clinical characteristics are less pronounced. In plain open-mouth radiographs and CT scans, the TMJ shows evidence of a non-sliding, but normally structured condyle—rotatory movements are, however, present (Nitzan *et al* 1997; Nitzan 2003; Sanroman 2004). In MRI, the disc appears stuck to the articular eminence and the condyle slides underneath it (Rao *et al* 1990; Sanroman 2004).

Case 8.1 Anchored Disc Phenomenon, 30-year-old Female Patient

Present complaint

Limited mouth opening. The patient reported that she cannot even bite a sandwich and must cut the food into small pieces. She also cannot chew on the left side due to pain.

History of present complaint

Three months prior to her referral she woke in the morning and could not open her mouth. Her dentist referred her to physiotherapy with no improvement. The patient claimed she had no joint clicking in the past.

General health

Healthy.

Patient evaluation

On the visual analogue scale (VAS, 10cm) her pain level was 7.8 when opening was forced. Pain was specifically located at her right TMJ. Dysfunction was graded 8 out of 10.

Clinical examination

Maximal mouth opening (MMO) was about 24mm with deviation to the right (see Fig. 8.7a). Upon forced passive opening pain was located in the right TMJ, but mouth opening remained unchanged. Lateral movements to the right were unrestricted but the patient felt she was unable to freely move her jaw to the left (see Fig. 8.7b). Protrusion was also restricted, with deviation to right. Upon palpation there was no TMJ pain, no masticatory muscles tenderness except for slight tenderness in her right external pterygoid. There was no clicking and pain was not generated upon right and left loading.

Imaging

Plain radiographs revealed normal anatomy. The condyle, however, demonstrated no sliding down the slope of the eminence. MRI demonstrated that at maximal opening the disc was stuck to the temporal bone and the condyle was only able to rotate under the stuck disc.

Diagnosis

The absence of a history of clicking, the sudden onset, the extremely limited mouth opening and the absolute resistance of the mandible to increase interincisal opening during active assistance suggested anchored disc phenomenon.

Treatment

Joint unloading by an interocclusal appliance followed by arthrocentesis with immediate rehabilitation of all joint movements. We now have four-year follow-up with no recurrence.

Discussion

It is important to begin by conservative therapy, such as unloading with an intraoral appliance, which may release the disc in 10% of patients. This is followed by arthrocentesis.

8.4.1. Pathogenesis of Anchored Disc Phenomenon

It has been suggested that the cause for limitation originates from a suction-cup effect, whereby the disc that clings to the articular eminence is responsible for the limitation of movement (Sanders 1986; Xu *et al* 2005). However, since the introduction of one needle into the upper joint space, which abolishes the vacuum, does not cure this limitation other adhesive forces between the disc and fossa have been suggested (Nitzan and Etsion 2002; Nitzan 2003; Sanroman 2004). Overloading of the joint is assumed to damage the normal lubrication of the joint (Fig. 8.4). Apparently, in the presence of suboptimal lubrication, adhesive forces can be generated between the pressed, denuded, smooth, elastic disc and the eminence (Nitzan and Etsion 2002; Nitzan 2003; Sanroman 2004). The disc might be in a normal or displaced position. Even a limited area of adhesion between the two opposing surfaces is capable of suddenly holding the disc from sliding down the slope of the eminence. Forced opening is not recommended, as the condyle is pulled away from the adhered disc. Such stretching of the joint's ligaments may traumatically disrupt the anatomical relationship between the condyle and the disc.

8.4.2. Treatment of ADP

Case 8.1 is a young woman with ADP that responded very well to arthrocentesis and joint unloading with good long-term stability (Fig. 8.7). Arthrocentesis neutralizes these adhesive forces, separates the flexible disc from the rigid surface of the eminence and enables smooth normal opening (Nitzan *et al* 1997; Sanroman 2004). Arthrocentesis should be enhanced by reducing joint loading and by physical therapy. The latter, which is not indicated as long as the disc is stuck, should be intensively used following disc release. In these circumstances, recurrence is rare, probably due to the awareness of the patient as well as the low likelihood that the two opposing articular surfaces will again become uncovered and adhere (Nitzan *et al* 1997).

8.5. TMJ Disorders Characterized by Inability to Close the Mouth

8.5.1. Open Lock versus TMJ Condylar Dislocation (Table 8.5)

Open lock is characterized by a sudden inability to close the mouth, and is usually released by the patient's manipulation. Mouth opening during open lock is usually less extreme than in condylar dislocation, and may range from 25 to 30mm (Nitzan 2002). In plain radiographs and CT scans, the condyle in 'open lock' is located under the eminence and not in front of it, as would be expected in condylar dislocation. MRIs show the condyle to be located in front of the lagging disc (Nitzan 2002). The cause for open lock probably involves diminished lubrication with increased friction between the disc and the eminence. The disc, which normally moves together with the condyle, lags behind it, and consequently the condyle slides under and in front of the disc and cannot return to its former position in the fossa; hence, the mouth remains open.

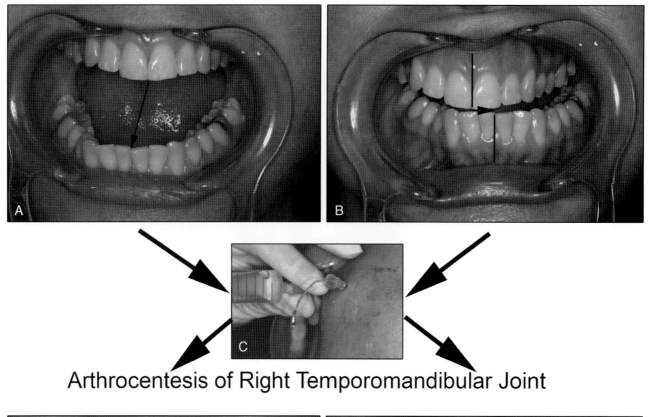

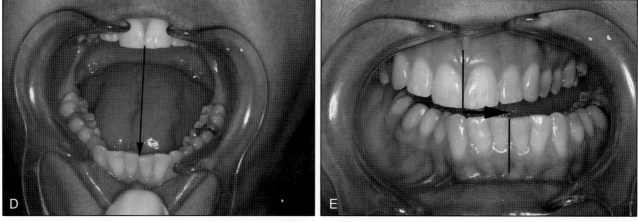

Arthrocentesis of Right Temporomandibular Joint

Fig. 8.7 • Patient with anchored disc phenomenon of the right temporomandibular joint. Prior to arthrocentesis mouth opening was limited and deviated to the affected side (A) and lateral excursion to the contralateral side was limited (B). Following superior joint space lavage (C) mouth opening improved markedly without deviation (D) and normal range of lateral excursion was regained (E). See Case 8.1.

Dislocation of the TMJ occurs when the mandibular condyle is displaced anteriorly beyond the articular eminence and the patient is unable to self-reduce the condyle. This is in contrast to subluxation, which is generally defined as a displacement of the condyle out of the glenoid fossa and anterosuperior to the articular eminence, which can be self-reduced by the patient (Shorey and Campbell 2000). There are multiple causes for dislocation that may be related to endogenous factors such as a lack of integrity of the joint ligaments or problems with the bony architecture of the joint surfaces (Shorey and Campbell 2000). Exogenous factors that may induce dislocation include trauma and imbalanced activity of the musculature acting on the joint, sometimes habitual or secondary to medications. Final diagnosis of either open lock or dislocation must be supported by imaging at the time of occurrence.

8.5.2. Treatment of Open Lock/Dislocation

For open lock non-surgical means are usually effective and if not, lavage of the upper compartment can restore sliding of the disc, allowing it and the condyle to move simultaneously. Preventing the condyle from moving in front of the disc provides relief, and with rare long-term recurrence.

For chronic dislocation injection of sclerosing solution (sodium morrhuate or sodium tetradecyl sulphate) has been suggested and induces scarring of the capsule and may prevent recurrence in some cases (Shorey and Campbell 2000). Similarly, injection of botulinum toxin to the lateral pterygoid muscle is claimed to be effective, but is by definition temporary. Surgical treatments for recurrent condylar dislocation include eminectomy (Guven 2005), capsule tightening, introduction of an obstacle

Table 8.5	Comparison between the Characteristics of Open Lock and Condylar Dislocation	

Characteristics	Open Lock	Condylar Dislocation
Age	Younger	Older
Occurrence	Spontaneous in joints with internal derangement	Maximal opening (yawning, shouting, neurogenic, neuroleptic drugs, joint laxity)
Maximal mouth opening during the event	Maximal opening with protrusion	>Maximal opening
Reduction	Difficult but self-corrected	Usually professional
Condyle location on radiographs	In front and inferior to eminence	In front and superior to eminence
Magnetic resonance imaging (open-mouth position)	Trapped condyle. Located in front of the lagging disc	Condyle located in front of the eminence
Treatment	Arthrocentesis and unloading	Surgery if recurrent

(e.g. bone) to prevent dislocation and surgical stripping of the lateral pterygoid muscle (Shorey and Campbell 2000).

9. TMJ Degeneration: Osteoarthritis (Tables 8.6, 8.7)

As in other synovial load-bearing joints the TMJ is subject to pathological overload or systemic disease that may lead to tissue breakdown, pain and dysfunction. There is some disagreement between the AAOP's and the RDC-TMD's classification of degenerative joint disease. The RDC-TMD clearly defines 'osteoarthrosis' as a noninflammatory asymptomatic disorder that causes degeneration of the TMJ structures (Table 8.7). The AAOP terms this entity 'primary osteoarthritis', probably in view of the fact that in most cases secondary synovitis develops rapidly (Israel *et al* 1998; Stegenga 2001). There are patients with clinical and radiographic signs of degenerative joint disease with minimal if any symptoms or signs; they probably represent a subacute or chronic form of osteoarthritis. The appearance of symptoms is associated with the identification of intra-articular inflammatory molecules (Holmlund *et al* 1991; Israel *et al* 1991). Accordingly we adopt the thinking that osteoarthritis is the most appropriate terminology (Stegenga 2001) and suggest that this simply be further characterized as with or without pain and/or dysfunction.

9.1. Epidemiology and Clinical Features, Case 8.2

Osteoarthritis (OA) increases with age and may be related to mechanical factors such as loss of molar support with shortening of the dental arch (Luder 2002). It is more common in women than in men, particularly after the age of 40–50. In one study about 10% of women and 5% of men aged 65 were found to have TMJ crepitation, compared to about 5 and 4%, respectively, in 35 year olds (Agerberg and Bergenholtz 1989). Radiographic evidence of OA is very common (14–50%) in asymptomatic individuals, mostly unilaterally, but only 8–16% will have clinically detectable disease (Sato *et al* 1996; Toure *et al* 2005). Both clinical and radiographic findings are found in about 5% of cases (Sato *et al* 1996; Lobbezoo *et al* 2004; Toure *et al* 2005). These figures are comparable to those found in other joints of the body (Cimmino *et al* 2005). Patients with OA or pain of the TMJ make up about 6% of clinic samples; most often these entities are seen together with muscle pain with (18%) or without (35%) disc displacements (Lobbezoo *et al* 2004).

In the acute painful phase of TMJ osteoarthritis, patients typically complain of early morning joint stiffness that lasts more than 30 minutes. This is accompanied by severe joint pain at rest, during jaw movement, difficulty in yawning, biting and chewing. Sometimes the symptoms are accompanied by a sensation of swelling in the TMJ area (Kopp 1985; Zarb and Carlsson 1999). On physical examination, there is painful limited mouth opening, lateral excursions in both directions induce pain in the affected joint (even if only one joint is affected) and attempts to protrude the jaw beyond the limits imposed by the disorder elicit considerable pain in the affected joint; see Case 8.2. Crepitation in the arthritic joint, with or without clicking, may occur during jaw movement. Palpation of the affected joint can evoke mild to severe pain. History of clicking is variable. In general, these patients do not present any distinctive description, complaining of all or some of the symptoms, with severity varying considerably from mild to severe (Zarb and Carlsson 1999). OA is not an easy diagnosis as patients often present with different combinations of signs and symptoms (Table 8.6).

Imaging of an osteoarthritic joint may show only mild changes; however, advanced stages typically show erosion of the cortical outline, loss of intra-articular space, osteophytes, marginal spurs, subcortical cysts, subchondral bone sclerosis, reduced joint space and a perforated disc, among other features (see Fig. 8.8) (Dolwick and Aufdemorte 1985; Israel *et al* 1997; Imhof *et al* 2000). Inconsistency may exist between the clinical symptoms and imaging: mild clinical disease might be associated with severe imaging appearance and vice versa. Indeed early osteoarthritis may not be detectable by radiographic imaging (Holmlund and Hellsing 1988; Brooks *et al* 1992; Brooks *et al* 1997; Zarb and Carlsson 1999) and conversely radiographic changes are present in many asymptomatic individuals (Ericson and Lundberg 1968; Holmlund and Hellsing 1988). MRI may show the presence of a joint effusion, particularly in painful joints (Takahashi *et al* 1999). Scintigraphy is useful to assess the degree of disease activity.

Table 8.6	Diagnostic Criteria and Symptomatology of Degenerative Joint Disease

Parameters	AAOP[a]: Primary Osteoarthritis[c]	RDC-TMD[b]: Osteoarthritis
Diagnostic signs	• TMJ pain on function • TMJ tenderness to palpation • No identifiable aetiology • Positive imaging findings	• Signs and symptoms of joint pain (arthralgia; see Table 8.2) • Coarse crepitus from affected TMJ (see Box 8.1), or • Positive imaging findings
Findings or comments	• Limited range of movement: – Deviation to affected side • Crepitus or multiple joint sounds	

Imaging	• Evidence of structural bony change:
	  – Subchondral sclerosis
	  – Osteophytes
	  – Erosion
	  – Joint space narrowing
		• Tomograms show:
		  – Cortical erosion, or
		  – Sclerosis, or
		  – Flattening, or
		  – Osteophytes

Authors' comments	• Osteoarthritis has an extremely variable clinical expression. It may present with no pain, minimal or no dysfunction and extensive radiographic degeneration only. Conversely there may be extreme pain and dysfunction in patients with minimal radiographic findings. These are difficult to classify with current criteria.	
Parameters	AAOP[a]: Secondary Osteoarthritis	RDC-TMD[b]: Secondary Osteoarthritis
Diagnostic signs	• As in primary • Documented disease or event associated with onset	• No clear criteria given. Dependent on rheumatologist's or other medical professional's diagnosis of polyarthritic condition.
Findings or comments	• As in primary	
Imaging	• As in primary	
Authors' comments	• See above. Secondary osteoarthritis may also occur after trauma, which is not discussed in this chapter.	

AAOP, American Academy of Orofacial Pain; RDC-TMD, Research Diagnostic Criteria Temporomandibular Disorders; TMJ, temporomandibular joint.

[a] Adapted from Okeson (1996).

[b] Adapted from Dworkin and LeResche (1992).

[c] The AAOP relates osteoarthritis as a noninflammatory condition although this is qualified by a statement that secondary synovitis is common. In contrast the RDC-TMD clearly define a noninflammatory degenerative disorder of the TMJ: osteoarthrosis; see Table 8.7.

Table 8.8 summarizes the differences between the clinical signs and symptoms, and imaging data of anchored disc phenomenon, disc displacement without reduction and osteoarthritis.

9.2. Specific Comments on the Pathogenesis of Osteoarthritis

Osteoarthritis involves the concomitant actions of inflammation, degeneration and attempts at repair. Degeneration is in essence a maladaptive response; a failure of the tissues to respond to the demands made of it. In osteoarthritis the usually well-kept balance between tissue synthesis (repair mechanisms) and breakdown (damage) is disturbed. Recent research has shown that osteoarthritis is much more complicated than previously thought

and the variable presentation is probably a result of the variety of factors linked with the disease. Awareness of these factors is essential for improving insight into the origin of the signs and symptoms and thereby the treatment approach.

As discussed earlier in the section on general pathophysiology, a number of processes may result from joint overloading (see Fig. 8.4). When overloading exceeds the joint's repair capacity a cascade of deterioration may be initiated. This may lead to disruption of the lubrication system, and wear of the articular cartilage that gradually penetrates the underlying bone (Mow and Ateshian 1997; Zarb and Carlsson 1999; Malemud *et al* 2003). Concomitantly, overloading is associated with a variety of mutilations to the subchondral bone leading to microfractures that induce subchondral bone sclerosis. When sclerosed,

Table 8.7	RDC-TMD Criteria for Osteoarthrosis of TMJ
Parameters	**RDC-TMD: Osteoarthrosis**
Diagnostic signs	• No signs and symptoms of joint pain (arthralgia; see Table 8.2) • Coarse crepitus (see Box 8.2) from affected TMJ, or • Positive imaging findings
Findings or comments	• There is no pain on function, loading or palpation

Imaging	• Tomograms show:
	  – Cortical erosion, or
	  – Sclerosis, or
	  – Flattening, or
	  – Osteophytes

Authors' comments	• As discussed in the text we opt not to use osteoarthrosis seeing as patients with osteoarthritis (OA) may be labile and frequently fluctuate between symptomatic and asymptomatic states. This probably reflects levels of inflammatory mediators within the joint and not separate diagnoses. We thus recommend the use of OA as a diagnosis with additional qualification as to the presence of pain or dysfunction as relevant; see text

RDC-TMD, Research Diagnostic Criteria Temporomandibular Disorders; TMJ, temporomandibular joint.
Adapted from Dworkin and LeResche (1992).

the subchondral bone does not provide the nutritional needs to the cartilage and does not function as an efficient shock absorber, both crucial for the integrity of the articular cartilage. It has been recently suggested that subsequent to the bony changes the cartilage is degraded and separates from the underlying bone. Other factors such as obesity and atheromatous disease may induce subchondral bone sclerosis and predispose the joint to damage.

9.2.1. Imbalance in Bone Physiology

The main radiologic features of OA are joint space narrowing and extensive remodelling of subchondral bone which is generally sclerotic. Bone changes may precede cartilage destruction and prominent alterations in subchondral bone suggest that this tissue plays a key role in the initiation of TMJ disease. Cartilage loss in knee osteoarthritis can often be predicted by the enhanced uptake of radioactive markers (scintigraphy) specifically by subchondral bone (Dieppe *et al* 1993). Moreover scintigraphic activity precedes episodes of radiographic degeneration. Bone cells, contrary to cartilage cells, are well supported by a capillary plexus. This, however, also exposes them to secondary effects of local or systemic disease that may affect local blood flow; see atheromatous disease below.

9.2.1.1. Bone Mass

It has been found that patients with OA have a significantly increased bone mass (Sinigaglia *et al* 2005). A high bone mass has been shown to play a role in the development of erosive changes in the TMJ (Flygare *et al* 1997). OA is characterized by an increase in material density in subchondral bone, constituting increased collagen matrix and abnormal mineralization (Martel-Pelletier *et al* 2006). Osteoarthritic bone of the femoral neck is significantly stiffer than that of controls (Li and Aspden 1997). On the one hand this results in relative protection from fractures but also in uncompliant subchondral bone structure that is inadequate support for the articular cartilage; shear forces are generated and cartilage damage with cleft formation and separation from bone occurs. Although the debate is ongoing (Cimmino and Parodi 2005; McDonald Blumer 2005), OA seems less common in patients with osteoporosis; possibly because osteoporosis renders the bone more flexible (Sinigaglia *et al* 2005). Cartilage separation results in the ability of cytokines, growth factors and prostaglandins produced by the subchondral bone tissue to cross through the bone–cartilage interface and damage the cartilage (Imhof *et al* 2000; Lajeunesse and Reboul 2003). In support, osteoarthritic subchondral bone has significantly increased levels of cytokines, inflammatory mediators and matrix metalloprotease activity (Mansell and Bailey 1998; Martel-Pelletier and Pelletier 2005). Recent data have shown that bone resorption pits in subchondral bone may release matrix metalloproteases derived from cells in bone marrow into the articular cartilage (Martel-Pelletier *et al* 2006).

9.2.2. Atheromatous Diseases

Atheromatous diseases are highly correlated with OA (Conaghan *et al* 2005), and compromised blood supply to the subchondral bone is a possible inducer of osteoarthritis. This provides an explanation for the occurrence of osteoarthritis in older patients with atheromatous diseases even in unloaded joints (Pufe *et al* 2004a). Hypoxia triggers the secretion of vasculo-endothelial growth factor (VEGF), which is suggested to initiate joint degradation, via subchondral bone sclerosis (Pufe *et al* 2004b; Tanaka *et al* 2005; Murata *et al* 2006). Correspondingly, when we injected VEGF intra-articularly in an animal model OA was induced (unpublished data).

9.2.3. Obesity

Obesity is a well-known risk factor for OA, thought to act via increased joint loading. However, increased OA of the hand in obese patients suggests that other, probably metabolic factors are at play (Cimmino and Parodi 2005). The hormone leptin, derived from adipocytes, may be key to this relationship. Leptin plays a major role in preventing obesity by effects at the hypothalamic level and leptin resistance is associated with obesity. Levels of leptin are increased in osteoblasts within

---

Case 8.2 TMJ Osteoarthritis, 45-year-old Man

Present complaint

Sudden severe pain in his right joint associated with severely limited mouth opening. He was unable to talk without suffering pain and eating had progressively become difficult.

History of present complaint

The patient, a lawyer in a specially demanding period, ran a normal but very intensive life until a month ago when sharp pain on the right side of the face had woken him up at night. Since then he could not bite or chew on the left side. Various medications such as analgesic nonsteroidal anti-inflammatories had been tried with no improvement. There was no history of clicking or trauma in the past. The patient reported no generalized joint pain and felt well. Recent laboratory tests (routine) revealed a normal differential blood count, liver function and electrolytes.

Medical history

Hypercholesterolaemia controlled with 20mg simvastatin daily.

Clinical evaluation

The patient evaluated his pain and dysfunction as 9 and 7.8, respectively, on a 10-cm VAS scale.

Clinical examination

Maximal mouth opening was 22mm with slight deviation to the right. Upon slight forced opening excruciating pain was generated in the right TMJ. Lateral movements to the right were unrestricted but were painful and limited to the left, both associated with severe pain in the right TMJ. Protrusion was limited with deviation to the right and severe pain on the right side. The patient had a deep overbite, a deviated dental midline (to the left) but a well-maintained dentition. Upon contralateral loading severe pain was generated in the right joint.

Imaging

A CT scan demonstrated typical degenerative changes on the right TMJ, limited movement and no widening of the intra-articular space (Fig. 8.8).

Diagnosis

The signs and symptoms are typical of osteoarthritis.

Treatment

Joint unloading and right TMJ arthrocentesis were followed by immediate improvement in mandibular movements (Fig. 8.9). Intensive physiotherapy was supported by analgesic medication.

Discussion

The purpose of the treatment is to aid the patient and provide optimal conditions for healing and restored function. This is performed by providing an IOA with anti-inflammatory medication: reduced internal and external load. These were able to control pain but only marginally improved maximal mouth opening. Arthrocentesis eliminates inflammatory products and is followed by immediate rehabilitation of movements. It is interesting that local anaesthesia applied prior to arthrocentesis eliminated pain but did not improve mouth opening. Physiotherapy is an essential component and maintains adequate function.

The severe degenerative changes demonstrated by the CT are not to be misinterpreted as contraindicating arthrocentesis: it is our experience that there is no correlation between the severity of the degeneration (by CT scan) and the results of arthrocentesis.

---

osteoarthritic subchondral bone (Martel-Pelletier *et al* 2006). Leptin exhibits, in synergy with other proinflammatory cytokines, a detrimental effect on articular cartilage cells by promoting nitric oxide synthesis (Otero *et al* 2006). A connection between obesity and TMJ has not been shown; this may be due to differential metabolic control of the TMJ relative to other joints (Luyten 1997).

9.2.4. Jaw Immobility

Immobilization is currently considered among the principal causes for joint deterioration mainly due to the absence of natural elimination of the virulent inflammatory core. Movements of the joint are necessary to induce fluctuating intra-articular pressures that function like a pump crucial for joint homeostasis.

Although most damage is associated with movement, immobilization of the joint is a dominant factor in joint deterioration. Interestingly, prolonged opening has led to osteoarthritis in mice (Fujisawa *et al* 2003), and immobilizing the joint in primates leads to marked thinning of the articular cartilage (Glineburg *et al* 1982).

Early and correct diagnosis associated with the appropriate treatment aiming to bring the joint back to normal movements is crucial. Adequate mobilization also avoids further complications such as ankylosis (see Fig. 8.3).

9.3. Treatment of Osteoarthritis

The physician's role is supportive, establishing ideal conditions for healing by unloading and enabling movement. As synovial joints are believed to be an adaptable organ our goal is to bring the symptomatic joint from an unadaptable state to an adaptable one, bearing in mind that we treat the patient and not the radiographic image. Especially in this

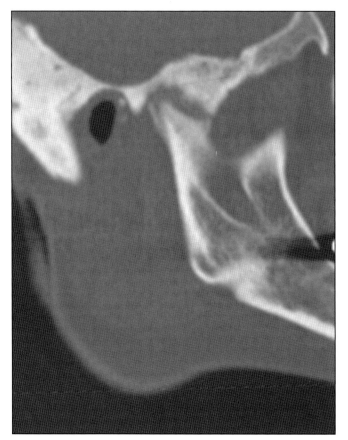

Fig. 8.8 • Section from computerized tomography showing osteoarthritis. The sagittal view shows the right temporomandibular joint. The head of the condyle is severely degenerated with flattening and osteophyte formation; see Case 8.2.

Table 8.8	Comparison between the Common Characteristics of the Anchored Disc Phenomenon, Disc Displacement without Reduction and Osteoarthritis		

Characteristics	Anchored Disc Phenomenon	Disc Displacement Without Reduction	Osteoarthritis
Occurrence	Sudden	Gradual	Sudden/gradual
Past clicks	No (30%)	Yes	No/Yes
Maximal mouth opening (mm)	15–25	30–45	10–30
Contralateral movement	Limited	Limited	Limited
Ipsilateral movement	Normal	Normal	Limited
Pain (self-assessment)	–	+	Severe to none
Dysfunction (self-assessment)	+	–	– to +++
Magnetic resonance imaging (open mouth position)	Disc stuck, located above and behind the condyle	Disc displaced-deformed, located in front of the condyle	Effusion +/– Adhesion +/– Disc displaced +/– Deformed disc +/– Perforated disc +/–
Effect of arthrocentesis	Excellent	Moderate	Very good (70%)
Occlusal changes	–	–	+ to +++

disorder, surgery should not be recommended unless non-surgical means have failed (Kopp 1985; Milam and Schmitz 1995; Nitzan 2003; Kurita *et al* 2004, 2006; Martinez Blanco *et al* 2004; Dimitroulis 2005b; Tanaka *et al* 2005). The prognosis of osteoarthritis following conservative management has been shown to be good and stable; although radiographic bone changes may show deterioration clinical signs and symptoms tend to improve (de Leeuw *et al* 1994, 1995a,b, 1996). Treatment should aim towards joint unloading, joint mobilization and pain control. Joint unloading is crucial for restoring lubrication and allowing healing. External loads may be reduced by modalities such as intraoral appliances, soft diet, and behavioural treatments. Reduction of 'internal' loading factors such as the inflammatory exudate may be attained by medication. Arthrocentesis mechanically rinses the joint and removes proinflammatory agents; this unloads, provides analgesia and releases adhesions, thus promoting joint mobility. Results are often dramatic (see Case 8.2, Figs. 8.8, 8.9).

To attain joint mobilization maximal pain control must be attained. Pain relief is rapidly achieved by pharmacological means (NSAIDs, analgesics; see below) or by joint unloading with IOA. Physiotherapy is a critical component essential for overcoming the acute stage of the disorder. Better functional performance allows for nutrition, efficient removal of waste and increased joint lubrication, thus establishing conditions that will allow healing of the TMJ constituents.

In our experience (Nitzan and Price 2001), arthrocentesis obviates the need for corrective surgery in 68.4% of patients that did not respond to other non-surgical treatment and were candidates for surgery. Following the arthrocentesis, maximal mouth opening increased from about 24 to 43 mm. Over a mean follow-up period of about 20 months (range 6–62 months), pain levels decreased substantially from VAS scores of about 7 to 2 and dysfunction levels were significantly improved. These outcomes are not perfect, but certainly suffice to obviate corrective surgery. However, in the remaining 31.6% of the cases similar symptoms were caused by joint pathologies such as bone spicules or fibrous ankylosis, which are not amenable to lavage (see Fig. 8.3). A similar rationale explains the effect of arthrocentesis in the treatment of TMJ rheumatoid arthritis and in other polyarthritides.

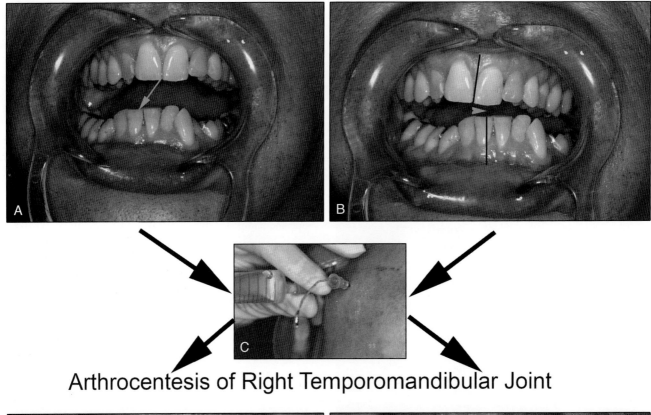

Arthrocentesis of Right Temporomandibular Joint

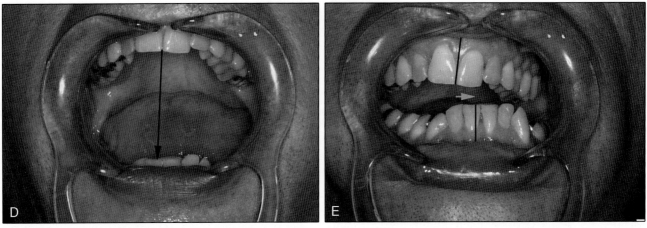

Fig. 8.9 • Patient with osteoarthritis of the right temporomandibular joint. Prior to arthrocentesis mouth opening was limited and deviated to the affected side (A) lateral excursion to the contralateral side was limited (B) and both caused severe pain. Following superior joint space lavage (C) mouth opening improved markedly without deviation (D) and normal range of lateral excursion was regained (E). See Case 8.2.

When arthrocentesis fails, surgical intervention is recommended; surgical arthroscopy, disc repair and repositioning, discectomy and, in very severe cases with marked loss of vertical dimension and malocclusion, joint replacement are required. Replacement is accomplished by autogenic bone or an artificial joint (see below).

9.4. Secondary Osteoarthritis

A number of systemic disorders may induce a degenerative process within the TMJ that is often clinically and radiologically indistinguishable from primary osteoarthritis. However, these entities are usually accompanied by symptoms associated with the systemic disease, such

as fatigue, pyrexia, anaemia and serology. In Table 8.9 we summarize salient features of systemic conditions that may induce TMJ pain and degeneration (Tegelberg and Kopp 1987, 1996; Celiker et al 1995; Yoshida et al 1998; Voog et al 2003; Helenius et al 2005, 2006).

9.5. Idiopathic Condylar Resorption (Condylysis)

Degenerative conditions of the condyle are usually primary and associated with increasing age and articular loading. Secondary osteoarthritis is related to a number of factors such as trauma or infection or due to systemic conditions that may involve the TMJ. Some cases have been reported following orthognathic surgery (Kerstens

Diagnosis	Laboratory Findings	Clinical
Table 8.9 Laboratory Findings of Osteoarthritis That May Involve the TMJ		
Rheumatoid		
Prevalence 2–2.5% Peak onset 40–60 years	Rheumatoid factor (70–80%) Antinuclear antibody (15%) Elevated ESR (90%) Mild anaemia (25%) HLA Dw5, HLA-DrW (50%)	Fatigue, weight loss, pyrexia. Bilateral joint pain (arthralgia) with crepitation. Open bite. Radiographic evidence of OA. TMJ involvement occurs in 50–75% of patients and signifies severe disease and usually not presenting symptom.
Psoriatic		
Prevalence 0.07% Peak onset 35–45 years	Seronegative. HLA-B27	Fatigue, weight loss, pyrexia, myalgia. Often unilateral pain of the TMJ. Psoriasis itself affects 1–2% of the population but arthritis is a rare complication and TMJ involvement even rarer.
Ankylosing spondylitis		
Prevalence 0.4–1.6% Peak onset 20–30 years	Seronegative. Elevated ESR (70%) HLA-B27	Joint pain, stiffness of TMJ that may result in ankylosis. TMJ involvement occurs in patients late in the disease
Reiter's syndrome		
Reactive to infection Peak onset 20–30 years	Seronegative	Fatigue, weight loss, pyrexia, lymphadenopathy. Acute unilateral joint pain.

TMJ, temporomandibular joint; OA, osteoarthritis; ESR, erythrocyte sedimentation rate.

et al 1990; Bouwman *et al* 1994) and prolonged steroid use has been associated with destructive joint disease.

However, there are cases, usually females aged 15–35 years, who present with condylar resorption with no apparent cause (Arnett *et al* 1996a,b). These have been termed idiopathic condylar resorption or condylysis (Okeson 1996); we adopt the former term. The patients complain of an anterior open bite and a variable degree of dysfunction. The presence of pain and sensitivity to pressure over the joints is inconsistent. Clinical findings also include a number of skeletal and occlusal features suggested to be involved in its pathogenesis (Wolford and Cardenas 1999). Radiography usually reveals bilateral condylar damage similar to that observed in OA, and scintigraphy is useful in assessing the current activity of bone destruction. By definition idiopathic condylar

resorption must be seronegative with no biochemical or haematological abnormalities.

The pathophysiology is poorly understood but the high predilection for females suggests that hormonal influences are important. Idiopathic condylar resorption may be a severe form of OA or be related to disturbed blood supply to subchondral bone, as observed in hip joints.

Treatment of idiopathic condylar resorption is largely empirical; it is a rare condition and there are no prospective studies. We suggest joint unloading with an IOA, the judicious use of analgesics or NSAIDs, and arthrocentesis during episodes of pain and active bone resorption. Severe facial deformity or an occlusion with significant dysfunction to the patient may indicate a need for surgery. Surgery may consist of orthognathic restoration or TMJ replacement, depending on the case. Orthognathic surgery is not associated with consistent results and usually leads to exacerbation or reinitiation of resorption (Merkx and Van Damme 1994; Huang *et al* 1997). However, good results for surgery have been described when patient selection includes evidence that disease progression is arrested, and there is adequate perioperative joint unloading (Arnett and Tamborello 1990). It is essential that candidate patients fully understand the risks.

10. Pain in the TMJ: Differential Diagnosis

Common pathologies within the joint that present with pain and/or dysfunction have been reviewed. However, the location of the TMJ in the midst of the skull with resultant referral of pain, often makes patient evaluation complex; see Chapter 1. Importantly, the differential diagnosis of pain *felt* in the TMJ, but not originating from the joint, includes a number of causes. Masticatory myofascial pain, a far more common condition, affecting the lateral and/or medial pterygoid and/or the masseter will often refer pain specifically to the TMJ (Chapter 7). Many other adjacent structures may refer pain to the TMJ area including intraoral pathology (Chapter 5), the ear (Chapter 6) and neurovascular (Chapters 9 and 10) or neuropathic syndromes (Chapter 11). In addition a variety of extra-articular systemic disorders may directly affect joint growth, anatomy and function; see Tables 8.1 and 8.9. Although rare, primary tumours (benign/malignant) may originate from TMJ structures and distant tumours may metastasize to the TMJ, presenting with joint pain or sensitivity (see also Chapter 14) (Nwoku and Koch 1974; Allias-Montmayeur *et al* 1997). Most tumours arising in the TMJ will be of bone or cartilage origin (Bavitz and Chewning 1990; Warner *et al* 2000). In any clinical evaluation careful data collection and examination are crucial for avoiding misdiagnosis; imaging is a complementary tool. Figure 8.10 is a simplified flow chart to aid clinicians in the diagnosis of painful TMJ disorders that may be accompanied by limited mouth opening and/or joint sounds.

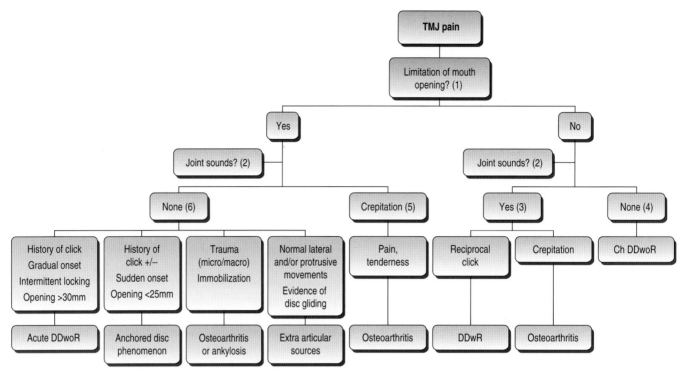

Fig. 8.10 • Flow diagram to aid in the diagnosis of painful temporomandibular joint disorders. A possible approach, as shown here (1), is to initially divide between patients with and without limitation of mouth opening (see text for definition). The presence of joint sounds (2) further subdivides these groups. In patients with no limitation in mouth opening and joint sounds (3) the quality may rapidly aid in diagnosis; crepitation is classical of osteoarthritis and reciprocal clicking of disc displacement with reduction (DDwR). No limitation of mouth opening in the absence of joint sounds (4) may be due to long-standing or chronic disc displacement without reduction (ChDDwoR). Limited mouth opening with crepitation is often present in active osteoarthritis (5); see also Case 8.2. The absence of joint sounds accompanied by limited mouth opening and a symptomatic TMJ is often difficult to diagnose (6). A history of clicking joints with a gradual onset of 'locking' or limitation of opening that is around 30 mm suggests acute disc displacement without reduction (AcDDwoR). In contrast an acute onset of limited mouth opening of less than 25 mm in a young patient with no history of clicks suggests anchored disc phenomenon (ADP). A history of clicks in the past does not exclude ADP. Macrotrauma, TMJ surgery or long-standing osteoarthritis that has been inadequately managed suggests that ankylosis is present (see Fig. 8.3). Extra-articular causes of limitation of mouth opening commonly include muscle disorders. Rare causes such as coronoid hyperplasia and tumours should be kept in mind (not shown).

11. Treatment of TMJ Disorders

Since the aetiology of TMJ disorders is considered multi-factorial, numerous forms of ostensibly targeted therapies have been designed. Modalities include mechanistic approaches such as orthotic or occlusal therapies, and biopsychosocial approaches that integrate behavioural therapies into the standard medical model of disease. Interestingly many of these interventions, alone or in combination, have an equally positive impact in reducing or eliminating patients' symptoms. Studies clearly show no superiority of any one treatment for patients with TMJ disorders; successful treatment outcomes typically follow a multimodal and often multidisciplinary approach.

Treatment of TMJ problems may be compared to the treatment of any other skeletal disorder. The ultimate goals are to decrease pain and increase function. Indeed, TMJ pain and/or dysfunction are the clearest indicators that treatment should be offered. Dysfunction includes limited mandibular range of motion and reduced functionality. However, it is important to clearly state the treatment objectives to the patient; elimination or alleviation of

pain and dysfunction may not always be accompanied by eradication of joint sounds. It is important to stress to the patient that long-term follow-up of clicking joints shows no significant deterioration in the vast majority of patients (Randolph *et al* 1990) and no advantage of surgical over non-surgical techniques in controlling deterioration (Greene and Laskin 1988). A conservative approach is therefore successful for most patients.

On the rare occasions when a patient complains of a disturbing joint sound even in the absence of pain or dysfunction surgical treatment may be offered; see below.

11.1. Non-surgical Options

Non-surgical treatment of painful, dysfunctional TMJs commonly relies on the use of patient education and awareness techniques, joint unloading by functional modification or appliances, physical therapy or manipulation (Jagger 1991; Nicolakis *et al* 2001), bite appliances (Ekberg 1998; Ekberg *et al* 1998; Ekberg and Nilner 2002), medications (Ekberg 1998) and cognitive behavioural therapy. Other less common modalities include warming (Dahlstrom 1992), soft laser (Fikackova *et al* 2006) and complementary or alternative medicine (Ernst and White 1999; DeBar *et al* 2003; see Chapter 17), but their efficacy is unclear. Because most patients with painful TMJs have a good prognosis the aim of treatment is palliative and supportive. Even in patients with DDwoR the use of a conservative approach is effective (Murakami *et al* 2002) and is in no way inferior to surgical intervention in controlling signs and symptoms (Schiffman *et al* 2007). However, patients with a history of a persistently limited mouth opening (<30mm) have been shown to be relatively resistant to non-surgical intervention (Iwase *et al* 2005).

11.1.1. Joint Unloading: Functional Behavioural Modification

In some patients clenching or other parafunctional habits (protrusion) may be associated with TMJ pain; behavioural modification to stop these will alleviate symptoms. In most cases of pain an initial period of rest and a soft diet is also useful. Rest, which is beneficial for any symptomatic synovial joint, is not totally relevant for the TMJ since it is involved in essentially daily functions such as eating, swallowing and speech. Moreover sleep parafunction is a major source of TMJ overloading and is not controllable by the patient, so appliances are indicated. The use of appliances is described below and more extensively in Chapter 7.

Enrolling the patient to actively participate in the treatment with the aim to identify and reduce potentially damaging parafunction is essential. This approach may be enhanced with the use of biofeedback and stress management (see Chapters 4 and 7).

11.1.2. Physical Therapy

Joint mobilization is essential to maintain its long-term function and mobility. Exercises can be taught by the treating physician but in difficult cases or when cooperation is not achieved it is essential to refer the patient to a professional physiotherapist. Exercises that we prescribe include passive and active symmetric movements in all directions (Nicolakis *et al* 2001); upon maximal movement further stretching exercises are recommended to increase range of motion. Exercises combined with anti-inflammatory drugs are an effective strategy (Yuasa and Kurita 2001). Careful follow-up and meticulous recording of the extent of motion is essential. In addition the patient should be actively involved in goal setting and follow-up.

11.1.3. Bite Appliances (see also Chapter 7)

In the short term parafunctional habits may be controlled with appliances or drugs and thus reduce joint loading, but habits tend to recur when appliances are removed or following long-term use (Solberg *et al* 1975; Sheikholeslam *et al* 1986; Rugh and Harlan 1988).

There is evidence to suggest that the use of stabilization is beneficial for reducing pain severity in patients with painful joint disorders, at rest and on palpation, when compared to no treatment (Ekberg 1998; Ekberg *et al* 2002; Forssell and Kalso 2004). Repositioning appliances have been advocated to treat internal derangements and to 'recapture' the disc. However, in the long term, clicks or abnormal disc positions tend to recur (Lundh *et al* 1985; Tallents *et al* 1990) and these appliances fail to recapture the disc in ID without reduction (Eberhard *et al* 2002). Indeed repositioning appliances have no significant benefit over stabilization appliances in the treatment of TMJ sounds (Tecco *et al* 2004) and may induce irreversible occlusal changes. Recent data suggest that flat centric splints will relieve clinical symptoms more efficiently than repositioning splints in patients with DDwoR (Schmitter *et al* 2005). In a randomized clinical trial, a group of patients with painful DDwR were treated with three types of bite plates; flat occlusal, canine-guided and non-occluding (Conti *et al* 2006). After six months all patients with occluding splints had significant improvement in pain with no difference between the type of guidance (Conti *et al* 2006). Interestingly the frequency of joint noises decreased over time, with no significant differences among the three groups. This effect has also been observed in non-treatment groups included in a similar study, suggesting natural fluctuation in the expression of clicks (Conti *et al* 2005).

Reduction of TMJ loading may be obtained by constructing an appliance with occlusal contacts in the posterior region only (Nitzan 1994). This type of interocclusal appliance reduces the pressure generated in the joint during active clenching by 81.2% (Nitzan 1994). The use of techniques to off-load the TMJ is not unlike the effect of different bandaging techniques as an adjunct to orthopaedic management.

It is imperative that patients are informed that intraoral appliances are a temporary means of management; long-term use is associated with uncontrolled changes in occlusion.

11.1.4. Medications

Most cases with TMJ pain will improve with the use of mild analgesics and NSAIDs. NSAIDs, both topically and systemically, have been shown to be effective in TMJ disorders (Ekberg 1998; Thie *et al* 2001; Di Rienzo Businco *et al* 2004). There are data suggesting that the nonspecific NSAIDs, such as naproxen, may be more effective than specific cyclooxygenase (COX)-2 inhibitors in the management of TMJ pain (Ta and Dionne 2004). Since naproxen has a better cardiovascular safety profile than COX-2 inhibitors, this would suggest their preferential use; see Chapter 15. In severe cases, the combination of initial steroid therapy followed by an NSAID was as effective as surgical or other management of DDwoR (Schiffman *et al* 2007).

In the absence of extensive and specific research on drug use in inflammatory TMJ disorders (List *et al* 2003) results of experimental models or of clinical trials of other joints affected by osteoarthritis may be extrapolated. For example, both acetaminophen and COX-2 inhibitors were able to reverse the behavioural effects of experimental TMJ inflammation in rats (Ahn *et al* 2005). Celecoxib (200–400mg/d) was compared to acetaminophen (slow release formulation 3990 mg/d) in patients with osteoarthritis in various sites (Yelland *et al* 2007). Paracetamol was found to be as effective as celecoxib by most patients (Yelland *et al* 2007). A systematic review on the treatment of osteoarthritis of the knee or hip concluded that acetaminophen in doses of about 4 g daily is clinically effective and superior to placebo (Towheed *et al* 2006). However, NSAIDs (e.g. ibuprofen 1200mg/d, diclofenac 75–150mg/d, celecoxib 200mg/d) improve pain, function and stiffness more than acetaminophen, especially in moderate to severe cases. Patients taking traditional NSAIDs were more likely to have adverse gastrointestinal effects but otherwise there was no major difference in side effects relative to acetaminophen. This would suggest that NSAIDs should also be employed in TMJ osteoarthritis; however, most of the studies were only about 6 weeks long (Towheed *et al* 2006). For long-term management the efficacy of NSAIDs must be countered with severe side effects on the gastrointestinal, renal and cardiovascular systems—factors that may favour the use of acetaminophen. Renal and cardiovascular risks are particularly relevant for the specific COX-2 inhibitors that also involve increased cost. Systemic side effects may be minimized by the use of topical application of diclofenac (see Chapter 16).

Taken together the data suggest that for short-term management of TMJ pain and osteoarthritis NSAIDs (naproxen, ibuprofen) are most likely to be effective, with minimal side effects. It is important to emphasize that renal and cardiovascular risks are increased within one month of NSAID use (see Chapter 15), so we suggest titrating clinical response and transferring patients at the earliest opportunity to other analgesics. Particularly in patients with medical comorbidity (cardiovascular, renal) acetaminophen is the drug of choice, although in patients with gastrointestinal problems NSAIDs may be used in conjunction with a proton pump inhibitor (consult the managing physician). For long-term management, the use of mild analgesics, such as acetaminophen, is effective for patients with TMJ pain and certainly safer. The advantages of mild analgesics over NSAIDs are discussed in Chapter 15. Rarely stronger analgesics such as mild opioids may be needed for short-term therapy in severe cases, or postoperatively. All the above medications, drug dosages, schedules and side effect profiles are extensively reviewed in Chapter 15. More recent data suggest that drugs specifically acting on cytokines may be clinically useful (Kopp *et al* 2005). Infliximab, an anti-TNF-α agent, was given systemically to patients with TMJ pain who reported significantly reduced pain levels (Kopp *et al* 2005).

When comorbid muscle pain is present the use of adjuvant analgesics is beneficial. These drugs include muscle relaxants (cyclobenzaprine), antidepressants (e.g.

amitriptyline) and anticonvulsants (gabapentin, clonazepam) and are reviewed in Chapter 16. The analgesic effects of antidepressants may account for their use in patients with articular disorders (Plesh *et al* 2000; Rizzatti-Barbosa *et al* 2003; Johansson Cahlin *et al* 2006). Based on two pilot studies, chondroitin sulfate or glucosamine hydrochloride are effective in TMJ pain (Nguyen *et al* 2001; Thie *et al* 2001); see also Chapter 17.

11.2. TMJ Surgery

Surgery of the temporomandibular joint plays a small but important role in the management of patients with TMJ disorders. The literature has shown that about 5% of patients with TMJ disorders require surgical intervention and a spectrum of invasive procedures, from simple arthrocentesis to more complex open joint surgical procedures, is available. Each surgical procedure should have strict criteria for which cases are most appropriate. However, each procedure has its enthusiastic supporters, and specific criteria for the most appropriate intervention in each diagnosis are lacking. Thus the literature is based more on observation than scientifically controlled studies. Recognizing that scientifically proven criteria are lacking we will discuss the criteria for each procedure, ranging from arthrocentesis to complex open joint surgery. The discussion will include indications, brief descriptions of techniques, outcomes and complications for each procedure.

11.2.1. Indications

Indications for surgery of the temporomandibular joint may be divided into relative and absolute (Dimitroulis 2005a,b). Absolute indications are reserved for those where surgery has an undisputed role such as tumours, growth anomalies and ankylosis of the TMJ.

Surgical intervention of the dysfunctional or painful joint must be based upon clearly defined criteria, such as:

1. Pain and/or dysfunction of such a magnitude as to constitute a disability to the patient;
2. Failure of non-surgical therapy to resolve the problem;
3. Documentation of TMJ intracapsular pathologic condition or anatomic derangement that is a major source of the patient's pain and/or dysfunction; and
4. Amenability of the condition to surgical intervention.

While the indications for surgery may appear clear, they are in fact, nonspecific. The first criterion, significant TMJ pain and dysfunction, may be the most important. What distinguishes the surgical candidate from the group of non-surgical patients is localization of the pain and dysfunction to the TMJ. The more localized the pain and dysfunction are to the TMJ, the better the prognosis for a successful surgical outcome. Conversely, the more diffuse the pain and dysfunction, the less likely surgical intervention will succeed. The decision for surgical intervention should be made based on clinical findings in conjunction with the impact of the pain and dysfunction on the well being of the patient, balanced against the prognosis if surgery is not performed. Surgical candidates should have localized, continuous TMJ pain that is moderate to severe, and becomes worse during mandibular function, i.e. talking or chewing. They may present limited movements with or without pain or other signs of dysfunction such as painful clicking, crepitation or locking of the TMJ.

The second criterion, refractory to non-surgical treatment, is also nonspecific. Temporomandibular disorders encompass a wide variety of aetiologies and complaints, and therefore, there is no clear consensus on a protocol for conservative or non-surgical treatment. None the less, most clinicians understand what non-surgical or conservative therapy involves. It typically includes a combination of patient education, medication, physical therapy, an occlusal appliance and possibly counselling or behavioural therapy. Most patients will respond successfully to this treatment, while others may see a reduction in symptoms over time, even in the absence of treatment. Therefore a surgical consideration should be reserved only for patients who fail to respond successfully over a reasonable period of time. It must also be stressed that not all patients who fail non-surgical treatment are surgical candidates. Surgical treatment must be limited to those who respond to the first criterion of pain and dysfunction arising from within the TMJ. Patients who have pain and dysfunction arising from the masticatory muscles or other non-TMJ sources are not surgical candidates and may be made worse by surgical intervention.

The third criterion, imaging evidence of disease, appears to be the most objective; however, imaging should not be interpreted in isolation. The correlation of disc derangement, dysfunction, and degeneration found on imaging with pain is poor (Kircos *et al* 1987b; Kozeniauskas and Ralph 1988). Therefore imaging should be used only to confirm and support the clinical findings. Surgery cannot be performed on the basis of imaging alone.

Surgical interventions include arthrocentesis, arthroscopy, condylotomy and open joint procedures such as disc repositioning and discectomy. Randomized clinical trials comparing these procedures do not exist, so the surgical procedure selected is based mostly on the surgeon's experience. Each procedure does have specific benefits as well as risks. Therefore, the procedure which has the highest potential for success with the lowest risks and most cost effectiveness should be chosen for the patient's specific problem.

Based on our experience arthrocentesis and arthroscopic lavage and lysis should be used for TMJ pain during function, intermittent clicking or limited opening (Kendell and Frost 1996). Condylotomy works best for TMJ pain with little or no restriction of opening and open TMJ surgery should be reserved for advanced cases of internal derangement and osteoarthrosis.

11.2.2. TMJ Arthrocentesis

In our view, arthrocentesis is probably the first surgical procedure that should be employed in patients with TMJ pain and dysfunction that have not responded to conservative therapy.

Studies on the effect of arthrocentesis on DDwoR have shown consistently improved mouth opening and decreased pain (Han *et al* 1999; Carvajal and Laskin 2000; Emshoff *et al* 2003b; Yura and Totsuka 2005). Our clinical experience suggests that range of jaw movements in DDwoR only improve marginally following arthrocentesis: interincisal opening may increase from about 32 to 36mm, and lateral excursions from 8 to 8.5mm. Pain and dysfunction levels are improved but response is unpredictable. These findings are expected as arthrocentesis and arthroscopic lavage are incapable of changing the disc's shape or position (Montgomery *et al* 1989; Moses and Poker 1989). The marked improvement described in the literature is probably in a group of patients that were not strictly defined and may include other disorders.

In a group of patients with disc displacements resistant to conservative therapy arthrocentesis was not significantly different to arthroscopy for decreasing patient reports of pain and increasing functional mobility of the mandible (Fridrich *et al* 1996). Since arthrocentesis is a simple outpatient procedure performed under local anaesthetic and is relatively safer than arthroscopy, it should be tried first.

11.2.2.1. Technique
Murakami et al (1987) were the first to offer a systematic description of TMJ arthrocentesis, which they termed 'manipulation technique followed by pumping and hydraulic pressure'. Arthrocentesis of the TMJ, as we present here, is a modification of the traditional method, and in which two needles instead of one are introduced into the upper joint space. This adaptation permits massive lavage of the joint, in addition to aspiration and injection (Nitzan et al 1991b).

The patient is seated inclined at a 45° angle, with the head turned to the unaffected side to provide an easy approach to the affected joint. After proper preparation of the target site, the external auditory meatus is blocked with cotton soaked in mineral oil. The points of needle insertion are marked on the skin, as follows. A line is drawn from the middle of the tragus to the outer canthus. The posterior entrance point is located along the canthotragal line, 10mm from the middle of the tragus and 2mm below the line (Fig. 8.11). The anterior point of entry is placed 10mm farther along the line and 8–10mm below it. These markings over the skin indicate the location of the articular fossa and the eminence of the TMJ. It is important that these points are used as guides; the precise location needs to be confirmed by careful examination of the patient's anatomy.

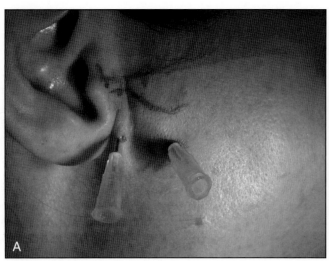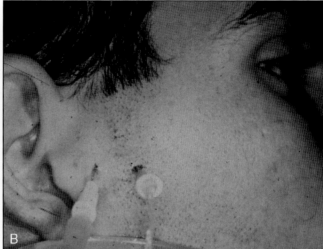

Fig. 8.11 • Arthrocentesis. Two needles are placed in the anterior and posterior recesses of the upper joint space (A). Irrigation is then performed (B) as described in the text.

Stages in arthrocentesis.

1. A local anaesthetic is injected at the planned entrance points, avoiding penetration into the joint and injection into the synovial fluid.
2. If samples of synovial fluid are needed for research or diagnostic assessment the procedure is continued by injecting 1 mL of lactated Ringer's solution into the superior compartment at the posterior point, and immediately aspirated. This procedure is repeated three times to obtain a sufficient amount of fluid for diagnostic and research purposes.
3. If the procedure is purely for therapeutic purposes stage 2 is omitted. Surface anaesthesia from stage 1 is then followed by injection of 2–3 mL bupivacaine 0.5% to distend the upper joint space and anaesthetize the adjacent tissues through the posterior point using a syringe with a 19-gauge needle. A second 19-gauge needle is then inserted into the distended compartment in the area of the articular eminence (anterior point of entry) to enable free flow of Ringer's solution through the superior compartment (Fig. 8.11). Slight adjustment of the needle position may be necessary. In cases of sluggish outflow, additional needles may be inserted into the distended compartment to enhance the transport of the solution. Zardeneta et al (1997) recommend a free flow of 100 mL of Ringer's solution, because denatured haemoglobin and various proteinases were recovered in this fraction. Later studies suggested that 300–400 mL should be used for the washout of bradykinin, IL-6 and proteins (Kaneyama et al 2004). A simplified procedure is one in which the second needle is inserted next to the first one, into the posterior rather than the anterior recess, and saline is then flushed through the upper compartment. During the lavage, the mandible is moved through opening, excursive and protrusive movements to facilitate lysis of adhesions (Segami et al 1990).

11.2.2.2. Mode of Action

By forcing apart the flexible disc from the fossa and by washing away degraded particles and inflammatory components arthrocentesis re-establishes joint movements and reduces both load and pain, which is the hallmark of joint health. Upon termination of the procedure and following the removal of one needle, medication can be injected into the joint space. Hyaluronic acid is an example of such a supplement of arthrocentesis (Alpaslan et al 2000; Xinmin and Jian 2005), the effectiveness of which is still debated (Shi et al 2003). The potency of hyaluronic acid will be minimal if inflammatory products in the affected joint are allowed to degrade it, but with the removal of the inflammatory products by arthrocentesis the hyaluronic acid remains intact and is probably more effective.

Reports on the elimination of products from the diseased TMJ by arthrocentesis suggest that this may be a major mode of action; see the earlier section on pathophysiology. Arthrocentesis is also an important diagnostic tool. Adhesions or osteophytes are not always unambiguously diagnosed by available imaging techniques as the causes of limitation or pain. Failure of lavage implies that surgical means may be required and are legitimate in order to release the joint and restore movement. Indeed, arthrocentesis is a prerequisite for most TMJ surgical intervention.

11.2.2.3. Complications

One should be aware that temporary facial weakness or paralysis, as a result of the use of a local anaesthetic, and/or swelling of the neighbouring tissues caused by perfusion of Ringer's solution might occur during arthrocentesis. Both signs are transient and disappear within hours. Numerous other complications as a result of arthrocentesis, including extradural haematoma, have been described. Correct diagnosis, appropriate treatment approach and careful surgical technique should prevent complications.

11.2.3. TMJ Arthroscopy

TMJ arthroscopy is a minimally invasive procedure but is, however, usually performed under general anaesthesia in the operating room. It is very much an equipment-dependent procedure that requires considerable manual dexterity on the part of the surgeon. TMJ arthroscopy now plays a major role in the surgical management of TMJ internal derangement and osteoarthrosis.

11.2.3.1. Technique

TMJ arthroscopy involves the placement of an arthroscopic telescope (1.8–2.6 mm in diameter) into the upper joint space (UJS) of the TMJ, and a camera is attached to the arthroscope in order to project the image onto a television monitor. The surgeon must conceptualize a three-dimensional space on a two-dimensional image. A second access instrument is placed approximately 10–15 mm in front of the arthroscope. This access point provides an outflow portal for irrigation and access for instrumentation of the joint space. The examination is started posteriorly by identifying the posterior attachment tissue. The synovial lining is inspected for the presence of inflammation such as increased capillary hyperaemia. The junction of the posterior band of the disc and posterior attachment tissues can be identified. Movement of the joint allows for the identification of clicking or restriction in movement of the disc. As the arthroscope is moved through the UJS the articular cartilage is inspected for the presence of degenerative changes such as softness, fibrillation or tears. The joint space is also inspected for the presence of adhesions, loose bodies or other pathology. The integrity of the disc or perforations of the disc or posterior attachment tissues can be identified. Although the lower joint space (LJS) is not usually examined, the presence of a perforation in the disc or posterior attachment may allow limited examination of the LJS and condyle. Although sophisticated operative techniques ranging from ablation of adhesions with lasers to plication of the disc have been developed, most surgeons limit the use of arthroscopy to lysis of adhesions and lavage of the UJS. Lysis of adhesions is accomplished most often by sweeping either the arthroscope or the irrigation cannula through the adhesions and tearing them. After completion of the examination the joint space is thoroughly irrigated to remove debris and small blood clots. The patient is usually discharged the same day after recovering from the anaesthesia. Postoperative care includes a non-chew soft diet for a few days, range of motion exercises continued for several days, an intraoral appliance and analgesics as necessary for pain control.

Multiple studies report 80–90% success rate with arthroscopic lysis and lavage for the management of patients with painful limited mouth opening (McCain et al 1992; Murakami et al 1998b, 2000; Reston and Turkelson 2003; Hall et al 2005; Smolka and Iizuka 2005; Schiffman et al 2007). The majority of patients have decreased pain and improved mouth opening. Murakami et al (1998b, 2000) have shown in studies with 5- and 10-year follow-up that arthroscopic lysis and lavage is successful for all stages of internal derangement, and that results are comparable to those obtained with open surgery procedures. Data from surgical arthroscopic techniques such as disc repositioning are difficult to interpret and it is unclear whether the outcomes are better than those obtained with simple lysis and lavage.

11.2.3.2. Mode of Action

Basically arthroscopy is a sophisticated method for lavage and lysis of adhesions in the TMJ (see above section on arthrocentesis). It offers the additional benefits of allowing the use of rotatory instruments, lasers and other microsurgical implements to modify anatomy, cauterize tissues, repair the disc and remove loose bodies.

11.2.3.3. Complications

The advantages of TMJ arthroscopy are that it is minimally invasive and causes less surgical trauma to the joint. Surgical complications are rare and mostly limited to reversible effects, some similar to those observed in arthrocentesis (Gonzalez-Garcia et al 2006). Patient recovery is rapid and healing time is shorter than with open surgical procedures. The disadvantages include the surgical limitations, the necessity for sophisticated equipment and a high level of training.

11.2.4. Modified Condylotomy

The modified TMJ condylotomy is the only TMJ surgical procedure that does not invade the joint structures. It is a modification of the transoral vertical ramus osteotomy used in orthognathic surgery. Although some authors recommend modified condylotomy as the surgical treatment of choice for all stages of TMJ internal derangement it seems to be most successful when used to treat painful TMJ internal derangement without reduced mouth opening (Hall et al 1993).

11.2.4.1. Mode of Action

The objective of the procedure is to surgically increase the joint space between the condyle and the fossa, thus allowing repositioning of the condyle anteriorly and inferiorly beneath the displaced disc.

Hall et al (1993) reported good pain relief in about 90% of 400 patients treated over a 9-year period with modified condylotomies. In follow-up studies 94% success in patients with disc displacement with reduction has been reported. Interestingly 72% of these patients had a normal disc position when evaluated with follow-up MRIs (Hall et al 2000a). This would suggest that the procedure is able to provide optimal conditions for the restoration of normal disc–condyle relationship. However, in a group of patients with disc displacement without reduction the success rate for modified condylotomy was slightly less at 88% (Hall et al 2000a).

11.2.4.2. Technique

The modified condylotomy is performed under general anaesthesia usually as an outpatient procedure but may require overnight stay in the hospital. An incision is made intraorally along the anterior border of the mandibular ramus. After exposure of the lateral aspect of the mandibular ramus a vertical cut is made posteriorly to the lingula from the coronoid notch to the mandibular angle. After mobilization of the condylar segment the medial pterygoid muscle is stripped from the segment. The mandible is then immobilized using maxillomandibular fixation (MMF). Although the surgery is simple, there is a period of postoperative rehabilitation involving 2–3 weeks of MMF followed by training elastics so that the occlusion is maintained.

11.2.4.3. Complications

The most significant potential complication of the modified condylotomy is excessive condylar sag, resulting in malocclusion. In one series of cases there was only a 4% complication rate which consisted primarily of minor occlusal discrepancies (Hall *et al* 2000b). Despite the simplicity of the procedure and its high success rate the procedure has not become widely used. The reasons for this are unclear but are most likely related to the necessity for MMF and the fear of excessive condylar sag resulting in an unstable condylar position with malocclusion.

11.2.5. Open Joint Surgery (Arthrotomy)

Open joint surgery is indicated for those patients with TMJ internal derangement and osteoarthritis who have failed to respond to simpler surgical procedures or have failed previous open surgery. In cases with previous surgery the surgeon must be very hesitant to perform repeated surgery because the success rate for this is very low; in fact after two surgeries, it may approach zero. The surgeon must be certain that the source of the pain and/or dysfunction is arising from within the joint. Severe mechanical interference such as loud, hard clicking or intermittent locking associated with loud, hard clicking is an indication to perform open surgery without first performing simpler procedures because experience indicates that simpler procedures are rarely successful in these cases.

Although the use of open joint surgery has decreased significantly it still has a small but important role in the surgical management of TMJ disorders. While other surgical procedures provide a limited range of options open TMJ surgery provides the surgeon with an unlimited scope of procedures ranging from simple debridement of the joint to removal of the disc. Disc repositioning procedures are less commonly performed today compared to the 1980s and 1990s, because most patients with discs that can be preserved are successfully treated with simpler procedures. Advanced cases of internal derangement which have degenerative discs and severe arthritic changes may require partial discectomy. Arthroplasty in the form of bone contouring of the articular eminence or condyle is

sometimes necessary, particularly with disc repositioning procedures.

Open joint surgery is performed under general anaesthesia in the hospital, and usually requires a one- to two-day stay. The most common surgical approach is via a preauricular incision. Incorporating the tragus of the ear into the incision line is often used for cosmetic purposes. Exposure of the capsule is carefully performed in order to protect the temporal branches of the facial nerve. After exposure of the capsule the UJS is entered, and it is inspected for the presence of adhesions. The contour and integrity of the fossa and eminence are evaluated and lastly the disc is visualized. Evaluation of the disc includes its colour, position, mobility, shape and integrity.

11.2.5.1. Disc Repositioning

If the disc is intact and can be repositioned without tension then disc repositioning can be performed by removing excess tissue from the posterior attachment tissues, repositioning the disc and stabilizing it with sutures. Bone recontouring of the glenoid fossa and/or articular eminence is generally performed, especially in cases of gross mechanical interference or advanced degenerative joint disease. The goal of disc repositioning surgery is the elimination of mechanical interferences to smooth joint function. After completion of the intra-articular procedures, the UJS is irrigated and the soft tissues are closed.

Exercises to improve range of motion are started immediately after the surgery. Continuation of postoperative conservative treatment is very important in order to assure a successful outcome. A soft non-chew diet is recommended for six weeks after the surgery.

The literature indicates that disc repositioning surgery is successful in 80–95% of cases; however, experience indicates that this may be an overestimate (Marciani and Ziegler 1983; Hall 1984; Piper 1989; Dolwick and Nitzan 1990, 1994). It has been found that while disc repositioning surgery significantly reduced pain and dysfunction in 51 subjects evaluated up to six years postoperatively, improvement in disc position was not maintained over the follow-up period for most patients (Montgomery *et al* 1992). Despite these findings the preservation of a healthy, freely mobile disc is justified.

11.2.5.2. Discectomy

A diseased or deformed disc that interferes with smooth function of the joint and cannot be repositioned should be removed. Only that portion of the disc which is diseased and deformed needs to be removed. The synovial tissues should be preserved as much as possible. After removal of the disc only minimal bone recontouring should be performed as exposure of bone marrow may result in heterotopic bone formation. Limitation caused by the heterotopic bone can be prevented by intensive physiotherapy. In order to minimize the risk of heterotopic bone formation the placement of an interpositional fat graft into the joint space is recommended. After completion of the intra-articular procedures, the joint space is irrigated and the soft tissues are closed.

The postoperative findings are the same after discectomy as described for disc repositioning. The postoperative recommendations are also the same except that a soft non-chew diet is recommended for six months.

Discectomy of the TMJ has the longest follow-up studies of any procedure for management of TMJ internal derangement. There are four studies with at least 30 years follow-up that report excellent reduction in pain and improvement in function in most patients (Silver 1984; Eriksson and Westesson 1985; Tolvanen *et al* 1988; Takaku and Toyoda 1994). Postoperative imaging studies of discectomy patients generally show significant changes in condylar morphology (Eriksson and Westesson 1985). These changes are thought to be adaptive changes and not degenerative. Despite the excellent long-term success associated with TMJ discectomy surgeons seem reluctant to perform this procedure.

Immediately after the surgery the patient may experience swelling in front of the ear and a slight change in occlusion and limited mouth opening, which usually resolves in about two weeks. All patients experience some numbness in front of the ear, which resolves in about six weeks. Patients normally have moderate discomfort, which lasts one to two weeks. The most significant complication associated with open surgery is facial nerve injury. While total facial nerve paralysis is possible, it is rare. Inability to raise the eyebrow is the most commonly observed finding and occurs in about 5% of cases, but usually resolves within three months. It is permanent in fewer than 1% of cases. Other complications are limited opening and minor occlusal changes. The complications associated with discectomy are similar to those associated with disc repositioning. The growth of heterotopic bone is more common after discectomy than other TMJ surgical procedures. This can be a significant complication which can result in complete ankylosis of the joint. The frequency of occurrence of heterotopic bone formation is unclear.

11.2.5.3. TMJ Replacement

A complete discussion of total TMJ replacement is beyond the scope of this chapter. The discussion will be limited to alloplastic total joint replacement in adult patients who have advanced degenerative joint disease, ankylosis or complications of previously preformed open surgery. The use of alloplastic materials to reconstruct or replace the diseased tissues of the TMJ caused disastrous results in the 1980s and 1990s. The use of Proplast-Teflon and Silastic implants caused significant foreign body reactions with severe destruction of the TMJ structures (Dolwick and Aufdemorte 1985; Heffez *et al* 1987; Westesson *et al* 1987; Kaplan *et al* 1988). This experience has led some surgeons to reject the use of alloplastic TMJ prostheses in favour of autologous tissues such as costochondral grafts for TMJ reconstruction (MacIntosh 2000). While there are advantages to using autologous tissues, recently developed alloplastic TMJ prostheses

provide safe and predictably successful reconstruction of the TMJ (Mercuri 2000; Quinn 2000).

Two basic prosthetic joints will be discussed: a patient-fitted prosthesis and stock prosthesis. A patient-fitted prosthesis is a custom-made implant which has been used for over 10 years (Mercuri 2000). The prosthesis consists of a glenoid fossa implant which has an articular surface made of high molecular weight polyethylene attached to a pure titanium mesh. The body of the condylar prosthesis is made of medical grade titanium alloy with a cobalt chromium molybdenum condylar head. The process for making the prosthesis requires that a head CT be obtained from which an acrylic model of the patient's skull can be made. The planned surgery is performed on the model. The prosthesis is designed on the model and sent to the surgeon for approval. After approval the patient's prosthesis is made using CAD CAM technology.

In contrast a stock prosthesis consists of a prefabricated implant available in various sizes: small, medium, and large for the fossa, and three lengths (45, 50 and 55 mm) for the condyle. The prosthesis includes a glenoid fossa component made of high molecular weight polyethylene and a condylar component made of cobalt chromium molybdenum alloy. The articular surface is the same on all three implants and only the flange varies in size.

The surgical placement is essentially the same for both implants. The surgery requires preauricular and retromandibular incisions for access to the TMJ and mandibular ramus. A gap arthroplasty is performed by removing either the diseased condyle or ankylosed bone. Generally a coronoidectomy is also performed. After the teeth are placed into maxillomandibular fixation the implants are fitted and secured using titanium screws. Stock implants are more difficult to place than the patient-fitted implants because the bony structures must be reshaped to fit the implants. The MMF is released, the occlusion is verified and the range of motion determined. If these are acceptable the wounds are irrigated, a fat graft is placed around the condyle and the soft tissues are closed.

The criteria used to determine success in complex, chronic TMJ pain patients are somewhat relative and as such precise success rates are difficult to determine. Successful outcome generally means that the patient has reduced pain levels, increased range of motion, improved function and an absence of surgical complications. Using these criteria the success rates are high for both prostheses.

Patients who have had multiple TMJ surgical procedures and who suffer from chronic pain generally experience about 50% pain reduction and gain 10–15 mm of mandibular opening. It should be emphasized that total TMJ replacement is not necessarily a solution to the management of chronic TMJ pain. The TMJ prosthesis can be used to predictably restore occlusion and increase range of motion but pain relief is variable. On the other hand, both TMJ prostheses predictably provide pain-free restoration of occlusion and range of motion for patients who have TMJ reconstruction for ankylosis, tumours or other conditions where pain is not an original component of the condition. This may suggest that the presence of pre-existing pain is a negative prognostic factor and may be related to plastic changes of the nervous system in persistent pain states (see Chapters 2 and 11).

The most significant complication following TMJ reconstruction with alloplastic implants is facial nerve injury. While uncommon it does occur more frequently than following routine open joint surgery, especially in patients with previous, multiple TMJ surgeries. The formation of heterotopic bone is a common complication, occurring in as many as 20% of the cases. Other complications such as infection, foreign body and allergic reactions, malocclusion and implant failure can occur but are rare. Complications requiring implant removal are unusual.

Unquestionably the patient-fitted prosthesis provides the best TMJ reconstruction. The surgery is easier to perform and the implants fit more accurately than a stock prosthesis. However, there is a need for both types of implants. Patient-fitted implants require 1–3 months to manufacture so immediate TMJ reconstruction is not possible. They are also more expensive than stock prosthesis. In addition, there are several situations in which two surgeries are necessary in order to use a patient-fitted prosthesis:

1. Patients who require significant mandibular repositioning to correct large malocclusions;
2. Patients with extensive bony ankylosis requiring large amounts of bone removal;
3. Patients with foreign bodies such as previously placed alloplastic TMJ prostheses that must be removed before an accurate CT can be obtained; and
4. Combination of 1 and 2.

When two surgeries are required it can be problematic to maintain the occlusion and function after the first surgery during the time the prosthesis is being constructed. Additionally two surgeries are inconvenient for the patient, prolong healing time, expose the patient to greater risks of complications and are more expensive. Stock joints can provide adequate reconstruction with a single operation in these situations. Conversely there are situations where a stock prosthesis cannot be used. These occur in patients who have extensive bone loss at either the lateral aspect of the fossa and articular eminence or the mandibular ramus, resulting in inadequate bone for placement of a stock prosthesis. There is great flexibility in the design of patient-fitted prosthesis which allows them to be adapted to a variety of complex clinical situations. The surgeon must be familiar with both types of prostheses so as to successfully meet the needs of the variety of TMJ patient conditions requiring TMJ replacement.

12. Conclusions

Complex referral patterns in the head and neck makes accurate diagnosis of TMJ-related pain difficult. Additionally diagnostic criteria are often not adhered to, leading to misdiagnosis of muscle-related pain as a TMJ disorder.

Most painful disorders of the TMJ may be successfully treated by conservative means. Surgical techniques include minimally invasive options such as arthrocentesis and arthroscopy, which have been shown to be highly effective in many patients resistant to conservative management. Relative indications for open surgical intervention include failed conservative therapy, and structural abnormalities causing pain and dysfunction. Open surgery allows for the most flexible treatment options but carries the greatest morbidity. However, open surgery is absolutely indicated for some TMJ disorders, mainly tumours and ankylosis. In a minority of cases prosthetic replacement of the TMJ may be needed and custom or stock options are available. It is essential that practitioners be familiar with all surgical techniques so as to be able to discuss options with the oral and maxillofacial surgeon involved. This will result in more optimal management of orofacial pain patients.

References

Abubaker AO, Raslan WF, Sotereanos GC (1993) Estrogen and progesterone receptors in temporomandibular joint discs of symptomatic and asymptomatic persons: a preliminary study. *J Oral Maxillofac Surg* **51**(10):1096–1100.

Abubaker AO, Hebda PC, Gunsolley JN (1996) Effects of sex hormones on protein and collagen content of the temporomandibular joint disc of the rat. *J Oral Maxillofac Surg* **54**(6):721–727; discussion 727–728.

Agerberg G, Bergenholtz A (1989) Craniomandibular disorders in adult populations of West Bothnia, Sweden. *Acta Odontol Scand* **47**(3):129–140.

Agerberg G, Inkapool I (1990) Craniomandibular disorders in an urban Swedish population. *J Craniomandib Disord* **4**(3): 154–164.

Ahn DK, Chae JM, Choi HS, *et al* (2005) Central cyclooxygenase inhibitors reduced IL-1beta-induced hyperalgesia in temporomandibular joint of freely moving rats. Pain **117**(1–2): 204–213.

Alexander CJ (2004) Idiopathic osteoarthritis: time to change paradigms? *Skeletal Radiol* **33**(6):321–324.

Allias-Montmayeur F, Durroux R, Dodart L, *et al* (1997) Tumours and pseudotumorous lesions of the temporomandibular joint: a diagnostic challenge. *J Laryngol Otol* **111**(8):776–781.

Almarza AJ, Athanasiou KA (2006) Evaluation of three growth factors in combinations of two for temporomandibular joint disc tissue engineering. *Arch Oral Biol* **51**(3):215–221.

Alpaslan C, Bilgihan A, Alpaslan GH, *et al* (2000) Effect of arthrocentesis and sodium hyaluronate injection on nitrite, nitrate, and thiobarbituric acid-reactive substance levels in the synovial fluid. *Oral Surg Oral Med Oral Pathol Oral Radiol Endod* **89**(6):686–690.

Alpaslan GH, Alpaslan C (2001) Efficacy of temporomandibular joint arthrocentesis with and without injection of sodium hyaluronate in treatment of internal derangements. *J Oral Maxillofac Surg* **59**(6):613–618; discussion 618–619.

Alstergren P, Kopp S (2000) Prostaglandin E2 in temporomandibular joint synovial fluid and its relation to pain and inflammatory disorders. *J Oral Maxillofac Surg* **58**(2): 180–186; discussion 186–188.

Alstergren P, Appelgren A, Appelgren B, *et al* (1995) Co-variation of neuropeptide Y, calcitonin gene-related peptide, substance P and neurokinin A in joint fluid from patients with temporomandibular joint arthritis. *Arch Oral Biol* **40**(2):127–135.

Ameye LG, Chee WS (2006) Osteoarthritis and nutrition. From nutraceuticals to functional foods: a systematic review of the scientific evidence. *Arthritis Res Ther* **8**(4):R127.

Appelgren A, Appelgren B, Kopp S, *et al* (1995) Neuropeptides in the arthritic TMJ and symptoms and signs from the stomatognathic system with special consideration to rheumatoid arthritis. *J Orofac Pain* **9**(3):215–225.

Appelgren A, Appelgren B, Kopp S, *et al* (1998) Substance P-associated increase of intra-articular temperature and pain threshold in the arthritic TMJ. *J Orofac Pain* **12**(2):101–107.

Arnett GW, Tamborello JA (1990) Progressive Class II development: female idiopathic condylar resorption. *Oral Maxillofac Clin North Am* **2**:699–716.

Arnett GW, Milam SB, Gottesman L (1996a) Progressive mandibular retrusion-idiopathic condylar resorption. Part II. *Am J Orthod Dentofacial Orthop* **110**(2):117–127.

Arnett GW, Milam SB, Gottesman L (1996b) Progressive mandibular retrusion–idiopathic condylar resorption. Part I. *Am J Orthod Dentofacial Orthop* **110**(1):8–15.

Baba K, Tsukiyama Y, Yamazaki M, *et al* (2001) . A review of temporomandibular disorder diagnostic techniques. *J Prosthet Dent* **86**(2):184–194.

Bavitz JB, Chewning LC (1990) Malignant disease as temporomandibular joint dysfunction: review of the literature and report of case. *J Am Dent Assoc* **120**(2):163–166.

Benito C, Casares G, Benito C (1998) TMJ static disk: correlation between clinical findings and pseudodynamic magnetic resonance images. *Cranio* **16**(4):242–251.

Bereiter DA, Shen S, Benetti AP (2002) Sex differences in amino acid release from rostral trigeminal subnucleus caudalis after acute injury to the TMJ region. *Pain* **98**(1-2):89–99.

Bewyer DC (1989) Biomechanical and physiologic processes leading to internal derangement with adhesion. *J Craniomandib Disord* **3**(1):44–49.

Blake DR, Merry P, Unsworth J, *et al* (1989) Hypoxic-reperfusion injury in the inflamed human joint. *Lancet* **1**(8633):289–293.

Bloebaum RD, Radley KM (1995) Three-dimensional surface analysis of young adult human articular cartilage. *J Anat* **187**(Pt 2):293–301.

Bouwman JP, Kerstens HC, Tuinzing DB (1994) Condylar resorption in orthognathic surgery. The role of intermaxillary fixation. *Oral Surg Oral Med Oral Pathol* **78**(2):138–141.

Boyd RL, Gibbs CH, Mahan PE, *et al* (1990) Temporomandibular joint forces measured at the condyle of Macaca arctoides. *Am J Orthod Dentofacial Orthop* **97**(6):472–479.

Brooks SL, Westesson PL, Eriksson L, *et al* (1992) Prevalence of osseous changes in the temporomandibular joint of asymptomatic persons without internal derangement. *Oral Surg Oral Med Oral Pathol* **73**(1):118–122.

Brooks SL, Brand JW, Gibbs SJ, *et al* (1997) Imaging of the temporomandibular joint: a position paper of the American Academy of Oral and Maxillofacial Radiology. *Oral Surg Oral Med Oral Pathol Oral Radiol Endod* **83**(5):609–618.

Broton JG, Hu JW, Sessle BJ (1988) Effects of temporomandibular joint stimulation on nociceptive and nonnociceptive neurons of the cat's trigeminal subnucleus caudalis (medullary dorsal horn). *J Neurophysiol* **59**(5):1575–1589.

Cai HX, Luo JM, Long X, *et al* (2006) Free-radical oxidation and superoxide dismutase activity in synovial fluid of patients with temporomandibular disorders. *J Orofac Pain* **20**(1):53–58.

Cairns BE, Sessle BJ, Hu JW (2001) Characteristics of glutamate-evoked temporomandibular joint afferent activity in the rat. *J Neurophysiol* **85**(6):2446–2454.

Carvajal WA, Laskin DM (2000) Long-term evaluation of arthrocentesis for the treatment of internal derangements of the temporomandibular joint. *J Oral Maxillofac Surg* **58**(8):852–855; discussion 856–857.

Celic R, Jerolimov V, Knezovic Zlataric D, *et al* (2003) Measurement of mandibular movements in patients with temporomandibular disorders and in asymptomatic subjects. *Coll Antropol* **27**(Suppl 2):43–49.

Celiker R, Gokce-Kutsal Y, Eryilmaz M (1995) Temporomandibular joint involvement in rheumatoid arthritis. Relationship with disease activity. *Scand J Rheumatol* **24**(1): 22–25.

Chen J, Xu L (1994) A finite element analysis of the human temporomandibular joint. *J Biomech Eng* **116**(4):401–407.

Choi BH, Yoo JH, Lee WY (1994) Comparison of magnetic resonance imaging before and after nonsurgical treatment of closed lock. *Oral Surg Oral Med Oral Pathol* **78**(3):301–305.

Cimmino MA, Parodi M (2005) Risk factors for osteoarthritis. *Semin Arthritis Rheum* **34**(6 Suppl 2):29–34.

Cimmino MA, Sarzi-Puttini P, Scarpa R, *et al* (2005) Clinical presentation of osteoarthritis in general practice: determinants of pain in Italian patients in the AMICA study. *Semin Arthritis Rheum* **35**(1 Suppl 1):17–23.

Clark JM, Norman AG, Kaab MJ, *et al* (1999) The surface contour of articular cartilage in an intact, loaded joint. *J Anat* **195** (Pt 1):45–56.

Clegg DO, Reda DJ, Harris CL, *et al* (2006) Glucosamine, chondroitin sulfate, and the two in combination for painful knee osteoarthritis. *N Engl J Med* **354**(8):795–808.

Conaghan PG, Vanharanta H, Dieppe PA (2005) Is progressive osteoarthritis an atheromatous vascular disease? *Ann Rheum Dis* **64**(11):1539–1541.

Conti PCR, Miranda JES, Conti ACCF, *et al* (2005) Partial time use of anterior repositioning splints in the management of TMJ pain and dysfunction: a one-year controlled study. *J Appl Oral Sci* **13**(4):345–350.

Conti PC, dos Santos CN, Kogawa EM, *et al* (2006) The treatment of painful temporomandibular joint clicking with oral splints: a randomized clinical trial. *J Am Dent Assoc* **137**(8):1108–1114.

Dahlstrom L (1992) Conservative treatment methods in craniomandibular disorder. *Swed Dent J* **16**(6):217–230.

Dan P, Nitzan DW, Dagan A, *et al* (1996) H_2O_2 renders cells accessible to lysis by exogenous phospholipase A2: a novel mechanism for cell damage in inflammatory processes. *FEBS Lett* **383**(1-2):75–78.

Davant TSt, Greene CS, Perry HT, *et al* (1993) A quantitative computer-assisted analysis of disc displacement in patients with internal derangement using sagittal view magnetic resonance imaging. *J Oral Maxillofac Surg* **51**(9):974–979; discussion 979–981.

Davidson JA, Metzinger SE, Tufaro AP, *et al* (2003) Clinical implications of the innervation of the temporomandibular joint. *J Craniofac Surg* **14**(2): 235–239.

DeBar LL, Vuckovic N, Schneider J, *et al* (2003) Use of complementary and alternative medicine for temporomandibular disorders. *J Orofac Pain* **17**(3):224–236.

de Bont LG, Liem RS, Boering G (1985) Ultrastructure of the articular cartilage of the mandibular condyle: aging and degeneration. *Oral Surg Oral Med Oral Pathol* **60**(6):631–641.

de Bont LG, Boering G, Liem RS, *et al* (1986) Osteoarthritis and internal derangement of the temporomandibular joint: a light microscopic study. *J Oral Maxillofac Surg* **44**(8):634–643.

De Kanter RJ, Truin GJ, Burgersdijk RC, *et al* (1993) Prevalence in the Dutch adult population and a meta-analysis of signs and symptoms of temporomandibular disorder. *J Dent Res* **72** (11):1509–1518.

de Leeuw R, Boering G, Stegenga B, *et al* (1994) Clinical signs of TMJ osteoarthrosis and internal derangement 30 years after nonsurgical treatment. *J Orofac Pain* **8**(1):18–24.

de Leeuw R, Boering G, Stegenga B, *et al* (1995a) Symptoms of temporomandibular joint osteoarthrosis and internal derangement 30 years after non-surgical treatment. *Cranio* **13**(2):81–88.

de Leeuw R, Boering G, Stegenga B, *et al* (1995b) Radiographic signs of temporomandibular joint osteoarthrosis and internal derangement 30 years after nonsurgical treatment. *Oral Surg Oral Med Oral Pathol Oral Radiol Endod* **79**(3):382–392.

de Leeuw R, Boering G, van der Kuijl B, *et al* (1996) Hard and soft tissue imaging of the temporomandibular joint 30 years after diagnosis of osteoarthrosis and internal derangement. *J Oral Maxillofac Surg* **54**(11):1270–1280; discussion 1280–1281.

Detamore MS, Athanasiou KA (2005) Evaluation of three growth factors for TMJ disc tissue engineering. *Ann Biomed Eng* **33**(3):383–390.

Diatchenko L, Slade GD, Nackley AG, *et al* (2005) Genetic basis for individual variations in pain perception and the development of a chronic pain condition. *Hum Mol Genet* **14**(1):135–143.

Dieppe P, Cushnaghan J, Young P, *et al* (1993) Prediction of the progression of joint space narrowing in osteoarthritis of the knee by bone scintigraphy. *Ann Rheum Dis* **52**(8):557–563.

Dijkgraaf LC, de Bont LG, Boering G, *et al* (1996) Structure of the normal synovial membrane of the temporomandibular joint: a review of the literature. *J Oral Maxillofac Surg* **54**(3):332–338.

Dijkgraaf LC, Zardeneta G, Cordewener FW, *et al* (2003) Crosslinking of fibrinogen and fibronectin by free radicals: a possible initial step in adhesion formation in osteoarthritis of the temporomandibular joint. *J Oral Maxillofac Surg* **61**(1):101–111.

Dimitroulis G (2005a) The role of surgery in the management of disorders of the temporomandibular joint: a critical review of the literature. Part 1. *Int J Oral Maxillofac Surg* **34**(2):107–113.

Dimitroulis G (2005b) The role of surgery in the management of disorders of the temporomandibular joint: a critical review of the literature. Part 2. *Int J Oral Maxillofac Surg* **34**(3):231–237.

Di Rienzo Businco L, Di Rienzo Businco A, D'Emilia M, *et al* (2004) Topical versus systemic diclofenac in the treatment of temporo-mandibular joint dysfunction symptoms. *Acta Otorhinolaryngol Ital* **24**(5):279–283.

Dolwick MF (1995) Intra-articular disc displacement. Part I: Its questionable role in temporomandibular joint pathology. *J Oral Maxillofac Surg* **53**(9):1069–1072.

Dolwick MF (2007) Temporomandibular joint surgery for internal derangement. *Dent Clin North Am* **51**(1):195–208, vii–viii.

Dolwick MF, Aufdemorte TB (1985) Silicone-induced foreign body reaction and lymphadenopathy after temporomandibular joint arthroplasty. *Oral Surg Oral Med Oral Pathol* **59**(5):449–452.

Dolwick MF, Dimitroulis G (1994) Is there a role for temporomandibular joint surgery? *Br J Oral Maxillofac Surg* **32**(5):307–313.

Dolwick MF, Nitzan DW (1990) TMJ disk surgery: 8-year follow-up evaluation. *Fortschr Kiefer Gesichtschir* **35**:162–163.

Dolwick MF, Nitzan DW (1994) The role of disc repositioning surgery for internal derangement of the temporomandibular joint. *Oral Maxillofac Clin North Am* **6**:271–275.

Dreessen D, Halata Z, Strasmann T (1990) Sensory innervation of the temporomandibular joint in the mouse. *Acta Anat (Basel)* **139**(2):154–160.

Dworkin SF, LeResche L (1992) Research diagnostic criteria for temporomandibular disorders: review, criteria, examinations and specifications, critique. *J Craniomandib Disord* **6**(4):301–355.

Dworkin SF, LeResche L, DeRouen T, *et al* (1990) Assessing clinical signs of temporomandibular disorders: reliability of clinical examiners. *J Prosthet Dent* **63**(5):574–579.

Dworkin SF, Sherman J, Mancl L, *et al* (2002) Reliability, validity, and clinical utility of the Research Diagnostic Criteria for Temporomandibular Disorders Axis II Scales: depression, non-specific physical symptoms, and graded chronic pain. *J Orofac Pain* **16**(3):207–220.

Eberhard D, Bantleon HP, Steger W (2002) The efficacy of anterior repositioning splint therapy studied by magnetic resonance imaging. *Eur J Orthod* **24**(4):343–352.

Ekberg E (1998) Treatment of temporomandibular disorders of arthrogeneous origin. Controlled double-blind studies of a non-steroidal anti-inflammatory drug and a stabilisation appliance. *Swed Dent J Suppl* **131**:1–57.

Ekberg E, Nilner M (2002) A 6- and 12-month follow-up of appliance therapy in TMD patients: a follow-up of a controlled trial. *Int J Prosthodont* **15**(6):564–570.

Ekberg EC, Vallon D, Nilner M (1998) Occlusal appliance therapy in patients with temporomandibular disorders. A double-blind controlled study in a short-term perspective. *Acta Odontol Scand* **56**(2):122–128.

Ekberg E, Vallon D, Nilner M (2002) Treatment outcome of headache after occlusal appliance therapy in a randomised controlled trial among patients with temporomandibular disorders of mainly arthrogenous origin. *Swed Dent J* **26**(3):115–124.

Eliav E, Teich S, Nitzan D, *et al* (2003) Facial arthralgia and myalgia: can they be differentiated by trigeminal sensory assessment? *Pain* **104**(3):481–490.

Emshoff R, Puffer P, Strobl H, *et al* (2000a) Effect of temporomandibular joint arthrocentesis on synovial fluid mediator level of tumor necrosis factor-alpha: implications for treatment outcome. *Int J Oral Maxillofac Surg* **29**(3):176–182.

Emshoff R, Rudisch A, Bosch R, *et al* (2000b) Effect of arthrocentesis and hydraulic distension on the temporomandibular joint disk position. *Oral Surg Oral Med Oral Pathol Oral Radiol Endod* **89**(3):271–277.

Emshoff R, Brandlmaier I, Bertram S, *et al* (2003a) Relative odds of temporomandibular joint pain as a function of magnetic resonance imaging findings of internal derangement, osteoarthrosis, effusion, and bone marrow edema. *Oral Surg Oral Med Oral Pathol Oral Radiol Endod* **95**(4):437–445.

Emshoff R, Rudisch A, Bosch R, *et al* (2003b) Prognostic indicators of the outcome of arthrocentesis: a short-term follow-up study. *Oral Surg Oral Med Oral Pathol Oral Radiol Endod* **96**(1):12–18.

Epstein JB, Rea A, Chahal O (2002) The use of bone scintigraphy in temporomandibular joint disorders. *Oral Dis* **8**(1):47–53.

Ericson S, Lundberg M (1968) Structural changes in the finger, wrist and temporomandiblar joints. A comparative radiologic study. *Acta Odontol Scand* **26**(2):111–126.

Eriksson L, Westesson PL (1985) Long-term evaluation of meniscectomy of the temporomandibular joint. *J Oral Maxillofac Surg* **43**(4):263–269.

Eriksson PO, Eriksson A, Ringqvist M, *et al* (1981) Special histochemical muscle-fibre characteristics of the human lateral pterygoid muscle. *Arch Oral Biol* **26**(6):495–507.

Ernst E, White AR (1999) Acupuncture as a treatment for temporomandibular joint dysfunction: a systematic review of randomized trials. *Arch Otolaryngol Head Neck Surg* **125** (3):269–272.

Eversole LR, Machado L (1985) Temporomandibular joint internal derangements and associated neuromuscular disorders. *J Am Dent Assoc* **110**(1):69–79.

Fikackova H, Dostalova T, Vosicka R, *et al* (2006) Arthralgia of the temporomandibular joint and low-level laser therapy. *Photomed Laser Surg* **24**(4):522–527.

Flake NM, Bonebreak DB, Gold MS (2005) Estrogen and inflammation increase the excitability of rat temporomandibular joint afferent neurons. *J Neurophysiol* **93**(3):1585–1597.

Flake NM, Hermanstyne TO, Gold MS (2006) Testosterone and estrogen have opposing actions on inflammation-induced plasma extravasation in the rat temporomandibular joint. *Am J Physiol Regul Integr Comp Physiol* **291**(2):R343–R348.

Flygare L, Hosoki H, Petersson A, *et al* (1997) Bone volume in human temporomandibular autopsy joints with and without erosive changes. *Acta Odontol Scand* **55**(3):167–172.

Forssell H, Kalso E (2004) Application of principles of evidence-based medicine to occlusal treatment for temporomandibular disorders: are there lessons to be learned? *J Orofac Pain* **18**(1):9–22; discussion 23–32.

Fridrich KL, Wise JM, Zeitler DL (1996) Prospective comparison of arthroscopy and arthrocentesis for temporomandibular joint disorders. *J Oral Maxillofac Surg* **54**(7):816–820; discussion 821.

Fujisawa T, Kuboki T, Kasai T, *et al* (2003) A repetitive, steady mouth opening induced an osteoarthritis-like lesion in the rabbit temporomandibular joint. *J Dent Res* **82**(9):731–735.

Fukuoka Y, Hagihara M, Nagatsu T, *et al* (1993) The relationship between collagen metabolism and temporomandibular joint osteoarthrosis in mice. *J Oral Maxillofac Surg* **51**(3):288–291.

Ghadially FN, Yong NK, Lalonde JM (1982) A transmission electron microscopic comparison of the articular surface of cartilage processed attached to bone and detached from bone. *J Anat* **135**(Pt 4):685–706.

Glineburg RW, Laskin DM, Blaustein DI (1982) The effects of immobilization on the primate temporomandibular joint: a histologic and histochemical study. *J Oral Maxillofac Surg* **40**(1):3–8.

Goldberg RJ, Katz J (2007) A meta-analysis of the analgesic effects of omega-3 polyunsaturated fatty acid supplementation for inflammatory joint pain. *Pain* **129**(1–2):210–223.

Gonzalez-Garcia R, Rodriguez-Campo FJ, Escorial-Hernandez V, *et al* (2006) Complications of temporomandibular joint arthroscopy: a retrospective analytic study of 670 arthroscopic procedures. *J Oral Maxillofac Surg* **64**(11):1587–1591.

Gotz W, Duhr S, Jager A (2005) Distribution of components of the insulin-like growth factor system in the temporomandibular joint of the aging mouse. *Growth Dev Aging* **69**(2):67–79.

Goudot P, Jaquinet AR, Hugonnet S, *et al* (2000) Improvement of pain and function after arthroscopy and arthrocentesis of the temporomandibular joint: a comparative study. *J Craniomaxillofac Surg* **28**(1):39–43.

Goulet JP, Clark GT (1990) Clinical TMJ examination methods. *J Calif Dent Assoc* **18**:25–33.

Greene CS, Laskin DM (1988) Long-term status of TMJ clicking in patients with myofascial pain and dysfunction. *J Am Dent Assoc* **117**(3):461–465.

Griffin CJ (1977) The prevalence of the lateral subcondylar tubercle of the mandible in fossil and recent man with particular reference to Anglo-Saxons. *Arch Oral Biol* **22** (10-11).633–639.

Guler N, Uckan S, Imirzaliogu P, *et al* (2005) Temporomandibular joint internal derangement: relationship between joint pain and MR grading of effusion and total protein concentration in the joint fluid. *Dentomaxillofac Radiol* **34**(3):175–181.

Guven O (2005) Inappropriate treatments in temporomandibular joint chronic recurrent dislocation: a literature review presenting three particular cases. *J Craniofac Surg* **16**(3):449–452.

Gynther GW, Holmlund AB, Reinholt FP (1994) Synovitis in internal derangement of the temporomandibular joint: correlation between arthroscopic and histologic findings. *J Oral Maxillofac Surg* **52**(9):913–917; discussion 918.

Gynther GW, Dijkgraaf LC, Reinholt FP, *et al* (1998) Synovial inflammation in arthroscopically obtained biopsy specimens from the temporomandibular joint: a review of the literature and a proposed histologic grading system. *J Oral Maxillofac Surg* **56**(11):1281–1286; discussion 1287.

Haeuchi Y, Matsumoto K, Ichikawa H, *et al* (1999) Immunohistochemical demonstration of neuropeptides in the articular disk of the human temporomandibular joint. *Cells Tissues Organs* **164**(4):205–211.

Hall D (1995) Intra-articular disc displacement. Part II: Its significant role in TMJ pathology. *J Oral Maxillofac Surg* **53**:1973.

Hall HD, Nickerson JW, Jr., McKenna SJ (1993) Modified condylotomy for treatment of the painful temporomandibular joint with a reducing disc. *J Oral Maxillofac Surg* **51**(2):133–142; discussion 143–134.

Hall HD, Navarro EZ, Gibbs SJ (2000a) Prospective study of modified condylotomy for treatment of nonreducing disk displacement. *Oral Surg Oral Med Oral Pathol Oral Radiol Endod* **89**(2):147–158.

Hall HD, Navarro EZ, Gibbs SJ (2000b) One- and three-year prospective outcome study of modified condylotomy for treatment of reducing disc displacement. *J Oral Maxillofac Surg* **58**(1):7–17; discussion 18.

Hall HD, Indresano AT, Kirk WS, *et al* (2005) Prospective multicenter comparison of 4 temporomandibular joint operations. *J Oral Maxillofac Surg* **63**(8):1174–1179.

Hall MB (1984) Meniscoplasty of the displaced temporomandibular joint meniscus without violating the inferior joint space. *J Oral Maxillofac Surg* **42**(12):788–792.

Hamada Y, Kondoh T, Holmlund AB, *et al* (2006) Inflammatory cytokines correlated with clinical outcome of temporomandibular joint irrigation in patients with chronic closed lock. *Oral Surg Oral Med Oral Pathol Oral Radiol Endod* **102**(5):596–601.

Han Z, Ha Q, Yang C (1999) [Arthrocentesis and lavage of TMJ for the treatment of anterior disc displacement without reduction]. *Zhonghua Kou Qiang Yi Xue Za Zhi* **34**(5):269–271.

Hardison JD, Okeson JP (1990) Comparison of three clinical techniques for evaluating joint sounds. *Cranio* **8**(4):307–311.

Haskin CL, Milam SB, Cameron IL (1995) Pathogenesis of degenerative joint disease in the human temporomandibular joint. *Crit Rev Oral Biol Med* **6**(3):248–277.

Heffez L, Mafee MF, Rosenberg H, *et al* (1987) CT evaluation of TMJ disc replacement with a Proplast-Teflon laminate. *J Oral Maxillofac Surg* **45**(8):657–665.

Helenius LM, Hallikainen D, Helenius I, *et al* (2005) Clinical and radiographic findings of the temporomandibular joint in patients with various rheumatic diseases. A case-control study. *Oral Surg Oral Med Oral Pathol Oral Radiol Endod* **99**(4):455–463.

Helenius LM, Tervahartiala P, Helenius I, *et al* (2006) Clinical, radiographic and MRI findings of the temporomandibular joint in patients with different rheumatic diseases. *Int J Oral Maxillofac Surg* **35**(11):983–989.

Henry CH, Wolford LM (2001) Substance P and mast cells: preliminary histologic analysis of the human temporomandibular joint. *Oral Surg Oral Med Oral Pathol Oral Radiol Endod* **92**(4):384–389.

Herring SW, Liu ZJ (2001) Loading of the temporomandibular joint: anatomical and in vivo evidence from the bones. *Cells Tissues Organs* **169**(3):193–200.

Hills BA (1996) Synovial surfactant and the hydrophobic articular surface. *J Rheumatol* **23**(8):1323–1325.

Hills BA (2000) Boundary lubrication in vivo. *Proc Inst Mech Eng [H]* **214**(1):83–94.

Hills BA, Butler BD (1984) Surfactants identified in synovial fluid and their ability to act as boundary lubricants. *Ann Rheum Dis* **43**(4):641–648.

Hills BA, Monds MK (1998) Enzymatic identification of the load-bearing boundary lubricant in the joint. *Br J Rheumatol* **37**(2): 137–142.

Holmlund A, Hellsing G (1988) Arthroscopy of the temporomandibular joint. A comparative study of arthroscopic and tomographic findings. *Int J Oral Maxillofac Surg* **17**(2): 128–133.

Holmlund A, Ekblom A, Hansson P, *et al* (1991) Concentrations of neuropeptides substance P, neurokinin A, calcitonin gene-related peptide, neuropeptide Y and vasoactive intestinal polypeptide in synovial fluid of the human temporomandibular joint. A correlation with symptoms, signs and arthroscopic findings. *Int J Oral Maxillofac Surg* **20**(4):228–231.

Huang YL, Pogrel MA, Kaban LB (1997) Diagnosis and management of condylar resorption. *J Oral Maxillofac Surg* **55**(2):114–119; discussion 119–120.

Huddleston Slater JJ, Lobbezoo F, Hofman N, *et al* (2005) Case report of a posterior disc displacement without and with reduction. *J Orofac Pain* **19**(4):337–342.

Imhof H, Sulzbacher I, Grampp S, *et al* (2000) Subchondral bone and cartilage disease: a rediscovered functional unit. *Invest Radiol* **35**(10):581–588.

Isacsson G, Linde C, Isberg A (1989) Subjective symptoms in patients with temporomandibular joint disk displacement versus patients with myogenic craniomandibular disorders. *J Prosthet Dent* **61**(1):70-77.

Isberg A, Isacsson G (1986) Tissue reactions associated with internal derangement of the temporomandibular joint. A radiographic, cryomorphologic, and histologic study. *Acta Odontol Scand* **44**(3):160-164.

Ishigaki S, Bessette RW, Maruyama T (1993) Vibration analysis of the temporomandibular joints with degenerative joint disease. *Cranio* **11**(4):276-283.

Israel HA, Saed-Nejad F, Ratcliffe A (1991) Early diagnosis of osteoarthrosis of the temporomandibular joint: correlation between arthroscopic diagnosis and keratan sulfate levels in the synovial fluid. *J Oral Maxillofac Surg* 49(7):708–711; discussion 712.

Israel HA, Diamond BE, Saed-Nejad F, *et al* (1997) Correlation between arthroscopic diagnosis of osteoarthritis and synovitis of the human temporomandibular joint and keratan sulfate levels in the synovial fluid. *J Oral Maxillofac Surg* 55(3):210–217; discussion 217–218.

Israel HA, Diamond B, Saed-Nejad F, *et al* (1998) Osteoarthritis and synovitis as major pathoses of the temporomandibular joint: comparison of clinical diagnosis with arthroscopic morphology. *J Oral Maxillofac Surg* 56(9):1023–1027; discussion 1028.

Iwase H, Sasaki T, Asakura S, *et al* (2005) Characterization of patients with disc displacement without reduction unresponsive to nonsurgical treatment: a preliminary study. *J Oral Maxillofac Surg* 63(8):1115–1122.

Iwata K, Tashiro A, Tsuboi Y, *et al* (1999) Medullary dorsal horn neuronal activity in rats with persistent temporomandibular joint and perioral inflammation. *J Neurophysiol* 82(3):1244–1253.

Jagger RG (1991) Mandibular manipulation of anterior disc displacement without reduction. *J Oral Rehabil* 18(6):497–500.

Johansson AS, Isberg A (1991) The anterosuperior insertion of the temporomandibular joint capsule and condylar mobility in joints with and without internal derangement: a double-contrast arthrotomographic investigation. *J Oral Maxillofac Surg* 49(11):1142–1148.

Johansson Cahlin B, Samuelsson N, Dahlstrom L (2006) Utilization of pharmaceuticals among patients with temporomandibular disorders: a controlled study. *Acta Odontol Scand* 64(3):187–192.

Kaneyama K, Segami N, Nishimura M, *et al* (2004) The ideal lavage volume for removing bradykinin, interleukin-6, and protein from the temporomandibular joint by arthrocentesis. *J Oral Maxillofac Surg* 62(6):657–661.

Kaneyama K, Segami N, Sato J, *et al* (2007) Prognostic factors in arthrocentesis of the temporomandibular joint: Comparison of bradykinin, leukotriene B4, prostaglandin E2, and substance P level in synovial fluid between successful and unsuccessful cases. *J Oral Maxillofac Surg* 65(2):242–247.

Kanyama M, Kuboki T, Kojima S, *et al* (2000) Matrix metalloproteinases and tissue inhibitors of metalloproteinases in synovial fluids of patients with temporomandibular joint osteoarthritis. *J Orofac Pain* 14(1):20–30.

Kaplan PA, Ruskin JD, Tu HK, *et al* (1988) Erosive arthritis of the temporomandibular joint caused by Teflon-Proplast implants: plain film features. *AJR Am J Roentgenol* 151(2):337–339.

Katzberg RW, Westesson PL, Tallents RH, *et al* (1996) Anatomic disorders of the temporomandibular joint disc in asymptomatic subjects. *J Oral Maxillofac Surg* 54(2):147–153; discussion 153–145.

Kawai Y, Kubota E, Okabe E (2000) Reactive oxygen species participation in experimentally induced arthritis of the temporomandibular joint in rats. *J Dent Res* 79(7):1489–1495.

Keeling SD, McGorray S, Wheeler TT, *et al* (1994) Risk factors associated with temporomandibular joint sounds in children 6 to 12 years of age. *Am J Orthod Dentofacial Orthop* 105(3):279–287.

Kendell BD, Frost DE (1996) Arthrocentesis. *Atlas Oral Maxillofac Surg Clin North Am* 4(2):1–14.

Kent JN, Block MS, Halpern J, *et al* (1993) Long-term results on VK partial and total temporomandibular joint systems. *J Long Term Eff Med Implants* 3(1):29–40.

Kerstens HC, Tuinzing DB, Golding RP, *et al* (1990) Condylar atrophy and osteoarthrosis after bimaxillary surgery. *Oral Surg Oral Med Oral Pathol* 69(3):274–280.

Kido MA, Kiyoshima T, Kondo T, *et al* (1993) Distribution of substance P and calcitonin gene-related peptide-like immunoreactive nerve fibers in the rat temporomandibular joint. *J Dent Res* 72(3):592–598.

Kido MA, Kiyoshima T, Ibuki T, *et al* (1995) A topographical and ultrastructural study of sensory trigeminal nerve endings in the rat temporomandibular joint as demonstrated by anterograde transport of wheat germ agglutinin-horseradish peroxidase (WGA-HRP). *J Dent Res* 74(7):1353–1359.

Kido MA, Zhang JQ, Muroya H, *et al* (2001) Topography and distribution of sympathetic nerve fibers in the rat temporomandibular joint: immunocytochemistry and ultrastructure. *Anat Embryol (Berl)* 203(5):357–366.

Kircos LT, Ortendahl DA, Mark AS (1987a) MRI of the TMJ disc in asymptomatic volunteers. *J Oral Maxillofac Surg* 54:852.

Kircos LT, Ortendahl DA, Mark AS, *et al* (1987b) Magnetic resonance imaging of the TMJ disc in asymptomatic volunteers. *J Oral Maxillofac Surg* 45(10):852–854.

Kononen M, Waltimo A, Nystrom M (1996) Does clicking in adolescence lead to painful temporomandibular joint locking? *Lancet* 347(9008):1080–1081.

Kopp S (1985) [Degenerative and inflammatory diseases of the temporomandibular joint]. *Schweiz Monatsschr Zahnmed* 95(10):950–962.

Kopp S (2001) Neuroendocrine, immune, and local responses related to temporomandibular disorders. *J Orofac Pain* 15(1): 9–28.

Kopp S, Alstergren P, Ernestam S, *et al* (2005) Reduction of temporomandibular joint pain after treatment with a combination of methotrexate and infliximab is associated with changes in synovial fluid and plasma cytokines in rheumatoid arthritis. *Cells Tissues Organs* 180(1):22–30.

Kozeniauskas JJ, Ralph WJ (1988) Bilateral arthrographic evaluation of unilateral temporomandibular joint pain and dysfunction. *J Prosthet Dent* 60(1):98–105.

Kurita H, Kojima Y, Nakatsuka A, *et al* (2004) Relationship between temporomandibular joint (TMJ)-related pain and morphological changes of the TMJ condyle in patients with temporomandibular disorders. *Dentomaxillofac Radiol* 33(5): 329–333.

Kurita H, Uehara S, Yokochi M, *et al* (2006) A long-term follow-up study of radiographically evident degenerative changes in the temporomandibular joint with different conditions of disk displacement. *Int J Oral Maxillofac Surg* 35(1):49–54.

Kurita K, Westesson PL, Sternby NH, *et al* (1989) Histologic features of the temporomandibular joint disk and posterior disk attachment: comparison of symptom-free persons with normally positioned disks and patients with internal derangement. *Oral Surg Oral Med Oral Pathol* 67(6):635–643.

Kurita K, Westesson PL, Yuasa H, *et al* (1998) Natural course of untreated symptomatic temporomandibular joint disc displacement without reduction. *J Dent Res* 77(2):361–365.

Lajeunesse D, Reboul P (2003) Subchondral bone in osteoarthritis: a biologic link with articular cartilage leading to abnormal remodeling. *Curr Opin Rheumatol* 15(5):628–633.

Lam DK, Sessle BJ, Cairns BE, *et al* (2005) Neural mechanisms of temporomandibular joint and masticatory muscle pain: A possible role for peripheral glutamate receptor mechanisms. *Pain Res Manag* 10(3):145–152.

Larheim TA (2005) Role of magnetic resonance imaging in the clinical diagnosis of the temporomandibular joint. *Cells Tissues Organs* 180(1):6–21.

Levine JD, Khasar SG, Green PG (2006) Neurogenic inflammation and arthritis. *Ann N Y Acad Sci* 1069:155–167.

Li B, Aspden RM (1997) Material properties of bone from the femoral neck and calcar femorale of patients with osteoporosis or osteoarthritis. *Osteoporos Int* 7(5):450–456.

List T, Axelsson S, Leijon G (2003) Pharmacologic interventions in the treatment of temporomandibular disorders, atypical facial pain, and burning mouth syndrome. A qualitative systematic review. *J Orofac Pain* 17(4):301–310.

Lobbezoo F, Drangsholt M, Peck C, *et al* (2004) Topical review: new insights into the pathology and diagnosis of disorders of the temporomandibular joint. *J Orofac Pain* 18(3):181–191.

Locker D, Slade G (1988) Prevalence of symptoms associated with temporomandibular disorders in a Canadian population. *Community Dent Oral Epidemiol* 16(5):310–313.

Luder HU (2002) Factors affecting degeneration in human temporomandibular joints as assessed histologically. *Eur J Oral Sci* **110**(2):106–113.

Luder HU, Bobst P, Schroeder HE (1993) Histometric study of synovial cavity dimensions of human temporomandibular joints with normal and anterior disc position. *J Orofac Pain* **7**:263–274.

Lundh H, Westesson PL, Kopp S, *et al* (1985) Anterior repositioning splint in the treatment of temporomandibular joints with reciprocal clicking: comparison with a flat occlusal splint and an untreated control group. *Oral Surg Oral Med Oral Pathol* **60**(2):131–136.

Lundh H, Westesson PL, Eriksson L, *et al* (1992) Temporomandibular joint disk displacement without reduction. Treatment with flat occlusal splint versus no treatment. *Oral Surg Oral Med Oral Pathol* **73**(6):655–658.

Luyten FP (1997) A scientific basis for the biologic regeneration of synovial joints. *Oral Surg Oral Med Oral Pathol Oral Radiol Endod* **83**(1):167–169.

McAlindon TE (2006) Nutraceuticals: do they work and when should we use them? *Best Pract Res Clin Rheumatol* **20**(1):99–115.

McCain JP, Sanders B, Koslin MG, *et al* (1992) Temporomandibular joint arthroscopy: a 6-year multicenter retrospective study of 4,831 joints. *J Oral Maxillofac Surg* **50**(9):926–930.

McDonald Blumer MH (2005) Bone mineral content versus bone density in a population with osteoarthritis: a new twist to the controversy? *J Rheumatol* **32**(10):1868–1869.

MacIntosh RB (2000) The use of autogenous tissues for temporomandibular joint reconstruction. *J Oral Maxillofac Surg* **58**(1):63–69.

Magnusson T, Egermark I, Carlsson GE (2000) A longitudinal epidemiologic study of signs and symptoms of temporomandibular disorders from 15 to 35 years of age. *J Orofac Pain* **14**(4):310–319.

Malemud CJ, Islam N, Haqqi TM (2003) Pathophysiological mechanisms in osteoarthritis lead to novel therapeutic strategies. *Cells Tissues Organs* **174**:34–48.

Manfredini D, Tognini F, Zampa V, *et al* (2003) Predictive value of clinical findings for temporomandibular joint effusion. *Oral Surg Oral Med Oral Pathol Oral Radiol Endod* **96**(5):521–526.

Mansell JP, Bailey AJ (1998) Abnormal cancellous bone collagen metabolism in osteoarthritis. *J Clin Invest* **101**(8):1596–1603.

Mao J, Stein RB, Osborn JW (1992) The size and distribution of fiber types in jaw muscles: a review. *J Craniomandib Disord* **6**(3):192–201.

Marchetti C, Bernasconi G, Reguzzoni M, *et al* (1997) The articular disc surface in different functional conditions of the human temporo-mandibular joint. *J Oral Pathol Med* **26**(6):278–282.

Marciani RD, Ziegler RC (1983) Temporomandibular joint surgery: a review of fifty-one operations. *Oral Surg Oral Med Oral Pathol* **56**(5):472–476.

Martel-Pelletier J, Pelletier JP (2005) New insights into the major pathophysiological processes responsible for the development of osteoarthritis. *Semin Arthritis Rheum* **34**(6 Suppl 2):6–8.

Martel-Pelletier J, Lajeunesse D, Fahmi H, *et al* (2006) New thoughts on the pathophysiology of osteoarthritis: one more step toward new therapeutic targets. *Curr Rheumatol Rep* **8**(1):30–36.

Martinez Blanco M, Bagan JV, Fons A, *et al* (2004) Osteoarthrosis of the temporomandibular joint. A clinical and radiological study of 16 patients. *Med Oral* **9**(2):110–115, 106–110.

Matsumoto K, Honda K, Ohshima M, *et al* (2006) Cytokine profile in synovial fluid from patients with internal derangement of the temporomandibular joint: a preliminary study. *Dentomaxillofac Radiol* **35**(6):432–441.

Mercuri LG (2000) The use of alloplastic prostheses for temporomandibular joint reconstruction. *J Oral Maxillofac Surg* **58**(1):70–75.

Mercuri LG, Wolford LM, Sanders B, *et al* (1995) Custom CAD/CAM total temporomandibular joint reconstruction system: preliminary multicenter report. *J Oral Maxillofac Surg* **53**(2): 106–115; discussion 115–116.

Merkx MA, Van Damme PA (1994) Condylar resorption after orthognathic surgery. Evaluation of treatment in 8 patients. *J Craniomaxillofac Surg* **22**(1): 53–58.

Merry P, Williams R, Cox N, *et al* (1991) Comparative study of intra-articular pressure dynamics in joints with acute traumatic and chronic inflammatory effusions: potential implications for hypoxic-reperfusion injury. *Ann Rheum Dis* **50**(12):917–920.

Milam SB, Schmitz JP (1995) Molecular biology of temporomandibular joint disorders: proposed mechanisms of disease. *J Oral Maxillofac Surg* **53**(12):1448–1454.

Montgomery MT, Van Sickels JE, Harms SE, *et al* (1989) Arthroscopic TMJ surgery: effects on signs, symptoms, and disc position. *J Oral Maxillofac Surg* **47**(12):1263–1271.

Montgomery MT, Gordon SM, Van Sickels JE, *et al* (1992) Changes in signs and symptoms following temporomandibular joint disc repositioning surgery. *J Oral Maxillofac Surg* **50**(4): 320–328.

Morrow D, Tallents RH, Katzberg RW, *et al* (1996) Relationship of other joint problems and anterior disc position in symptomatic TMD patients and in asymptomatic volunteers. *J Orofac Pain* **10**(1):15–20.

Moses JJ, Poker ID (1989) TMJ arthroscopic surgery: an analysis of 237 patients. *J Oral Maxillofac Surg* **47**(8):790–794.

Mow VC, Ateshian GA (1997) Lubrication and wear of diarthrodial joints. In: Mow VC, Hayes WC (eds) *Basic Orthopaedic Biomechanics*, 2nd edn. Philadelphia: Lippincott-Raven, pp 275–315.

Murakami KI, Iizuka T, Matsuki M, *et al* (1987) Recapturing the persistent anteriorly displaced disk by mandibular manipulation after pumping and hydraulic pressure to the upper joint cavity of the temporomandibular joint. *Cranio* **5**(1):17–24.

Murakami K, Segami N, Fujimura K, *et al* (1991) Correlation between pain and synovitis in patients with internal derangement of the temporomandibular joint. *J Oral Maxillofac Surg* **49**(11):1159–1161; discussion 1162.

Murakami KI, Shibata T, Kubota E, *et al* (1998a) Intra-articular levels of prostaglandin E2, hyaluronic acid, and chondroitin-4 and -6 sulfates in the temporomandibular joint synovial fluid of patients with internal derangement. *J Oral Maxillofac Surg* **56**(2):199–203.

Murakami KI, Tsuboi Y, Bessho K, *et al* (1998b) Outcome of arthroscopic surgery to the temporomandibular joint correlates with stage of internal derangement: five-year follow-up study. *Br J Oral Maxillofac Surg* **36**(1):30–34.

Murakami K, Segami N, Okamoto M, *et al* (2000) Outcome of arthroscopic surgery for internal derangement of the temporomandibular joint: long-term results covering 10 years. *J Craniomaxillofac Surg* **28**(5):264–271.

Murakami K, Kaneshita S, Kanoh C, *et al* (2002) Ten-year outcome of nonsurgical treatment for the internal derangement of the temporomandibular joint with closed lock. *Oral Surg Oral Med Oral Pathol Oral Radiol Endod* **94**(5): 572–575.

Murata M, Yudoh K, Nakamura H, *et al* (2006) Distinct signaling pathways are involved in hypoxia- and IL-1-induced VEGF expression in human articular chondrocytes. *J Orthop Res* **24**(7):1544–1554.

Nguyen P, Mohamed SE, Gardiner D, *et al* (2001) A randomized double-blind clinical trial of the effect of chondroitin sulfate and glucosamine hydrochloride on temporomandibular joint disorders: a pilot study. *Cranio* **19**(2):130–139.

Nicolakis P, Erdogmus B, Kopf A, *et al* (2001) Effectiveness of exercise therapy in patients with internal derangement of the temporomandibular joint. *J Oral Rehabil* **28**(12):1158–1164.

Nitzan DW (1994) Intraarticular pressure in the functioning human temporomandibular joint and its alteration by uniform elevation of the occlusal plane. *J Oral Maxillofac Surg* **52**(7):671–679; discussion 679–680.

Nitzan DW (2001) The process of lubrication impairment and its involvement in temporomandibular joint disc displacement: a theoretical concept. *J Oral Maxillofac Surg* **59**(1):36–45.

Nitzan DW (2002) Temporomandibular joint "open lock" versus condylar dislocation: signs and symptoms, imaging, treatment, and pathogenesis. *J Oral Maxillofac Surg* **60**(5):506–511; discussion 512–513.

Nitzan DW (2003) 'Friction and adhesive forces'–possible underlying causes for temporomandibular joint internal derangement. *Cells Tissues Organs* **174**(1-2):6–16.

Nitzan DW, Dolwick MF (1991) An alternative explanation for the genesis of closed-lock symptoms in the internal derangement process. *J Oral Maxillofac Surg* **49**(8):810–815; discussion 815–816.

Nitzan DW, Etsion I (2002) Adhesive force: the underlying cause of the disc anchorage to the fossa and/or eminence in the temporomandibular joint–a new concept. *Int J Oral Maxillofac Surg* **31**(1):94–99.

Nitzan DW, Price A (2001) The use of arthrocentesis for the treatment of osteoarthritic temporomandibular joints. *J Oral Maxillofac Surg* **59**(10):1154–1159; discussion 1160.

Nitzan DW, Dolwick MF, Heft MW (1990) Arthroscopic lavage and lysis of the temporomandibular joint: a change in perspective. *J Oral Maxillofac Surg* **48**(8):798–801; discussion 802.

Nitzan DW, Dolwick FM, Marmary Y (1991a) The value of arthrography in the decision-making process regarding surgery for internal derangement of the temporomandibular joint. *J Oral Maxillofac Surg* **49**(4):375–379; discussion 379–380.

Nitzan DW, Dolwick MF, Martinez GA (1991b) Temporomandibular joint arthrocentesis: a simplified treatment for severe, limited mouth opening. *J Oral Maxillofac Surg* **49**(11):1163–1167; discussion 1168–1170.

Nitzan DW, Samson B, Better H (1997) Long-term outcome of arthrocentesis for sudden-onset, persistent, severe closed lock of the temporomandibular joint. *J Oral Maxillofac Surg* **55**(2): 151–157; discussion 157–158.

Nitzan DW, Nitzan U, Dan P, *et al* (2001) The role of hyaluronic acid in protecting surface-active phospholipids from lysis by exogenous phospholipase A(2). *Rheumatology (Oxford)* **40**(3):336–340.

Nitzan DW, Goldfarb A, Gati I, *et al* (2002) Changes in the reducing power of synovial fluid from temporomandibular joints with "anchored disc phenomenon." *J Oral Maxillofac Surg* **60**(7):735–740.

Nwoku AL, Koch H (1974) The temporomandibular joint: a rare localisation for bone tumours. *J Maxillofac Surg* **2**(2-3):113–119.

Ogura N, Tobe M, Sakamaki H, *et al* (2002) Interleukin-1 beta induces interleukin-6 mRNA expression and protein production in synovial cells from human temporomandibular joint. *J Oral Pathol Med* **31**(6):353–360.

Ogura N, Tobe M, Sakamaki H, *et al* (2005) Tumor necrosis factor-alpha increases chemokine gene expression and production in synovial fibroblasts from human temporomandibular joint. *J Oral Pathol Med* **34**(6):357–363.

Ogus H (1981) *Common Disorders of the Temporomandibular Joint*. Bristol: Wright.

Ogus H (1987) The mandibular joint: internal rearrangement. *Br J Oral Maxillofac Surg* **25**(3):218–226.

Ohnuki T, Fukuda M, Nakata A, *et al* (2006) Evaluation of the position, mobility, and morphology of the disc by MRI before and after four different treatments for temporomandibular joint disorders. *Dentomaxillofac Radiol* **35**(2):103–109.

Okamoto K, Hirata H, Takeshita S, *et al* (2003) Response properties of TMJ units in superficial laminae at the spinomedullary junction of female rats vary over the estrous cycle. *J Neurophysiol* **89**(3):1467–1477.

Okeson JP (1996) *Orofacial Pain: Guidelines for Assessment, Classification, and Management*. The American Academy of Orofacial Pain. Chicago: Quintessence Publishing.

Olesen J, Bousser M-G, Diener HC, *et al* (2004) The International Classification of Headache Disorders, 2nd Edition. *Cephalalgia* **24**(suppl 1):24–150.

Otero M, Lago R, Gomez R, *et al* (2006) Towards a pro-inflammatory and immunomodulatory emerging role of leptin. *Rheumatology (Oxford)* **45**(8):944–950.

Paesani D, Westesson PL, Hatala MP, *et al* (1992) Accuracy of clinical diagnosis for TMJ internal derangement and arthrosis. *Oral Surg Oral Med Oral Pathol* **73**(3):360–363.

Pereira FJ Jr, Lundh H, Westesson PL, *et al* (1994a) Clinical findings related to morphologic changes in TMJ autopsy specimens. *Oral Surg Oral Med Oral Pathol* **78**(3):288–295.

Pereira FJ Jr, Lundh H, Westesson PL (1994b) Morphologic changes in the temporomandibular joint in different age groups. An autopsy investigation. *Oral Surg Oral Med Oral Pathol* **78**(3):279–287.

Pereira FJ, Lundh H, Eriksson L, *et al* (1996) Microscopic changes in the retrodiscal tissues of painful temporomandibular joints. *J Oral Maxillofac Surg* **54**(4):461–468; discussion 469.

Peroz I, Tai S (2002) Masticatory performance in patients with anterior disk displacement without reduction in comparison with symptom-free volunteers. *Eur J Oral Sci* **110**(5):341–344.

Piper MA (1989) Microscopic disc preservation surgery of the temporomandibular joint. *Oral Maxillofac Clinic North Am* **1**:279–302.

Plesh O, Curtis D, Levine J, *et al* (2000) Amitriptyline treatment of chronic pain in patients with temporomandibular disorders. *J Oral Rehabil* **27**(10):834–841.

Prinz JF (1998a) Correlation of the characteristics of temporomandibular joint and tooth contact sounds. *J Oral Rehabil* **25**(3):194–198.

Prinz JF (1998b) Resonant characteristics of the human head in relation to temporomandibular joint sounds. *J Oral Rehabil* **25**(12):954–960.

Pufe T, Harde V, Petersen W, *et al* (2004a) Vascular endothelial growth factor (VEGF) induces matrix metalloproteinase expression in immortalized chondrocytes. *J Pathol* **202**(3): 367–374.

Pufe T, Lemke A, Kurz B, *et al* (2004b) Mechanical overload induces VEGF in cartilage discs via hypoxia-inducible factor. *Am J Pathol* **164**(1):185–192.

Puri V, Cui L, Liverman CS, *et al* (2005) Ovarian steroids regulate neuropeptides in the trigeminal ganglion. *Neuropeptides* **39**(4):409–417.

Quinn PD (2000) Alloplastic reconstruction of the temporomandibular joint. *Sel Read Oral Maxillofac Surg* **7**:1.

Rachamim E, Better H, Dagan A, *et al* (2001) Electron microscopic demonstration and biochemical extraction of phospholipids from TMJ synovial fluid and articular surfaces. *J Oral Maxillofac Surg* **59**:1326–1332.

Randolph CS, Greene CS, Moretti R, *et al* (1990) Conservative management of temporomandibular disorders: a posttreatment comparison between patients from a university clinic and from private practice. *Am J Orthod Dentofacial Orthop* **98**(1):77–82.

Rao VM, Farole A, Karasick D (1990) Temporomandibular joint dysfunction: correlation of MR imaging, arthrography, and arthroscopy. *Radiology* **174**(3 Pt 1):663–667.

Rasmussen OC (1981) Description of population and progress of symptoms in a longitudinal study of temporomandibular arthropathy. *J Dent Res* **89**:196–203.

Ratcliffe A, Israel HA, Saed-Nejad F, *et al* (1998) Proteoglycans in the synovial fluid of the temporomandibular joint as an indicator of changes in cartilage metabolism during primary and secondary osteoarthritis. *J Oral Maxillofac Surg* **56**(2):204–208.

Reston JT, Turkelson CM (2003) Meta-analysis of surgical treatments for temporomandibular articular disorders. *J Oral Maxillofac Surg* **61**(1): 3–10; discussion 10–12.

Rizzatti-Barbosa CM, Nogueira MT, de Andrade ED, *et al* (2003) Clinical evaluation of amitriptyline for the control of chronic pain caused by temporomandibular joint disorders. *Cranio* **21**(3):221–225.

Roberts C, Katzberg RW, Tallents RH, *et al* (1991) The clinical predictability of internal derangements of the temporomandibular joint. *Oral Surg Oral Med Oral Pathol* **71**(4):412–414.

Rodrigues LL, Oliveira MC, Pelegrini-da-Silva A, *et al* (2006) Peripheral sympathetic component of the temporomandibular joint inflammatory pain in rats. *J Pain* **7**(12):929–936.

Rossomando EF, White LB, Hadjimichael J, *et al* (1992) Immunomagnetic separation of tumor necrosis factor alpha. I. Batch procedure for human temporomandibular fluid. *J Chromatogr* **583**(1):11–18.

Rugh JD, Harlan J (1988) Nocturnal bruxism and temporomandibular disorders. *Adv Neurol* **49**:329–341.

Sanders B (1986) Arthroscopic surgery of the temporomandibular joint: treatment of internal derangement with persistent closed lock. *Oral Surg Oral Med Oral Pathol* **62**(4):361–372.

Sanroman JF (2004) Closed lock (MRI fixed disc): a comparison of arthrocentesis and arthroscopy. *Int J Oral Maxillofac Surg* **33**(4):344–348.

Sarzi-Puttini P, Cimmino MA, Scarpa R, *et al* (2005) Osteoarthritis: an overview of the disease and its treatment strategies. *Semin Arthritis Rheum* **35**(1 Suppl 1):1–10.

Sato H, Osterberg T, Ahlqwist M, *et al* (1996) Association between radiographic findings in the mandibular condyle and temporomandibular dysfunction in an elderly population. *Acta Odontol Scand* **54**(6):384–390.

Sato J, Segami N, Kaneyama K, *et al* (2004) Relationship of calcitonin gene-related peptide in synovial tissues and temporomandibular joint pain in humans. *Oral Surg Oral Med Oral Pathol Oral Radiol Endod* **98**(5):533–540.

Sato S, Goto S, Kawamura H, *et al* (1997) The natural course of nonreducing disc displacement of the TMJ: relationship of clinical findings at initial visit to outcome after 12 months without treatment. *J Orofac Pain* **11**(4): 315–320.

Sato S, Sakamoto M, Kawamura H, *et al* (1999) Long-term changes in clinical signs and symptoms and disc position and morphology in patients with nonreducing disc displacement in the temporomandibular joint. *J Oral Maxillofac Surg* **57**(1):23–29; discussion 29–30.

Sato S, Goto S, Nasu F, *et al* (2003) Natural course of disc displacement with reduction of the temporomandibular joint: changes in clinical signs and symptoms. *J Oral Maxillofac Surg* **61**(1):32–34.

Scapino RP (1983) Histopathology associated with malposition of the human temporomandibular joint disc. *Oral Surg Oral Med Oral Pathol* **55**(4):382–397.

Scapino RP (1991) The posterior attachment: its structure, function, and appearance in TMJ imaging studies. Part 1. *J Craniomandib Disord* **5**(2):83–95.

Schiffman EL, Look JO, Hodges JS, *et al* (2007) Randomized effectiveness study of four therapeutic strategies for TMJ closed lock. *J Dent Res* **86**(1):58–63.

Schmitter M, Zahran M, Duc JM, *et al* (2005) Conservative therapy in patients with anterior disc displacement without reduction using 2 common splints: a randomized clinical trial. *J Oral Maxillofac Surg* **63**(9):1295–1303.

Schwarz IM, Hills BA (1998) Surface-active phospholipid as the lubricating component of lubricin. *Br J Rheumatol* **37**(1):21–26.

Segami N, Murakami K, Iizuka T (1990) Arthrographic evaluation of disk position following mandibular manipulation technique for internal derangement with closed lock of the temporomandibular joint. *J Craniomandib Disord* **4**(2):99–108.

Sessle BJ, Hu JW (1991) Mechanisms of pain arising from articular tissues. *Can J Physiol Pharmacol* **69**(5):617–626.

Shankland WE, 2nd (1998) The effects of glucosamine and chondroitin sulfate on osteoarthritis of the TMJ: a preliminary report of 50 patients. *Cranio* **16**(4):230–235.

Sheets DW, Jr., Okamoto T, Dijkgraaf LC, *et al* (2006) Free radical damage in facsimile synovium: correlation with adhesion formation in osteoarthritic TMJs. *J Prosthodont* **15**(1):9–19.

Sheikholeslam A, Holmgren K, Riise C (1986) A clinical and electromyographic study of the long-term effects of an occlusal splint on the temporal and masseter muscles in patients with functional disorders and nocturnal bruxism. *J Oral Rehabil* **13**(2):137–145.

Shi Z, Guo C, Awad M (2003) Hyaluronate for temporomandibular joint disorders. *Cochrane Database Syst Rev* (1):CD002970.

Shinoda C, Takaku S (2000) Interleukin-1 beta, interleukin-6, and tissue inhibitor of metalloproteinase-1 in the synovial fluid of the temporomandibular joint with respect to cartilage destruction. *Oral Dis* **6**(6):383–390.

Shinoda M, Honda T, Ozaki N, *et al* (2003) Nerve terminals extend into the temporomandibular joint of adjuvant arthritic rats. *Eur J Pain* **7**(6):493–505.

Shorey CW, Campbell JH (2000) Dislocation of the temporomandibular joint. *Oral Surg Oral Med Oral Pathol Oral Radiol Endod* **89**(6):662–668.

Silver CM (1984) Long-term results of meniscectomy of the temporomandibular joint. *Cranio* **3**(1):46–57.

Sindelar BJ, Herring SW (2005) Soft tissue mechanics of the temporomandibular joint. *Cells Tissues Organs* **180**(1):36–43.

Sinigaglia L, Varenna M, Casari S (2005) Bone involvement in osteoarthritis. *Semin Arthritis Rheum* **34**(6 Suppl 2):44–46.

Smolka W, Iizuka T (2005) Arthroscopic lysis and lavage in different stages of internal derangement of the temporomandibular joint: correlation of preoperative staging to arthroscopic findings and treatment outcome. *J Oral Maxillofac Surg* **63**(4):471–478.

Solberg WK, Clark GT, Rugh JD (1975) Nocturnal electromyographic evaluation of bruxism patients undergoing short term splint therapy. *J Oral Rehabil* **2**(3):215–223.

Stegenga B (2001) Osteoarthritis of the temporomandibular joint organ and its relationship to disc displacement. *J Orofac Pain* **15**(3):193–205.

Stegenga B, de Bont LG, Boering G, *et al* (1991) Tissue responses to degenerative changes in the temporomandibular joint: a review. *J Oral Maxillofac Surg* **49**(10):1079–1088.

Swann DA, Slayter HS, Silver FH (1981) The molecular structure of lubricating glycoprotein-I, the boundary lubricant for articular cartilage. *J Biol Chem* **256**(11):5921–5925.

Ta LE, Dionne RA (2004) Treatment of painful temporomandibular joints with a cyclooxygenase-2 inhibitor: a randomized placebo-controlled comparison of celecoxib to naproxen. *Pain* **111**(1-2):13–21.

Takahashi T, Kondoh T, Kamei K, *et al* (1996) Elevated levels of nitric oxide in synovial fluid from patients with temporomandibular disorders. *Oral Surg Oral Med Oral Pathol Oral Radiol Endod* **82**(5):505–509.

Takahashi T, Nagai H, Seki H, *et al* (1999) Relationship between joint effusion, joint pain, and protein levels in joint lavage fluid of patients with internal derangement and osteoarthritis of the temporomandibular joint. *J Oral Maxillofac Surg* **57**(10): 1187–1193; discussion 1193–1194.

Takaku S, Toyoda T (1994) Long-term evaluation of discectomy of the temporomandibular joint. *J Oral Maxillofac Surg* **52**(7): 722–726; discussion 727–728.

Takatsuka S, Yoshida K, Ueki K, *et al* (2005) Disc and condyle translation in patients with temporomandibular disorder. *Oral Surg Oral Med Oral Pathol Oral Radiol Endod* **99**(5):614–621.

Takeda M, Tanimoto T, Ikeda M, *et al* (2005) Temporomandibular joint inflammation potentiates the excitability of trigeminal root ganglion neurons innervating the facial skin in rats. *J Neurophysiol* **93**(5):2723–2738.

Takeuchi Y, Zeredo JL, Fujiyama R, *et al* (2004) Effects of experimentally induced inflammation on temporomandibular joint nociceptors in rats. *Neurosci Lett* **354**(2):172–174.

Tallents RH, Katzberg RW, Macher DJ, *et al* (1990) Use of protrusive splint therapy in anterior disk displacement of the temporomandibular joint: a 1- to 3-year follow-up. *J Prosthet Dent* **63**(3):336–341.

Tallents RH, Katzberg RW, Murphy W, *et al* (1996) Magnetic resonance imaging findings in asymptomatic volunteers and symptomatic patients with temporomandibular disorders. *J Prosthet Dent* **75**(5):529–533.

Tanaka E, Kawai N, Tanaka M, *et al* (2004) The frictional coefficient of the temporomandibular joint and its dependency on the magnitude and duration of joint loading. *J Dent Res* **83**(5):404–407.

Tanaka E, Aoyama J, Miyauchi M, *et al* (2005) Vascular endothelial growth factor plays an important autocrine/paracrine role in the progression of osteoarthritis. *Histochem Cell Biol* **123**(3):275–281.

Tasaki MM, Westesson PL, Isberg AM, *et al* (1996) Classification and prevalence of temporomandibular joint disk displacement in patients and symptom-free volunteers. *Am J Orthod Dentofacial Orthop* **109**(3):249–262.

Tecco S, Festa F, Salini V, *et al* (2004) Treatment of joint pain and joint noises associated with a recent TMJ internal derangement: a comparison of an anterior repositioning splint, a full-arch maxillary stabilization splint, and an untreated control group. *Cranio* **22**(3):209–219.

Tegelberg A, Kopp S (1987) Subjective symptoms from the stomatognathic system in individuals with rheumatoid arthritis and osteoarthrosis. *Swed Dent J* **11**(1-2):11–22.

Tegelberg A, Kopp S (1996) A 3-year follow-up of temporomandibular disorders in rheumatoid arthritis and ankylosing spondylitis. *Acta Odontol Scand* **54**(1):14–18.

Thie NM, Prasad NG, Major PW (2001) Evaluation of glucosamine sulfate compared to ibuprofen for the treatment of temporomandibular joint osteoarthritis: a randomized double blind controlled 3 month clinical trial. *J Rheumatol* **28**(6):1347–1355.

Thonar EJ, Lenz ME, Klintworth GK, *et al* (1985) Quantification of keratan sulfate in blood as a marker of cartilage catabolism. *Arthritis Rheum* **28**(12):1367–1376.

Tolvanen M, Oikarinen VJ, Wolf J (1988) A 30-year follow-up study of temporomandibular joint meniscectomies: a report on five patients. *Br J Oral Maxillofac Surg* **26**(4):311–316.

Toolson GA, Sadowsky C (1991) An evaluation of the relationship between temporomandibular joint sounds and mandibular movements. *J Craniomandib Disord* **5**(3):187–196.

Toure G, Duboucher C, Vacher C (2005) Anatomical modifications of the temporomandibular joint during ageing. *Surg Radiol Anat* **27**(1):51–55.

Towheed TE, Maxwell L, Judd MG, *et al* (2006) Acetaminophen for osteoarthritis. *Cochrane Database Syst Rev* (1):CD004257.

Uddman R, Grunditz T, Kato J, *et al* (1998) Distribution and origin of nerve fibers in the rat temporomandibular joint capsule. *Anat Embryol (Berl)* **197**(4):273–282.

Undt G, Murakami K, Rasse M, *et al* (2006) Open versus arthroscopic surgery for internal derangement of the temporomandibular joint: a retrospective study comparing two centres' results using the Jaw Pain and Function Questionnaire. *J Craniomaxillofac Surg* **34**(4):234–241.

van der Kraan PM, van den Berg WB (2000) Anabolic and destructive mediators in osteoarthritis. *Curr Opin Clin Nutr Metab Care* **3**(3):205–211.

Voog U, Alstergren P, Eliasson S, *et al* (2003) Inflammatory mediators and radiographic changes in temporomandibular joints of patients with rheumatoid arthritis. *Acta Odontol Scand* **61**(1):57–64.

Ward DM, Behrents RG, Goldberg JS (1990) Temporomandibular synovial fluid pressure response to altered mandibular positions. *Am J Orthod Dentofacial Orthop* **98**(1):22–28.

Warner BF, Luna MA, Robert Newland T (2000) Temporomandibular joint neoplasms and pseudotumors. *Adv Anat Pathol* **7**(6):365–381.

Westesson PL, Rohlin M (1984) Internal derangement related to osteoarthrosis in temporomandibular joint autopsy specimens. *Oral Surg Oral Med Oral Pathol* **57**(1):17–22.

Westesson PL, Eriksson L, Lindstrom C (1987) Destructive lesions of the mandibular condyle following discectomy with temporary silicone implant. *Oral Surg Oral Med Oral Pathol* **63**(2):143–150.

Westesson PL, Kurita K, Eriksson L, *et al* (1989) Cryosectional observations of functional anatomy of the temporomandibular joint. *Oral Surg Oral Med Oral Pathol* **68**(3):247–251.

Westling L (1992) Temporomandibular joint dysfunction and systemic joint laxity. *Swed Dent J Suppl* **81**:1–79.

Widmalm SE, Brooks SL, Sano T, *et al* (2006) Limitation of the diagnostic value of MR images for diagnosing temporomandibular joint disorders. *Dentomaxillofac Radiol* **35**(5):334–338.

Wilkes C (1989) Internal derangement of the TMJ. *Arch Otolaryngol Head Neck Surg* **115**:469.

Wolford LM, Cardenas L (1999) Idiopathic condylar resorption: diagnosis, treatment protocol, and outcomes. *Am J Orthod Dentofacial Orthop* **116**(6):667–677.

Xinmin Y, Jian H (2005) Treatment of temporomandibular joint osteoarthritis with viscosupplementation and arthrocentesis on rabbit model. *Oral Surg Oral Med Oral Pathol Oral Radiol Endod* **100**(3):e35–e38.

Xu Y, Zhang ZG, Zheng YH (2005) [Measurement and analysis of the intra-articular pressure in temporomandibular joint with sudden-onset, severe closed lock]. *Hua Xi Kou Qiang Yi Xue Za Zhi* **23**(1):41–42.

Yap AU, Dworkin SF, Chua EK, *et al* (2003) Prevalence of temporomandibular disorder subtypes, psychologic distress, and psychosocial dysfunction in Asian patients. *J Orofac Pain* **17**(1):21–28.

Yelland MJ, Nikles CJ, McNairn N, *et al* (2007) Celecoxib compared with sustained-release paracetamol for osteoarthritis: a series of n-of-1 trials. *Rheumatology (Oxford)* **46**:135–140.

Yoshida A, Higuchi Y, Kondo M, *et al* (1998) Range of motion of the temporomandibular joint in rheumatoid arthritis: relationship to the severity of disease. *Cranio* **16**(3):162–167.

Yoshida H, Fujita S, Nishida M, *et al* (1999) The expression of substance P in human temporomandibular joint samples: an immunohistochemical study. *J Oral Rehabil* **26**(4):338–344.

Yoshida K, Takatsuka S, Hatada E, *et al* (2006) Expression of matrix metalloproteinases and aggrecanase in the synovial fluids of patients with symptomatic temporomandibular disorders. *Oral Surg Oral Med Oral Pathol Oral Radiol Endod* **102**(1):22–27.

Yuasa H, Kurita K (2001) Randomized clinical trial of primary treatment for temporomandibular joint disk displacement without reduction and without osseous changes: a combination of NSAIDs and mouth-opening exercise versus no treatment. *Oral Surg Oral Med Oral Pathol Oral Radiol Endod* **91**(6):671–675.

Yura S, Totsuka Y (2005) Relationship between effectiveness of arthrocentesis under sufficient pressure and conditions of the temporomandibular joint. *J Oral Maxillofac Surg* **63**(2):225–228.

Zarb GA, Carlsson GE (1999) Temporomandibular disorders: osteoarthritis. *J Orofac Pain* **13**(4):295–306.

Zardeneta G, Milam SB, Schmitz JP (1997) Elution of proteins by continuous temporomandibular joint arthrocentesis. *J Oral Maxillofac Surg* **55**(7):709–716; discussion 716–707.

Zardeneta G, Milam SB, Lee T, *et al* (1998) Detection and preliminary characterization of matrix metalloproteinase activity in temporomandibular joint lavage fluid. *Int J Oral Maxillofac Surg* **27**(5):397–403.

Zardeneta G, Milam SB, Schmitz JP (2000) Iron-dependent generation of free radicals: plausible mechanisms in the progressive deterioration of the temporomandibular joint. *J Oral Maxillofac Surg* **58**(3):302–308; discussion 309.

Zea-Aragon Z, Terada N, Ohtsuki K, *et al* (2005) Immunohistochemical localization of phosphatidylcholine in rat mandibular condylar surface and lower joint cavity by cryotechniques. *Histol Histopathol* **20**(2):531–536.

CHAPTER 9

Migraine and possible facial variants
(neurovascular orofacial pain)

Yair Sharav and Rafael Benoliel

1. Introduction

Chapters 9 and 10 deal with primary neurovascular cranio-facial pain (NVCP) and their orofacial clinical equivalents. NVCP includes the migraines, trigeminal autonomic cephalgias (TACs) and hemicrania continua (HC). The term neurovascular emphasizes the aetiology of the pain considered to result, at least partly, from an interaction between the nervous and vascular systems (Goadsby 2001). The TACs is a novel group appearing in the most recent International Headache Society's (IHS) classification (Olesen *et al* 2004a) and includes cluster headache (CH), paroxysmal hemicrania (PH) and short-lasting neuralgiform headache attacks with conjunctival injection and tearing (SUNCT); these will be discussed in the following chapter along with HC.

Common clinical features of NVCPs include pain that is unilateral, episodic, severe and pulsatile, causes waking from sleep and is often accompanied by local autonomic signs usually ocular (tearing, redness), nasal (rhinorrhea, congestion), local swelling or redness. Accompanying systemic signs such as nausea, vomiting and photo- or phonophobia are also observed.

However, although sharing many signs and symptoms, NVCPs are clearly classified based on well-defined criteria of location, attack frequency, duration, accompanying signs or symptoms and treatment response.

Referral of pain to oral structures is very common in NVCPs and pain quality often resembles dental pathologies so that patients with NVCP are often encountered in orofacial pain clinics. We collected cases with NVCP and,

applying IHS criteria, diagnosed 15% as migraine without aura, 22% as episodic cluster headache and 11% as paroxysmal hemicrania, leaving 52% as unclassifiable and later grouped by us into an entity termed neurovascular orofacial pain (NVOP) (Benoliel *et al* 1997). Taking into account the population prevalence rates of the entities involved, it is apparent that migraine patients approach orofacial pain specialists less than TAC patients do. This is probably due to the referral patterns of the syndromes involved.

Migraines and TACs are classically located around the ocular and frontal regions. However, primary neurovascular type pain in the lower two-thirds of the face has been reported in the literature (Benoliel *et al* 1997; Penarrocha *et al* 2004). These patients are not easily classified with IHS criteria and have been termed facial migraine, lower-half-facial migraine or vascular orofacial pain (Benoliel *et al* 1997; Daudia and Jones 2002; Penarrocha *et al* 2004; Lance and Goadsby 2005). Based on these reports we suggest an additional diagnostic subentity to the classification of primary NVCP, namely neurovascular orofacial pain (Benoliel *et al* 1997; Sharav 1999). The mechanisms and clinical manifestations of NVOP may be related to the pathophysiology of migraine and/or TACs and understanding these entities is therefore crucial.

2. Migraine

Migraine is a common primary headache with an additional number of rarer related syndromes; see Table 9.1 (Olesen *et al* 2004a). The combination of a high prevalence, severe pain and debilitating neurological symptoms

Table 9.1	International Headache Society's (IHS) Classification of Migraine Subtypes	

Category	Classification	Notes
1.1	**Migraine without aura**	Detailed in text
1.2	**Migraine with aura**	Detailed in text
1.2.1	Typical aura with migraine headache	Detailed in text
1.2.2	Typical aura with non-migraine headache	Aura may accompany headaches other than migraine
1.2.3	Typical aura without headache	Aura that occurs with no headache
1.2.4	Familial hemiplegic migraine	Familial migraine with unilateral motor symptoms
1.2.5	Sporadic hemiplegic migraine	Non-familial appearance of 1.2.4
1.2.6	Basilar-type migraine	Migraine with aura symptoms clearly of brainstem origin, or from both hemispheres
1.3	**Childhood periodic syndromes that are common precursors of migraine**	
1.3.1	Cyclical vomiting	Vomiting/nausea accompanied by pallor. Self-limiting condition
1.3.2	Abdominal migraine	Episodic midline abdominal pain, moderate to severe and lasting 1–72 hours. Associated with vasomotor symptoms, nausea/vomiting
1.3.3	Benign paroxysmal vertigo of childhood	Recurrent and brief vertigo, spontaneous resolution
1.4	**Retinal migraine**	Repeated monocular visual disturbances (may include blindness) preceding migraine without aura
1.5	**Complications of migraine**	
1.5.1	Chronic migraine	Detailed in text
1.5.2	Status migrainosus	Migraine attack lasting >72 hours
1.5.3	Persistent aura without infarction	Long-lasting (>1 week) aura symptoms without evidence of brain infarct (neuroimaging)
1.5.4	Migrainous infarction	One or more migraine aura symptoms accompanying an ischaemic brain lesion (neuroimaging)
1.5.5	Migraine-triggered seizure	Epileptic seizure triggered by migraine
1.6	**Probable migraine**	Headaches or related symptomatology missing a feature that otherwise would classify it as a disorder from 1.1–1.5
1.6.1	Probable migraine without aura	
1.6.2	Probable migraine with aura	
1.6.3	Probable chronic migraine	

Criteria adapted from Olesen *et al* (2004a), with permission.

increases the social impact of migraine to that beyond other primary headaches. The two most common types of migraine headaches are migraine without aura (MWA) and migraine with aura (MA), often confused in the clinic and in the literature (Olesen 2000). In this section we will describe MWA, MA and chronic migraine (CM).

The clinical features of the headache phase in MWA and in MA are very similar and are described under the section for MWA. Features specific to MA are discussed under that section.

2.1. Migraine Without Aura

2.1.1. Clinical Features

MWA, previously termed common migraine or hemicrania simplex, is the most common form of migraine (Olesen *et al* 2004a). MWA is a disease affecting the young with an onset before the age of 20 years in about half of the cases (Steiner *et al* 2003).

Case example. Case 9.1 is MWA and classic in its presentation and clinical behaviour. This particular case would be difficult to confuse with tension-type headache (TTH; see below). However, confusion with the TACs due to some autonomic activation and its periorbital location could easily occur (Chapter 10, differential diagnosis).

Location. Headache is typically unilateral with no side preference, but is reported bilaterally in some patients (Rasmussen *et al* 1991a; Rasmussen and Olesen 1992a; Kelman 2005). Migraine that occurs persistently on the same side (side-locked migraine) has been observed in up to half of migraineurs (Kelman 2005).

A single location is rarely encountered and commonly migraines occur in the ocular, temporal and frontal regions (Kelman 2005). Other areas often involved are the occipital and neck regions whilst the vertex and diffuse location are rarer (Kelman 2005) (see Fig. 9.1) Clinical impressions suggest that 3% of migraine and TTH patients in a neurology clinic complain of intraoral pain (Bussone and Tullo 2005), and in our experience this is even more

Case 9.1 Migraine Without Aura, 41-year-old Female

Present complaint

Strong pain (VAS 8) around the eye, forehead and upper teeth (Fig. 9.3). Usually the pain is unilateral (left) side but side shift does occur. Pain is throbbing often with superimposed sharp pain and lasts from 9 to 48 hours, depending on whether she can rest and on response to treatment. Rarely, she suffers a milder bilateral headache that is pressing in quality and located frontally and occipitally.

History of present complaint

Similar though milder unilateral pain attacks began at the age of 15 (frequency 1/2–3 months). Over the years the pain became stronger and more frequent particularly during stressful periods. At the time of examination frequency had increased dramatically. Pain is menstrually related. During some attacks she feels a throbbing pain in the ipsilateral molars.

Premonitory signs include repeated yawning and tiredness. Pain is accompanied by photophobia, phonophobia, nausea and when intense pain is present also ipsilateral ptosis and nasal congestion. During attacks she is unable to brush her hair as this is very painful. On resolution of symptoms, she feels very tired.

Interictal jabs of severe pain (ice pick) around the left eye occur with no warning signs and independent of migraine. These are very severe (VAS 9), last seconds and occur either in clusters or individually (see Fig. 9.2).

Physical examination

Pericranial muscle tenderness (bilateral) was present with no limitation of jaw movement; cranial nerve examination was normal. Interoral exam (including bite-wing radiographs) revealed no dental or other pathology.

Relevant medical history

Hypothyroidism since age 35, takes 50 μg Eltroxin. Oral contraceptive pill (5 years) with no change in headache parameters. Mother suffered from severe migraines up till menopause.

Diagnosis

Migraine without aura. Infrequent tension-type headache (TTH), with pericranial muscle tenderness.

Diagnostic and treatment considerations

The early onset and associated family history are typical of migraine. Due to the change in headache frequency patient underwent a brain CT, which was normal. The long duration, premonitory signs, accompanying features and the headache resolution phase make migraine without aura the most likely diagnosis. The intraoral pain is secondary to migraine as we excluded a dental source. A pain diary confirmed that the headaches were menstrually related, with few attacks in between (Fig. 9.2). The patient also reported infrequent (2–3/month) attacks of very sharp short-lasting pain around the eye, but not within a migraine. The bilateral headaches were rarer and matched a diagnosis of TTH; these responded to mild analgesics. Abortive therapy was initiated with sumatriptan that caused intolerable side effects—similar results were obtained with rizatriptan. The patient also reported only mild resolution of symptoms with the triptans employed. Soluble aspirin (1 g stat) produced significant reduction in pain intensity and duration in about 70% of attacks. Similar results were obtained with naproxen sodium (775 mg stat). The patient has thus far opted to remain on abortive therapy and refuses prophylactic therapy.

common in orofacial pain clinics due to biased patient referral. A migraine-like headache is reported to occur in the lower half of the face (Lance and Goadsby 2005) but remains unclassified by the IHS. This entity will be discussed in detail below under the section on neurovascular orofacial pain.

Quality. Typically pain is throbbing or pulsating (47–82%) but may be occasionally pressing (Table 9.2; Rasmussen *et al* 1991a; Russell *et al* 1996; Stewart *et al* 2003). Pain intensity is moderate to severe and on average a visual analogue scale (VAS) rating of 7.5 is reported (Steiner *et al* 2003). However, pain intensity is not uniform; mild to moderate (VAS 3–6) and moderate to severe (VAS 7–8) pain is reported by about 40% of migraneurs each and 15% report very severe pain (VAS 9–10) (Stewart *et al* 2003). Some patients (24%) describe exacerbations of pain within an attack (Stewart *et al* 2003). Others report interictal short, sharp periorbital pain, often described as icepick pains (Rasmussen and Olesen 1992b).

A feature of MWA is that it is almost invariably (95%) aggravated by routine physical activity such as walking or climbing stairs (Rasmussen *et al* 1991a; Russell *et al* 1996). Many patients report that even moving the head, coughing or breath holding will accentuate headaches.

Temporal pattern. Headache development is often insidious and from a mild nonspecific ache to a typical migraine may take 0.5–2 hours (Zagami and Rasmussen 2000). Migraine is a periodic headache lasting 4–72 hours, and longer lasting attacks are considered 'status migrainosus' (Olesen *et al* 2004a). In about half of migraineurs pain duration was 5–24 hours and a third reported pain lasting more than 25 hours (Stewart *et al* 2003). In a small number (16.4%) duration was less than 5 hours (Solomon *et al* 1985; Stewart *et al* 2003).

For most migraineurs in the population headache frequency is less than one per month (Rasmussen *et al* 1991b; Pryse-Phillips *et al* 1992; Steiner *et al* 2003). However, attack frequency varies considerably from 6–12 per

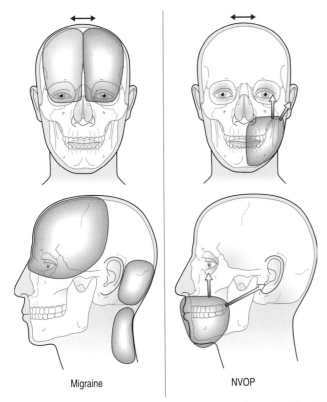

Migraine   NVOP

Fig. 9.1 • Pain location in migraine and neurovascular orofacial pain (NVOP). Migraine pain is typically periorbital and frontotemporal with referral to suboccipital and neck regions, usually unilateral but may be bilateral in up to 30% of cases (this has been marked by a lighter shaded area contralaterally). NVOP is characterized by its location in the lower two-thirds of the face with intraoral and perioral areas frequently involved as primary sites. Two-headed arrow above diagram indicates side shift occurrences in specific headache.

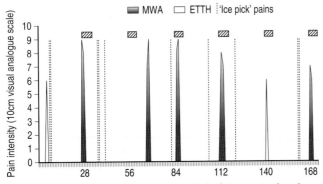

Fig. 9.2 • Case 9.1's pain diary over a period of 6 menstrual cycles. Note that the migraines without aura (MWA) are menstrually related but not exclusively; MWA occurs at other points of the menstrual cycle and not at every menstruation (marked by hatched rectangles) and generally lasts for the better part of 1–2 days. On rare occasions she suffers a bilateral dull headache of shorter duration and less severe with no accompanying signs (see day 140) and these are infrequent episodic tension-type headaches (ETTH). Additionally she experiences sharp, severe jabs of momentary pain around the eye ('icepick' pain): marked by vertical line.

year (46%) to 1–2 per month (20%), up to 2–4 per month (16%) (Stewart *et al* 2003). Clinic populations report more frequent headaches with a third suffering more than 4 attacks monthly (Magnusson and Becker 2003). MWA has a higher average attack frequency and is usually more debilitating than MA. Seasonal or cyclic patterns have

been associated with migraine attacks, often correlating with light hours (Fox and Davis 1998; Alstadhaug *et al* 2005).

Decreased quality of life between attacks (interictally) has been recognized in migraine patients (Cavallini *et al* 1995; Steiner 2000). Although comorbidity can partially explain some of the disability, migraineurs report significant interictal behavioural symptoms such as reduced activity, reduced vigour and a higher level of sleepiness (Stronks *et al* 2004).

A minority (15.6%) of migraineurs describe daily or near-daily headaches (Stewart *et al* 2003) and according to the IHS classification such frequent migraine attacks are distinguished as *chronic migraine*, as described below.

Associated signs. On average 50% of migraineurs vomit during an attack, 80% report nausea and more than 80% of migraineurs report photo- or phonophobia (Rasmussen *et al* 1991a; Rasmussen and Olesen 1992a). Associated signs are more prominent and common in severe headaches (Rasmussen *et al* 1991a; Russell *et al* 1992). However, not all headaches are accompanied by the same signs, even within patients. For example, nausea and photo- or phonophobia accompany more than half of headache episodes in only a third or fewer of migraineurs (Stewart *et al* 2003).

Migraine may present with ipsilateral autonomic signs (AS), most usually lacrimation (~50%), demonstrating significant correlation with unilateral and severe attacks (Barbanti *et al* 2002; Kaup *et al* 2003).

Premonitory symptoms and headache resolution phase. Many migraineurs will report some type of premonitory symptom before some or all headaches and these may accurately predict migraine onset by days or hours (Giffin *et al* 2003; Kelman 2004a). The most common symptoms are tiredness, difficulty in concentration and stiff neck. Additionally hyper- or hypoactivity, depression, food craving and repetitive yawning are reported. Some of the following signs have been found to be relatively reliable in predicting headache: speech difficulty, reading/writing difficulty, yawning, emotional changes, blurred vision and phonophobia (Giffin *et al* 2003). A high percentage of patients may report photo- and phonophobia and nausea in the premonitory phase (Giffin *et al* 2003) but it is important to stress that most premonitory signs are actually part of the migraine complex and not a trigger.

The headache resolution phase is gradual in most patients, with similar signs to those observed in the premonitory phase (Giffin *et al* 2003). Common symptoms include mood changes, muscle weakness, tiredness and reduced appetite that last 23 hours on average but may continue for up to 2 days (Giffin *et al* 2003).

2.1.2. Migraine Triggers

Several factors, termed triggers or precipitating factors, have been reported as initiators of individual attacks in migraineurs (Table 9.3; Martin and Behbehani 2001). One

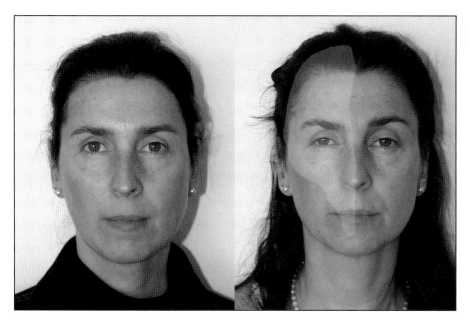

or more such factors are reported by up to 90% of migraineurs (Rasmussen 1993; Chabriat *et al* 1999). However, only a subgroup of migraineurs reacts to specific triggers and individual migraineurs do not always get a headache with the same precipitant. Many studies found that anxiety and stress are the most common precipitants but as stress is also a prodromal sign, care must be exercised in interpretation (Rasmussen 1993; Spierings *et al* 2001).

Other common triggers include foods (e.g. chocolate, cheese), alcoholic beverages (e.g. wine), menstruation, sensory stimuli, fatigue and changes in weather. Often a patient will report more than one factor that may act together or individually (Rasmussen 1993; Chabriat *et al* 1999).

Although precipitants are accepted as clinically relevant there is a paucity of research that conclusively and consistently links most of these to migraine (Breslau and Rasmussen 2001). Moreover many precipitating factors may not differentiate tension-type headache from migraine. Interestingly precipitants were identical between the two groups and largely induced more severe headaches in migraineurs (Chabriat *et al* 1999). However, fatigue, sleeping difficulties, foods and drinks, menstruation, weather changes, smells, smoke and light have been significantly associated with migraine (Karli *et al* 2005).

Dietary. Foods and drinks are significantly and consistently related to headache onset in migraineurs (Chabriat *et al* 1999). The frequency of dietary trigger factors reported by migraine patients varies widely from 7 to 44% (Robbins 1994). The most consistent are chocolate, cheese, fruit and alcoholic beverages. However, double-blind studies of chocolate as a migraine trigger have been inconclusive (Gibb *et al* 1991; Marcus *et al* 1997). Food sensitivity is not consistently able to differentiate between patients with migraine or tension-type headache (Savi *et al* 2002); however, although foods trigger both headache types chocolate and cheese seem highly related to migraine (Smetana 2000). Alcoholic drinks precipitate headache in

many migraineurs and many principally identify red wine (Rasmussen 1993; Peatfield 1995).

Migraine and sleep. The relationship between sleep and headaches is well established (Dodick *et al* 2003; Rains and Poceta 2005). Many migraineurs report that sleeping, even for a couple of hours, will abolish headache and frequently migraine patients either choose or feel forced to go to sleep to relieve headaches (Kelman and Rains 2005). Moreover a lack of sleep will often induce migraines and disturbed or excessive sleep can trigger a headache. The sleep association and inherent periodicity of migraine headaches suggests involvement of central sites in biological rhythm. In humans these are located in the posterior hypothalamic grey, an area termed the suprachiasmatic nucleus (Leone and Bussone 1993). Nearly two-thirds of migraineurs report symptoms suggestive of hypothalamic dysfunction and disturbed sleep patterns are present during nights preceding headache (Goder *et al* 2001). Additionally, many (71%) patients reported at least occasionally being woken from sleep by a migraine (Kelman and Rains 2005). Migraines are more likely to occur during periods of rapid eye movement (REM) sleep and with morning arousals (Dodick *et al* 2003).

Migraine and the menstrual cycle. Oestrogen has long been considered to play a role in headache. In addition to its better known functions, oestrogen is a central neuromodulator (Ceccarelli *et al* 2004) and its withdrawal can induce headache: 'oestrogen withdrawal headache' (Olesen *et al* 2004a). Furthermore many women report improvement or resolution of migraine headaches during late pregnancy (Russell *et al* 1996; Rasmussen 2001). Since gender differences persist past menopause other major influences on migraine headaches are clearly involved.

Variations in hormone levels during puberty, menstruation, menopause or exogenous hormones (contraceptives, hormone replacement) are associated with migraine onset and changes in headache pattern (more in MWA than in MA). Oral contraceptives worsen

Table 9.2 Diagnostic Criteria for Migraine without Aura

Diagnostic Criteria		Notes
A	At least 5 attacks fulfilling criteria B-D	Individuals who otherwise meet criteria for migraine without aura but have had fewer than 5 attacks should be coded *probable* migraine without aura.
B	Headache attacks lasting 4–72 hours (untreated or unsuccessfully treated)	When the patient falls asleep during migraine and wakes up without it, duration of the attack is calculated until the time of awakening.
C	Headache has at least two of the following characteristics: 1. Unilateral location 2. Pulsating quality 3. Moderate or severe pain intensity 4. Aggravation by or causing avoidance of routine physical activity	Migraine headache is commonly bilateral in young children. Occipital headache in children is rare and calls for diagnostic caution; many cases are attributable to structural lesions. *Pulsating* means throbbing or varying with the heart beat.
D	During headache at least one of the following occurs: 1. Nausea and/or vomiting 2. Photo- and phonophobia	In young children, photo- and phonophobia may be inferred from their behaviour.
E	Not attributed to another disorder	History and physical examination do not suggest any structural lesion or other disorders, or such disorder is ruled out by appropriate investigation, or the attacks do not occur for the first time in close temporal relation to the disorder.

Criteria adapted from Olesen *et al* (2004a), with permission.

Table 9.3 Common Migraine Triggers

Group	Example
Endogenous factors	
Hormonal changes	Menstruation (4) Contraceptive pill Hormone replacement therapy
Fatigue (1)	
Mental	Stress (2) Cessation of stress ('weekend headache')
Exogenous factors	
Alcoholic beverages (3)	Red wine Beer
Foodstuffs (3)	Chocolate Cheese Hot Dogs
Drugs Chemical additives	Nitrites Monosodium glutamate Aspartame Caffeine (or withdrawal) Amines: e.g. histamine, phenylethylamine (PEA), tyramine
Strong or flickering lights	
Weather changes (5)	
Head trauma	Footballer's headache
Behavioural	
Missed meals Oversleeping Physical exertion	

Numbers in parentheses rate the most common precipitants according to frequency reported: 1 = most frequent, 5 = least. Some of the factors have overlapping mechanisms; e.g. wine contains alcohol and nitrites, some cheeses contain tyramine.

MWA more often than MA but with no significant change in treatment response (Granella *et al* 2004). Headaches, in general, are very common around menstruation and in the population up to a quarter of women report menstrually related migraine (Couturier *et al* 2003; Martin *et al* 2005). In the clinic, however, over half of female patients report menstruation as a common migraine precipitant occurring more in MWA (Robbins 1994; Chabriat *et al* 1999; Granella *et al* 2000). Indeed MWA often has a prominent menstrual relation, and in the IHS classification has been subclassified in the appendix as *pure menstrual migraine* and *menstrually related migraine* (Olesen *et al* 2004a). Pure menstrual migraine is classified as headache fulfilling criteria for MWA with attacks occurring exclusively from 2 days prior to 2 days following onset of endometrial bleeding in a normal menstrual cycle or after withdrawal of OCP; it is proposed that it may respond better to hormone replacement (Olesen *et al* 2004a). Menstrually related migraine is classified as headache fulfilling criteria for MWA with attacks occurring in two-thirds of menstrual cycles from 2 days prior to 2 days following menstruation and additionally at other times of the cycle. Menstrually related migraine headaches are significantly longer and more severe and resistant to abortive treatment than attacks at any other time of the menstrual cycle and therefore induce increased work-related disability (Granella *et al* 2004).

Oestrogen receptors have been localized to brain in regions involved in migraine pathogenesis and migraine-linked variation has been demonstrated in the oestrogen SR1 gene, suggesting a role in migraine susceptibility

(Colson *et al* 2004). The neuropeptides galanin and neuropeptide Y are involved in the neuronal response to trigeminal nerve injury. These peptides have been shown to be modulated during the natural oestrous cycle in trigeminal ganglia, suggesting hormonal regulation of these peptides (Puri *et al* 2005). This cyclic influence on trigeminal ganglion peptides may contribute to oestrogen-related changes in trigeminal excitability and headache.

2.2. Migraine with Aura

Previously used terms were classic or classical migraine, ophthalmic, hemiparaesthetic, hemiplegic or aphasic migraine, migraine accompagnee and complicated migraine (Olesen *et al* 2004a). Typical aura with migraine headache is the most common migraine syndrome associated with aura (see Table 9.4).

MA is a recurrent disorder manifesting in attacks of reversible focal neurological symptoms that usually develop gradually over 5–20 minutes and last for less than 60 minutes. These neurological symptoms (the aura) are reported by about 40% of migraineurs and are followed in about 10 minutes by a headache fulfilling the criteria for MWA (Kelman 2004b). In most cases headache will follow the aura (93%), and in a minority headache and aura will occur simultaneously (4%) or the aura will follow headache (3%) (Russell and Olesen 1996). Less commonly, the headache lacks migrainous features or is indeed completely absent. We limit our discussion in this section to *typical aura with migraine headache.*

The typical aura consists of visual and/or sensory and/or speech symptoms. It develops gradually and lasts no longer than an hour. The focal neurological symptoms that usually precede or sometimes accompany the headache consist of one or more of the following: visual disturbances, unilateral paraesthesia and/or numbness, unilateral weakness, aphasia or unclassifiable speech difficulty (Olesen *et al* 2004a). In a large population-based study (Russell and Olesen 1996) visual symptoms were most frequent (99%), followed by sensory (31%), aphasic (18%) and motor (6%) symptoms. When several types of aura symptoms were reported, visual aura was invariably present (Russell and Olesen 1996; Kelman 2004b). The typical visual aura starts as a flickering, uncoloured, zigzag line in the centre of the visual field and affects the central vision — a fortification spectrum. Areas of lost vision (scotomata) may also be observed at this stage. The area progresses towards the periphery of one hemifield and often leaves a residual scotoma.

Next in frequency are sensory disturbances (pins and needles) affecting a variable part of one side of the body and face. The typical sensory aura is unilateral, starts in the hand, progresses towards the arm and then affects the face and tongue. Less frequent are speech disturbances, usually dysphasic but often hard to categorize. The typical motor aura is half-sided and affects the hand

Table 9.4	Diagnostic Criteria for Typical Aura with Migraine Headache	
Diagnostic Criteria		**Notes**
A	At least 2 attacks fulfilling criteria B–D	
B	Aura consisting of at least one of the following but no motor weakness: 1. Fully reversible visual symptoms including positive features (i.e. flickering lights, spots or lines) and/or negative features (i.e. loss of vision) 2. Fully reversible sensory symptoms including positive features (i.e. pins and needles) and/or negative features (i.e. numbness) 3. Fully reversible dysphasic speech disturbances	If includes motor weakness code as *familial or sporadic hemiplegic migraine.* Don't mistake sensory loss for weakness. Symptoms usually follow one another in succession beginning with visual, then sensory symptoms and dysphasia, but the reverse and other orders have been noted.
C	At least two of the following: 1. Homonymous visual symptoms and/or unilateral sensory symptoms 2. At least one aura symptom develops gradually over 5 minutes and/or different aura symptoms occur in succession over 5 minutes 3. Each symptom lasts >5 and <60 minutes	Additional loss or blurring of central vision may occur
D	Headache fulfilling criteria B–D for *migraine without aura* begins during the aura or follows aura within 60 minutes	
E	Not attributed to another disorder	History and physical examination do not suggest any structural lesion or other disorders, or such disorder is ruled out by appropriate investigation, or the attacks do not occur for the first time in close temporal relation to the disorder.

Criteria adapted from Olesen *et al* (2004a) with permission.

and arm. Complete reversibility characterizes a headache-associated aura; the visual, sensory and aphasic auras rarely last >1 hour, while in many cases the motor aura may persist (Russell and Olesen 1996). Diagnostic criteria for typical aura with migraine headache are presented in Table 9.4.

2.3. Migraine without Aura and Migraine with Aura: Separate Entities?

Whether MA and MWA are part of a continuum or distinct entities has been much disputed (Olesen and Cutrer 2000). The continuum theory is based on the clinical co-occurrence of MA and MWA, the similarity between MA and MWA during the prodrome, the headache and the resolution phases and the similar therapeutic response. Clinical observations also suggest that one form may transform into the other (Olesen 2000). However, clinical, epidemiological, pathophysiological and genetic findings suggest that MA and MWA are distinct (Russell and Olesen 1995; Russell *et al* 1996). The co-occurrence of MA and MWA is no more than a random occurrence (Russell *et al* 2002). Moreover, headaches in MA are less severe and shorter than in MWA and in MWA a hormonal influence is clearer (Russell *et al* 1996; Granella *et al* 2000). In a population-based twin sample it was found that unilateral headache, photophobia and a shorter duration were associated with MA whilst nausea was more common in MWA (Kallela *et al* 1999).

Dilatation of large inter- and extracranial arteries occurs in both forms during an attack, but regional cerebral blood flow (rCBF) changes are present only in MA (Olesen 2000). Finally imaging and biochemical studies suggest that these are two distinct entities (Russell *et al* 1996; Zeller *et al* 2005).

2.4. Differential Diagnosis

The clinical overlap between MWA and tension type headaches is prominent, but the overall profile of signs and symptoms differs (Table 9.5). The similarities may at times be very marked and some believe them to be clinical phenotypes of a common pathophysiology — the convergence hypothesis (Cady *et al* 2002). Mild nausea and photo- and phonophobia form part of the TTH phenotype and diagnosis may often be difficult. However, these signs are usually more severe and frequent in MWA; therefore routinely grading them in the clinic (mild, moderate, severe) is recommended (Iversen *et al* 1990; Rasmussen *et al* 1991a; Koseoglu *et al* 2003).

TTH is mostly bilateral whilst MWA is largely unilateral, although bilateral migraine and unilateral TTH may be observed in significant proportions (Koseoglu *et al* 2003; Kelman 2005). Pain is consistently more intense in migraine than in TTH and may be a sensitive marker (Rasmussen *et al* 1991a; Zebenholzer *et al* 2000). Similarly attack duration in MWA is usually longer than in episodic TTH but may overlap particularly as migraine attacks of <5 hours have been observed (Solomon *et al* 1985; Stewart *et al* 2003). Local autonomic signs (e.g. lacrimation) may occur in migraine to a higher degree than previously considered and this has not been reported in TTH. Classically TTH is not considered to be exacerbated by physical activity whilst MWA is. However,

| Table 9.5 | Differentiating Signs and Symptoms for Migraine without Aura (MWA) and Episodic Tension-Type Headache (ETTH). | |

Parameter	MWA	ETTH
Location	Unilateral	Bilateral
Quality	Throbbing	Aching/ pressing
Severity	Moderate to severe	Mild to moderate
Duration	4–72 hours	30 mins–7 days
Physical activity aggravates pain	Yes	Occasionally
Photo- and phonophobia	May have both	Only one
Anorexia	Yes	Yes
Nausea, vomiting	May have both	None
Associated autonomic signs	In severe attacks	None
Wakes from sleep	Yes	No
Menstrual trigger	High association	Low association

reports of TTH aggravated by exercise have appeared (Pryse-Phillips *et al* 1992; Koseoglu *et al* 2003).

A careful history and assessment of individual pain characteristics will usually facilitate correct diagnosis (Zebenholzer *et al* 2000). Routine use of pain diaries and careful reassessment will identify misdiagnosed cases.

Secondary migraine. Headaches with migraine characteristics may occur for the first time in close approximation to a primary organic cause (Campbell and Sakai 2000). Vascular disorders such as transient ischaemic attacks, thromboembolic stroke, intracranial haematoma, subarachnoid haemorrhage and arterial hypertension may cause migraine-like headaches. Intracranial tumours and infections may also cause migraine-like headaches. Many of these are sudden onset headaches or are accompanied by atypical neurological signs and symptoms and need referral for imaging and neurological management. Indications for neuroimaging in headaches are discussed in Chapter 1. Neurovascular type headaches following head and neck trauma have been described (Baandrup and Jensen 2005).

Very often cervicogenic headache is similar in its clinical presentation to that seen in migraine and other neurovascular headaches. This entity is described in detail in Chapter 13 and is also discussed with TACs in Chapter 10.

2.5. Chronic Migraine (CM)

Epidemiological studies demonstrate that 2–2.5% of the general population has chronic migraine (CM). A proportion of migraineurs (15.6%) describe daily or near-daily headaches

(Stewart *et al* 2003). Recent evidence suggests that a sub-group of migraine sufferers may have a clinically progressive disease in which migraine episodes increase in frequency over time (Lipton and Pan 2004; Lipton and Bigal 2005). Longitudinal epidemiologic studies showed that over the course of one year 3–14 % of individuals with episodic headache progressed to chronic daily headache (CDH) (Scher *et al* 2003; Katsarava *et al* 2004). Additionally MWA is most prone to accelerate with frequent use of symptomatic medication, resulting in a new headache termed *medication-overuse headache; see Chapter 13* (Olesen *et al* 2004a).

Case example. The patient described in Case 9.2 had a typical history of episodic headaches that over a period of 2–3 years became CM. Response to pharmacotherapy was very good and long-term follow-up has shown improvement in disability and consistent pain relief. Compare the case to that described under chronic type NVOP.

Limited data are at our disposal to predict which patients will progress from episodic to CM (Lipton and Bigal 2005). Clear risk factors are prior head trauma (Couch and Bearss 2001) and drug abuse (Katsarava *et al* 2004); but these would be currently subclassified into relevant diagnoses. The risk increases significantly in Caucasians, with obesity and a high baseline headache frequency (Scher *et al* 2003; Katsarava *et al* 2004).

CM is defined as a headache that occurs on more than 15 days monthly for more than 3 months in the absence of medication overuse (Olesen *et al* 2004a). The headache must meet criteria C and D for MWA (Table 9.2) and not be secondary to another disorder. Most cases with CM seem to begin as episodic migraine and *transform* into chronicity (Mathew *et al* 1987; Solomon *et al* 1992). Indeed many patients report episodic migraine that around age 30–40 became increasingly frequent although this may not always be easy to recall. Particularly in females CM is still accompanied by migrainous features (e.g. nausea, photophobia), although of decreasing intensity. Menstrual relation and other triggers may still be

---

Case 9.2 Chronic Migraine, 41-year-old Female

Present complaint

Continuous headache over the eye and frontotemporal region (Fig. 9.4). Unilateral (usually right) but may also be bilateral in the same areas. Character is pressing and dull often with a pulsating quality and may wake in the early morning. Pain intensity is mostly constant (VAS 5–6), with frequent exacerbations of VAS 7–8. When pain exacerbates it is accompanied by photo/phonophobia and often nasal congestion. Pain refers to ipsilateral maxilla and feels like a toothache.

History of present complaint

Twenty-six-year history of episodic migraine without aura (MWA), successfully treated with nonspecific abortive medications (largely NSAIDs). Mean attack frequency for MWA had been 2–3 per month. About 2–3 years ago frequency increased and was successfully treated with propranolol. However, the patient had stopped medication about 2 years ago. A short time following this, over a period of some months, frequency had gradually increased to a point where she was rarely free from headaches and suffered constant pain of variable intensity. In addition to daily pain the patient reported significant social and work disability; she was currently unemployed due to the headaches.

Physical examination

Pericranial and masticatory muscle tenderness present bilaterally.

Relevant medical history

Eight months previously epidermoid cyst removal via craniotomy. Treated with carbamazepine postoperatively with no change in chronic headache pattern.

Diagnosis

Chronic daily headache; chronic migraine (transformed migraine).

Diagnostic and treatment considerations

Primary chronic daily headaches includes chronic migraine, chronic tension-type headache, hemicrania continua and new daily persistent headache. Often the subentities are difficult to distinguish and a definitive diagnosis is based on the history and treatment response. A trial of indomethacin up to 100 mg daily had not provided relief, suggesting that this was not hemicrania continua. A common secondary cause would be analgesic abuse headache but our patient had no history of such drug abuse. In this case post-traumatic headache is not relevant due to the fact that the craniotomy had been performed well after (>1 year) the onset of chronic migraine and surgery had not altered the headache pattern in any way. We initiated therapy with valproic acid starting at 200 mg daily and escalating every 3 days by 200 mg to a maintenance dose of 600 mg daily in 3 doses. The effect was remarkable: pain relief occurred very rapidly (Fig. 9.5) and the patient returned to useful part-time employment within 2 months of therapy. We have been able to follow up this patient for 4 years (2.5 years are shown in graph) and with occasional dose titrations (400–800 mg/d) of valproic acid have maintained long-term relief of pain and disability. Note that occasional exacerbations in pain do occur but overall a VAS of <2.5 has been obtained. The follow-up suggested that 800 mg was superior to 600 mg valproic acid in providing pain relief but was accompanied by increased side effects so that the patient preferred a 600-mg maintenance dose.

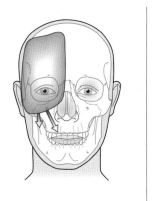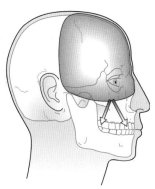

Fig. 9.4 • Case 9.2; pain location.

prominent, and severe typical migraine attacks occur superimposed on the chronic headache (Srikiatkhachorn and Phanthumchinda 1997; Krymchantowski and Moreira 2001). Classically the headache location is bilateral in the frontotemporal region, but up to half may be strictly unilateral (Spierings et al 1998; Krymchantowski and Moreira 2001). Headache is mostly mild to moderate with a dull and pressing quality (Krymchantowski and Moreira 2001). Truly continuous headache is observed in under half of patients, and although most patients do not awaken with a headache many will develop it during early morning. Night-time arousals due to headache were reported particularly by women (Spierings et al 1998; Krymchantowski and Moreira 2001).

Anxiety and depression seem to be very common in CM patients, affecting from one-third to nearly 90% of patients (Krymchantowski and Moreira 2001). Hypothalamic dysfunction has also been found in chronic migraine (Peres et al 2001).

3. Migraine Epidemiology

In individuals up to 64 years of age, the average annual incidence rate was 3.4–3.7 per 1000 person-years, affecting twice as many women as men (Stang et al 1992; Rasmussen 2001). New cases of migraine are uncommon among males but relatively common among females in their late 20s with the highest rates found in the 25–34 years age group (males 6.5, females 22.8 per 1000) (Stewart et al 1991; Lyngberg et al 2005). Among both males and females under the age of 30 years, the incidence rate for migraine with visual aura appears to peak earlier than MWA (Stewart et al 1991). Both MA and MWA peak earlier in boys, which explains why in childhood males have a higher prevalence of migraine than girls (Lipton and Bigal 2005). However, the incidence of migraine has been studied less extensively than its prevalence (Lipton and Bigal 2005).

Prevalence studies in Western countries show that migraine affects approximately 10–12% of the adult population, but figures are not always consistent (Rasmussen et al 1991b; Henry et al 1992; Stewart et al 1992; O'Brien et al 1994). In both men and women, the overall prevalence of migraine has been found highest from age 30–40 years (Lipton and Bigal 2005). The prevalence is consistently higher in females (18%) than in males (6%) (Lipton et al 2001a). No sex differences are apparent until age 11; above that a female preponderance appears, possibly linked to female hormones.

In most studies MWA is slightly more prevalent than MA (Rasmussen and Olesen 1992a). The 1-year prevalence of MA is 2–5.8% (males 1.3–4%, females 6–9%) (Rasmussen and Olesen 1992a; Steiner et al 2003). Lifetime prevalences for MA in over 1000 respondents in the USA were 3.4% for males and 7.4% for females (Breslau et al 1991).

Between 1981 and 1989 a 60% increase in the prevalence of migraine in the United States was observed; from 25.8 to 41 per 1000 person-years (Centers for Disease Control 1991). This increase may reflect improved diagnosis and awareness rather than a real prevalence increase. Race differences have been demonstrated in epidemiological studies of migraine, suggesting altered genetic susceptibility (Breslau and Rasmussen 2001). In general, African and Asian countries show prevalence rates lower than those of North America or European countries. This has been replicated in race-based studies in North America where Caucasians showed rates higher than those of African or Asian Americans (Stewart et al 1996a).

Fig. 9.5 • Mean weekly visual analogue scale rating (VAS) for Case 9.2. Since initiation of therapy with valproic acid a marked and relatively rapid improvement was observed. Note that exacerbations do occur even on prophylactic regimens and some dose response is apparent with 800mg being more efficient than 600 mg. Arrows and figures in mg denote duration and dosage of valproic acid.

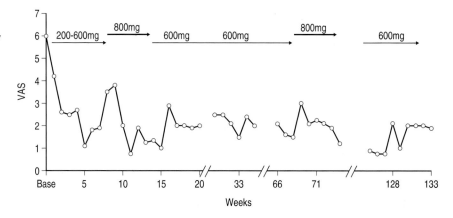

4. Migraines and Disability

The World Health Organization (WHO) (Murthy *et al* 2001) ranks migraine nineteenth amongst disability-inducing diseases in both men and women. In women migraine is ranked twelfth, attesting to the severe effects migraine exerts in females. Eighty percent of migraineurs report disability secondary to headaches and more than half of the attacks result in significant interference with daily activities (Steiner *et al* 2003; MacGregor *et al* 2004). The high prevalence during the most productive years of life imposes a substantial cost in lost workdays (Steiner *et al* 2003; Lipton and Bigal 2005). It has been estimated that 5.7 workdays/year are lost for every working or student migraineur, although most of this effect is produced by the most disabled 10% (Steiner *et al* 2003). Migraineurs report significantly reduced work efficiency (40 to >50%) due to headache with a greater impact on productivity (Stewart *et al* 1996b; Von Korff *et al* 1998). Indeed it has been estimated that more than 25 million work- or school-days are lost worldwide on a yearly basis due to migraine headaches (Murthy *et al* 2001; Steiner *et al* 2003).

Pain diaries may be used to assess headache disability but these give data only on headache frequency and intensity. A recommended approach is to apply the migraine disability assessment (MIDAS) questionnaire that is simple to use and has been shown to capture unique information relating to the disabling consequences of headache beyond frequency and intensity (Stewart *et al* 2000, 2003).

5. Migraine Comorbidity

Several disorders have been associated with migraine both in community and in patient samples (Merikangas and Rasmussen 2000; Scher *et al* 2005). Strong evidence suggests a relation between migraine and depression or anxiety, stroke (particularly in MA with smoking), other pain syndromes and allergies. Less substantial is the link between migraine and asthma, cardiovascular disease (including mitral valve prolapse), gastrointestinal disorders and epilepsy. The exact mechanisms involved are not entirely clear.

6. Genetics

There is up to a twofold increase of MWA amongst first-degree relatives of probands suffering MWA and a four-fold increase in MA (Russell and Olesen 1995; Stewart *et al* 1997). Twin studies in MWA and in MA reveal a maximum proband concordance rate of 50% in monozygotic and dizygotic twins (higher in females) (Gervil *et al* 1999; Ulrich *et al* 1999). These and other studies of inheritance factors emphasize that both MWA and MA are caused by the combined effects of environment and genetics and suggest a multifactorial inheritance pattern (Ferrari and Russell 2000).

A severe form of MA is linked to an autosomal dominant disease termed familial hemiplegic migraine (FHM). Migraineurs with FHM present with transient attacks of spreading neurologic phenomena including hemiparesis and some FHM families may display cerebellar degeneration or seizures. About half of FHM families' genotype has been linked to a mis-sense mutation on chromosome 19p13 (FHM1) (Joutel *et al* 1993; Ophoff *et al* 1994), others to chromosome 1q21 (FHM2) or 1q23 (Ducros *et al* 1997) and some to none of these, suggesting at least a third gene. The specific FHM site on chromosome 19p13 encodes the brain expressed voltage gated a-1A Ca^{2+}-channel sub-unit gene, CACNA1A (Ophoff *et al* 1996). In FHM2, mutations have been found in the ATP1A2 gene essential for maintaining sodium gradients that facilitate intercellular Ca^{2+} export (De Fusco *et al* 2003; Vanmolkot *et al* 2003). These loci may give rise to abnormal channel dynamics and altered levels of excitability in migraineurs. They may also affect the threshold for the initiation of cortical spreading depression (CSD) in migraine patients, a phenomenon linked to migraine aura and capable of initiating trigeminal nociceptor activity.

The identification of mutations on the CACNA1A gene in FHM led to the hypothesis that other migraine variants may be also attributable to polymorphisms or mutations in this gene. A nearby but distinct locus was found in families with MA (Jones *et al* 2001). However, recent studies suggest that multiple receptor polymorphisms and multigene inheritance are involved in migraine (Mochi *et al* 2003; Estevez and Gardner 2004).

7. Pathophysiology

Historically migraine was considered to be a vascular phenomenon: the aura was due to transient ischaemia secondary to vasoconstriction and the headache was secondary to rebound vasodilatation and mechanical activation of perivascular nociceptors (Goadsby *et al* 2002). Current evidence, however, does not support this hypothesis. Magnetic resonance angiography has clearly shown that changes in flow or vessel diameter in migraine (and in cluster headache) are a *result* of pain in the trigeminal ophthalmic division (Weiller *et al* 1995; May *et al* 1998a, 2001; Bahra *et al* 2001). Brainstem areas activated in migraine, but not in tension-type headache or controls, include the periaqueductal grey, the locus coeruleus and the dorsal raphe nucleus (Weiller *et al* 1995; Bahra *et al* 2001). These areas are involved in the sensory modulation of craniovascular afferents. The migraine aura has been experimentally linked to a wave of oligaemia spreading slowly (2–6 mm/min) across the cortex (Sanchez del Rio *et al* 1999). A short hyperaemic phase precedes oligaemia and correlates, in migraine patients, with aura signs such as flashing lights (Hadjikhani *et al* 2001). However, the oligaemia persists throughout the headache phase and is probably a reaction to depressed neuronal function (Cutrer *et al* 1998). Finally the local oxygen supply is adequate (Cao *et al* 2002) and migraine headaches may be experimentally induced with no changes in vessel diameter (Kruuse *et al* 2003) so that taken together the data refute the vascular hypothesis. Migraine is therefore considered to arise from a primary brain dysfunction that leads to activation and sensitization of the trigeminovascular system.

In order to understand the pathophysiology of migraine we must appreciate the role of the various elements involved. Peripherally these include the anatomy of the trigeminovascular system and the physiology of neurogenic inflammation with plasma extravasation. Centrally, the processing of signals in the trigeminal nucleus (particularly the trigeminocervical complex) and the contribution of cortical structures, brainstem and diencephalic modulatory systems that control trigeminal pain processing are considered key elements (Goadsby 2005a).

7.1. The Trigeminovascular System

The trigeminovascular system consists of trigeminal neurons (largely from the ophthalmic division) and the blood vessels (usually cerebral) they innervate (Fig. 9.6). The bipolar cell bodies of these neurons are located in the trigeminal ganglion (TG). The peripheral axons synapse with cranial structures and craniofacial blood vessels (particularly the pain-producing large cranial vessels), whereas the centrally projecting fibres synapse in the

trigeminal nucleus caudalis and the upper two cervical divisions, the trigeminocervical complex (Goadsby and Hoskin 1997). A plexus of mainly unmyelinated fibres that arise from the ophthalmic division of the trigeminal fibres and the upper cervical dorsal roots surrounds the cerebral and pial vessels, the large venous sinuses and the dura mater. These fibres contain substance P (SP) and calcitonin gene-related peptide (CGRP), released when the trigeminal ganglion is stimulated (Uddman *et al* 1985; Goadsby *et al* 1988a). Nerve fibres are distinguishable on the basis of their neuropeptide content; sensory fibres are rich in SP, CGRP, nitric oxide (NO) and neurokinin A; parasympathetic fibres contain vasoactive intestinal polypeptide (VIP) and NO; and sympathetic fibres express neuropeptide-Y (Tajti *et al* 1999a,b). These peptides (NO, SP, CGRP, VIP) induce vasodilatation and plasma extravasation and are released into the blood stream; they may therefore be assayed as indicators of trigeminal and autonomic nerve fibre activation.

7.2. Neurogenic Inflammation

Neurogenic inflammation occurs when trigeminal afferents are stimulated antidromically and release vasoactive neuropeptides that induce mast cell degranulation and plasma extravasation. Because of similarities with the reactive inflammatory response it has been termed neurogenic or 'sterile' inflammation. Activation of trigeminal nociceptors and neurogenic inflammation may occur peripherally or centrally. Neuropeptide release will further activate trigeminal afferents, inducing sensitization.

Neurogenic inflammation in the trigeminovascular system of the dura and other craniofacial structures is considered to play a central role in the initiation of neurovascular type headaches. However, there is no conclusive evidence that neurogenic inflammation occurs in humans with migraine (Goadsby 2005a).

The main function of trigeminal afferents is the transduction of information from the craniofacial areas to the central nervous system (CNS). However, additional efferent roles important in wound healing and homeostasis via peripherally released neurotransmitters have become apparent. Stimulation of peripheral trigeminal nerves leads to antidromic neuropeptide release at the periphery. These neuropeptides include SP, CGRP and neurokinin A (NKA), the most potent vasodilator being CGRP. The fibres releasing these neuropeptides are characteristic of thin, unmyelinated C fibres. When released, the neuropeptides initiate a cascade of events including mast cell degranulation, platelet aggregation, vasodilatation and plasma extravasation (Izumi 1999), i.e. neurogenic inflammation (Fig. 9.6).

Similarly, stimulation of the TG in cats induces the release of SP and CGRP into the cranial circulation (Goadsby *et al* 1988b). Stimulation of the TG or the superior sagittal sinus will induce a cerebral vasodilatatory

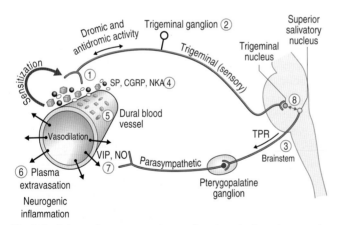

Fig. 9.6 • Schematic representation at the trigeminal-cerebrovascular junction (1). Cell bodies of cerebrovascular and other orofacial nociceptors reside in the trigeminal ganglion (2) with their second-order neurons in trigeminal nucleus caudalis (3). Neurogenic inflammation: vasoactive peptides such as calcitonin gene-related peptide (CGRP), substance P (SP) and neurokinin A (NKA) are released from trigeminal C fibres (4) following antidromic activation, possibly secondary to brainstem dysfunction. These peptides bind to receptors (5) and induce vasodilation (6), plasma extravasation and further nociceptor activation. Although rare, local autonomic signs such as lacrimation have been reported in migraine. This is thought to be secondary to reflex parasympathetic activation (the trigeminoparasympathetic reflex, TPR) mediated by connections between the trigeminal system and the superior salivatory nucleus (8, SSN) at brainstem level (see also Chapter 10). Similar processes may also occur within oral and dental tissues, leading to a primary neurovascular orofacial pain syndrome.

response and a concomitant increase in rCBF. Clinically this has been observed during thermocoagulation of the human TG by dermatomal facial flushing accompanied by an increase in local temperature (Drummond et al 1983). Concomitant increases in levels of SP and CGRP occur in the external jugular vein but not in the peripheral circulation (Schon et al 1987; Goadsby et al 1988b). A decrease in carotid artery resistance accompanied by increased facial temperatures also occurs following TG stimulation in experimental animals (Lambert et al 1984; Goadsby et al 1986). Electrical stimulation of the trigeminal ganglion leads to increases in extracerebral blood flow and local release of SP, CGRP and vasoactive VIP (May and Goadsby 1999).

Although to date there are no strong supporting human data, indirect support may be drawn from experiments, suggesting that migraine pain may be secondary to neurogenic inflammation (Moskowitz 1990). During attacks of migraine, CH and CPH plasma levels of CGRP are elevated, indicating trigeminal nociceptor activation (Goadsby and Edvinsson 1996). Furthermore it has been recently shown that nitroglycerin-triggered migraine is also associated with CGRP release (Juhasz et al 2003). Sumatriptan, an anti-migraine drug, blocks the plasma extravasation associated with neurogenic inflammation (Moskowitz and Cutrer 1993) and reduces elevated CGRP levels in parallel to headache relief (Goadsby and Edvinsson 1993). Moreover intravenous administration of CGRP induces headache and migraine in migraineurs (Lassen et al 2002) and a highly specific CGRP antagonist is effective in the treatment of migraine attacks (Olesen et al 2004b). Taken together these studies clearly establish the important role of CGRP in migraine and suggest that it is released secondary to trigeminal nerve activation (neurogenic inflammation).

It is important to note at this point that the observed vasodilatatory effect is thought also to be partly mediated by reflex activation of the parasympathetic system and the release of VIP (Fig. 9.6; Goadsby and Edvinsson 1994). Noxious stimulation of the superior sagittal sinus induces activity in neurons of the superior salivatory nucleus (Knight et al 2005), an important relay in the cranial parasympathetic outflow to the lacrimal and nasal glands. Reflex activation would therefore induce AS such as reported by migraineurs during severe headaches and by TAC patients. This reflex activation is particularly important in understanding TAC and is therefore discussed in Chapter 10.

The role of NO in headaches has received much attention (Thomsen and Olesen 2001; Goadsby 2005b). Nitroglycerin, an NO prodrug, reliably induces CH and migraine headache associated with CGRP release (Juhasz et al 2003), indistinguishable or very similar to spontaneous attacks (Ashina et al 2004; Sances et al 2004). Plasma nitrate levels are elevated interictally in CH and migraine patients, suggesting a basal dysfunction in NO metabolism and supporting the involvement of NO in

neurovascular headaches (D'Amico et al 2002; Costa et al 2003). NO synthase inhibitors have been shown experimentally to attenuate neuronal activation in the trigeminocervical complex following sagittal sinus stimulation (Hoskin et al 1999a), and clinically to relieve migraine headache (Lassen et al 1997). The data thus support a prominent role for NO in the pain associated with neurovascular headaches.

In summary, while it is generally accepted that initiation of a sterile inflammatory response would cause pain, it is not clear what initiates this process. Some studies suggest that CSD may be a sufficient stimulus to activate trigeminal neurons (Bolay et al 2002) and brainstem areas are increasingly being proposed as candidate generators in migraine (see below). Whether neurogenic inflammation is sufficient or requires other stimulators or promoters is similarly unclear. Blockade of neurogenic plasma protein extravasation is not completely predictive of antimigraine efficacy in humans as evidenced by the failure in clinical trials of SP antagonists (Diener 2003; Goadsby 2005a).

7.3. The Trigeminocervical Complex

Activation of meningeal trigeminovascular afferents activates second-order neurons in trigeminal nucleus caudalis and upper two cervical divisions (together the trigeminocervical complex). Following meningeal irritation, neuronal activation is detected in the trigeminal nucleus caudalis (Nozaki et al 1992) and stimulation of the superior sagittal sinus activates neurons in the trigeminocervical complex in the cat (Kaube et al 1993a), thus accounting for the referral of pain to the neck so commonly observed in the clinic. Stimulation of a lateralized structure, the middle meningeal artery, activates neurons bilaterally in both cat and monkey brain (Hoskin et al 1999b), a finding that is consistent with the fact that up to one-third of patients complain of bilateral pain. Experimental pharmacological evidence suggests that abortive antimigraine drugs such as ergots, acetylsalicylic acid and triptans act at these second-order neurons and reduce neuronal activity (Goadsby 2005a). Neuronal inhibition via 5HT receptors can occur at two levels: prejunctional, which will inhibit neuropeptide release from primary afferents and inhibit neurotransmission (Buzzi et al 1991; Buzzi and Moskowitz 1991), and postjunctional, which inhibits neurons in trigeminal nucleus caudalis (Kaube et al 1993b). This activity may reflect 5HT-1B, 5HT-1D or 5HT-1F receptor agonist action, or a combination of these (Goadsby and Classey 2003). There is solid evidence for the synthesis of 5-HT1D and 5-HT1F receptors in human TG (Rebeck et al 1994; Bouchelet et al 1996) and these locate to small and medium-sized neurons often co-localizing with glutamate and CGRP (Bonaventure et al 1998; Ma 2001; Ma et al 2001). Thus 5-HT1D and 5-HT1F receptors are in a prime location to inhibit release of neuropeptides intimately involved in the pathogenesis of migraine. Furthermore, the demonstration that some part of this action is postsynaptic offers the future prospect of highly anatomically localized treatment options (Goadsby 2005a). Unfortunately 5HT-1B receptors are also found on coronary arteries, accounting for the cardiovascular side effects of triptans.

Following transmission in the caudal brainstem, information is relayed rostrally to pain-related areas such as the brainstem periaqueductal grey (PAG) and the thalamus. The PAG is involved in craniovascular pain perception through ascending projections to the thalamus and descending inhibitory modulation of nociceptor activity (Knight and Goadsby 2001). Trigeminal nociceptors from both dural and facial areas are modulated by the PAG (Bartsch et al 2004). Capsaicin application to the superior sagittal sinus has shown that trigeminal projections with a high degree of nociceptive input are processed particularly in neurons of the ventroposteromedial thalamus and in its ventral periphery (Zagami and Lambert 1991). Human imaging studies have confirmed activation of thalamus contralateral to pain in acute migraine (Afridi et al 2005a,b; Bahra et al 2001).

7.4. Central Pain Activation and Modulation

Figure 9.6 summarizes the brainstem regions, the neurovascular interaction and higher brain centres thought to underlie pain in migraine and NVOP.

Central nervous system activation may be a primary event triggering trigeminal nociceptor activity and peripheral pain sensation at the vascular bed (Moskowitz et al 1993). A nociceptive stimulus to the rat cortex induces blood flow changes reminiscent of CSD (Bolay et al 2002) known to be involved in the human migraine aura (Hadjikhani et al 2001). Activation of trigeminal neurons in subnucleus caudalis was detected secondary to this accompanied by vasodilatation and plasma extravasation, all attenuated by trigeminal nerve section (Bolay et al 2002). An SP-receptor antagonist also attenuated plasma extravasation, supporting that this phenomenon is under sensory-nerve control. Parasympathetic nerve section attenuated vasodilatation but not plasma extravasation (Bolay et al 2002). In summary a central noxious event activated trigeminal afferents (i.e. pain) with reflex parasympathetic activation. These induced vasodilatation and neurogenic inflammation (increased nociceptor activation and ensuing sensitization), establishing a model that explains pain, vasodilatation and other AS in neurovascular headaches. Plasma extravasation was thus clearly shown to be under trigeminal nerve control whilst vasodilatation seemed to be dependent on intact trigeminal and parasympathetic systems, suggesting involvement of a trigeminoparasympathetic reflex (TPR). However, there is no evidence for CSD in MWA, CH or other NVCPs, although this may yet be identified in other cortical areas. Alternatively, based on current knowledge,

other brain regions may be active such as the brainstem in migraine and the hypothalamus in CH.

During MWA, human positron emission tomographic (PET) studies demonstrate activation of the PAG in the region of the dorsal raphe nucleus, the dorsal pons and near the locus coeruleus (Afridi et al 2005a,b; Weiller et al 1995). These areas are active immediately after successful treatment of the headache but not interictally (Weiller et al 1995). Activation of 5-HT-1B/1D receptors, by local injection of naratriptan into ventrolateral PAG produces selective inhibition of trigeminovascular nociceptive afferent input but not facial afferents (Bartsch et al 2004). This finding may have important consequences for the treatment of other neurovascular pains located in the orofacial region such as CH and NVOP. Migraine-like headaches are induced when PAG areas are electrically stimulated (Raskin et al 1987; Veloso et al 1998), or triggered by structural pathologies affecting the PAG (Haas et al 1993; Goadsby 2002). Iron homeostasis in the PAG has been demonstrated to be progressively impaired in MA, MWA and chronic headache (Welch et al 2001). These results support the hypothesis that the PAG is a major element in the pathophysiology of migraine attacks, possibly acting as a central generator or as a permissive dysfunctional control of trigeminovascular nociception. Blockade of calcium channels in the PAG significantly enhances trigeminal nociception linking dysfunctional ion channels and disrupted PAG modulation in migraine pathophysiology (Knight et al 2002).

Interestingly brainstem activation was observed contralateral (Weiller et al 1995), ipsilateral (Afridi et al 2005b) and left-sided (Afridi et al 2005a) but due to study limitations the issue of brainstem activation and headache laterality is unsolved. These same brainstem structures are active in CM, further linking its pathophysiology to that of MWA (Matharu et al 2004). Since brainstem areas are activated specifically in migraines and not in CH (May et al 1998a, 2000) or experimental pain (May et al 1998b) brainstem activation is considered central to migraine pathophysiology. Therefore migraine is likely to involve a disorder of brainstem areas associated with modulation of sensory processing (Afridi et al 2005a). Based on the findings that the structure of the hypothalamus is changed in CH (May et al 1999) the possibility that migraineurs' brain structure is altered has been studied with PET but no differences were found (Matharu et al 2003).

Although there are still unanswered questions there have been great advances in the understanding of migraine pathophysiology. The role of neurogenic inflammation is unclear; however, it is apparent that some form of central sensitization takes place during migraine (Burstein et al 2000). Observed widespread allodynia is consistent with third-order neuronal sensitization such as in thalamic neurons clearly supporting a CNS component to the pathophysiology of migraine (Burstein et al 2000, 2004). The establishment of sensitization is a crucial negative factor in determining the outcome of triptan treatment (Burstein *et al* 2004). This finding has therefore led to a change in treatment philosophy so that early and aggressive intervention is advised; migraine attacks in humans treated with triptans prior to the onset of allodynia respond significantly better than those with allodynia (Waeber and Moskowitz 2003; Burstein *et al* 2004).

The source of pain in migraine is likely to be a combination of direct factors, i.e. activation of the nociceptors of pain producing intracranial structures together with a reduction in the functioning of the endogenous pain control pathways that normally modulate pain (Goadsby *et al* 1991; Goadsby 2005a). This may manifest as hyperexcitability of which there is accumulating evidence in migraineurs (Welch 2003).

8. Treatment

There is currently no cure for migraine, but adequate control can be achieved for the majority of cases. Patient education and symptomatic and prophylactic treatments are the essential cornerstones of successful treatment in all headaches (Dodick *et al* 2000).

Patient education includes provision of accurate and comprehensible information about the disorder and explaining the importance of contributing factors such as sleep, diet and other lifestyle practices that may precipitate attacks (Pryse-Phillips *et al* 1998). Some patients may, for health or personal reasons or due to intolerable side effects, prefer non-pharmacologic therapies such as stress-management training, acupuncture and physical therapy (Campbell *et al* 2000). Often combining modalities with each other or with pharmacologic agents may improve outcome (Campbell *et al* 2000). Based on current understanding of the pathophysiologic processes involved in migraine the pharmacotherapeutic emphasis is no longer on altering vascular tone but on stabilizing involved neuromodulatory systems.

Pharmacological treatment can be abortive (acute, symptomatic) or preventive (chronic, prophylactic). Abortive treatment is taken during or just prior to attack onset with the aim of stopping the pain attack whilst prophylactic medication is taken on a daily basis in order to reduce the severity, duration and frequency of migraine attacks. Despite the severe disability associated with migraine up to half of migraineurs will not seek medical advice and self-medicate (Lipton *et al* 2002; MacGregor *et al* 2003). The most common medications (22–54%) are simple over-the-counter (OTC) analgesics (Lipton *et al* 2002; MacGregor *et al* 2003). Even after physician consultation, only 3–19% are prescribed triptans and overall less than half of migraineurs are satisfied with their current treatment (MacGregor *et al* 2003). It is therefore important to thoroughly assess the patient's response to therapy. Often nonspecific medication may be rated as satisfactory but a trial of triptans results in improved quality of life. Indeed patient satisfaction with triptans is significantly higher than with conventional first-line medications (Robbins 2002). Alternative management strategies employed by patients include avoidance of trigger factors, stress management, relaxation therapy, regular exercise and herbal/homeopathic remedies (MacGregor *et al* 2003). Particularly bed rest is commonly employed (62%) to supplement care (MacGregor *et al* 2003), suggesting that patients are not optimally managed.

All treatment strategies are based on accurate diagnosis and good baseline data. Patients may often need to manage a pain diary and return for re-assessment before definitive therapy is initiated. In the following section we review drug therapies for migraine and whenever relevant quote figures for number needed to treat (NNT) and number needed to harm (NNH); see Chapters 15 and 16.

8.1. Abortive Treatment

Abortive therapy is usually utilized when there are less than four attacks per month but may be augmented with prophylactic medications in special circumstances. Additionally abortive drugs are often used to supplement prophylactic regimens that do not totally eradicate headaches; in these situations the drugs are often referred to as 'escape' medications. The major goals of abortive therapy are to rapidly (<2 hours) relieve headache with no recurrence, cause minimal (or no) side effects, restore function and reduce additional medication use (Matchar *et al* 2000; Diamond and Cady 2005). An attempt should also be made at identifying individuals at risk and preventing disease progression into chronic migraine (Diamond and Cady 2005). Many therapies not only relieve headache, but also alleviate associated symptoms such as nausea (Goadsby *et al* 2002). Acute migraine therapy can be strategically approached in three ways: step care within attack, step care between attacks and stratified care (Lipton *et al* 2000a; Diamond and Cady 2005). In step care, the first-line medication will often be a relatively inexpensive analgesic with a good safety profile. Nonresponders are 'stepped up' to a more specific drug (e.g. a triptan) in a stepped fashion till a satisfactory outcome is obtained. This strategy can be applied within a single attack (step care within attack) or between a number of attacks (step care between attacks). Usually treatment escalates over time from simple analgesics to combination medications (e.g. analgesic plus antiemetics) to migraine-specific drugs (e.g. triptans) as necessary. In stratified care, initial treatment is selected based on assessment of severity of attacks and associated disability. Stratified care provides a significantly better and faster clinical outcome and is more cost effective than the two other strategies (Lipton *et al* 2000a; Sculpher *et al* 2002).

8.1.1. Nonspecific Medication

The preference of the patient, including cost and past experience as well as any contraindications, must be taken into consideration (Goadsby *et al* 2002). Efficacy of abortive therapy is maximized when an appropriate dose is initiated as early in the course of the attack as possible. Analgesics and anti-inflammatory drugs are to be considered first, and if these are not effective triptans should be utilized. Rarely opioids, preferably as an intranasal spray, may be considered. Fixed drug combinations (FDC) are also available; some contain ergot derivatives combined with other medications such as caffeine, codeine and antiemetics and may be sufficient for many cases (Loder 2005). No uniform data on efficacy of oral ergot formulations are available, and these are less commonly utilized since the triptans became available. Parenteral ergot formulations although effective are impractical for routine use. However, trials with intranasal dihydroergotamine (2mg) reveal a significant positive effect at 30 minutes (NNT 2.4 (1.9–3.5)) (Tfelt-Hansen and Saxena 2000). Analgesics such as 1000 mg aspirin preferably as an effervescent tablet or ibuprofen (400*–800mg, *NNT 7.5 (4.5–22)) are good first-line alternatives in the acute treatment of migraine (Matchar *et al* 2000; Morillo 2004; Diener *et al* 2005). For patients unable to take NSAIDs 1000 mg paracetamol may be effective (NNT 5.2 (3.8–9.2)) (Moore *et al* 2003). Combination analgesics may be superior to single drugs but results may be inconsistent. For mild to moderate headaches FDCs such as aspirin with acetaminophen and caffeine (AAC) with an NNT of 3.9 (3.2–4.8) may provide excellent response rates, superior to sumatriptan 50 mg (Matchar *et al* 2000; Diener *et al* 2005; Goldstein *et al* 2005). Aspirin with the antiemetic metoclopramide (NNT 3.5 (2.8–4.4)) or acetaminophen with codeine also have proven clinical efficacy (Matchar *et al* 2000; Tfelt-Hansen and McEwen 2000). If these fail, 550–825 mg naproxen sodium, or 50–100 mg diclofenac can be tried (Matchar *et al* 2000; Tfelt-Hansen and McEwen 2000). Most of these analgesics and NSAIDs can be obtained OTC and are associated with improper dosing or timing, leading to treatment failure, abuse and the risk of serious side effects such as gastric complications or withdrawal/abuse headaches. A summary of the more commonly used abortive treatments for migraine is presented in Table 9.6.

8.1.2. Triptans

Triptans (selective 5-HT$_{1B/1D}$ receptor agonists) have become the drug of choice when specific agents for abortive treatment of migraine are needed to relieve pain and associated signs (Matchar *et al* 2000; Silberstein 2000). Indeed triptans are the most widely employed (64%) prescription drug for migraine in the United States (Diamond and Cady 2005). Response to triptans is not, however, considered pathognomonic of migraine; patients with TTH and CH also respond. Triptans are thought to act at a number of sites both peripherally and centrally; see Chapter 16.

The introduction of sumatriptan represented a remarkable advancement in the treatment and research of migraine headache. It stimulated the development of

Table 9.6 Some of the Common Abortive Treatments for Migraine

Class	Drugs	Initial Oral Dose (mg)
Analgesics	Aspirin	500–1000
Combinations	Aspirin and	500–600
	Paracetamol and	200–400
	Caffeine	50–200
	Paracetamol and	400
	Codeine	25
Ergot alkaloids	Dihydroergotamine NS	2
NSAIDs: Non specific	Naproxen sodium	550–825
	Ibuprofen	400–800
	Diclofenac	50–100
Selective COX-2 inhibitors	Rofecoxib	25–50
Triptans (5HT agonist)	Sumatriptan	50–100
	Sumatriptan NS	20 (1 NS metered dose)
	Sumatriptan SC	6
	Naratriptan	2.5
	Eletriptan	40
	Rizatriptan	10
	Zolmitriptan	2.5
	Zolmitriptan NS	2.5 (1 NS metered dose)
Opioids	Butorphanol NS	1–2 metered doses

NS, nasal spray; SC, subcutaneous injection; NSAIDs, nonsteroidal anti-inflammatory drugs.

several second-generation agents such as zolmitriptan, naratriptan, rizatriptan, almotriptan, eletriptan and frova-triptan (Tfelt-Hansen *et al* 2000). Eletriptan, naratriptan, rizatriptan and zolmitriptan display increased stability to first-pass metabolic inactivation by monoamine oxidase as well as decreased hydrophilicity, resulting in a two- to fivefold increase in oral bioavailability relative to sumatriptan (Millson *et al* 2000). Rizatriptan and zolmitriptan are also available in a rapidly dissolving wafer formulation, which can be taken without water, a particular advantage in patients with nausea (Dahlof *et al* 1999). Unfortunately these new drugs are not superior in parameters such as speed of onset and recurrence rates (Dahlof *et al* 2002). Sumatriptan nasal spray (20mg) is significantly better than placebo but the difference is modest (NNT 6.7), inconsistent and the taste unpleasant (Dahlof 2003). More recently sumatriptan has been combined with naproxen, providing superior results to either drug alone (Smith *et al* 2005). Zolmitriptan 5 mg intranasal spray (NNT 2.85 (2.5–3.2)) has a rapid onset (15 minutes) with good tolerability and is the drug of choice for this route of administration (Dodick *et al* 2005). A summary of the triptan's efficacy

Table 9.7	The Triptans (5HT Agonists): Summary of Efficacy and Side Effect Profile		
Drug/Route	**Dose (mg)**	**NNT**	**NNH**
Sumatriptan	50	3.87	23.38
Sumatriptan SC	6	2.64	3.25
Naratriptan	2.5	6.49	−98.50
Rizatriptan	10	3.15	7.10
Zolmitriptan	2.5	5.92	26.82

Efficacy: pain free at 2 hours: side effect profiles: all adverse effects.

and adverse effects as measured by NNTs and NNHs is shown in Table 9.7. Some triptans have the potential for significant drug interactions, such as sumatriptan, rizatriptan and zolmitriptan with MAO inhibitors; zolmitriptan with cimetidine; and eletriptan with P-glycoprotein pump inhibitors (Tepper *et al* 2003). Other interactions should be considered with medications such as propranolol, serotonin selective reuptake inhibitors (SSRIs) and ergot derivatives (Ferrari 2003).

8.1.2.1. Side Effects and Safety
The most frequent adverse events are dizziness, somnolescence, nausea, fatigue, chest symptoms and paraesthesias (Ferrari *et al* 2001; Goadsby *et al* 2002). Adverse events occur less frequently with naratriptan and almotriptan than with rizatriptan, sumatriptan, zolmitriptan and eletriptan, and the tolerability profile of almotriptan 12.5 mg resembles that of placebo (Dahlof *et al* 2002). A sensation of chest tightness is a well-documented adverse effect with sumatriptan and occurs in 3–5% of patients (Dahlof *et al* 1994). These symptoms often mimic the pain of myocardial infarction, but are not associated with ECG changes and are not due to coronary vasoconstriction or cardiac ischaemia (Dahlof and Mathew 1998). In a PET study, subcutaneous sumatriptan (6 mg) did not affect myocardial perfusion in a group of subjects without cardiovascular disease (Lewis *et al* 1997). Although sumatriptan has an acceptable risk–benefit ratio, very rare but serious cardiovascular adverse events contraindicate the use of triptans in patients with coronary artery disease (Welch *et al* 2000; Dahlof *et al* 2002; Goadsby *et al* 2002). Almotriptan and naratriptan appear to have fewer chest symptoms than sumatriptan or zolmitriptan, but do not confer superior cardiovascular safety (Dahlof *et al* 2002; Goadsby *et al* 2002). Particularly, the possible interaction between triptans and prophylactic drugs such as propranolol (Ferrari 2003) should be considered; see later. Many migraineurs will be taking antidepressants, particularly SSRIs, due to comorbidity

of migraine and depression (Tepper *et al* 2003). The serotonin syndrome is a potential complication when co-prescribing triptans with SSRIs; however, this seems to be very rare (Putnam *et al* 1999).

Efficacy and side effects may not be similar across patients and clinicians need to be familiar with a number of triptans (Ferrari *et al* 2002). Differences between the triptans may be clinically significant and expert recommendation suggests that rizatriptan 10 mg will consistently provide rapid relief (Ferrari *et al* 2002; Dodick *et al* 2004). The newer almotriptan (12.5 mg) has good efficacy and tolerability whilst eletriptan will provide high efficacy with low recurrence but low tolerability (Ferrari *et al* 2002). These three triptans are currently considered the drugs of choice (Dodick *et al* 2004). A good starting point is low doses of rizatriptan (5 mg) or eletriptan (40 mg) with titration as necessary. Sumatriptan remains the most versatile drug with oral, intranasal, subcutaneous (SC) and rectal formulations. Indeed the SC format provides the most consistent and efficacious relief from migraine but with a high frequency of side effects and the need to self-inject (Table 9.7).

8.2. Prophylactic Treatment

Although 25% of migraineurs suffer >3 headaches monthly, many with severe disability, it is surprising that only 5% receive prophylactic treatment (Lipton *et al* 2001b, 2002). The goals of migraine preventive therapy are to reduce attack frequency, severity and duration, to enhance responsiveness to treatment of acute attacks (synergy) and to improve or restore function and reduce disability (Ramadan *et al* 2000). Indications that warrant prophylactic treatment include 4 or more attacks monthly, ≥2 attacks/month that induce disability for ≥3 days, contraindication or ineffectiveness of abortive therapies, use of abortive medications more than twice weekly and in special circumstances, e.g. specific professions or lifestyles, and headaches that induce disruption of routine (Ramadan *et al* 2000; Silberstein *et al* 2000). There is evidence that repeated headaches lead to permanent CNS changes and early, aggressive treatment of frequent migraine is indicated (Welch *et al* 2001; Loder and Biondi 2005). Efficient prophylaxis may therefore prevent disease progression into chronic migraine (Silberstein 2005).

Drugs that have documented high efficacy and mild to moderate adverse events include β-blockers, amitriptyline and divalproex (Table 9.8; Ramadan *et al* 2000; Chronicle and Mulleners 2004). Drugs that have lower documented efficacy and mild to moderate adverse events include selective SSRIs, calcium channel antagonists, gabapentin, topiramate, riboflavin and NSAIDs (Silberstein and Goadsby 2002). The choice of prophylactic medicine is influenced by medical contraindications, possible side effects and the need to treat comorbidities such as insomnia, tension-type headache, depression and hypertension (Silberstein and

Table 9.8 Choice of Migraine Preventive Treatment

Drug	Dose (mg)	Adverse Events	Contraindications	Relative Indications
Propranolol (SR)	80–240	Bradycardia Hypotension Fatigue Sleep disturbances Dyspepsia Depression	Asthma Depression Cardiac failure Raynaud's Diabetes	Hypertension Angina
Amitriptyline	10–50	Sedation Weight gain Dry mouth Blurred vision Constipation Urinary retention	Mania Urinary retention Heart block	Insomnia Anxiety Depression TTH Other chronic pains
Sodium valproate	500–1000	Nausea, vomiting Alopecia Tremor Weight gain/loss	Liver disease Bleeding disorder	Mania Epilepsy Anxiety

The three most effective and commonly used drugs are presented. Choice is influenced by adverse events, comorbidity and relative indications; see Fig. 9.7. The efficacy of all three drugs is similar. TTH, tension-type headache.

Goadsby 2002). Cost is an additional consideration in a long-term prophylactic schedule; amitriptyline is relatively cheap, whilst propranolol (especially the slow release preparation) is 3–4 times and divalproex about 15 times more expensive than amitriptyline (Ramadan *et al* 1997).

In view of evidence that the migraine brain is hyperexcitable (Welch 2003) major aims of prophylactic agents are suppression of neuronal hyperexcitability and enhancement of antinociceptive mechanisms (Ramadan 2004). However, our understanding of the mechanisms of migraine prophylaxis is limited, with no unifying molecular-based concept for drugs of many different therapeutic classes. There are multiple potential mechanisms for prophylactic drugs to exert their effects, and a change in the function of voltage-regulated sodium and calcium ion channels leading to neuronal stability has been recently suggested as a possible unifying hypothesis (Cohen 2005).

8.2.1. Principles of Preventive Therapy

In clinical practice a patient may have to test a number of migraine preventive drugs for a full therapeutic trial (2–6 months) before the drug of choice is found. The patient should understand the process and aims of therapy, and the patient's preferences should be taken into account and full cooperation obtained. Treatment objectives and drug side effects should be carefully described and the patient's expectations should be addressed. Comorbidity should be considered when choosing the most appropriate drug (see Table 9.8 and Fig. 9.7). In general the drug should be started at a low dose and titrated up until a therapeutic

effect is reached or side effects become intolerable. There are interindividual variations in pharmacokinetics, and therefore fixed dosing may lead to poor compliance and is not recommended (Dahlof 2002). It is important to re-evaluate therapy: if the headache is well controlled slowly taper, and if possible discontinue the drug. Many patients experience continued relief with a lower dose and others may not require it at all (Silberstein and Goadsby 2002). Breakthrough headache is not an indication to alter therapy (Silberstein *et al* 2001); long-term assessment of response is essential; see Case 9.2. Women of childbearing potential must be informed of potential risks of relevant drugs to conception or the fetus with consideration to the risk–benefit value of prophylaxis.

Three main drug groups are currently considered most effective, with relatively few and minor side effects: β-adrenoceptor blocking drugs, tricyclic antidepressants and anticonvulsants (Table 9.8; Silberstein and Goadsby 2002). On average two-thirds of patients will experience a 50% reduction in headache frequency (albeit with significant side effects) on most preventive therapies (Goadsby 2005c), with a somewhat better rate for sodium valproate (Dahlof 2002).

8.2.2. β-Adrenergic Blockers

This is the most widely used class of drugs in the prophylaxis of migraine (Loder and Biondi 2005). There is consistent evidence for the efficacy of propranolol 120–240 mg daily with no significant correlation between dose and clinical outcome (Morey 2000; Linde and Rossnagel 2004). Based on a meta-analysis propranolol prophylaxis

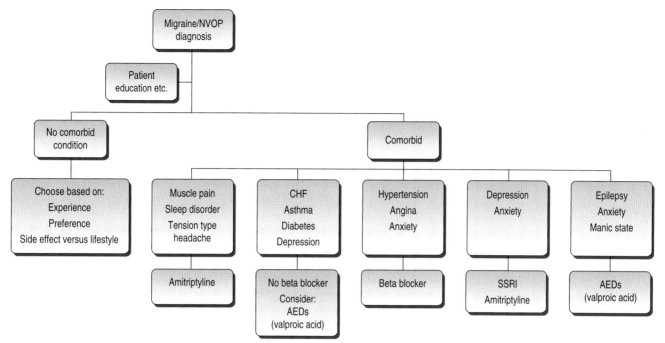

Fig. 9.7 • Preventive treatment of migraine and neurovascular orofacial pain (NVOP); effects of comorbidity. CHF, congestive heart failure; AED, antiepileptic drugs; SSRI, selective serotonin reuptake inhibitors.

has an NNT of 3.3 for a significant reduction in migraine activity (Holroyd *et al* 1991). It is unclear whether these effects are stable after stopping propranolol (Linde and Rossnagel 2004). Most studies show no significant difference between different β-blockers; clinical efficacy correlates solely with an absence of partial sympathomimetic effect (Silberstein and Goadsby 2002). Propranolol and amitriptyline are equally effective in migraine prophylaxis (Ziegler *et al* 1987) but propranolol is more efficacious in patients with migraine alone whilst amitriptyline is superior for patients with migraine and tension-type headache (Mathew 1981). Initial doses are 80mg of the slow release preparation and 40–80mg of the standard formulation; these are then titrated according to side effects versus treatment response and may reach 240mg daily (see Chapter 16). If no response is achieved within 4–6 weeks at the maximum dosage therapy should be gradually discontinued over a 2-week period. However, the efficacy of propranolol may increase progressively between 3 and 12 months of therapy. A longer trial period is therefore indicated, particularly in patients with a partial response (Diamond *et al* 1982).

The mechanisms of action of β-blockers in migraine prevention are not fully understood. However, propranolol possesses several properties likely to be involved and these are discussed in Chapter 16.

Adverse events most commonly reported in clinical trials with β-blockers were fatigue, depression, nausea, dizziness and insomnia, but are usually fairly well tolerated. Congestive heart failure, asthma and insulin-dependent diabetes are contraindications to the use of non-selective β-blockers (Silberstein and Goadsby 2002). Atenolol is a selective β1 blocker with fewer side effects

than propranolol, but its effectiveness in migraine prophylaxis is debatable (Forssman *et al* 1983). In patients on escape medication with zolmitriptan an interaction with a metabolite of propranolol mandates a dosage reduction of zolmitriptan to 5mg (Millson *et al* 2000).

8.2.3. Antidepressants

Sedative effects of antidepressant drugs make them an attractive option in patients with sleep problems, and comorbidity with depression or tension-type headache often indicates their use. Pooling treatment outcomes for chronic headaches, a meta-analysis found an NNT of 3.2 (2.5–4.3) for all antidepressant drugs (Tomkins *et al* 2001). Tricyclic antidepressants (TCAs) and serotonin blockers (e.g. pizotifen) were equally effective whilst results for SSRIs were less certain (Tomkins *et al* 2001). Amitriptyline, a TCA, is a serotonin and noradrenaline reuptake inhibitor (SNRI), and its efficacy in migraine treatment has been shown to be independent of its antidepressant action (Couch and Hassanein 1979). Thus the optimum dosage for two-thirds of subjects was less than 50mg per day (Gomersall and Stuart 1973), and in our experience a dose of 25–35mg at bedtime is often effective. We usually initiate therapy with 10mg at bedtime and titrate according to response and side effects. Response is normally seen within 10 days but may take much longer (Silberstein *et al* 2001). Clinical studies indicate that amitriptyline is the only antidepressant that has shown consistent efficacy in the prevention of migraine (Silberstein 2000; Tomkins *et al* 2001).

Recently venlafaxine, a structurally novel antidepressant was compared in a double-blind crossover design to amitriptyline in the prophylactic treatment of migraine (Bulut *et al* 2004). Amitriptyline (75 mg/d) and venlafaxine (150 mg/d) reduced the frequency, duration and severity of migraine attacks significantly but with no difference between them. Venlafaxine has mechanisms of action similar to amitriptyline but with fewer side effects; sedation, dry mouth and difficulty in concentration were higher in the amitriptyline group. However, the dose of amitriptyline used in the study (75 mg) was higher than that used in common practice. Furthermore the fixed dosing employed is not advised. The mechanisms involved in the effect of amitriptyline in headaches are discussed in Chapter 16.

8.2.4. Anticonvulsants

Placebo-controlled studies clearly point to anticonvulsant medication as increasingly recommended for migraine prevention (Chronicle and Mulleners 2004; Young *et al* 2004). Meta-analysis of published studies suggests that anticonvulsants significantly reduce migraine frequency by about 1–2 attacks per month, with an overall NNT of 3.8 (3.2–4.6) (Chronicle and Mulleners 2004). Of the anticonvulsants, the related compounds sodium valproate and valproic acid have been the most extensively studied (Chronicle and Mulleners 2004). Divalproex sodium is a stable coordination complex comprised of sodium valproate and valproic acid in a 1:1 molar ratio. Valproic acid has been widely used for migraine prevention with high rates of efficacy (45–86%) significantly superior to placebo (Klapper 1997; Freitag *et al* 2001). Treatment with valproic acid, although very effective in reducing frequency of attacks, may not reduce the peak intensity or duration of the migraine attacks (Rothrock 1997). Divalproex sodium is found to be effective at an initial dose of 500 mg, although some patients may benefit from higher doses (Klapper 1997). An extended release form is available with comparable efficacy to the standard formulation with adverse effect rates comparable to placebo (Silberstein and Goadsby 2002). Sodium valproate has an NNT of 3.1 (1.0–8.9) and divalproex sodium 4.8 (3.5–7.4) (Chronicle and Mulleners 2004). When the prophylactic effect on MWA was compared between divalproex and propranolol no significant difference was found between the two drugs over 3 months (Kaniecki 1997). For both sodium valproate and divalproex the most common side effect is nausea (NNH 6.6 (5–9.8)); vomiting and gastrointestinal distress are also frequent and are dose-related. Fatigue, tremor, weight gain and dizziness are rare (<8%) and are also dose-related; at 1500 mg/d of valproic acid dizziness and tremor were particularly pronounced (Klapper 1997; Chronicle and Mulleners 2004). Safety and efficacy of divalproex during 6 years of use revealed no hepatotoxicity and negligible weight gain (Freitag *et al* 2001).

Overall evidence from multiple well-designed clinical trials has been sufficient to establish divalproex sodium as a first-line prophylactic therapy for migraine. The effect of another anticonvulsant, gabapentin (NNT 3.3 (2.1–8.4)), on the prevention of migraine was less favourable than valproic acid, with conflicting evidence on its efficacy (Silberstein and Goadsby 2002; Chronicle and Mulleners 2004). Recently, 100 mg/d of topiramate was found to significantly reduce the frequency of migraine attacks and the quantity of symptomatic drugs, with an NNT of 3.5 (2.8–4.9) (Chronicle and Mulleners 2004). Dose-related side effects are common; at a dose of 100 mg daily the most common unwanted effect of topiramate is paraesthesias (NNH 2.4 (2.0–2.8)) (Chronicle and Mulleners 2004). Less frequent (<9%) events include taste disturbance, weight loss, language problems and anorexia (Chronicle and Mulleners 2004). Paraesthesias are transient and if bothersome respond to potassium supplementation. The mechanisms via which anticonvulsants exert their actions in pain and headache are discussed in Chapter 16.

Monotherapy is the recommended prophylactic approach but when standard medications are ineffective polytherapy may be considered; e.g. combining sodium valproate and a β-blocker has been successfully employed (Pascual *et al* 2003). Newer antiepileptic drugs such as levetiracetam and zonisamide have been successful in open trials (Drake *et al* 2004; Miller 2004). Botulinum toxin induces muscle paralysis and early trials suggested efficacy in the treatment and prevention of migraine (Tepper *et al* 2004). However, later RCTs have questioned these results so that its use in migraine is unclear (Evers *et al* 2004).

8.2.5. Managing Chronic Migraine

Daily or nearly daily headache indicates a prophylactic regimen and it is advisable to first withdraw all acute medications (Saper *et al* 2005). Traditionally the same prophylactics have been employed as in frequent MWA, including amitriptyline, β-blockers and anticonvulsants. Anticonvulsants have emerged as one of the most useful; valproic acid, topiramate and gabapentin have all been successfully tested (Freitag *et al* 2001; Silvestrini *et al* 2003; Spira and Beran 2003).

8.3. Migraine Therapy in Pregnancy

Epidemiologically women in their reproductive years are the most predominant migraineurs. Migraine attacks may subside during pregnancy particularly towards the third trimester. However, migraines commonly occur during the first trimester at the time of fetal organogenesis and require careful management (Sances *et al* 2003; Fox *et al* 2005). For example, ergot alkaloids are contraindicated whilst opioids and codeine have no teratogenic hazard. The use of aspirin during the first two trimesters seems safe but all NSAIDs should be avoided in the third trimester due to the danger of premature closure of the ductus arteriosus and pulmonary hypertension in the neonate (Fox *et al* 2005). Paracetamol, if efficacious in the specific patient, is a safe alternative. Sumatriptan does not increase rates of spontaneous abortions or fetal malformation but has been associated with preterm delivery. Prophylaxis is not advised but if unavoidable should be begun only in the second trimester and propranolol is the drug recommended (Fox *et al* 2005). Expert review of these cases is essential and we routinely refer relevant cases for teratologic guidance.

8.4. Migraine in the Child and Adolescent

Migraines are very common in these age groups but diagnosis may be more difficult due to problems in obtaining an accurate history. Recommendations for the acute treatment of migraine in children under 6 years include ibuprofen (effective) and acetaminophen (probably effective) (Lewis *et al* 2004). For adolescents over 12 years of age, acute treatment of migraine with sumatriptan nasal spray is recommended. Preventive therapy with flunarizine is probably effective (unavailable in the USA). Unfortunately the data concerning amitriptyline, divalproex sodium and topiramate are insufficient and conflicting concerning propranolol. For a problem so prevalent in children and adolescents, there is a surprising lack of evidence.

9. Prognosis

Migraine is a chronic illness and although some may suffer increased attacks as they reach middle age, many will report long-term remissions (Bille 1997; Lipton *et al* 2000b). Morever it seems that the age progression of migraine for many patients is favourable with a reduction in headache frequency, intensity and associated symptoms (Mattsson *et al* 2000). This may not be expressed in disability reduction due to age-related impaired coping abilities. When patients with MA were studied, about one-third had been attack-free in the past 5 years and up to 40% reported less severe and less frequent attacks each (Cologno *et al* 1998; Eriksen *et al* 2004). Favourable prognostic factors were short duration of migraine (from onset in years), male gender and a solely visual aura (Eriksen *et al* 2004).

A small group of patients will develop increased frequency of migraine headache with reduced intensity, ultimately transforming into chronic migraine (Mathew *et al* 1987).

10. Future Avenues

The management of migraine is in the midst of far-reaching changes because of advancements in neuroimaging, genomics, pharmacogenomics and molecular biology techniques. The discovery of the genes underlying FHM

suggests that migraine may involve at least one or more channelopathies and will lead to new therapeutic targets for headache.

11. Facial Pain with Neurovascular Features; Facial Migraine, Neurovascular Orofacial Pain (NVOP)

Aberrant migraine locations are not recognized by the IHS or the International Association for the Study of Pain (IASP). The IASP classifies atypical odontalgia which many consider to be a neurovascular type pain. However, the clinical reality is unquestionable; many patients present with a primary lower facial pain characterized by classical neurovascular features, including AS, nausea and photo- or phonophobia (Benoliel *et al* 1997; Daudia and Jones 2002; Penarrocha *et al* 2004).

Theoretically migraine mechanisms may present in the facial or oral region and neurogenic inflammation in the orofacial region is examined below. NVOP shares many of the signs and symptoms common to migraine and TACs and some may consider this a migraine or CH variant but the relationship is as yet unclear. The rationale for introducing NVOP is based on specific features that segregate it from other primary neurovascular-type craniofacial pain and justify a unique diagnosis, particularly its intraoral and perioral location (i.e. second and third divisions of the trigeminal nerve) (Benoliel *et al* 1997). Furthermore, primary orofacial pain of neurovascular origin is of great diagnostic and therapeutic importance. NVOP patients often present with dental symptomatology (thermal hypersensitivity) and the similarities with dental pulpitis have obviously caused diagnostic difficulties (Benoliel *et al* 1997; Czerninsky *et al* 1999). A clear classification and terminology will avoid misdiagnosis and dental mutilation.

11.1. Clinical Features of Facial Migraine/ Neurovascular Orofacial Pain

Location. The vast majority of patients (93%) report unilateral pain. Pain occurs primarily at an intraoral site, usually around the alveolar process (62%), but may be associated with a mucosal site (32%) (Benoliel *et al* 1997; Peñarrocha *et al* 2004). In 35% of cases pain referral was to perioral structures (lips, chin etc), to the periorbital region (usually infraorbital) in 35% and to the periauricular region in 30% (Fig. 9.3; Benoliel *et al* 1997).

Quality and temporal pattern. NVOP is characterized by moderate to strong, episodic pain (Benoliel *et al* 1997; Czerninsky *et al* 1999; Peñarrocha *et al* 2004). In 48% of cases the pain throbs, and in 35% woke the patient from sleep (Benoliel *et al* 1997). Pain may last from minutes to hours (45–72% of cases) or more rarely continues for >24 hours (28–55% of cases) (Benoliel *et al* 1997;

Peñarrocha *et al* 2004). Many cases are characterized by a chronic high–frequency pattern.

Accompanying phenomena. Pain can be accompanied by various local AS, and these were found in 36% of cases (Penarrocha *et al* 2004). Specifically tearing (10%), nasal congestion (7%), a feeling of swelling or fullness (7%) particularly in the cheek and a complaint of excessive sweating (7%) were reported (Benoliel *et al* 1997). Other phenomena such as photo- or phonophobia (14%) and nausea (24%) have been observed (Benoliel *et al* 1997; Penarrocha *et al* 2004). Often patients report dental hypersensitivity to cold leading to diagnostic confusion (Czerninsky *et al* 1999). Based on the above we suggest diagnostic criteria as outlined in Table 9.9.

Recently we have found that the combination of perioral facial pain, throbbing quality, autonomic and/or systemic features and attack duration of over 60 minutes resulted in a positive predictive value of 0.71 and a negative predictive value of 0.95 (Benoliel *et al* 2008).

Case examples. Our clinical experience suggests that two temporal patterns are common: an episodic and chronic form. Case 9.3 suffered high-frequency pain lasting up to one hour that was in some ways similar to an atypical PH. However, treatment with indomethacin was unsuccessful whilst propranolol provided long-term relief. The patient shown in Case 9.4 is representative of a 'chronic type' NVOP. A constant throbbing low-grade pain is present with severe exacerbations accompanied by migrainous features. Etodolac (a COX-2 inhibitor, Chapter 15) and analgesic combination drugs were unsuccessful. Rizatriptan provided rapid relief of attacks and due to the high frequency observed in pain diaries and to the background pain prophylactic therapy was indicated. Note the similarities to chronic daily headache, particularly HC and chronic migraine. Case 9.3 is an 'episodic type' NVOP: pain attacks clearly spaced apart with no background pain. Due to the high frequency preventive therapy was also employed.

Epidemiology. The onset of NVOP is around 35–50 years of age, and it affects females more often than males (3–10:1) (Benoliel *et al* 1997; Peñarrocha *et al* 2004). Time to diagnosis was on average 34–101 months (range 1–528 months), attesting to the diagnostic difficulties presented by these patients (Benoliel *et al* 1997; Peñarrocha *et al* 2004). Often patients have a positive history of migraine (Peñarrocha *et al* 2004). In 38–45% of cases the pain was diagnosed as secondary to dental pathology and patients underwent dental treatment with no success (Benoliel *et al* 1997; Peñarrocha *et al* 2004). Some cases (36%) underwent repeated extractions in the same quadrant (Peñarrocha *et al* 2004).

Treatment. Low-dose amitriptyline, β-blockers and ergotamine have been successful in NVOP (Benoliel *et al* 1997; Czerninsky *et al* 1999; Penarrocha *et al* 2004). No trials with triptans have appeared in the literature. The drugs and guidelines outlined in the migraine treatment section are relevant for NVOP, as is the treatment algorithm (Fig. 9.3).

Table 9.9	Suggested Criteria for Neurovascular Orofacial Pain (NVOP)	
Diagnostic criteria		**Notes**
A	At least 5 attacks of facial pain fulfilling criteria B–E	
B	Severe, unilateral oral and/or perioral pain	May refer to orbital and/or temporal regions. Side shift may occur; rarely bilateral cases are reported.
C	At least one of the following characteristics: 1. Toothache with no local pathology 2. Throbbing 3. Wakes	Frequently painful vital teeth will be hypersensitive to cold stimuli. Some of the teeth in the painful region may have undergone root canal therapy with no long-lasting pain relief.
D	Episodic attacks lasting 60 minutes to >24 hours	Chronic unremitting cases that may result in subclassification into episodic and chronic forms have been observed.
E	Accompanied by at least one of the following: 1. Ipsilateral lacrimation and/or conjunctival injection 2. Ipsilateral rhinorrhea and/or nasal congestion 3. Ipsilateral cheek swelling 4. Photo- and/or phonophobia 5. Nausea and/or vomiting	
F	Not attributed to another disorder	Dental pathology may be very difficult to differentiate and needs careful assessment.

Benoliel *et al* 2008

11.2. Differential Diagnosis

Due to the dental thermal hypersensitivity observed in NVOP the differential diagnosis would include irreversible pulpitis and cold stimulus, or 'ice cream' headache. Cold stimulus headache occurs particularly in individuals with a history of migraine and is not associated with dental pathology; see Table 9.10 (Fuh *et al* 2003). Pain follows the passage of cold material over the palate and posterior pharyngeal wall, and does not originate in the teeth. It is postulated that incoming impulses due to cold cause disinhibition of central pain pathways. Application of ice to the palate or to the posterior pharyngeal mucosa produces facial pain in the mid-frontal region or around the ears; referred probably by the trigeminal and glossopharyngeal nerves respectively. No treatment other than sensible caution is needed. Although

Case 9.3 Neurovascular Orofacial Pain (Episodic Type); 21-year-old Female

Present complaint

Strong paroxysmal pain in the right mandibular area; pain is spontaneous and causes the patient to wake from sleep. Six to seven attacks occur within 24 hours, each lasting from 20 to 60 minutes. Pain is typically evoked by ingestion of cold and hot drinks.

History of present complaint

Pain started about 5 months ago and its frequency, intensity and duration have increased with time. Pain responded minimally to analgesics. Patient was previously diagnosed with paroxysmal hemicrania and prescribed indomethacin with no response.

Physical examination

Oral structures and the masticatory system were normal. No caries lesions were detected on physical and X-ray examinations (Fig. 9.8). Cold application evoked strong pain, lasting about 30 s after application (overshoot), from most right mandibular teeth (#41 to #46) and the adjacent vestibular area.

Relevant medical history

Healthy. No history of migraine.

Diagnosis

Neurovascular orofacial pain (NVOP).

Diagnostic and treatment considerations

The type of pain, duration and frequency were highly suggestive of paroxysmal hemicrania. However, lack of response to indomethacin and the very high sensitivity of the teeth to cold application led us to the diagnosis of NVOP. The patient was started on 80 mg of slow-release propranolol that was increased within 3 days to 160 mg/d. There was a marked improvement in pain within 1 week; the spontaneous pain almost completely disappeared, and did not wake the patient.

Upon examination a week after drug initiation the teeth were still sensitive to cold but with no overshoot. Patient was followed-up for another 6 months; the dosage was adjusted to 80 mg/d and the patient became symptom-free at 4 weeks after initiation of treatment.

Certain points typical to this case should be emphasized:
(a) the quick response to propranolol (1 week);
(b) the cold allodynia of not only the teeth but also the adjacent vestibular area, and
(c) the high daily frequency (6–7/d) and short duration (20–60 min) of attacks not typical of migraine.

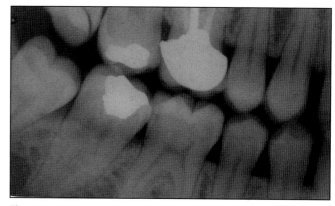

Fig. 9.8 • Bite-wing radiograph of Case 9.3. Very high sensitivity, with overshoot, to cold application of all right mandibular teeth and adjacent vestibular area was found. However, no local pathology was identified.

and may be a manifestation of migraine or CH at atypical locations or a discrete diagnostic entity (Benoliel *et al* 1997; Penarrocha *et al* 2004).

It is tempting to retain the term 'lower-half migraine' (Penarrocha *et al* 2004). Many of these lower-half migraines may, however, be a distinct subdiagnosis and deserve classification (Benoliel *et al* 1997). Furthermore while TACs and migraine have been linked to the ophthalmic division of the trigeminal nerve no similar syndromes have been described for the second and third divisions. The paucity of AS in NVOP (10%) relative to TACs (62–91%) and migraine (41–46%) may be a reflection of this basic difference. Indeed, until recently no attempt had been made to characterize or categorize these patients (Benoliel *et al* 1997; Penarrocha *et al* 2004). We suggest the term be updated to neurovascular orofacial pain in keeping with current thought on the mechanisms underlying migraines and TACs. Although exhibiting some similarities to primary neurovascular headaches there are enough differentiating factors to distinctly classify NVOP. The most prominent characteristic is its location: oral and perioral (Benoliel *et al* 1997; Czerninsky *et al* 1999; Penarrocha *et al* 2004) or midface (Daudia and Jones 2002). Since NVOP is considered a migraine variant one would expect to see the majority of patients with longer pain attacks, a younger onset and more photo- and phonophobia and nausea (Benoliel *et al* 1997). The similarities to the CH group are limited by the fact that there is an overwhelming female preponderance and treatment response is not similar. Treatment of NVOP with classical antimigraine drugs has been successful, which firmly establishes an association between NVOP and migraine (Benoliel *et al* 1997; Czerninsky *et al* 1999; Penarrocha *et al* 2004). A summary of migraine and NVOP features is presented in Table 9.10. The throbbing quality, paucity of AS, long attack duration and chronic pattern observed in NVOP is similar to that observed in HC. However, clinically we have found these cases do not respond to indomethacin, thus refuting the possible relation. NVOP is characterized by a chronic pain pattern and many of these patients describe a history of episodic migraine, suggesting a possible link to chronic

initially pulpal pain may resemble NVCPs careful history and examination should easily differentiate between them (Table 9.11).

11.3. Nosological Issues

Facial migraine is referred to in the literature and in headache texts (Daudia and Jones 2002; Perry *et al* 2004; Lance and Goadsby 2005). Descriptions of perioral pain with distinct neurovascular type features have been reported

Case 9.4 Neurovascular Orofacial Pain (Chronic Type); 24-year-old Female

Present complaint

Strong (VAS 5–9.5), pulsating pain in the posterior-mandibular area, sometimes on the right side and sometimes on the left, but never bilateral. When pain is very strong it usually radiates to the temporal area (Fig. 9.9). Pain causes patient to wake from sleep, and may be associated with nausea, dizziness and sometimes vomiting.

History of present complaint

Pain started about 2 years ago. Pain appears from once a week to once a month. Each pain attack lasts from half a day to 4 days and is not related to menstrual period. When in an attack, chewing increases pain, and so does physical activity. Since the pain started she has been wearing a bite-guard, and arthrocentesis was performed on both TM joints. None of these treatments eased her pain.

Physical examination

Both right and left masseters and sternomastoid muscles were very tender to palpation. Mouth opening was normal (46 mm) and both TMJs were not tender to palpation and moved freely. No tenderness was detected from other masticatory or pericranial muscles, including the temporalis.

Relevant medical history

For the past couple of years patient has been on fluvoxamine 100 mg/d for anxiety and depressive episodes. Takes zopiclone 3.75 mg at bedtime to aid sleep onset. Multiple allergies, suspected asthma.

Diagnosis

Neurovascular orofacial pain.

Diagnostic and treatment considerations

While the symptomatology of this patient is similar to migraine without aura, the strict confinement of the pain to the mandibular area justifies a distinct diagnosis of neurovascular orofacial pain. Unfortunately, because of the pain location the patient was mistreated with a bite-guard and arthrocentesis of the TMJ. The continuous nature suggests similarity to chronic migraine.

Initially our patient had reported that the pain was episodic in nature and we started treatment with an abortive strategy. Nonspecific abortives were unsuccessful including etodolac 600 mg and an analgesic-antiemetic combination (Migraleve: buclizine 6.25 mg, paracetamol 500 mg, codeine 8 mg, dioctylsodium sulphosuccinate 10 mg). We resorted to rizatriptan 10 mg, which proved very effective in shortening attacks, but caused a lot of dizziness and tiredness; hence we reduced the dose to 5 mg. The pain diary revealed interictal low-grade background pain and a high frequency of attacks (Fig. 9.10) so we decided to start the patient also on a prophylactic regimen of slow-release divalproex. This was preferred over amitriptyline due to the fact that the patient was already on an SSRI, and propranolol was contraindicated due to the possibility of asthma.

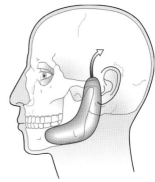

Fig. 9.9 • Pain location; Case 9.4

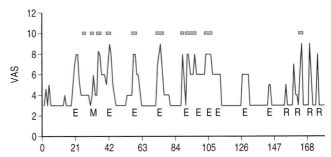

Fig. 9.10 • Mean daily VAS for Case 9.4. The patient suffered constant low-grade background pain (VAS 3). Superimposed on these are exacerbations of moderate-severe pain (VAS 6–8). The grey rectangles above the plot show when the patient was woken by nocturnal pain. Patient tried abortive therapies with etodolac (E), migraleve (M), and rizatriptan (R). Only rizatriptan significantly shortened attack duration. Due to the high frequency of attacks patient was started on divalproex sustained release.

migraine (Benoliel *et al* 1997; Penarrocha *et al* 2004). However, pain in NVOP is largely unilateral and throbbing, and exacerbations of pain are not characterized by more prominent or typical migrainous features as in chronic migraine.

The IASP defines atypical odontalgia (AO) as a severe, throbbing tooth pain without major pathology; see Chapter 11 (Merskey and Bogduk 1994). The high incidence of pulsatile, episodic pain that migrates and changes sides suggests a neurovascular-type pain (Schnurr and Brooke 1992) and neurovascular or migrainous toothache has been interchangeably used for AO (Okeson 2005). However, AO has been referred to as phantom toothache, implying a traumatic neuropathic mechanism (Vickers *et al* 1998). In appropriate cases the term NVOP is less ambiguous.

11.4. Pathophysiology of Neurovascular Orofacial Pain

The pathophysiology of NVOP may be based on migraine. If so, we need to analyse the possibility that neurogenic inflammation occurs in the oral and perioral tissues and consider its possible role in the phenotype of NVOP.

Table 9.10	Differential Diagnosis: Migraine and Neurovascular Orofacial Pain (NVOP)	
	Migraine	**NVOP**
Onset (age)	20–40	40–50
M:F	1:2	1:2.5
Location (mostly unilateral)	Forehead, temple	Intraoral/ lower face
Duration	Hours to days	Mins. to hours
Time course	Periodic/chronic	Periodic/chronic
Character of pain	Throbbing Deep Continuous	Throbbing Paroxysmal
Pain intensity	Moderate to severe	Moderate to severe
Precipitating factors	Stress, hunger menstrual period, etc.	Sometimes cold foods
Associated signs	Nausea, photophobia, visual aura	Cheek swelling and redness, tearing
Treatment (abortive)	NSAIDs Triptans	NSAIDs Triptans (?)
Treatment: (prophylactic)	Amitriptyline β-blockers Valproate	Amitriptyline β-blockers

NSAIDs, nonsteroidal anti inflammatory drugs.

Table 9.11	Craniofacial Pain in Response to Cold Ingestion; Comparative Features		
Parameter	NVOP	Irr P.	Cold Stim HA
History of:			
Migraine	+	–	+
Past endodontics	+	–	–
Autonomic/systemic signs	+	–	–
Treatment/effectiveness:			
Endodontics	–	++	–
NSAIDs	+	+/–	–
Amitriptyline	++	–	–
β-adrenergic blocker	++	–	–
Clinical signs: Teeth			
Hypersensitive to cold	+	++	–[a]
Tender to percussion	–	++(80%)	–
Change location/side shift	+	–	–
Carious (clinical/ radiological)	–	++	–
Soft tissues			
Swelling	+	–	–
Redness	+	–	–

NVOP, neurovascular orofacial pain; Irr P, irreversible pulpitis; Cold Stim HA, cold stimulus headache.
[a] Pain induced by cold application to palatal and pharyngeal mucosa.

11.4.1. Neurogenic Inflammation in Oral Tissues and the Dental Pulp

Nerve fibres entering the dental pulp have been identified as unmyelinated C fibres and autonomic nerves, myelinated Aδ and Aβ fibres; see Chapters 2 and 5. Nerve fibres exhibiting SP and CGRP positive immunoreactivity are present in the dental pulp and oral mucosa in several species including humans (Tajti *et al* 1999b; Uddman *et al* 1999). Analysis of human dental pulp revealed significantly greater expression of CGRP, SP and VIP in permanent teeth relative to deciduous counterparts (Rodd and Boissonade 2002). This may explain the lack of children in reports of NVOP (Benoliel *et al* 1997; Penarrocha *et al* 2004). In rat dental pulp, CGRP-immunoreactive nerves and nerve terminals containing many granular vesicles supply both arterioles and postcapillary venules (Iijima and Zhang 2002). The anatomical substrate for neurovascular tooth pain is therefore present.

Application of SP to dental pulp and salivary glands induced plasma extravasation, and SP infusion to the craniofacial circulation induced plasma extravasation in oral mucosa (Fazekas *et al* 1992; Gyorfi *et al* 1995). Following antidromic electrical nerve stimulation, neurogenic inflammation has been demonstrated in the dental pulp of dogs and in the dental pulp, lower lip and oral mucosa of rats (Inoki *et al* 1973; Fazekas *et al* 1990; Izumi and Karita 1991; Ohkubo *et al* 1993). This effect is not attenuated following sympathectomy (Komorowski *et al* 1996). Involvement of adjacent teeth suggests that collateral C-fibre innervation exists within the pulps of molar teeth in the same dental quadrant (Komorowski *et al* 1996) and may partly explain referral patterns in primary NVOP.

Since neurogenic inflammation in the trigeminovascular system seems to play a central role in the genesis of NVCPs the same mechanism could function in the oral mucosa and teeth. It has been postulated that the trigeminovascular system causes some of its effects by neurovascular activation within the space limited by the skull; a closed system that may rapidly lead to pressure build-up and increased nociceptor activation. This system is replicated in the dental pulp that is similarly confined by the surrounding dental hard tissues and it is feasible that pressure build-up plays a role in intrapulpal nociceptor activation. For example, Aδ fibres have been shown to be sensitive to the increased intrapulpal pressure following plasma extravasation (Kim 1990; Byers and Narhi 1999). However, homeostatic mechanisms limit pressure build-up in the pulp following antidromic stimulation (Heyeraas and Kvinnsland 1992), probably by reabsorption into the circulation. This may explain clinical observations that despite pulpitis-like symptoms in teeth of patients with NVOP, spontaneous pulp necrosis is rare. The TPR in the orofacial region is examined in Chapter 10 on TACs.

12. Conclusions

Migraine is a common and debilitating condition with a clear but complex genetic component. Clinical presentation is heterogeneous with features that include neurologic disturbances, alterations in sensory sensitivity, mood changes and autonomic dysfunction. Research suggests that episodic dysfunction of brainstem regions may play a key role in migraine pain as either central generators or faulty modulation, particularly the periaqueductal grey, a pain-inhibiting structure. This leads to activation and sensitization of the trigeminovascular system. These studies have relied on advanced neuroimaging that may therefore evolve into a diagnostic test. Accumulated evidence also points to a state of neuronal excitation in migraineurs. The nosologic status of primary NVCP in the lower face is at present unclear. We suggest that this entity be referred to as neurovascular orofacial pain, a descriptive term that stresses the anatomical location and suspected mechanism of this type of pain. The relationship between NVOP and migraine needs more research in order to clarify common mechanisms and response to therapy.

References

Afridi SK, Giffin NJ, Kaube H, *et al* (2005a) A positron emission tomographic study in spontaneous migraine. *Arch Neurol* **62**(8):1270–1275.

Afridi SK, Matharu MS, Lee L, *et al* (2005b) A PET study exploring the laterality of brainstem activation in migraine using glyceryl trinitrate. *Brain* **128**(Pt 4):932–939.

Alstadhaug KB, Salvesen R, Bekkelund SI (2005) Seasonal variation in migraine. *Cephalalgia* **25**(10):811–816.

Ashina M, Simonsen H, Bendtsen L, *et al* (2004) Glyceryl trinitrate may trigger endogenous nitric oxide production in patients with chronic tension-type headache. *Cephalalgia* **24**(11):967–972.

Baandrup L, Jensen R (2005) Chronic post-traumatic headache–a clinical analysis in relation to the International Headache Classification 2nd Edition. *Cephalalgia* **25**(2):132–138.

Bahra A, Matharu MS, Buchel C, *et al* (2001) Brainstem activation specific to migraine headache. *Lancet* **357**(9261):1016–1017.

Barbanti P, Fabbrini G, Pesare M, *et al* (2002) Unilateral cranial autonomic symptoms in migraine. *Cephalalgia* **22**(4):256–259.

Bartsch T, Knight YE, Goadsby PJ (2004) Activation of 5-HT(1B/1D) receptor in the periaqueductal gray inhibits nociception. *Ann Neurol* **56**(3):371–381.

Benoliel R, Elishoov H, Sharav Y (1997) Orofacial pain with vascular-type features. *Oral Surg Oral Med Oral Pathol Oral Radiol Endod* **84**(5):506–512.

Benoliel R, Birman N, Eliav E *et al* (2008) The International Headache Society classification: accurate diagnosis of orofacial pain? *Cephalalgia* [in press].

Bille B (1997) A 40-year follow-up of school children with migraine. *Cephalalgia* **17**(4):488–491; discussion 487.

Bolay H, Reuter U, Dunn AK, *et al* (2002) Intrinsic brain activity triggers trigeminal meningeal afferents in a migraine model. *Nat Med* **8**(2):136–142.

Bonaventure P, Voorn P, Luyten WH, *et al* (1998) 5HT1B and 5HT1D receptor mRNA differential co-localization with peptide mRNA in the guinea pig trigeminal ganglion. *Neuroreport* **9**(4):641–645.

Bouchelet I, Cohen Z, Case B, *et al* (1996) Differential expression of sumatriptan-sensitive 5-hydroxytryptamine receptors in human trigeminal ganglia and cerebral blood vessels. *Mol Pharmacol* **50**(2):219–223.

Breslau N, Rasmussen BK (2001) The impact of migraine: epidemiology, risk factors, and co-morbidities. *Neurology* **56**(6 Suppl 1):S4–S12.

Breslau N, Davis GC, Andreski P (1991) Migraine, psychiatric disorders, and suicide attempts: an epidemiologic study of young adults. *Psychiatry Res* **37**(1):11–23.

Bulut S, Berilgen MS, Baran A, *et al* (2004) Venlafaxine versus amitriptyline in the prophylactic treatment of migraine: randomized, double-blind, crossover study. *Clin Neurol Neurosurg* **107**(1):44–48.

Burstein R, Cutrer MF, Yarnitsky D (2000) The development of cutaneous allodynia during a migraine attack clinical evidence for the sequential recruitment of spinal and supraspinal nociceptive neurons in migraine. *Brain* **123** (Pt 8):1703–1709.

Burstein R, Collins B, Jakubowski M (2004) Defeating migraine pain with triptans: a race against the development of cutaneous allodynia. *Ann Neurol* **55**(1):19–26.

Bussone G, Tullo V (2005) Reflections on the nosology of craniofacial pain syndromes. *Neurol Sci* **26**(Suppl 2):S61–S64.

Buzzi MG, Moskowitz MA (1991) Evidence for 5-HT1B/1D receptors mediating the antimigraine effect of sumatriptan and dihydroergotamine. *Cephalalgia* **11**(4):165–168.

Buzzi MG, Carter WB, Shimizu T, *et al* (1991) Dihydroergotamine and sumatriptan attenuate levels of CGRP in plasma in rat superior sagittal sinus during electrical stimulation of the trigeminal ganglion. *Neuropharmacology* **30**(11):1193–1200.

Byers MR, Narhi MV (1999) Dental injury models: experimental tools for understanding neuroinflammatory interactions and polymodal nociceptor functions. *Crit Rev Oral Biol Med* **10**(1):4–39.

Cady R, Schreiber C, Farmer K, *et al* (2002) Primary headaches: a convergence hypothesis. *Headache* **42**(3):204–216.

Campbell JK, Sakai F (2000) The migraines; diagnosis and differential diagnosis. In: Olesen J, Tfelt-Hansen P, Welch KMA (eds) *The Headaches*, 2nd edn. Philadelphia: Lippincott Williams and Wilkins.

Campbell JK, Keith J, Penzien DB, *et al* (2000) *US Headache Consortium: Evidenced-Based Guidelines for Migraine Headache: Behavioral and Physical Treatments.* Available at: http://www.aan.com/professionals/practice/pdfs/gl0089.pdf. October 2005.

Cao Y, Aurora SK, Nagesh V, *et al* (2002) Functional MRI-BOLD of brainstem structures during visually triggered migraine. *Neurology* **59**(1):72–78.

Cavallini A, Micieli G, Bussone G, *et al* (1995) Headache and quality of life. *Headache* **35**(1):29–35.

Ceccarelli I, Fiorenzani P, Grasso G, *et al* (2004) Estrogen and mu-opioid receptor antagonists counteract the 17 beta-estradiol-induced licking increase and interferon-gamma reduction occurring during the formalin test in male rats. *Pain* **111**(1-2):181–190.

Centers for Disease Control (1991) Current Trends Prevalence of Chronic Migraine Headaches - United States, 1980–1989. *Morbidity and Mortality Weekly Report* **40**(20):331, 337–338. Available at: http://www.cdc.gov/mmwr/preview/mmwrhtml/00001982.htm

Chabriat H, Danchot J, Michel P, et al (1999) Precipitating factors of headache. A prospective study in a national control-matched survey in migraineurs and nonmigraineurs. *Headache* **39**(5):335–338.

Chronicle E, Mulleners W (2004) Anticonvulsant drugs for migraine prophylaxis. *Cochrane Database Syst Rev* (3):CD003226.

Cohen GL (2005) Migraine prophylactic drugs work via ion channels. *Med Hypotheses* **65**(1):114–122.

Cologno D, Torelli P, Manzoni GC (1998) Migraine with aura: a review of 81 patients at 10-20 years' follow-up. *Cephalalgia* **18**(10):690–696.

Colson NJ, Lea RA, Quinlan S, et al (2004) The estrogen receptor 1 G594A polymorphism is associated with migraine susceptibility in two independent case/control groups. *Neurogenetics* **5**(2):129–133.

Costa A, Ravaglia S, Sances G, et al (2003) Nitric oxide pathway and response to nitroglycerin in cluster headache patients: plasma nitrite and citrulline levels. *Cephalalgia* **23**(6):407–413.

Couch JR, Bearss C (2001) Chronic daily headache in the posttrauma syndrome: relation to extent of head injury. *Headache* **41**(6):559–564.

Couch JR, Hassanein RS (1979) Amitriptyline in migraine prophylaxis. *Arch Neurol* **36**(11):695–699.

Couturier EG, Bomhof MA, Neven AK, et al (2003) Menstrual migraine in a representative Dutch population sample: prevalence, disability and treatment. *Cephalalgia* **23**(4):302–308.

Cutrer FM, Sorensen AG, Weisskoff RM, et al (1998) Perfusion-weighted imaging defects during spontaneous migrainous aura. *Ann Neurol* **43**(1):25–31.

Czerninsky R, Benoliel R, Sharav Y (1999) Odontalgia in vascular orofacial pain. *J Orofac Pain* **13**(3):196–200.

Dahlof CGH (2002) Management of primary headaches: current and future aspects. In: Giamberardino MA (ed) *Pain – An Updated Review: Refresher Course*. Seattle: IASP Press, pp 85–112.

Dahlof C (2003) Clinical applications of new therapeutic deliveries in migraine. *Neurology* **61**(8 Suppl 4):S31–S34.

Dahlof CG, Mathew N (1998) Cardiovascular safety of 5HT1B/1D agonists–is there a cause for concern? *Cephalalgia* **18**(8):539–545.

Dahlof C, Ekbom K, Persson L (1994) Clinical experiences from Sweden on the use of subcutaneously administered sumatriptan in migraine and cluster headache. *Arch Neurol* **51**(12):1256–1261.

Dahlof CG, Rapoport AM, Sheftell FD, et al (1999) Rizatriptan in the treatment of migraine. *Clin Ther* **21**(11):1823–1836; discussion 1821.

Dahlof CG, Dodick D, Dowson AJ, et al (2002) How does almotriptan compare with other triptans? A review of data from placebo-controlled clinical trials. *Headache* **42**(2):99–113.

D'Amico D, Ferraris A, Leone M, et al (2002) Increased plasma nitrites in migraine and cluster headache patients in interictal period: basal hyperactivity of L-arginine-NO pathway? *Cephalalgia* **22**(1):33–36.

Daudia AT, Jones NS (2002) Facial migraine in a rhinological setting. *Clin Otolaryngol Allied Sci* **27**(6):521–525.

De Fusco M, Marconi R, Silvestri L, et al (2003) Haploinsufficiency of ATP1A2 encoding the Na+/K+ pump alpha2 subunit associated with familial hemiplegic migraine type 2. *Nat Genet* **33**(2):192–196.

Diamond M, Cady R (2005) Initiating and optimizing acute therapy for migraine: the role of patient-centered stratified care. *Am J Med* **118** (Suppl 1):18S–27S.

Diamond S, Kudrow L, Stevens J, et al (1982) Long-term study of propranolol in the treatment of migraine. *Headache* **22**(6):268–271.

Diener HC (2003) RPR100893, a substance-P antagonist, is not effective in the treatment of migraine attacks. *Cephalalgia* **23**(3):183–185.

Diener H, Pfaffenrath V, Pageler L, et al (2005) The fixed combination of acetylsalicylic acid, paracetamol and caffeine is more effective than single substances and dual combination for the treatment of headache: a multicentre, randomized, double-blind, single-dose, placebo-controlled parallel group study. *Cephalalgia* **25**(10):776–787.

Dodick DW, Rozen TD, Goadsby PJ, et al (2000) Cluster headache. *Cephalalgia* **20**(9):787–803.

Dodick DW, Eross EJ, Parish JM, et al (2003) Clinical, anatomical, and physiologic relationship between sleep and headache. *Headache* **43**(3):282–292.

Dodick DW, Lipton RB, Ferrari MD, et al (2004) Prioritizing treatment attributes and their impact on selecting an oral triptan: results from the TRIPSTAR Project. *Curr Pain Headache Rep* **8**(6):435–442.

Dodick D, Brandes J, Elkind A, et al (2005) Speed of onset, efficacy and tolerability of zolmitriptan nasal spray in the acute treatment of migraine: a randomised, double-blind, placebo-controlled study. *CNS Drugs* **19**(2):125–136.

Drake ME Jr, Greathouse NI, Renner JB, et al (2004) Open-label zonisamide for refractory migraine. *Clin Neuropharmacol* **27**(6):278–280.

Drummond PD, Gonski A, Lance JW (1983) Facial flushing after thermocoagulation of the Gasserian ganglion. *J Neurol Neurosurg Psychiatry* **46**(7):611–616.

Ducros A, Joutel A, Vahedi K, et al (1997) Mapping of a second locus for familial hemiplegic migraine to 1q21-q23 and evidence of further heterogeneity. *Ann Neurol* **42**(6):885–890.

Eriksen MK, Thomsen LL, Russell MB (2004) Prognosis of migraine with aura. *Cephalalgia* **24**(1):18–22.

Estevez M, Gardner KL (2004) Update on the genetics of migraine. *Hum Genet* **114**(3):225–235.

Evers S, Vollmer-Haase J, Schwaag S, et al (2004) Botulinum toxin A in the prophylactic treatment of migraine–a randomized, double-blind, placebo-controlled study. *Cephalalgia* **24**(10):838–843.

Fazekas A, Vindisch K, Posch E, et al (1990) Experimentally-induced neurogenic inflammation in the rat oral mucosa. *J Periodontal Res* **25**(5):276–282.

Fazekas A, Gyorfi A, Irmes F, et al (1992) Effect of substance P administration on vascular permeability in the rat dental pulp and submandibular gland. *Proc Finn Dent Soc* **88** (Suppl 1):481–486.

Ferrari MD (2003) Current perspectives on effective migraine treatments: are small clinical differences important for patients? *Drugs Today (Barc)* **39**(Suppl D):37–41.

Ferrari MD, Russell MB (2000) Genetics of migraine. In: Olesen J, Tfelt-Hansen P, Welch KMA (eds) *The Headaches*, 2nd edn. Philadelphia: Lippincott Williams and Wilkins, pp 241–254.

Ferrari MD, Roon KI, Lipton RB, et al (2001) Oral triptans (serotonin 5-HT(1B/1D) agonists) in acute migraine treatment: a meta-analysis of 53 trials. *Lancet* **358**(9294):1668–1675.

Ferrari MD, Goadsby PJ, Roon KI, et al (2002) Triptans (serotonin, 5-HT1B/1D agonists) in migraine: detailed results and methods of a meta-analysis of 53 trials. *Cephalalgia* **22**(8):633–658.

Forssman B, Lindblad CJ, Zbornikova V (1983) Atenolol for migraine prophylaxis. *Headache* **23**(4):188–190.

Fox AW, Davis RL (1998) Migraine chronobiology. *Headache* **38**(6):436–441.

Fox AW, Diamond ML, Spierings EL (2005) Migraine during pregnancy: options for therapy. *CNS Drugs* **19**(6):465–481.

Freitag FG, Diamond S, Diamond ML, et al (2001) Divalproex in the long-term treatment of chronic daily headache. *Headache* **41**(3):271–278.

Fuh JL, Wang SJ, Lu SR, et al (2003) Ice-cream headache–a large survey of 8359 adolescents. *Cephalalgia* **23**(10):977–981.

Gervil M, Ulrich V, Kaprio J, et al (1999) The relative role of genetic and environmental factors in migraine without aura. *Neurology* **53**(5):995-999.

Gibb CM, Davies PT, Glover V, et al (1991) Chocolate is a migraine-provoking agent. *Cephalalgia* **11**(2):93–95.

Giffin NJ, Ruggiero L, Lipton RB, *et al* (2003) Premonitory symptoms in migraine: an electronic diary study. *Neurology* **60**(6):935–940.

Goadsby PJ (2001) Neuroimaging in headache. *Microsc Res Tech* **53**(3):179–187.

Goadsby PJ (2002) Neurovascular headache and a midbrain vascular malformation: evidence for a role of the brainstem in chronic migraine. *Cephalalgia* **22**(2):107–111.

Goadsby PJ (2005a) Migraine pathophysiology. *Headache* **45** (Suppl 1):S14–S24.

Goadsby PJ (2005b) New targets in the acute treatment of headache. *Curr Opin Neurol* **18**(3):283–288.

Goadsby PJ (2005c) Advances in the understanding of headache. *Br Med Bull* **73–74**:83–92.

Goadsby PJ, Classey JD (2003) Evidence for serotonin (5-HT)1B, 5-HT1D and 5-HT1F receptor inhibitory effects on trigeminal neurons with craniovascular input. *Neuroscience* **122**(2):491–498.

Goadsby PJ, Edvinsson L (1993) The trigeminovascular system and migraine: studies characterizing cerebrovascular and neuropeptide changes seen in humans and cats. *Ann Neurol* **33**(1):48–56.

Goadsby PJ, Edvinsson L (1994) Human in vivo evidence for trigeminovascular activation in cluster headache. Neuropeptide changes and effects of acute attacks therapies. *Brain* **117**(Pt 3):427–434.

Goadsby PJ, Edvinsson L (1996) Neuropeptide changes in a case of chronic paroxysmal hemicrania–evidence for trigemino-parasympathetic activation. *Cephalalgia* **16**(6):448–450.

Goadsby PJ, Hoskin KL (1997) The distribution of trigeminovascular afferents in the nonhuman primate brain Macaca nemestrina: a c-fos immunocytochemical study. *J Anat* **190** (Pt 3):367–375.

Goadsby PJ, Lambert GA, Lance JW (1986) Stimulation of the trigeminal ganglion increases flow in the extracerebral but not the cerebral circulation of the monkey. *Brain Res* **381** (1):63–67.

Goadsby PJ, Edvinsson L, Ekman R (1988a) Release of vasoactive peptides in the extracerebral circulation of humans and the cat during activation of the trigeminovascular system. *Ann Neurol* **23**(2):193–196.

Goadsby PJ, Edvinsson L, Ekman R (1988b) Release of vasoactive peptides in the extracerebral circulation of humans and the cat during activation of the trigeminovascular system. *Ann Neurol* **23**(2):193–196.

Goadsby PJ, Zagami AS, Lambert GA (1991) Neural processing of craniovascular pain: a synthesis of the central structures involved in migraine. *Headache* **31**(6):365–371.

Goadsby PJ, Lipton RB, Ferrari MD (2002) Migraine—current understanding and treatment. *N Engl J Med* **346**(4):257–270.

Goder R, Fritzer G, Kapsokalyvas A, *et al* (2001) Polysomnographic findings in nights preceding a migraine attack. *Cephalalgia* **21**(1):31–37.

Goldstein J, Silberstein SD, Saper JR, *et al* (2005) Acetaminophen, aspirin, and caffeine versus sumatriptan succinate in the early treatment of migraine: results from the ASSET trial. *Headache* **45** (8):973–982.

Gomersall JD, Stuart A (1973) Amitriptyline in migraine prophylaxis. Changes in pattern of attacks during a controlled clinical trial. *J Neurol Neurosurg Psychiatry* **36**(4):684–690.

Granella F, Sances G, Pucci E, *et al* (2000) Migraine with aura and reproductive life events: a case control study. *Cephalalgia* **20**(8):701–707.

Granella F, Sances G, Allais G, *et al* (2004) Characteristics of menstrual and nonmenstrual attacks in women with menstrually related migraine referred to headache centres. *Cephalalgia* **24**(9):707–716.

Gyorfi A, Fazekas A, Irmes F, *et al* (1995) Effect of substance P administration on vascular permeability in the rat oral mucosa and sublingual gland. *J Periodontal Res* **30**(3):181–185.

Haas DC, Kent PF, Friedman DI (1993) Headache caused by a single lesion of multiple sclerosis in the periaqueductal gray area. *Headache* **33**(8):452–455.

Hadjikhani N, Sanchez Del Rio M, Wu O, *et al* (2001) Mechanisms of migraine aura revealed by functional MRI in human visual cortex. *Proc Natl Acad Sci U S A* **98**(8):4687–4692.

Henry P, Michel P, Brochet B, *et al* (1992) A nationwide survey of migraine in France: prevalence and clinical features in adults. GRIM. *Cephalalgia* **12**(4):229–237; discussion 186.

Heyeraas KJ, Kvinnsland I (1992) Tissue pressure and blood flow in pulpal inflammation. *Proc Finn Dent Soc* **88** (Suppl 1): 393–401.

Holroyd KA, Penzien DB, Cordingley GE (1991) Propranolol in the management of recurrent migraine: a meta-analytic review. *Headache* **31**(5):333–340.

Hoskin KL, Bulmer DC, Goadsby PJ (1999a) Fos expression in the trigeminocervical complex of the cat after stimulation of the superior sagittal sinus is reduced by L-NAME. *Neurosci Lett* **266**(3):173–176.

Hoskin KL, Zagami AS, Goadsby PJ (1999b) Stimulation of the middle meningeal artery leads to Fos expression in the trigeminocervical nucleus: a comparative study of monkey and cat. *J Anat* **194** (Pt 4):579–588.

Iijima T, Zhang JQ (2002) Three-dimensional wall structure and the innervation of dental pulp blood vessels. *Microsc Res Tech* **56**(1):32–41.

Inoki R, Toyoda T, Yamamoto I (1973) Elaboration of a bradykinin-like substance in dog's canine pulp during electrical stimulation and its inhibition by narcotic and nonnarcotic analgesics. *Naunyn Schmiedebergs Arch Pharmacol* **279**(4):387–398.

Iversen HK, Langemark M, Andersson PG, *et al* (1990) Clinical characteristics of migraine and episodic tension-type headache in relation to old and new diagnostic criteria. *Headache* **30**(8):514–519.

Izumi H (1999) Nervous control of blood flow in the orofacial region. *Pharmacol Ther* **81**(2):141–161.

Izumi H, Karita K (1991) Vasodilator responses following intracranial stimulation of the trigeminal, facial and glossopharyngeal nerves in the cat gingiva. *Brain Res* **560**(1-2):71–75.

Jones KW, Ehm MG, Pericak-Vance MA, *et al* (2001) Migraine with aura susceptibility locus on chromosome 19p13 is distinct from the familial hemiplegic migraine locus. *Genomics* **78**(3):150–154.

Joutel A, Bousser MG, Biousse V, *et al* (1993) A gene for familial hemiplegic migraine maps to chromosome 19. *Nat Genet* **5**(1):40–45.

Juhasz G, Zsombok T, Modos EA, *et al* (2003) NO-induced migraine attack: strong increase in plasma calcitonin gene-related peptide (CGRP) concentration and negative correlation with platelet serotonin release. *Pain* **106**(3):461–470.

Kallela M, Wessman M, Farkkila M, *et al* (1999) Clinical characteristics of migraine in a population-based twin sample: similarities and differences between migraine with and without aura. *Cephalalgia* **19**(3):151–158.

Kaniecki RG (1997) A comparison of divalproex with propranolol and placebo for the prophylaxis of migraine without aura. *Arch Neurol* **54**(9):1141–1145.

Karli N, Zarifoglu M, Calisir N, *et al* (2005) Comparison of pre-headache phases and trigger factors of migraine and episodic tension-type headache: do they share similar clinical pathophysiology? *Cephalalgia* **25**(6):444–451.

Katsarava Z, Schneeweiss S, Kurth T, *et al* (2004) Incidence and predictors for chronicity of headache in patients with episodic migraine. *Neurology* **62**(5):788–790.

Kaube H, Keay KA, Hoskin KL, *et al* (1993a) Expression of c-Fos-like immunoreactivity in the caudal medulla and upper cervical spinal cord following stimulation of the superior sagittal sinus in the cat. *Brain Res* **629**(1):95–102.

Kaube H, Hoskin KL, Goadsby PJ (1993b) Inhibition by sumatriptan of central trigeminal neurones only after blood-brain barrier disruption. *Br J Pharmacol* **109**(3):788–792.

Kaup AO, Mathew NT, Levyman C, *et al* (2003) 'Side locked' migraine and trigeminal autonomic cephalgias: evidence for clinical overlap. *Cephalalgia* **23**(1):43–49.

Kelman L (2004a) The premonitory symptoms (prodrome): a tertiary care study of 893 migraineurs. *Headache* **44**(9):865–872.

Kelman L (2004b) The aura: a tertiary care study of 952 migraine patients. *Cephalalgia* **24**(9):728–734.

Kelman L (2005) Migraine pain location: a tertiary care study of 1283 migraineurs. *Headache* **45**(8):1038–1047.

Kelman L, Rains JC (2005) Headache and sleep: examination of sleep patterns and complaints in a large clinical sample of migraineurs. *Headache* **45**(7):904–910.

Kim S (1990) Neurovascular interactions in the dental pulp in health and inflammation. *J Endod* **16**(2):48–53.

Klapper J (1997) Divalproex sodium in migraine prophylaxis: a dose-controlled study. *Cephalalgia* **17**(2):103–108.

Knight YE, Goadsby PJ (2001) The periaqueductal grey matter modulates trigeminovascular input: a role in migraine? *Neuroscience* **106**(4):793–800.

Knight YE, Bartsch T, Kaube H, et al (2002) P/Q-type calcium-channel blockade in the periaqueductal gray facilitates trigeminal nociception: a functional genetic link for migraine? *J Neurosci* **22**(5):RC213.

Knight YE, Classey JD, Lasalandra MP, et al (2005) Patterns of fos expression in the rostral medulla and caudal pons evoked by noxious craniovascular stimulation and periaqueductal gray stimulation in the cat. *Brain Res* **1045**(1-2):1–11.

Komorowski RC, Torneck CD, Hu JW (1996) Neurogenic inflammation and tooth pulp innervation pattern in sympathectomized rats. *J Endod* **22**(8):414–417.

Koseoglu E, Nacar M, Talaslioglu A, et al (2003) Epidemiological and clinical characteristics of migraine and tension type headache in 1146 females in Kayseri, Turkey. *Cephalalgia* **23**(5):381–388.

Kruuse C, Thomsen LL, Birk S, et al (2003) Migraine can be induced by sildenafil without changes in middle cerebral artery diameter. *Brain* **126**(Pt 1):241–247.

Krymchantowski AV, Moreira PF (2001) Clinical presentation of transformed migraine: possible differences among male and female patients. *Cephalalgia* **21**(5):558–566.

Lambert GA, Bogduk N, Goadsby PJ, et al (1984) Decreased carotid arterial resistance in cats in response to trigeminal stimulation. J Neurosurg **61**(2):307–315.

Lance JW, Goadsby PJ (2005) *Mechanism and management of headache*, 7th edn. Philadelphia, Elsevier.

Lassen LH, Ashina M, Christiansen I, et al (1997) Nitric oxide synthase inhibition in migraine. *Lancet* **349**(9049):401–402.

Lassen LH, Haderslev PA, Jacobsen VB, et al (2002) CGRP may play a causative role in migraine. *Cephalalgia* **22**(1):54–61.

Leone M, Bussone G (1993) A review of hormonal findings in cluster headache. Evidence for hypothalamic involvement. *Cephalalgia* **13**(5):309–317.

Lewis D, Ashwal S, Hershey A, et al (2004) Practice parameter: pharmacological treatment of migraine headache in children and adolescents: report of the American Academy of Neurology Quality Standards Subcommittee and the Practice Committee of the Child Neurology Society. *Neurology* **63**(12):2215-2224.

Lewis PJ, Barrington SF, Marsden PK, et al (1997) A study of the effects of sumatriptan on myocardial perfusion in healthy female migraineurs using 13NH3 positron emission tomography. *Neurology* **48**(6):1542–1550.

Linde K, Rossnagel K (2004) Propranolol for migraine prophylaxis. *Cochrane Database Syst Rev* (2):CD003225.

Lipton RB, Bigal ME (2005) Migraine: epidemiology, impact, and risk factors for progression. *Headache* **45**(Suppl 1):S3–S13.

Lipton RB, Pan J (2004) Is migraine a progressive brain disease? *JAMA* **291**(4):493–494.

Lipton RB, Stewart WF, Stone AM, et al (2000a) Stratified care vs step care strategies for migraine: the Disability in Strategies of Care (DISC) Study: A randomized trial. *JAMA* **284**(20):2599–2605.

Lipton RB, Stewart WF, Scher AI (2000b) Epidemiology of migraine. In: Diener HC (ed) *Treatment of Migraine and Other Headaches*. Basel: Karger, pp 2–15.

Lipton RB, Stewart WF, Diamond S, et al (2001a) Prevalence and burden of migraine in the United States: data from the American Migraine Study II. *Headache* **41**(7):646–657.

Lipton RB, Diamond S, Reed M, et al (2001b) Migraine diagnosis and treatment: results from the American Migraine Study II. *Headache* **41**(7):638–645.

Lipton RB, Scher AI, Kolodner K, et al (2002) Migraine in the United States: epidemiology and patterns of health care use. *Neurology* **58**(6):885–894.

Loder E (2005) Fixed drug combinations for the acute treatment of migraine: place in therapy. *CNS Drugs* **19**(9):769–784.

Loder E, Biondi D (2005) General principles of migraine management: the changing role of prevention. *Headache* **45**(Suppl 1):S33–S47.

Lyngberg AC, Rasmussen BK, Jorgensen T, et al (2005) Incidence of primary headache: a Danish epidemiologic follow-up study. *Am J Epidemiol* **161**(11):1066–1073.

Ma QP (2001) Co-localization of 5-HT(1B/1D/1F) receptors and glutamate in trigeminal ganglia in rats. *Neuroreport* **12**(8):1589–1591.

Ma QP, Hill R, Sirinathsinghji D (2001) Colocalization of CGRP with 5-HT1B/1D receptors and substance P in trigeminal ganglion neurons in rats. *Eur J Neurosci* **13**(11):2099–2104.

MacGregor EA, Brandes J, Eikermann A (2003) Migraine prevalence and treatment patterns: the global Migraine and Zolmitriptan Evaluation survey. *Headache* **43**(1):19–26.

MacGregor EA, Brandes J, Eikermann A, et al (2004) Impact of migraine on patients and their families: the Migraine And Zolmitriptan Evaluation (MAZE) survey–Phase III. *Curr Med Res Opin* **20**(7):1143–1150.

Magnusson JE, Becker WJ (2003) Migraine frequency and intensity: relationship with disability and psychological factors. *Headache* **43**(10):1049–1059.

Marcus DA, Scharff L, Turk D, et al (1997) A double-blind provocative study of chocolate as a trigger of headache. *Cephalalgia* **17**(8):855–862; discussion 800.

Martin VT, Behbehani MM (2001) Toward a rational understanding of migraine trigger factors. *Med Clin North Am* **85**(4):911–941.

Martin VT, Wernke S, Mandell K, et al (2005) Defining the relationship between ovarian hormones and migraine headache. *Headache* **45**(9):1190–1201.

Matchar DB, Young WB, Rosenberg JH, et al (2000) *US Headache Consortium: Evidence-Based Guidelines for Migraine Headache in the Primary Care Setting: Pharmacological Management of Acute Attacks*. American Academy of Neurology. Available at: http://www.aan.com/professionals/practice/pdfs/gl0087.pdf. October 2005.

Matharu MS, Good CD, May A, et al (2003) No change in the structure of the brain in migraine: a voxel-based morphometric study. *Eur J Neurol* **10**(1):53-57.

Matharu MS, Bartsch T, Ward N, et al (2004) Central neuromodulation in chronic migraine patients with suboccipital stimulators: a PET study. *Brain* **127**(Pt 1):220–230.

Mathew NT (1981) Prophylaxis of migraine and mixed headache. A randomized controlled study. *Headache* **21**(3):105–109.

Mathew NT, Reuveni U, Perez F (1987) Transformed or evolutive migraine. *Headache* **27**(2):102–106.

Mattsson P, Svardsudd K, Lundberg PO, et al (2000) The prevalence of migraine in women aged 40-74 years: a population-based study. *Cephalalgia* **20**(10):893–899.

May A, Goadsby PJ (1999) The trigeminovascular system in humans: pathophysiologic implications for primary headache syndromes of the neural influences on the cerebral circulation. *J Cereb Blood Flow Metab* **19**(2):115–127.

May A, Bahra A, Buchel C, et al (1998a) Hypothalamic activation in cluster headache attacks. *Lancet* **352**(9124):275–278.

May A, Kaube H, Buchel C, et al (1998b) Experimental cranial pain elicited by capsaicin: a PET study. *Pain* **74**(1):61–66.

May A, Ashburner J, Buchel C, et al (1999) Correlation between structural and functional changes in brain in an idiopathic headache syndrome. *Nat Med* **5**(7):836–838.

May A, Bahra A, Buchel C, *et al* (2000) PET and MRA findings in cluster headache and MRA in experimental pain. *Neurology* **55**(9):1328–1335.

May A, Buchel C, Turner R, *et al* (2001) Magnetic resonance angiography in facial and other pain: neurovascular mechanisms of trigeminal sensation. *J Cereb Blood Flow Metab* **21**(10):1171–1176.

Merikangas KR, Rasmussen BK (2000) Migraine comorbidity. In: Olesen J, Tfelt-Hansen P, Welch KMA (eds) *The Headaches*, 2nd edn. Philadelphia: Lippincott Williams and Wilkins, pp 235–240.

Merskey H, Bogduk N (1994) *Classification of Chronic Pain: Descriptions of Chronic Pain Syndromes and Definition of Pain Terms*, 2nd edn. Seattle: IASP Press.

Miller GS (2004) Efficacy and safety of levetiracetam in pediatric migraine. *Headache* **44**(3):238–243.

Millson DS, Tepper SJ, Rapoport AM (2000) Migraine pharmacotherapy with oral triptans: a rational approach to clinical management. *Expert Opin Pharmacother* **1**(3):391–404.

Mochi M, Cevoli S, Cortelli P, *et al* (2003) A genetic association study of migraine with dopamine receptor 4, dopamine transporter and dopamine-beta-hydroxylase genes. *Neurol Sci* **23**(6):301–305.

Moore A, Edwards J, Barden J, *et al* (2003) *Bandolier's Little Book of Pain*. Oxford: Oxford University Press.

Morey SS (2000) Guidelines on migraine: part 5. Recommendations for specific prophylactic drugs. *Am Fam Physician* **62**(11):2535–2539.

Morillo LE (2004) Migraine headache. *Clin Evid* (11):1696–1719.

Moskowitz MA (1990) Basic mechanisms in vascular headache. *Neurol Clin* **8**(4):801–815.

Moskowitz MA, Cutrer FM (1993) SUMATRIPTAN: a receptor-targeted treatment for migraine. *Annu Rev Med* **44**:145–154.

Moskowitz MA, Nozaki K, Kraig RP (1993) Neocortical spreading depression provokes the expression of c-fos protein-like immunoreactivity within trigeminal nucleus caudalis via trigeminovascular mechanisms. *J Neurosci* **13**(3):1167–1177.

Murthy RS, Bertolote JM, Epping-Jordan J, *et al* (2001) The World Health Report 2001. Mental health: new understanding, new hope. WHO Library, Geneva.

Nozaki K, Boccalini P, Moskowitz MA (1992) Expression of c-fos-like immunoreactivity in brainstem after meningeal irritation by blood in the subarachnoid space. *Neuroscience* **49**(3):669–680.

O'Brien B, Goeree R, Streiner D (1994) Prevalence of migraine headache in Canada: a population-based survey. *Int J Epidemiol* **23**(5):1020–1026.

Ohkubo T, Shibata M, Yamada Y, *et al* (1993) Role of substance P in neurogenic inflammation in the rat incisor pulp and the lower lip. *Arch Oral Biol* **38**(2):151–158.

Okeson JP (2005) Vascular and neurovascular pains. In: Okeson JP *Bell's Orofacial Pains*, 6th edn. Chicago: Quintessence Publishing, pp 401–448.

Olesen J (2000) The migraines: introduction. In: Olesen J, Tfelt-Hansen P, Welch KMA (eds) *The Headaches*, 2nd edn. Philadelphia: Lippincott Williams & Wilkins, pp 223–225.

Olesen J, Cutrer FM (2000) Migraine with aura and its subforms. In: Olesen J, Tfelt-Hansen P, Welch KMA (eds) *The Headaches*, 2nd edn. Philadelphia: Lippincott Williams & Wilkins, pp 345–363.

Olesen J, Bousser M-G, Diener HC, *et al* (2004a) The International Classification of Headache Disorders, 2nd Edition. *Cephalalgia* **24** (suppl 1):24–150.

Olesen J, Diener HC, Husstedt IW, *et al* (2004b) Calcitonin gene-related peptide receptor antagonist BIBN 4096 BS for the acute treatment of migraine. *N Engl J Med* **350**(11):1104–1110.

Ophoff RA, van Eijk R, Sandkuijl LA, *et al* (1994) Genetic heterogeneity of familial hemiplegic migraine. *Genomics* **22**(1):21–26.

Ophoff RA, Terwindt GM, Vergouwe MN, *et al* (1996) Familial hemiplegic migraine and episodic ataxia type-2 are caused by mutations in the Ca2+ channel gene CACNL1A4. *Cell* **87**(3):543–552.

Pascual J, Leira R, Lainez JM (2003) Combined therapy for migraine prevention? Clinical experience with a beta-blocker plus sodium valproate in 52 resistant migraine patients. *Cephalalgia* **23**(10):961–962.

Peatfield RC (1995) Relationships between food, wine, and beer-precipitated migrainous headaches. *Headache* **35**(6):355–357.

Peñarrocha M, Bandres A, Penarrocha M, *et al* (2004) Lower-half facial migraine: a report of 11 cases. *J Oral Maxillofac Surg* **62**(12):1453–1456.

Peres MF, Sanchez del Rio M, Seabra ML, *et al* (2001) Hypothalamic involvement in chronic migraine. *J Neurol Neurosurg Psychiatry* **71**(6):747–751.

Perry BF, Login IS, Kountakis SE (2004) Nonrhinologic headache in a tertiary rhinology practice. *Otolaryngol Head Neck Surg* **130**(4):449–452.

Pryse-Phillips W, Findlay H, Tugwell P, *et al* (1992) A Canadian population survey on the clinical, epidemiologic and societal impact of migraine and tension-type headache. *Can J Neurol Sci* **19**(3):333–339.

Pryse-Phillips WE, Dodick DW, Edmeads JG, *et al* (1998) Guidelines for the nonpharmacologic management of migraine in clinical practice. Canadian Headache Society. *CMAJ* **159**(1):47–54.

Puri V, Cui L, Liverman CS, *et al* (2005) Ovarian steroids regulate neuropeptides in the trigeminal ganglion. *Neuropeptides* **39**(4):409–417.

Putnam GP, O'Quinn S, Bolden-Watson CP, *et al* (1999) Migraine polypharmacy and the tolerability of sumatriptan: a large-scale, prospective study. *Cephalalgia* **19**(7):668–675.

Rains JC, Poceta JS (2005) Sleep-related headache syndromes. *Semin Neurol* **25**(1):69–80.

Ramadan NM (2004) Prophylactic migraine therapy: mechanisms and evidence. *Curr Pain Headache Rep* **8**(2):91–95.

Ramadan NM, Schultz LL, Gilkey SJ (1997) Migraine prophylactic drugs: proof of efficacy, utilization and cost. *Cephalalgia* **17**(2):73–80.

Ramadan NM, Silberstein SD, Freitag FG, *et al* (2000) *US Headache Consortium: Evidence-Based Guidelines for Migraine Headache in the Primary Care Setting: Pharmacological Management for Prevention of Migraine*. American Academy of Neurology. Available at: http://www.aan.com/professionals/practice/pdfs/gl0090.pdf. October 2005.

Raskin NH, Hosobuchi Y, Lamb S (1987) Headache may arise from perturbation of brain. *Headache* **27**(8):416–420.

Rasmussen BK (1993) Migraine and tension-type headache in a general population: precipitating factors, female hormones, sleep pattern and relation to lifestyle. *Pain* **53**(1):65–72.

Rasmussen BK (2001) Epidemiology of headache. *Cephalalgia* **21**(7):774–777.

Rasmussen BK, Olesen J (1992a) Migraine with aura and migraine without aura: an epidemiological study. *Cephalalgia* **12**(4):221–228; discussion 186.

Rasmussen BK, Olesen J (1992b) Symptomatic and nonsymptomatic headaches in a general population. *Neurology* **42**(6):1225–1231.

Rasmussen BK, Jensen R, Olesen J (1991a) A population-based analysis of the diagnostic criteria of the International Headache Society. *Cephalalgia* **11**(3):129–134.

Rasmussen BK, Jensen R, Schroll M, *et al* (1991b) Epidemiology of headache in a general population–a prevalence study. *J Clin Epidemiol* **44**(11):1147–1157.

Rebeck GW, Maynard KI, Hyman BT, *et al* (1994) Selective 5-HT1D alpha serotonin receptor gene expression in trigeminal ganglia: implications for antimigraine drug development. *Proc Natl Acad Sci U S A* **91**(9):3666-3669.

Robbins L (1994) Precipitating factors in migraine: a retrospective review of 494 patients. *Headache* **34**(4):214–216.

Robbins L (2002) Triptans versus analgesics. *Headache* **42**(9):903–907.

Rodd HD, Boissonade FM (2002) Comparative immunohistochemical analysis of the peptidergic innervation of human primary and permanent tooth pulp. *Arch Oral Biol* **47**(5):375–385.

Rothrock JF (1997) Successful treatment of persistent migraine aura with divalproex sodium. *Neurology* **48**(1):261–262.

Russell MB, Olesen J (1995) Increased familial risk and evidence of genetic factor in migraine. *BMJ* **311**(7004):541–544.

Russell MB, Olesen J (1996) A nosographic analysis of the migraine aura in a general population. *Brain* **119** (Pt 2):355–361.

Russell MB, Rasmussen BK, Brennum J, *et al* (1992) Presentation of a new instrument: the diagnostic headache diary. *Cephalalgia* **12**(6):369–374.

Russell MB, Rasmussen BK, Fenger K, *et al* (1996) Migraine without aura and migraine with aura are distinct clinical entities: a study of four hundred and eighty-four male and female migraineurs from the general population. *Cephalalgia* **16** (4):239–245.

Russell MB, Ulrich V, Gervil M, *et al* (2002) Migraine without aura and migraine with aura are distinct disorders. A population-based twin survey. *Headache* **42**(5):332–336.

Sances G, Granella F, Nappi RE, *et al* (2003) Course of migraine during pregnancy and postpartum: a prospective study. *Cephalalgia* **23**(3):197–205.

Sances G, Tassorelli C, Pucci E, *et al* (2004) Reliability of the nitroglycerin provocative test in the diagnosis of neurovascular headaches. *Cephalalgia* **24**(2):110–119.

Sanchez del Rio M, Bakker D, Wu O, *et al* (1999) Perfusion weighted imaging during migraine: spontaneous visual aura and headache. *Cephalalgia* **19**(8):701–707.

Saper JR, Dodick D, Gladstone JP (2005) Management of chronic daily headache: challenges in clinical practice. *Headache* **45** (Suppl 1):S74–S85.

Savi L, Rainero I, Valfre W, *et al* (2002) Food and headache attacks. A comparison of patients with migraine and tension-type headache. *Panminerva Med* **44**(1):27–31.

Scher AI, Stewart WF, Ricci JA, *et al* (2003) Factors associated with the onset and remission of chronic daily headache in a population-based study. *Pain* **106**(1-2):81–89.

Scher AI, Bigal ME, Lipton RB (2005) Comorbidity of migraine. *Curr Opin Neurol* **18**(3):305–310.

Schnurr RF, Brooke RI (1992) Atypical odontalgia. Update and comment on long-term follow-up. *Oral Surg Oral Med Oral Pathol* **73**(4):445–448.

Schon H, Thomas DT, Jewkes DA, *et al* (1987) Failure to detect plasma neuropeptide release during trigeminal thermocoagulation. *J Neurol Neurosurg Psychiatry* **50**(5):642–643.

Sculpher M, Millson D, Meddis D, *et al* (2002) Cost-effectiveness analysis of stratified versus stepped care strategies for acute treatment of migraine: The Disability in Strategies for Care (DISC) Study. *Pharmacoeconomics* **20**(2):91–100.

Sharav Y (1999) Orofacial pain. In: Wall PD, Melzack R (eds) *Textbook of Pain*, 4th edn. Edinburgh: Churchill Livingstone, pp 711–738.

Silberstein SD (2000) Practice parameter: evidence-based guidelines for migraine headache (an evidence-based review): report of the Quality Standards Subcommittee of the American Academy of Neurology. *Neurology* **55**(6):754–762.

Silberstein SD (2005) Preventive treatment of headaches. *Curr Opin Neurol* **18**(3):289–292.

Silberstein SD, Goadsby PJ (2002) Migraine: preventive treatment. *Cephalalgia* **22**(7):491–512.

Silberstein SD, Goadsby PJ, Lipton RB (2000) Management of migraine: an algorithmic approach. *Neurology* **55**(9 Suppl 2): S46–S52.

Silberstein SD, Saper JR, Freitag FG (2001) Migraine: Diagnosis and treatment. In: Silberstein SD, Lipton RB, Dalessio DJ (eds) *Wolff's Headache and Other Head Pains*, 7th edn. Oxford: Oxford University Press, pp 121–237.

Silvestrini M, Bartolini M, Coccia M, *et al* (2003) Topiramate in the treatment of chronic migraine. *Cephalalgia* **23**(8):820–824.

Smetana GW (2000) The diagnostic value of historical features in primary headache syndromes: a comprehensive review. *Arch Intern Med* **160**(18):2729–2737.

Smith TR, Sunshine A, Stark SR, *et al* (2005) Sumatriptan and naproxen sodium for the acute treatment of migraine. *Headache* **45**(8):983–991.

Solomon S, Karfunkel P, Guglielmo KM (1985) Migraine-cluster headache syndrome. *Headache* **25**(5):236–239.

Solomon S, Lipton RB, Newman LC (1992) Clinical features of chronic daily headache. *Headache* **32**(7):325–329.

Spierings EL, Schroevers M, Honkoop PC, *et al* (1998) Presentation of chronic daily headache: a clinical study. *Headache* **38**(3): 191–196.

Spierings EL, Ranke AH, Honkoop PC (2001) Precipitating and aggravating factors of migraine versus tension-type headache. *Headache* **41**(6):554–558.

Spira PJ, Beran RG (2003) Gabapentin in the prophylaxis of chronic daily headache: a randomized, placebo-controlled study. *Neurology* **61**(12):1753–1759.

Srikiatkhachorn A, Phanthumchinda K (1997) Prevalence and clinical features of chronic daily headache in a headache clinic. *Headache* **37**(5):277–280.

Stang PE, Yanagihara PA, Swanson JW, *et al* (1992) Incidence of migraine headache: a population-based study in Olmsted County, Minnesota. *Neurology* **42**(9):1657–1662.

Steiner TJ (2000) Headache burdens and bearers. *Funct Neurol* **15** (Suppl 3):219–223.

Steiner TJ, Scher AI, Stewart WF, *et al* (2003) The prevalence and disability burden of adult migraine in England and their relationships to age, gender and ethnicity. *Cephalalgia* **23** (7):519–527.

Stewart WF, Linet MS, Celentano DD, *et al* (1991) Age- and sex-specific incidence rates of migraine with and without visual aura. *Am J Epidemiol* **134**(10):1111–1120.

Stewart WF, Lipton RB, Celentano DD, *et al* (1992) Prevalence of migraine headache in the United States. Relation to age, income, race, and other sociodemographic factors. *JAMA* **267**(1):64–69.

Stewart WF, Lipton RB, Liberman J (1996a) Variation in migraine prevalence by race. *Neurology* **47**(1):52–59.

Stewart WF, Lipton RB, Simon D (1996b) Work-related disability: results from the American migraine study. *Cephalalgia* **16**(4): 231–238; discussion 215.

Stewart WF, Staffa J, Lipton RB, *et al* (1997) Familial risk of migraine: a population-based study. *Ann Neurol* **41**(2):166–172.

Stewart WF, Lipton RB, Kolodner KB, *et al* (2000) Validity of the Migraine Disability Assessment (MIDAS) score in comparison to a diary-based measure in a population sample of migraine sufferers. *Pain* **88**(1):41–52.

Stewart WF, Lipton RB, Kolodner K (2003) Migraine disability assessment (MIDAS) score: relation to headache frequency, pain intensity, and headache symptoms. *Headache* **43**(3): 258–265.

Stronks DL, Tulen JH, Bussmann JB, *et al* (2004) Interictal daily functioning in migraine. *Cephalalgia* **24**(4):271–279.

Tajti J, Moller S, Uddman R, *et al* (1999a) The human superior cervical ganglion: neuropeptides and peptide receptors. *Neurosci Lett* **263**(2-3):121–124.

Tajti J, Uddman R, Moller S, *et al* (1999b) Messenger molecules and receptor mRNA in the human trigeminal ganglion. *J Auton Nerv Syst* **76**(2-3):176–183.

Tepper S, Allen C, Sanders D, *et al* (2003) Coprescription of triptans with potentially interacting medications: a cohort study involving 240,268 patients. *Headache* **43**(1):44–48.

Tepper SJ, Bigal ME, Sheftell FD, *et al* (2004) Botulinum neurotoxin type A in the preventive treatment of refractory headache: a review of 100 consecutive cases. *Headache* **44**(8):794–800.

Tfelt-Hansen P, McEwen J (2000) Nonsteroidal antiinflammatory drugs in the acute treatment of migraine. In: Olesen J, Tfelt-Hansen P, Welch KMA (eds) *The Headaches*, 2nd edn. Philadelphia: Lippincott Williams and Wilkins, pp 391–397.

Tfelt-Hansen P, Saxena PR (2000). Ergot alkaloids in the acute treatment of migraine. In: Olesen J, Tfelt-Hansen P, Welch KMA (eds) *The Headaches*, 2nd edn. Philadelphia: Lippincott Williams and Wilkins, pp 399–409.

Tfelt-Hansen P, De Vries P, Saxena PR (2000) Triptans in migraine: a comparative review of pharmacology, pharmacokinetics and efficacy. *Drugs* **60**(6):1259–1287.

Thomsen LL, Olesen J (2001) Nitric oxide in primary headaches. *Curr Opin Neurol* **14**(3):315–321.

Tomkins GE, Jackson JL, O'Malley PG, *et al* (2001) Treatment of chronic headache with antidepressants: a meta-analysis. *Am J Med* **111**(1):54–63.

Uddman R, Edvinsson L, Ekman R, *et al* (1985) Innervation of the feline cerebral vasculature by nerve fibers containing calcitonin gene-related peptide: trigeminal origin and co-existence with substance P. *Neurosci Lett* **62**(1):131–136.

Uddman R, Kato J, Lindgren P, *et al* (1999) Expression of calcitonin gene-related peptide-1 receptor mRNA in human tooth pulp and trigeminal ganglion. *Arch Oral Biol* **44**(1):1–6.

Ulrich V, Gervil M, Kyvik KO, *et al* (1999) Evidence of a genetic factor in migraine with aura: a population-based Danish twin study. *Ann Neurol* **45**(2):242–246.

Vanmolkot KR, Kors EE, Hottenga JJ, *et al* (2003) Novel mutations in the Na+, K+-ATPase pump gene ATP1A2 associated with familial hemiplegic migraine and benign familial infantile convulsions. *Ann Neurol* **54**(3):360–366.

Veloso F, Kumar K, Toth C (1998) Headache secondary to deep brain implantation. *Headache* **38**(7):507–515.

Vickers ER, Cousins MJ, Walker S, *et al* (1998) Analysis of 50 patients with atypical odontalgia. A preliminary report on pharmacological procedures for diagnosis and treatment. *Oral Surg Oral Med Oral Pathol Oral Radiol Endod* **85**(1):24–32.

Von Korff M, Stewart WF, Simon DJ, *et al* (1998) Migraine and reduced work performance: a population-based diary study. *Neurology* **50**(6):1741–1745.

Waeber C, Moskowitz MA (2003) Therapeutic implications of central and peripheral neurologic mechanisms in migraine. *Neurology* **61**(8 Suppl 4):S9–S20.

Weiller C, May A, Limmroth V, *et al* (1995) Brain stem activation in spontaneous human migraine attacks. *Nat Med* **1**(7):658–660.

Welch KM (2003) Contemporary concepts of migraine pathogenesis. *Neurology* **61**(8 Suppl 4):S2–S8.

Welch KM, Mathew NT, Stone P, *et al* (2000) Tolerability of sumatriptan: clinical trials and post-marketing experience. *Cephalalgia* **20**(8):687–695.

Welch KM, Nagesh V, Aurora SK, *et al* (2001) Periaqueductal gray matter dysfunction in migraine: cause or the burden of illness? *Headache* **41**(7):629–637.

Young WB, Siow HC, Silberstein SD (2004) Anticonvulsants in migraine. *Curr Pain Headache Rep* **8**(3):244–250.

Zagami AS, Lambert GA (1991) Craniovascular application of capsaicin activates nociceptive thalamic neurones in the cat. *Neurosci Lett* **121**(1–2):187–190.

Zagami AS, Rasmussen BK (2000) Symptomatology of migraine. In: Olesen J, Tfelt-Hansen P, Welch KMA (eds) *The Headaches*, 2nd edn. Philadelphia: Lippincott Williams and Wilkins, pp 337–343.

Zebenholzer K, Wober C, Kienbacher C, *et al* (2000) Migrainous disorder and headache of the tension-type not fulfilling the criteria: a follow-up study in children and adolescents. *Cephalalgia* **20**(7):611–616.

Zeller JA, Lindner V, Frahm K, *et al* (2005) Platelet activation and platelet-leucocyte interaction in patients with migraine. Subtype differences and influence of triptans. *Cephalalgia* **25**(7):536–541.

Ziegler DK, Hurwitz A, Hassanein RS, *et al* (1987) Migraine prophylaxis. A comparison of propranolol and amitriptyline. *Arch Neurol* **44**(5):486–489.

CHAPTER 10

The trigeminal autonomic cephalgias (TACs)

Rafael Benoliel and Yair Sharav

1. Introduction

The International Headache Society's (IHS) most recent classification introduces the trigeminal autonomic cephalgias (TACs), a group that includes cluster headache (CH), paroxysmal hemicrania (PH) and short-lasting neuralgiform headache attacks with conjunctival injection and tearing (SUNCT); see Table 10.1 (Olesen *et al* 2004). TACs are characterized by a shared clinical phenotype of trigeminal pain accompanied by prominent autonomic signs (AS) suggesting a common pathophysiology. Hemicrania continua (HC), although classified separately by the IHS, is thought to be related to TACs and is described in this chapter (Olesen *et al* 2004).

Common diagnostic features of TACs include episodic pain that is unilateral, pulsatile or sharp, is of severe intensity, that wakes from sleep and is accompanied by autonomic phenomena include tearing and rhinorrhea (Goadsby and Lipton 1997; Benoliel and Sharav 1998a,b; Dodick *et al* 2000; Benoliel *et al* 2002; Olesen *et al* 2004). However, TACs have been classified based on well-defined criteria of location, attack frequency, duration and accompanying signs and symptoms with an individual and distinctive response to therapy (Olesen *et al* 2004).

Pain quality in TACs and dental pulpitis are similar and dentists are often the first healthcare providers consulted (Benoliel *et al* 1997; van Vliet *et al* 2003a; Bahra and Goadsby 2004). Incorrect diagnosis may lead to dental treatment that is both misguided and unjustified. Primary intraoral pain of neurovascular origin is rare but there are clinical data that support the existence of a primary intraoral syndrome (Benoliel *et al* 1997; Penarrocha *et al* 2004). This entity, termed neurovascular orofacial pain (NVOP), has been described in detail in Chapter 9 where the possibility that NVOP is a migraine-related syndrome was examined. In this chapter we describe the TACs and examine the alternative possibility that NVOP is a TAC variant.

2. Cluster Headache

Cluster headache (CH) is essentially the archetypal TAC with severe pain and major autonomic activation (Olesen *et al* 2004). Pain in CH is probably the most severe of the primary headaches and approaches that for trigeminal neuralgia with cases even considering suicide (Dodick *et al* 2000; Torelli and Manzoni 2003).

2.1. Clinical Features

CH attacks tend to occur in clusters that last for a variable period of time (weeks to years) (Dodick *et al* 2000). Based on the distinct temporal patterns of these cluster periods two clinical presentations of CH are described. Most CH patients (80–85%) suffer from the episodic type (Rasmussen 1999) characterized by considerable pain-free periods between clusters. The IHS defines episodic as 'at least 2 cluster periods lasting 7–365 days and separated by pain-free periods of ≥1 month'. In chronic CH repeated attacks recur over more than a year without remission or with remission periods lasting less than one month. Interictal pain may also be present between attacks or between clusters (van Vliet *et al* 2003a). Of the 15% of patients with chronic CH, in two-thirds it usually begins as such and in the remaining evolves from the episodic form (Rasmussen 1999). Up to half of chronic CH patients report transition to an episodic pattern (Krabbe 1991; Manzoni *et al* 1991a). Over the course of the disease, attack duration tends to lengthen in both episodic and chronic CH whilst concomitantly frequency tends to increase in episodic and decrease in chronic CH (Black *et al* 2006).

Table 10.1	International Headache Society's (IHS) Classification of Trigeminal Autonomic Cephalgias (TACs) and Other Primary Headaches

Code 3. Cluster HA and other TACs

Cluster HA	Episodic	3.1.2
	Chronic	3.1.3
Paroxysmal Hemicrania	Episodic	3.2.1
	Chronic	3.2.1
SUNCT		3.3
SUNA[a]	Episodic	A3.3.1
	Chronic	A3.3.2

Code 4. Other primary headaches

Primary stabbing HA		4.1
Primary cough HA		4.2
Primary HA associated with sexual activity		4.4
	Preorgasmic HA	4.4.1
	Orgasmic HA	4.4.2
Hypnic HA		4.5
Primary thunderclap HA		4.6
Hemicrania Continua		4.7
New daily persistent HA		4.8

[a]In IHS appendix, not in main classification.
Adapted from Olesen *et al* (2004) with permission.

Clinical example. Examine Case 10.1. Note the prominent AS that are particularly pronounced in this case whilst in other TACs they may be subtler (Fig. 10.1). Relative to other TACs the pattern is low-frequency, long-lasting headaches with a nocturnal occurrence (Fig. 10.5A).

Despite dramatic symptomatology, CH often remains misdiagnosed for long periods. Studies have shown that the median interval between the first episode and final diagnosis is 3 years: 34–45% had consulted a dentist and 27–33% an otolaryngologist before the diagnosis was accurately established (van Vliet *et al* 2003a; Bahra and Goadsby 2004). Among factors that increase the diagnostic delay were the presence of photophobia or phonophobia, nausea, an episodic attack pattern and a young onset age, which are signs more typical of migraine. The IHS diagnostic criteria for CH are summarized in Table 10.2 (Olesen *et al* 2004).

Location. CH is strictly unilateral but attacks may change sides in about 20% of cases (Dodick *et al* 2000; Black *et al* 2006). Attacks that alternate sides are more common between clusters than between attacks in the same cluster (Dodick *et al* 2000). Peak pain intensity in

CH is classically felt periorbitally or in the eye (Dodick *et al* 2000; Bahra *et al* 2002). 'Lower' and 'upper' subtypes of CH have been reported; pain in lower CH is ocular, temporal and suboccipital with radiation to the teeth, jaws and neck and is therefore highly relevant for dentists (Dodick *et al* 2000; Cademartiri *et al* 2002). Intra/perioral radiation of pain includes the jaws (37%), teeth (maxillary 50%, mandibular 32%) and the cheeks (45%) (Bahra *et al* 2002; van Vliet *et al* 2003a). In upper CH pain is periorbital but radiates to the forehead and temporal and parietal regions (Dodick *et al* 2000).

Quality. CH is severe and rated as 8–10 on a 10-point visual analogue scale (VAS) by >85% of patients (Dodick *et al* 2000; Torelli and Manzoni 2003; Olesen *et al* 2004). Nearly all patients describe their pain either as throbbing or as neuralgic (sharp, boring, burning, stabbing, piercing) (Torelli and Manzoni 2003; Black *et al* 2006). A small number describe combined characteristics of 'neuralgic' with throbbing. Many patients describe the pain as a 'hot poker' or a 'stabbing' feeling in the eye (Dodick *et al* 2000; Bahra *et al* 2002). The extensive array of descriptors used by patients attests to the wide variety of presentation (Torelli and Manzoni 2003). In addition, sudden jabs of intense pain are often felt and may be an integral part of some CH variants (Black *et al* 2006).

Temporal pattern of individual attacks. Peak intensity is usually reached within 9–10 minutes of onset but may develop rapidly, within 3 minutes (Russell 1981; Torelli and Manzoni 2003). Most attacks last 30 minutes to 1 hour (average 45–90 minutes, range 15–180 minutes) but rarely may last from 3 to 48 hours (Russell 1981; Dodick *et al* 2000; van Vliet *et al* 2003a). See Fig. 10.5A and compare the duration of attacks with other TACs (PH and SUNCT) and with migraine (Chapter 9).

Cluster periods. Episodic CH commonly occurs at least once daily for a period of weeks (Ekbom 1970). At low frequencies, CH attacks tend to occur at the same time of day or night with surprising clockwise regularity (Manzoni *et al* 1983; Dodick *et al* 2000). Active periods (average 6–12 weeks) are followed by a temporary remission or an inactive period that may last from weeks to years (average 12 months). Attacks tend to be shorter and less severe at the beginning and towards the end of each cluster period (Black *et al* 2006). Particularly at the initial onset of CH, active periods are seasonal, occurring around spring or autumn (Kudrow 1987; Dodick *et al* 2000). Correlation between daylight hours and CH occurrence and frequency has also been noted (Manzoni *et al* 1991b). However, as CH develops, the active periods become less predictable and variations in the length of both active and inactive periods are apparent (Dodick *et al* 2000).

Remission periods in many patients may increase with time and active CH beyond the age of 65–75 is rare so that long-term prognosis may be good (Ekbom and Hardebo 2002; Black *et al* 2006). Following a first CH attack, a quarter of cases were found to have no further recurrence over a mean follow-up of 8 years (Sjostrand *et al* 2000) and

Case 10.1 Cluster Headache, 29 year-old Male

Present complaint

Attacks of extremely severe pain (VAS 9) periorbitally radiating to the ipsilateral temple, cheek and maxillary molars. Pain is stabbing and sometimes throbbing. Most attacks last 30–60 minutes but he has suffered more prolonged attacks of up to 4 hours.

History of present complaint

For the past 11 years he has suffered repeated pain attacks that have often woken him from sleep in the early hours of the morning. These occur during specific periods lasting 2–14 weeks but at other times, for up to 6 months, he does not suffer from any pain whatsoever. Once an attack begins he is unable to continue working and becomes irritated and extremely agitated.

Attacks are accompanied by ipsilateral tearing, rhinorrhoea and ptosis (Fig. 10.1). The longer lasting attacks are very often accompanied by nausea and photophobia. The patient reported onset of pain in the waiting room; the pain was preceded by a strange sensation around the right cheek and eye (twinges) and rapidly (<5 min) reached peak intensity with clear local signs.

Physical examination

Head and neck examination between attacks was unremarkable. During attacks the findings described under Fig. 10.1 were present.

Relevant medical history

None.

Diagnosis

A tentative diagnosis of episodic cluster headache was made and the patient was instructed to use oxygen (5 L/min) as abortive therapy.

Diagnostic and treatment considerations

At follow up the patient reported that O_2 was very effective in either eradicating or significantly reducing pain attacks (see Fig. 10.5A). However, despite relatively easy access to O_2 he often found it took too long to obtain and requested alternative therapy. Preventive treatment with verapamil was offered but the patient was unwilling to be on permanent medication; therefore sumatriptan 6 mg SC was prescribed with excellent response.

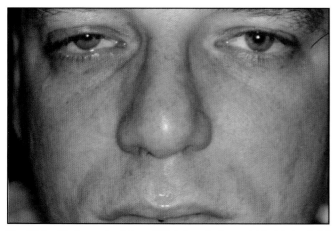

Fig. 10.1 • Photograph of Case 10.1 taken during a right-sided painful attack. Note the ipsilateral ptosis and miosis. Additionally there is obvious ipsilateral lacrimation and rhinorrhoea (see upper lip).

since only the one attack occurred they would not be classified as CH (Olesen *et al* 2004). The majority (65%) of patients had subsequent episodic attacks, most within 3–5 years (Sjostrand *et al* 2000).

Frequency of nocturnal CH is high (51–73%) and pain awakens patients 90 minutes after sleep initiation, at about the onset of rapid eye movement (REM) sleep (see Case 10.1 's pain diary, Fig. 10.5A) (Bahra *et al* 2002). An association between episodic CH and REM sleep has been shown, less so with chronic CH (Pfaffenrath *et al* 1986). Sleep deprivation, resulting from high-frequency attacks, leads to early-onset REM often triggering further attacks. Severity of nocturnal pain is no different to that occurring during the day (Dodick *et al* 2000). Patients with CH demonstrate a greater percentage of obstructive sleep apnoea (58.3%) than a control group (14.3%) or the general population (2–4%) (Chervin *et al* 2000). Treatment of one entity frequently improves the other.

Triggers. Alcohol, even in small amounts, may precipitate CH attacks during active cluster periods (Levi *et al* 1992). CH patients, particularly those who evolve into chronic CH, are high consumers of alcohol and tobacco (Torelli *et al* 2000). Dietary factors are unimportant in CH.

Nitroglycerin provocative test. Nitroglycerin (NG) administration provokes headaches in CH patients during active clusters and has been considered diagnostic. However, NG will induce headaches in CH patients, in migraineurs and in chronic tension-type headache (TTH) sufferers and is therefore not specific (Sances *et al* 2004).

Associated autonomic signs. Ipsilateral AS are very common in CH with lacrimation being the most frequent, occurring in up to 90% of cases (Ekbom 1990; Bahra *et al* 2002). About 50–75% may have conjunctival injection, nasal congestion, ptosis and/or miosis and rhinorrhea (see Case 10.1, Fig. 10.1) (Ekbom 1990; Bahra *et al* 2002). AS are transient and resolve with the headache but rarely

Table 10.2 Diagnostic Criteria for Cluster Headache (CH)

	Diagnostic Criteria	Notes
A	At least 5 attacks fulfilling criteria B–D	Attacks usually occur in clusters lasting weeks/months separated by months/years. Age at onset 20–40 years, male:female ratio is 5:1
B	Severe to very severe unilateral orbital, supraorbital and/or temporal regions pain lasting 15–180 minutes if untreated	During less than half of the time course, attacks may be less severe and/or shorter/longer. Interictal pain or discomfort may occur. During active periods attacks may be provoked by alcohol, histamine or nitroglycerin. During the worst attacks patients are usually unable to lie down and become characteristically agitated (e.g. pace the floor).
C	Headache is accompanied by at least one of the following: 1. Ipsilateral conjunctival injection and/or lacrimation 2. Ipsilateral nasal congestion and/or rhinorrhoea 3. Ipsilateral eyelid oedema 4. Ipsilateral forehead and facial sweating 5. Ipsilateral miosis and/or ptosis 6. A sense of restlessness or agitation	Cases where autonomic signs appear with no headache and vice versa have been reported.
D	Attacks frequency ranges from one every other day to 8 per day	During less than half of the time attacks may be less frequent *Episodic:* At least 2 cluster periods lasting 7–365 days and separated by pain-free periods of ≥1 month *Chronic:* Attacks recur over >1 year without remission periods or with remission periods lasting <1 month.
E	Not attributed to another disorder	4% of patients with pituitary tumour suffer from CH

Adapted from Olesen *et al* (2004) with permission.

ptosis and miosis (partial Horner's syndrome) may persist. Rarely forehead sweating may be observed in severe attacks. Lower CH patients were found to report not only a higher overall rate of AS, but also a higher predominance of nasal congestion, ptosis and forehead and facial sweating (Cademartiri *et al* 2002). Intensity of AS may be related to pain severity; i.e. in patients with weaker CH attacks mild or no AS may occur (Drummond 1990; Goadsby *et al* 2001). Temperature difference between the orbits increases with increasing severity of pain and CH with AS is significantly more painful independent of pain location (Saper *et al* 2002; Martins *et al* 2005). However, a small number of CH of patients (3–6%) may not have AS during attacks and this may make diagnosis difficult (Torelli *et al* 2001; Martins *et al* 2005).

Associated systemic features. Migrainous features including photophobia (56%), phonophobia (43%), nausea (41%), vomiting (24%) and more rarely gustatory, olfactory, ocular and behavioural phenomena are common in CH attacks (Nappi *et al* 1992; Wheeler 1998; Bahra *et al* 2002). Rarely patients may complain of concomitant ipsilateral limb pain that may alternate sides. CH associated with transient hemiparesis also accompanied by visual symptoms, photo- and phonophobia and nausea has been reported (Siow *et al* 2002). This clinical phenotype is strikingly similar to side-locked migraine.

Changes in cardiovascular parameters include increases and decreases in heart rate at onset and during

attacks, respectively, and arrhythmias. Increases in both systolic and diastolic blood pressure have been reported. These changes are probably mediated by connections between the trigeminal and the parabrachial nuclei involved in autonomic control of cardiovascular function (Allen *et al* 1996).

Prodromata and premonitory symptoms. In CH patients specific symptoms may occur minutes to days before pain onset (Raimondi 2001; Bahra *et al* 2002; Torelli and Manzoni 2003). Prodromes precede headache onset by minutes and are reported by almost all patients (Torelli and Manzoni 2003). Local prodromes include AS and mild pain or non-painful sensations in the area that subsequently becomes painful, e.g. twinges, pressure, tingling and a pulsating feeling (Torelli and Manzoni 2003). Additionally blurred vision, sensitivity to smells, nausea, dyspepsia, hunger, irritability, tiredness and tenseness are described (Blau and Engel 1998). Symptoms specific to the oral cavity include dry mouth, metallic taste and feeling tightness in the teeth. General psychic symptoms are also common (Torelli and Manzoni 2003). Premonitory symptoms may predict CH days before onset and are reported in 40% of CH cases (Torelli and Manzoni 2003). These may be similar to those experienced by migraineurs and include body numbness, neck pain, irritability, lethargy and sleepiness (Blau and Engel 1998). 'Aura-like' symptoms are found in 14% of cases (Bahra *et al* 2002; Langedijk *et al* 2005).

Patient behaviour. Restlessness during attacks is so frequent (>80%) that it has been included as a CH diagnostic criterion (Torelli and Manzoni 2003; Olesen *et al* 2004). Patients appear agitated, continually move around and change body position and this is particularly prominent during severe attacks (Russell 1981), in sharp contrast to the quiet-seeking behaviour observed in migraine.

2.2. Secondary CH

Symptomatic CH is common and has been described as a result of inflammatory orbital myositis, inflammatory myeloblastic pseudotumour of the posterior fossa, sphenoidal aspergillosis and multiple sclerosis (Matharu *et al* 2003a; Trucco *et al* 2004). Vascular lesions with CH symptomatology may occur in carotid artery dissection, arteriovenous malformation of the middle cerebellar artery and vertebral artery injury. CH secondary to post-traumatic head injury is commonly observed (37%) (Manzoni 1999a). Cases of CH with onset following tooth extraction have recently been published (Penarrocha *et al* 2001; Soros *et al* 2001) but the importance of such peripheral nerve lesions in the aetiology of CH is unclear and needs further research.

In patients with pituitary tumour 4% were found to suffer from CH (Levy *et al* 2005). Non-metastatic and brain-metastasized lung cancer have presented with cluster headache (Tajti *et al* 1996; Sarlani *et al* 2003a). Careful review of such cases reveals that 'tell-tale' signs were often present in the neurologic examination and in the behaviour, presentation and symptomatology of the headaches (Carter 2004).

2.3. Epidemiology

Several studies of the general population show that CH is a relatively rare syndrome that affects men about five times more than women (Ekbom *et al* 2002; Tonon *et al* 2002). Based on epidemiological data, the closest approximation to actual CH prevalence is proposed to be 0.30%: 0.45% for males and 0.15% for females (Manzoni 1999b; Rasmussen 1999). More recently a higher proportion of female sufferers has been reported with a male:female ratio of 2.1–3.5:1 (Dodick *et al* 2000; Ekbom *et al* 2002). This has been postulated to be associated with the increase of alcohol and tobacco abuse amongst females but the exact reasons are unclear. The clinical characteristics of CH in women are similar to those in men although with some differentiating features. Typical age of onset in men is around the third decade whilst peak onset in women is bimodal in the second (major) and the fifth to sixth (minor) decades (Rozen *et al* 2001). In females mean attack duration is shorter, miosis and ptosis are less common and nausea and vomiting are more frequent than in males (Rozen *et al* 2001).

2.4. Genetics

First-degree relatives of CH patients are up to 39 times and second-degree relatives 8 times more likely to have CH than the general population (Leone *et al* 2001; Russell 2004). A family history is present in 0.8–7% of CH patients (F > M) and accumulated evidence indicates that CH is inherited (Russell *et al* 1996; El Amrani *et al* 2002). There is also high concordance in monozygotic and dizygotic twins (Schuh-Hofer *et al* 2003). CH is likely to have an autosomal dominant gene with low penetrance and present in 3–4% of males and 7–10% of females, but autosomal recessive or multifactorial inheritance may also occur (Russell *et al* 1996).

Co-occurrence of CH and migraine suggests common inheritance; however, the incidence of migraine in CH patients is not significantly different to that observed in the general population (Kudrow and Kudrow 1994; Bahra *et al* 2002; Lipton and Bigal 2005). Moreover no mutations of the calcium channel gene (CACNA1A) implicated in migraine were found in CH (Haan *et al* 2001; Sjostrand *et al* 2001). Actions of the nitric oxide synthase (NOS) enzyme induce NO release, a molecule important in CH's aetiology, but no significant NOS polymorphism associations have been found (Sjostrand *et al* 2002). The circadian rhythm of CH suggests that the genes involved (clock genes) may display polymorphisms, but again no significant associations between genotype and phenotype were observed (Rainero *et al* 2005). The neuropeptide hypocretin is found exclusively in the posterolateral hypothalamus, an area highly associated with CH. Moreover functions of hypocretin include pain modulation (Bartsch *et al* 2004) and regulation of the sleep–wake cycle. A significant association between a polymorphism in the hypocretin receptor 2 gene and CH suggests an aetiologic role (Rainero *et al* 2004).

2.5. Pathophysiology

The three major features of CH and most TACs are trigeminal pain, rhythmicity and autonomic signs. Specific features of distinct diagnoses are discussed in later sections.

2.5.1. Pain and Rhythmicity

Central to the pathophysiology of neurovascular headaches is the trigeminovascular system, described in Chapter 9. The distribution of pain in TACs implicates activity of the trigeminal nerve, particularly the ophthalmic branch. Peripheral nerve activation explains pain and may initiate some of the autonomic manifestations. Such activation was thought to originate from dilated blood vessels that stimulate trigeminal nociceptors directly, a hypothesis refuted by research findings (see Chapter 9). There is, however, some evidence that an inflammatory process in the cavernous sinus and its tributary veins, an area of sensory and autonomic fibre convergence, is involved in the aetiology of CH. This would peripherally activate both the trigeminal nerve and the autonomic nervous system, leading to pain and autonomic signs (Hardebo 1991,

1994). Nociceptor activation may be further increased by pressure build-up on surrounding tissues such as in the bony carotid canal, enclosed oral structures or the pterygopalatine fossa or as a result of obstructed venous flow occurring in the cavernous sinus (Benoliel *et al* 1997; Waldenlind and Goadsby 2006). Headache and local AS would resolve together with the inflammation. This theory relies on findings of abnormal orbital phlebography in patients with CH and on the fact that nitroglycerin and other vasodilators can induce CH (Hannerz 1991). However, certain features of TACs are not easily explained by a peripheral mechanism: gender predilections, unilaterality of the symptoms, sleep association and particularly in CH the circadian rhythmicity of attacks. Moreover, the frequency and pattern of pathologic findings at orbital phlebography in cervicogenic headache, migraine, and tension-type headache are similar to those in cluster headache. It seems likely that the vascular changes are an epiphenomenon of activation of the trigeminovascular system (Goadsby and Duckworth 1987; May and Goadsby 1999) and current thinking is that primary headaches occur with no substantial peripheral pathology (Ekbom and Hardebo 2002; Goadsby *et al* 2002).

The periodicity and sleep association in TACs suggest involvement of central sites involved in the control of the human 'biological clock'. In humans these are located in the posterior hypothalamic grey, an area termed the suprachiasmatic nucleus (Leone and Bussone 1993). Hypothalamic regulation of the endocrine system involves rhythmic and phasic homeostatic modulation of the hypophyseal hormones and melatonin. Measuring changes in these hormones is an attractive way to examine hypothalamic involvement in headache. Lowered concentrations of testosterone in males with CH were the first indications of hypothalamic involvement (Romiti *et al* 1983). However, other studies have found lowered levels only in chronic CH and this may be a secondary effect (Murialdo *et al* 1989). Melatonin is produced by the pineal gland, which receives sympathetic innervation from the hypothalamus and autonomic centres of the thoracic spinal cord, the sympathetic cervical plexus and the carotid plexus. The principal external stimulus for the rhythmic production of melatonin is light intensity. This input reaches the suprachiasmatic nucleus of the hypothalamus via a direct pathway from the retina. In man, melatonin levels are low during the day and increase during the hours of darkness. Studies of melatonin in CH patients found that 24-hour production was reduced and its pattern altered during the cluster period compared to normal subjects (Waldenlind *et al* 1987). This finding links to descriptions of CH variations with daylight hours, partly explaining the seasonal timing of active cluster periods. Twenty-four-hour cortisol production was also significantly increased in the cluster period, indicating hypothalamic–pituitary–adrenal axis hyperactivity (Facchinetti *et al* 1986; Waldenlind *et al* 1987). Based on such hypothalamic dysfunction, testosterone and a gonadotropin-releasing hormone analogue

have been applied therapeutically with varying success (Nicolodi *et al* 1993).

The role of the hypothalamus in CH has been elegantly confirmed by functional and morphometric neuroimaging. During attacks of CH, SUNCT and HC, but not in experimental pain there is marked activation in the ipsilateral ventral hypothalamic grey (May *et al* 1998a,b, 1999a, 2000; Matharu *et al* 2004). Activation in migraine is seen largely in brainstem structures, whilst in HC activation of the posterior hypothalamus is paralleled by activation in the dorsal rostral pons, supporting the clinical phenotype of HC: an overlap of TAC and migraine symptomatology (Weiller *et al* 1995; Matharu *et al* 2004; Afridi *et al* 2005). Within headaches and interictally, positron emission tomography (PET) morphometric studies reveal a significant structural difference (increased volume) in the inferior posterior hypothalamus of CH patients (May *et al* 1999b). The morphometric and functional images identify the same area in the inferior posterior hypothalamus (May *et al* 1998a, 1999b).

The hypothalamus is connected to the parasympathetic pterygopalatine ganglion and receives inputs from the sensory trigeminal nuclei. The hypothalamus also connects with the medullary dorsal reticular nucleus, a supraspinal system that gives origin to a descending projection that facilitates pain perception. Experimental data suggest involvement of the posterior hypothalamus in the modulation of nociceptive processing in rodents and humans (Manning and Franklin 1998; Leone *et al* 2005). The ventromedial hypothalamus is also active in nociceptive pathways, so that the hypothalamus is in a prime position to initiate and 'manage' the TACs. Activation from brain areas other than the hypothalamus may also be a primary event triggering headache; for example, a nociceptive stimulus to the rat cortex induces trigeminal activation and plasma extravasation; see Chapter 9 (Bolay *et al* 2002).

Recent case descriptions of continued tearing with no pain in CH patients following surgical section of the trigeminal nerve further establish the role of central mechanisms in the TAC phenotype (Lin and Dodick 2005). Moreover a 59-year-old man with a 14-year history of left-sided CH underwent surgical section of the ipsilateral trigeminal root but continued to suffer *both* headaches and AS (Matharu and Goadsby 2002a). Clearly in this case central nervous system (CNS) structures only were necessary to induce CH and express the full phenotype; therefore pain need not originate peripherally.

2.5.2. Trigeminoparasympathetic Reflex

The blood vessels of craniofacial tissues are innervated by three sets of nerves: the cranial parasympathetic, the superior cervical sympathetic and the trigeminal sensory nerves. Cranial parasympathetic fibres arise in the superior salivatory nucleus (SSN) and innervate part of the craniofacial structures via the oculomotor, facial, glossopharyngeal or vagal nerves. These efferents synapse in the ciliary, pterygopalatine, submandibular, lingual or otic ganglia and postganglionic fibres project to specific craniofacial targets such as the lacrimal, nasal mucosa and salivary glands as well as the craniofacial vasculature. Parasympathetic stimulation induces lacrimation and rhinorrhea as observed in TACs. Indeed activity of the parasympathetic system in CH and chronic paroxysmal hemicrania (CPH) is confirmed by elevated plasma vasoactive intestinal peptide (VIP) levels; in migraine this occurs only if AS are present (Goadsby and Edvinsson 1994, 1996).

Painful experimental stimuli in areas innervated by trigeminal nerve divisions 1 and 2 will cause ipsilateral lacrimation and local sweating, signs similar to those observed in TACs (Drummond 1992, 1995; Frese *et al* 2003). Following trigeminal nerve stimulation decreased carotid artery resistance was observed, an effect blocked by trigeminal section (Lambert *et al* 1984). These effects are largely considered secondary to initiation of a parasympathetic reflex via trigeminal nerve activation: the trigeminoparasympathetic reflex (TPR). In TACs the afferent limb of the TPR is the ophthalmic branch of the trigeminal nerve and the efferent is the facial nerve. Stimulation of the facial nerve and of parasympathetic fibres induces an increased regional cerebral blood flow (rCBF), confirming the efferent role of the parasympathetic nervous system in the TPR (Goadsby 1989; Suzuki *et al* 1990). Existence of a TPR is established by anatomical and functional connections at brainstem level between the trigeminal complex and the SSN (Spencer *et al* 1990; Knight *et al* 2005).

Interruption of the efferent branch of the TPR by sectioning the facial nerve produces an 80% reduction of vascular dilatation (Goadsby *et al* 1984). The remaining effect is thought to be induced by antidromic activation of trigeminal neurons and neurogenic inflammatory effects. These two processes, TPR and neurogenic inflammation, are thought central to the pathophysiology of neurovascular headaches and occur simultaneously. Neurogenic inflammation has been extensively described in Chapter 9.

The TPR is thought to be actively modulated by higher centres. Injection of a γ-aminobutyric acid (GABA) antagonist intravenously elicits a parasympathetic response similar to a reflex and supports the existence of a tonically active GABA-mediated inhibition of the TPR (Izumi 1999). Furthermore electrical stimulation of the anterior hypothalamus attenuates lip vasodilatation in response to lingual nerve stimulation, an effect abolished by administration of a GABA antagonist (Izumi 1999). This suggests a role for hypothalamic modulation of orofacial TPR; it has been proposed that the TPR may be pathologically disinhibited.

2.5.3. The Trigeminoparasympathetic Reflex in the Orofacial Region

Neurovascular orofacial pain may be related pathophysiologically to migraine. Alternatively NVOP may be related to TACs or both as in HC. We therefore examine the possibility that the TPR may be initiated from oral structures.

Experimentally the TPR has been shown in animals after stimulation of the lingual nerve (Mizuta and Izumi 2004). Stimulation of the infraorbital nerve and the maxillary buccal gingiva in cats (Izumi 1999) and painful stimulation of tooth pulp in humans induce an increase in ipsilateral lip blood flow (Kemppainen *et al* 1994). Reflex salivation secondary to experimental lingual nerve stimulation has been reported and has also been observed in patients with craniofacial pain (Rasmussen 1991; Takahashi *et al* 1995).

An oral TPR activated by intradermatomal stimuli is therefore apparent (Izumi 1999). However, some cases of NVOP present with tearing and mandibular pain (Benoliel *et al* 1997), i.e. cross-dermatomal activation of the TPR. Cross-dermatomal activation has been experimentally demonstrated; electrical stimuli to the infraorbital nerve induce vasodilatation in the ipsilateral *lower* lip of cats (Izumi 1999). Such cross-dermatomal reflexes could therefore explain clinical reports of lacrimation in mandibular and maxillary pain syndromes, for example, in NVOP of mandibular teeth (Benoliel *et al* 1997; Benoliel and Sharav 1998c). However, there is no experimental evidence of ocular AS following peripheral stimuli to the mandibular region. Capsaicin injected into the forehead induced a rapid ipsilateral autonomic response, but injection of capsaicin into the mandibular region (third trigeminal division) did not (Frese *et al* 2003). In mild to moderate experimental pain in the mandibular branches of the trigeminal nerve we found no reflex lacrimation (unpublished observations). Experimental ophthalmic pain will induce vasodilatation in the internal carotid artery whilst mandibular pain will not (May *et al* 2001). From these data we conclude that cases with pain in the distribution of the mandibular divisions accompanied by ocular AS such as lacrimation are not driven via peripheral activation of the TPR and central mechanisms are therefore likely candidates. This may also explain the relative paucity of AS in NVOP.

2.5.4. Neurogenic Inflammation

The pain in cluster headache may be associated with a perivascular neurogenic inflammatory process (Gobel *et al* 2000) of the internal carotid artery in its bony canal or, as supported by findings, of increased intraocular pressure within the confines of the eye (Pareja *et al* 1996a). An orbital 'vasculitis' has been suggested in the aetiology of CPH and CH (Hannerz 1991).

Trigeminal and autonomic activation, as evidenced by increased levels of CGRP and VIP in the cranial circulation, is present in CPH (Goadsby and Edvinsson 1996). Similar neuropeptide changes, including increased levels of NO, are seen in CH and suggest a shared underlying pathophysiology within TACs (D'Amico *et al* 2002; Costa *et al*

2003). Moreover successful treatment with indomethacin normalizes levels of both CGRP and VIP in CPH and oxygen administration reverses the elevation of CGRP in CH (Goadsby and Edvinsson 1994, 1996). Neurogenic inflammatory mechanisms have been reviewed in Chapter 9.

2.5.5. 'Neuropathic' Mechanisms

Attacks of PH and SUNCT may be mechanically activated, often with a short latency, implicating neurogenic transmission (Pareja and Cuadrado 2005). In PH, 10% of cases report a clear trigger mechanism; usually neck movement and SUNCT patients demonstrate trigeminal neuralgia-like triggers (Pareja *et al* 1994; Lain *et al* 2000; Boes *et al* 2006). Moreover reports of successful therapy in CH and SUNCT by microvascular decompression that is successful in trigeminal neuralgia suggests that in some cases neuropathic mechanisms may be involved (Lovely *et al* 1998; Lagares *et al* 2005). Initiation of CH by traumatic events such as head injury and dental extractions suggests a role for nerve injury in the aetiology of TACs (Penarrocha *et al* 2001; Soros *et al* 2001).

Taken together current data suggest that CH and other TACs are conditions whose pathophysiological basis is in the hypothalamic grey matter that drives the initiation of the clinical phenotype. The involvement of peripheral mechanisms is unclear.

2.5.6. Specific Aspects of CH Pathophysiology

It has been proposed that in CH trigeminal nociceptor activation occurs secondary to ophthalmic artery vasodilatation. Evidence for increased blood flow in the cavernous sinus (and thus the carotid artery) during CH has suggested that this area may be the origin of pain (May *et al* 1998a). However, studies fail to show pathological changes in the area of the cavernous sinus (Sjaastad and Rinck 1990) and orbital phlebography studies demonstrate identical results in a number of other headaches including SUNCT, migraine, tension-type headache and PH (Hannerz *et al* 1992; Antonaci 1994). Flow changes are therefore not central to the generation of pain in CH and may be secondary to trigeminal activation (Dodick *et al* 2000), as in migraine (Chapter 9).

Neuropeptide changes in the cranial circulation observed in CH support the hypothesis that there is antidromic trigeminal and reflex parasympathetic activation. Jugular blood levels of CGRP, VIP and nitrate (indicative of NO) are raised during CH attacks while there is no change in neuropeptide Y or SP (Goadsby and Edvinsson 1994; D'Amico *et al* 2002; Costa *et al* 2003). Treatment with both oxygen and subcutaneous sumatriptan reduced the CGRP level to normal (Goadsby and Edvinsson 1994). Observed ptosis and miosis, suggestive of sympathetic dysfunction, may be secondary to neuropaxic effects of carotid oedema on the sympathetic plexus or may signify a generalized sympathetic dysfunction. Indeed, a

dysfunction in the central control of the autonomic system in CH and PH has been proposed (Boes *et al* 2006). However, autonomic dysfunction as a driving force in CH does not explain pain that may occur in CH with no AS and vice versa. A schematic summary of CH pathophysiology is shown in Fig. 10.2.

2.6. CH Treatment

A combination of patient education, symptomatic treatment and prophylactic regimens is the essential cornerstone of successful treatment in all headaches (Dodick *et al* 2000). Based on attack patterns patients should be instructed to avoid daytime naps, alcoholic beverages and other triggers such as volatile substances (e.g. paints). Altitude hypoxaemia may trigger an attack during active periods but may be pharmacologically prevented (Dodick *et al* 2000). A clear explanation of mechanisms, treatment options and prognosis is essential.

2.6.1. Abortive

Rapid symptomatic relief may be obtained with oxygen inhalation. Oxygen at 7–10 L per minute for 15 minutes will provide relief in about 70% of cases, number needed to treat (NNT) 2.04 (Kudrow 1981; Fogan 1985). The

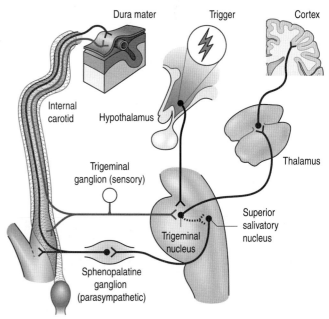

Fig. 10.2 • Cluster headache (CH)—pain and autonomic mechanisms. Schematic representation of major areas involved in CH. Neuroimaging studies implicate the hypothalamus as central to the pathogenesis of CH. Trigeminal activation will result in neurogenic inflammation at peripheral sites such as dural blood vessels, (vasodilatation, plasma extravasation, pain, swelling). At brainstem level connections exist to the superior salivatory nucleus (SSN), which is therefore stimulated with subsequent activation of the parasympathetic nervous system leading to autonomic signs (vasodilatation, tearing, rhinorrhoea), termed the trigeminoparasympathetic reflex. It is thought that vasodilatation causes neuropraxic injury to the perivascular sympathetic plexus speckled area (grid), inducing sympathetic dysfunction that is clinically observed as ptosis and miosis.

response rates in males are higher (87%) than in older chronic CH patients (57%) and in females (59%) (Kudrow 1981; Rozen 2004). Higher flow rates (15 L/min) may be successful in previously resistant cases (Rozen 2004) and hyperbaric oxygen is also effective but is more difficult for patients to access.

Subcutaneous (SC) sumatriptan and more recently via intranasal (IN) spray is effective in the acute treatment of cluster headache with few side effects even with prolonged usage and high dosing (Ekbom et al 1995; Centonze et al 2000a; van Vliet et al 2003b). In open-label studies SC sumatriptan (6 mg) is effective in 76–100% of cases within 15 minutes of administration (Ekbom et al 1995; Gobel et al 1998) but is slightly less effective in chronic CH (Gobel et al 1998). Based on two placebo controlled studies SC sumatriptan (6 mg) has an NNT of about 2.2 (SCHSG 1991; Ekbom et al 1993). Sumatriptan (20 mg) IN is less effective but is more amenable despite its unpleasant taste (NNT 3.45) (Hardebo and Dahlof 1998; van Vliet et al 2003b). There have been reports that use of sumatriptan may lead to increased frequency of CH attacks (Rossi et al 2004). Oral zolmitriptan 10 mg is effective in episodic but not in chronic CH, and although more tolerable is inferior to sumatriptan (NNT 5) (Bahra et al 2000). Dihydroergotamine has been successfully used in CH by intravenous administration but is impractical (Mather et al 1991). Oral ergot formulations have also been used but absorption may not be rapid enough to be effective and nasal inhalation seems only to reduce attack intensity (Andersson and Jespersen 1986). Intranasal lidocaine may be effective but is generally considered as adjunctive therapy (Robbins 1995). SC sumatriptan is currently the most effective abortive therapy (Table 10.3).

2.6.2. Prophylactic

During prolonged periods of active episodic and chronic CH continuous abortive therapy is impractical and may be associated with unacceptable side effects. Corticosteroids are effective prophylactic agents and although the evidence base is weak their obvious clinical efficacy justifies trial therapy for a limited period in selected patients (Antonaci et al 2005; Shapiro 2005). Prevention is often initiated with verapamil (Dodick et al 2000) that is efficacious for long-term management of episodic and chronic CH (Bussone et al 1990; Leone et al 2000). For chronic CH lithium carbonate is an established prophylactic therapy that may induce remission. Lithium has been shown to be as efficient as verapamil albeit with more side effects (Bussone et al 1990) and requires monitoring of serum concentrations due its narrow therapeutic window. Methysergide was an effective therapy but its use has been terminated due to potential fibrotic complications. Anticonvulsant drugs have also been tested in CH with mixed success; valproic acid may be efficacious particularly in CH with migrainous features and topiramate is associated with clinical improvement (Wheeler 1998; Forderreuther et al 2002; Leone 2004). Prophylactic agents are summarized in Table 10.4, for chronic CH in Table 10.5.

2.6.3. CH Refractory to Pharmacotherapy

Medically resistant CH is a distressing condition; up to 10–20% patients remain with excruciating pain unresponsive to a number of therapies (May 2005). Some patients may respond to medical therapy but suffer intolerable side effects that severely compromise their quality of life. In these situations surgical intervention or deep brain stimulation may be considered. Relevant neurosurgical treatments are discussed in Chapter 13. Procedures may be aimed at the trigeminal ganglion or nerve, the sphenopalatine ganglion and the superior petrosal nerve. Microvascular decompression and trigeminal nerve root resection as in the management of trigeminal neuralgia have also been employed. However, some patients will remain symptomatic following these procedures (Matharu and Goadsby

Table 10.3	Selected Abortive Pharmacological Treatment Options for Episodic Cluster Headache		
Agent	**Dose**	**Comments**	**Side Effects**
Oxygen (inhaled via face mask)	5–15 L/min for 15 min	First line but cumbersome. Hyperbaric oxygen also efficacious but impractical	None
Sumatriptan	6–12 mg SC	First line, fast and efficacious. 12 mg as effective as 6 mg but with more side effects. Marginally less effective in chronic CH.	Contraindicated in IHD or HBP. Fatigue Nausea/vomiting Chest symptoms Skin reactions over puncture wound
	20 mg intra nasal	Less effective but easier to use	None
Dihydroergotamine	0.5–1 mg intra nasal (bilateral)	Reduces severity but not frequency	None
Lidocaine	1 mL of 4–10% solution applied intra nasal on cotton pledget bilaterally	Pain is decreased but not enough studies. Needs to be inserted deep near pterygopalatine foramen	Bitter taste

Table 10.4 Prophylactic Treatment of Episodic Cluster Headache

Agent	Dose	Comments	Side Effects
Verapamil	160–480 mg/d (PO)	First-line treatment Perform baseline ECG	Hypotension, bradycardia, heart block, dizziness and fatigue
Prednisone	50–80 mg/d (PO)	Good for initial therapy till e.g. verapamil takes effect. Prolonged use not recommended due to side effects. Taper over 10–21 days.	Increased appetite, nervousness, hyperglycaemia, insomnia, headaches
Valproic acid	600–2000 mg/d (PO)	Efficacious in patients with pronounced migrainous features. Monitor liver function.	Nausea, dizziness, dyspepsia, thrombocytopenia
Topiramate	25–200 mg/d (PO)	Increase by 25 mg/d every 5 days	Cognitive effects, paraesthesias, dizziness
Gabapentin	900 mg/d (PO)	Few studies but promising results	Drowsiness
Melatonin	9–10 mg/d nocte (PO)	Few studies	None

Table 10.5 Treatment of Chronic Cluster Headache

Agent	Dose	Comments	Side Effects
Verapamil	360–480 mg/d (PO)	First-line treatment. Perform baseline ECG	Hypotension, bradycardia, heart block, dizziness and fatigue
Lithium carbonate	300–900 mg (PO)	Requires monitoring of renal and thyroid function, and of serum concentrations (best at 0.4–0.8 mEq/L)	Weakness, nausea, tremor, slurred speech, blurred vision. Side effects >verapamil.

2002a). Thus, patient selection for surgery needs to include careful assessment and considerations; see Table 10.6. Occipital nerve blocks and deep brain stimulation have provided pain relief in some cases and seem to be a logical option prior to surgery (Peres *et al* 2002a; Kinney *et al* 2003; Ambrosini *et al* 2005). The hypothalamus is considered central to the pathogenesis of CH and stimulation of posterior inferior hypothalamic areas has resulted in excellent pain control (Leone *et al* 2004a; Schoenen *et al* 2005). Strict selection criteria include the following:

- Long-lasting (>2 years) unilateral chronic CH has been accurately diagnosed;
- Pharmacotherapy has been exhausted;
- The patient's medical, neurological and psychological profiles do not contraindicate surgery or electrode stimulation;
- Neuroimaging studies are normal; and
- The patient does not smoke or consume alcohol (Leone *et al* 2004b).

3. Paroxysmal Hemicrania

Paroxysmal hemicrania was first described in 1974 (Sjaastad and Dale 1974) and was thought initially to be

a rare variant of cluster headache (Blau and Engel 1990). However, a separate category for PH was created based on a number of features that distinguish it from CH.

Table 10.6 Assessment of Intractable CH Prior to Surgery

1. Rule out or reassess organic pathology.

2. Reassess diagnosis versus other entities such as:
   a. Side-locked migraine
   b. Paroxysmal hemicrania
   c. SUNCT

3. Review pharmacotherapy
   a. Adequate monotherapy
      i. Have the front-line drugs all been tested?
      ii. At adequate dosing/duration?
   b. Adequate polytherapy as above?

4. Consider referral
   a. Reassessment and diagnosis
   b. For in-patient treatment with IV medication

5. Is the patient fit for neurosurgery?
   a. Medically
   b. Psychologically

6. Patients with strictly unilateral pain are best candidates.
   a. Pain that has alternated sides is a poor prognostic factor.

7. Patient must understand that surgical failure is a possibility and attacks or autonomic signs or both may continue

3.1. Clinical Features

Case example. Examine Case 10.2. Notice how similar pain location is in CH, PH and indeed across all TACs. In this case duration and frequency were typical. Referral of pain to dental structures is very common and often leads to misguided dental treatment. Indomethacin very often causes gastric side effects and in these cases combination with an antacid is indicated.

Location. Pain occurs typically in the temporal, periauricular, periorbital and maxillary areas (Boes and Dodick 2002; Boes *et al* 2006). Extratrigeminal (occipital) distribution of pain in PH is rare (Dodick 1998; Boes and Dodick 2002). However, referral to the shoulder, neck and arm is quite common (Boes and Dodick 2002; Boes *et al* 2006). Pain is unilateral and in extremely rare circumstances may become bilateral (Boes and Dodick 2002; Bingel and Weiller 2005; Matharu and Goadsby 2005; Boes *et al* 2006). Strong pain may cross the midline (Sjaastad and Dale 1976) but the vast majority of attacks in PH do not change sides (Antonaci and Sjaastad 1989; Boes and Dodick 2002).

Quality and temporal pattern. The attacks in PH are short, average duration of 13–29 minutes but may last nearly an hour and are usually sharp and excruciating (Boes and Dodick 2002). Often a number of descriptors are employed by one patient including throbbing, stabbing, sharp or boring (Benoliel and Sharav 1998a; Boes and Dodick 2002; Sarlani *et al* 2003b; Boes *et al* 2006). Pain onset is rapid and mostly peaks in less than 5 minutes (Boes and Dodick 2002).

Frequency is high; about 8 attacks per 24 hours but with as many as 30 (Antonaci and Sjaastad 1989; Boes *et al* 2006). Lower frequencies of 1–5 attacks per 24 hours have also been reported (Boes and Dodick 2002). The temporal similarity to CH behaviour has led to the term 'modified cluster pattern' that describes the frequent attacks of PH (Boes *et al* 2006). More recently a seasonal pattern of attacks in PH patients has been described (Veloso *et al* 2001; Siow 2004).

The first reported cases of PH were of a continuous nature and were categorized as chronic PH. Only a scant number of PHs behaved episodically (Boes and Dodick 2002) and many of these eventually developed into a chronic form (CPH:EPH=4:1) (Antonaci and Sjaastad 1989).

A high number of patients (30%) report nocturnal attacks of PH that cause them to wake from sleep (Antonaci and Sjaastad 1989). Like most neurovascular-type craniofacial pain, PH is considered to be REM sleep-related (Sahota and Dexter 1990).

Accompanying phenomena. AS may occur bilaterally but are more pronounced on the symptomatic side. The most commonly seen are ipsilateral lacrimation (62%), nasal congestion (42%), conjunctival injection and rhinorrhoea (36% each) (Goadsby and Lipton 1997; Benoliel and Sharav 1998a; Sarlani *et al* 2003b). Heart rate changes (bradycardia, tachycardia, extrasystoles), increased local sweating and salivation are not common (Boes *et al*

Case 10.2 Paroxysmal Hemicrania, a 56-year-old Male

Present complaint

Left facial pain, excruciating (VAS 9) and sharp. Located periorbitally, periauricularly and radiating to the neck (Fig. 10.3). Onset may be preceded by pain over the ipsilateral premolar and molar teeth and adjoining alveolar bone. The pain could awaken the patient from sleep but also occurred equally frequently throughout the day. Attacks lasted up to 15 minutes (Fig. 10.5B).

History of present complaint

Began 12 months previously and occurred frequently with an approximate maximum of up to 6 attacks daily and a minimum of 3 per day, with increasing frequency over the past few months (Fig. 10.5B). The pain was invariably accompanied by conjunctival injection, nasal congestion and occasional ptosis.

Dental treatment had included extraction of a left lower molar with no change in pain character or quality. Computerized tomography (CT) of the TMJs was normal as were two full sets of full-mouth intraoral periapical films.

Physical examination

No relevant findings.

Relevant medical history

None.

Diagnosis

Trigeminal autonomic cephalgia: paroxysmal hemicrania.

Diagnostic and treatment considerations

This case caused difficulty due to pain often beginning intraorally.

Because of the extensive reports on organic pathology underlying paroxysmal hemicrania the patient was referred for a CT scan of the head which was normal. Indomethacin, 75 mg daily, provided significant relief. Per-schedule antacids were added due to dyspepsia; however, any attempt at reducing the indomethacin caused pain relapse. The patient continues to take indomethacin for pain relief.

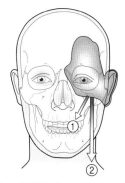

Fig. 10.3 • Patient (Case 10.2) indicated pain primarily in periorbital and periauricular area and radiating to the teeth and neck (1 and 2, respectively).

2006). Pain in PH is not considered secondary to autonomic activation as pain continues despite these phenomena being blocked (Pareja 1995).

IHS diagnostic criteria for PH are shown in Table 10.7.

Table 10.7 Diagnostic Criteria for Paroxysmal Hemicrania (PH)

	Diagnostic Criteria	Notes
A	At least 20 attacks fulfilling criteria B–D	Onset is usually in adulthood, although childhood cases are reported. Unlike cluster headache there is no male predominance.
B	Attacks of severe unilateral orbital, supraorbital or temporal pain lasting 2–30 minutes	Attacks are similar to CH but are shorter lasting and more frequent
C	Headache is accompanied by at least one of the following: 1. Ipsilateral conjunctival injection and/or lacrimation 2. Ipsilateral nasal congestion and/or rhinorrhoea 3. Ipsilateral eyelid oedema 4. Ipsilateral forehead and facial sweating 5. Ipsilateral miosis and/or ptosis	
D	Attack frequency above 5 per day for more than half of the time, although periods with lower frequency may occur	During less than half of the time attacks may be less frequent. *Episodic type* has attacks occurring in periods lasting 7 days to 1 year separated by pain-free periods >1 month. *Chronic type* has attacks occurring for more than 1 year without remission or with remission lasting less than 1 month.
E	Attacks are prevented completely by therapeutic doses of indomethacin	To rule out incomplete response indomethacin should be used in a dose of 150 mg/d or more orally or rectally, or >100 mg by injection, but for maintenance smaller doses are often sufficient.
F	Not attributed to another disorder	It has been suggested that CPH secondary to organic disease may be the rule rather than the exception and requires careful work-up in these cases.

Adapted from Olesen *et al* (2004) with permission.

3.2. Epidemiology

PH is rare and large population-based studies are needed to accurately assess its prevalence. Based on CH figures and patient populations, the prevalence of PH has been estimated to be 0.021–0.07% (Boes *et al* 2006). It has been suggested that PH is more common than previously thought and as it shares many clinical characteristics with dental pain will frequently be seen in orofacial pain clinics (Benoliel *et al* 1997).

Family history of any of the neurovascular-type headaches was examined in PH patients, with no significantly increased prevalence found (Boes *et al* 2006). No other familial association has been found in PH patients. Initial reported cases were largely female but in a recent review (Boes and Dodick 2002) the female:male ratio was 1.6:1 and it has been predicted that as more cases are reported there will be a 1:1 ratio (Boes *et al* 2006).

Mean age of onset is usually 34–41 years (most 30–40 years), with an average illness duration of 13 years (Antonaci and Sjaastad 1989; Kudrow and Kudrow 1989; Boes and Dodick 2002). Children aged 6 and adults aged 81 years have been reported. The episodic form is considered to have an earlier mean age of onset (27 years) than the chronic form (37 years) (Antonaci and Sjaastad 1989).

3.3. Secondary Paroxysmal Hemicrania

Many cases with CPH (22%) report head and neck trauma (Antonaci and Sjaastad 1989). However, this prevalence is no different to that found in CH or migraine (Boes *et al* 2006).

Malignancy, CNS disease and benign tumours have been implicated in secondary PH (Trucco *et al* 2004). A case of parotid gland epidermoid carcinoma with cerebral metastasis causing PH has been reported (Mariano da Silva *et al* 2004).

In two literature reviews (Antonaci and Sjaastad 1989; Trucco *et al* 2004) systemic diseases were common in PH, including connective tissue disease and thrombocytopenia. Thus it has been suggested that CPH secondary to organic disease may be the rule rather than the exception and requires careful work-up in these cases (Gatzonis *et al* 1996).

3.4. Paroxysmal Hemicrania's Absolute Response to Indomethacin

PH's response to indomethacin is absolute (Antonaci *et al* 2003) but the mechanism is poorly understood and it seems not entirely dependent on inhibition of cyclooxygenase activity. However, indomethacin has inhibitory effects on the central nociceptive system and has also been shown to reduce rCBF in experimental animals and humans; see Chapter 15. An interaction between indomethacin and NO, involved in headache pathogenesis, has been proposed (Castellano *et al* 1998). Findings from an experimental pain model suggest that an interaction between indomethacin and local NO synthesis is involved in the antinociceptive effects of indomethacin (Ventura-Martinez *et al* 2004). It is likely that the therapeutic effect of indomethacin in PH involves these mechanisms.

The inclusion of an absolute indomethacin response as part of PH's criteria has been questioned but its usefulness outweighs any disadvantage. Most cases respond within 24 hours, but 3 days at 75 mg followed, if needed, by 150 mg for a further 3 days is recommended as trial therapy (Pareja and Sjaastad 1996). High persistent dosage requirements may indicate underlying pathology (Sjaastad *et al* 1995). Prognosis in PH is good and long-term remission has been reported (Sjaastad and Antonaci 1987). Indomethacin-resistant PH has been treated with calcium channel blockers, naproxen and carbamazepine (Benoliel and Sharav 1998a). Acetazolamide, a diuretic with anticonvulsant properties, reduces intraocular pressure and is partially effective in PH (Warner *et al* 1994). Sumatriptan, beneficial in both CH and migraine, is relatively ineffective in PH (Dahlof 1993). A summary of therapies for PH, SUNCT and HC is shown in Table 10.8.

4. Short-Lasting, Unilateral, Neuralgiform Headache Attacks with Conjunctival Injection and Tearing (SUNCT)

SUNCT syndrome was first reported in 1978 and is a unilateral headache/facial pain characterized by brief paroxysmal attacks accompanied by ipsilateral local AS, usually conjunctival injection and lacrimation (Sjaastad *et al* 1989). The similarities of this syndrome to trigeminal neuralgia (TN) are marked, particularly the triggering mechanism and many believed SUNCT to be a TN variant (Sjaastad and Kruszewski 1992). AS are typical of neurovascular-type pains and not usually associated with

neuralgias (Goadsby and Lipton 1997). Therefore some clinicians considered SUNCT to be a subtype of cluster headache. However, because of particular features, SUNCT is believed to be a separate disorder and is currently classified by the IHS as a TAC (Olesen *et al* 2004).

4.1. Clinical Features

Case example. The patient described in Case 10.3 clearly shows the difficulty in differentiating between SUNCT and TN of the ophthalmic branch. TN with lacrimation is a particularly difficult differential (see Chapter 12).

Location. Pain is unilateral with no obvious side predilection and located in the temporal, auricular and occipital regions (Benoliel and Sharav 1998b; Pareja and Cuadrado 2005). It typically appears in the ocular and periocular regions (Sjaastad *et al* 1989; Pareja and Sjaastad 1997). Pain spreading across the midline or changing sides is rare (Pareja and Cuadrado 2005).

Quality. SUNCT is considered as a moderate to severe pain syndrome (Pareja and Cuadrado 2005) and is usually less severe than TN. It is rarely pulsatile, usually stabbing and sometimes electric or burning (Pareja *et al* 1994; Pareja and Sjaastad 1997; Matharu *et al* 2003b).

Temporal pattern. Multiple attacks occur usually during daytime with less than 2% occurring at night (Pareja *et al* 1996b). A bimodal distribution of attacks occurring in the morning and late afternoon has been observed, but the pattern of SUNCT attacks is usually irregular, unlike CH (Pareja *et al* 1996b). Remissions have been observed and may last for several months (Pareja and Sjaastad 1997; Benoliel and Sharav 1998b; Pareja *et al* 2002a).

Each attack lasts from 15–120 s with a mean duration of about 1 minute but longer lasting attacks of 250 or 600 s and even 2–3 hours have been reported (Pareja *et al* 1996b; Montes *et al* 2001). Frequency ranges from several daily to many per hour with an average of 28 per day (Fig. 10.5) (Sjaastad *et al* 1991; Pareja *et al* 1996b). A 'cluster-like' pattern has been reported with active and inactive episodes but is variably present (Sjaastad *et al* 1989). 'SUNCT status', pain lasting for the better part of the day for 1–3 days, may occur but is rare (Pareja *et al* 1996c). Low-grade background pain or local discomfort may also be part of SUNCT (Pareja *et al* 1996c).

Table 10.8	Pharmacotherapy of PH, SUNCT and HC		
Headache	**Drug of Choice**	**Dose (route)**	**2nd Line**
PH	Indomethacin	75–225 mg/d (PO)	Other NSAIDs Verapamil Acetazolamide
SUNCT	Lamotrigine	100–300 mg/d (PO)	Gabapentin 900–2700 mg/d Topiramate 50–200 mg/d
HC	Indomethacin	25–300 mg/d (PO)	Other NSAIDs Piroxicam-beta-cyclodextrin

Case 10.3 SUNCT, a 57-year-old Male

Present complaint

Severe periorbital pain (Fig. 10.4) with an electric, spasm-like quality that severely interfered with normal activity. At least 10 attacks/day (usually more) with duration of up to 3–5 minutes (very rarely more; Fig. 10.5C). The pain referred to the left temporal area and intraorally. Pain could be induced by mechanical stimulation around the lips (such as shaving and eating) and by intraoral stimuli such as tooth brushing. However, the vast majority of attacks were spontaneous with no clear trigger preceding onset and were always accompanied by ipsilateral lacrimation.

History of present complaint

Attacks had begun 1.5 years previously. Pain did not waken patient from sleep. Neurological examination and brain CT scan were normal. In the past the patient had received carbamazepine, baclofen and amitriptyline in adequate doses with no pain relief and was recently worsening.

Physical examination

Normal. Blood chemistry and haematology were within normal limits.

Relevant medical history

None.

Diagnosis

Trigeminal autonomic cephalgia: SUNCT.

Diagnostic and treatment considerations

The occasionally longer attacks are not typical of SUNCT and trial treatment with indomethacin 75 mg daily was therefore initiated. Four weeks later the patient returned complaining of strong pain and lacrimation, although there was improvement. The dose was therefore increased to 150 mg indomethacin daily with no change. Clonazepam 0.5 mg to aid in sleep helped him during nights but the diurnal pain was unaffected. An MRI of the brain was normal.

A period of spontaneous remission followed for some weeks but unfortunately the pain returned. The patient was then prescribed lamotrigine 100–200 mg daily, and although this was partially successful it was considered clinically significant by the patient.

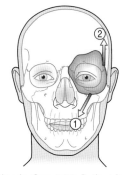

Fig. 10.4 • Pain location in Case 10.3. Patient indicated pain primarily in periorbital area and radiating to the teeth and temporal areas (arrows 1 and 2, respectively).

Triggering. Pain in SUNCT may be triggered by light mechanical stimuli in the areas innervated by the trigeminal nerve but with a short latency till pain onset (Pareja and Sjaastad 1994). Extratrigeminal triggers including neck movements have also been shown to precipitate attacks (Becser and Berky 1995). Alcohol is not usually reported to worsen pain (Pareja and Sjaastad 1994; Goadsby and Lipton 1997). In contrast to TN no refractory period has been demonstrated in SUNCT and is a major differentiating sign (Pareja *et al* 1994; Benoliel and Sharav 1998b,c; Lain *et al* 2000).

Accompanying phenomena. By definition SUNCT is accompanied by marked ipsilateral conjunctival injection and lacrimation (Merskey and Bogduk 1994; Olesen *et al* 2004) that appear rapidly with onset of pain (Pareja and Cuadrado 2005). Nasal stuffiness and rhinorrhoea are common whilst sweating may accompany attacks but is rarer and often subclinical (Sjaastad *et al* 1989; Kruszewski *et al* 1993).

Associated phenomena. Respiratory studies have indicated that SUNCT patients hyperventilate during attacks. Heart rate was found to decrease during attacks in 2 SUNCT patients. Some cardiovascular changes occurred before pain onset and were probably not in response to pain. Increased intraocular pressure with increased facial temperature periocularly has been reported (Sjaastad *et al* 1992). Orbital phlebography studies show abnormalities on the painful side and may indicate venous vasculitis (Kruszewski 1992). Imaging studies during attacks are essentially normal, but cerebral blood flow may be abnormal in SUNCT (Shen and Johnsen 1994). Diagnostic criteria as defined by the IHS are shown in Table 10.9A (Olesen *et al* 2004).

4.2. Short-Lasting, Unilateral, Neuralgiform Headache Attacks with Cranial Autonomic Features (SUNA)

This is a novel diagnostic entity included in the IHS classification's appendix. Essentially two criteria differentiate it from SUNCT: SUNA may be accompanied by any autonomic sign (nasal congestion, etc.), and attack duration is extended up to 10 minutes (Olesen *et al* 2004). A case of SUNA in a female child has been reported (Volcy *et al* 2005). Suggested criteria for SUNA as they appear in the appendix of the IHS's classification are shown in Table 10.9B (Olesen *et al* 2004).

4.3. Epidemiology

It is possible that the clinical similarities with TN and even CH leads to the misdiagnosis of many cases (Pareja and Cuadrado 2005). SUNCT may therefore be more common than estimates based on the sparse case reports. Cases of all ages have been reported from childhood to old age with a mean onset of about 50 years (D'Andrea and Granella 2001; Pareja and Cuadrado 2005).

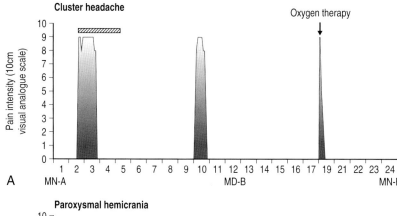

Cluster headache

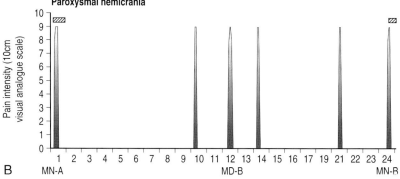

Paroxysmal hemicrania

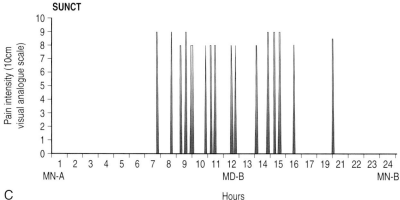

SUNCT

Fig. 10.5 • Graphic representation of Case 10.1, 10.2 and 10.3's pain diaries over a 24-hour period (midnight (MN) on day A to midnight on day B).
(A) Cluster headache (Case 10.1). Pain duration varies from 45 to 90 minutes and frequency over this period is 3 per 24 hours with one attack waking him about 2 hours after sleep onset (hatched rectangles above). Pain intensity is severe (VAS 8–9). The third attack (at 17.00) occurred when access to oxygen was available and inhalation rapidly aborted the attack. (B) Episodic paroxysmal hemicrania (Case 10.2). Pain duration varies from 10 to 15 minutes and frequency over this period is 6 per 24 hours with two attacks waking from sleep (grey rectangles above). Pain intensity is moderate to severe (VAS 7–9). (C) Short-lasting unilateral neuralgiform headache attacks with conjunctival injection and tearing (SUNCT, Case 10.3). Pain duration varies from 3 to 5 minutes to a rare duration of 10 minutes. Frequency over this period is 16 per 24 hours with no attacks waking from sleep. Pain intensity is moderate to severe (VAS 9–10).

A male:female ratio of 7:1 was reported in 1998 (Benoliel and Sharav 1998b) but with more female cases appearing, SUNCT is currently considered only slightly more common in males (Pareja and Cuadrado 2005).

SUNCT occurring in siblings has recently been presented as 'familial SUNCT' (Gantenbein and Goadsby 2005) and raises the possibility that SUNCT together with migraine, CH and possibly other TACs will eventually be considered to be of genetic predisposition.

4.4. Symptomatic SUNCT

Diagnoses in symptomatic SUNCT include brainstem infarction, cerebellopontine arteriovenous malformations, cerebellopontine astrocytoma or other tumours, cavernous hemangioma of the brainstem, cavernous sinus tumour, extraorbital cystic mass and neurofibromatosis (Trucco *et al* 2004; Pareja and Cuadrado 2005). Post-traumatic SUNCT, including eye trauma, have been reported (Pareja and Cuadrado 2005; Putzki *et al* 2005). Rare

reports include SUNCT related to HIV and to osteogenesis imperfecta (Trucco *et al* 2004). In a series of pituitary tumour patients, 5% were found to suffer from SUNCT (Levy *et al* 2005). These lesions are diagnosable with magnetic resonance imagining (MRI) and all SUNCT patients should therefore be referred for appropriate imaging (Pareja and Cuadrado 2005).

4.5. SUNCT Treatment

A distinct factor in SUNCT is its absolute resistance to both anti-neuralgic and anti-vascular drug therapy (Pareja *et al* 1995). Similar to CH, SUNCT may also respond to steroids (Pareja *et al* 1995). Recently a case of SUNCT responsive to verapamil has been described (Narbone *et al* 2005), which is in sharp contrast to past reports of a possible worsening of SUNCT secondary to verapamil (Jimenez-Huete *et al* 2002). Anticonvulsant drugs may produce some improvement; SUNCT may initially be responsive to carbamazepine with some reduction in attack frequency and severity (Matharu

Table 10.9A Diagnostic Criteria for SUNCT

	Diagnostic Criteria	Notes
A	At least 20 attacks fulfilling criteria B–D.	SUNCT may coexist with trigeminal neuralgia; in such patients there is overlap of signs and symptoms and the differentiation is clinically difficult.
B	Attacks of unilateral orbital, supraorbital or temporal stabbing pain lasting 5–240 s.	This the shortest of the TACs.
C	Pain is accompanied by ipsilateral conjunctival injection and lacrimation.	Patients may be seen with only one of conjunctival injection or tearing, or other cranial autonomic symptoms such as nasal congestion, rhinorrhoea or eyelid oedema (see SUNA below)
D	Attacks occur with a frequency from 3 to 200 per day.	
E	Not attributed to another disorder.	Most common mimics of SUNCT are lesions in the posterior fossa or involving the pituitary gland.

Adapted from Olesen *et al* (2004) with permission.

Table 10.9B Suggested Criteria for SUNA

A history of ≥20 pain attacks fulfilling the following criteria:
- Unilateral
- Lasting 2 s to 10 min
- Located in orbital, supraorbital or temporal regions
- Stabbing or pulsating

- Accompanied by one of the following:
  - Ipsilateral conjunctival injection and/or lacrimation
  - Nasal congestion and/or rhinorrhoea
  - Eyelid oedema
- A frequency of ≥1 per day for more than half the time
- No refractory period follows attacks triggered from trigger areas
- Not attributed to another disorder

Episodic SUNA:
- At least 2 attack periods lasting (if untreated) from 7 days to 1 year and separated by pain-free remission periods of ≥1 month

Chronic SUNA:
- Recurring over >1 year without remission periods or with remission periods lasting <1 month

Adapted from Olesen *et al* (2004) with permission.

et al 2003b; Pareja and Cuadrado 2005). There have been reports of SUNCT responding to treatment with relatively new anticonvulsants such as topiramate, gabapentin and lamotrigine (Matharu *et al* 2003b; Pareja and Cuadrado 2005). Lamotrigine is emerging as the treatment of choice and is currently recommended as initial therapy; see Table 10.8. Gabapentin and topiramate have been advised as second-line agents in patients who fail a trial of lamotrigine (Matharu *et al* 2003b).

Cases of SUNCT associated with trigeminal nerve compression and with a vascular malformation in the cerebellopontine angle have been reported (Morales *et al* 1994; Koseoglu *et al* 2005). Moreover case reports of surgical microvascular decompression and percutaneous trigeminal ganglion compression for SUNCT as performed for TN have appeared (Morales-Asin *et al* 2000; Lagares *et al* 2005). A number of cases with SUNCT remain asymptomatic after microvascular decompression.

5. Hemicrania Continua

HC was initially considered a 'primary chronic daily headache', clearly reflecting its temporal pattern. Other primary chronic daily headaches are transformed migraine, chronic tension-type headache and new daily persistent headache; see Chapters 7 and 9. However, as HC was further documented, many claimed that this headache entity belonged to the TACs (Pareja *et al* 2001). Indeed in the latest IHS classification, HC has been classified in group 4 (other primary headaches) but is tagged on to the TACs (Olesen *et al* 2004).

5.1. Clinical Features

Case example. Case 10.4 is an excellent example of HC with good long-term follow up. The pain is constant with mild autonomic and migrainous features that become very prominent during exacerbations. Indomethacin is consistently effective. Failed treatments included amitriptyline, propranolol and carbamazepine.

Location. The vast majority of cases are unilateral with no definite side preponderance noted and few bilateral cases have been reported (Bordini *et al* 1991; Benoliel *et al* 2002). Although very rare, pain can also change sides (Newman *et al* 1992a). Pain is generally felt in the frontal and temporal regions and periorbitally (Bordini *et al* 1991; Newman *et al* 1994). Some patients (18%) will describe a distinct ocular sensation mimicking a foreign body (or sand), that may accompany or precede the headaches (Benoliel *et al* 2002).

Quality. Pain is described as throbbing in about a third of cases and this may be a constant feature of the pain or

Case 10.4 Hemicrania Continua, a 30-year-old Female

Present complaint

Continuous pain on the right side of the face and head (Fig. 10.6). The intensity of the pain was usually moderate (VAS 5–6) with occasional exacerbations (VAS 7–8) that did not have a 'jabs and jolts' quality. A throbbing, pressure-like quality was associated with the pain that sometimes awakened her from sleep, usually in the early morning.

History of present complaint

Pain had begun approximately 2 years previously as a continuous headache. There were no accompanying autonomic or systemic signs. Pain was also felt unilaterally intraorally in the upper first and second molar area. Dental treatment had been ineffective in relieving the pain. Paracetamol in doses of 1–2 g/d provided partial relief.

No abnormal findings on neurological, ENT and dental examination. Haematological and biochemical blood screening were within normal limits. Computerized scanning of the head, paranasal sinuses and TMJs and dental radiographs showed no pathology. Doppler examination of carotid blood flow was normal.

Past treatments had included propranolol, diazepam, ergotamine combinations, and intensive physiotherapy with no significant improvement. Diclofenac sodium had initially reduced pain intensity but had become ineffective within approximately 10 days.

Physical examination

Mild masticatory and neck muscle tenderness ipsilateral to the pain with no limitation of mouth opening or neck movements.

Relevant medical history

None.

Diagnosis

Chronic daily headache; hemicrania continua.

Diagnostic and treatment considerations

The referral pattern caused confusion with dental pain and the muscle tenderness falsely indicated a musculoskeletal disorder.

Pain description is typical of a chronic daily headache. Because of the combination of musculoskeletal and vascular-type features treatment was initiated with amitriptyline starting at 10 mg and increasing to 35 mg at bedtime. Four weeks later the patient was seen again with no change in pain frequency or intensity.

The salient features of the pain included the following:

1. Unilateral, including half the head and face;
2. Continuous, with a throbbing, sometimes pressure-like quality;
3. Fluctuating, from moderate to severe;
4. Not accompanied by autonomic signs; and
5. Able to waken the patient.

These features suggested a diagnosis of hemicrania continua. The patient began indomethacin 75 mg daily in three doses, and reduced the amitriptyline to 10 mg daily. At her next review appointment, 3 weeks later, the patient reported significant reduction in pain intensity and frequency on 50 mg indomethacin (see Fig. 10.7). Relief had begun rapidly and within 2 days she was essentially pain-free. Gastrointestinal symptoms had been avoided with omeprazole 20 mg daily. The patient had continued pain relief and reported that any attempt to reduce the dose resulted in headaches.

Long-term review

The patient did not attend for follow-up for about 6 months. She had attempted to stop the indomethacin as she wanted to get pregnant. All such attempts induced headache recurrence. Three months previously she had attended a neurologist's clinic and had been treated with IM steroids with no improvement. A further trial with propranolol slow release (80 mg) followed by carbamazepine (200–800 mg) had provided no pain relief.

Without indomethacin she reported that she still suffered moderate headaches (VAS 5–6) that rapidly responded to initiation of therapy (VAS 0–2). About 7 weeks prior to her attendance she began experiencing severe exacerbations of unilateral headaches (VAS 9–10) accompanied by nausea and ipsilateral autonomic signs (lacrimation, nasal congestion, eyelid oedema). These attacks could last 36–48 hours. During the first 3 weeks she suffered one attack and subsequently these became weekly (Fig. 10.7).

The patient was instructed to cease the carbamazepine and re-initiate indomethacin 25 mg 3 times daily. Over a period of 11 weeks the patient continued to take indomethacin and reported substantial improvement in baseline pain and the exacerbations became less frequent, shorter in duration and less intense (Fig. 10.7).

appear as pain intensity increases (Peres *et al* 2001a; Benoliel *et al* 2002). Other common pain descriptors at baseline include 'dull' and 'pressure' whilst in exacerbations 'stabbing' is common in addition to 'throbbing' (Peres *et al* 2001a). Exacerbations are also distinguishable in that they

are totally disabling in about 40% of patients (Peres *et al* 2001a). In addition many patients report a sharp pain similar to the condition of 'jabs and jolts' (Peres *et al* 2001a).

Severity is graded as moderate (VAS 4.7) by most patients (Peres *et al* 2001a) and characterized in many cases

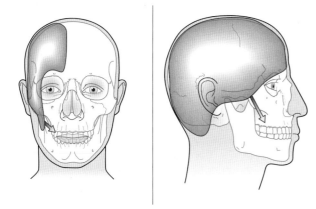

Fig. 10.6 • Case 10.4; pain location.

(74%) by fluctuations in pain severity (Benoliel *et al* 2002). Exacerbations often result in severe pain (VAS 9.3) lasting 30 minutes to 10 hours and even up to 2–5 days (Peres *et al* 2001a; Benoliel *et al* 2002). During an exacerbation, the features of HC in most cases (approx. 70%) are indistinguishable from migraine (Peres *et al* 2001a).

Temporal pattern. Two forms of HC have been described, remitting and continuous. The remitting form is characterized by headache that can last for some days followed by a pain-free period lasting from 2 to 15 days. This pattern is initially present in about half of the patients, in the rest pain is continuous from its onset (Peres *et al* 2001a; Benoliel *et al* 2002). One-third of remitting cases become continuous following a mean duration of 7.8 years (Peres *et al* 2001a; Benoliel *et al* 2002). Nocturnal attacks were reported in up to half of patients and some patients report that if awakened for other reasons the pain was invariably present (Peres *et al* 2001a; Benoliel *et al* 2002).

Precipitating or aggravating factors. A variety of factors such as bending over, menses, strong odours and stress have been reported to provoke or worsen the pain (Peres *et al* 2001a; Benoliel *et al* 2002). These are reminiscent of migraine but are not consistent features of HC. Some cases may clearly identify alcohol as a provoking or aggravating factor (Peres *et al* 2001a; Benoliel *et al* 2002).

Physical and laboratory findings. HC is not usually accompanied by notable pathology or other abnormalities

(Benoliel *et al* 2002). Most published cases of HC with computerized scanning of the head, neurological and other physical examination, haematology and serum biochemistry were all normal. However, the clinician must be aware that cases of HC secondary to pathology or systemic disease have been reported (Trucco *et al* 2004).

Accompanying phenomena. There is usually a paucity of AS that accompany the continuous pain (Rapoport and Bigal 2003). However, during exacerbation AS commonly appear singly or in various combinations, but are still relatively mild. This strengthens the hypothesis that activation of AS is dependent on pain severity. The most common signs present in 30–40% of patients are photophobia, nausea, conjunctival injection, phonophobia and tearing (Benoliel *et al* 2002). During exacerbations up to 60% of patients display qualities such as photophobia, phonophobia, nausea and more rarely vomiting (Peres *et al* 2001a). HC with aura has also been described further linking HC to migraine pathophysiology (Peres *et al* 2002b). More rarely (15–18%) nasal stuffiness or rhinorrhoea, vomiting or ptosis may also be reported (Benoliel *et al* 2002). These features establish the HC phenotype as straddling both TACs and migraine. The IHS criteria for HC are presented in Table 10.10 (Olesen *et al* 2004).

5.2. Epidemiology

Most cases reported are female (F:M ratio=2–2.8:1) with a mean age of onset of 28–33 years (range 5–67 years) (Peres *et al* 2001a; Benoliel *et al* 2002). There is no significant difference observed in mean onset age between cases that had begun as remitting (32±2.8 years) and those that had begun as continuous (34±2.6 years) (Benoliel *et al* 2002).

5.3. Secondary Hemicrania Continua

Three cases of HC complicated or caused by medication abuse have been reported (Benoliel *et al* 2002). Two abused ergotamine and one acetaminophen and cessation of the drug eliminated or reduced headaches. HC secondary to a mesenchymal tumour in the sphenoid bone has been reported (Benoliel *et al* 2002).

Fig. 10.7 • Pain diary representing mean weekly visual analogue scale in Case 10.4. Following initial diagnosis and indomethacin treatment there was rapid improvement (weeks 1–19). She was then lost to follow-up for about 6 months. Pain had returned and treatment with propranolol and carbamazepine was unsuccessful (weeks 43–50). Reinstatement of indomethacin was successful (week 52).

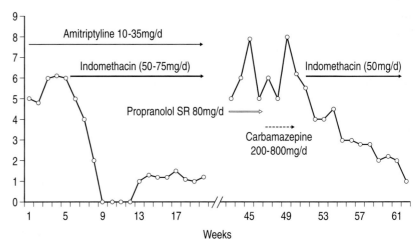

Table 10.10 Diagnostic Criteria for Hemicrania Continua (HC)

	Diagnostic Criteria	Notes
A	Headache for >3 months fulfilling criteria B–D	Unlike other TACs or migraine, no sleep association reported
B	All of the following characteristics 1. Unilateral pain with no side shift 2. Daily and continuous, without pain-free periods 3. Moderate intensity, but with exacerbations of severe pain	Rare cases of remission are reported
C	At least one of the following autonomic features occurs during exacerbations and ipsilateral to the side of pain 1. Conjunctival injection and/or lacrimation 2. Nasal congestion and/or rhinorrhoea 3. Ptosis and/or miosis	During exacerbation HC is distinctly similar to migraine
D	Complete response to therapeutic doses of indomethacin	
E	Not attributed to another disorder	Some cases reported secondary to analgesic and ergot abuse, and may not be reversible

Adapted from Olesen *et al* (2004) with permission.

Some patients with HC report a history of mild to moderate head trauma and surgery (Lay and Newman 1999; Evans and Lay 2000). The patients met the IHS criteria for chronic post-traumatic headache and displayed clinical signs typical of HC. Furthermore treatment with indomethacin, with doses up to 200 mg daily, was successful in all cases.

5.4. Pathophysiology of Hemicrania Continua

The relative rarity of HC has made studying its pathophysiology difficult. The sporadic appearance of AS and the throbbing pain quality suggest that HC, at least partly, may share some mechanisms of neurovascular-type pains (Goadsby and Lipton 1997). Nonspecific findings in orbital phlebography confirm a limited role for the regional vasculature (Antonaci 1994). Various autonomic parameters were studied in cases of HC and only a subclinical ipsilateral sympathetic dysfunction was found (Sjaastad *et al* 1984; Antonaci *et al* 1992). Functional neuroimaging in HC demonstrates activation of both the posterior hypothalamus and the dorsal rostral pons (Matharu *et al* 2004). Posterior hypothalamic and brainstem activation are considered markers of TACs and migrainous syndromes respectively, thus linking HC to the pathophysiology of both CH and migraine and mirroring HC's clinical phenotype (overlap of TACs and migraine). A lowered pain threshold was found in HC patients than in controls but may be a result rather than a cause of long-standing headaches (Antonaci *et al* 1994).

5.5. Hemicrania Continua: Treatment

Indomethacin is usually totally effective in HC and is included as part of its definition (Olesen *et al* 2004). The vast majority (68%) of reported cases have indeed responded to indomethacin (Peres *et al* 2001a). The results are dramatic with a rapid onset of relief occurring within hours or 1–2 days often with a dose–response (Pareja and Sjaastad 1996; Benoliel *et al* 2002). When 50 mg indomethacin was given intramuscularly in 12 HC patients complete pain relief occurred within 73 minutes and lasted for 13 hours; this has been proposed as the diagnostic 'Indotest' (Antonaci *et al* 1998a). However, the occurrence of indomethacin-resistant HC is a possibility although it may be a reflection of inadequate dosing (Newman *et al* 1992b).

Other NSAIDs are less effective, although aspirin, ibuprofen, piroxicam-beta-cyclodextrin, diclofenac, COX-2 inhibitors and paracetamol have provided partial relief (Benoliel *et al* 2002; Peres and Silberstein 2002). Following a case that responded well to piroxicam-beta-cyclodextrin (Trucco *et al* 1992) an open study on 6 patients with HC was performed (Sjaastad and Antonaci 1995). In 4 patients a complete response was observed and although the authors conclude that piroxicam-beta-cyclodextrin is inferior to indomethacin in HC its better tolerability may offer a good alternative for selected cases. The triptans seem ineffective in HC (Bordini *et al* 1991). An open trial on 7 HC patients using 6 mg of subcutaneous sumatriptan has shown partial but clinically doubtful efficacy (Antonaci *et al* 1998b).

6. Differential Diagnosis of TACs and Other Neurovascular Craniofacial Pain

Historically new diagnoses in neurovascular headaches have tended to be conservatively classified as subtypes of recognized entities. Cluster headache was initially considered a migraine subtype, whilst paroxysmal hemicrania and hemicrania continua were thought of as CH variants. Cervicogenic headache was thought an HC subtype and SUNCT a transformation or severe form of TN or a CH variant. This tendency is at least partly explained by the clinical overlap between these entities.

The similarities between all the neurovascular-type headaches in general and the TACs in particular may cause diagnostic difficulties in the clinic. Patients rarely present with all criteria as listed in the IHS classification (Olesen et al 2004). Moreover, descriptions of cases with coexisting headaches (Evers et al 1999; Centonze et al 2000b; Lisotto et al 2003) and reports of possible transformation of diagnoses within individual patients (Bouhassira et al 1994) suggest common pathophysiological mechanisms with a spectrum of clinical expression. Furthermore there is substantial overlap in some of the ostensibly distinct diagnostic features (Fuad and Jones 2002; Buzzi and Formisano 2003; Kaup et al 2003).

In this section we review the differential diagnosis of TACs versus other similar craniofacial pain syndromes, both primary and secondary. Additionally we provide an overview of the differential diagnosis within the spectrum of the TACs.

6.1. Entities Relevant to Differential Diagnosis

6.1.1. Orofacial Pathology

The connection between peripheral orofacial pathology and TACs is complex. Peripheral activation of the trigeminovascular system by local pathology (e.g. sinus disease), resulting in neurogenic inflammation, may exacerbate PH. Cases of CH that may have begun following extractions have also been described and may involve a similar mechanism.

The main problem is, however, the referral patterns of TACs that often involve orofacial structures and at times may primarily present in intraoral or unusual facial sites. Thus, CH and PH have caused misdiagnosis as dental pain, leading to unnecessary dental interventions (Benoliel and Sharav 1998a; van Vliet et al 2003a; Bahra and Goadsby 2004). Pain that radiates to structures within the mouth is very common in primary neurovascular-type pains so patients may point to the mouth and teeth as the sources of pain (Benoliel et al 1997; Benoliel and Sharav 1998a). Some TACs are characterized by short, repeated and severe pain that may be pulsatile and similar to the inflammatory symptoms of pulpitis (Antonaci and Sjaastad 1989; Benoliel et al 1997, 2002; Benoliel and Sharav 1998a,b). Up to 15% of PH patients (and more rarely in HC) report pain with a quality similar to that of dental pain; many had undergone unnecessary treatment (Benoliel and Sharav 1998a). Although both TACs and dental pain may be throbbing, the latter is usually evoked. Even continuous dental pains such as in dental abscesses are aggravated by mastication and have clear

signs. Thorough clinical and radiological dental evaluation usually eliminates a dental cause in these cases.

Referral patterns of migraines include the areas over the paranasal sinuses and migraine is a common diagnosis in otolaryngology settings; see Chapter 6. Similarly cluster headaches are often seen by ENT surgeons and erroneously diagnosed as sinus pathology; see Chapter 6 (Bahra et al 2002; van Vliet et al 2003a).

Up to 10% of patients with PH have pain triggered by neck movement (Sjaastad et al 1979), causing confusion with musculoskeletal pain syndromes. Some of the cases reported (Benoliel and Sharav 1998a) demonstrated ipsilateral masticatory muscle tenderness and although confusing this is consistent with findings in other primary neurovascular-type headaches such as migraine, particularly chronic migraine; see Chapter 9. HC patients may also describe pain that refers to the jaw, ear and mastoid (Trucco et al 1992) and could be confused with pain arising from temporomandibular disorders (TMDs). However, although HC and TMDs are both continuous TMDs rarely wake the patient from sleep and are not throbbing in character.

Regional tumours may cause TACs and have been discussed under individual entities. It is important to bear in mind that although headache induced by tumour is rare, they may affect 0.8–5.9% of facial pain patients (Bullitt et al 1986; Cheng et al 1993).

6.1.2. Trigeminal Neuralgia

Differential diagnosis in 'classical' TN versus TAC cases should not be difficult. However, TN may be preceded by a 'pretrigeminal neuralgia' syndrome with atypical features such as long-lasting, throbbing pain that may be diagnostically confusing (Chapter 12). There are also reports of TN with parasympathetic activation and specifically with vascular activation. More recently trigeminal neuralgia affecting the ophthalmic, maxillary or mandibular branches accompanied by lacrimation has been reported (Sjaastad et al 1997; Benoliel and Sharav 1998c; Pareja et al 2002b). Indeed the sole presence of lacrimation in this type of TN versus the multiple AS in SUNCT may be a distinct diagnostic feature (Pareja et al 2002b). Cases diagnosed as TN with lacrimation may be 'misdiagnosed' SUNCT (Sjaastad and Kruszewski 1992). Alternatively it is possible that AS will occur above a certain pain threshold so that many primary headaches, if painful enough, will present with lacrimation.

At present SUNCT is distinguished by resistance to classical anti-neuralgic therapy, the invariable presence of AS and the absence of a refractory period—a typical TN phenomenon (Pareja and Cuadrado 2005). SUNCT is usually located periorbitally whilst TN with lacrimation has been reported in maxillary and mandibular distributions. Both isolated first branch TN and SUNCT are extremely rare. Triggering of short, severe pain attacks may also be observed in PH and can cause confusion with TN. Although the sex distribution is similar, age of onset is somewhat later (50–60 years) in TN. Nocturnal attacks, common in PH, are not typical of TN which also does not usually wake from sleep. Although cases of PH responding to carbamazepine have been reported, this is rare (Evers and Husstedt 1996). In summary the major differentiating features between TACs (particularly SUNCT) and TN are very short attack duration in TN, on average 10 times shorter than in SUNCT (Sjaastad *et al* 1997; Pareja *et al* 2005); TN has a clear refractory period; TN is predominantly located in the areas of the second and third trigeminal dermatomes; and carbamazepine although very effective in TN is largely ineffective in TACs.

6.1.3. Combination Syndromes

The combination of CH and TN in cluster-tic syndrome (CTS), although very rare, may cause particular diagnostic difficulties. Neck movements may precipitate pain in CTS (40%) and an atypical form of CTS has been described with very short attacks that make CTS disturbingly similar to PH and even SUNCT (Alberca and Ochoa 1994). As in SUNCT, carbamazepine alleviates but does not eliminate pain in CTS. PH has been associated with TN in a 'CPH-tic' syndrome (Zukerman *et al* 2000; Boes *et al* 2003). Mixed attacks have also been described and may cause confusion with SUNCT; however, the CPH-tic syndrome components are individually responsive to treatment (Boes *et al* 2003).

6.1.4. Cervicogenic Headache

Cervicogenic headache is a unilateral headache that originates in the neck or back of the head and spreads anteriorly to the frontotemporal area; see Chapter 13. Pain in cervicogenic headache is usually episodic but

may become chronic and accompanied by mild AS. These clinical signs are similar to those seen in HC. However, in cervicogenic headache there are additional signs referable to the neck, including restricted motion, occipital nerve tenderness and often radiological signs of neck pathology that follow a history of trauma (e.g. whiplash). A case with typical indomethacin-responsive HC that required consistently high (225–275 mg/d) indomethacin doses was reported (Sjaastad *et al* 1995). The patient finally underwent neck surgery for disc protrusion causing C7 nerve compression, resulting in a dramatic reduction in indomethacin requirements. This case stresses the similarities between the two headache types, but since the HC continued after surgery we assume both headaches occurred concomitantly. High indomethacin requirements should always alert the physician to underlying pathology.

6.2. Differential Diagnosis within Neurovascular Craniofacial Pain (NVCP)

6.2.1. Quality and Location (Fig. 10.8, Table 10.11)

Pain quality across neurovascular headaches is often throbbing, but some entities may be distinctly different; SUNCT, for example, is more often stabbing or electrical. The pain qualities that best distinguish CH from other vascular headaches are the presence of punctate pressure and thermal sensations and the absence of dull pain (Jerome *et al* 1988). It is commonly accepted that CH pain severity is higher than that of migraine and similar to that of TN and SUNCT.

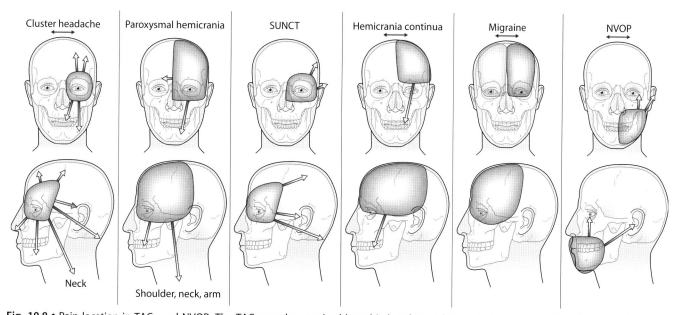

Fig. 10.8 • Pain location in TACs and NVOP. The TACs are characterized by orbital and periorbital pain. In paroxysmal hemicrania and hemicrania continua large adjacent areas are affected. Migraine is largely unilateral but may be bilateral in up to 30% of cases (this has been marked by a lighter shaded area contralaterally). Neurovascular orofacial pain (NVOP) is characterized by its location in the lower two-thirds of the face with intraoral and perioral areas frequently involved as primary sites. Two-headed arrow above diagram indicates side shift occurs in specific headache.

Table 10.11 Typical Clinical Features in Unilateral Headaches with Autonomic Signs

Parameter	Migraine	CH	CPH	SUNCT	NVOP	HC	TN
Demographics							
Onset age (yrs)	20–30	30–40[a]	30–40	40–50	40–50	30–40	50–60
Gender ratio (M:F)	1:3	5:1	1:2	9:1	1:3	1:2	1:2
Family history	60%	0.8–7%	None	?	?	—	None
Prevalence/1000	100–150	3	0.3–2.1	R[b]	R	R	0.043
Signs and symptoms							
Pain duration	4 h–3 d	15 min–3 h	2–30 min	5–240 s	45 min–12 h	Days	<120 s (pre-TN)
Sleep association	REM, III/IV	REM	REM	–	+	+	–
Awakens subjects	+	+	+	–	+	+	+/–
Time/frequency	Early morning	51%	33%	<2%	35%	30–50%	—
Frequency	1–4/m	1/2 d–8/d	5–40/d	3–200/d	Chronic	Chronic	↑[c]
Changes sides	Yes	Maybe	Rare	No	Yes	No	No
Intensity	++	+++	++	++++	++	+/++	++++
Paroxysmal	+	+	+	+	+	–	+
Throbbing	++	+(30%)	+/–	–	++	–^[d]	–(pre-TN)
Location	Forehead	Orbital	Upper	Orbital	Lower	Half	II>III>I
Remission	Pregnancy	Months–years	Unusual	+/–	–/?	–	Weeks to years
Triggering							
Touch	–	–	–	+	–	–	++
Neck	–	–	+(10%)	+	–	–	–
Alcohol	Delayed	+	+/–	+/–	–	+	–
Others (e.g. foods/stress)	+	–	–	–	–	+	–

CH, cluster headache; CPH, chronic paroxysmal hemicrania; SUNCT, short-lasting unilateral neuralgiform headache attacks with conjunctival injection and tearing; NVOP, neurovascular orofacial pain; HC, hemicrania continua; TN, trigeminal neuralgia; pre-TN, pre-trigeminal neuralgia.
[a] Onset in women differs; see text.
[b] R, rare.
[c] ↑ usually related to triggering events, but of normally high frequency.
[d] ^ increased during exacerbations.

Location is a complex issue in the diagnosis of headaches. The pain origin and patterns of referral are particularly similar in TACs and are characterized by orbital and periorbital pain that may radiate to the frontal and temporal regions (Fig. 10.8, Cases 10.1 to 10.3). These findings are not surprising in view of the common trigeminovascular system involved in all the primary neurovascular headaches. However, in PH 95% of cases report pain at sites outside the orbital region whilst 63% of CH patients report orbital pain (Zidverc-Trajkovic et al 2005).

No side shift or bilateral tendency is seen in PH though it is common in CH. Migraine may be side-locked in 15.1% of patients with aura and in 16.9% of cases without (Leone et al 1993). Unilateral, side-locked migraine may therefore be confusing; the location and accompanying AS are common features with TACs (Kaup et al 2003).

6.2.2. Temporal Patterns (Fig. 10.9, Table 10.11)

The temporal pattern for each headache is clearly defined in the IHS classification (Olesen et al 2004). Examine Cases 10.1 to 10.4; these are classical cases and the differences in duration and frequency are striking. The plotting of information from pain diaries is sometimes invaluable in diagnosing complicated cases.

However, there is often substantial overlap between TAC behaviour. Thus a prolonged SUNCT attack may

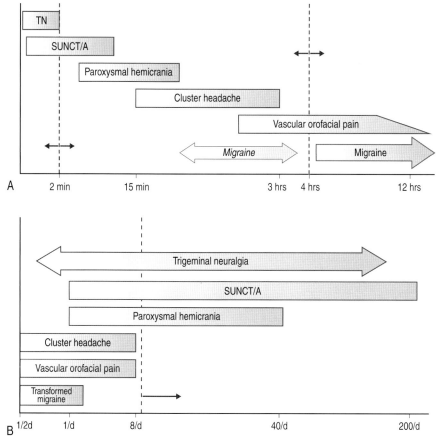

Fig. 10.9 • Duration (A) and frequency (B) in neurovascular headaches and trigeminal neuralgia. The International Headache Society (Olesen *et al* 2004) clearly defines pain duration and frequency but there is considerable overlap. Duration overlap occurs particularly in headaches lasting from 2 minutes to 4 hours; beyond these limits (dotted lines) diagnosis is relatively limited (see text). It is important to note that migraines may occasionally last less than 4 hours (migraine in double arrow) and cluster headache has been reported to last up to 48 hours. The short-lasting headaches (trigeminal neuralgia, SUNCT, paroxysmal hemicrania) are very frequent (>8 per day, dotted line) with considerable overlap. Similarly, the long-lasting headaches overlap in the frequency of attacks. TN (shown in double arrow) is often triggered but is usually of high frequency. TN, trigeminal neuralgia; SUNCT/A, short-lasting unilateral neuralgiform headache attacks with conjunctival injection and tearing/autonomic signs.

be just as lengthy as a short PH attack that similarly may, at the other end of the spectrum, overlap with short CH attacks (Fig. 10.9, Table 10.11). In comparative studies the mean duration of CH was significantly longer than that observed in PH (Zidverc-Trajkovic *et al* 2005). Duration of attack in PH has been found to be of high diagnostic value (Boes and Dodick 2002; Boes 2005). Relatively short migraine attacks (Stewart *et al* 2003) may occur and when dealing with a patient suffering from chronic migraine with autonomic features differentiation from TACs or HC may be difficult (Kaup *et al* 2003).

Unilateral headache with ipsilateral AS lasting less than 2 minutes is highly likely to be SUNCT or SUNA; TN accompanied by AS would be a second differential. Headaches accompanied by AS lasting more than 4 hours are highly likely to be migraine, or a migraine variant with AS especially in the upper third of the head (Dora 2003; Kaup *et al* 2003). Lower half headache with similar signs would likely be NVOP or lower half migraine (Benoliel *et al* 1997; Penarrocha *et al* 2004). More rarely CH may last for up to 48 hours (van Vliet *et al* 2003a). Two clear extremes in duration therefore become apparent: 2 minutes or less and 4 hours or more (see Fig. 10.9).

Although PH may wake (31%), CH is much more frequent at night (50%) and SUNCT is rarely nocturnal.

Similar overlap within the TACs is also evident with headache frequency (Fig. 10.9B, Table 10.6). Although high frequency is characteristic of PH frequent CH may be confusing (Zidverc-Trajkovic *et al* 2005). Additionally,

migraine attacks may 'cluster' or behave cyclically and overlap with more sustained CH attacks (Fox and Davis 1998; Salvesen and Bekkelund 2000). Indeed the typical clustering or seasonal pattern of CH is often observed in other headaches including HC and PH (Peres *et al* 2001b; Veloso *et al* 2001; Siow 2004). The majority of PH cases are characterized by chronic patterns that will differentiate them from the predominantly episodic nature of CH (Zidverc-Trajkovic *et al* 2005).

The high potential frequency of SUNCT/SUNA and PH attacks will no doubt cause confusion with TN in borderline cases. Triggering is a particular feature of TN but may also occur in SUNCT and even in PH; pain is triggered by neck movement in CPH and may thus cause difficulty vis-à-vis SUNCT.

6.2.3. Accompanying Signs (Table 10.12)

TACs may often occur with no or little AS and conversely AS may occur with no headache (Leone *et al* 2002). However, the presence of AS is common in all TACs and differences rely more on their number and intensity. Across all TACs lacrimation is the sign most often reported and is also observed in selected TN cases, making it of poor predictive value (Fig. 10.10). Similarly other severe headaches such as migraine may present with some degree of AS. Migraine with ipsilateral AS has been described in up to 45.5% of cases. The most common is lacrimation, the occurrence of which is

Table 10.12 Accompanying Signs and Treatment Response in Unilateral Headaches with Autonomic Signs

Parameter	Migraine	CH	CPH	SUNCT/A	NVOP	HC	TN
Autonomic signs	+	+++	++	+++	+/-	+/-	+/- -
Lacrimation (%)	41[a]	84–91	62	+	10	12–53	5–31
Conj injn (%)	[a]	58–77	36	+	7	12–32	?
Nasal congn (%)	14[b]	48–72	42	+	7	9–21	?
Rhinorrhoea (%)	[b]	43–72	36	+	7	10–12	?
Flushing (%)	+	–	–		+	2.9	+
Ptosis/miosis (%)	–	57–74	–	–	–	2–28	–
Ocular + nasal (%)	46[c]						
Systemic signs (%)	> 80	24–56	–	–	38	50	–
Treatment response							
Analgesics	+	+/-	–	–	+	–	–
Carbamazepine	–	–	–	–	–	–	++
Valproic acid	+	+/-	–	–	?	–	–
Lamotrigine	–	–	–	+	?	–	+/-
Indomethacin	–	–	++	–	–	++	–
Sumatriptan	++	++	+/-	–	+	–	–
Amitriptyline	+	–	–	–	+	–	–
Steroids	–	+	–	–	?	–	–
β-Blockers	+	–	–	–	+	–	–
Ca^{2+}-blockers	+	+	+(cases)	–	–	–	–

CH, cluster headache; CPH, chronic paroxysmal hemicrania; SUNCT, short-lasting unilateral neuralgiform headache attacks with conjunctival injection and tearing; NVOP, neurovascular orofacial pain; HC, hemicrania continua; TN, trigeminal neuralgia; AEDs, antiepileptic drugs.
Autonomic signs in HC refer to baseline and exacerbation studies.
[a] Specific ocular symptoms and
[b] specific nasal symptoms: numbers for migraine were reported together.
[c] Combination of all ocular and nasal symptoms in migraine patients.

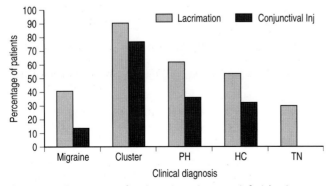

Fig. 10.10 • Percentage of patients in various craniofacial pain syndromes that report lacrimation or conjunctival injection. Although these signs are considered of high diagnostic value they are clearly nonspecific in their appearance.

significantly associated with unilateral, severe headaches (Barbanti *et al* 2002).

The extreme restlessness seen in CH patients is rarely observed to the same extent in other TACs. Migraine is associated with a number of signs thought to be of high positive predictive value such as aura, occasional hemiplegia, nausea, vomiting and photo- and phonophobia (Smetana 2000). However, CH with some of these signs has been reported (Bahra *et al* 2002; Langedijk *et al* 2005) and similarly exacerbations of HC often present with migrainous-type features (Peres *et al* 2001a, 2002b).

CH and SUNCT occur predominantly in males whilst PH is more evenly distributed and migraine is a classically female syndrome.

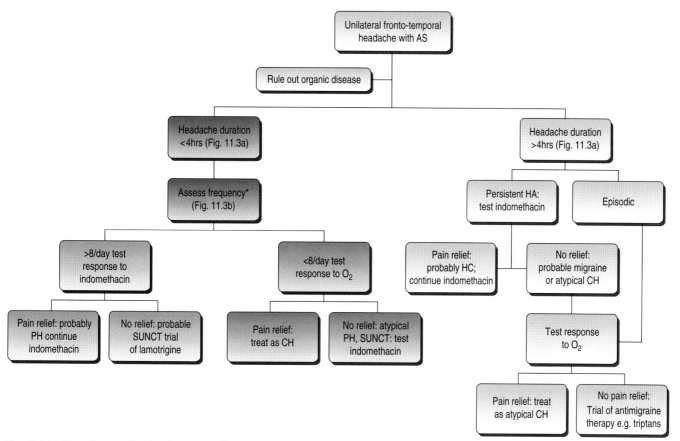

Fig. 10.11 • Flow diagram for the diagnosis of headaches with autonomic signs (use with Fig. 11.3). Preliminary diagnosis is based on location and accompanying autonomic signs (AS). This is followed by duration, frequency and treatment response particularly to oxygen and indomethacin. Bear in mind that high-frequency triggered facial pain may also be trigeminal neuralgia with autonomic signs; see text and Chapter 14. AS, autonomic signs; HA, headache; O₂, oxygen; PH, paroxysmal hemicrania; SUNCT, short-lasting unilateral neuralgiform headache attacks with conjunctival injection and tearing; CH, cluster headache.

Overlaps, although rare, are clearly apparent. The pain history and pain diary remain central to accurate diagnosis and it is indeed the overall combination of signs, symptoms and behaviour that lead the astute clinician to the correct diagnosis.

6.2.4. Treatment Response

TACs are different in their response to therapy (see Table 10.8) and we often rely on this as a final endorsement of the diagnosis. For example, response to abortive oxygen, lithium or verapamil would suggest a diagnosis of CH. A positive indomethacin response is considered highly indicative that the patient suffers from PH or HC (Boes 2005).

However, some overlap does occur in treatment response; for example, migraine and CH may respond to indomethacin whilst PH and HC may not. Atypical cases of CH may not only respond to indomethacin but also present with unusual features.

In borderline cases, reaching an exact diagnosis may be academic and it is often best to commence therapy under a tentative diagnosis of TAC and exploit treatment response and follow-up. Based on initial grouping by duration and frequency the clinician is often able to reach an accurate working diagnosis; see algorithm in Fig. 10.11. In unclear TAC cases it has been suggested that a trial of indomethacin is indicated (Matharu and Goadsby 2002b). However, due to the low prevalence of PH and HC the best approach is to instigate indomethacin treatment in patients with > 5 attacks daily and/or with attack duration of <30 minutes (Matharu and Goadsby 2002b).

References

Afridi SK, Matharu MS, Lee L, *et al* (2005) A PET study exploring the laterality of brainstem activation in migraine using glyceryl trinitrate. *Brain* **128**(Pt 4):932–939.

Alberca R, Ochoa JJ (1994) Cluster tic syndrome. *Neurology* **44**(6): 996–999.

Allen GV, Barbrick B, Esser MJ (1996) Trigeminal-parabrachial connections: possible pathway for nociception-induced cardiovascular reflex responses. *Brain Res* **715**(1–2):125–135.

Ambrosini A, Vandenheede M, Rossi P, *et al* (2005) Suboccipital injection with a mixture of rapid- and long-acting steroids in cluster headache: a double-blind placebo-controlled study. *Pain* **118**(1–2):92–96.

Andersson PG, Jespersen LT (1986) Dihydroergotamine nasal spray in the treatment of attacks of cluster headache. A double-blind trial versus placebo. *Cephalalgia* **6**(1):51–54.

Antonaci F (1994) Chronic paroxysmal hemicrania and hemicrania continua: orbital phlebography and MRI studies. *Headache* **34**(1):32–34.

Antonaci F, Sjaastad O (1989) Chronic paroxysmal hemicrania (CPH): a review of the clinical manifestations. *Headache* 29(10):648–656.

Antonaci F, Sand T, Sjaastad O (1992) Hemicrania continua and chronic paroxysmal hemicrania: a comparison of pupillometric findings. *Funct Neurol* 7(5):385–389.

Antonaci F, Sandrini G, Danilov A, *et al* (1994) Neurophysiological studies in chronic paroxysmal hemicrania and hemicrania continua. *Headache* 34(8):479–483.

Antonaci F, Pareja JA, Caminero AB, *et al* (1998a) Chronic paroxysmal hemicrania and hemicrania continua. Parenteral indomethacin: the 'indotest'. *Headache* 38(2):122–128.

Antonaci F, Pareja JA, Caminero AB, *et al* (1998b) Chronic paroxysmal hemicrania and hemicrania continua: lack of efficacy of sumatriptan. *Headache* 38(3):197–200.

Antonaci F, Costa A, Ghirmai S, *et al* (2003) Parenteral indomethacin (the INDOTEST) in cluster headache. *Cephalalgia* 23(3):193–196.

Antonaci F, Costa A, Candeloro E, *et al* (2005) Single high-dose steroid treatment in episodic cluster headache. *Cephalalgia* 25(4):290–295.

Bahra A, Goadsby PJ (2004). Diagnostic delays and mis-management in cluster headache. *Acta Neurol Scand* 109(3): 175–179.

Bahra A, Gawel MJ, Hardebo JE, *et al* (2000) Oral zolmitriptan is effective in the acute treatment of cluster headache. *Neurology* 54(9):1832–1839.

Bahra A, May A, Goadsby PJ (2002) Cluster headache: a prospective clinical study with diagnostic implications. *Neurology* 58(3):354–361.

Barbanti P, Fabbrini G, Pesare M, *et al* (2002) Unilateral cranial autonomic symptoms in migraine. *Cephalalgia* 22(4):256–259.

Bartsch T, Levy MJ, Knight YE, *et al* (2004) Differential modulation of nociceptive dural input to [hypocretin] orexin A and B receptor activation in the posterior hypothalamic area. *Pain* 109(3):367–378.

Becser N, Berky M (1995) SUNCT syndrome: a Hungarian case. *Headache* 35(3):158–160.

Benoliel R, Sharav Y (1998a) Paroxysmal hemicrania. Case studies and review of the literature. *Oral Surg Oral Med Oral Pathol Oral Radiol Endod* 85(3):285–292.

Benoliel R, Sharav Y (1998b) SUNCT syndrome: case report and literature review. *Oral Surg Oral Med Oral Pathol Oral Radiol Endod* 85(2):158–161.

Benoliel R, Sharav Y (1998c) Trigeminal neuralgia with lacrimation or SUNCT syndrome? *Cephalalgia* 18(2):85–90.

Benoliel R, Elishoov H, Sharav Y (1997) Orofacial pain with vascular-type features. *Oral Surg Oral Med Oral Pathol Oral Radiol Endod* 84(5):506–512.

Benoliel R, Robinson S, Eliav E, *et al* (2002) Hemicrania continua. *J Orofac Pain* 16(4):317–325.

Bingel U, Weiller C (2005) An unusual indomethacin-sensitive headache: a case of bilateral episodic paroxysmal hemicrania without autonomic symptoms? *Cephalalgia* 25(2):148–150.

Black DF, Bordini CA, Russell D (2006) Symptomatology of cluster headache. In: Olesen J, Goadsby PJ, Ramadan NM, *et al* (eds) *The Headaches*, 3rd edn. Philadelphia: Lippincott Williams & Wilkins, pp 789–796.

Blau JN, Engel H (1990) Episodic paroxysmal hemicrania: a further case and review of the literature. *J Neurol Neurosurg Psychiatry* 53(4):343–344.

Blau JN, Engel HO (1998) Premonitory and prodromal symptoms in cluster headache. *Cephalalgia* 18(2):91–93; discussion 71–92.

Boes C (2005) Differentiating paroxysmal hemicrania from cluster headache. *Cephalalgia* 25(4):241–243.

Boes CJ, Dodick DW (2002) Refining the clinical spectrum of chronic paroxysmal hemicrania: a review of 74 patients. *Headache* 42(8):699–708.

Boes CJ, Matharu MS, Goadsby PJ (2003) The paroxysmal hemicrania-tic syndrome. *Cephalalgia* 23(1):24–28.

Boes CJ, Vincent M, Russell D (2006) Chronic paroxysmal hemicrania. In: Olesen J, Goadsby PJ, Ramadan NM, *et al* (eds)

The Headaches, 3rd edn. Philadelphia: Lippincott Williams & Wilkins, pp 815–822.

Bolay H, Reuter U, Dunn AK, *et al* (2002) Intrinsic brain activity triggers trigeminal meningeal afferents in a migraine model. *Nat Med* 8(2):136–142.

Bordini C, Antonaci F, Stovner LJ, *et al* (1991) 'Hemicrania continua': a clinical review. *Headache* 31(1):20–26.

Bouhassira D, Attal N, Esteve M, *et al* (1994) 'SUNCT' syndrome. A case of transformation from trigeminal neuralgia? *Cephalalgia* 14(2):168–170.

Bullitt E, Tew JM, Boyd J (1986) Intracranial tumors in patients with facial pain. *J Neurosurg* 64(6):865–871.

Bussone G, Leone M, Peccarisi C, *et al* (1990) Double blind comparison of lithium and verapamil in cluster headache prophylaxis. *Headache* 30(7):411–417.

Buzzi MG, Formisano R (2003) A patient with cluster headache responsive to indomethacin: any relationship with chronic paroxysmal hemicrania? *Cephalalgia* 23(5):401–404.

Cademartiri C, Torelli P, Cologno D, *et al* (2002) Upper and lower cluster headache: clinical and pathogenetic observations in 608 patients. *Headache* 42(7):630–637.

Carter DM (2004) Cluster headache mimics. *Curr Pain Headache Rep* 8(2):133–139.

Castellano AE, Micieli G, Bellantonio P, *et al* (1998) Indomethacin increases the effect of isosorbide dinitrate on cerebral hemodynamic in migraine patients: pathogenetic and therapeutic implications. *Cephalalgia* 18(9):622–630.

Centonze V, Bassi A, Causarano V, *et al* (2000a) Sumatriptan overuse in episodic cluster headache: lack of adverse events, rebound syndromes, drug dependence and tachyphylaxis. *Funct Neurol* 15(3):167–170.

Centonze V, Bassi A, Causarano V, *et al* (2000b) Simultaneous occurrence of ipsilateral cluster headache and chronic paroxysmal hemicrania: a case report. *Headache* 40(1):54–56.

Cheng TM, Cascino TL, Onofrio BM (1993) Comprehensive study of diagnosis and treatment of trigeminal neuralgia secondary to tumors. *Neurology* 43(11):2298–2302.

Chervin RD, Zallek SN, Lin X, *et al* (2000) Timing patterns of cluster headaches and association with symptoms of obstructive sleep apnea. *Sleep Res Online* 3(3):107–112.

Costa A, Ravaglia S, Sances G, *et al* (2003) Nitric oxide pathway and response to nitroglycerin in cluster headache patients: plasma nitrite and citrulline levels. *Cephalalgia* 23(6): 407–413.

Dahlof C (1993) Subcutaneous sumatriptan does not abort attacks of chronic paroxysmal hemicrania (CPH). *Headache* 33(4):201–202.

D'Amico D, Ferraris A, Leone M, *et al* (2002) Increased plasma nitrites in migraine and cluster headache patients in interictal period: basal hyperactivity of L-arginine-NO pathway? *Cephalalgia* 22(1):33–36.

D'Andrea G, Granella F (2001) SUNCT syndrome: the first case in childhood. Short-lasting unilateral neuralgiform headache attacks with conjunctival injection and tearing. *Cephalalgia* 21(6):701–702.

Dodick DW (1998) Extratrigeminal episodic paroxysmal hemicrania. Further clinical evidence of functionally relevant brain stem connections. *Headache* 38(10):794–798.

Dodick DW, Rozen TD, Goadsby PJ, *et al* (2000) Cluster headache. *Cephalalgia* 20(9):787–803.

Dora B (2003) Migraine with cranial autonomic features and strict unilaterality. *Cephalalgia* 23(7):561–562.

Drummond PD (1990) Dissociation between pain and autonomic disturbances in cluster headache. *Headache* 30(8):505–508.

Drummond PD (1992) The mechanism of facial sweating and cutaneous vascular responses to painful stimulation of the eye. *Brain* 115 (Pt 5):1417–1428.

Drummond PD (1995) Lacrimation and cutaneous vasodilatation in the face induced by painful stimulation of the nasal ala and upper lip. *J Auton Nerv Syst* 51(2):109–116.

Ekbom K (1970) A clinical comparison of cluster headache and migraine. *Acta Neurol Scand* Suppl 41:1–48.

Ekbom K (1990) Evaluation of clinical criteria for cluster headache with special reference to the classification of the International Headache Society. *Cephalalgia* **10**(4):195–197.

Ekbom K, Hardebo JE (2002) Cluster headache: aetiology, diagnosis and management. *Drugs* **62**(1):61–69.

Ekbom K, Monstad I, Prusinski A, *et al* (1993) Subcutaneous sumatriptan in the acute treatment of cluster headache: a dose comparison study. The Sumatriptan Cluster Headache Study Group. *Acta Neurol Scand* **88**(1):63–69.

Ekbom K, Krabbe A, Micieli G, *et al* (1995) Cluster headache attacks treated for up to three months with subcutaneous sumatriptan (6 mg). Sumatriptan Cluster Headache Long-term Study Group. *Cephalalgia* **15**(3):230–236.

Ekbom K, Svensson DA, Traff H, *et al* (2002) Age at onset and sex ratio in cluster headache: observations over three decades. *Cephalalgia* **22**(2):94–100.

El Amrani M, Ducros A, Boulan P, *et al* (2002) Familial cluster headache: a series of 186 index patients. *Headache* **42**(10): 974–977.

Evans RW, Lay CL (2000) Posttraumatic hemicrania continua? *Headache* **40**(9):761–762.

Evers S, Husstedt IW (1996) Alternatives in drug treatment of chronic paroxysmal hemicrania. *Headache* **36**(7):429–432.

Evers S, Bahra A, Goadsby PJ (1999) Coincidence of familial hemiplegic migraine and hemicrania continua? A case report. *Cephalalgia* **19**(5):533–535.

Facchinetti F, Nappi G, Cicoli C, *et al* (1986) Reduced testosterone levels in cluster headache: a stress-related phenomenon? *Cephalalgia* **6**(1):29–34

Fogan L (1985) Treatment of cluster headache. A double-blind comparison of oxygen v air inhalation. *Arch Neurol* **42**(4): 362–363.

Forderreuther S, Mayer M, Straube A (2002) Treatment of cluster headache with topiramate: effects and side-effects in five patients. *Cephalalgia* **22**(3):186–189.

Fox AW, Davis RL (1998) Migraine chronobiology. *Headache* **38**(6):436–441.

Frese A, Evers S, May A (2003) Autonomic activation in experimental trigeminal pain. *Cephalalgia* **23**(1):67–68.

Fuad F, Jones NS (2002) Paroxysmal hemicrania and cluster headache: two discrete entities or is there an overlap? *Clin Otolaryngol* **27**(6):472–479.

Gantenbein AR, Goadsby PJ (2005) Familial SUNCT. *Cephalalgia* **25**(6):457–459.

Gatzonis S, Mitsikostas DD, Ilias A, *et al* (1996) Two more secondary headaches mimicking chronic paroxysmal hemicrania. Is this the exception or the rule? *Headache* **36**(8):511–513.

Goadsby PJ (1989) Effect of stimulation of facial nerve on regional cerebral blood flow and glucose utilization in cats. *Am J Physiol* **257**(3 Pt 2):R517–R521.

Goadsby PJ, Duckworth JW (1987) Effect of stimulation of trigeminal ganglion on regional cerebral blood flow in cats. *Am J Physiol* **253**(2 Pt 2):R270–R274.

Goadsby PJ, Edvinsson L (1994) Human in vivo evidence for trigeminovascular activation in cluster headache. Neuropeptide changes and effects of acute attacks therapies. *Brain* **117**(Pt 3):427–434.

Goadsby PJ, Edvinsson L (1996) Neuropeptide changes in a case of chronic paroxysmal hemicrania–evidence for trigemino-parasympathetic activation. *Cephalalgia* **16**(6):448–450.

Goadsby PJ, Lipton RB (1997) A review of paroxysmal hemicranias, SUNCT syndrome and other short- lasting headaches with autonomic feature, including new cases. *Brain* **120**(Pt 1):193–209.

Goadsby PJ, Lambert GA, Lance JW (1984) The peripheral pathway for extracranial vasodilatation in the cat. *J Auton Nerv Syst* **10**(2):145–155.

Goadsby PJ, Matharu MS, Boes CJ (2001) SUNCT syndrome or trigeminal neuralgia with lacrimation. *Cephalalgia* **21**(2): 82–83.

Goadsby PJ, Lipton RB, Ferrari MD (2002) Migraine–current understanding and treatment. *N Engl J Med* **346**(4):257–270.

Gobel H, Lindner V, Heinze A, *et al* (1998) Acute therapy for cluster headache with sumatriptan: findings of a one-year long-term study. *Neurology* **51**(3):908–911.

Gobel H, Czech N, Heinze-Kuhn K, *et al* (2000) Evidence of regional protein plasma extravasation in cluster headache using Tc-99m albumin SPECT. *Cephalalgia* **20**(4):287.

Haan J, van Vliet JA, Kors EE, *et al* (2001) No involvement of the calcium channel gene (CACNA1A) in a family with cluster headache. *Cephalalgia* **21**(10):959–962.

Hannerz J (1991) Orbital phlebography and signs of inflammation in episodic and chronic cluster headache. *Headache* **31**(8): 540–542.

Hannerz J, Greitz D, Hansson P, *et al* (1992) SUNCT may be another manifestation of orbital venous vasculitis. *Headache* **32**(8):384–389.

Hardebo JE (1991) On pain mechanisms in cluster headache. *Headache* **31**(2):91–106.

Hardebo JE (1994) How cluster headache is explained as an intracavernous inflammatory process lesioning sympathetic fibers. *Headache* **34**(3):125–131.

Hardebo JE, Dahlof C (1998) Sumatriptan nasal spray (20 mg/dose) in the acute treatment of cluster headache. *Cephalalgia* **18**(7):487–489.

Izumi H (1999) Nervous control of blood flow in the orofacial region. *Pharmacol Ther* **81**(2):141–161.

Jerome A, Holroyd KA, Theofanous AG, *et al* (1988) Cluster headache pain vs. other vascular headache pain: differences revealed with two approaches to the McGill Pain Questionnaire. *Pain* **34**(1):35–42.

Jimenez-Huete A, Franch O, Pareja JA (2002) SUNCT syndrome: priming of symptomatic periods and worsening of symptoms by treatment with calcium channel blockers. *Cephalalgia* **22**(10): 812–814.

Kaup AO, Mathew NT, Levyman C, *et al* (2003) 'Side locked' migraine and trigeminal autonomic cephalgias: evidence for clinical overlap. *Cephalalgia* **23**(1):43–49.

Kemppainen P, Leppanen H, Jyvasjarvi E, *et al* (1994) Blood flow increase in the orofacial area of humans induced by painful stimulation. *Brain Res Bull* **33**(6):655–662.

Kinney MA, Wilson JL, Carmichael SW, *et al* (2003) Prolonged facial hypesthesia resulting from greater occipital nerve block. *Clin Anat* **16**(4):362–365.

Knight YE, Classey JD, Lasalandra MP, *et al* (2005) Patterns of fos expression in the rostral medulla and caudal pons evoked by noxious craniovascular stimulation and periaqueductal gray stimulation in the cat. *Brain Res* **1045**(1-2):1–11.

Koseoglu E, Karaman Y, Kucuk S, *et al* (2005) SUNCT syndrome associated with compression of trigeminal nerve. *Cephalalgia* **25**(6):473–475.

Krabbe A (1991) The prognosis of cluster headache. A long-term observation of 226 cluster headache patients. *Cephalalgia* (Suppl 11):250–251.

Kruszewski P (1992) Shortlasting, unilateral, neuralgiform headache attacks with conjunctival injection and tearing (SUNCT syndrome): V. Orbital phlebography. *Cephalalgia* **12**(6):387–389.

Kruszewski P, Zhao JM, Shen JM, *et al* (1993) SUNCT syndrome: forehead sweating pattern. *Cephalalgia* **13**(2):108–113.

Kudrow DB, Kudrow L (1989) Successful aspirin prophylaxis in a child with chronic paroxysmal hemicrania. *Headache* **29**(5): 280–281.

Kudrow L (1981) Response of cluster headache attacks to oxygen inhalation. *Headache* **21**(1):1–4.

Kudrow L (1987) The cyclic relationship of natural illumination to cluster period frequency. *Cephalalgia* **7**(Suppl 6):76–78.

Kudrow L, Kudrow DB (1994) Inheritance of cluster headache and its possible link to migraine. *Headache* **34**(7):400–407.

Lagares A, Gomez PA, Perez-Nunez A, *et al* (2005) Short-lasting unilateral neuralgiform headache with conjunctival injection and tearing syndrome treated with microvascular decompression of the trigeminal nerve: case report. *Neurosurgery* **56**(2):E413; discussion E413.

Lain AH, Caminero AB, Pareja JA (2000) SUNCT syndrome; absence of refractory periods and modulation of attack duration by lengthening of the trigger stimuli. *Cephalalgia* **20**(7):671–673.

Lambert GA, Bogduk N, Goadsby PJ, *et al* (1984) Decreased carotid arterial resistance in cats in response to trigeminal stimulation. *J Neurosurg* **61**(2):307–315.

Langedijk M, van der Naalt J, Luijckx GJ, *et al* (2005) Cluster-like headache aura status. *Headache* **45**(1):80–81.

Lay CL, Newman LC (1999) Posttraumatic hemicrania continua. *Headache* **39**:275–279.

Leone M (2004) Chronic cluster headache: new and emerging treatment options. *Curr Pain Headache Rep* **8**(5):347–352.

Leone M, Bussone G (1993) A review of hormonal findings in cluster headache. Evidence for hypothalamic involvement. *Cephalalgia* **13**(5):309–317.

Leone M, D'Amico D, Frediani F, *et al* (1993) Clinical considerations on side-locked unilaterality in long-lasting primary headaches. *Headache* **33**(7):381–384.

Leone M, D'Amico D, Frediani F, *et al* (2000) Verapamil in the prophylaxis of episodic cluster headache: a double-blind study versus placebo. *Neurology* **54**(6):1382–1385.

Leone M, Russell MB, Rigamonti A, *et al* (2001) Increased familial risk of cluster headache. *Neurology* **56**(9):1233–1236.

Leone M, Rigamonti A, Bussone G (2002) Cluster headache sine headache: two new cases in one family. *Cephalalgia* **22**(1):12–14.

Leone M, Franzini A, Broggi G, *et al* (2004a) Long-term follow-up of bilateral hypothalamic stimulation for intractable cluster headache. *Brain* **127**(Pt 10):2259–2264.

Leone M, May A, Franzini A, *et al* (2004b) Deep brain stimulation for intractable chronic cluster headache: proposals for patient selection. *Cephalalgia* **24**(11):934–937.

Leone M, Franzini A, D'Andrea G, *et al* (2005) Deep brain stimulation to relieve drug-resistant SUNCT. *Ann Neurol* **57**(6):924–927.

Levi R, Edman GV, Ekbom K, *et al* (1992) Episodic cluster headache. II: High tobacco and alcohol consumption in males. *Headache* **32**(4):184–187.

Levy MJ, Matharu MS, Meeran K, *et al* (2005) The clinical characteristics of headache in patients with pituitary tumours. *Brain* **128**(Pt 8):1921–1930.

Lin H, Dodick DW (2005) Tearing without pain after trigeminal root section for cluster headache. *Neurology* **65**(10):1650–1651.

Lipton RB, Bigal ME (2005) Migraine: epidemiology, impact, and risk factors for progression. *Headache* **45**(Suppl 1):S3–S13.

Lisotto C, Mainardi F, Maggioni F, *et al* (2003) Hemicrania continua with contralateral episodic cluster headache: a case report. *Cephalalgia* **23**(9):929–930.

Lovely TJ, Kotsiakis X, Jannetta PJ (1998) The surgical management of chronic cluster headache. *Headache* **38**(8):590–594.

Manning BH, Franklin KB (1998) Morphine analgesia in the formalin test: reversal by microinjection of quaternary naloxone into the posterior hypothalamic area or periaqueductal gray. *Behav Brain Res* **92**(1):97–102.

Manzoni GC (1999a) Cluster headache and lifestyle: remarks on a population of 374 male patients. *Cephalalgia* **19**(2):88–94.

Manzoni GC (1999b) Epidemiological and clinical aspects of cluster headache: relation with the migrainous syndrome. *Ital J Neurol Sci* **20**(2 Suppl):S4–S6.

Manzoni GC, Terzano MG, Bono G, *et al* (1983) Cluster headache—clinical findings in 180 patients. *Cephalalgia* **3**(1):21–30.

Manzoni GC, Micieli G, Granella F, *et al* (1991a) Cluster headache—course over ten years in 189 patients. *Cephalalgia* **11**(4):169–174.

Manzoni GC, Micieli G, Zanferrari C, *et al* (1991b) Cluster headache. Recent developments in clinical characterization and pathogenesis. *Acta Neurol (Napoli)* **13**(6):506–513.

Mariano da Silva H, Benevides-Luz I, Santos AC, *et al* (2004) Chronic paroxysmal hemicrania as a manifestation of intracranial parotid gland carcinoma metastasis–a case report. *Cephalalgia* **24**(3):223–227.

Martins IP, Gouveia RG, Parreira E (2005) Cluster headache without autonomic symptoms: why is it different? *Headache* **45**(3):190–195.

Matharu MS, Goadsby PJ (2002a) Persistence of attacks of cluster headache after trigeminal nerve root section. *Brain* **125**(Pt 5):976–984.

Matharu MS, Goadsby PJ (2002b) Trigeminal autonomic cephalgias. *J Neurol Neurosurg Psychiatry* **72**(Suppl 2):ii19–ii26.

Matharu MS, Goadsby PJ (2005) Bilateral paroxysmal hemicrania or bilateral paroxysmal cephalalgia, another novel indomethacin-responsive primary headache syndrome? *Cephalalgia* **25**(2):79–81.

Matharu MS, Boes CJ, Goadsby PJ (2003a) Management of trigeminal autonomic cephalgias and hemicrania continua. *Drugs* **63**(16):1637–1677.

Matharu MS, Cohen AS, Boes CJ, *et al* (2003b) Short-lasting unilateral neuralgiform headache with conjunctival injection and tearing syndrome: a review. *Curr Pain Headache Rep* **7**(4):308–318.

Matharu MS, Cohen AS, McGonigle DJ, *et al* (2004) Posterior hypothalamic and brainstem activation in hemicrania continua. *Headache* **44**(8):747–761.

Mather PJ, Silberstein SD, Schulman EA, *et al* (1991) The treatment of cluster headache with repetitive intravenous dihydroergotamine. *Headache* **31**(8):525–532.

May A (2005) Cluster headache: pathogenesis, diagnosis, and management. *Lancet* **366**(9488):843–855.

May A, Goadsby PJ (1999) The trigeminovascular system in humans: pathophysiologic implications for primary headache syndromes of the neural influences on the cerebral circulation. *J Cereb Blood Flow Metab* **19**(2):115–127.

May A, Bahra A, Buchel C, *et al* (1998a) Hypothalamic activation in cluster headache attacks. *Lancet* **352**(9124):275–278.

May A, Kaube H, Buchel C, *et al* (1998b) Experimental cranial pain elicited by capsaicin: a PET study. *Pain* **74**(1):61–66.

May A, Bahra A, Buchel C, *et al* (1999a) Functional magnetic resonance imaging in spontaneous attacks of SUNCT: short-lasting neuralgiform headache with conjunctival injection and tearing. *Ann Neurol* **46**(5):791–794.

May A, Ashburner J, Buchel C, *et al* (1999b) Correlation between structural and functional changes in brain in an idiopathic headache syndrome. *Nat Med* **5**(7):836–838.

May A, Bahra A, Buchel C, *et al* (2000) PET and MRA findings in cluster headache and MRA in experimental pain. *Neurology* **55**(9):1328–1335.

May A, Buchel C, Turner R, *et al* (2001) Magnetic resonance angiography in facial and other pain: neurovascular mechanisms of trigeminal sensation. *J Cereb Blood Flow Metab* **21**(10):1171–1176.

Merskey H, Bogduk N (1994). *Classification of chronic pain: descriptions of chronic pain syndromes and definition of pain terms*, 2 edn. IASP Press: Seattle.

Mizuta K, Izumi H (2004) Bulbar pathway for contralateral lingual nerve-evoked reflex vasodilatation in cat palate. *Brain Res* **1020**(1-2):86–94.

Montes E, Alberca R, Lozano P, *et al* (2001) Statuslike SUNCT in two young women. *Headache* **41**(8):826–829.

Morales-Asin F, Espada F, Lopez-Obarrio LA, *et al* (2000) A SUNCT case with response to surgical treatment. *Cephalalgia* **20**(1):67–68.

Morales F, Mostacero E, Marta J, *et al* (1994) Vascular malformation of the cerebellopontine angle associated with 'SUNCT' syndrome. *Cephalalgia* **14**(4):301–302.

Murialdo G, Fanciullacci M, Nicolodi M, *et al* (1989) Cluster headache in the male: sex steroid pattern and gonadotropic response to luteinizing hormone releasing hormone. *Cephalalgia* **9**(2):91–98.

Nappi G, Micieli G, Cavallini A, *et al* (1992) Accompanying symptoms of cluster attacks: their relevance to the diagnostic criteria. *Cephalalgia* **12**(3):165–168.

Narbone MC, Gangemi S, Abbate M (2005) A case of SUNCT syndrome responsive to verapamil. *Cephalalgia* **25**(6):476–478.

Newman LC, Lipton RB, Russell M, et al (1992a) Hemicrania continua: attacks may alternate sides [see comments]. Headache 32(5):237–238.

Newman LC, Gordon ML, Lipton RB, et al (1992b) Episodic paroxysmal hemicrania: two new cases and a literature review. Neurology 42(5):964–966.

Newman LC, Lipton RB, Solomon S (1994) Hemicrania continua: ten new cases and a review of the literature. Neurology 44(11):2111–2114.

Nicolodi M, Sicuteri F, Poggioni M (1993) Hypothalamic modulation of nociception and reproduction in cluster headache. I. Therapeutic trials of leuprolide. Cephalalgia 13(4):253–257.

Olesen J, Bousser M-G, Diener HC, et al (2004) The International Classification of Headache Disorders, 2nd Edition. Cephalalgia 24(Suppl 1):24–150.

Pareja JA (1995) Chronic paroxysmal hemicrania: dissociation of the pain and autonomic features. Headache 35(2):111–113.

Pareja JA, Cuadrado ML (2005) SUNCT syndrome: an update. Expert Opin Pharmacother 6(4):591–599.

Pareja JA, Sjaastad O (1994) SUNCT syndrome in the female. Headache 34(4):217–220.

Pareja J, Sjaastad O (1996) Chronic paroxysmal hemicrania and hemicrania continua. Interval between indomethacin administration and response. Headache 36(1):20–23.

Pareja JA, Sjaastad O (1997) SUNCT syndrome. A clinical review. Headache 37(4):195–202.

Pareja JA, Pareja J, Palomo T, et al (1994) SUNCT syndrome: repetitive and overlapping attacks. Headache 34(2):114–116.

Pareja JA, Kruszewski P, Sjaastad O (1995) SUNCT syndrome: trials of drugs and anesthetic blockades. Headache 35(3):138–142.

Pareja JA, White LR, Sjaastad O (1996a) Pathophysiology of headaches with a prominent vascular component. Pain Res Manage 1(2):93–108.

Pareja JA, Shen JM, Kruszewski P, et al (1996b) SUNCT syndrome: duration, frequency, and temporal distribution of attacks. Headache 36(3):161–165.

Pareja JA, Caballero V, Sjaastad O (1996c) SUNCT syndrome. Statuslike pattern. Headache 36(10):622–624.

Pareja JA, Vincent M, Antonaci F, et al (2001) Hemicrania continua: diagnostic criteria and nosologic status. Cephalalgia 21(9):874–877.

Pareja JA, Caminero AB, Sjaastad O (2002a) SUNCT syndrome: diagnosis and treatment. CNS Drugs 16(6):373–383.

Pareja JA, Baron M, Gili P, et al (2002b) Objective assessment of autonomic signs during triggered first division trigeminal neuralgia. Cephalalgia 22(4):251–255.

Pareja JA, Cuadrado ML, Caminero AB, et al (2005) Duration of attacks of first division trigeminal neuralgia. Cephalalgia 25(4):305–308.

Penarrocha M, Bandres A, Penarrocha MA, et al (2001) Relationship between oral surgical and endodontic procedures and episodic cluster headache. Oral Surg Oral Med Oral Pathol Oral Radiol Endod 92(5):499–502.

Penarrocha M, Bandres A, Penarrocha M, et al (2004) Lower-half facial migraine: a report of 11 cases. J Oral Maxillofac Surg 62(12):1453–1456.

Peres MF, Silberstein SD (2002) Hemicrania continua responds to cyclooxygenase-2 inhibitors. Headache 42(6):530–531.

Peres MF, Silberstein SD, Nahmias S, et al (2001a) Hemicrania continua is not that rare. Neurology 57(6):948–951.

Peres MF, Stiles MA, Oshinsky M, et al (2001b) Remitting form of hemicrania continua with seasonal pattern. Headache 41(6):592–594.

Peres MF, Stiles MA, Siow HC, et al (2002a) Greater occipital nerve blockade for cluster headache. Cephalalgia 22(7):520–522.

Peres MF, Siow HC, Rozen TD (2002b) Hemicrania continua with aura. Cephalalgia 22(3):246–248.

Pfaffenrath V, Pollmann W, Ruther E, et al (1986) Onset of nocturnal attacks of chronic cluster headache in relation to sleep stages. Acta Neurol Scand 73(4):403–407.

Putzki N, Nirkko A, Diener HC (2005) Trigeminal autonomic cephalalgias: a case of post-traumatic SUNCT syndrome? Cephalalgia 25(5):395–397.

Raimondi E (2001) Premonitory symptoms in cluster headache. Curr Pain Headache Rep 5(1):55–59.

Rainero I, Gallone S, Valfre W, et al (2004) A polymorphism of the hypocretin receptor 2 gene is associated with cluster headache. Neurology 63(7):1286–1288.

Rainero I, Rivoiro C, Gallone S, et al (2005) Lack of association between the 3092 T-C clock gene polymorphism and cluster headache. Cephalalgia 25(11):1078–1081.

Rapoport AM, Bigal ME (2003) Hemicrania continua: clinical and nosographic update. Neurol Sci 24(Suppl 2):S118–S121.

Rasmussen P (1991) Facial pain. IV. A prospective study of 1052 patients with a view of: precipitating factors, associated symptoms, objective psychiatric and neurological symptoms. Acta Neurochir (Wien) 108(3-4):100–109.

Rasmussen BK (1999). Epidemiology of cluster headache. In: Olesen J, Goadsby P (eds) Cluster Headaches and Related Conditions. Oxford: Oxford University Press, pp 23–26.

Robbins L (1995) Intranasal lidocaine for cluster headache. Headache 35(2):83–84.

Romiti A, Martelletti P, Gallo MF, et al (1983) Low plasma testosterone levels in cluster headache. Cephalalgia 3(1):41–44.

Rossi P, Lorenzo GD, Formisano R, et al (2004) Subcutaneous sumatriptan induces changes in frequency pattern in cluster headache patients. Headache 44(7):713–718.

Rozen TD (2004) High oxygen flow rates for cluster headache. Neurology 63(3).593.

Rozen TD, Niknam RM, Shechter AL, et al (2001) Cluster headache in women: clinical characteristics and comparison with cluster headache in men. J Neurol Neurosurg Psychiatry 70(5):613–617.

Russell D (1981) Cluster headache: severity and temporal profiles of attacks and patient activity prior to and during attacks. Cephalalgia 1(4):209–216.

Russell MB (2004) Epidemiology and genetics of cluster headache. Lancet Neurol 3(5):279–283.

Russell MB, Andersson PG, Iselius L (1996) Cluster headache is an inherited disorder in some families. Headache 36(10):608–612.

Sahota PK, Dexter JD (1990) Sleep and headache syndromes: a clinical review. Headache 30(2):80–84.

Salvesen R, Bekkelund SI (2000) Migraine, as compared to other headaches, is worse during midnight-sun summer than during polar night. A questionnaire study in an Arctic population. Headache 40(10):824–829.

Sances G, Tassorelli C, Pucci E, et al (2004) Reliability of the nitroglycerin provocative test in the diagnosis of neurovascular headaches. Cephalalgia 24(2):110–119.

Saper JR, Klapper J, Mathew NT, et al (2002) Intranasal civamide for the treatment of episodic cluster headaches. Arch Neurol 59(6):990–994.

Sarlani E, Schwartz AH, Greenspan JD, et al (2003a) Facial pain as first manifestation of lung cancer: a case of lung cancer-related cluster headache and a review of the literature. J Orofac Pain 17(3):262–267.

Sarlani E, Schwartz AH, Greenspan JD, et al (2003b) Chronic paroxysmal hemicrania: a case report and review of the literature. J Orofac Pain 17(1):74–78.

Schoenen J, Di Clemente L, Vandenheede M, et al (2005) Hypothalamic stimulation in chronic cluster headache: a pilot study of efficacy and mode of action. Brain 128(Pt 4):940–947.

SCHSG TSCHSG (1991) Treatment of acute cluster headache with sumatriptan. N Engl J Med 325(5):322–326.

Schuh-Hofer S, Meisel A, Reuter U, et al (2003) Monozygotic twin sisters suffering from cluster headache and migraine without aura. Neurology 60(11):1864–1865.

Shapiro RE (2005) Corticosteroid treatment in cluster headache: evidence, rationale, and practice. Curr Pain Headache Rep 9(2):126–131.

Shen JM, Johnsen HJ (1994) SUNCT syndrome: estimation of cerebral blood flow velocity with transcranial Doppler ultrasonography. Headache 34(1):25–31.

Siow HC (2004) Seasonal episodic paroxysmal hemicrania responding to cyclooxygenase-2 inhibitors. *Cephalalgia* **24**(5): 414–415.

Siow HC, Young WB, Peres MF, *et al* (2002) Hemiplegic cluster. *Headache* **42**(2):136–139.

Sjaastad O, Antonaci F (1987) Chronic paroxysmal hemicrania: a case report. Long-lasting remission in the chronic stage. *Cephalalgia* **7**(3):203–205.

Sjaastad O, Antonaci F (1995) A piroxicam derivative partly effective in chronic paroxysmal hemicrania and hemicrania continua. *Headache* **35**(9):549–550.

Sjaastad O, Dale I (1974) Evidence for a new, treatable headache entity. *Headache* **14**(2):105–108.

Sjaastad O, Dale I (1976) A new Clinical headache entity 'chronic paroxysmal hemicrania' 2. *Acta Neurol Scand* **54**(2):140–159.

Sjaastad O, Kruszewski P (1992) Trigeminal neuralgia and 'SUNCT' syndrome: similarities and differences in the clinical pictures. An overview. *Funct Neurol* **7**(2):103–107.

Sjaastad O, Rinck P (1990) Cluster headache: MRI studies of the cavernous sinus and the base of the brain. *Headache* **30**(6): 350–351.

Sjaastad O, Egge K, Horven I, *et al* (1979) Chronic paroxysmal hemicranial: mechanical precipitation of attacks. *Headache* **19**(1):31–36.

Sjaastad O, Spierings EL, Saunte C, *et al* (1984) 'Hemicrania continua.' An indomethacin responsive headache. II. Autonomic function studies. *Cephalalgia* **4**(4):265–273.

Sjaastad O, Saunte C, Salvesen R, *et al* (1989) Shortlasting unilateral neuralgiform headache attacks with conjunctival injection, tearing, sweating, and rhinorrhea. *Cephalalgia* **9**(2): 147–156.

Sjaastad O, Zhao JM, Kruszewski P, *et al* (1991) Short-lasting unilateral neuralgiform headache attacks with conjunctival injection, tearing, etc. (SUNCT): III. Another Norwegian case. *Headache* **31**(3):175–177.

Sjaastad O, Kruszewski P, Fostad K, *et al* (1992) SUNCT syndrome: VII. Ocular and related variables. *Headache* **32**(10):489–495.

Sjaastad O, Stovner LJ, Stolt-Nielsen A, *et al* (1995) CPH and hemicrania continua: requirements of high indomethacin dosages—an ominous sign? *Headache* **35**(6):363–367.

Sjaastad O, Pareja JA, Zukerman E, *et al* (1997) Trigeminal neuralgia. Clinical manifestations of first division involvement. *Headache* **37**(6):346–357.

Sjostrand C, Waldenlind E, Ekbom K (2000) A follow-up study of 60 patients after an assumed first period of cluster headache. *Cephalalgia* **20**(7):653–657.

Sjostrand C, Giedratis V, Ekbom K, *et al* (2001) CACNA1A gene polymorphisms in cluster headache. *Cephalalgia* **21**(10):953–958.

Sjostrand C, Modin H, Masterman T, *et al* (2002) Analysis of nitric oxide synthase genes in cluster headache. *Cephalalgia* **22**(9): 758–764.

Smetana GW (2000) The diagnostic value of historical features in primary headache syndromes: a comprehensive review. *Arch Intern Med* **160**(18):2729–2737.

Soros P, Frese A, Husstedt IW, *et al* (2001) Cluster headache after dental extraction: implications for the pathogenesis of cluster headache? *Cephalalgia* **21**(5):619–622.

Spencer SE, Sawyer WB, Wada H, *et al* (1990) CNS projections to the pterygopalatine parasympathetic preganglionic neurons in the rat: a retrograde transneuronal viral cell body labeling study. *Brain Res* **534**(1-2):149–169.

Stewart WF, Lipton RB, Kolodner K (2003) Migraine disability assessment (MIDAS) score: relation to headache frequency, pain intensity, and headache symptoms. *Headache* **43**(3): 258–265.

Suzuki N, Hardebo JE, Kahrstrom J, *et al* (1990) Selective electrical stimulation of postganglionic cerebrovascular parasympathetic nerve fibers originating from the sphenopalatine ganglion enhances cortical blood flow in the rat. *J Cereb Blood Flow Metab* **10**(3):383–391.

Tajti J, Sas K, Szok D, *et al* (1996) Clusterlike headache as a first sign of brain metastases of lung cancer. *Headache* **36**(4):259–260.

Takahashi H, Izumi H, Karita K (1995) Parasympathetic reflex salivary secretion in the cat parotid gland. *Jpn J Physiol* **45**(3): 475–490.

Tonon C, Guttmann S, Volpini M, *et al* (2002) Prevalence and incidence of cluster headache in the Republic of San Marino. *Neurology* **58**(9):1407–1409.

Torelli P, Manzoni GC (2003) Pain and behaviour in cluster headache. A prospective study and review of the literature. *Funct Neurol* **18**(4):205–210.

Torelli P, Cologno D, Cademartiri C, *et al* (2000) Possible predictive factors in the evolution of episodic to chronic cluster headache. *Headache* **40**(10):798–808.

Torelli P, Cologno D, Cademartiri C, *et al* (2001) Application of the International Headache Society classification criteria in 652 cluster headache patients. *Cephalalgia* **21**(2):145–150.

Trucco M, Antonaci F, Sandrini G (1992) Hemicrania continua: a case responsive to piroxicam-beta-cyclodextrin. *Headache* **32**(1):39–40.

Trucco M, Mainardi F, Maggioni F, *et al* (2004) Chronic paroxysmal hemicrania, hemicrania continua and SUNCT syndrome in association with other pathologies: a review. *Cephalalgia* **24**(3):173–184.

van Vliet JA, Bahra A, Martin V, *et al* (2003a) Intranasal sumatriptan in cluster headache: randomized placebo-controlled double-blind study. *Neurology* **60**(4):630–633.

van Vliet JA, Eekers PJ, Haan J, *et al* (2003b) Features involved in the diagnostic delay of cluster headache. *J Neurol Neurosurg Psychiatry* **74**(8):1123–1125.

Veloso GG, Kaup AO, Peres MF, *et al* (2001) Episodic paroxysmal hemicrania with seasonal variation: case report and the EPH-cluster headache continuum hypothesis. *Arq Neuropsiquiatr* **59**(4):944–947.

Ventura-Martinez R, Deciga-Campos M, Diaz-Reval MI, *et al* (2004) Peripheral involvement of the nitric oxide-cGMP pathway in the indomethacin-induced antinociception in rat. *Eur J Pharmacol* **503**(1-3):43–48.

Volcy M, Tepper SJ, Rapoport AM, *et al* (2005) Short-lasting unilateral neuralgiform headache attacks with cranial autonomic symptoms (SUNA)–a case report. *Cephalalgia* **25**(6):470–472.

Waldenlind E, Gustafsson SA, Ekbom K, *et al* (1987) Circadian secretion of cortisol and melatonin in cluster headache during active cluster periods and remission. *J Neurol Neurosurg Psychiatry* **50**(2):207–213.

Waldenlind E, Goadsby PJ (2006) Synthesis of cluster headache pathophysiology. In: Olesen J, Goadsby PJ, Ramadan NM, *et al*. (eds) *The Headaches*, 3rd edn. Philadelphia: Lippincott Williams and Wilkins, pp 783–787.

Warner JS, Wamil AW, McLean MJ (1994) Acetazolamide for the treatment of chronic paroxysmal hemicrania. *Headache* **34**(10): 597–599.

Weiller C, May A, Limmroth V, *et al* (1995) Brain stem activation in spontaneous human migraine attacks. *Nat Med* **1**(7):658–660.

Wheeler SD (1998) Significance of migrainous features in cluster headache: divalproex responsiveness. *Headache* **38**(7):547–551.

Zidverc-Trajkovic J, Pavlovic AM, Mijajlovic M, *et al* (2005) Cluster headache and paroxysmal hemicrania: differential diagnosis. *Cephalalgia* **25**(4):244–248.

Zukerman E, Peres MF, Kaup AO, *et al* (2000) Chronic paroxysmal hemicrania-tic syndrome. *Neurology* **54**(7):1524–1526.

CHAPTER 11

Neuropathic orofacial pain

Rafael Benoliel, Gary M Heir and Eli Eliav

1. Introduction

Pain initiated by a primary lesion or dysfunction of the nervous system is defined as neuropathic pain (NP) (Merskey and Bogduk 1994). However, NP may be an idiopathic process reflecting abnormal sensory processing in the peripheral (PNS) or central nervous system (CNS) but with no clearly associated pathological lesion (Merskey and Bogduk 1994). Secondary NPs appear following physical insult or disease affecting the PNS or CNS. Although secondary NP may be due to ongoing disease, healed injury may leave the nervous system in a pathological state as in painful post-traumatic neuropathies.

When affecting the orofacial region NP may be termed neuropathic orofacial pain (NOP) and includes a heterogeneous group of entities. Based on symptomatology NOP may be divided into two broad categories, paroxysmal and continuous (Okeson 1996). Paroxysmal neuropathies such as trigeminal neuralgia are characterized by short electrical or sharp pain. Continuous pain, sometimes of a burning quality, is characteristic of post-traumatic neuropathy or of inflammation in nerve structures (neuritis). This chapter describes the common NOPs, neuritis of the trigeminal nerve, and discusses their differential diagnosis. Rarer cranial neuralgias are not described (see Table 11.1).

1.1. Clinical Approach to Neuropathic Pain

Symptomatology of NP may include touch-evoked or stimulus-dependent pain that may be constant or intermittent. Additionally there may be spontaneous or stimulus-independent pain (Dworkin *et al* 2003). Sensory symptoms may be positive (e.g. hyperalgesia) and/or negative (e.g. numbness) and these should be assessed and recorded using universally accepted terminology (Merskey and Bogduk 1994). Some of these signs and symptoms (thermal/mechanical allodynia) are frequently associated with NP (Rasmussen *et al* 2004). However, the translation of symptomatology into pathophysiological mechanisms and their extrapolation to treatment may be difficult and till now has not resulted in improved treatment outcomes. Quantitative sensory testing (QST) provides accurate and reproducible data that are extremely valuable for patient assessment, treatment and research; see Chapter 3. When advanced QST apparatus is unavailable a simple pin, blunt instruments, warmed and cooled implements and cotton wool may be employed. The mapping of affected areas and photographic documentation adds information as to the dermatomal distribution of the sensory changes and should form part of patient evaluation and follow-up.

1.2. Classification of Neuropathic Orofacial Pain

There is no current classification system that satisfies the needs of the majority of clinicians dealing with NOP. The International Headache Society (IHS) and the International Association for the Study of Pain (IASP) clearly classify a number of conditions but are neither broad enough nor specific enough for orofacial pain clinics (Merskey and Bogduk 1994; Olesen *et al* 2004). The American Academy of Orofacial Pain (AAOP) classifies many of the NOPs and is probably the most clinically useful (Okeson 1996).

The problems with classification of NP are not limited to the orofacial region and more specific definitions have been called for, with many supporting a mechanism-based classification. We have outlined a possible classification of NOP in Table 11.2.

Table 11.1 Other Cranial Neuralgias and Central Causes of Facial Pain

IHS Classification	Name	Comments
13.4	Superior laryngeal neuralgia	Rare disorder characterized by severe pain in the lateral aspect of the throat, submandibular region and underneath the ear, precipitated by swallowing, shouting or turning the head. Local anaesthetic block relieves pain and nerve section is curative.
13.5 13.6	Nasociliary neuralgia[a] Supraorbital neuralgia[a]	Rare conditions in which touching the outer aspect of one nostril (13.5) or the areas supplied by the supraorbital nerve (13.6) causes a lancinating pain. Local anaesthetic block relieves pain and nerve section is curative.
13.7	Other terminal branch neuralgias	Injury or entrapment of peripheral branches of the trigeminal nerve other than in 13.5-6. Local anaesthetic block relieves pain and nerve section is curative.
13.8	Occipital neuralgia	Paroxysmal jabbing pain in the distribution of the greater, lesser or third occipital nerves. May be accompanied by hypoaesthesia or dysaesthesia of the affected area. Commonly associated with tenderness over the affected nerve. Local anaesthetic block temporarily relieves pain.
13.12	Constant pain caused by compression, irritation or distortion of cranial nerves or upper cervical roots by structural lesions	Due to a lesion directly compromising afferent fibres in nerves of head and neck. Sensory deficit may be present.
13.13	Optic neuritis	Pain behind one or both eyes accompanied by impairment of central vision caused by demyelination of the optic nerve.
13.14	Ocular diabetic neuropathy	Eye and forehead pain associated with paresis of ≥ 1 ocular cranial nerves (usually III), in a patient with diabetes mellitus.
13.17	Ophthalmoplegic 'migraine'	Recurrent headaches with migrainous characteristics and paresis of ≥ 1 ocular cranial nerves (usually III), with no intracranial lesion other than MRI changes in the affected nerve.
13.19	Other cranial neuralgia or other centrally mediated facial pain	

Based on Olesen *et al* (2004) with permission.

[a] These are branches of the trigeminal nerve and may theoretically be considered subtypes of trigeminal neuralgia.

1.3. Neuropathic Pain: Epidemiology and Impact

Neuropathic pain, including NOP, is believed to be prevalent. However, there is a lack of accurate data to support this, partly due to inconsistent definitions and clinical criteria. In primary medical care settings the prevalence of neuropathic pain is between 2 and 11% (Clark 2002; Hasselstrom *et al* 2002; Koleva *et al* 2005). Out of 300 consecutive patients seen in our orofacial pain clinic 21% were diagnosed as NOP, most of whom suffered from painful traumatic neuropathy (10%) or classical trigeminal neuralgia (9%, unpublished data). One recent study examined the prevalence of 'pain of predominantly neuropathic origin' using a questionnaire and revealed

that about 8% of a British population suffered from neuropathic-like pain (Torrance *et al* 2006). This is probably an overestimation but does reflect a prevalence higher than previously accepted. The epidemiology of four common neuropathic conditions, postherpetic neuralgia, trigeminal neuralgia, phantom limb pain and painful diabetic neuropathy, is around 83.8 per 100000 person years (Hall *et al* 2006). Increased life expectancy and disease survival rates will increase the prevalence of age-associated neuropathic pain syndromes such as trigeminal neuralgia or AIDS-related or diabetic neuropathies.

Neuropathic pain and its treatment lead to impaired quality of life, reduced employment and productivity and extensive usage of healthcare facilities (Meyer-Rosberg *et al* 2001; McDermott *et al* 2006). Chronic

Table 11.2	Proposed Classification of Painful Neuropathies Affecting the Orofacial Region

Idiopathic	Secondary
Classical trigeminal neuralgia *(Nasociliary and supraorbital)	Symptomatic trigeminal neuralgia
Classical glossopharyngeal neuralgia	Symptomatic glossopharyngeal neuralgia
Nervus intermedius neuralgia	
	Neck tongue syndrome
	Tolosa hunt syndrome
Atypical odontalgia	Painful post-traumatic neuropathies Peripheral • CRPS I • CRPS II Central • CPSP
Neuralgias of regional nerves: • Superior laryngeal • Occipital	
	Neuritis
Primary BMD	Secondary BMD

The use of the term idiopathic circumvents problems with conditions often but not always associated with specific aetiologies, for example trigeminal neuralgia or atypical odontalgia, but may not necessarily be always primary. CRPS, chronic regional pain syndrome; CPSP, central post-stroke pain; BMD, burning mouth disorder.

[a] Includes nasociliary and supraorbital despite the different clinical presentation and treatment relative to trigeminal neuralgia (see Table 11.1).

Table 11.3	Diagnostic Criteria for Classical Trigeminal Neuralgia

	Diagnostic Criteria	Notes
A	Paroxysmal attacks of pain lasting from a fraction of a second to 2 minutes, affecting one or more divisions of the trigeminal nerve and fulfilling criteria B and C.	Pain is mostly unilateral and does not cross the midline. It is very rarely bilateral, which may indicate disease (e.g. multiple sclerosis). Most patients suffer pain in the distribution of the second or third division or both. Interictally there is usually no pain but some cases have low-grade background pain. Periods of remission from days to years may occur.
B	Pain has at least one of the following characteristics: 1. Intense, sharp, superficial or stabbing 2. Precipitated from trigger areas or by trigger factors.	Many cases will describe their pain as 'electrical'. Pain may be accompanied by spasm of the facial muscles. Following an attack a refractory period occurs where pain cannot be triggered. Triggers are usually innocuous stimuli (touch, wind, shaving) but may also be temperature, noise, lights and taste. A short gap between trigger and pain may be observed (latency).
C	Attacks are stereotyped in the individual patient.	Attack duration, distribution, etc., may vary between patients but are highly consistent within cases. Trigger points may, however, change location within the same patient.
D	There is no clinically evident neurological deficit.	Sensory testing may reveal mild deficits in the distribution of the trigeminal nerve.
E	Not attributed to another disorder.	Other causes are ruled out by history, physical examination and special investigations. Compression of the nerve root by a vascular malformation (tortuous or aberrant vessels) is considered 'classical'.

Based on Olesen et al (2004) with permission.

neuropathies are characterized by pain of moderate to severe intensity. Treatment often requires long-term prescription medications that have significant side effects (McDermott *et al* 2006). The use of nonsteroidal analgesics and opioids is particularly common whilst antiepileptic drugs (AED) and tricyclic antidepressants (TCA) are relatively uncommon (McDermott *et al* 2006). This is surprising in view of the higher effectiveness of AEDs and TCAs in neuropathic pain and suggests that patients may not be seeking treatment or are inadequately managed. It is not unusual for patients to turn to alternative medicine and many report the use of vitamins and supplements; see Chapter 17 (McDermott *et al* 2006).

2. Trigeminal Neuralgia

2.1. Introduction and Definition

Trigeminal neuralgia (TN) is an excruciating short-lasting, unilateral facial pain with clear classification criteria (Table 11.3). The diagnostic criteria published by the IHS recognize two subsets of TN: a classical (previously idiopathic or primary) type that may be unrelated to pathology and a symptomatic (or secondary) form that is related to a variety of clear pathologies including

Table 11.4 Diagnostic Criteria for Symptomatic Trigeminal Neuralgia

	Diagnostic Criteria	Notes
A	Paroxysmal attacks of pain lasting from a fraction of a second to 2 minutes, with or without persistence of aching between paroxysms, affecting one or more divisions of the trigeminal nerve and fulfilling criteria B and C.	Pain will affect the distribution adjacent to the pathology. Bilateral pain may indicate multiple sclerosis, particularly in younger patients. Interictally there are usually more reports of background pain than in classical trigeminal neuralgia.
B	Pain has at least one of the following characteristics: 1. Intense, sharp, superficial or stabbing 2. Precipitated from trigger areas or by trigger factors.	See Table 11.3; however, no refractory period occurs as in classical TN. Sensory deficits may be clinically apparent and may also be accompanied by other cranial nerve dysfunction.
C	Attacks are stereotyped in the individual patient.	A progressive pattern in duration, spread, associated neurologic deficits and intensity may be evident.
D	A causative lesion, other than vascular compression, has been demonstrated by special investigations and/or posterior fossa exploration.	

Based on Olesen *et al* (2004) with permission.

tumours, cysts, viral infection, trauma and systemic disease such as multiple sclerosis; see Table 11.4 (Olesen *et al* 2004). Recent evidence suggests that many, but not all cases of classical TN (CTN) result from compression of the trigeminal nerve root by a vascular malformation. It is for this reason the IHS has opted for the term classical and not primary and includes cases with vascular malformation. The vast majority (>85%) of TN patients are diagnosed as CTN. Unrecognized by any current classification are atypical TN cases that present with most but not all diagnostic criteria.

2.2. Clinical Features of TN

The diagnosis of TN is based on a thorough history and characteristic clinical signs and symptoms. In typical cases TN should be a reasonably straightforward diagnosis. However, patient surveys reveal that most TN cases suffer from misdiagnosis. Because of its location and paroxysmal nature TN has often been confused with dental pathology, leading to unnecessary dental treatment (Mitchell 1980; Taha *et al* 1995; Bowsher 2000; de Siqueira

et al 2004). Clinical signs may vary depending on the stage at which the patient attends. In primary care the undiagnosed patient is common and will be both emotionally distressed and in severe pain. Cases that have been initially diagnosed but are requesting a second opinion more usually attend specialist centres and may be symptomless. Relapsed CTN patients in active treatment tend to return to their treating physician and are usually suffering from less severe pain. Each case demands careful history-taking to enable adequate management.

Case example. The elderly patient described in Case 11.1 had a typical history of classical TN with an onset some days previously.

Location. TN is a unilateral facial pain syndrome (Olesen *et al* 2004). Bilateral cases have been reported in 1–4% of cases but one side usually precedes the onset of pain on the contralateral side by years (Katusic *et al* 1990; Rasmussen 1991a; Tacconi and Miles 2000; Kuncz *et al* 2006). Reviews of case series suggest that the right side is involved more often; however, this is inconsistent and as no correlation has been found with age, gender or handedness the clinical significance is doubtful (Katusic *et al* 1990; Rasmussen 1991a). Pain location is usually described according to the major branches of the

Case 11.1 Trigeminal Neuralgia, an 81-year-old Female

Present complaint

Pain for the past 3 months. Increasing in frequency and severity. Pain occurs spontaneously or following touch over the lower left face. Eating or drinking can also induce pain.

History of present complaint

Similar pain had occurred for short periods of time about a year and 2 years ago with no treatment.

Physical examination

Cranial nerves intact. Edentulous. Panoramic radiograph showed no pathology. Pain was easily triggered by lightly touching the face. The resulting pain lasted for less than 2 minutes and was excruciating (see Fig. 11.1).

Relevant medical history

Healthy.

Diagnosis

Classical trigeminal neuralgia (CTN).

Diagnostic and treatment considerations

The presentation is typical of CTN. The prevalence of CTN increases with age and is therefore not a surprising event in an octogenarian. Treatment was with carbamazepine titrated slowly from 100–200 mg/d and increased till response (in this case 600 mg/d). The patient was pain-free within 72 hours. Computerized tomographic brain imaging revealed no pathology. Liver function tests remained normal during follow-up and carbamazepine levels were within the therapeutic range. Some months later there was breakthrough pain and the carbamazepine dose was increased to 800 mg/d, providing pain relief.

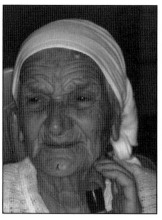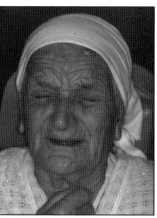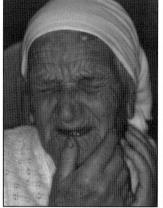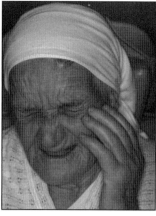

Base   Trigger ──────────────────────────→ 8 seconds

Fig. 11.1 • Case 11.1: Patient with recent onset of severe trigeminal pain; signs and symptoms were typical of trigeminal neuralgia. Attacks could be reproduced (triggered) in the clinic by gently touching the lower lip. Response to pharmacotherapy with carbamazepine was very rapid and the patient was pain-free by 72 hours. Note the guarding position of the patient's hand, the rapid onset of pain and the accompanying facial tic.

trigeminal nerve; 36–42% of cases report pain in one branch. In 16–18% of patients the singly affected nerve will be the maxillary or the mandibular branch whilst the ophthalmic is affected singly in only about 2% of cases (Rasmussen 1991a). Most commonly the maxillary and mandibular branches are affected together (35%) and all three branches are involved in 14% of patients. The jaws are therefore involved in most cases, explaining why CTN patients so often seek help from dentists. Pain radiation is generally within the dermatome of origin (Rasmussen 1991a).

Although the location, intensity and triggers of TN vary across patients they are highly *stereotyped* within individual TN patients; i.e. each attack is similar in location, duration and intensity.

Quality. Pain in TN is most often described as paroxysmal, shooting, sharp, piercing, stabbing or electrical in nature (70–95%) (Benoliel and Sharav 1998; Zakrzewska *et al* 1999; de Siqueira *et al* 2004; Sato *et al* 2004). Some TN patients (4–35%) may describe two types of pain: paroxysmal attacks of short sharp pain superimposed on a dull background pain of varying duration (Katusic *et al* 1990; Rasmussen 1990). Background pain may be described as dull, throbbing and burning (Zakrzewska *et al* 1999; Nurmikko and Eldridge 2001). There are indications that patients with prominent background pain have detectable sensory loss and may be poorer candidates for successful surgical intervention (Nurmikko and Eldridge 2001; Haines and Chittum 2003). Pain severity in TN is extreme with ratings of 9–10 on a 10-cm visual analogue scale (VAS) (Zakrzewska *et al* 1999; Bowsher 2000).

Triggering. The diagnostic criteria for TN include the premise that pain may be precipitated by light touch in *trigger* areas or initiated by trigger factors. How innocuous stimuli result in the excruciating pain felt by patients with TN is an intriguing feature. A short gap between stimulation of a trigger area and pain onset may be

observed and is termed *latency*. TN attacks are often spontaneous and trigger areas are not always present or clinically identifiable – 40–50% of TN patients may not report a clear trigger (Rasmussen 1991b; Sato *et al* 2004). Trigger areas are usually in the distribution of the affected trigeminal branch, particularly around the lips but may be extratrigeminal (Bowsher 2000) or multiple and may even change location (Dubner *et al* 1987).

The triggering stimuli are innocuous and include talking (76%), chewing (74%), touch (65%), temperature (cold 48%, heat 1%), wind and shaving (Rasmussen 1991b; Bowsher 2000). Data suggest that intraoral TN triggers and pain are more often associated with the gingivae (Bowsher 2000; de Siqueira *et al* 2004). The triggering of TN-like pain by gustatory stimuli is an interesting phenomenon that has been described as both primary and secondary (postsurgical) pain syndromes (Sharav *et al* 1991; Scrivani *et al* 1998). The initiation of pain by sweet or salty foods is usually associated with dental pathology so that these cases present a difficult diagnosis (see Chapter 5). Trigger-like areas may be detected in about 9% of other orofacial pain syndromes so that this is suggestive but not pathognomonic (Rasmussen 1991b; Sato *et al* 2004).

Trigger factors are distinct from trigger areas and include noise, lights and stress (Rasmussen 1991b; Bowsher 2000). These may also occur in up to 60% of other orofacial pain patients (Rasmussen 1991b; Sato *et al* 2004) but the rapid, severe, electric-like pain that occurs in TN should distinguish it from other pain syndromes.

Temporal pattern. Individual attacks are characterized by a rapid onset and peak (see Fig. 11.1), then subsidence, lasting overall from 10 seconds up to 2 minutes (Benoliel and Sharav 1998; Pareja *et al* 2002). This is followed by a *refractory period* whose duration is related to the intensity of the TN attack; during this time pain is impossible or extremely difficult to trigger (Kugelberg and Lindblom 1959). Attacks occur mostly during the day, but there are few reports of nocturnal TN (Rasmussen 1990).

TN may begin abruptly or via a rarer preceding syndrome termed pre-TN described below (Mitchell 1980; Fromm *et al* 1990). Long-term follow-up of TN patients reveals that there are well-defined periods of pain attacks variably followed by periods of remission that may last from weeks to years (Rushton and Macdonald 1957; Katusic *et al* 1990; Rasmussen 1990). The median active period is reported at about 49 days followed by remission of some months (36%), weeks (16%) or even days (16%). Only 6% may look forward to remissions of more than a year and about 20% may suffer from incessant attacks. Following a first attack of TN it has been calculated that 65% of patients will suffer a second attack within 5 years and 77% within 10 years (Katusic *et al* 1990).

About 90% of TN cases report increased attack frequency and severity (Bowsher 2000; Zakrzewska and Patsalos 2002). A progressive and increasing resistance to pharmacological and surgical treatment is common so that TN is a progressive disease with a poor prognosis (Fromm 1989; Zakrzewska and Lopez 2004). For example, initial response to carbamazepine is around 70% but after 5–16 years the response rate is around 20% with 44% of patients requiring drug combinations or alternative medication (Taylor *et al* 1981). Long-term follow-up of oxcarbazepine-treated TN cases demonstrated a high failure rate necessitating surgery (Zakrzewska and Patsalos 2002). Supporting the progressive nature of TN is the fact that microvascular decompression (MVD) has a significantly reduced prognosis in long-standing TN (>7 years) (Broggi *et al* 2000).

Associated sensory and motor signs. Sensory disturbances such as hypoaesthesia are rare but occur in some patients with TN (Nurmikko 1991; Bowsher *et al* 1997). These may be more readily detected when employing sophisticated examination techniques (see Chapter 3) but may go unnoticed in gross examinations. Preoperative sensory loss is a negative predictor for the long-term outcome of MVD (Tyler-Kabara *et al* 2002). Reflex and evoked potential studies reveal nociceptive fibre dysfunction in TN and electrophysiological testing is able to accurately diagnose symptomatic TN (Cruccu *et al* 2006). Following successful MVD, nerve conduction properties return to normal (Leandri *et al* 1998) but clinical improvement is often delayed (Love and Coakham 2001).

Accompanying the pain of TN is a classic contraction of the facial musculature, hence the terms *tic douloureux, tic convulsif* (see Fig. 11.1). Hemifacial spasm, probably secondary to vascular compression of the facial nerve root, is found in about 1% of TN cases and is more frequent in patients with vertebrobasilar artery compression (Linskey *et al* 1994).

Accompanying autonomic signs. Characteristically lacrimation is not considered a diagnostic sign of neuropathic-type pain but has been observed in CTN patients (see Chapters 9 and 10) (Rasmussen 1991b). However, lacrimation and rhinorrhoea have been reported in CTN (Rasmussen 1991b). Patients with TN and lacrimation have been described in ophthalmic (Sjaastad *et al* 1997), maxillary and mandibular branch CTN (Benoliel and Sharav 1998). The question arises whether these are cases of TN with lacrimation, short-lasting neuralgiform headache attacks with conjunctival injection and tearing (SUNCT) or one of the other unilateral headache syndromes accompanied by lacrimation (Chapter 10). This is discussed later under differential diagnosis. However, the appearance of lacrimation or tearing in TN is highly inconsistent. In other headaches the occurrence of parasympathetic activation has been linked to pain severity. If so, then when TN is severe trigeminal autonomic activation may occur (see Chapter 10).

Vascular activity in TN may be inferred from reports of facial flushing (vasodilatation) and swelling in TN (Dubner *et al* 1987; Nurmikko *et al* 2000). Autonomic dysfunction is suggested by the increased salivation seen in cases of TN affecting the mandibular nerve (Rasmussen 1991b) and by a case of cardiac arrest in association with TN (Gottesman *et al* 1996).

Investigations. There are no specific special tests that are absolutely diagnostic in TN. A thorough cranial nerve examination should be routine. Imaging techniques such as magnetic resonance tomographic angiography (MRTA) may indicate neurovascular compression (see Pathophysiology below) and electrophysiological testing offers promise in diagnosing symptomatic TN cases. More sophisticated techniques such as three-dimensional magnetic resonance imaging (MRI) with constructive interference in steady state sequence has shown superiority over MRTA in detecting venular compressions (Yoshino *et al* 2003). Published evidence suggests that all TN patients should undergo imaging (CT or MRI) at least once during diagnosis and therapy (Yang *et al* 1996; Goh *et al* 2001). A thorough clinical evaluation and adequate oral radiographs (bite-wings, full mouth periapicals, panoramic) of oral structures are essential to rule out pathology.

All patients to be treated with anticonvulsants need baseline and follow-up of haematological, electrolyte and liver function tests (see Chapter 16).

Quality of life (QoL). The severity and progressive nature of TN has resulted in patients committing suicide; however, CTN of itself does not alter life expectancy (Rothman and Monson 1973). QoL is much reduced in TN patients as either a direct effect of the pain or secondary to side effects of the drugs employed (Bowsher 2000; Zakrzewska 2001). Patients with TN are often depressed and anxious and successful surgical treatment often relieves their suffering (Zakrzewska *et al* 1999). These patients therefore need support and understanding.

2.3. Unusual Trigeminal Neuralgia Presentations

Up to 30% of TN patients report atypical features (Nurmikko and Eldridge 2001; Sato *et al* 2004). In most cases the symptomatology is distinctly similar to that of TN so that diagnosis is usually straightforward. Additionally the natural history of CTN in some cases indicates that it may begin in an atypical fashion that is termed pretrigeminal neuralgia. The clinical features of pretrigeminal neuralgia are, however, extremely uncharacteristic of CTN and highly variable.

2.3.1. Atypical Trigeminal Neuralgia

A number of patients may present with longer TN pain attacks or with a constant background pain that makes them 'atypical'. Diagnostic criteria have been proposed for atypical TN but these have not been adopted by the IASP, IHS or the AAOP (Nurmikko and Eldridge 2001). In a recent study, microvascular decompression (see below and Chapter 12) provided absolute postoperative pain relief in CTN for 80% of cases and for 47% of atypical TN cases (Tyler-Kabara et al 2002). Long-term follow-up (>5 years) revealed excellent results in 75% of classical and 35% of atypical TN cases. The definition of such a subclassification would therefore be advantageous in establishing whether such a diagnosis is justified and for the assessment of long-term prognosis and treatment outcomes.

2.3.2. Pretrigeminal Neuralgia

An early form of TN termed 'pretrigeminal neuralgia' (PTN) has been described (Mitchell 1980; Fromm et al 1990). PTN has been reported in 18% of TN patients and is characterized by a dull continuous pain in one of the jaws that lasts from days to years (Mitchell 1980). As the process continues PTN becomes more typical with characteristic flashes of pain. Thermal stimuli may cause triggering at a relatively higher rate and a throbbing quality to PTN pain mimicking dental pathology is sometimes present (Mitchell 1980). Indeed these qualities combined with the success of regional anaesthesia have led to misdiagnosis of PTN as pain of dental origin. PTN is, however, highly responsive to anticonvulsant therapy and careful dental assessment should help differentiate it. Our clinical experience confirms that there are cases with highly atypical features that respond to carbamazepine and develop into TN. However, the lack of clear and consistent diagnostic criteria makes this a problematic entity to recognize; it is usually diagnosed when all other possibilities are exhausted or in retrospect once CTN develops (Okeson 1996).

2.4. TN Comorbidity

2.4.1. Combination Syndromes

Trigeminal neuralgia most often occurs as a single pain syndrome. However, it has been reported rarely to occur with cluster headache and with paroxysmal hemicrania; these are termed cluster-tic and chronic paroxysmal hemicrania-tic syndromes respectively (see Differential Diagnosis and Chapter 10).

2.4.2. Hypertension

The presence of hypertension has been found to increase the risk of TN by a factor of 2.1 in females and 1.5 in males (Katusic et al 1990; de Siqueira et al 2004). The presence of hypertension in these cases has been linked with arterial compression of the ventrolateral aspect of the rostral medulla in the region of the left glossopharyngeal and vagus nerve roots.

2.4.3. Other Neuralgias

As many as 11.5% of patients with glossopharyngeal neuralgia were also diagnosed with TN (Rushton et al 1981). Although in only 9 cases did the two forms of neuralgia occur simultaneously, the high prevalence suggests some pathophysiological association (see below).

2.5. Symptomatic TN
2.5.1. Multiple Sclerosis

Multiple sclerosis (MS) is a common disabling disease affecting individuals between the ages of 20 and 40. The typical MRI picture includes periventricular lesions either in the cerebral hemispheres or infratentorially. Spinal cord lesions are also extremely common. The neuropathology is characterized by perivenous inflammation, neuronal demyelination and ultimately gliosis. Cerebrospinal fluid demonstrates positive oligoclonal bands and an elevated IgG index and synthesis rate. Evoked potentials aid in the diagnosis of MS but may be abnormal in other inflammatory conditions of the CNS. MS patients often present with paraesthesias, numbness, motor weakness and a painful optic neuritis characterized by visual blurring. Over half of MS patients will report some type of pain during the course of their disease (Osterberg et al 2005). Over a quarter will suffer central pain that is bilateral, constant, aching, burning or pricking.

Multiple sclerosis increases the risk of developing TN by a factor of 20 (Katusic et al 1990). Clinical signs predictive of MS in TN patients are bilateral pain (14% in MS) and young age (Meaney et al 1995a; De Simone et al 2005). Very rarely does TN herald the onset of MS; this was observed in only 0.3% of MS cases (Jensen et al 1982; Hooge and Redekop 1995). Usually TN develops in a diagnosed case of MS, on average about 12 years after the onset of MS, and occurs in 1.5–4.9% of MS cases (Jensen et al 1982; Hooge and Redekop 1995; Osterberg et al 2005). Non-facial pain may be a presenting symptom of MS in 5.5% of cases, alone or in combination with other signs.

TN in MS may be due to demyelination of the trigeminal nerve. Additionally findings of neurovascular compression of the nerve root and positive outcome of microvascular decompression for these cases suggest that vascular malformations may also contribute to the appearance of TN in MS (Broggi et al 2004).

2.5.2. Tumours

Trigeminal nerve dysfunction has been observed in 33% of patients with middle and posterior cranial fossa tumours but in only 13% were these presenting symptoms (Puca *et al* 1995). About 10% of cases with intracranial tumours suffered from TN-like symptomatology (Puca and Meglio 1993; Puca *et al* 1993). Posterior fossa tumours and meningiomas are most likely to cause TN-like symptoms (Bullitt *et al* 1986; Cheng *et al* 1993; Puca and Meglio 1993; Puca *et al* 1993, 1995). Cerebellopontine angle tumours (e.g. acoustic neuromas; see Chapter 12) may also cause TN and this diagnosis is more likely when the patient is young and suffers pain in more than one trigeminal branch (Yang *et al* 1996). In TN patients under the age of 29 years the prevalence of intracranial tumour or MS is extremely high (approx. 100%) but subsequently decreases with increasing age (Yang *et al* 1996). Specifically 10–13.4% of TN patients may suffer from intracranial tumours and MRI is the most sensitive diagnostic technique (Cheng *et al* 1993; Nomura *et al* 1994). A reduced corneal reflex and hypaesthesia were typical of cranial masses (Nomura *et al* 1994). Most of these patients are younger than expected for cases of TN and develop subtle or frank neurological deficits but 2% had CTN with no significant sensory aberration (Cheng *et al* 1993). The data stress the importance of thorough cranial nerve examination and indicate that all TN patients need imaging studies.

2.6. Differential Diagnosis

2.6.1. Dental

TN may mimic dental pain and a quarter of cases will initially consult a dentist (Rasmussen 1990; Taha *et al* 1995; de Siqueira *et al* 2004). Unfortunately TN is often misdiagnosed and 33–65% of cases may undergo unwarranted dental interventions; up to 12% may be eventually rendered edentulous (Main *et al* 1992; Taha *et al* 1995; Bowsher 2000). The numbers of TN cases with extensive and misguided dental interventions suggest a lack of awareness of many dentists of the features of CTN (Fig. 11.2). Thorough clinical and radiographic dental examinations are essential. Invasive dental treatment must not be performed when no positive anamnestic, clinical and radiographic signs indicate it.

2.6.2. SUNCT and Cluster-Tic Syndrome

The differential diagnosis of TN with lacrimation includes SUNCT and an atypical (shorter) cluster-tic syndrome (CTS); see Table 11.5, Fig. 11.3. SUNCT syndrome is extensively discussed in Chapter 10 and combines characteristics of neuralgiform pain with vascular-type signs, such as lacrimation.

Mechanical precipitation of attacks are a hallmark of TN, but are seen also in SUNCT (Pareja and Cuadrado

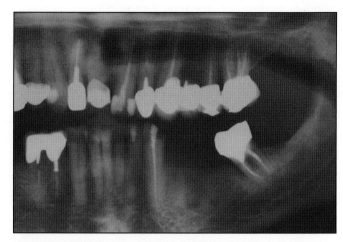

Fig. 11.2 • Patient diagnosed with left-sided trigeminal neuralgia who had undergone extensive dental treatment (multiple root canal therapies, extractions) in the upper and lower quadrants aimed at relieving the pain.

2005). Refractory periods are considered typical of TN but so far they have been unreported in SUNCT patients (Pareja and Cuadrado 2005). Supraorbital nerve blockade has been relatively unsuccessful in SUNCT (Pareja and Cuadrado 2005), whilst nerve blocks are effective in TN cases with lacrimation (Benoliel and Sharav 1998). TN will initially respond to carbamazepine whilst SUNCT syndrome is characterized by resistance to a wide range of drugs from its onset (Pareja and Cuadrado 2005). Recent neuroimaging findings of hypothalamic involvement in SUNCT suggest that it is related to the trigeminal autonomic cephalgias; see Chapter 10 (May *et al* 1999).

In CTS both cluster headache and TN usually appear on the same side, and both respond favourably to carbamazepine therapy (Alberca and Ochoa 1994; Merskey and Bogduk 1994). Most CTS patients are females and although onset may be at any age it seems slightly more common between 40 and 50 years (Alberca and Ochoa 1994). Chronic paroxysmal hemicrania-tic syndrome has been reported (Goadsby and Lipton 2001; Boes *et al* 2003). The classical characteristics of both pain entities occur together on the same side and may be controlled with indomethacin (Hannerz 1993).

2.7. TN Epidemiology

Lifetime prevalence figures suggest there are around 70 TN cases per 100000 population and that therefore TN is a rare condition (MacDonald *et al* 2000). The crude annual incidence of TN is 4.3–8 per 100000, higher in females (5.7) than in males (2.5). However, in the >80 year olds, males have a very high incidence of 45 per 100000 (Katusic *et al* 1991a; MacDonald *et al* 2000; Zakrzewska 2003). Peak incidence begins at 50–60 years and increases with age; in 60–69 year olds it is 17.5 per 100000 whilst in >80 year-olds it is 25.9 per 100000 (Katusic *et al* 1990; Zakrzewska 2003). TN is extremely rare in children.

Parameter	PH	CTS	SUNCT	TN
Demographics				
Age	30–40	40–50	40–50	50–60
Pain duration (minutes)	2–30	<45	<4	<2 (> in pre-TN)
Severity	++	+++	++	++++
Paroxysmal	+	+	+	+
Throbbing	+/−	+	−	− (pre-TN +)
Location	Hemicrania	Orbital	Orbital	Vb>Vc>Va
Wakes	+	+/−	−	+/−
Frequency (/24 h)	15	6–40	20–80	=Triggering[a]
Triggering				
Touch	−	+	+	+
Neck	+	+ (40%)	+	−
Alcohol	+/−	+	+/−	−
Autonomic signs	+	+	+	+/−
Response to:				
Carbamazepine	−	+/−	−	++
Indomethacin	++	−	−	−
Steroids	−	+/−	−	−
Lamotrigine	−	−	+	+/−

Table 11.5 Typical Clinical Features of Unilateral Headaches Relevant to the Differential Diagnosis of Trigeminal Neuralgia

Data from Benoliel and Sharav (1998).

PH, paroxysmal hemicrania; CTS, cluster-tic syndrome; SUNCT, short-lasting unilateral neuralgiform headache attacks with conjunctival injection and tearing; TN, trigeminal neuralgia; pre-TN, pretrigeminal neuralgia. V, trigeminal dermatomes: a, ophthalmic; b, maxillary; c, mandibular.
[a] Usually related to triggering events, but of normally high frequency.

2.8. Pathophysiology

There are several lines of evidence pointing to compression of the trigeminal root at or near the dorsal root entry zone (DREZ) by a blood vessel as a major causative or contributing factor (Love and Coakham 2001; Nurmikko and Eldridge 2001). The DREZ is the point where the peripheral and central myelin sheaths of Schwann cells and astrocytes meet. The compression is often arterial but may be venous or combined (Barker et al 1996a; Matsushima et al 2004). Imaging methods and surgical observations confirm a high rate of vascular compression of the nerve in TN patients (Masur et al 1995; Meaney et al 1995a,b; Boecher-Schwarz et al 1998). In a recent high-quality study, identification of neurovascular compression employing sophisticated imaging techniques predicted the symptomatic side in 78% of patients (Anderson et al 2006). Decompression of the nerve leads to prolonged pain relief (see Chapter 12) and reversal of sensory loss in many patients (Barker et al 1996b; Taha and Tew 1996; Miles et al 1997; McLaughlin et al 1999). Further support is obtained from cadaver studies where 91% of TN patients had a vessel in contact with the trigeminal nerve adjacent to the brainstem, most with a demonstrable groove (Hamlyn 1997a). Grooving or deformation of the nerve is considered essential for the induction of pain (Kuroiwa et al 1996).

Biopsy specimens of trigeminal roots demonstrate pathological changes such as axonal loss and demyelination (Devor et al 2002a; Love and Coakham 2001). Within zones of demyelination, groups of axons were often closely apposed without an intervening glial process. The location of the zone of demyelination matches the point of vascular indentation and extends about 2 mm in each direction (Love and Coakham 2001). Juxtaposed axons have also been demonstrated in MS patients with TN. Additionally the trigeminal ganglion of TN patients demonstrates degenerative hypermyelination and microneuromata with no significant damage to neuronal soma; the initiating event is, however, unclear (Beaver 1967; Kerr 1967).

In TN the pain trigger is often innocuous stimulation that usually does not induce pain. How then is the

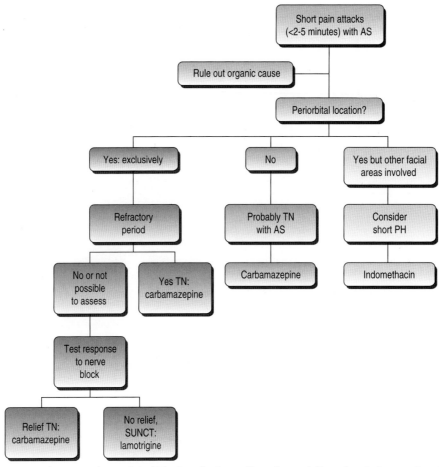

Fig. 11.3 • Differential diagnosis of trigeminal neuralgia (TN), short-lasting unilateral neuralgiform headache attacks with conjunctival injection and tearing (SUNCT) and atypical trigeminal autonomic cephalgias (TACs).

trigeminal system altered so that light mechanical touch results in pain? Following nerve injury there is an increased proportion of neurons with subthreshold oscillations (pacemaker activity) that bring the neuron close to its firing threshold. These neurons often generate ectopic discharges spontaneously or following external stimuli (Amir *et al* 1999; Liu *et al* 2000). These ectopic discharges often last a number of seconds and are termed 'after-discharge'. Stimulation of the peripheral nerve (particularly Aβ fibres) or the dorsal root produces a transient depolarization in passive neighbouring C-fibre neurons in the same ganglion (Amir and Devor 2000). In experimental setups about 90% of neurons sampled responded with this 'cross-depolarization'. In injured nerves this cross-depolarization leads to prolonged activity in neighbouring neurons (crossed-afterdischarge). These findings demonstrate a mechanism by which afferent nociceptors could be stimulated by activity in low-threshold mechanoreceptors, particularly in the event of nerve injury. Moreover the data explain the explosive and disproportionate pain response experienced by TN patients. The ignition hypothesis was formulated based on these findings (Devor *et al* 2002b). According to the hypothesis, injury renders axons and axotomized somata hyperexcitable, resulting in synchronized afterdischarge activity,

cross-excitation of nociceptors and pain paroxysms. CNS neuroplasticity will no doubt occur in the presence of such peripheral changes and will ultimately affect the clinical phenotype and response to therapy. The ignition hypothesis seems to explain many of the phenomena in TN but awaits definitive proof.

Interestingly some cases of TN have no vascular contact in the DREZ on operation (Broggi *et al* 2004). Moreover cadavers with no history of TN demonstrate vascular contacts in up to 14% of cases, albeit with minimal grooving (Hamlyn 1997a,b). Pain is reported in some patients who did not appear to have a severe compressive injury at surgical exposure and it is therefore probable that additional mechanisms are at play (Devor *et al* 2002a).

2.9. Treatment

TN is a progressive disease and eventually dose escalation or addition of drugs to obtain synergism is common. The improved morbidity rates of neurosurgical techniques such as MVD coupled with high efficacy rates suggest that many patients may benefit from surgery, possibly at an earlier stage. We will no doubt need to rethink our treatment approach as data accumulate. At present medical management is the mainstay of most TN patients; even for surgical candidates medical therapy is essential preoperatively and is often needed postoperatively, albeit in reduced doses (Nurmikko and Eldridge 2001).

2.9.1. Pharmacological

This section deals with the indications and selection of drugs for TN; the pharmacology and modes of action of these drugs are reviewed in Chapter 16. Carbamazepine is highly efficacious in TN and is usually the first drug tested. The number needed to treat (NNT) for any pain relief for carbamazepine in TN is 1.9 (95% confidence intervals (CI) 1.4–2.8) and for significant effectiveness is 2.6 (CI 2–3.4) (Wiffen et al 2005a,c). Its success in TN has been extrapolated to serve as a diagnostic test. However, up to 30% of patients may be initially resistant and up to 50% become refractory to carbamazepine therapy (Taylor et al 1981; Sato et al 2004). Oxcarbazepine, a carbamazepine derivative, is efficacious in TN with less side effects but patients will also develop resistance (Zakrzewska and Patsalos 2002). Baclofen has been successfully used in TN with some recommending it as first-line therapy. Because of its low side effect profile baclofen may be titrated to relatively high doses (80 mg/d) with an NNT of 1.4 (1–2.6) (Fromm et al 1984). Moreover a strong synergistic effect with both carbamazepine and phenytoin has been reported, making baclofen suitable for combined therapy (Fromm et al 1984; Fromm 1994). Phenytoin was the first drug for TN and is prescribed at 150–200 mg twice daily but has a relatively low success rate (25%). Side effects such as drowsiness and dizziness occur in 10% of patients even at low doses. However, phenytoin is synergistic with carbamazepine, and is therefore still used as add-on therapy (Fromm 1989). Gingival hyperplasia is a common dental complication of phenytoin. Clonazepam, at doses ranging from 3 to 8 mg daily, may provide some relief in TN, but side effects are very common and limiting. The newer anticonvulsants have fewer side effects and have been shown to be effective for some cases either as mono- or add-on therapy. Topiramate has been shown to be both effective and ineffective for TN and additionally has significant side effects (Zvartau-Hind et al 2000; Gilron et al 2001). Lamotrigine is effective (Lunardi et al 1997) and has been rigorously tested as add-on therapy with an NNT of 2.1 (CI 1.3–6.1) (Zakrzewska et al 1997). Gabapentin has not been rigorously tested in TN but for postherpetic neuralgia demonstrates an NNT for effectiveness of 3.9 (CI 3–5.7) and may be useful in selected TN cases (Wiffen et al 2005b).

Based on the current evidence we initiate therapy with carbamazepine and transfer patients at the earliest opportunity to the controlled release formulation that has fewer side effects. If carbamazepine continues to cause troublesome side effects we reduce the dose and add baclofen. Alternatively oxcarbazepine or add-on therapy with lamotrigine may be tried. In refractory cases gabapentin is probably the most promising drug (Solaro et al 2000). Pregabalin, topiramate or even the 'older' anticonvulsants valproate and phenytoin may be tried in recalcitrant cases (Cheshire 2002; Sindrup and Jensen 2002); see Table 11.6.

It is important to appreciate that even in successfully treated patients exacerbations (breakthrough pain) may occur and require temporary dose adjustment; in extreme cases in-patient care with intravenous phenytoin may be needed (Sindrup and Jensen 2002). Medically resistant cases who are physically able to withstand neurosurgery particularly with typical CTN are prime candidates for surgery.

Table 11.6	Drugs Commonly Used in the Treatment of Trigeminal Neuralgia				
Drug	**Initial Dose (mg)**	**Target Dose (mg)**[a]	**Dose Increase (titration)**[a]	**Schedule**	**Evidence**
Carbamazepine	100–200	1200	100–200 mg/2 d	×3–4/d	A
Carbamazepine-CR	200–400	1200	Usually transfer from regular format at equivalent dose	×2/d	A
Oxcarbazepine	300	1200–2400	300–600 mg/wk	×3/d	B
Baclofen	5–15	30–60	5 mg/3 d	×3/d	A
Clonazepam	0.25–0.5	1–4	0.25 mg/wk	Bedtime	C
Gabapentin	300	900–2400	300 mg/1–2 d	×3/d	B
Pregabalin	150	300–600	50 mg/2–3 d	×2–3/d	C
Lamotrigine	25	400–600	25–50 mg/wk	×1–2/d	A[b]
Topiramate	25	100	25 mg/wk	×2/d	C

CR, controlled release. Evidence for efficacy rated A (best), B (moderate), or C (low).
[a] Titrate according to response and side effects.
[b] Evidence for efficacy based on study using lamotrigine as add-on therapy.

2.9.2. Surgical

Since the neurosurgical approach to TN is described in Chapter 12, only the clinical effects are summarized here. The decision to opt for surgery is based on response to and side effects from medical treatment, the patient's age and profession and the surgical facilities and expertise available. The candidate must be in a physical condition that will allow safe general anaesthesia and neurosurgery. Patients require concise and clear explanations of the alternative neurosurgical procedures.

Surgery may be aimed peripherally at the affected nerve or centrally at the trigeminal ganglion or the posterior fossa. Any surgical procedure seems to have a better prognosis when carried out as a first procedure particularly on patients with typical CTN; in MVD best effects are obtained when performed within 7 years of TN onset (Broggi *et al* 2000).

2.9.2.1. Peripheral Procedures

Nerve blocks which we have employed to permit patients to eat or be involved in important personal activities, may provide some hours of absolute pain relief in TN. Peripheral procedures all aim at inducing nerve damage and therefore carry the attendant risk of developing dysaesthesia. Reported early success rates for neurectomy are conflicting (50–64%) and involve relatively small series with short-term follow-up (Peters and Nurmikko 2002). Moreover peripheral neurectomy may lead to neuropathic pain and is therefore not recommended. Cryotherapy of peripheral branches may give pain relief for 6 months (Pradel *et al* 2002). Pain recurrence after cryotherapy was usually in the original site (80%) and repeated cryotherapy often produced better results. However, up to one-third may develop atypical facial pain after cryotherapy and this technique is therefore not recommended (Zakrzewska 1991). Alcohol injections have been used but are painful and fibrosis makes repeat injections technically difficult. Complications may include full-thickness skin or mucosal ulceration, cranial nerve palsies, herpes zoster reactivation and bony necrosis (Peters and Nurmikko 2002). Pain control after alcohol block lasts just over one year and there have been reports of post-injection neuropathic pain (Fardy *et al* 1994). A 60% success rate at 24 months following peripheral glycerol injection has been reported but others report pain relapse by 7 months (Fardy *et al* 1994; Erdem and Alkan 2001). Reinjection is, however, possible with reportedly good results (Erdem and Alkan 2001).

In summary high recurrence and complication rates in peripheral procedures give no benefit over ganglion-level procedures. Peripheral procedures should be reserved for emergency use or in patients with significant medical problems that make other procedures unsafe (Peters and Nurmikko 2002).

2.9.2.2. Central Procedures

Percutaneous trigeminal rhizotomy. Three techniques may be used: radiofrequency rhizolysis, glycerol injection or balloon compression; see Chapter 12. The basis of these techniques is that controlled heat (69–90 °C), a neurotoxin or ischaemic and mechanical damage respectively will selectively ablate nociceptors (Aδ, C) whilst sparing mechanoreceptors (Aβ). The ability of these modalities to selectively damage nociceptive fibres has been questioned and patients often experience sensory loss of all fibres (Hakanson 1997).

These three modalities give approximately equal initial pain relief (around 90%) but are each associated with different rates of recurrence and complications (see Figs 11.4, 11.5). Overall radiofrequency rhizolysis consistently provides the highest rates of pain relief but is associated with high frequencies of facial and corneal numbness (Taha and Tew 1996; Lopez *et al* 2004).

Microvascular decompression. The procedure is based on the hypothesis that proximity between the intracerebral arteries and the trigeminal nerve root may allow pulsatile stimulation to cause chronic demyelination leading to

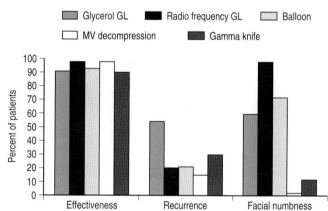

Fig. 11.4 • Effectiveness, recurrence and side effects of surgical and radiofrequency interventions used in the treatment of trigeminal neuralgia.

Data from Taha and Tew (1996), Kalkanis *et al* (2003), Lim and Ayiku (2004) and Henson *et al* (2005).

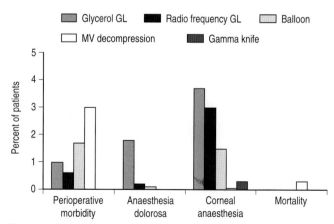

Fig. 11.5 • Complications and side effects of surgical and radiofrequency interventions used in the treatment of trigeminal neuralgia.

Data from Taha and Tew (1996), Kalkanis *et al* (2003), Lim and Ayiku (2004) and Henson *et al* (2005).

trigeminal neuralgia (Jannetta 1967). Thus separating between them may offer a permanent cure. The relatively high surgical morbidity (10%) reported in 1996 (Taha and Tew 1996) declined to about 0.3–3% in 2003 (Kalkanis *et al* 2003), making MVD a more attractive option. However, mortality remains a risk in MVD (Kalkanis *et al* 2003). Complication rates are lowest in high-volume hospitals and when the surgeon performs a large number of MVDs yearly (Kalkanis *et al* 2003). Long-term follow-up reveals that after 10 years 30–40% of patients that underwent MVD will experience a relapse (Burchiel *et al* 1988; Barker *et al* 1996a). Notwithstanding, MVD is at present the most cost-effective surgical approach to CTN (Pollock and Ecker 2005). Patient satisfaction with MVD is very high, particularly if this is their first intervention for TN (Zakrzewska *et al* 2005a).

Gamma knife. Gamma knife stereotactic radiosurgery (GKS) is a minimally invasive technique that is becoming common practice for the treatment of TN. The technique precisely delivers radiosurgical doses of 70–90 Gray units and relies on accurate MRI sequencing. The isocentre is the trigeminal nerve root at the point of vascular compression as mapped by MRI. Alternatively, if no compressing vessels are identified, the site of exit of the trigeminal nerve from the pons or other preselected position on the trigeminal nerve is treated. When GKS was compared with glycerol rhizotomy it was concluded that despite greater facial numbness and a higher failure rate glycerol provided more rapid pain relief than GKS. Indeed in some reports GKS is associated with delay before pain relief (Jawahar *et al* 2005). However, GKS showed better long-term pain relief with less treatment-related morbidity than glycerol rhizotomy and may be indicated in patients that are poor candidates for MVD (Lim and Ayiku 2004; Henson *et al* 2005). Although posterior fossa surgery (MVD or partial nerve section) was shown superior to GKS over a mean follow-up duration of about 2 years (Lim and Ayiku 2004; Pollock 2005) there are reports that GKS may be a more efficient primary intervention and the procedure of choice for recurrent CTN (Sanchez-Mejia *et al* 2005). There are insufficient data at present to assess the long-term outcomes or complications of GKS, particularly the unknown effects of radiation in the area of the trigeminal root. Moreover since gamma knife radiosurgery units are rare in most centres, the choice of treatment technique is restricted to percutaneous and MVD techniques.

2.10. Summary

Trigeminal neuralgia has a good initial response to almost all treatments but a predictable relapse of up to 40–50% over 15 years. Periods of pain relief are shortest for peripheral procedures, intermediate for drug therapy or rhizotomies and longest for MVD. Accumulating evidence suggests that for healthy patients with typical TN, surgery should be performed sooner rather than later; 7 years seems the current cutoff point and beyond that the success of MVD declines.

TN is distressing and patients often need support; the education of partners and close family is essential. The Trigeminal Neuralgia Association (http://www.tna-support.org) is an excellent resource and publishes an interesting lay person's guide on TN, *Striking Back!*

3. Glossopharyngeal Neuralgia

3.1. Introduction and Definition

Glossopharyngeal neuralgia (GN) is a rare condition similar in presentation to TN. GN affects the throat or periauricular area corresponding to the distribution of auricular and pharyngeal branches of the vagus and glossopharyngeal nerves. This accounts for the alternative term used: vagoglossopharyngeal neuralgia. The characteristic pain location may direct affected cases to other medical specialists such as otolaryngologists. Although similarities with TN are prominent, GN is characterized by a milder natural history with the majority of patients going into remission. However, because of its location and features GN is a difficult diagnosis and adequate treatment is often delayed for some years (Patel *et al* 2002).

3.2. Clinical Features of GN (Table 11.7)

Location. The glossopharyngeal (IXth) nerve has two main sensory branches: the auricular (tympanic) that supplies the mastoid, auricle and external meatus and the pharyngeal that innervates the pharyngeal mucosa. The pharyngeal branches together with vagal (Xth) afferents also innervate the base of the tongue, tonsil and soft palate. Pain distribution is therefore in the posterior part of the tongue, tonsillar fossa, pharynx and the angle of the lower jaw and/or the ear (Olesen *et al* 2004). Based on primary location and particular referral patterns two anatomical variants have been described for GN: a 'pharyngeal' and a 'tympanic' form. Pain in pharyngeal-GN is usually located in the pharynx, tonsil, soft palate or posterior tongue base and radiates upwards to the inner ear, or the angle of the mandible. It may also radiate to involve the eye, nose, maxilla or shoulder and even the tip of the tongue.

Tympanic GN is characterized by pain that either remains confined to or markedly predominates in the ear but may subsequently radiate to the pharynx; these cases may pose serious differential diagnostic dilemmas vis-à-vis geniculate neuralgia (see below). The left side is usually affected more often than the right but the clinical significance of this is unclear (Patel *et al* 2002). Bilaterality is not uncommon and occurs in 12–25% of patients (Rushton *et al* 1981; Katusic *et al* 1991b).

Quality and severity. Pain is usually described as sharp, stabbing, shooting or lancinating. Some patients may report a scratching or foreign body sensation in the throat

Table 11.7 Diagnostic Criteria for Classical and Symptomatic Glossopharyngeal Neuralgia (GN)

	Classic (A–E)	Symptomatic (A–D)	Notes
A	Paroxysmal attacks of facial pain lasting from a fraction of a second to 2 min and fulfilling criteria B and C.	Paroxysmal attacks of facial pain lasting from a fraction of a second to 2 min, with or without persistence of aching between paroxysms, and fulfilling criteria B and C.	Remission as has been described for TN.
B	Pain has all of the following characteristics: 1. Unilateral location 2. Distribution within the posterior part of the tongue, tonsillar fossa, pharynx or beneath the angle of the lower jaw and/or in the ear 3. Sharp, stabbing and severe 4. Precipitated by swallowing, chewing, talking, coughing and/or yawning.	As in classic.	Many cases will describe their pain as 'electrical'. Pain may additionally be experienced in the auricular and pharyngeal branches of the vagus nerve.
C	Attacks are stereotyped in the individual patient.	As in classic.	Attack duration, distribution, etc. may vary between patients but are highly consistent within cases.
D	There is no clinically evident neurological deficit.	A causative lesion has been demonstrated by special investigations and/or surgery.	Sensory testing may reveal mild deficits in the distribution of the trigeminal nerve.
E	Not attributed to another disorder.	Not relevant.	For classic GN, other causes are ruled out by history, physical examination and special investigations.

TN, trigeminal neuralgia. Based on Olesen *et al* (2004) with permission.

(Rushton *et al* 1981). An atypical form with prominent burning and long-lasting pain has been described (Resnick *et al* 1995). Attacks of GN are commonly mild but may vary in intensity to excruciating (Rushton *et al* 1981; Katusic *et al* 1991b). Features of pain attacks are stereotyped within patients (Olesen *et al* 2004). There is usually no warning sign of an oncoming attack but some cases report pre-attack discomfort in the throat or ear (Bruyn 1983).

Triggering. Typically GN trigger areas are located in the tonsillar region and posterior pharynx and are activated by swallowing, chewing, talking, coughing and/or yawning (Minagar and Sheremata 2000; Olesen *et al* 2004). Sneezing, clearing the throat, touching the gingiva or oral mucosa, blowing the nose and rubbing the ear or around it often trigger pain (Katusic *et al* 1991b; Minagar and Sheremata 2000). Topical analgesia to trigger areas will eliminate both trigger and pain (Rushton *et al* 1981).

Temporal pattern. Pain usually lasts from 8 to 50 s, but may continue for a few minutes. The IHS criteria require pain of less than 2 min but the validity of this has been untested. Atypical cases with pain paroxysms lasting 4–40 minutes and cases with longer-lasting attacks consisting of continuous series of paroxysms have been described (Ekbom and Westerberg 1966). Frequency of paroxysms may be from 5 to 12 every hour, but may occasionally reach 150–200 attacks per day. Following an individual attack further stimuli are incapable of inducing pain: a refractory period (Olesen *et al* 2004).

Attacks may occur in clusters lasting weeks to months, then relapse for up to a number of years (Olesen *et al* 2004). Spontaneous remissions were noted in 74% of patients, but 17% had no periods of pain relief (Rushton *et al* 1981). In two-thirds of cases there may be only one attack and the average annual recurrence rate for a second episode is low (3.6%) (Rushton *et al* 1981; Katusic *et al* 1991b).

Associated signs. GN is reported to induce syncope, probably mediated by functional central connections between visceral afferents of cranial nerves (IX and X) and autonomic medullary nuclei (Odeh and Oliven 1994). Cardiac arrhythmias are common, particularly bradycardia (Ferrante *et al* 1995). Uncontrollable coughing has been reported in 8% of cases (Rushton *et al* 1981). The pain-paroxysms may also be associated with either ipsilateral dryness of the oral cavity or considerably increased salivation. Rarely pain may radiate to the eye and cause lacrimation.

Investigations. The relative rarity of GN has prevented high-quality studies on predictive value of special tests. Imaging of the head and neck to rule out pathology is indicated. An electrocardiogram should be performed prior to and after treatment. Preoperative MRTA is recommended to locate possible neurovascular contacts.

3.3. Symptomatic GN

A significant association between GN and MS has been reported (Minagar and Sheremata 2000). Four of 8000 MS patients (i.e. 0.05%) developed GN over a follow-up period of 20 years, which although of a lower incidence resembles the pattern for TN (Minagar and Sheremata 2000). Regional infectious or inflammatory processes may mimic GN. Cerebellopontine angle or pontine lesions may cause GN-like symptoms (Huynh-Le *et al* 2004). Tonsillar carcinoma invading the parapharyngeal space and other regional tumours (tongue, oropharyngeal) may cause GN (Pfendler 1997). Post-traumatic GN is relatively rare but has been reported (Webb *et al* 2000).

3.4. Differential Diagnosis

The most common differential is TN particularly when pain of GN spreads to trigeminal dermatomes. Moreover the co-occurrence of TN and GN is common and expected to occur in 10-12% of GN patients (Rushton *et al* 1981). Bradycardia, clustering of attacks and very rarely the spread of pain to the eye with lacrimation may cause confusion with cluster headache; see Chapter 10 (Rushton *et al* 1981; Katusic *et al* 1991b).

3.5. Epidemiology of GN

GN is extremely rare; the annual crude incidence is about 0.7 per 100 000 for both sexes (0.9–1.1 in men and 0.5 in women) (Rushton *et al* 1981; Katusic *et al* 1991b). Mean age at onset is 64 years and GN is more common in patients older than 50 years (57%), but may occur in patients aged 13–50 (Rushton *et al* 1981; Katusic *et al* 1991b). Age-specific rates increase slightly with age, peaking at around 40–60 years (Katusic *et al* 1991b).

3.6. Pathophysiology of GN

The pathophysiology is uncertain but is considered to probably be secondary to compression of the nerve root by a blood vessel. GN cases demonstrate nerve compression on MRI and on surgical exposure (Fischbach *et al* 2003). Biopsy of the nerve from a patient with GN revealed large patches of demyelinated axons in close membrane-to-membrane apposition to one another and zones of less severe myelin damage (Devor *et al* 2002c). These morphological changes are similar to those observed in patients with trigeminal neuralgia and suggest shared pathophysiological processes.

3.7. Treatment

Therapy for GN has largely been based on successful pharmacological and surgical treatments for TN. Life threatening arrhythmias may require cardiac pacing.

3.7.1. Pharmacological

Carbamazepine is usually successful and is the favoured medication (Rushton *et al* 1981). Alternatives are similar to those used for TN: baclofen, oxcarbazepine, gabapentin, lamotrigine and phenytoin (Rozen 2004).

3.7.2. Surgical

Patients with GN successfully treated with anticonvulsants may become resistant, in which case there is a clear indication for surgery. In the past surgeries consisted of extracranial avulsion of the glossopharyngeal nerve or intracranial section at the jugular foramen. Subsequently section of the glossopharyngeal nerve, the upper rootlets of the vagus nerve and the fifth cranial nerve (if TN was also present) provided good relief of pain in over 50% of patients (Rushton *et al* 1981; Taha and Tew 1995). More recently MVD and GKS have been successfully applied to patients with GN (Stieber *et al* 2005). MVD induced immediate and complete relief of pain in 80–95% of GN patients with stable long-term results (Patel *et al* 2002; Sampson *et al* 2004). Permanent neurological deficits are rare (approx. 10%) and may include mild hoarseness and/or dysphagia, or facial nerve paresis. MVD carries morbidity and mortality risks but is considered a relatively safe procedure; see above under TN.

4. Nervus Intermedius Neuralgia

The intermedius nerve is a small sensory branch of the facial nerve that innervates the skin overlying the mastoid process and the external meatus. The cell bodies of the sensory afferents are located in the geniculate ganglion; hence the alternative term for nervus intermedius neuralgia (NIN) is 'geniculate neuralgia'.

NIN is centred directly in the ear, and often felt deep within the ear (Pulec 2002; Olesen *et al* 2004). Pain is described as sharp, stabbing and paroxysmal and lasts seconds to minutes. NIN may, however, be of a gradual onset and persistent nature (Pulec 2002; Olesen *et al* 2004). A trigger point in the posterior wall of the auditory canal may be present but is difficult to verify. NIN is extremely rare with an uncertain pathogenesis but may be secondary to herpes zoster infection (see below) together with facial palsy, ipsilateral loss of taste and herpetic vesicles in the auditory canal and is then termed Ramsay Hunt syndrome (see Chapter 6).

In one study the nerve was examined under electron microscopy revealing nonspecific myelin sheath delamination (Pulec 2002). However, the exact mechanisms in NIN are unclear at present.

Treatment. Anticonvulsant pharmacotherapy should be tried as for TN. In resistant cases or in patients with intolerable side effects surgery may be necessary. Findings indicate that excision of the nervus intermedius and geniculate ganglion can be routinely performed without causing facial paralysis and that it is an effective definitive treatment for intractable geniculate neuralgia (Pulec 2002). The greater petrosal nerve is usually sectioned so that the ipsilateral eye remains tearless (Pulec 2002). In some cases NIN may be accompanied by symptoms suggestive of TN and/or GN and these cases are managed by combined nerve section and MVD (Lovely and Jannetta 1997).

5. Facial Pain Associated with Herpes Zoster

5.1. Acute Herpes Zoster

Acute herpes zoster (HZ) or shingles is actually a reactivation of latent varicella virus infection and may occur decades after the primary infection. HZ is a disease of the dorsal root ganglion and therefore induces a dermatomal vesicular eruption. The exact mechanisms underlying viral reactivation and the subsequent appearance of acute HZ are unknown. In immunocompromised patients the clinical presentation may be more severe with numerous vesicles that take longer to heal. Diagnosis of HZ is based on the clinical presentation described below; see also Table 11.8. Definitive diagnosis may be obtained by identification of viral DNA from vesicular fluid employing the polymerase chain reaction.

5.1.1. Clinical Features

Location. The most common location is the thoracic, followed by the lumbar region (Goh and Khoo 1997). Trigeminal and cervical nerves are affected in 8–28% and 13–23% of cases, respectively (Goh and Khoo 1997; Haanpaa *et al* 1999). The ophthalmic branch is affected in over 80% of the trigeminal cases, particularly in elderly males and may cause keratitis, which is sight-threatening. The vesicles and pain are dermatomal and unilateral and will appear intraorally when the maxillary or mandibular branch of the trigeminal nerve is affected. The case shown in Fig. 11.6 developed maxillary and mandibular HZ; vesicles are apparent unilaterally on the lips, and have broken down, leaving ulcers on the intraoral mucosa.

Quality and severity. Pain is usually described as constant but in one series over a quarter reported superimposed lancinating pains (Haanpaa *et al* 1999). In some patients

Table 11.8 Diagnostic Criteria for Head or Facial Pain Attributed to Herpes Zoster

	Diagnostic Criteria		
	Acute Herpes Zoster	**Postherpetic Neuralgia**	**Notes**
A	Head or facial pain in the distribution of a nerve division and fulfilling criteria C and D.		Facial herpes zoster mostly affects the ophthalmic branch.
B	Herpetic eruption in the territory of the same nerve.		Involvement of the geniculate ganglion causes an eruption in the external auditory meatus and may also present with facial palsy (Ramsay Hunt syndrome; see Chapter 6).
C	Pain precedes herpetic eruption by <7 days.[a]		Herpes zoster infection is common in immunocompromised individuals and very common in lymphomas.
D	Pain resolves within 3 months.	Pain persists after 3 months.	Postherpetic neuralgia is usually more common in patients >60 years old.

Based on Olesen *et al* (2004) with permission.
[a] In postherpetic neuralgia this information is usually obtained from the history.

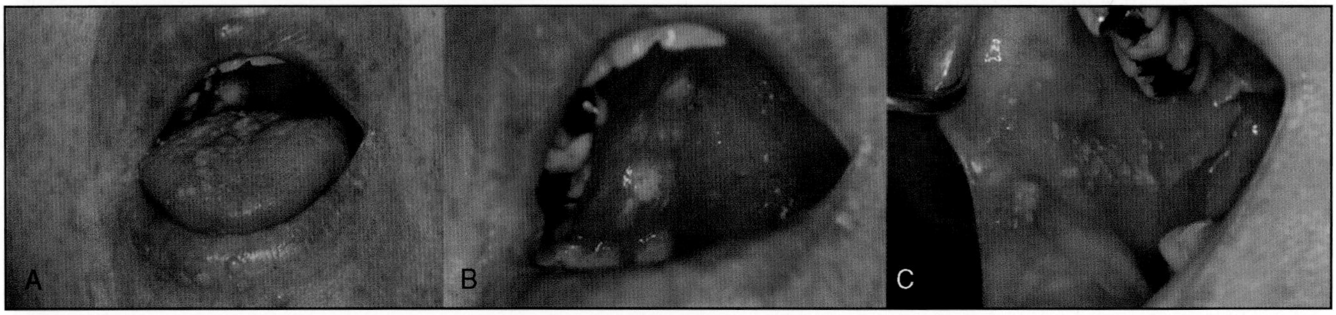

Fig. 11.6 • Acute herpes zoster. Intact vesicles are apparent on the lips (A). Most of the intraoral vesicles have ruptured leaving ulcerations. The tongue and circumoral region (A), palate (B) and buccal (C) mucosa were all affected unilaterally.

evoked (stimulus-dependent) pain may also be present and may be the prominent feature (Nurmikko and Bowsher 1990; Haanpaa *et al* 1999). Descriptors of pain at rash onset include burning (26%), stabbing (15%), shooting (15%), tingling (10%) and aching (9%) (Goh and Khoo 1997). Severity may be moderate to severe (VAS 6.2), but up to 25% of patients may report no pain (Goh and Khoo 1997; Haanpaa *et al* 1999; Dworkin *et al* 2001). High pain severity correlates with an increased incidence of postherpetic neuralgia (PHN) (Haanpaa *et al* 1999; Dworkin *et al* 2001).

Temporal pattern and associated signs. Acute HZ begins with a prodrome of pain, headache, itching and malaise (Goh and Khoo 1997; Haanpaa *et al* 1999; Volpi *et al* 2005). Pain usually precedes the acute stage by 2–3 days (<7) and may continue for up to 3–6 months with varying intensity (Haanpaa *et al* 1999; Volpi *et al* 2005). The acute stage is characterized by a red maculopapular rash that develops into a vesicular eruption over a period of 3–5 days; these usually dry out over a further 7–10 days. Complete healing may last one month (Loeser 1986; Portenoy *et al* 1986). Very rarely dermatomal pain occurs with no rash: *zoster sine herpete* (Gilden *et al* 1994).

Mechanical allodynia and disturbed sensory thresholds are often seen and these usually spread to adjacent dermatomes and may also occur bilaterally (Haanpaa *et al* 1999).

5.1.2. Epidemiology

Every year approximately 0.1–0.5% of people will develop HZ: 0.02% in children <5 years old, 0.06% between ages 15 and 19, 0.25% between 20 and 50 and up to 1% in subjects over the age of 80 (Guess *et al* 1985). The overall lifetime risk of HZ is 10–20% and more than 50% in patients over the age of 80 (Ragozzino *et al* 1982).

5.1.3. Pathophysiology

Viral replication induces epithelial cell degeneration characterized by ballooning, followed by invasion of giant cells. Rarely necrosis and bleeding may be observed. The vesicles subsequently become cloudy as polymorphonucleocytes, fibrin and degenerated cells appear; subsequently these rupture and release infectious contents.

Following HZ infection, dorsal root ganglia (DRGs) demonstrate cell degeneration, satellitosis and lymphocytic infiltration of the nerve root. Viral DNA is found in most thoracic and trigeminal ganglial cells examined. Spread within the spinal cord involves adjacent segments (bilaterally) and accounts for the distribution of sensory changes and hyperalgesia observed. In severe cases the spinal ventral horn may be involved with resultant paralysis.

5.1.4. Treatment

Therapy is directed at controlling pain, accelerating healing and reducing the risk of complications such as dissemination, PHN and local secondary infection (Volpi *et al* 2005). When antivirals (acyclovir, famcyclovir, valacyclovir) are initiated early (<72 hours from onset of rash), particularly in patients >50 years old, they decrease rash duration, pain severity and the incidence of PHN (Dworkin *et al* 2001; Schmader 2001). Table 11.9 summarizes antiviral medications and dosages. Fever and pain should be controlled initially by analgesics such as paracetamol but for stronger pain opioids are effective. Amitriptyline and gabapentin will provide analgesia (see Chapter 16); amitriptyline may shorten illness duration and provides added protection from PHN (Bowsher 1997; BSSI 1995).

Vaccinating at-risk individuals such as the elderly and infirm may be an efficacious technique to prevent HZ and PHN. A randomized, double-blind, placebo-controlled trial of an investigational live attenuated varicella zoster virus vaccine showed that the zoster vaccine markedly reduced morbidity from herpes zoster and postherpetic neuralgia among older adults (Oxman *et al* 2005).

5.2. Postherpetic Trigeminal Neuralgia

A proportion (16–22%) of acute HZ patients will report pain 3–6 months after initial onset, but by one year only

Table 11.9	Antiviral Drugs Used in the Treatment of Herpes Zoster That Also Reduce Incidence of Postherpetic Neuralgia			
Drug	**Dosage (mg)**	**Times daily**	**Duration (days)**	**Comments**
Acyclovir	800	5	7–10	Side effects may include headache and nausea. Patients must
Valacyclovir	1000	3	7	maintain fluid intake to prevent renal drug deposition. May require dose adjustment in renal dysfunction and elderly. Precaution in immunocompromised patients as cases of severe thrombotic thrombocytopenic purpura have been reported.
Famcyclovir	250–500[a]	3	7	Most common side effects are headache and nausea. Elimination is impaired in renal dysfunction.

[a] Recommended dosage in the USA.

5–10% continue to suffer pain. Several risk factors for persistent pain have emerged and include advanced age, severe prodromal pain, severe acute pain and severe rash (Jung *et al* 2004). Of these age >50 and pain VAS ratings of >5 were independently shown to predict PHN at 3 months post HZ (Coen *et al* 2006). In the older age group (>60 years) 50% or more will continue to suffer pain lasting more than one year.

The exact definition of when acute HZ-associated pain becomes PHN is disputed and ranges between 1 and 6 months after lesion crusting. This has led to the suggestion that pain occurring after HZ infection be classified as a continuum and termed 'zoster-associated pain' or ZAP. However, this classification leaves unresolved the evidence supporting that acute HZ and PHN are separate and different entities. There is wide acceptance that pain lasting less than 30 days is acute HZ and for more than 120 days is 'chronic' or PHN.

5.2.1. Clinical Features

PHN is a direct complication of acute HZ and will therefore localize to the affected dermatomes, usually the ophthalmic branch (22%) of the trigeminal nerve (Bowsher 1996). Pale sometimes red/purple scars may remain in the affected area and these are usually hypoaesthetic or anaesthetic; paradoxically these areas may exhibit allodynia and hyperalgesia (Fig. 11.7). The descriptors used for PHN are similar to those for acute HZ: burning, throbbing, stabbing, shooting or sharp (Dworkin and Portenoy 1996). The allodynic areas are often described by patients as tender (Dworkin and Portenoy 1996). The presence of burning pain is significantly higher in patients that did not receive antiviral therapy in the acute HZ stage (Bowsher 1996). Itching of affected areas is more common in trigeminal dermatomes and may be very prominent and extremely bothersome (Bowsher 1996; Oaklander *et al* 2003). Most patients with PHN will suffer from allodynia and exhibit deficits for temperature and pinprick sensation (Bowsher 1996). Indeed itching may often be subjectively graded as worse

than pain (Bowsher 1996). PHN is usually severe with VAS ratings of 8 but is characterized by fluctuations from moderate background pain to excruciating, superimposed lancinating pains (Bowsher 1996; Dworkin and Portenoy 1996).

5.2.2. Pathophysiology

PHN is considered to be pathophysiologically separate from acute HZ. This is based on the findings of sensory deficits and spinal cord changes in PHN that are absent in patients with healed acute HZ and no pain (Nurmikko and Bowsher 1990; Watson *et al* 1991; Bowsher 1996).

PHN is a neuropathic pain syndrome resulting from viral-induced nerve injury; scarring of sensory ganglia and peripheral nerves and loss of large myelinated fibres are commonly found in PHN patients (Watson *et al* 1991). Two processes, peripherally generated pain by irritable nociceptors and centrally generated pain secondary to nerve injury, have been suggested (Nurmikko and Haanpaa 2005). The clinical phenotype will be affected by the degree that each process plays in individual patients.

Skin biopsies from affected and contralateral sites demonstrate bilateral peripheral nerve damage (Oaklander *et al* 1998). PHN occurred in patients with the least epidermal neurites remaining after acute HZ, suggesting pain secondary to nerve injury (Oaklander *et al* 1998). Virus is not usually recovered from spinal cord of PHN patients, suggesting that an infective process is not actively involved (Bowsher 1996). Postmortem examination of an ophthalmic PHN patient revealed severe peripheral nerve pathology that involved also the contralateral side (Dostrovsky 2000). However, the trigeminal ganglion and trigeminal root were unaffected. It is possible that PHN is a disease that progresses from the periphery to central structures. Ongoing activity in peripheral nociceptors has been shown to be important in the early stages (<1 year) of PHN, whereas central mechanisms may become prominent in later stages (Pappagallo *et al* 2000).

5.2.3. Treatment

Early treatment of established PHN is essential as it improves prognosis (Bowsher 1996). Ophthalmic PHN per se seems to have the worst prognosis (Bowsher 1996). Evidence-based treatment options for PHN include tricyclic antidepressant drugs, gabapentin, pregabalin, opioids and topical lidocaine patches; see Chapters 15, 16 (Dubinsky *et al* 2004). Lidocaine patches are very effective with a mean NNT of 2 (CI 1.4–3.3). Topical aspirin or capsaicin may be effective with marginal clinical benefit (Watson *et al* 1993; Dubinsky *et al* 2004). For PHN the overall NNT for effectiveness of antidepressants compared with placebo was 2.20 (CI 1.7–3.13) (Saarto and Wiffen 2005). Specifically for amitriptyline NNTs of 1.6–3.2 have been reported (CI 1.2–2.4) (Max *et al* 1988). NNTs for opioids range from 2.5 to 3 and some patients may prefer opioids over TCAs (Raja

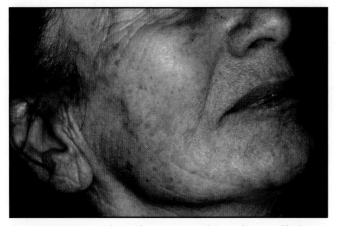

Fig. 11.7 • Patient with postherpetic neuralgia in the mandibular branch of the trigeminal nerve. The area anterior to the ear and lateral to the mouth shows purplish scars that were very sensitive to touch.

et al 2002; Hempenstall et al 2005). Gabapentin is beneficial with NNTs of 3.9–4.39 (Hempenstall et al 2005; Wiffen et al 2005b). Pregabalin is a relatively new drug of proven efficacy in PHN with NNTs of 3.3–4.93 (Hempenstall et al 2005; van Seventer et al 2006). Tramadol may provide a reasonable alternative with an NNT of 4.7 (Boureau et al 2003).

More invasive modalities include epidural and intrathecal steroids and a variety of neurosurgical techniques (Watson and Oaklander 2002). The most promising surgical intervention seems to be DREZ lesion (see Chapter 12) which provides relief in 59% of treated cases (Friedman and Nashold 1984). CNS stimulation may also provide pain relief.

6. Central Causes of Facial Pain

Central pain (CP) may be caused by direct damage as in stroke and spinal cord trauma or secondary to centrally occurring diseases such as epilepsy, Parkinson's disease and MS. Pain due to MS has been discussed earlier under trigeminal neuralgia. Anaesthesia dolorosa, sometimes termed deafferentation pain (see discussion on the true meaning of the term in Chapter 2), denotes pain after lesions of the nervous system and is associated with decreased sensation. The IASP relate to anaesthesia dolorosa as a symptom and define it as pain in an area or region which is anaesthetic (Merskey and Bogduk 1994). Painful peripheral traumatic neuropathies involve central mechanisms but are not strictly speaking CPs and are therefore dealt with in the section on traumatic neuropathies.

6.1. Central Post-Stroke Pain (CPSP)

CPSP is characterized by constant or paroxysmal pain accompanied by sensory abnormalities, decreased perception and often allodynia; see Table 11.10.

6.1.1. Clinical Features and Treatment

Depending on the extent and location of the lesion motor impairment and a variety of sensory symptoms may accompany pain (Bowsher et al 1998). Pain onset is usually within one month but may take up to 3 years (Leijon et al 1989). According to IHS criteria, however, symptom onset must be within 6 months of a stroke to be classified as CPSP (Table 11.10) (Olesen et al 2004). Symptoms include pain and/or dysaesthesia in one half of the face, associated with loss of sensation to pinprick, temperature and/or touch (Olesen et al 2004). Sensory dysfunction occurs in over half of cases and correlates with the presence of pain (Andersen et al 1995; MacGowan et al 1997; Fitzek et al 2001). The most common pain descriptors for CPSP are burning, aching, pricking and lacerating (Andersen et al 1995; Bowsher et al 1998). Burning pain is most common, except among patients with thalamic

stroke who more often describe lacerating pain (Leijon et al 1989; Andersen et al 1995). Pain frequency varies but intensity is usually moderate to severe and increased by external stimuli, most commonly movement, light touch and cold (Leijon et al 1989; Andersen et al 1995; Fitzek et al 2001). Dysaesthesia is the most common abnormal sensation and may be evoked or constant (Nicholson 2004). Sensory impairment (temperature) is present in the majority of cases (Leijon et al 1989). Muscle spasticity is present in about 60% of CPSP patients.

Facial pain is common in brainstem lesions and may cause constant burning or paroxysmal sharp pain (Chia and Shen 1993; Fitzek et al 2001). In 65 patients with brainstem infarcts, 12 had lateral medullary infarcts of which 50% had ipsilateral facial pain with or without accompanying body pain. The facial pain was mostly located periorbitally and was described as burning or hot, stinging and pressure-like. Persistent pain with superimposed attacks was reported by 25%, and 42% had only paroxysmal pain lasting seconds to minutes (Fitzek et al 2001). Ipsilaterally there was sensory dysfunction and corneal reflexes were abolished in all facial pain patients. Facial pain was highly correlated to lesions of the lower medulla (Fitzek et al 2001).

Amitriptyline is effective in CPSP as is the anticonvulsant lamotrigine and these should be considered first

Table 11.10 Diagnostic Criteria for Central Post Stroke Pain

	Diagnostic Criteria	Notes
A	Pain and dysaesthesia in one half of the face, associated with loss of sensation to pinprick, temperature and/or touch and fulfilling criteria C and D.	Thalamic lesions are often involved. Depending on the site of the lesion other areas may be affected both in sensory and motor components. Pain and sensory disturbance are resistant to therapy.
B	One or more of the following: 1. History of sudden onset, suggesting a vascular lesion (stroke) 2. Demonstration by CT or MRI of a vascular lesion in an appropriate site	Diagnosis is often made retrospectively in a patient with a history of stroke and facial pain that started afterwards.
C	Pain and dysaesthesia develop within 6 months after stroke.	
D	Not explicable by a lesion of the trigeminal nerve.	

CT, computerized tomography; MRI, magnetic resonance imaging. Based on Olesen et al (2004) with permission.

(Vestergaard *et al* 2001; Saarto and Wiffen 2005; Frese *et al* 2006). Gabapentin and the Na channel blocker mexiletine are good second choices. Short-term relief may be obtained with intravenous lidocaine or propofol (Frese *et al* 2006). Post-stroke patients are often not good candidates for tricyclic antidepressants and therefore the anticonvulsants are indicated (Finnerup *et al* 2005).

6.1.2. Pathophysiology

Damage to pain pathways in the thalamus was thought to initiate CP, hence the alternative term thalamic pain. CPSP is often linked with lesions of the ventrocaudal thalamic nuclei and particularly within the ventroposterior inferior nucleus. Later studies suggested that spinothalamic pathways and cortical processing play a significant role in CPSP (Leijon *et al* 1989; Bowsher *et al* 1998; Frese *et al* 2006). However, many patients with post-stroke damage to spinothalamic pathways do not develop pain, so other factors must be involved. The pain of CPSP is thought to occur due to ectopic activity in damaged circuits induced by the stroke and an imbalance in facilitatory and inhibitory pathways (Canavero and Bonicalzi 1998).

6.1.3. Epidemiology

CPSP is quite common; 8.4–11% of all stroke and 25% of brainstem infarct patients develop pain over a 6- to 12-month follow-up period (Andersen *et al* 1995; MacGowan *et al* 1997; Nicholson 2004).

7. Burning Mouth Syndrome/Disorder

Burning mouth syndrome (BMS) is a poorly understood pain condition that is most probably neuropathic with a central component. The condition is also known as stomatodynia, oral dysaesthesia or stomatopyrosis and is characterized by a burning mucosal pain with no major visible signs, often accompanied by dysgeusia and xerostomia; thus the term 'syndrome' is used. Some investigators argue against the term BMS altogether as there is no indication that this is indeed a syndrome. Burning mouth disorder (BMD) has been suggested as a reasonable alternative until there is more information regarding aetiology and thus will be used in this section (Rhodus *et al* 2003a). Although clear diagnostic criteria have been proposed these should be field-tested and validated; see Table 11.11 (Woda and Pionchon 1999; Olesen *et al* 2004). Future classifications of BMD should include criteria of oral pain or dysaesthesia of a burning quality with no major paroxysmal character of >3 months duration or of a recurrent pattern. Symptoms should be present during most of the day and clinical and/or radiographic examination does not reveal any obvious cause (Woda and Pionchon 1999).

Table 11.11 IHS Diagnostic Criteria for Burning Mouth Syndrome

	Diagnostic Criteria	Notes
A	Pain in the mouth present daily and persisting most of the day.	Some areas are particularly prone: e.g. tongue tip and lips. Concomitant complaints may include dry mouth, paraesthesia and taste disturbance. Usually affects post-menopausal women.
B	Oral mucosa is of normal appearance.	Erosive or ulcerative mucosal diseases commonly induce burning.
C	Local and systemic diseases have been excluded.	Regional musculoskeletal disorders should be ruled out.

Based on Olesen et al (2004) with permission.

BMD may be subclassified into 'primary BMD' or essential/idiopathic BMD for which a neuropathological cause is likely, and 'secondary BMD', resulting from local or systemic pathological conditions (Scala *et al* 2003). By definition primary BMD cannot be attributed to any systemic or local cause (Woda and Pionchon 1999; Rhodus *et al* 2003a).

BMD is unfortunately characterized by resistance to a wide range of treatments and is one of the most challenging management problems in the field of orofacial pain.

7.1. Epidemiology

Due to often vague criteria the exact prevalence of BMD is unclear. However, it seems that BMD is most common in post-menopausal women and reported prevalence rates in general populations vary from 0.7 to 15% (Forman and Settle 1990a,b; Zakrzewska *et al* 2005b). In a US country-wide survey of residents aged 18 and older BMD-like symptoms were reported by 0.7% of all adults, 0.8% by women and 0.6% by men (Lipton *et al* 1993). In middle aged and elderly women BMD was reported by 4.6% (Hakeberg *et al* 1997). In Europe, the population prevalence of BMD was estimated to be 13–15% (Tammiala-Salonen *et al* 1993; Femiano 2002a), but in one study about half had an oral disease that could cause symptoms (Tammiala-Salonen *et al* 1993). In men, no BMD was found in patients under the age of 40. In the 40–49 age group a prevalence of 0.7% was found that increased to 3.6% in the 50–69 age group (Bergdahl and Bergdahl 1999). In women no BMD was found in patients under the age of 30. In the 30–39 age group the prevalence was 0.6% and increased to 12.2% in the 50–69 age group (Bergdahl and Bergdahl 1999).

7.2. Clinical Features

Location. The tongue, usually the anterior two-thirds, is the primary location of the burning complaint in the majority of cases (Bergdahl and Bergdahl 1999). However, usually more than one site is involved and in addition to the tongue the hard palate, lips and gingivae are frequently painful (Lamey *et al* 1996).

Quality and severity. The pain intensity varies from mild to severe; VAS scores reported range from 5 to 7 but may reach 8–10 (Danhauer *et al* 2002; Gremeau-Richard *et al* 2004; Petruzzi *et al* 2004). The most common terms used to describe the pain quality are burning or hot (Ship *et al* 1995).

Temporal pattern. BMD is typically of spontaneous onset and lasts from months to several years (Rhodus *et al* 2003a,b; Zakrzewska *et al* 2005b). Although a chronic unremitting pattern is usual, spontaneous remission of BMD has been reported in 3% of patients about 5 years after onset (Sardella *et al* 2006). Partial remission has been reported in about one-half to two-thirds of patients 6–7 years after onset (Bergdahl and Bergdahl 1999). The pain pattern may be irregular but some patients may complain that pain increases towards the end of the day (Gorsky *et al* 1991).

Associated signs. More than two-thirds of the patients complain of altered taste sensation (dysgeusia) accompanying the burning sensation; in many cases the alteration is described as a spontaneous metallic taste (Grushka and Sessle 1988; Mott *et al* 1993).

A possible association to anxiety, depression and personality disorders is described in the literature particularly in post-menopausal women (Gorsky *et al* 1991; Bergdahl and Bergdahl 1999; Scala *et al* 2003), but it is unclear whether pain initiated the psychological disorder or vice versa (Al Quran 2004; Maina *et al* 2005). Approximately 21% of BMD patients presented personality profiles that indicated a likelihood of significant psychologic distress requiring further evaluation by a relevant health professional (Carlson *et al* 2000). However, as a group BMD patients have shown no evidence for significant clinical depression, anxiety and somatization (Carlson *et al* 2000). Moreover BMD patients report fewer disruptions in normal activities as a result of their pain compared to other chronic pain patients (Carlson *et al* 2000). This suggests that although there are a minority of BMD patients with significant distress the vast majority cope better than most chronic pain patients (Carlson *et al* 2000). A further study on BMD patients revealed characteristics common among those with chronic pain conditions, including significantly higher adverse early life experiences than in healthy controls: depression, anxiety, cancer phobia, gastrointestinal problems and chronic fatigue (Lamey *et al* 2005).

Secondary BMD. Oral and perioral burning sensation accompanying local or systemic factors or diseases is classified as secondary BMD (SBMD) (Scala *et al* 2003). Local factors and diseases known to induce SBMD include oral candidiasis, galvanism, lichen planus, allergies, hyposalivation and xerostomia (Vitkov *et al* 2003). Systemic disorders known to induce SBMD include hormonal changes, nutritional abnormalities (e.g. vitamin B_{12}, folic acid or iron deficiencies), diabetes mellitus, drugs (directly or indirectly), autoimmune diseases and emotional stress (Scala *et al* 2003). Successful treatment aimed at the primary disease will usually (but not invariably) alleviate the burning sensation in SBMD patients (Danhauer *et al* 2002).

7.3. Pathophysiology

There are various regional and local phenomena that have been associated with idiopathic BMD; these include reduced parotid gland function (Lamey *et al* 2001) and altered salivary composition but not salivary flow rate reduction (Granot and Nagler 2005). BMD patients generally exhibit greater vasoreactivity, suggesting involvement of the autonomic nervous system (Heckmann *et al* 2001). Current evidence supports two main theories: a sensory neuropathy that may be peripheral and/or central or a disturbance in a balance between the gustatory and sensory systems.

Taste sensation of the anterior two-thirds of the tongue is supplied by the chorda tympani nerve, a branch of the facial nerve. Other sensory modalities such as mechanical and thermal sensations are supplied by the lingual nerve, a branch of the mandibular division of the trigeminal nerve. Inhibitory influences between the two systems are thought to maintain a 'sensory balance' in the tongue. Hypothetically, altered chorda tympani dysfunction can disrupt the equilibrium with the lingual nerve, leading to lingual nerve hyperfunction and burning sensation.

Data suggest that individuals who suffer from BMD are likely to be 'supertasters' (can taste the bitter compound phenylthiocarbamide) and have large numbers of fungiform papillae; these are innervated mostly (75%) by the trigeminal and partly (25%) by the chorda tympani nerve (Femiano 2004). BMD and supertasting may result from hyperactivity of the sensory component of the trigeminal nerve following loss of central inhibition as a result of damage to the chorda tympani (Grushka *et al* 2003; Femiano 2004). Indeed chorda tympani nerve hypofunction was demonstrated by employing the electrogustatory test in BMD patients (Eliav *et al* 2007). Sweet taste detection threshold is higher in BMD patients, suggesting altered taste sensation (Grushka and Sessle 1988). Topical anaesthetic applied to the tongue reduced dysgeusia but affected the pain component differentially; pain decreased, increased or remained unchanged in subgroups of cases (Formaker *et al* 1998). Furthermore, in a study on patients with BMD lower intensity ratings to salt and sweet stimuli were reported and are consistent with damage to the taste pathway (Formaker and Frank 2000). However, this was found in female but not in male subjects. Based on these accumulating data it has been suggested that BMD involves CNS and PNS pathologies induced by damage to the taste system at the level of the chorda tympani nerve (Bartoshuk *et al* 2005). This damage results in reduced inhibition of the trigeminal nerve that in turn leads to an intensified response to oral irritants and eventually to oral phantom pain. The exact mechanisms and interactions are, however, obscure and the evidence is unclear.

BMD as a sensory neuropathy is suggested by findings that sensory threshold in the tongue was significantly higher in patients than in controls. Sensory assessment in BMD patients revealed reduced thermal pain tolerance and elevated pain detection thresholds (Grushka *et al* 1987; Svensson *et al* 1993). BMD patients perceived significantly more pain from mechanical stimulation that lasted longer and was described more intricately than in controls (Ito *et al* 2002). Additionally, BMD cases have significantly elevated thermal sensory thresholds, decreased pain scores for tonic heat pain and an increased level of somatization (Granot and Nagler 2005). Taken together these data suggest the presence of sensory nerve damage and indicate strong affective/motivational components to BMD. BMD cases have a significantly lower density of epithelial nerve fibres in the anterior two-thirds of the tongue with some correlation with the duration of symptoms. Epithelial and subpapillary nerve fibres showed diffuse morphological changes reflecting axonal degeneration, suggesting a trigeminal small-fibre sensory neuropathy (Lauria *et al* 2005). Combining QST and blink reflex recordings in BMD patients suggests the existence of several diagnostic subgroups (Forssell *et al* 2002). About a fifth of patients may have trigeminal neuropathy or brainstem pathology and a further fifth had increased excitability of the blink reflex, with deficient habituation of one of its components. In about three-quarters of the patients one or more sensory thresholds were abnormal, most with hypoaesthesia, indicating neuronal dysfunction. Only 10% had normal findings in both tests. Altered blink reflex and/or thermal hypoaesthesia was found in 89% of BMD patients (Jaaskelainen *et al* 1997; Forssell *et al* 2002). Application of a local anaesthetic solution on a BMD patient's tongues reduced phantom dysgeusia but did not reduce the burning sensation and in 40% of cases the pain was aggravated (Formaker *et al* 1998; Formaker and Frank 2000).

Overall these changes reflect a regional small-fibre idiopathic neuropathy affecting sensory and autonomic pathways and resulting in both disturbed oral sensation and inconsistently altered salivary secretion in BMD. The findings support the definition of BMD as an oral dysaesthesia or neuropathic pain.

Central dysfunction of pain modulatory systems in BMD has been suggested. In BMD patients presynaptic dysfunction of the nigrostriatal dopaminergic system, involved in central pain modulation, has been shown by positron emission tomography (PET) (Hagelberg *et al*

2003). A recent functional imaging study suggests that hypoactivity of the thalamus and brain may be involved in BMD (Albuquerque *et al* 2006). The authors, however, advise caution in interpreting these findings in view of the small sample size and heterogeneity.

Physiological levels of oestrogens are neuroprotective in the nigrostriatal dopaminergic system so that their decline with menopause may partly explain the age and gender predilection of this disorder (Gajjar *et al* 2003). Moreover recent findings suggest that oestrogen receptors found in trigeminal neurons modulate nociceptive responses (Puri *et al* 2005) and may offer a valuable link in explaining the female preponderance observed in BMD patient populations.

7.4. Treatment

Management of patients with BMD is difficult; patients report seeing numerous clinicians and undergoing batteries of special tests in the search for an underlying but elusive physical cause. Although there is no one accepted treatment for BMD, this condition should be treated as a neuropathic pain.

Topical therapies may be useful particularly in elderly, medically compromised patients. Topical clonazepam (sucking and spitting 1mg three times daily for 2 weeks) was effective in reducing pain intensity only in a subgroup of BMD patients, with some carryover effect at 6 months (Gremeau-Richard *et al* 2004). Mouthwashes with 0.15% benzydamine or lactoperoxidase are ineffective in BMD patients (Sardella *et al* 1999; Femiano 2002b). Topical anaesthetics may decrease or increase pain so that this is not a predictable mode of therapy (Formaker *et al* 1998).

Reduction in pain following treatment with benzodiazepines, e.g. clonazepam and diazepam (Gorsky *et al* 1991; Grushka *et al* 1998; Woda *et al* 1998), or low-dose tricyclic antidepressants (Pinto *et al* 2003) appears as case reports. Multiple studies consistently demonstrate the prolonged benefit of a 2-month course of 600mg daily of alpha lipoic acid (e.g. Femiano and Scully 2002; Femiano *et al* 2004a); but these studies await replication and confirmation. Systemic capsaicin (0.25% capsule 3/d for 30 d) demonstrated beneficial effects on reducing BMD pain intensity (Petruzzi *et al* 2004). However, as the authors note, conclusions should be tempered by the facts that the sample size was small and the study duration short (Petruzzi *et al* 2004). Moreover significant gastric pain was reported by over 30% of cases. One single-blind study compared the atypical antipsychotic amisulpride to the selective serotonin reuptake inhibitors (SSRIs) paroxetine and sertraline (Maina *et al* 2002). The results suggest that all these may be equally effective treatments for BMD and confirm previous work on SSRIs (Van Houdenhove and Joostens 1995). However, amisulpride had a shorter response time and was associated with better compliance within the first week of treatment as compared to SSRIs. Therapy-resistant BMD has been associated with underlying psychological distress and these patients may particularly benefit from cognitive behavioural therapy (CBT) (Bergdahl *et al* 1995). CBT has been successfully supplemented with alpha lipoic acid (Femiano *et al* 2004b). Evidence-based management of BMD is therefore based on topical clonazepam, systemic SSRI, alpha lipoic acid and CBT. Widespread clinical practice for BMD and for neuropathic pains would support a trial for selected cases using topical therapies such as lidocaine, doxepin or capsaicin. Similarly systemic therapies would include TCAs, selective noradrenaline and serotonin reuptake inhibitors, anticonvulsants, opioids and benzodiazepines.

8. Traumatic Orofacial Neuropathies

8.1. Introduction

The lack of a comprehensive classification for neuropathic orofacial pain is particularly prominent in trigeminal post-traumatic neuropathies. Post-traumatic neuropathies may involve partial nerve injuries and are not always complete injuries. The current IHS classification only includes 'anaesthesia dolorosa', which insinuates a complete denervation injury (Olesen *et al* 2004). The AAOP lists post-traumatic and postsurgical trigeminal neuropathies in the differential diagnosis of NOP but there are no suggested working criteria (Okeson 1996). Peripheral traumatic trigeminal neuropathies are often accompanied by some form of sensory deficit or aberration and may be painful. Thus we suggest 'painful traumatic trigeminal neuropathy' when accompanied by pain and 'traumatic trigeminal neuropathy' when only sensory dysfunction is present.

Considering the number of surgical interventions performed by dentists the incidence of painful trigeminal traumatic neuropathies is either surprisingly low or largely undiagnosed. However, some patients develop and complain of chronic pain following negligible trauma such as root canal therapy or following considerable trauma such as fractures of the facial skeleton (Benoliel *et al* 2005; Polycarpou *et al* 2005). The lack of a consistent classification severely limits our ability to assess the typical clinical features and treatment responses across a wide range of published cases.

Various terms describing this entity abound in the literature; phantom tooth pain and atypical odontalgia or atypical facial pains are probably also traumatic neuropathies. Orofacial complex regional pain syndrome (CRPS) is a further post-traumatic entity whose occurrence in the orofacial region is unclear (see below).

Major trauma to branches of the trigeminal nerve may result in chronic pain. Chronic pain which continues following blunt macrotrauma (e.g. road traffic accidents) may be difficult to diagnose as there may be no tangible physical signs. The problem is confounded by the fact that the severity of the original injury may have no bearing on the

intensity of the resultant persistent pain, with significant disability occurring even after minor trauma. Moreover major trauma often induces more than one pain syndrome in the same patient (Benoliel *et al* 1994).

8.1.1. Epidemiology of Traumatic Trigeminal Neuropathies

Due to the lack of universally accepted criteria it is difficult to assess the incidence of pain or sensory loss after trigeminal injury. Following zygomatic complex fractures residual, mild hypoaesthesia of the infraorbital nerve is common but chronic neuropathic pain developed in only 1 out of 30 patients (3.3%) followed up for 6 months (Benoliel *et al* 2005). This compares with about 5–17% in other body regions (Macrae 2001; Beniczky *et al* 2005).

Following dental implant surgery 1–8% and following orthognathic surgery 5–30% of patients may remain with permanent sensory dysfunction but the incidence of chronic pain is unclear (Gregg 2000; Walton 2000; Cheung and Lo 2002). In the patient shown in Figs. 11.8A–C, chronic neuropathic pain occurred following nerve injury from dental implants. The left mental nerve region (marked by a black line in Fig. 11.8A) was hypoaesthetic to electrical and thermal stimuli, indicating frank nerve damage. The implants were impinging on the inferior alveolar nerve (Fig. 11.8B). Removal of the implants in this case (Fig. 11.8C) did not improve the paraesthesia or the pain.

Third molar extractions are associated with transient hypoaesthesia (Eliav and Gracely 1998; Barron *et al* 2004). Disturbed sensation may remain in the lingual or inferior alveolar nerve for varying periods and has been found in 0.3–1% of cases (Carmichael and McGowan 1992; Robinson and Smith 1996; Valmaseda-Castellon *et al* 2001). However, long-term follow-up (combined) of over 1900 cases failed to demonstrate any chronic neuropathic pain cases (Valmaseda-Castellon *et al* 2000; Berge 2002). Lingual nerve damage is rarer than inferior alveolar nerve injuries (Gomes *et al* 2005; Robert *et al* 2005; Queral-Godoy *et al* 2006) but may commonly occur in certain extraction techniques particularly with nerve retraction and may reach 4% (Fried *et al* 2001). Patient complaints of tongue dysaesthesia after injury may remain in a small group of patients (0.5%). This variably correlates with the presence of histologic chronic inflammation, suggesting that the use of anti-inflammatory agents may be beneficial at late stages (Fried *et al* 2001; Vora *et al* 2005).

Persistent pain after successful endodontics was found to occur in 3–13% of cases (Marbach *et al* 1982; Lobb *et al* 1996; Polycarpou *et al* 2005), whilst surgical endodontics resulted in chronic neuropathic pain in 5% of cases (Campbell *et al* 1990). Factors significantly associated with persistent pain were long duration of preoperative pain, marked symptomatology from the tooth, previous chronic pain problems or a history of painful treatment in the orofacial region, and female gender (Polycarpou

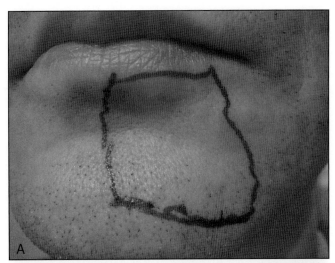
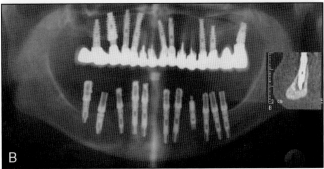
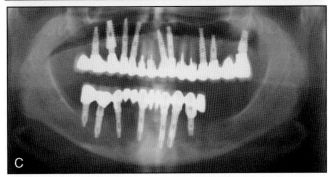

Fig. 11.8 • Pain and neurosensory deficit following dental implants. (A) Area of pain and disturbed sensation. (B) Initial implant placement. Inset is a CT section of an implant causing nerve damage. (C) Implants in the affected quadrant were removed but no change in pain or numbness was achieved.

et al 2005). The fact that preoperative pain parameters were important suggests that some form of sensitization may have occurred predisposing to chronic pain.

8.2. Clinical Features

Neural damage or disease can induce pain originating in a peripheral nerve (peripheral neuropathy), in a ganglion (ganglionopathy), in a dorsal root (radiculopathy) or from the CNS (central neuropathic pain). Probably the most common precipitating event is trauma, but infection (AIDs), metabolic abnormalities (diabetes), malnutrition, vascular abnormalities (trigeminal neuralgia), infarction (CPSP), neurotoxins, radiation and autoimmune disease

are also implicated. However, even following identical injuries onset of neuropathic pain and its characteristics vary from patient to patient. Such variability is probably due to a combination of environmental, psychosocial and genetic factors. A further consideration is that, relative to spinal nerves, the trigeminal nerve may show subtle differences in the pathophysiological events that may lead to pain (Benoliel *et al* 2001; Fried *et al* 2001). Most often in orofacial pain clinics, reported onset has a clear association with craniofacial or oral trauma (Benoliel *et al* 1994, 2005). However, pain may often begin following minor dental interventions (Polycarpou *et al* 2005).

Painful neuropathies often present with a clinical phenotype involving combinations of spontaneous and evoked pain and of positive (e.g. dysaesthesia) and negative symptomatology (e.g. numbness). Pain is of moderate to severe intensity and usually burning but may possess paroxysmal qualities. Pain is unilateral and may be precisely located to the dermatome of the affected nerve with demonstrable sensory dysfunction, particularly if a major nerve branch (e.g. infraorbital, inferior alveolar) has been injured. The pain may be diffuse and spread across dermatomes, but in our experience rarely if ever crosses the midline. Patients may complain of swelling or a feeling of swelling, foreign body, hot or cold, local redness or flushing. Based on the above we have compiled a preliminary set of criteria for painful traumatic trigeminal neuropathies; see Table 11.12. These may hopefully lead to discussion on a wide scale and the establishment of internationally accepted criteria.

8.3. Possible Syndromes of Painful Traumatic Trigeminal Neuropathy

8.3.1. Persistent Idiopathic Facial Pain (Previous Term: Atypical Facial Pain)

The original term, atypical facial pain (AFP), is a historical counterpart to the 'typical' presentation of trigeminal neuralgia. It is essentially employed when no other diagnosis is feasible and has therefore tended to include a heterogeneous group of patients. Some AFP cases have responded to triptans, suggesting migraine-like mechanisms (al Balawi *et al* 1996) whilst in another study they were ineffective (Harrison *et al* 1997). As knowledge and diagnostic skills accumulated many AFP cases were classified as chronic myofascial pain, traumatic neuropathy, pre- or atypical trigeminal neuralgia, facial migraine or neurovascular orofacial pain. It is likely that much of the collected data on AFP represents a neuropathic condition and many AFP patients demonstrate some degree of sensory dysfunction (Jaaskelainen *et al* 1999).

The latest IHS criteria for persistent idiopathic facial pain (PIFP) include the presence of daily or near daily pain that is initially confined but may subsequently spread. The pain is not associated with sensory loss and cannot be attributed to any other pathological process. This is a rather loose definition that has not been field-tested and may

Table 11.12	Proposed Diagnostic Criteria for Painful Traumatic Trigeminal Neuropathy	
	Diagnostic Criteria	**Notes**
A	Touch-evoked (stimulus-dependent) or spontaneous, paroxysmal pain affecting one or more divisions of the trigeminal nerve that: 1. Lasts from a fraction of a second to minutes. 2. Is constant (>8 h/d, >15 d/month).[a]	Pain is mostly unilateral and does not cross the midline. Paroxysmal pain may be described as electrical or stabbing. Constant pain is usually burning.
B	Develops within 3 months of a clear traumatic event to the painful area. Fulfils criteria C and E **or** D and E	Trauma, surgery, invasive dental treatment.
C	At least one clinically evident positive neuropathic sign: 1. Hyperalgesia 2. Allodynia 3. Swelling or flushing	Must be a constant feature and repeatable.
D	At least one demonstrable negative neurological deficit such as: 1. Anaesthesia 2. Hypoaesthesia	If area is amenable quantitative sensory testing will reveal deficits in the distribution of the trigeminal nerve.
E	Not attributed to another disorder.	Other causes are ruled out by history, physical examination and special investigations if necessary.

[a] Constant pain may also have superimposed episodes of paroxysmal pain.

misleadingly allow the classification of a large number of chronic facial pain disorders. Till specific data on PIFP accumulate we describe in brief the features of AFP.

8.3.1.1. Clinical Features

Pain is usually poorly localized, radiating and mostly unilateral although up to 40% of cases may describe bilateral pain (Mock *et al* 1985; Rasmussen 1990; Pfaffenrath *et al* 1993). AFP is commonly described as burning, throbbing and often stabbing (Melzack *et al* 1986; Pfaffenrath *et al* 1993). Severity is mild to severe and rated approximately 7 on a VAS (Agostoni *et al* 2005). Most patients report long-lasting (years) chronic daily pain although there have been reports of pain-free periods (Mock *et al* 1985; Rasmussen 1990; Pfaffenrath *et al* 1993). Pain onset is often associated with surgical or other invasive procedures (Pfaffenrath *et al* 1993). Although there should be no sensory deficits these have been reported in up to 60% of cases (Pfaffenrath *et al* 1993; Jaaskelainen *et al* 1999). The lack of a clear pathophysiological basis precludes the

establishment of a treatment protocol. The use of tricyclic antidepressants and anticonvulsants may be beneficial.

8.3.2. Atypical Odontalgia

The IASP has defined atypical odontalgia (AO) as a severe throbbing pain in the tooth without major pathology (Merskey and Bogduk 1994). The question whether AO is a neurovascular or neuropathic syndrome is the source of controversy and some consider AO a subentity of AFP. The incidence of pain that is pulsatile, episodic and migrating suggests that this may be a vascular-type pain (Brooke 1980; Graff-Radford and Solberg 1992). However, many AO cases present with neuropathic symptomatology such as continuous, burning pain and many report trauma as the initiating event. Indeed, AO has been referred to as phantom toothache, supporting a neuropathic aetiology (Marbach 1993). This has led most researchers to conclude that AO is a neuropathic syndrome (Schnurr and Brooke 1992; Vickers and Cousins 2000; Melis *et al* 2003; BaadHansen *et al* 2006).

It is possible that cases with neurovascular or other undiagnosed orofacial pain (see Chapter 9) metamorphose into and coexist with trigeminal neuropathy as a result of nerve injury from repeated dental interventions aimed at pain relief. This theory is supported by findings that chronic orofacial pain patients undergo extensive but often misguided surgical interventions (Israel *et al* 2003; Merrill 2004). A history of previous regional invasive procedures was found in 38 of 120 patients (32%). Procedures performed included endodontics (30%), extractions (27%), apicoectomies (12%), temporomandibular joint (TMJ) surgery (6%), neurolysis (5%), orthognathic surgery (3%) and debridement of bone cavities (2%). Surgical intervention clearly exacerbated pain in 21 of 38 patients (55%) who had undergone surgery. However, a multidisciplinary group of experts diagnosed these cases as myofascial pain (50%), atypical facial neuralgia (40%), TMJ synovitis (14%), TMJ osteoarthritis (12%), trigeminal neuralgia (10%) and TMJ fibrosis (2%) with many having more than one diagnosis (Israel *et al* 2003). Gross misdiagnosis leading to serious sequelae and delay of necessary treatment occurred in 6 of 120 patients (5%) (Israel *et al* 2003).

8.3.3. Complex Regional Pain Syndrome

Complex regional pain syndrome (CRPS) has been previously termed sympathetically maintained pain, reflex sympathetic dystrophy or causalgia. These early terms were based on observations of the clinical phenotype that often suggested involvement of the sympathetic nervous system. However, the link between nociceptive neurons and postganglionic sympathetic activity is inconstant, with sympathetic blocks sometimes altering the syndrome at least temporarily and sometimes not (Stanton-Hicks 2003). Adrenergic mechanisms in some form do appear to be involved in some of these conditions but measurements of sympathetic responses have often shown normal results (Janig and Baron 2003, 2004). The current terminology attempts to solve these issues and is not suggestive of suspected aetiologic mechanisms.

CRPSs are painful disorders that develop as a consequence of injury. Two subtypes have been defined by the IASP (see Table 11.13): CRPS I, previously reflex sympathetic dystrophy, and CRPS II, previously causalgia (Merskey and Bogduk 1994). Both these entities present with spontaneous pain accompanied by allodynia and hyperalgesia that are not limited to dermatomal regions (Janig and Baron 2004). Additional signs include oedema, abnormal blood flow in the skin and abnormal sudomotor activity. CRPS I may develop as a consequence of remote trauma or after relatively minor local trauma such as sprains or surgery. These result in minor or no identifiable nerve lesion with disproportionate pain. The less frequent form, CRPS II, is characterized by a substantiated injury to a major nerve and is therefore a neuropathic pain syndrome by definition. In both of these syndromes there may be clinical evidence to support the involvement of the sympathetic nervous system in which case the term 'sympathetically maintained pain' is added. This is not, however, a prerequisite for the diagnosis of CRPS.

8.3.3.1. Clinical Features

Pain and sensory disturbances. Pain is usually of a burning or pricking character felt deep within the most distal part of the affected limb (Baron and Wasner 2001). Three-quarters of patients will describe pain at rest, and movement or joint pressure will elicit or worsen pain (Birklein 2005). Reduced sensitivity to thermal and mechanical stimuli is usually present and may spread to involve the adjacent body quadrant or even half of the body, suggesting central sensitization (Rommel et al 2001). These patients usually suffer more severe pain and longer illness duration than patients with localized sensory abnormalities (Thimineur et al 1998; Rommel et al 2001). Hyperalgesia to cold is more common in CRPS II patients (Birklein 2005). Other sensory abnormalities include allodynia and hyperalgesia not restricted to nerve territories (Sieweke et al 1999; Maleki et al 2000). Paraesthesias are rare but about one-third will complain of a foreign, neglect-type feeling in the affected limb (Galer and Jensen 1999).

Motor signs. Weakness of the affected site is observed in over three-quarters of patients and may initially be due to guarding behaviour (Birklein 2005). Contraction and fibrosis may be seen and tremor occurs in up to half of cases (Birklein 2005). In CRPS II focal dystonia (abnormal muscle tone) or myoclonus (involuntary muscle contraction) may be observed.

Autonomic signs. During the acute stage over 80% have oedema and there is cutaneous vasodilatation with the skin appearing red (Birklein 2005). In the chronic stages this may subsequently reverse into vasoconstriction resulting in cold bluish skin (Wasner et al 2002). Differences in skin temperature at any stage will usually be >1 °C. Increased sweating is observed in over half of cases.

Other changes. Trophic phenomena affect about half of patients. Over time atrophic changes appear in skin, nails and muscles.

Treatment. Therapy should be aimed at restoration of function and reduction of pain. Depending on the disease stage and symptomatology steroids and sympathetic blocks may be indicated. Antidepressants and anticonvulsants may relieve neuropathic pain components and opioids should be tried if these fail (Birklein 2005).

8.3.3.2. CRPS in the Orofacial Region

The historical dependence on sympathetic involvement for the diagnosis of CRPS has probably prevented the identification and documentation of head and neck cases. Thus the cases reported have relied on cervical sympathectomy, clonidine, guanethidine and stellate ganglion blockade to confirm CRPS (Melis et al 2002). The IASP criteria would probably allow a large number of post-traumatic orofacial pain patients to be diagnosed as CRPS. However, some of the criteria listed in Table 11.13 are rarely if ever observed in post-traumatic orofacial pain. For example, trophic changes and atrophy of skin are unreported in the trigeminal region and motor disturbances are rare. The other criteria listed are distinctly similar to those described in atypical facial pain, atypical odontalgia and clear post-trauma cases. The particular

Table 11.13 Complex Regional Pain Syndrome (CRPS)

Criterion	CRPS I	CRPS II
Initiating mechanism	Noxious event	
Nerve lesion	None demonstrable	Demonstrable
Location	Distal aspect of the affected extremity	
Distribution	Not limited to dermatome of single nerve	
Pain	Spontaneous, burning	
Sensory phenomena	Hyperalgesia and allodynia not limited to nerve territory	
Motor signs	Impaired motor function / Tremor	
Autonomic signs	Skin blood flow changes / Oedema / Sudomotor abnormalities	
Exacerbated	Movement, touch, stress	
Associated signs	Initial trophic changes / Atrophy of skin and nails / Guarding behaviour	
Others	No other diagnosis reasonable	

Data from Merskey and Bogduk (1994) and Birklein (2005).

clinical phenotype may reflect the trigeminal system's differential response to trauma (Fried *et al* 2001).

8.4. Pathophysiology of Painful Traumatic Neuropathies

The pathophysiology of painful inflammatory or traumatic neuropathies involves a cascade of events in nervous system function. These events include alterations in functional, biochemical and physical characteristics, collectively termed neuronal plasticity. The events occurring after nerve injury that may lead to chronic pain are the focus of ongoing research and have been reviewed (Woolf and Salter 2000; Ji and Woolf 2001; Julius and Basbaum 2001; Scholz and Woolf 2002; Devor 2005).

In the subsequent section we examine various selected aspects of these events; see also Chapter 2. Inflammation at sites of injury is the first event that triggers the onset of neuronal changes and may be the initiating factor in many painful neuropathies. The establishment of ectopic activity probably underlies the presence of spontaneous pain and increased mechanical sensitivity in inflammatory and traumatic neuropathic syndromes. Phenotypic changes in Aβ mechanoreceptors endow them with properties of nociceptors such that peripheral innocuous stimuli are interpreted

centrally as pain, thus leading to the clinical complaint of allodynia. The sympathetic nervous system modulates pain and in traumatic neuropathies interacts with sensory neurons and their cell bodies to increase nerve sensitivity and pain. These peripheral events are accompanied or followed by changes in the CNS that serve to perpetuate chronic pain. More recently the roles of central glial cells and peripheral satellite glia have been recognized as active in chronic pain conditions. These events are overviewed below (see also Fig. 11.9).

8.4.1. Tissue Injury and Inflammation

The 'inflammatory soup' is a mixture of bioactive molecules produced in response to a variety of stimuli and tissue injury that may directly activate or indirectly sensitize nociceptors (see also Chapter 15). In consequence nociceptors display altered activity that may be spontaneous (i.e. not stimulus-induced) or as a response to normally subthreshold stimuli, i.e. increased sensitivity. These changes are reversible and are mediated by surface receptors on neurons. This change in receptor sensitivity, called peripheral sensitization, which may manifest as hyperalgesia (increased pain to a normally painful stimulus) and/or allodynia (ordinarily nonpainful stimuli

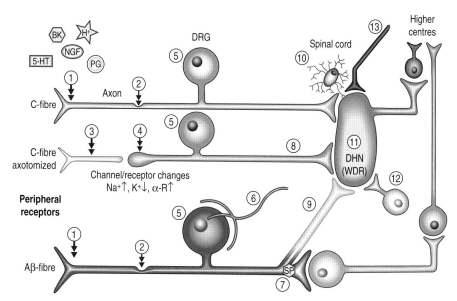

Fig. 11.9 • Peripheral and central nervous system changes in chronic pain. Peripheral sensitization: Tissue damage (1) releases inflammatory mediators, e.g. bradykinin (BK), nerve growth factor (NGF), serotonin (5-HT), prostaglandins (PG) and protons (H+). This 'inflammatory soup' of bioactive molecules induces increased sensitivity of peripheral nociceptors leading to allodynia and hyperalgesia. Axonal injury (2), e.g. transection, crush or chronic pressure and inflammation induce increases in sodium (Na+) and α-adrenoreceptors (α-R), initiating ectopic activity and increased sensitivity. Axotomy results in death of the distal part of the nerve (3) and if the proximal section survives there is healing with neuroma formation (4). Some of the neurons will, however, die. This activity leads to altered gene expression in the neuronal cell bodies located in the ganglia (DRG) (5). Nerve injury may lead to sympathetic nerve fibre sprouting (6), particularly around the larger DRG cells. The modulating effects of satellite glial cells in DRGs have recently been demonstrated. Aβ fibres undergo a phenotypic change (7) and express neurotransmitters associated with nociceptors, e.g. substance P (SP). Injury-induced C-fibre degeneration (8) may result, allowing Aβ fibres to sprout from deep to superficial dorsal horn layers (9), augmenting allodynia. Primary afferents and dorsal horn neurons activate glial cells in the dorsal horn (10), and these compromise opioid analgesia, enhance dorsal-horn-neuron and primary afferent activity and excitability. Persistent nociceptive input results in the sensitization of wide dynamic range (WDR) dorsal horn neurons (DHN; 11), excitation of adjacent neurons (central sensitization) and activation of glial cells. Glutamate-induced excitotoxicity reduces the number of inhibitory interneurons, augmenting excitation (12). Persistent pain initiates descending modulation, which in pathological states tends towards facilitation (13).

induce pain) develops rapidly. For example, pain in irreversible pulpitis is spontaneous and application of cold, normally mildly painful, now induces extreme pain (hyperalgesia). Tooth sensitivity to percussion seen in periapical periodontitis is an example of allodynia.

The importance of inflammation following nerve injury in the initiation of neuropathic pain has become apparent (Eliav et al 1999; Benoliel et al 2002a; Watkins and Maier 2002). In the trigeminal system, structures often lie within closed spaces (e.g. inferior alveolar canal) and pressure build-up secondary to inflammation may induce frank nerve damage (Benoliel et al 2002a). This would support aggressive treatment of inflammation affecting the trigeminal nerve.

8.4.2. Nerve Injury, Inflammation and Ectopic Activity

Following traumatic tissue damage an inflammatory response is initiated, crucial to the onset of neuropathic pain. Even perineural inflammation with no axonal nerve damage of the nerve trunk elevates spontaneous activity (usually observed only after nerve injury) and induces mechanosensitivity in myelinated axons (Eliav et al 2001). Thus the sole presence of inflammation can induce ectopic activity and spontaneous pain.

If, as a consequence of trauma, neuronal tissue is severely injured (e.g. transection), cell death may be induced. However, if the proximal stump survives, healing involves disorganized sprouting of nerve fibres that form a neuroma (Fried et al 2001). Neuroma formation is often dependent on the degree of nerve damage and always occurs when the perineurium is cut, whilst an intact perineurium (as in crush injuries) may permit improved healing. However, milder injuries such as nerve constriction or compression may also cause regions of neuroma formation and focal demyelination. These regions are characterized by ectopic discharge, partially caused by upregulation of specific sodium and calcium channels and downregulation of potassium channels (Fried et al 2001). Ectopic activity is also seen in the cell bodies of injured nerves in the dorsal root or trigeminal ganglia. These phenomena partly explain spontaneous neuropathic pain. Additionally, ectopic activity in neuromas is enhanced by mechanical and chemical stimulation; thus pain is experienced when neuromas are touched. Experimentally, trigeminal nerve neuromas (in myelinated and unmyelinated axons) are less active than sciatic nerve neuromas (Tal and Devor 1992). Similarly, mechanosensitivity and acute injury discharge in trigeminal neuromas were minimal, suggesting relative resistance of the trigeminal nerve to trauma-induced hyperactivity.

8.4.3. Phenotypic Changes

Neuropeptide expression is altered in the trigeminal ganglion following nerve injury and suggests functional modification. For example, Aβ fibres usually transmit innocuous stimuli, but catalyzed by inflammation or injury a phenotypic change results in the expression of substance P. Thus Aβ fibres acquire the ability to induce painful sensations in response to peripheral stimulation and may underlie the phenomenon of allodynia.

8.4.4. Novel Sensitivity to Catecholamines

Patients may report increased pain during periods of stress or anxiety that are characterized by increased sympathetic activity. This may be due to upregulation of α-adrenoreceptors in the dorsal root ganglion and the site of injury that induce sensitivity to circulating catecholamines. Additionally, basket-like sprouting of sympathetic fibres occurs around the neuronal cell bodies within the dorsal root ganglion, augmenting sensory–sympathetic interactions. This phenomenon has not, however, been experimentally detected in the trigeminal ganglion and may explain the relative rarity of sympathetically maintained craniofacial pain (Benoliel et al 2001).

8.4.5. Central Changes

Central changes or plasticity are triggered by the barrage of activity from primary afferents transmitted to dorsal horn neurons (DHNs). Repeated primary nociceptive afferent input increasingly depolarizes DHNs, resulting in amplified responses, a phenomenon termed 'wind up'. Prolonged DHN depolarization ultimately results in the phosphorylation and sensitization of the N-methyl D-aspartate (NMDA) receptor (NMDAr), a calcium channel normally blocked by a magnesium ion. NMDAr activation removes the magnesium ion plug and allows calcium ions into the DHN, initiating a variety of intracellular events. Although NMDAr activation will not elicit nociception of itself, it will enhance neuronal excitability; its activation is thought important in the establishment of central sensitization. In addition to the NMDAr, other calcium channels (L-, P- and N-type) are activated by repeated pain stimuli leading to increases in intracellular calcium and DHN hypersensitivity (Salter 2005). DHN hypersensitivity manifests as hypersensitivity and/or allodynia.

Hypersensitivity may induce activation of adjacent DHNs, directly (possibly by diffusion of neurotransmitters) and by the unmasking of silent inter-DHN connections. This increases the receptive field so that pain is felt in areas not normally innervated by the involved peripheral nerve. Clinically, sensitivity of uninjured areas in the vicinity of the injury is detectable; this is termed secondary hyperalgesia. In a patient suffering from severe facial pain (e.g. irreversible pulpitis), these changes account for increased pain and its spread to adjacent structures of the face. The early changes in neuronal excitability are activity-dependent and are thus amenable to therapy by controlling peripheral nociceptive input. However, with continuing stimuli, long-term changes are initiated in the DRG and DHNs; these changes involve modified gene expression and transcription, as well as downregulation of repressor mechanisms, resulting in further excitability.

Some months following nerve injury neuronal death is observed, mainly in C fibres. Withdrawal of injured C-fibre terminals from lamina I/II may allow sprouting of Aβ fibres from deeper lamina, augmenting pain induced by light touch; however, the occurrence of Aβ sprouting has been questioned (Sah *et al* 2003). Nerve injury may also cause structural changes in the dorsal horn; excitotoxic cell death is thought to deplete inhibitory interneurons and increase pain, although this does not seem necessary to allow development of persistent pain (Polgar *et al* 2005). Supraspinal modification of peripheral signals is an essential part of balanced nociception and in inflammatory or neuropathic pain states there is evidence for decreased inhibition with increased facilitation.

The above events show how the progressive malfunctioning of the nervous system establishes conditions for chronic pain and increases the difficulty of therapeutic interventions.

8.4.6. Glial Cells, Satellite Glial Cells and Pain

Recent research implicates spinal cord glial cells in the initiation and maintenance of chronic pain. Glia express receptors and transporter proteins for many neurotransmitters, so they are well equipped to participate in pain modulation (Watkins *et al* 2007). In response to neuronal signals glia are able to release excitatory molecules, including proinflammatory cytokines, glutamate, nitric oxide and prostaglandins, which enhance DHN hyperexcitability and neurotransmitter release from primary afferents (Watkins *et al* 2007). More recently glia have been shown to compromise the efficacy of opioid analgesia (Watkins *et al* 2007).

Glial cell activation does not change normal responses to acute pain, but it interferes with pathological pain. Bacteria and viruses also activate glial cells; this may explain the pain and allodynia often associated with some systemic infections (e.g. acquired immunodeficiency syndrome; see Chapter 14). The possible involvement of glial cells in the initiation and maintenance of chronic neuropathic pain has recently been reviewed (Watkins *et al* 2007). Because glial cells are involved in pathological pain but not in acute nociceptive responses, they are an attractive future therapeutic target.

In a similar fashion, peripherally situated satellite glial cells (in sensory ganglia such as trigeminal ganglion) are thought to be able to interact with neurons and may play a role in changes following nerve injury (Hanani 2005; Dublin and Hanani 2007).

8.4.7. Syndrome-Specific Mechanisms

8.4.7.1. Macrotrauma to the Head and Face
Peripheral nerve injury has been implicated in posttraumatic headache and facial pain. This may take the form of paroxysmal neuralgic-type pain or the chronic deafferentation-type (burning) pain seen in other nerve injuries. Nerve entrapment in scar tissue or direct nerve injury with aberrant regeneration and abnormal nerve activity due to neuroma formation as seen in other traumatic neuropathic conditions may be the peripheral pathological basis.

Early direct CNS mechanisms are also possibly involved; following relatively minor head trauma progressive and extensive axonal injury due to widespread shearing occurs and is commonly known as diffuse axonal injury; see also Chapter 13 (Inglese *et al* 2005; Povlishock and Katz 2005).

8.4.7.2. Pathophysiology of CRPS
In addition to the sequence of events described earlier that follow nerve injury, research has suggested particular processes are important in CRPS. Neurogenic inflammation can explain the presence of oedema, increased blood flow and skin temperature and the early trophic changes observed. Evidence exists for upregulated neuropeptide release and their impaired inactivation (exaggerated response) in CRPS patients (Birklein 2005). Concomitant release of neuropeptides centrally would induce sensitization. The effect of sympathetic blocks in some CRPS patients suggests involvement of the sympathetic nervous system; this may be based on adrenoreceptor upregulation and/or sensory sympathetic coupling in DRG (see above). Genetic susceptibility may explain why some patients develop CRPS whilst others do not (van de Beek *et al* 2003).

8.5. Treatment of Painful Traumatic Trigeminal Neuropathies

The inescapable progression of events after nerve or extensive tissue damage suggests that intervention is most effective within a specific time frame. Prevention is a primary objective but is not always attainable so early treatment is essential.

8.5.1. Strategies for Preventing Neuropathic Pain

Preemptive analgesia is a strategy whereby preoperative treatment is designed to prevent central sensitization. Success in preventing the injury-associated afferent barrage and resultant central sensitization by using local anaesthetic blocks during surgery, although theoretically well based, has been inconsistent. Indeed, the whole area of preemptive analgesia has not as yet produced significantly better pain management on a wide scale. The use of epidural local anaesthetics or morphine has been unsuccessful in the prevention of postamputation stump pain (Woolf and Chong 1993; Woolf and Mannion 1999). The lack of success may be partly a result of weak study design, including inadequate management of the initial sensory barrage and insufficient treatment duration (Kelly *et al* 2001a,b). Some strategies, however, seem to be beneficial. The use of preoperative anaesthetic blocks has resulted in less postoperative pain compared with no local anaesthesia at all, but no protocol has as yet received wide acceptance (Kelly *et al* 2001a,b).

8.5.2. Strategies for Established Painful Traumatic Trigeminal Neuropathies

The available evidence confirms that the mainstays of NP treatment remain the AEDs and the TCAs; see Chapter 16 (Finnerup *et al* 2005). The usual endpoint in drug trials has generally been a 50% reduction in pain intensity (Sindrup and Jensen 2001). However, research has shown that about a 30% reduction represents meaningful pain relief for NP patients (Farrar *et al* 2001).

The role of surgery in the management of traumatic trigeminal neuropathies is unclear. In our clinical experience most cases that have undergone peripheral surgical procedures for traumatic trigeminal neuropathy have ended up with *more* pain. The literature reveals that some cases have been treated with peripheral glycerol injections with some success but we have found no prospective controlled trials. Thus we advise patients not to undergo further surgery, but this has not been rigorously tested. We found no prospective trials in the literature on central procedures aimed at the trigeminal ganglion or the DREZ for the treatment of such cases. Anecdotal evidence suggests that central procedures may be useful for recalcitrant cases (Abdennebi *et al* 1993). In a mixed group of patients with craniofacial pain, some with post-traumatic neuropathic pain, DREZ operations were reported to significantly alleviate symptoms; 67% rated relief as good to excellent after one year (Bullard and Nashold 1997). In 17 patients with intractable atypical facial pain who underwent neurosurgical procedures, 16 enjoyed moderate to good improvement in pain control (Kanpolat *et al* 2005). The authors suggest that the primary choice of operation should be minimally invasive, such as a trigeminal tractotomy–nucleotomy. Trigeminal DREZ operation, which affects a larger area, may subsequently be performed for failures (Kanpolat *et al* 2005).

AEDs for the treatment of painful neuropathies exhibit varied NNTs (Wiffen *et al* 2005a). Phenytoin (NNT=2) is superior to both carbamazepine (NNT=3.3) and gabapentin (NNT=3.8), but as a group AEDs are inferior to the TCAs in the management of painful polyneuropathies (Sindrup and Jensen 2001). For trigeminal neuralgia, however, anticonvulsants remain the drugs of choice, particularly carbamazepine with an NNT for substantial relief of 2.6 (Sindrup and Jensen 2001; Wiffen *et al* 2005a). Based on the efficacy of pregabalin and gabapentin in peripheral neuropathies (PHN or diabetic neuropathy) they may also be good treatment options in traumatic neuropathy.

Analgesic trials with TCAs reveal that drugs with mixed serotonin/noradrenaline (e.g. imipramine and amitriptyline) or specific noradrenaline reuptake inhibition

(e.g. nortriptyline) are superior to the SSRIs, such as fluoxetine or paroxetine (Saarto and Wiffen 2005). Calculations of the NNT show that TCAs such as amitriptyline benefit approximately every other patient (NNT=2.2) suffering from painful polyneuropathies (Beniczky *et al* 2005). With careful dose titration, an NNT of 1.4 for imipramine may be attained in the treatment of traumatic neuropathies (Sindrup and Jensen 2001). In contrast, SSRIs have an NNT of 7 in painful polyneuropathies. Venlafaxine has an NNT of around 4 for painful polyneuropathy and duloxetine has an NNT of 4.1 for diabetic neuropathy; both have fewer side effects than the TCAs and may be attractive alternatives; see Chapter 16 (Finnerup *et al* 2005).

The Na channel-blocking agent mexiletine may be useful in traumatic neuropathies (NNT 2.2 (1.3–8.7)) but has been largely ineffective in other neuropathic pains (Finnerup *et al* 2005).

Based on a large literature review and on our clinical experience TCAs or gabapentin/pregabalin would be the first drugs indicated in peripheral neuropathy (Fig. 11.10) (Finnerup *et al* 2005). The excellent NNTs for TCAs are counterbalanced by the better side effect profile of the newer anticonvulsants. This is particularly important since response in NP is dose dependent. In patients initiated on amitriptyline with problematic side effects imipramine, desipramine or venlafaxine should be tried. If these fail or are contraindicated the anticonvulsants gabapentin and pregabalin offer the best chances for success. Similarly in patients started on gabapentin, treatment failure is an indication for a trial of TCAs. Alternatively if TCAs or gabapentin are only partly successful, combination therapy with their counterparts should be considered, e.g. venlafaxine and gabapentin, gabapentin and morphine; see below (Finnerup *et al* 2005). Third-line monotherapy or add-on therapy may be attained with opioids or tramadol. Based on their efficacy in PHN and diabetic neuropathy, newer agents such as pregabalin and duloxetine may prove useful and are discussed in Chapter 16.

8.5.2.1. Combination Therapies

Therapy of neuropathic pain with any one of the established drug groups (TCAs, anticonvulsants, opioids) leads to improved quality of life, sleep and improved mood. However, these results are directly related to the primary endpoint, which is significant pain relief. Pain intensity is reduced by 20–40% in only a subset of responders and is usually accompanied by significant side effects, particularly at the higher doses often required in neuropathic pain (McQuay *et al* 1996; Duhmke *et al* 2004; Rowbotham *et al* 2004; Eisenberg *et al* 2005). Neuropathic pain (e.g. PHN, post-traumatic) involves multiple mechanisms at various sites with a complex interaction between them. Theoretically the use of drugs with different modes and sites of action may lead to improved efficacy with reduced side effects. This combination approach to neuropathic pain

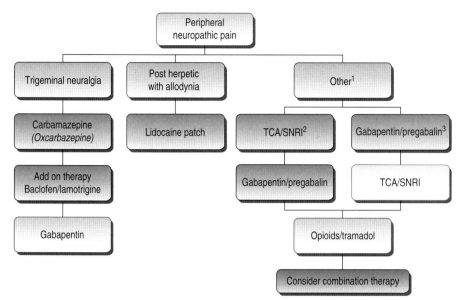

Fig. 11.10 • Treatment algorithm for peripheral neuropathic pain. (1) The choice between tricyclic antidepressants (TCAs) or selective noradrenaline reuptake inhibitors (SNRIs) versus the use of gabapentin (GBP) or pregabalin (PGB) is based on the medical profile and other patient-based variables (profession, comorbidities). TCAs are more effective than GBP/PGB but have significantly more side effects. (2) SNRIs have not been as extensively tested as TCAs but seem less effective for neuropathic pain. (3) Patients initiated on GBP or PGB but not responding to treatment may not be medically suitable for second-line therapy with TCAs/SNRIs. In these cases the patient is transferred directly to opioids singly or together with GBP.

Data from Dubinsky et al (2004), Finnerup et al (2005) and Wiffen et al (2005a,b), that on combination therapies from Simpson (2001) and Gilron et al (2005).

although not well based on scientific evidence seems common clinical practice but scarce clinical data have been published. The combination of gabapentin and morphine produced significant analgesia in patients with neuropathic pain (PHN and diabetic neuropathy) at a dose lower than that of each drug separately (Gilron *et al* 2005). In patients with painful diabetic neuropathy who did not respond to gabapentin monotherapy, the addition of venlafaxine in a double-blind fashion resulted in significant pain improvement (Simpson 2001).

In summary the data presented above emphasize that there are no universally effective therapies; some patients will respond and others will not. Nonresponders may, however, respond to another drug, a different drug class or combinations.

8.5.3. Specific Targets for the Treatment of Neuropathic Pain

Based on their sensitivity to tetrodotoxin (TTX), Na channels have been subclassified as TTX-resistant or TTX-sensitive. Upregulation of a TTX-sensitive Na channel after nerve injury makes this an attractive molecular target (Black *et al* 2001). Indeed many of the drugs successful with neuropathic pain (TCAs, AEDs) have significant Na channel-blocking properties (see Chapter 16). Surprisingly, however, the available drugs that have largely Na channel-blocking properties (local anaesthetics such as lidocaine and antiarrhythmics such as mexiletine) are inefficient in the treatment of neuropathic pain. Initial clinical trials on the successful effects of TTX in the treatment of opioid-resistant cancer pain have been reported (Nitu *et al* 2003), but severe nausea and facial paraesthesia were reported. Concomitant advances in pharmaceuticals and molecular characterization of pain-specific Na channels along the neuraxis may result in the production of attractive drugs for neuropathic pain.

Animal studies have established the important role of the NMDA receptor in the induction and maintenance of neuropathic pain. Most of the available NMDA antagonists have severe clinical side effects that preclude their routine use. The NMDAr is made up of a number of subunits; amongst these the NR2B has been successfully blocked, leading to neuroprotection and antiallodynic effects with fewer side effects (Chizh *et al* 2001). NMDAr activation requires the presence of glycine that binds to a specific site on the receptor. An attractive approach with fewer side effects has been to try and block the glycine site, thus reducing NMDAr activation (Leeson and Iversen 1994). Similarly the development of specific Ca channel modulators shows promise in the management of NP (Dickinson *et al* 2003).

The input from primary afferents to DHNs triggers intracellular signalling cascades, which increase spinal cord excitability. The cascade begins with neurotransmitter–receptor interactions and involves a number of intracellular molecules. Molecular targeting may be a novel strategy for the treatment of neuropathic pain (Ji and Woolf 2001). One such intracellular molecule, protein kinase C, plays an important role in receptor modification and in the regulation of injury-induced pain hypersensitivity (Basbaum 1999). Mice that lack an isoform of protein kinase C display intact nociceptive pain responses but experience reduced pain from a neuropathic or inflammatory insult. Such a molecular target would leave good pain and abolish bad pain. The actions of cholecystokinin, an excitatory modulator of pain, on its receptor are antagonized by the drugs proglumide and devazepide. In clinical trials, these drugs have proved beneficial in the management of chronic pain with mild side effects (taste impairment with proglumide) (Nitu *et al* 2003).

Another novel approach may be to interfere with the phenotypic changes and dorsal horn reorganization after nerve injury via intrathecal application of various neurotrophins (Hunt and Mantyh 2001). Recombinant nerve growth factor is in clinical trials for the control of painful neuropathies associated with diabetes and sensory neuropathies associated with AIDS (Nitu *et al* 2003; Sah *et al* 2003).

9. Neuropathy Secondary to Neuritis

The involvement of inflammation in various neuropathic pain syndromes has been increasingly recognized. Neuritis is defined as inflammation of nerve or nerves. Several animal models demonstrated that perineural inflammation along the nerve trunk can produce pain and aberrant sensations in the nerve distal end even in the absence of frank axonal damage (Eliav *et al* 1999; Chacur *et al* 2001; Benoliel *et al* 2002b). In other words, inflammation anywhere along a nerve can be a source of pain in the organ supplied by the nerve. Inflammation may affect the nerve either by direct pressure induced by the accompanying oedema or via mediator secretion (mainly cytokines) (DeLeo *et al* 1997; Zelenka *et al* 2005). Both processes can induce nerve damage if allowed to persist (Eliav *et al* 2004a). Additional studies have characterized the symptoms accompanying this condition and revealed tactile allodynia with a dominant role for myelinated nerve fibres (Neumann *et al* 1996; Eliav *et al* 2004b).

The term neuritis is often used in the medical literature with no apparent evidence of inflammation, but with signs and symptoms that may suggest neural inflammation. Treatment with anti-inflammatory medication such as steroids can be beneficial since perineural and neural inflammation have a role in most of the neuronal pathologies and may accompany various conditions such as trauma, infection, malignancy or autoimmune conditions. The term peripheral neuritis was used commonly to describe generalized neuropathies related to chemical poisoning, autoimmunity and alcohol and nutritional deficiencies that may have an inflammatory component. At present neuritis is used to describe localized nerve pathologies secondary to inflammation. Optic neuritis is inflammation or demyelination of the optic nerve and is also known as retrobulbar neuritis. It has been estimated that about 55% of people with MS will have at least one episode of optic neuritis, frequently as the first symptom. Optic neuritis is generally experienced as an acute blurring, greying or loss of vision, most often in only one eye and may be accompanied by pain. Loss of vision usually reaches its maximum extent within a few days, and generally improves within 4–12 weeks without treatment (Arnold 2005; Balcer 2006). Vestibular neuritis, thought to be a viral infection of the vestibular nerve, is a disorder of the vestibular system without an associated auditory deficit or other CNS disease. Unilateral disease may induce vertigo (Strupp and Brandt 1999).

In the orofacial region, dental and other invasive procedures can generate temporary perineural inflammation, usually asymptomatic. However, misplaced implants or periapical inflammation can produce chronic symptoms. Other conditions such as temporomandibular joint pathologies (Eliav *et al* 2003), paranasal sinusitis (Benoliel *et al* 2006) or even malignancies (Eliav *et al* 2002) can induce symptomatic perineural inflammation, pain and other aberrant sensations.

The involvement of inflammation in a clinical painful neuropathy is a clear indication for anti-inflammatory therapy. In mild cases or in cases where surgical or endodontic therapy is planned to further relieve inflammation we use standard NSAIDs (for example, ibuprofen 400mg tds, diclofenac 100mg 1/d, etodolac 400mg tds, etrocoxib 120 mg/d). Severe cases with marked pain and/or sensory changes, or in milder cases where adjuvant therapy is impractical the use of steroids may be warranted (prednisone 40–60mg initially then tapered over 7–10 days, dexamethasone 12mg initially then similarly tapered).

Acknowledgements

We thank Professors Marshal Devor and Michael Tal for their input in the preparation of this chapter.

References

Abdennebi B, Bouatta F, Bougatene B (1993) [Nucleotomy of the spinal trigeminal nucleus. Apropos of 2 post-traumatic neuralgia with surgical treatment]. *Neurochirurgie* **39**(4): 231–234.

Agostoni E, Frigerio R, Santoro P (2005) Atypical facial pain: clinical considerations and differential diagnosis. *Neurol Sci* **26**(Suppl 2):S71–S74.

al Balawi S, Tariq M, Feinmann C (1996) A double-blind, placebo-controlled, crossover study to evaluate the efficacy of subcutaneous sumatriptan in the treatment of atypical facial pain. *Int J Neurosci* **86**(3–4):301–309.

Alberca R, Ochoa JJ (1994) Cluster tic syndrome. *Neurology* **44**(6): 996–999.

Albuquerque RJ, de Leeuw R, Carlson CR, *et al* (2006) Cerebral activation during thermal stimulation of patients who have burning mouth disorder: an fMRI study. *Pain* **122**(3): 223–234.

Al Quran FA (2004) Psychological profile in burning mouth syndrome. *Oral Surg Oral Med Oral Pathol Oral Radiol Endod* **97**(3):339–344.

Amir R, Devor M (2000) Functional cross-excitation between afferent A- and C-neurons in dorsal root ganglia. *Neuroscience* **95**(1):189–195.

Amir R, Michaelis M, Devor M (1999) Membrane potential oscillations in dorsal root ganglion neurons: role in normal electrogenesis and neuropathic pain. *J Neurosci* **19**(19): 8589–8596.

Andersen G, Vestergaard K, Ingeman-Nielsen M, *et al* (1995) Incidence of central post-stroke pain. *Pain* **61**(2):187–193.

Anderson VC, Berryhill PC, Sandquist MA, *et al* (2006) High-resolution three-dimensional magnetic resonance angiography and three-dimensional spoiled gradient-recalled imaging in the evaluation of neurovascular compression in patients with trigeminal neuralgia: a double-blind pilot study. *Neurosurgery* **58**(4):666–673; discussion 666–673.

Arnold AC (2005) Evolving management of optic neuritis and multiple sclerosis. *Am J Ophthalmol* **139**(6):1101–1108.

Baad-Hansen L, List T, Kaube H, et al (2006) Blink reflexes in patients with atypical odontalgia and matched healthy controls. Exp Brain Res 172(4):498–506.

Balcer LJ (2006) Clinical practice. Optic neuritis. N Engl J Med 354(12):1273–1280.

Barker FG 2nd, Jannetta PJ, Bissonette DJ, et al (1996a) The long-term outcome of microvascular decompression for trigeminal neuralgia. N Engl J Med 334(17):1077–1083.

Barker FG 2nd, Jannetta PJ, Babu RP, et al (1996b) Long-term outcome after operation for trigeminal neuralgia in patients with posterior fossa tumors. J Neurosurg 84(5):818–825.

Baron R, Wasner G (2001) Complex regional pain syndromes. Curr Pain Headache Rep 5(2):114–123.

Barron RP, Benoliel R, Zeltser R, et al (2004) Effect of dexamethasone and dipyrone on lingual and inferior alveolar nerve hypersensitivity following third molar extractions: preliminary report. J Orofac Pain 18(1):62–68.

Bartoshuk LM, Snyder DJ, Grushka M, et al (2005) Taste damage: previously unsuspected consequences. Chem Senses 30(Suppl 1): i218–i219.

Basbaum AI (1999) Distinct neurochemichal features of acute and persistent pain. Proc Natl Acad Sci USA 96:7739–7743.

Beaver DL (1967) Electron microscopy of the gasserian ganglion in trigeminal neuralgia. J Neurosurg 26(1 Suppl):138–150.

Beniczky S, Tajti J, Timea Varga E, et al (2005) Evidence-based pharmacological treatment of neuropathic pain syndromes. J Neural Transm 112(6):735–749.

Benoliel R, Sharav Y (1998) Trigeminal neuralgia with lacrimation or SUNCT syndrome? Cephalalgia 18(2):85–90.

Benoliel R, Eliav E, Elishoov H, et al (1994) Diagnosis and treatment of persistent pain after trauma to the head and neck. J Oral Maxillofac Surg 52(11): 1138–1147; discussion 1147–1148.

Benoliel R, Eliav E, Tal M (2001) No sympathetic nerve sprouting in rat trigeminal ganglion following painful and non-painful infraorbital nerve neuropathy. Neurosci Lett 297(3): 151–154.

Benoliel R, Wilensky A, Tal M, et al (2002a) Application of a pro-inflammatory agent to the orbital portion of the rat infraorbital nerve induces changes indicative of ongoing trigeminal pain. Pain 99(3):567–578.

Benoliel R, Eliav E, Tal M (2002b) Strain-dependent modification of neuropathic pain behaviour in the rat hindpaw by a priming painful trigeminal nerve injury. Pain 97(3):203–212.

Benoliel R, Birenboim R, Regev E, et al (2005) Neurosensory changes in the infraorbital nerve following zygomatic fractures. Oral Surg Oral Med Oral Pathol Oral Radiol Endod 99(6):657–665.

Benoliel R, Quek S, Biron A, et al (2006) Trigeminal neurosensory changes following acute and chronic paranasal sinusitis. Quintessence Int 37(6):437–443.

Bergdahl M, Bergdahl J (1999) Burning mouth syndrome: prevalence and associated factors. J Oral Pathol Med 28 (8):350–354.

Bergdahl J, Anneroth G, Perris H (1995) Cognitive therapy in the treatment of patients with resistant burning mouth syndrome: a controlled study. J Oral Pathol Med 24(5):213–215.

Berge TI (2002) Incidence of chronic neuropathic pain subsequent to surgical removal of impacted third molars. Acta Odontol Scand 60(2):108–112.

Birklein F (2005) Complex regional pain syndrome. J Neurol 252(2):131–138.

Black JA, Dib-Haj S, Cummins TR, et al (2001) Sodium channels as therapeutic targets in neuropathic pain. In: Hansson PT, Fields HL, Hill RG, et al (eds) Neuropathic Pain: Pathophysiology and Treatment. Seattle: IASP Press, pp 19–36.

Boecher-Schwarz HG, Bruehl K, Kessel G, et al (1998) Sensitivity and specificity of MRA in the diagnosis of neurovascular compression in patients with trigeminal neuralgia. A correlation of MRA and surgical findings. Neuroradiology 40(2):88–95.

Boes CJ, Matharu MS, Goadsby PJ (2003) The paroxysmal hemicrania-tic syndrome. Cephalalgia 23(1):24–28.

Boureau F, Legallicier P, Kabir-Ahmadi M (2003) Tramadol in post-herpetic neuralgia: a randomized, double-blind, placebo-controlled trial. Pain 104(1-2):323–331.

Bowsher D (1996) Postherpetic neuralgia and its treatment: a retrospective survey of 191 patients. J Pain Symptom Manage 12(5):290–299.

Bowsher D (1997) The effects of pre-emptive treatment of postherpetic neuralgia with amitriptyline: a randomized, double-blind, placebo-controlled trial. J Pain Symptom Manage 13(6):327–331.

Bowsher D (2000) Trigeminal neuralgia: a symptomatic study of 126 successive patients with and without previous interventions. Pain Clinic 12(2):93–98.

Bowsher D, Miles JB, Haggett CE, et al (1997) Trigeminal neuralgia: a quantitative sensory perception threshold study in patients who had not undergone previous invasive procedures. J Neurosurg 86(2):190–192.

Bowsher D, Leijon G, Thuomas KA (1998) Central poststroke pain: correlation of MRI with clinical pain characteristics and sensory abnormalities. Neurology 51(5):1352–1358.

Broggi G, Ferroli P, Franzini A, et al (2000) Microvascular decompression for trigeminal neuralgia: comments on a series of 250 cases, including 10 patients with multiple sclerosis. J Neurol Neurosurg Psychiatry 68(1):59–64.

Broggi G, Ferroli P, Franzini A, et al (2004) Operative findings and outcomes of microvascular decompression for trigeminal neuralgia in 35 patients affected by multiple sclerosis. Neurosurgery 55(4):830–838; discussion 838–839.

Brooke RI (1980) Atypical odontalgia. A report of twenty-two cases. Oral Surg Oral Med Oral Pathol 49(3):196–199.

Bruyn GW (1983) Glossopharyngeal neuralgia. Cephalalgia 3(3):143–157.

BSSI (1995) Guidelines for the management of shingles. report of a working group of the British Society for the Study of Infection (BSSI). J Infect 30(3):193–200.

Bullard DE, Nashold BS Jr (1997) The caudalis DREZ for facial pain. Stereotact Funct Neurosurg 68(1-4 Pt 1):168–174.

Bullitt E, Tew JM, Boyd J (1986) Intracranial tumors in patients with facial pain. J Neurosurg 64(6):865–871.

Burchiel KJ, Clarke H, Haglund M, et al (1988) Long-term efficacy of microvascular decompression in trigeminal neuralgia. J Neurosurg 69(1):35–38.

Campbell RL, Parks KW, Dodds RN (1990) Chronic facial pain associated with endodontic therapy. Oral Surg Oral Med Oral Pathol 69(3):287–290.

Canavero S, Bonicalzi V (1998) The neurochemistry of central pain: evidence from clinical studies, hypothesis and therapeutic implications. Pain 74(2-3):109–114.

Carlson CR, Miller CS, Reid KI (2000) Psychosocial profiles of patients with burning mouth syndrome. J Orofac Pain 14(1): 59–64.

Carmichael FA, McGowan DA (1992) Incidence of nerve damage following third molar removal: a West of Scotland Oral Surgery Research Group study. Br J Oral Maxillofac Surg 30(2): 78–82.

Chacur M, Milligan ED, Gazda LS, et al (2001) A new model of sciatic inflammatory neuritis (SIN): induction of unilateral and bilateral mechanical allodynia following acute unilateral peri-sciatic immune activation in rats. Pain 94(3):231–244.

Cheng TM, Cascino TL, Onofrio BM (1993) Comprehensive study of diagnosis and treatment of trigeminal neuralgia secondary to tumors. Neurology 43(11):2298–2302.

Cheshire WP Jr (2002) Defining the role for gabapentin in the treatment of trigeminal neuralgia: a retrospective study. J Pain 3(2):137–142.

Cheung LK, Lo J (2002) The long-term clinical morbidity of mandibular step osteotomy. Int J Adult Orthodon Orthognath Surg 17(4):283–290.

Chia LG, Shen WC (1993) Wallenberg's lateral medullary syndrome with loss of pain and temperature sensation on the contralateral face: clinical, MRI and electrophysiological studies. J Neurol 240(8):462–467.

Chizh BA, Headley PM, Tzschentke TM (2001) NMDA receptor antagonists as analgesics: focus on the NR2B subtype. *Trends Pharmacol Sci* **22**(12):636–642.

Clark JD (2002) Chronic pain prevalence and analgesic prescribing in a general medical population. *J Pain Symptom Manage* **23**(2): 131–137.

Coen PG, Scott F, Leedham-Green M, et al (2006) Predicting and preventing post-herpetic neuralgia: Are current risk factors useful in clinical practice? *Eur J Pain* **10**(8):695–700.

Cruccu G, Biasiotta A, Galeotti F, et al (2006) Diagnostic accuracy of trigeminal reflex testing in trigeminal neuralgia. *Neurology* **66**(1):139–141.

Danhauer SC, Miller CS, Rhodus NL, et al (2002) Impact of criteria-based diagnosis of burning mouth syndrome on treatment outcome. *J Orofac Pain* **16**(4):305–311.

DeLeo JA, Colburn RW, Rickman AJ (1997) Cytokine and growth factor immunohistochemical spinal profiles in two animal models of mononeuropathy. *Brain Res* **759**(1):50–57.

De Simone R, Marano E, Brescia Morra V, et al (2005) A clinical comparison of trigeminal neuralgic pain in patients with and without underlying multiple sclerosis. *Neurol Sci* **26**(Suppl 2): s150–s151.

de Siqueira SR, Nobrega JC, Valle LB, et al (2004) Idiopathic trigeminal neuralgia: clinical aspects and dental procedures. *Oral Surg Oral Med Oral Pathol Oral Radiol Endod* **98**(3):311–315.

Devor M (2005) Response of nerves to injury in relation to neuropathic pain. In: Koltzenburg M, McMahon SB (eds) *Wall and Melzack's Textbook of Pain*. Edinburgh: Churchill Livingstone.

Devor M, Govrin-Lippmann R, Rappaport ZH (2002a) Mechanism of trigeminal neuralgia: an ultrastructural analysis of trigeminal root specimens obtained during microvascular decompression surgery. *J Neurosurg* **96**(3):532–543.

Devor M, Amir R, Rappaport ZH (2002b) Pathophysiology of trigeminal neuralgia: the ignition hypothesis. *Clin J Pain* **18**(1): 4–13.

Devor M, Govrin-Lippmann R, Rappaport ZH, et al (2002c) Cranial root injury in glossopharyngeal neuralgia: electron microscopic observations. *Case report. J Neurosurg* **96**(3): 603–606.

Dickinson T, Lee K, Spanswick D, et al (2003) Leading the charge-pioneering treatments in the fight against neuropathic pain. *Trends Pharmacol Sci* **24**(11):555–557.

Dostrovsky JO (2000) Trigeminal postherpetic neuralgia postmortem: clinically unilateral, pathologically bilateral. In: Devor M, Rowbotham MC, Wiesenfeld-Hallin Z (eds) *Proceedings of the 9th World Congress on Pain*. Seattle: IASP Press, pp 733–739.

Dubinsky RM, Kabbani H, El-Chami Z, et al (2004) Practice parameter: treatment of postherpetic neuralgia: an evidence-based report of the Quality Standards Subcommittee of the American Academy of Neurology. *Neurology* **63**(6): 959–965.

Dublin P, Hanani M (2007) Satellite glial cells in sensory ganglia: their possible contribution to inflammatory pain. *Brain Behav Immun* **21**(5):592–598.

Dubner R, Sharav Y, Gracely RH, et al (1987) Idiopathic trigeminal neuralgia: sensory features and pain mechanisms. *Pain* **31**(1): 23–33.

Duhmke RM, Cornblath DD, Hollingshead JR (2004) Tramadol for neuropathic pain. *Cochrane Database Syst Rev* (2):CD003726.

Dworkin RH, Portenoy RK (1996) Pain and its persistence in herpes zoster. *Pain* **67**(2-3):241–251.

Dworkin RH, Nagasako EM, Johnson RW, et al (2001) Acute pain in herpes zoster: the famciclovir database project. *Pain* **94**(1): 113–119.

Dworkin RH, Backonja M, Rowbotham MC, et al (2003) Advances in neuropathic pain: diagnosis, mechanisms, and treatment recommendations. *Arch Neurol* **60**(11):1524–1534.

Eisenberg E, McNicol ED, Carr DB (2005) Efficacy and safety of opioid agonists in the treatment of neuropathic pain of nonmalignant origin: systematic review and meta-analysis of randomized controlled trials. *JAMA* **293**(24):3043–3052.

Ekbom KA, Westerberg CE (1966) Carbamazepine in glossopharyngeal neuralgia. *Arch Neurol* **14**(6):595–596.

Eliav E, Gracely RH (1998) Sensory changes in the territory of the lingual and inferior alveolar nerves following lower third molar extraction. *Pain* **77**(2):191–199.

Eliav E, Herzberg U, Ruda MA, et al (1999) Neuropathic pain from an experimental neuritis of the rat sciatic nerve. *Pain* **83**(2):169–182.

Eliav E, Benoliel R, Tal M (2001) Inflammation with no axonal damage of the rat saphenous nerve trunk induces ectopic discharge and mechanosensitivity in myelinated axons. *Neurosci Lett* **311**(1):49–52.

Eliav E, Teich S, Benoliel R, et al (2002) Large myelinated nerve fiber hypersensitivity in oral malignancy. *Oral Surg Oral Med Oral Pathol Oral Radiol Endod* **94**(1):45–50.

Eliav E, Teich S, Nitzan D, et al (2003) Facial arthralgia and myalgia: can they be differentiated by trigeminal sensory assessment? *Pain* **104**(3):481–490.

Eliav E, Tal M, Benoliel R (2004a) Experimental malignancy in the rat induces early hypersensitivity indicative of neuritis. *Pain* **110**(3):727–737.

Eliav E, Gracely RH, Nahlieli O, et al (2004b) Quantitative sensory testing in trigeminal nerve damage assessment. *J Orofac Pain* **18**(4):339–344.

Eliav E, Kamran B, Schaham R, et al (2007) Evidence for chorda tympani dysfunction in burning mouth syndrome patients. *J Am Dent Assoc* **138**(5):628–633.

Erdem E, Alkan A (2001) Peripheral glycerol injections in the treatment of idiopathic trigeminal neuralgia: retrospective analysis of 157 cases. *J Oral Maxillofac Surg* **59**(10):1176–1180.

Fardy MJ, Zakrzewska JM, Patton DW (1994) Peripheral surgical techniques for the management of trigeminal neuralgia–alcohol and glycerol injections. *Acta Neurochir (Wien)* **129**(3-4):181–184; discussion 185.

Farrar JT, Young JP Jr, LaMoreaux L, et al (2001) Clinical importance of changes in chronic pain intensity measured on an 11-point numerical pain rating scale. *Pain* **94**(2):149–158.

Femiano F (2002a) [Statistical survey of afferent pathologies during a 5-year study in the Oral Pathology Department at the Second University of Naples]. *Minerva Stomatol* **51**(3):73–78.

Femiano F (2002b) Burning mouth syndrome (BMS): an open trial of comparative efficacy of alpha-lipoic acid (thioctic acid) with other therapies. *Minerva Stomatol* **51**(9):405–409.

Femiano F (2004) Damage to taste system and oral pain: burning mouth syndrome. *Minerva Stomatol* **53**(9):471–478.

Femiano F, Scully C (2002) Burning mouth syndrome (BMS): double blind controlled study of alpha-lipoic acid (thioctic acid) therapy. *J Oral Pathol Med* **31**(5):267–269.

Femiano F, Gombos F, Scully C (2004a) Burning mouth syndrome: the efficacy of lipoic acid on subgroups. *J Eur Acad Dermatol Venereol* **18**(6):676–678.

Femiano F, Gombos F, Scully C (2004b) Burning mouth syndrome: open trial of psychotherapy alone, medication with alpha-lipoic acid (thioctic acid), and combination therapy. *Med Oral* **9**(1):8–13.

Ferrante L, Artico M, Nardacci B, et al (1995) Glossopharyngeal neuralgia with cardiac syncope. *Neurosurgery* **36**(1):58–63; discussion 63.

Finnerup NB, Otto M, McQuay HJ, et al (2005) Algorithm for neuropathic pain treatment: an evidence based proposal. *Pain* **118**(3):289–305.

Fischbach F, Lehmann TN, Ricke J, et al (2003) Vascular compression in glossopharyngeal neuralgia: demonstration by high-resolution MRI at 3 tesla. *Neuroradiology* **45**(11):810–811.

Fitzek S, Baumgartner U, Fitzek C, et al (2001) Mechanisms and predictors of chronic facial pain in lateral medullary infarction. *Ann Neurol* **49**(4):493–500.

Formaker BK, Frank ME (2000) Taste function in patients with oral burning. *Chem Senses* **25**(5):575–581.

Formaker BK, Mott AE, Frank ME (1998) The effects of topical anesthesia on oral burning in burning mouth syndrome. *Ann N Y Acad Sci* **855**:776–780.

Forman R, Settle RG (1990a) Burning mouth symptoms: a clinical review, Part I. *Compendium* **11**(2):74, 76, 78 passim.

Forman R, Settle RG (1990b) Burning mouth symptoms, Part II: A clinical review. *Compendium* **11**(3):140, 142, 144 passim.

Forssell H, Jaaskelainen S, Tenovuo O, *et al* (2002) Sensory dysfunction in burning mouth syndrome. *Pain* **99**(1-2):41–47.

Frese A, Husstedt IW, Ringelstein EB, *et al* (2006) Pharmacologic treatment of central post-stroke pain. *Clin J Pain* **22**(3):252–260.

Fried K, Bongenhielm U, Boissonade FM, *et al* (2001) Nerve injury-induced pain in the trigeminal system. *Neuroscientist* **7** (2):155–165.

Friedman AH, Nashold BS, Jr (1984) Dorsal root entry zone lesions for the treatment of postherpetic neuralgia. *Neurosurgery* **15**(6): 969–970.

Fromm GH (1989) The pharmacology of trigeminal neuralgia. *Clin Neuropharmacol* **12**(3):185–194.

Fromm GH (1994) Baclofen as an adjuvant analgesic. *J Pain Symptom Manage* **9**(8):500–509.

Fromm GH, Terrence CF, Chattha AS (1984) Baclofen in the treatment of trigeminal neuralgia: double-blind study and long-term follow-up. *Ann Neurol* **15**(3):240–244.

Fromm GH, Graff-Radford SB, Terrence CF, *et al* (1990) Pre-trigeminal neuralgia. *Neurology* **40**(10):1493–1495.

Gajjar TM, Anderson LI, Dluzen DE (2003) Acute effects of estrogen upon methamphetamine induced neurotoxicity of the nigrostriatal dopaminergic system. *J Neural Transm* **110**(11): 1215–1224.

Galer BS, Jensen M (1999) Neglect-like symptoms in complex regional pain syndrome: results of a self-administered survey. *J Pain Symptom Manage* **18**(3):213–217.

Gilden DH, Wright RR, Schneck SA, *et al* (1994) Zoster sine herpete, a clinical variant. *Ann Neurol* **35**(5):530–533.

Gilron I, Booher SL, Rowan JS, *et al* (2001) Topiramate in trigeminal neuralgia: a randomized, placebo-controlled multiple crossover pilot study. *Clin Neuropharmacol* **24**(2): 109–112.

Gilron I, Bailey JM, Tu D, *et al* (2005) Morphine, gabapentin, or their combination for neuropathic pain. *N Engl J Med* **352**(13): 1324–1334.

Goadsby PJ, Lipton RB (2001) Paroxysmal hemicrania-tic syndrome. *Headache* **41**(6):608–609.

Goh BT, Poon CY, Peck RH (2001) The importance of routine magnetic resonance imaging in trigeminal neuralgia diagnosis. *Oral Surg Oral Med Oral Pathol Oral Radiol Endod* **92**(4):424–429.

Goh CL, Khoo L (1997) A retrospective study of the clinical presentation and outcome of herpes zoster in a tertiary dermatology outpatient referral clinic. *Int J Dermatol* **36**(9): 667–672.

Gomes AC, Vasconcelos BC, de Oliveira e Silva ED, *et al* (2005) Lingual nerve damage after mandibular third molar surgery: a randomized clinical trial. *J Oral Maxillofac Surg* **63**(10): 1443–1446.

Gorsky M, Silverman S, Jr., Chinn H (1991) Clinical characteristics and management outcome in the burning mouth syndrome. An open study of 130 patients. *Oral Surg Oral Med Oral Pathol* **72**(2):192–195.

Gottesman MH, Ibrahim B, Elfenbein AS, *et al* (1996) Cardiac arrest caused by trigeminal neuralgia. *Headache* **36**(6):392–394.

Graff-Radford SB, Solberg WK (1992) Atypical odontalgia. *J Craniomandib Disord* **6**(4):260–265.

Granot M, Nagler RM (2005) Association between regional idiopathic neuropathy and salivary involvement as the possible mechanism for oral sensory complaints. *J Pain* **6**(9):581–587.

Gregg JM (2000) Neuropathic complications of mandibular implant surgery: review and case presentations. *Ann R Australas Coll Dent Surg* **15**:176–180.

Gremeau-Richard C, Woda A, Navez ML, *et al* (2004) Topical clonazepam in stomatodynia: a randomised placebo-controlled study. *Pain* **108**(1-2):51–57.

Grushka M, Sessle B (1988) Taste dysfunction in burning mouth syndrome. *Gerodontics* **4**(5):256–258.

Grushka M, Sessle BJ, Howley TP (1987) Psychophysical assessment of tactile, pain and thermal sensory functions in burning mouth syndrome. *Pain* **28**(2):169–184.

Grushka M, Epstein J, Mott A (1998) An open-label, dose escalation pilot study of the effect of clonazepam in burning mouth syndrome. *Oral Surg Oral Med Oral Pathol Oral Radiol Endod* **86**(5):557–561.

Grushka M, Epstein JB, Gorsky M (2003) Burning mouth syndrome and other oral sensory disorders: a unifying hypothesis. *Pain Res Manag* **8**(3):133–135.

Guess HA, Broughton DD, Melton LJ 3rd, *et al* (1985) Epidemiology of herpes zoster in children and adolescents: a population-based study. *Pediatrics* **76**(4):512–517.

Haanpaa M, Laippala P, Nurmikko T (1999) Pain and somatosensory dysfunction in acute herpes zoster. *Clin J Pain* **15**(2):78–84.

Hagelberg N, Forssell H, Rinne JO, *et al* (2003) Striatal dopamine D1 and D2 receptors in burning mouth syndrome. *Pain* **101** (1-2):149–154.

Haines SJ, Chittum CJ (2003) Which operation for trigeminal neuralgia? *Pract Neurol* **3**:30–35.

Hakanson S (1997) Comparison of surgical treatments for trigeminal neuralgia: reevaluation of radiofrequency rhizotomy. *Neurosurgery* **40**(5):1106–1107.

Hakeberg M, Berggren U, Hagglin C, *et al* (1997) Reported burning mouth symptoms among middle-aged and elderly women. *Eur J Oral Sci* **105**(6):539–543.

Hall GC, Carroll D, Parry D, *et al* (2006) Epidemiology and treatment of neuropathic pain: the UK primary care perspective. *Pain* **122**(1-2):156–162.

Hamlyn PJ (1997a) Neurovascular relationships in the posterior cranial fossa, with special reference to trigeminal neuralgia. 2. Neurovascular compression of the trigeminal nerve in cadaveric controls and patients with trigeminal neuralgia: quantification and influence of method. *Clin Anat* **10**(6): 380–388.

Hamlyn PJ (1997b) Neurovascular relationships in the posterior cranial fossa, with special reference to trigeminal neuralgia. 1. Review of the literature and development of a new method of vascular injection-filling in cadaveric controls. *Clin Anat* **10**(6): 371–379.

Hanani M (2005) Satellite glial cells in sensory ganglia: from form to function. *Brain Res Brain Res Rev* **48**(3):457–476.

Hannerz J (1993) Trigeminal neuralgia with chronic paroxysmal hemicrania: the CPH-tic syndrome. *Cephalalgia* **13**(5):361–364.

Harrison SD, Balawi SA, Feinmann C, *et al* (1997) Atypical facial pain: a double-blind placebo-controlled crossover pilot study of subcutaneous sumatriptan. *Eur Neuropsychopharmacol* **7** (2):83–88.

Hasselstrom J, Liu-Palmgren J, Rasjo-Wraak G (2002) Prevalence of pain in general practice. *Eur J Pain* **6**(5):375–385.

Heckmann SM, Heckmann JG, Hilz MJ, *et al* (2001) Oral mucosal blood flow in patients with burning mouth syndrome. *Pain* **90**(3):281–286.

Hempenstall K, Nurmikko TJ, Johnson RW, *et al* (2005) Analgesic therapy in postherpetic neuralgia: a quantitative systematic review. *PLoS Med* **2**(7):e164.

Henson CF, Goldman HW, Rosenwasser RH, *et al* (2005) Glycerol rhizotomy versus gamma knife radiosurgery for the treatment of trigeminal neuralgia: an analysis of patients treated at one institution. *Int J Radiat Oncol Biol Phys* **63**(1):82–90.

Hooge JP, Redekop WK (1995) Trigeminal neuralgia in multiple sclerosis. *Neurology* **45**(7):1294–1296.

Hunt SP, Mantyh PW (2001) The molecular dynamics of pain control. *Nat Rev Neurosci* **2**(2):83–91.

Huynh-Le P, Matsushima T, Hisada K, *et al* (2004) Glossopharyngeal neuralgia due to an epidermoid tumour in the cerebellopontine angle. *J Clin Neurosci* **11**(7):758–760.

Inglese M, Makani S, Johnson G, *et al* (2005) Diffuse axonal injury in mild traumatic brain injury: a diffusion tensor imaging study. *J Neurosurg* **103**(2):298–303.

Israel HA, Ward JD, Horrell B, *et al* (2003) Oral and maxillofacial surgery in patients with chronic orofacial pain. *J Oral Maxillofac Surg* **61**(6):662–667.

Ito M, Kurita K, Ito T, *et al* (2002) Pain threshold and pain recovery after experimental stimulation in patients with burning mouth syndrome. *Psychiatry Clin Neurosci* **56**(2):161–168.

Jaaskelainen SK, Forssell H, Tenovuo O (1997) Abnormalities of the blink reflex in burning mouth syndrome. *Pain* **73**(3):455–460.

Jaaskelainen SK, Forssell H, Tenovuo O (1999) Electrophysiological testing of the trigeminofacial system: aid in the diagnosis of atypical facial pain. *Pain* **80**(1-2):191–200.

Janig W, Baron R (2003) Complex regional pain syndrome: mystery explained? *Lancet Neurol* **2**(11):687–697.

Janig W, Baron R (2004) Experimental approach to CRPS. *Pain* **108**(1-2):3–7.

Jannetta PJ (1967) Arterial compression of the trigeminal nerve at the pons in patients with trigeminal neuralgia. *J Neurosurg* **26**(1):Suppl:159–162.

Jawahar A, Wadhwa R, Berk C, *et al* (2005) Assessment of pain control, quality of life, and predictors of success after gamma knife surgery for the treatment of trigeminal neuralgia. *Neurosurg Focus* **18**(5):E8.

Jensen TS, Rasmussen P, Reske-Nielsen E (1982) Association of trigeminal neuralgia with multiple sclerosis: clinical and pathological features. *Acta Neurol Scand* **65**(3):182–189.

Ji RR, Woolf CJ (2001) Neuronal plasticity and signal transduction in nociceptive neurons: implications for the initiation and maintenance of pathological pain. *Neurobiol Dis* **8**(1):1–10.

Julius D, Basbaum AI (2001) Molecular mechanisms of nociception. *Nature* **413**(6852):203–210.

Jung BF, Johnson RW, Griffin DR, *et al* (2004) Risk factors for postherpetic neuralgia in patients with herpes zoster. *Neurology* **62**(9):1545–1551.

Kalkanis SN, Eskandar EN, Carter BS, *et al* (2003) Microvascular decompression surgery in the United States, 1996 to 2000: mortality rates, morbidity rates, and the effects of hospital and surgeon volumes. *Neurosurgery* **52**(6):1251–1261; discussion 1261–1262.

Kanpolat Y, Savas A, Ugur HC, *et al* (2005) The trigeminal tract and nucleus procedures in treatment of atypical facial pain. *Surg Neurol* **64**(Suppl 2):S96–S100; discussion S100–S101.

Katusic S, Beard CM, Bergstralh E, *et al* (1990) Incidence and clinical features of trigeminal neuralgia, Rochester, Minnesota, 1945-1984. *Ann Neurol* **27**(1):89–95.

Katusic S, Williams DB, Beard CM, *et al* (1991a) Epidemiology and clinical features of idiopathic trigeminal neuralgia and glossopharyngeal neuralgia: similarities and differences, Rochester, Minnesota, 1945-1984. *Neuroepidemiology* **10**(5-6):276–281.

Katusic S, Williams DB, Beard CM, *et al* (1991b) Incidence and clinical features of glossopharyngeal neuralgia, Rochester, Minnesota, 1945-1984. *Neuroepidemiology* **10**(5-6):266–275.

Kelly DJ, Ahmad M, Brull SJ (2001a) Preemptive analgesia II: recent advances and current trends. *Can J Anaesth* **48**(11):1091–1101.

Kelly DJ, Ahmad M, Brull SJ (2001b) Preemptive analgesia I: physiological pathways and pharmacological modalities. *Can J Anaesth* **48**(10):1000–1010.

Kerr FW (1967) Pathology of trigeminal neuralgia: light and electron microscopic observations. *J Neurosurg* **26**(Suppl 1):151–156.

Koleva D, Krulichova I, Bertolini G, *et al* (2005) Pain in primary care: an Italian survey. *Eur J Public Health* **15**(5):475–479.

Kugelberg E, Lindblom U (1959) The mechanism of the pain in trigeminal neuralgia. *J Neurol Neurosurg Psychiatry* **22**(1):36–43.

Kuncz A, Voros E, Barzo P, *et al* (2006) Comparison of clinical symptoms and magnetic resonance angiographic (MRA) results in patients with trigeminal neuralgia and persistent idiopathic facial pain. Medium-term outcome after microvascular decompression of cases with positive MRA findings. *Cephalalgia* **26**(3):266–276.

Kuroiwa T, Matsumoto S, Kato A, *et al* (1996) MR imaging of idiopathic trigeminal neuralgia: correlation with non-surgical therapy. *Radiat Med* **14**(5):235–239.

Lamey PJ, Hobson RS, Orchardson R (1996) Perception of stimulus size in patients with burning mouth syndrome. *J Oral Pathol Med* **25**(8):420–423.

Lamey PJ, Murray BM, Eddie SA, *et al* (2001) The secretion of parotid saliva as stimulated by 10% citric acid is not related to precipitating factors in burning mouth syndrome. *J Oral Pathol Med* **30**(2):121–124.

Lamey PJ, Freeman R, Eddie SA, *et al* (2005) Vulnerability and presenting symptoms in burning mouth syndrome. *Oral Surg Oral Med Oral Pathol Oral Radiol Endod* **99**(1):48–54.

Lauria G, Majorana A, Borgna M, *et al* (2005) Trigeminal small-fiber sensory neuropathy causes burning mouth syndrome. *Pain* **115**(3):332–337.

Leandri M, Eldridge P, Miles J (1998) Recovery of nerve conduction following microvascular decompression for trigeminal neuralgia. *Neurology* **51**(6):1641–1646.

Leeson PD, Iversen LL (1994) The glycine site on the NMDA receptor: structure-activity relationships and therapeutic potential. *J Med Chem* **37**(24):4053–4067.

Leijon G, Boivie J, Johansson I (1989) Central post-stroke pain–neurological symptoms and pain characteristics. *Pain* **36**(1):13–25.

Lim JNW, Ayiku L (2004) The clinical efficacy and safety of stereotactic radiosurgery (gamma knife) in the treatment of trigeminal neuralgia. National Institute for Clinical Excellence (NICE). Available at: http://www.nice.org.uk/page.aspx?o=ip173systematicreview. Accessed September 2006.

Linskey ME, Jho HD, Jannetta PJ (1994) Microvascular decompression for trigeminal neuralgia caused by vertebrobasilar compression. *J Neurosurg* **81**(1):1–9.

Lipton JA, Ship JA, Larach-Robinson D (1993) Estimated prevalence and distribution of reported orofacial pain in the United States. *J Am Dent Assoc* **124**(10):115–121.

Liu CN, Michaelis M, Amir R, *et al* (2000) Spinal nerve injury enhances subthreshold membrane potential oscillations in DRG neurons: relation to neuropathic pain. *J Neurophysiol* **84**(1):205–215.

Lobb WK, Zakariasen KL, McGrath PJ (1996) Endodontic treatment outcomes: do patients perceive problems? *J Am Dent Assoc* **127**(5):597–600.

Loeser JD (1986) Herpes zoster and postherpetic neuralgia. *Pain* **25**(2):149–164.

Lopez BC, Hamlyn PJ, Zakrzewska JM (2004) Systematic review of ablative neurosurgical techniques for the treatment of trigeminal neuralgia. *Neurosurgery* **54**(4):973–982; discussion 982–983.

Love S, Coakham HB (2001) Trigeminal neuralgia: pathology and pathogenesis. *Brain* **124**(Pt 12):2347–2360.

Lovely TJ, Jannetta PJ (1997) Surgical management of geniculate neuralgia. *Am J Otol* **18**(4):512–517.

Lunardi G, Leandri M, Albano C, *et al* (1997) Clinical effectiveness of lamotrigine and plasma levels in essential and symptomatic trigeminal neuralgia. *Neurology* **48**(6):1714–1717.

McDermott AM, Toelle TR, Rowbotham DJ, *et al* (2006) The burden of neuropathic pain: results from a cross-sectional survey. *Eur J Pain* **10**(2):127–135.

MacDonald BK, Cockerell OC, Sander JW, *et al* (2000) The incidence and lifetime prevalence of neurological disorders in a prospective community-based study in the UK. *Brain* **123** (Pt 4):665–676.

MacGowan DJ, Janal MN, Clark WC, *et al* (1997) Central poststroke pain and Wallenberg's lateral medullary infarction: frequency, character, and determinants in 63 patients. *Neurology* **49**(1):120–125.

McLaughlin MR, Jannetta PJ, Clyde BL, *et al* (1999) Microvascular decompression of cranial nerves: lessons learned after 4400 operations. *J Neurosurg* **90**(1):1–8.

McQuay HJ, Tramer M, Nye BA, *et al* (1996) A systematic review of antidepressants in neuropathic pain. *Pain* **68**(2-3):217–227.

Macrae WA (2001) Chronic pain after surgery. *Br J Anaesth* **87** (1):88–98.

Main JH, Jordan RC, Barewal R (1992) Facial neuralgias: a clinical review of 34 cases. *J Can Dent Assoc* **58**(9):752–755.

Maina G, Vitalucci A, Gandolfo S, *et al* (2002) Comparative efficacy of SSRIs and amisulpride in burning mouth syndrome: a single-blind study. *J Clin Psychiatry* **63**(1):38–43.

Maina G, Albert U, Gandolfo S, *et al* (2005) Personality disorders in patients with burning mouth syndrome. *J Personal Disord* **19**(1):84–93.

Maleki J, LeBel AA, Bennett GJ, *et al* (2000) Patterns of spread in complex regional pain syndrome, type I (reflex sympathetic dystrophy). *Pain* **88**(3):259–266.

Marbach JJ (1993) Is phantom tooth pain a deafferentation (neuropathic) syndrome? Part I: Evidence derived from pathophysiology and treatment. *Oral Surg Oral Med Oral Pathol* **75**(1):95–105.

Marbach JJ, Hulbrock J, Hohn C, *et al* (1982) Incidence of phantom tooth pain: an atypical facial neuralgia. *Oral Surg Oral Med Oral Pathol* **53**(2):190–193.

Masur H, Papke K, Bongartz G, *et al* (1995) The significance of three-dimensional MR-defined neurovascular compression for the pathogenesis of trigeminal neuralgia. *J Neurol* **242**(2): 93–98.

Matsushima T, Huynh-Le P, Miyazono M (2004) Trigeminal neuralgia caused by venous compression. *Neurosurgery* **55**(2): 334–337; discussion 338–339.

Max MB, Schafer SC, Culnane M, *et al* (1988) Amitriptyline, but not lorazepam, relieves postherpetic neuralgia. *Neurology* **38**(9):1427–1432.

May A, Bahra A, Buchel C, *et al* (1999) Functional magnetic resonance imaging in spontaneous attacks of SUNCT: short-lasting neuralgiform headache with conjunctival injection and tearing. *Ann Neurol* **46**(5):791–794.

Meaney JF, Watt JW, Eldridge PR, *et al* (1995a) Association between trigeminal neuralgia and multiple sclerosis: role of magnetic resonance imaging. *J Neurol Neurosurg Psychiatry* **59**(3):253–259.

Meaney JF, Eldridge PR, Dunn LT, *et al* (1995b) Demonstration of neurovascular compression in trigeminal neuralgia with magnetic resonance imaging. Comparison with surgical findings in 52 consecutive operative cases. *J Neurosurg* **83**(5): 799–805.

Melis M, Zawawi K, al-Badawi E, *et al* (2002) Complex regional pain syndrome in the head and neck: a review of the literature. *J Orofac Pain* **16**(2):93–104.

Melis M, Lobo SL, Ceneviz C, *et al* (2003) Atypical odontalgia: a review of the literature. *Headache* **43**(10):1060–1074.

Melzack R, Terrence C, Fromm G, *et al* (1986) Trigeminal neuralgia and atypical facial pain: use of the McGill Pain Questionnaire for discrimination and diagnosis. *Pain* **27**(3):297–302.

Merrill RL (2004) Intraoral neuropathy. *Curr Pain Headache Rep* **8**(5):341–346.

Merskey H, Bogduk N (1994) *Classification of Chronic Pain: Descriptions of Chronic Pain Syndromes and Definition of Pain Terms*, 2nd edn. Seattle: IASP Press.

Meyer-Rosberg K, Kvarnstrom A, Kinnman E, *et al* (2001) Peripheral neuropathic pain–a multidimensional burden for patients. *Eur J Pain* **5**(4):379–389.

Miles JB, Eldridge PR, Haggett CE, *et al* (1997) Sensory effects of microvascular decompression in trigeminal neuralgia. *J Neurosurg* **86**(2):193–196.

Minagar A, Sheremata WA (2000) Glossopharyngeal neuralgia and MS. *Neurology* **54**(6):1368–1370.

Mitchell RG (1980) Pre-trigeminal neuralgia. *Br Dent J* **149**(6): 167–170.

Mock D, Frydman W, Gordon AS (1985) Atypical facial pain: a retrospective study. *Oral Surg Oral Med Oral Pathol* **59**(5): 472–474.

Mott AE, Grushka M, Sessle BJ (1993) Diagnosis and management of taste disorders and burning mouth syndrome. *Dent Clin North Am* **37**(1):33–71.

Neumann S, Doubell TP, Leslie T, *et al* (1996) Inflammatory pain hypersensitivity mediated by phenotypic switch in myelinated primary sensory neurons. *Nature* **384**(6607): 360–364.

Nicholson BD (2004) Evaluation and treatment of central pain syndromes. *Neurology* **62**(5 Suppl 2):S30–S36.

Nitu AN, Wallihan R, Skljarevski V, *et al* (2003) Emerging trends in the pharmacotherapy of chronic pain. *Expert Opin Investig Drugs* **12**(4):545–559.

Nomura T, Ikezaki K, Matsushima T, *et al* (1994) Trigeminal neuralgia: differentiation between intracranial mass lesions and ordinary vascular compression as causative lesions. *Neurosurg Rev* **17**(1):51–57.

Nurmikko TJ (1991) Altered cutaneous sensation in trigeminal neuralgia. *Arch Neurol* **48**(5):523–527.

Nurmikko T, Bowsher D (1990) Somatosensory findings in postherpetic neuralgia. *J Neurol Neurosurg Psychiatry* **53**(2): 135–141.

Nurmikko TJ, Eldridge PR (2001) Trigeminal neuralgia–pathophysiology, diagnosis and current treatment. *Br J Anaesth* **87**(1):117–132.

Nurmikko TJ, Haanpaa M (2005) Treatment of postherpetic neuralgia. *Curr Pain Headache Rep* **9**(3):161–167.

Nurmikko TJ, Haggett CE, Miles J (2000) Neurogenic vasodilation in trigeminal neuralgia. In: Devor M, Rowbotham MC, Wiesenfeld-Hallin Z (eds) *Proceedings of the 9th World Congress of Pain*. Seattle: IASP Press, pp 747–755.

Oaklander AL, Romans K, Horasek S, *et al* (1998) Unilateral postherpetic neuralgia is associated with bilateral sensory neuron damage. *Ann Neurol* **44**(5):789–795.

Oaklander AL, Bowsher D, Galer B, *et al* (2003) Herpes zoster itch: preliminary epidemiologic data. *J Pain* **4**(6): 338–343.

Odeh M, Oliven A (1994) Glossopharyngeal neuralgia associated with cardiac syncope and weight loss. *Arch Otolaryngol Head Neck Surg* **120**(11):1283–1286.

Okeson JP (1996) *Orofacial Pain: Guidelines for Assessment, Classification, and Management*. The American Academy of Orofacial Pain. Illinois: Quintessence Publishing.

Olesen J, Bousser M-G, Diener HC, *et al* (2004) The International Classification of Headache Disorders, 2nd edition. *Cephalalgia* **24**(Suppl 1):24–150.

Osterberg A, Boivie J, Thuomas KA (2005) Central pain in multiple sclerosis–prevalence and clinical characteristics. *Eur J Pain* **9**(5):531–542.

Oxman MN, Levin MJ, Johnson GR, *et al* (2005) A vaccine to prevent herpes zoster and postherpetic neuralgia in older adults. *N Engl J Med* **352**(22):2271–2284.

Pappagallo M, Oaklander AL, Quatrano-Piacentini AL, *et al* (2000) Heterogeneous patterns of sensory dysfunction in postherpetic neuralgia suggest multiple pathophysiologic mechanisms. *Anesthesiology* **92**(3):691–698.

Pareja JA, Cuadrado ML (2005) SUNCT syndrome: an update. *Expert Opin Pharmacother* **6**(4):591–599.

Pareja JA, Baron M, Gili P, *et al* (2002) Objective assessment of autonomic signs during triggered first division trigeminal neuralgia. *Cephalalgia* **22**(4):251–255.

Patel A, Kassam A, Horowitz M, *et al* (2002) Microvascular decompression in the management of glossopharyngeal neuralgia: analysis of 217 cases. *Neurosurgery* **50**(4):705–710; discussion 710–711.

Peters G, Nurmikko TJ (2002) Peripheral and gasserian ganglion-level procedures for the treatment of trigeminal neuralgia. *Clin J Pain* **18**(1):28–34.

Petruzzi M, Lauritano D, De Benedittis M, *et al* (2004) Systemic capsaicin for burning mouth syndrome: short-term results of a pilot study. *J Oral Pathol Med* **33**(2):111–114.

Pfaffenrath V, Rath M, Pollmann W, *et al* (1993) Atypical facial pain–application of the IHS criteria in a clinical sample. *Cephalalgia* **13**(Suppl 12):84–88.

Pfendler DF (1997) Glossopharyngeal neuralgia with tongue carcinoma. *Arch Otolaryngol Head Neck Surg* **123**(6):658.

Pinto A, Sollecito TP, DeRossi SS (2003) Burning mouth syndrome. A retrospective analysis of clinical characteristics and treatment outcomes. *N Y State Dent J* **69**(3):18–24.

Polgar E, Hughes DI, Arham AZ, *et al* (2005) Loss of neurons from laminas I-III of the spinal dorsal horn is not required for development of tactile allodynia in the spared nerve injury model of neuropathic pain. *J Neurosci* **25**(28):6658–6666.

Pollock BE (2005) Comparison of posterior fossa exploration and stereotactic radiosurgery in patients with previously nonsurgically treated idiopathic trigeminal neuralgia. *Neurosurg Focus* **18**(5):E6.

Pollock BE, Ecker RD (2005) A Prospective Cost-Effectiveness Study of Trigeminal Neuralgia Surgery. *Clin J Pain* **21**(4): 317–322.

Polycarpou N, Ng YL, Canavan D, *et al* (2005) Prevalence of persistent pain after endodontic treatment and factors affecting its occurrence in cases with complete radiographic healing. *Int Endod J* **38**(3):169–178.

Portenoy RK, Duma C, Foley KM (1986) Acute herpetic and postherpetic neuralgia: clinical review and current management. *Ann Neurol* **20**(6):651-664.

Povlishock JT, Katz DI (2005) Update of neuropathology and neurological recovery after traumatic brain injury. *J Head Trauma Rehabil* **20**(1):76–94.

Pradel W, Hlawitschka M, Eckelt U, *et al* (2002) Cryosurgical treatment of genuine trigeminal neuralgia. *Br J Oral Maxillofac Surg* **40**(3):244–247.

Puca A, Meglio M (1993) Typical trigeminal neuralgia associated with posterior cranial fossa tumors. *Ital J Neurol Sci* **14**(7): 549–552.

Puca A, Meglio M, Tamburrini G, *et al* (1993) Trigeminal involvement in intracranial tumours. Anatomical and clinical observations on 73 patients. *Acta Neurochir (Wien)* **125**(1-4): 47–51.

Puca A, Meglio M, Vari R, *et al* (1995) Evaluation of fifth nerve dysfunction in 136 patients with middle and posterior cranial fossae tumors. *Eur Neurol* **35**(1):33–37.

Pulec JL (2002) Geniculate neuralgia: long-term results of surgical treatment. *Ear Nose Throat J* **81**(1):30–33.

Puri V, Cui L, Liverman CS, *et al* (2005) Ovarian steroids regulate neuropeptides in the trigeminal ganglion. *Neuropeptides* **39**(4): 409–417.

Queral-Godoy E, Figueiredo R, Valmaseda-Castellon E, *et al* (2006) Frequency and evolution of lingual nerve lesions following lower third molar extraction. *J Oral Maxillofac Surg* **64**(3): 402–407.

Ragozzino MW, Melton LJ 3rd, Kurland LT, *et al* (1982) Population-based study of herpes zoster and its sequelae. *Medicine (Baltimore)* **61**(5):310–316.

Raja SN, Haythornthwaite JA, Pappagallo M, *et al* (2002) Opioids versus antidepressants in postherpetic neuralgia: a randomized, placebo-controlled trial. *Neurology* **59**(7): 1015–1021.

Rasmussen P (1990) Facial pain. II. A prospective survey of 1052 patients with a view of: character of the attacks, onset, course, and character of pain. *Acta Neurochir (Wien)* **107**(3-4): 121–128.

Rasmussen P (1991a) Facial pain. III. A prospective study of the localization of facial pain in 1052 patients. *Acta Neurochir (Wien)* **108**(1-2):53–63.

Rasmussen P (1991b) Facial pain. IV. A prospective study of 1052 patients with a view of: precipitating factors, associated symptoms, objective psychiatric and neurological symptoms. *Acta Neurochir (Wien)* **108**(3-4):100–109.

Rasmussen PV, Sindrup SH, Jensen TS, *et al* (2004) Symptoms and signs in patients with suspected neuropathic pain. *Pain* **110**(1-2):461–469.

Resnick DK, Jannetta PJ, Bissonnette D, *et al* (1995) Microvascular decompression for glossopharyngeal neuralgia. *Neurosurgery* **36**(1):64–68; discussion 68–69.

Rhodus NL, Carlson CR, Miller CS (2003a) Burning mouth (syndrome) disorder. *Quintessence Int* **34**(8):587–593.

Rhodus NL, Fricton J, Carlson P, *et al* (2003b) Oral symptoms associated with fibromyalgia syndrome. *J Rheumatol* **30**(8): 1841–1845.

Robert RC, Bacchetti P, Pogrel MA (2005) Frequency of trigeminal nerve injuries following third molar removal. *J Oral Maxillofac Surg* **63**(6):732–735; discussion 736.

Robinson PP, Smith KG (1996) Lingual nerve damage during lower third molar removal: a comparison of two surgical methods. *Br Dent J* **180**(12):456–461.

Rommel O, Malin JP, Zenz M, *et al* (2001) Quantitative sensory testing, neurophysiological and psychological examination in patients with complex regional pain syndrome and hemisensory deficits. *Pain* **93**(3):279–293.

Rothman KJ, Monson RR (1973) Survival in trigeminal neuralgia. *J Chronic Dis* **26**(5):303–309.

Rowbotham MC, Goli V, Kunz NR, *et al* (2004) Venlafaxine extended release in the treatment of painful diabetic neuropathy: a double-blind, placebo-controlled study. *Pain* **110**(3):697–706.

Rozen TD (2004) Trigeminal neuralgia and glossopharyngeal neuralgia. *Neurol Clin* **22**(1):185–206.

Rushton JG, Macdonald HN (1957) Trigeminal neuralgia; special considerations of nonsurgical treatment. *J Am Med Assoc* **165**(5):437–440.

Rushton JG, Stevens JC, Miller RH (1981) Glossopharyngeal (vagoglossopharyngeal) neuralgia: a study of 217 cases. *Arch Neurol* **38**(4):201–205.

Saarto T, Wiffen PJ (2005) Antidepressants for neuropathic pain. *Cochrane Database Syst Rev* (3):CD005454.

Sah DW, Ossipov MH, Porreca F (2003) Neurotrophic factors as novel therapeutics for neuropathic pain. *Nat Rev Drug Discov* **2**(6):460–472.

Salter MW (2005) Cellular signalling pathways of spinal pain neuroplasticity as targets for analgesic development. *Curr Top Med Chem* **5**(6):557–567.

Sampson JH, Grossi PM, Asaoka K, *et al* (2004) Microvascular decompression for glossopharyngeal neuralgia: long-term effectiveness and complication avoidance. *Neurosurgery* **54**(4): 884–889; discussion 889–890.

Sanchez-Mejia RO, Limbo M, Cheng JS, *et al* (2005) Recurrent or refractory trigeminal neuralgia after microvascular decompression, radiofrequency ablation, or radiosurgery. *Neurosurg Focus* **18**(5):e12.

Sardella A, Uglietti D, Demarosi F, *et al* (1999) Benzydamine hydrochloride oral rinses in management of burning mouth syndrome. A clinical trial. *Oral Surg Oral Med Oral Pathol Oral Radiol Endod* **88**(6):683–686.

Sardella A, Lodi G, Demarosi F, *et al* (2006) Burning mouth syndrome: a retrospective study investigating spontaneous remission and response to treatments. *Oral Dis* **12**(2):152–155.

Sato J, Saitoh T, Notani K, *et al* (2004) Diagnostic significance of carbamazepine and trigger zones in trigeminal neuralgia. *Oral Surg Oral Med Oral Pathol Oral Radiol Endod* **97**(1):18–22.

Scala A, Checchi L, Montevecchi M, *et al* (2003) Update on burning mouth syndrome: overview and patient management. *Crit Rev Oral Biol Med* **14**(4):275–291.

Schmader K (2001) Herpes zoster in older adults. *Clin Infect Dis* **32**(10): 1481–1486.

Schnurr RF, Brooke RI (1992) Atypical odontalgia. Update and comment on long-term follow-up. *Oral Surg Oral Med Oral Pathol* **73**(4):445–448.

Scholz J, Woolf CJ (2002) Can we conquer pain? *Nat Neurosci* **5**(Suppl):1062–1067.

Scrivani SJ, Keith DA, Kulich R, *et al* (1998) Posttraumatic gustatory neuralgia: a clinical model of trigeminal neuropathic pain. *J Orofac Pain* **12**(4):287–292.

Sharav Y, Benoliel R, Schnarch A, *et al* (1991) Idiopathic trigeminal pain associated with gustatory stimuli. *Pain* **44**(2):171–174.

Ship JA, Grushka M, Lipton JA, *et al* (1995) Burning mouth syndrome: an update. *J Am Dent Assoc* **126**(7):842–853.

Sieweke N, Birklein F, Riedl B, *et al* (1999) Patterns of hyperalgesia in complex regional pain syndrome. *Pain* **80**(1-2):171–177.

Simpson DA (2001) Gabapentin and venlafaxine for the treatment of painful diabetic neuropathy. *J Clin Neuromusc Disease* **3**:53–62.

Sindrup SH, Jensen TS (2001) Antidepressants in the treatment of neuropathic pain. In: Hanson PT, Fields HL, Hill RG, *et al* (eds) *Neuropathic Pain: Pathophysiology and Treatment*. Seattle: IASP Press, pp 169–183.

Sindrup SH, Jensen TS (2002) Pharmacotherapy of trigeminal neuralgia. *Clin J Pain* **18**(1):22–27.

Sjaastad O, Pareja JA, Zukerman E, *et al* (1997) Trigeminal neuralgia. Clinical manifestations of first division involvement. *Headache* **37**(6):346–357.

Solaro C, Messmer Uccelli M, Uccelli A, *et al* (2000) Low-dose gabapentin combined with either lamotrigine or carbamazepine can be useful therapies for trigeminal neuralgia in multiple sclerosis. *Eur Neurol* **44**(1):45–48.

Stanton-Hicks M (2003) Complex regional pain syndrome. *Anesthesiol Clin North America* **21**(4):733–744.

Stieber VW, Bourland JD, Ellis TL (2005) Glossopharyngeal neuralgia treated with gamma knife surgery: treatment outcome and failure analysis. Case report. *J Neurosurg* **102**(Suppl):155–157.

Strupp M, Brandt T (1999) Vestibular neuritis. *Adv Otorhinolaryngol* **55**:111–136.

Svensson P, Bjerring P, Arendt-Nielsen L, *et al* (1993) Sensory and pain thresholds to orofacial argon laser stimulation in patients with chronic burning mouth syndrome. *Clin J Pain* **9**(3): 207–215.

Tacconi L, Miles JB (2000) Bilateral trigeminal neuralgia: a therapeutic dilemma. *Br J Neurosurg* **14**(1):33–39.

Taha JM, Tew JM Jr (1995) Long-term results of surgical treatment of idiopathic neuralgias of the glossopharyngeal and vagal nerves. *Neurosurgery* **36**(5):926–930; discussion 930–931.

Taha JM, Tew JM Jr (1996) Comparison of surgical treatments for trigeminal neuralgia: reevaluation of radiofrequency rhizotomy. *Neurosurgery* **38**(5):865–871.

Taha JM, Tew JM Jr, Buncher CR (1995) A prospective 15-year follow up of 154 consecutive patients with trigeminal neuralgia treated by percutaneous stereotactic radiofrequency thermal rhizotomy. *J Neurosurg* **83**(6):989–993.

Tal M, Devor M (1992) Ectopic discharge in injured nerves: comparison of trigeminal and somatic afferents. *Brain Res* **579**(1):148–151.

Tammiala-Salonen T, Hiidenkari T, Parvinen T (1993) Burning mouth in a Finnish adult population. *Community Dent Oral Epidemiol* **21**(2):67–71.

Taylor JC, Brauer S, Espir ML (1981) Long-term treatment of trigeminal neuralgia with carbamazepine. *Postgrad Med J* **57**(663):16–18.

Thimineur M, Sood P, Kravitz E, *et al* (1998) Central nervous system abnormalities in complex regional pain syndrome (CRPS): clinical and quantitative evidence of medullary dysfunction. *Clin J Pain* **14**(3):256-267.

Torrance N, Smith BH, Bennett MI, *et al* (2006) The epidemiology of chronic pain of predominantly neuropathic origin. Results from a general population survey. *J Pain* **7**(4):281–289.

Tyler-Kabara EC, Kassam AB, Horowitz MH, *et al* (2002) Predictors of outcome in surgically managed patients with typical and atypical trigeminal neuralgia: comparison of results following microvascular decompression. *J Neurosurg* **96**(3): 527–531.

Valmaseda-Castellon E, Berini-Aytes L, Gay-Escoda C (2000) Lingual nerve damage after third lower molar surgical extraction. *Oral Surg Oral Med Oral Pathol Oral Radiol Endod* **90**(5):567–573.

Valmaseda-Castellon E, Berini-Aytes L, Gay-Escoda C (2001) Inferior alveolar nerve damage after lower third molar surgical extraction: a prospective study of 1117 surgical extractions. *Oral Surg Oral Med Oral Pathol Oral Radiol Endod* **92**(4):377–383.

van de Beek WJ, Roep BO, van der Slik AR, *et al* (2003) Susceptibility loci for complex regional pain syndrome. *Pain* **103**(1-2):93–97.

Van Houdenhove B, Joostens P (1995) Burning mouth syndrome. Successful treatment with combined psychotherapy and psychopharmacotherapy. *Gen Hosp Psychiatry* **17**(5):385–388.

van Seventer R, Feister HA, Young JP Jr, *et al* (2006) Efficacy and tolerability of twice-daily pregabalin for treating pain and related sleep interference in postherpetic neuralgia: a 13-week, randomized trial. *Curr Med Res Opin* **22**(2):375–384.

Vestergaard K, Andersen G, Gottrup H, *et al* (2001) Lamotrigine for central poststroke pain: a randomized controlled trial. *Neurology* **56**(2):184–190.

Vickers ER, Cousins MJ (2000) Neuropathic orofacial pain part 1–prevalence and pathophysiology. *Aust Endod J* **26**(1):19–26.

Vitkov L, Weitgasser R, Hannig M, *et al* (2003) Candida-induced stomatopyrosis and its relation to diabetes mellitus. *J Oral Pathol Med* **32**(1):46–50.

Volpi A, Gross G, Hercogova J, *et al* (2005) Current management of herpes zoster: the European view. *Am J Clin Dermatol* **6**(5): 317–325.

Vora AR, Loescher AR, Boissonade FM, *et al* (2005) Ultrastructural characteristics of axons in traumatic neuromas of the human lingual nerve. *J Orofac Pain* **19**(1):22–33.

Walton JN (2000) Altered sensation associated with implants in the anterior mandible: a prospective study. *J Prosthet Dent* **83**(4):443–449.

Wasner G, Schattschneider J, Baron R (2002) Skin temperature side differences–a diagnostic tool for CRPS? *Pain* **98**(1-2):19–26.

Watkins LR, Maier SF (2002) Beyond neurons: evidence that immune and glial cells contribute to pathological pain states. *Physiol Rev* **82**(4):981–1011.

Watkins LR, Hutchinson MR, Ledeboer A, *et al* (2007) Norman Cousins Lecture. Glia as the 'bad guys': implications for improving clinical pain control and the clinical utility of opioids. *Brain Behav Immun* **21**(2):131–146.

Watson CP, Oaklander AL (2002) Postherpetic neuralgia. *Pain Practice* **2**(4):295–307.

Watson CP, Deck JH, Morshead C, *et al* (1991) Post-herpetic neuralgia: further post-mortem studies of cases with and without pain. *Pain* **44**(2):105–117.

Watson CP, Tyler KL, Bickers DR, *et al* (1993) A randomized vehicle-controlled trial of topical capsaicin in the treatment of postherpetic neuralgia. *Clin Ther* **15**(3):510–526.

Webb CJ, Makura ZG, McCormick MS (2000) Glossopharyngeal neuralgia following foreign body impaction in the neck. *J Laryngol Otol* **114**(1):70–72.

Wiffen P, Collins S, McQuay H, *et al* (2005a) Anticonvulsant drugs for acute and chronic pain. *Cochrane Database Syst Rev* (3): CD001133.

Wiffen PJ, McQuay HJ, Edwards JE, *et al* (2005b) Gabapentin for acute and chronic pain. *Cochrane Database Syst Rev* (3): CD005452.

Wiffen PJ, McQuay HJ, Moore RA (2005c) Carbamazepine for acute and chronic pain. *Cochrane Database Syst Rev* (3): CD005451.

Woda A, Pionchon P (1999) A unified concept of idiopathic orofacial pain: clinical features. *J Orofac Pain* **13**(3):172–184; discussion 185–195.

Woda A, Navez ML, Picard P, *et al* (1998) A possible therapeutic solution for stomatodynia (burning mouth syndrome). *J Orofac Pain* **12**(4):272–278.

Woolf CJ, Chong MS (1993) Preemptive analgesia–treating postoperative pain by preventing the establishment of central sensitization. *Anesth Analg* **77**(2):362–379.

Woolf CJ, Mannion RJ (1999) Neuropathic pain: aetiology, symptoms, mechanisms, and management. *Lancet* **353**(9168): 1959–1964.

Woolf CJ, Salter MW (2000) Neuronal plasticity: increasing the gain in pain. *Science* **288**(5472):1765–1769.

Yang J, Simonson TM, Ruprecht A, *et al* (1996) Magnetic resonance imaging used to assess patients with trigeminal neuralgia. *Oral Surg Oral Med Oral Pathol Oral Radiol Endod* **81**(3):343–350.

Yoshino N, Akimoto H, Yamada I, *et al* (2003) Trigeminal neuralgia: evaluation of neuralgic manifestation and site of neurovascular compression with 3D CISS MR imaging and MR angiography. *Radiology* **228**(2):539–545.

Zakrzewska JM (1991) Cryotherapy for trigeminal neuralgia: a 10 year audit. *Br J Oral Maxillofac Surg* **29**(1):1–4.

Zakrzewska JM (2001) Consumer views on management of trigeminal neuralgia. *Headache* **41**(4):369–376.

Zakrzewska JM (2003) Trigeminal neuralgia. *Clin Evid* (9): 1490–1498.

Zakrzewska JM, Lopez BC (2004) Trigeminal neuralgia. *Clin Evid* (12):1880–1890.

Zakrzewska JM, Patsalos PN (2002) Long-term cohort study comparing medical (oxcarbazepine) and surgical management of intractable trigeminal neuralgia. *Pain* **95**(3): 259–266.

Zakrzewska JM, Chaudhry Z, Nurmikko TJ, *et al* (1997) Lamotrigine (lamictal) in refractory trigeminal neuralgia: results from a double-blind placebo controlled crossover trial. *Pain* **73**(2):223–230.

Zakrzewska JM, Jassim S, Bulman JS (1999) A prospective, longitudinal study on patients with trigeminal neuralgia who underwent radiofrequency thermocoagulation of the Gasserian ganglion. *Pain* **79**(1):51–58.

Zakrzewska JM, Lopez BC, Kim SE, *et al* (2005a) Patient reports of satisfaction after microvascular decompression and partial sensory rhizotomy for trigeminal neuralgia. *Neurosurgery* **56**(6):1304–1311; discussion 1311–1312.

Zakrzewska JM, Forssell H, Glenny AM (2005b) Interventions for the treatment of burning mouth syndrome. *Cochrane Database Syst Rev* (1):CD002779.

Zelenka M, Schafers M, Sommer C (2005) Intraneural injection of interleukin-1beta and tumor necrosis factor-alpha into rat sciatic nerve at physiological doses induces signs of neuropathic pain. *Pain* **116**(3):257–263.

Zvartau-Hind M, Din MU, Gilani A, *et al* (2000) Topiramate relieves refractory trigeminal neuralgia in MS patients. *Neurology* **55**(10):1587–1588.

CHAPTER 12

Neurosurgical aspects of orofacial pain

Zvi Harry Rappaport

1. Introduction

Neurosurgical therapy is considered for the treatment of patients with orofacial pain when more conservative measures are deemed to have failed or when the pain is a symptom of a neurosurgically treatable disease process. There are also data to support the improved prognosis of early surgical intervention in suitable cases—this has been discussed in Chapter 11. It is of paramount importance to establish the appropriate diagnosis prior to considering surgical therapy, as the type of procedure chosen and the likely success of outcome are diagnosis dependent (Burchiel 2003). From a neurosurgical viewpoint the temporal pattern of the pain and its anatomic distribution are important features in diagnosis. The temporal pattern may be divided into paroxysmal, paroxysmal superimposed on a constant pain and continuous pain without paroxysms. Neurosurgical interventions are by far more successful in paroxysmal than in continuous neuropathic pains; this is similar to the results of medical therapy (see Chapter 11). Similarly, anatomical distribution affects outcome. If the pain is localized to known anatomical distribution surgery can be directed to the appropriate structure. Diffuse non-anatomical or bilateral pain syndromes do not offer a successful surgical target. Finally a sensory facial examination is of prognostic importance (see Chapter 3). Sensory hypoaesthesia accompanying pain is detrimental to surgical outcome, unless a structural compressive lesion is present. When these principles are followed it becomes clear that trigeminal, glossopharyngeal and nervus intermedius neuralgias are the main diagnoses responding to surgical therapy, while surgery has a limited role in ill-defined atypical facial pain syndromes. Neuropathic pain may be symptomatic of a mass lesion or vascular disease which requires life-saving intervention. When these are treated neurosurgically, the pain is usually, but not always, ameliorated.

2. Intracranial Sources of Orofacial Pain

2.1. Vascular

Vascular compression of cranial nerves has emerged as the leading treatable aetiology for orofacial neuralgic pain (Moller 1998, 1999). Pathological studies have demonstrated changes in myelination within the compressed nerve root (Devor *et al* 2002a,b) that are compatible with a neurophysiological understanding of the pain mechanism (Devor *et al* 2002c).

However, other rarer vascular causes of facial pain have been described. These include arteriovenous malformations (Ito *et al* 1996; Karibe *et al* 2004), dural arteriovenous fistulae (Ito *et al* 1996) and intracavernous aneurysms (Linskey *et al* 1990). These lesions can be visualized by magnetic resonance imaging/angiography (MRI/MRA). Cerebral vasculitis may be associated with headache, but rarely with facial pain (Younger 2004). Carotid and vertebral artery dissections occur mainly in the neck, but may also be intracranial in location (see Chapter 13). Pain phenomena include Raeder's paratrigeminal neuralgia, facial paraesthesia and orbital pain (Selky and Pascuzzi 1995; Saeed *et al* 2000; Mainardi *et al* 2002). Associated neurological signs such as Horner's syndrome, cranial nerve findings and transient ischaemic attacks may suggest the correct diagnosis. Primary neurovascular craniofacial pain syndromes are described in Chapters 9 and 10.

2.2. Neoplastic

2.2.1. Incidence

Intracranial tumours give rise to orofacial pain when involving the trigeminal or glossopharyngeal root. Approximately 7% of patients with trigeminal neuralgia suffer from a mass lesion along the course of the nerve root (secondary trigeminal neuralgia). Therefore a brain imaging study should be performed on all patients suffering from trigeminal pain, before embarking on a therapeutic programme (Goh *et al* 2001). As the age of the patient decreases, the likelihood of a tumour or multiple sclerosis causing the trigeminal symptoms becomes greater. In patients younger than 40 with trigeminal neuralgia these aetiologies may represent the majority (Yang *et al* 1996). The average age of patients with trigeminal neuralgia secondary to tumours in Goh's (Goh *et al* 2001) series was 53 years.

2.2.2. Tumour types

While typical trigeminal neuralgia is possible in this context, most cases of facial pain secondary to mass lesions cause some degree of facial numbness. Typical lesions that cause trigeminal pain include meningiomas (Samii *et al* 1997), schwannomas such as trigeminal and acoustic neuromas (Dolenc 1994; Barker *et al* 1996a; Matsuka *et al* 2000) and epidermoid cysts (Rappaport 1985; Meng *et al* 2005). Meningiomas involving the trigeminal root are the most frequently encountered mass lesion causing trigeminal symptomatology with acoustic neuromas in second place. The tumour should be resected with the usual microneurosurgical techniques. Pain relief can be achieved in the majority of patients (Barker *et al* 1996a). When the tumour intimately involves the trigeminal root and has already caused hypaesthesia, neuropathic pain may persist after resection of the lesion (Samii *et al* 1997). Trigeminal pain due to circumscribed tumours in strategic locations such as the cavernous sinus or the petrous apex can respond favourably to radiosurgery (Pollock *et al* 2000).

2.3. Other

Inflammatory lesions of the cavernous sinus cause intra- and supraorbital pain (Forderreuther and Straube 1999). Associated ocular signs allow for anatomical localization and diagnosis. Pachymeningitis (Yamamoto *et al* 2000) and sarcoidosis (Quinones-Hinojosa *et al* 2003) can involve the trigeminal root and its branches, giving rise to facial pain. Finally in malignant disease both cerebral spinal fluid (CSF) carcinomatosis (Lee *et al* 2005) and sellar and parasellar metastases are associated with facial pain and neurological symptomatology (Yi *et al* 2000). Neurosurgical biopsy of the lesion may be required to arrive at the correct diagnosis.

3. Neurosurgical Interventions for Orofacial Pain

3.1. Trigeminal Neuralgia

Of all chronic pain syndromes trigeminal neuralgia is one of the most gratifying conditions to treat; see Case 12.1.

Virtually all patients will respond at least initially to drug therapy, e.g. carbamazepine; see Chapter 11. Because of drug intolerance, side effects or drug failure, approximately half of the patients will eventually require neurosurgical intervention. Three categories of interventional therapy are available: peripheral neurectomy, percutaneous rhizotomy and microvascular root decompression or rhizotomy via a craniotomy approach. Stimulation of the trigeminal root is an investigational procedure and is uncommonly utilized in cases of refractory facial pain (Young 1995). Gamma knife radiation therapy for trigeminal neuralgia has been introduced more recently but is associated with a longer latency period until pain relief sets in. Moreover long-term follow-up is only currently being compiled so its place in the future management of trigeminal neuralgia is unclear (Regis *et al* 2001; McNatt *et al* 2005; Sheehan *et al* 2005).

3.1.1. Peripheral Neurectomy

In elderly fragile patients peripheral neurectomy especially of the supraorbital and infraorbital nerves provides effective pain relief lasting for approximately 12 months (Murali and Rovit 1996; Oturai *et al* 1996). Local dense anaesthesia, the development of dysaesthesiae and the rather rapid return of the pain in most treated patients make this procedure unattractive for the patient with a longer life expectancy.

3.1.2. Percutaneous Trigeminal Rhizotomy

Three methods are commonly used: radiofrequency (RF) rhizolysis (Moraci *et al* 1992; Taha and Tew 1996; Broggi *et al* 2005), retrogasserian glycerol injection (Gomori and Rappaport 1985; Jho and Lunsford 1997; Kondziolka and Lunsford 2005; Pollock 2005) and trigeminal root balloon compression (Brown and Gouda 1997). A percutaneous puncture of the foramen ovale is performed under fluoroscopic guidance by inserting a spinal needle or guide with an indwelling stylet at a point approximately 3 cm lateral to the angle of the mouth (Fig. 12.1). Partial damage to the nerve root and ganglion is achieved by heating with an RF electrode introduced through the guide, chemically by injecting glycerol through the needle or by compression with a balloon catheter being inserted through the guide.

RF rhizolysis is the most senior of the three percutaneous procedures. The endpoint of the procedure is arrived at when an area of decreased sensation is produced in the painful area of the face. Patient cooperation during the stimulation testing procedure is important and is not readily obtained in some elderly patients. The recurrence rate is lower than that in the other two procedures; however the incidence of painful dysaesthesia is greater. For ophthalmic branch neuralgia, the risk of corneal hypaesthesia is somewhat higher than with the alternative procedures (Sweet 1988; Gybels and Sweet 1989).

Case 12.1 Trigeminal Neuralgia Treated by MVD Operation, 49-year-old Female

Present complaint

Patient complained of daily severe knife-like pain attacks in her right face. A trigger point was identified around the angle of the mouth from which the pain shot up to the temple on the same side. The attacks could be continuous for several hours. Speaking and chewing triggered the attack. She had recently increased her dosage of carbamazepine to 1000 mg with the addition of baclofen 10 mg t.i.d. without affecting the pain severity. As a result of the daily attacks, she had stopped working and refused to leave the house, except for frequenting the hospital's emergency room, where she received injections of narcotics.

History of present complaint

Five years ago the patient underwent a root canal procedure in her right upper jaw. She remembers suffering from intermittent pain in the area for several months afterwards. The pain subsided spontaneously but 18 months ago she suddenly developed the painful attacks from which she now suffers. At the time they were less frequent, limited in time, and over a smaller area of her face. She was started on carbamazepine, 200 mg b.i.d., which relieved her attacks for 2 months only. After the pain resumed her dosage was gradually elevated to the present level. Two months ago, baclofen was added, without effect.

Physical examination

Her physical and neurological examination, including facial sensation, was normal. During the examination she had a painful attack. Her right face winced, and she became immobile for several seconds. Pressing her right cheek seemed to lessen the intensity of the pain.

Diagnostic examinations

A cranial MRI scan was performed. Non-specific white matter bright spots were seen in the cerebrum on the T2 scan. In the posterior fossa the right trigeminal root was crossed by a vessel shadow at its entrance to the brainstem (Fig. 12.3). A diagnostic evaluation for multiple sclerosis was negative.

Treatment considerations

The patient was referred for neurosurgical consultation. She refused to consider increasing her medication levels, as she felt that they made her groggy. Considering her age and the positive MRI scan a microvascular decompression procedure was recommended.

Operation

The patient was operated on under general anaesthesia in the supine position with her head turned to the left. Surgical exposure for MVD was performed as described above. The cerebellum was gently retracted to allow visualization of the upper cerebellopontine angle. The arachnoid over the trigeminal nerve was opened while preserving the petrosal vein intact. An artery was seen crossing and indenting the trigeminal root at its entry site into the brainstem. The artery was lifted off the nerve. We saw a greyish discolouration of the nerve root at the site of the vascular contact (Fig. 12.2). A small fluff of Teflon felt was inserted between the nerve root and the artery to prevent renewed contact. The wound was closed in a routine fashion. The operation was performed in 90 minutes skin-to-skin.

Postoperative follow-up

The patient woke up from surgery without facial pain. She had an uncomplicated postoperative course and remained neurologically intact. Her medications were not renewed. She was discharged from the hospital after 48 hours. Three years following surgery she has remained without pain.

Glycerol rhizolysis does not require patient cooperation and has a lower incidence of facial dysaesthesia. As its recurrence rate is higher (70% of patients pain free at 1-year follow-up) than that of RF rhizolysis, repeat procedures may be necessary but increase the risk of subsequent dysaesthesia (Rappaport and Gomori 1988).

Balloon compression of the trigeminal root has a success rate intermediate between the previous two procedures. It results in a higher incidence of masticator muscle dysfunction. As a large bore needle must be used for insertion, general anaesthesia may be required, making it less appealing in the author's view (Fraioli *et al* 1989).

All three procedures are ablative in nature. As in any procedure that causes damage to the nervous system the danger of developing dysaesthesia and deafferentation pain exists. For the younger patient without significant medical risks a microvascular decompression procedure may be more appropriate for the long term as it treats the structural cause of the pain-producing pathology without damaging the nerve root (Rappaport 1996; Taha and Tew 1996; Broggi *et al* 2005).

3.1.3. Microvascular Decompression (MVD)

Most cases of trigeminal neuralgia are caused by vascular compression of the trigeminal root entry zone at the pons (Jannetta 1976). It is, however, important to exclude other causes of trigeminal neuralgia such as tumours

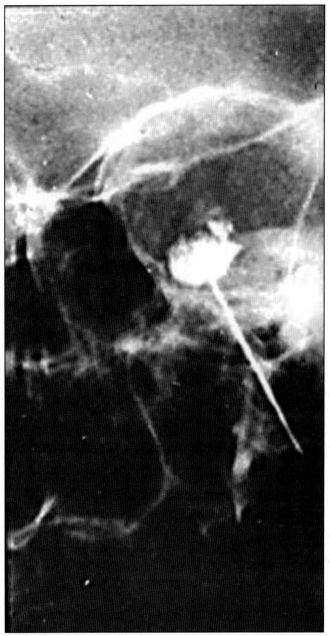

Fig. 12.1 • A lateral fluoroscopic view of the trigeminal cistern following contrast agent injection: the spinal needle used for the injection enters the cistern via the foramen ovale.

contacts. Arterial loops that knuckle into the root will frequently cause local discolouration of the root, implying secondary demyelination (Fig. 12.2) (Devor *et al* 2002a). The vessel loop is moved from the root and kept at a distance by a Teflon pledget. In about 10% of cases no arterial contact can be found despite a diligent exploration. Even if a significant venous contact is present, it is preferable to perform a partial sensory rhizotomy to ensure pain relief. The patient can usually be discharged from the hospital two to three days after surgery.

The advantage of this operation lies in the resolution of the causative pathology and cessation of the pain without causing nerve root damage. Sensory deafferentation phenomena are thereby avoided. The initial success rate is in the order of 90% and the recurrence rate is in the order of 2% per year (Sindou and Mertens 1993; Barker *et al* 1996b; Lovely and Jannetta 1997a). These outcome results are better than those obtained in percutaneous rhizotomy. The outcome is dependent on the zeal and the skill with which the surgeon can find the offending artery. In cases where no definite arterial compression is visualized, a topographically appropriate partial sensory rhizotomy is performed (Bederson and Wilson 1989; Klun 1992; Delitala *et al* 2001). Newer techniques of rhizotomy such as a partial crush of the root or interfibre dissection may lead to an acceptable level of dysaesthesia (Zakrzewska *et al* 2005). These results for MVD surgery refer to patients with typical trigeminal neuralgia.

When atypical features such as a poorly defined trigger zone, a background of burning pain and sensory loss are present, only about half the patients achieve a long-term satisfactory outcome (Tyler-Kabara *et al* 2002).

The morbidity of the surgery should be within 4%. This low morbidity and virtually zero mortality are achieved by limiting the operation to patients less than 70 years of age and who do not suffer from major systemic diseases. In the older, high-risk patient, the percutaneous procedures would be more appropriate (Rappaport 1996).

3.1.4. Gamma Knife Radiosurgery

Gamma knife radiosurgery has become a popular technique for the treatment of trigeminal neuralgia in recent years due to its relative non-invasiveness. The procedure involves the fixation under local anaesthesia of a stereotactic frame to the head of the patient, MRI imaging while in the frame and computer simulation of the radiosurgical treatment. Thus the technique is more cumbersome, labour-intensive and expensive than the more established percutaneous procedures. The onset of pain relief has a latency of at least several weeks and is therefore not attractive to patients with severe pain (Henson *et al* 2005). With a 40–60% pain recurrence rate at 1 year and a 6–18% rate of dysaesthesia, the procedure does not seem to offer an advantage over the percutaneous procedures (Kondziolka *et al* 1996; McNatt *et al* 2005; Sheehan *et al* 2005).

compressing the trigeminal root (7% of cases) or multiple sclerosis (2% of cases) by performing an MRI scan prior to surgery.

The operation is performed under general anaesthesia (see Case 12.1). A linear incision is performed behind the ear on the side of the pain. A 20 mm craniotomy is performed at the angle between the transverse and sigmoid sinus. Following dural opening the operative microscope is brought into the field and CSF is allowed to egress. There is very little need for cerebellar retraction if the patient is well anaesthetized and properly positioned. The arachnoid over the trigeminal root is opened and the root is carefully examined for possible arterial

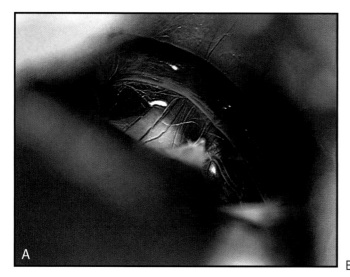

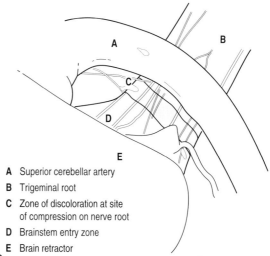

A Superior cerebellar artery
B Trigeminal root
C Zone of discoloration at site
of compression on nerve root
D Brainstem entry zone
E Brain retractor

Fig. 12.2 • A view of the right trigeminal root through the operating microscope. An arterial loop of the superior cerebellar artery has been lifted off the root. There is a band-like greyish discolouration of the root where it had been compressed close to its entrance to the brainstem. In (B) the picture is represented in diagrammatic form with the anatomical landmarks identified.

3.1.5. Timing and Choice of Neurosurgical Procedure in Trigeminal Neuralgia

Trigeminal neuralgia responds readily to medical therapy. Invasive therapy should only be considered following the failure of an adequate trial of medication. If the patient stops responding to carbamazepine or suffers from side effects that affect his quality of life, he may be switched to gabapentin or lamotrigine, occasionally in combination with baclofen (Chapters 11 and 16). If the patient remains symptomatic despite medical therapy, invasive therapy should be considered sooner rather than later. Chronic compression of the trigeminal nerve root may over time lead to neuropathic pain or atypical trigeminal neuralgia, which responds less well to any type of therapy (Tyler-Kabara et al 2002; Li et al 2004).

There is a general consensus among neurosurgeons that the MVD is the procedure of choice in the non-elderly and medically low-risk patient (Rappaport 1996; Javadpour et al 2003; Broggi et al 2005). Modern high-Tesla MRI scanners can often delineate the relevant artery compressing the trigeminal root (Fig. 12.3) (Voros et al 2001; Fukuda et al 2003). The high rates of long-term pain relief with the absence of neuropathic disturbances that accompany alternative destructive procedures of the root make MVD especially attractive for the younger patient.

In the elderly or medically infirm, a palliative percutaneous rhizolysis should be performed. There are differences of opinion which of the three commonly used procedures—retrogasserian glycerol injection, RF rhizolysis or balloon compression—should be preferred (Sweet 1988; Moraci et al 1992; Broggi et al 2005; Kondziolka and Lunsford 2005). Personally, this author prefers glycerol rhizolysis owing to its technical simplicity and its not requiring patient cooperation as with the RF

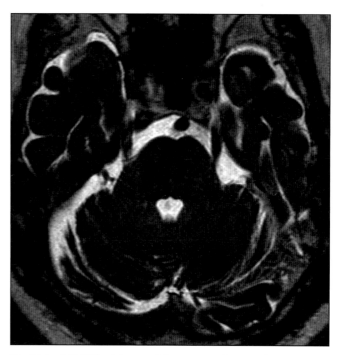

Fig. 12.3 • A T2 MRI axial scan of the posterior fossa, at the level of the trigeminal roots. A vessel is seen crossing the right trigeminal root, whereas the left trigeminal root is free of a vascular contact.

procedure. Following the glycerol procedure some 40% of patients have sustained pain relief without noticeable hypaesthesia, whereas in the RF procedure, sensory loss is the endpoint of the thermal lesion in all cases. There is, however, a trade-off. Following glycerol rhizolysis only about 55% of patients are pain free at 5 years, some 10–15% less than with RF. The ease of performing a repeat glycerol injection when pain does recur, however, outweighs in this author's view the increased incidence of hypaesthesia and dysaesthesia following the more aggressive RF rhizolysis. Using these two procedures, this author sees little need for the balloon compression technique, which requires deeper sedation of the patient due to the large bore needle used and which has a higher incidence of potentially more serious side effects without providing significantly better outcomes.

3.1.6. Trigeminal Neuralgia Secondary to Multiple Sclerosis

The incidence of trigeminal neuralgia in multiple sclerosis patients is 2%. While in the majority of multiple sclerosis patients the neuralgia is associated with reduction of facial sensation, at the beginning of the process hypaesthesia may be absent. In the absence of typical neurological symptomatology early in the course of the disease the MRI picture is pathognomonic of multiple sclerosis. Following failure of medical therapy the interventional options are similar to those in typical trigeminal neuralgia. If the MRI scan shows a typical vascular loop compressing the trigeminal root, an MVD procedure may be considered (Resnick *et al* 1996; Eldridge *et al* 2003; Broggi *et al* 2004). Given that only 50% of patients have long-term postoperative pain relief, a partial sensory rhizotomy should be added to the procedure unless the vessel pathology is very prominent.

The more standard procedure is a percutaneous rhizotomy. Glycerol rhizolysis may achieve a 50% success rate at 1 year with repeat treatment necessary (Pickett *et al* 2005). RF rhizolysis has a similar recurrence rate (Berk *et al* 2003).

4. Glossopharyngeal Neuralgia

Patients with glossopharyngeal neuralgia present with a frequency of less than 1% when compared to trigeminal neuralgia sufferers. Their clinical manifestations, moreover, are more variable. Generally pain is felt unilaterally in the throat region while swallowing or speaking. Autonomic manifestations such as syncope or bradycardia leading even to asystole are the most dramatic manifestations of the syndrome. Surgical therapy in medically refractory patients can be expected to lead to good results in a high percentage of patients. Classically a glossopharyngeal open rhizotomy is performed with the addition of an upper third vagal rhizotomy. Complications include difficulty in swallowing with or without hoarseness (Gybels and Sweet 1989). In the 1970s percutaneous RF rhizotomy via the pars nervosa of the jugular foramen gained popularity and became the procedure of choice. Bradycardia and vocal cord paralysis are the risks of this procedure (Taha and Tew 1995a). As with trigeminal neuralgia, MVD has been successful in relieving glossopharyngeal neuralgia pain, as the vascular aetiology and pathological picture have been found to be similar (Devor *et al* 2002b). Some authors routinely perform a rhizotomy following the vascular decompression (Taha and Tew 1995a). Others have found that this is not necessary and have achieved long-term pain relief in over 75% of patients

with minimal permanent side effects (Sindou and Mertens 1993; Resnick *et al* 1995; Kondo 1998). Percutaneous computed tomography (CT)-guided RF trigeminal nucleotomy-tractotomy has more recently been described as useful for complex cases (Kanpolat *et al* 1998). Very few centres, however, have experience with this technique.

5. Geniculate Neuralgia

Geniculate neuralgia involves the sensory distribution of the seventh cranial nerve (facial nerve) via the nervus intermedius (of Wrisberg). The painful attacks are centred within the ear canal and are sharp and stabbing in nature. A dull background pain may persist for several hours after an attack (Pulec 2002). Affected patients tend to be younger than in trigeminal and glossopharyngeal neuralgia. When seen together with hemifacial spasm the term 'tic convulsive' has been used (Yeh and Tew 1984). The established surgical therapy is section of the nervus intermedius either via a middle fossa approach (Pulec 2002) or in conjunction with an MVD of the adjacent cranial nerves (Lovely and Jannetta 1997b). A favourable outcome may be expected in up to 90% of cases.

6. Trigeminal Autonomic Cephalalgias (see Chapter 10)

Of the trigeminal autonomic cephalalgias, chronic cluster headaches unresponsive to medication have attracted surgical therapeutic attempts. RF ablation of the sphenopalatine ganglion has been useful in episodic cluster headaches, but unsuccessful in chronic patients (Sanders and Zuurmond 1997). Trigeminal rhizotomy may lead to corneal anaesthesia and has an inconsistent beneficial effect (Morgenlander and Wilkins 1990). It is doubtful whether section of the nervus intermedius improves outcome (Morgenlander and Wilkins 1990; Rowed 1990), though combining it with MVD of the trigeminal root has shown beneficial results (Lovely *et al* 1998).

Percutaneous RF trigeminal rhizotomy is a less invasive procedure and has been successfully used for pain around the eye. Major pain in the malar and temporal area responded poorly (Taha and Tew 1995b). Considering the disabling consequences of the accompanying corneal hypaesthesia, glycerol trigeminal rhizolysis may be the initial invasive procedure of choice (Hassenbusch *et al* 1991).

7. Persistent Idiopathic Facial Pain (Atypical Facial Pain)

Atypical facial pain has recently been renamed as persistent idiopathic facial pain and is a poorly defined clinical entity that has a large variety of potential causes (see Chapter 11). It is one of the most difficult chronic pain entities to treat. Consequently, patients have been sub-jected to a large variety of surgical procedures ranging from local neurectomies to cerebral ablative procedures (Gybels and Sweet 1989). Success rates have varied greatly, reflecting the lack of homogeneity of the patient population. Surgical procedures should not be performed if the pathophysiology of the pain syndrome remains obscure. In cases of trigeminal neuropathic pain, stimula-tion of the trigeminal root via a transoval percutaneously implanted electrode has shown some success, relieving pain in about half of the treated patients (Young 1995). Movement and breakage of the electrode during mastica-tion limits the technical success rate of the procedure. Thus it has had very limited popularity.

RF lesions to the nucleus caudalis dorsal root entry zone (DREZ) have been advocated for otherwise intractable facial pain syndromes. A posterior fossa craniotomy and upper cervical laminectomy are performed and thermal lesions of the nucleus are made from the level of the obex down to the C2 level of the spinal cord (Gorecki and Nashold 1995; Bullard and Nashold 1997). Given the high incidence of neurological complications (ipsilateral arm ataxia due to spinocerebellar tract injury and ipsilateral lower limb weakness from the pyramidal tract), this proce-dure should probably be reserved for pain secondary to malignancy only.

Percutaneous trigeminal tractotomy–nucleotomy is performed under CT guidance by inserting an RF elec-trode between the occiput and the lamina of C1 into the posterolateral spinal cord. It has an incidence of undesir-able neurological side effects lower than that of open pro-cedures but also has more limited applicability (Kanpolat et al 1998). In a recent series of 17 cases with atypical facial pain treated by this method only 7 were deemed to have had a 'good' long-term response (Kanpolat et al 2005). The categorization of the pain type that shows the best response is as yet unclear and the surgical experience is as yet quite limited. It remains an interesting option for severe cases.

Motor cortex stimulation has been utilized over the past several years in a variety of central pain conditions (Tirakotai et al 2004). The motor cortex is visualized on an MRI scan transferred to a neuronavigation system in the operating room. A limited craniotomy is performed over the appropriate area and the position of the motor cortex is confirmed by intraoperative electrical stimula-tion. The electrode is then implanted at this site and attached to a supraclavicular generator. For atypical facial pain, the electrode would be implanted over the facial motor cortex (Rainov and Heidecke 2003). In a recent series (Brown and Pilitsis 2005), motor cortex stimulation was applied in 10 patients with facial pain due to posther-petic neuralgia, surgical trigeminal injury and a medul-lary infarct. Following trial stimulation 8 systems were implanted. At 10-month mean follow-up patients had a 75% decrease in their pain, which had been present for a mean of 6 years preoperatively. In their literature review, the authors found that 29 (76%) of 38 patients with neuropathic facial pain treated with motor cortex stimulation achieved greater than 50% pain relief (Brown and Pilitsis 2005). These encouraging results, if more widely confirmed, open a therapeutic window for a most difficult class of patients.

8. Conclusion

Structural lesions of the central and peripheral nervous system are not infrequent causes of orofacial pain that may be relieved by neurosurgical intervention. Paroxys-mal pain in an anatomical neural distribution such as in trigeminal neuralgia is the most responsive type of pain to neurosurgical procedures. Destructive lesions of the nervous system may be required in the more diffuse chronic pain conditions, but entail potential complica-tions and have a lower success rate. Electrical stimulation is an attractive alternative that has the advantage of being reversible. The role of such procedures as motor cortex stimulation in the treatment of intractable chronic orofa-cial pain syndromes is still under investigation.

References

Barker FG, Jannetta PJ, Babu RP et al (1996a) Long-term outcome after operation for trigeminal neuralgia in patients with posterior fossa tumors. J Neurosurg 84:818–825.

Barker FG, Jannetta PJ, Bissonette DJ, et al (1996b) The long-term outcome of microvascular decompression for trigeminal neuralgia. N Engl J Med 334:1077–1083.

Bederson JB, Wilson CB (1989) Evaluation of microvascular decompression and partial sensory rhizotomy in 252 cases of trigeminal neuralgia. J Neurosurg 71:359–367.

Berk C, Constantoyannis C, Honey CR (2003) The treatment of trigeminal neuralgia in patients with multiple sclerosis using percutaneous radiofrequency rhizotomy. Can J Neurol Sci 30:220–223.

Broggi G, Ferroli P, Franzini A, et al (2004) Operative findings and outcomes of microvascular decompression for trigeminal neuralgia in 35 patients affected by multiple sclerosis. Neurosurgery 55:830–838.

Broggi G, Ferroli P, Franzini A, et al (2005) The role of surgery in the treatment of typical and atypical facial pain. Neurol Sci 26 (Suppl 2):S95–S100.

Brown JA, Gouda JJ (1997) Percutaneous balloon compression of the trigeminal nerve. Neurosurg Clin N Am 8:53–62.

Brown JA, Pilitsis JG (2005) Motor cortex stimulation for central and neuropathic facial pain: a prospective study of 10 patients and observations of enhanced sensory and motor function during stimulation. Neurosurgery 56:290–297.

Bullard DE, Nashold BS Jr (1997) The caudalis DREZ for facial pain. Stereotact Funct Neurosurg 68:168–174.

Burchiel KJ (2003) A new classification for facial pain. Neurosurgery 53:1164–1166.

Delitala A, Brunori A, Chiappetta F (2001) Microsurgical posterior fossa exploration for trigeminal neuralgia: a study on 48 cases. Minim Invasive Neurosurg 44:152–156.

Devor M, Govrin-Lippmann R, Rappaport ZH (2002a) Mechanism of trigeminal neuralgia: an ultrastructural analysis of trigeminal root specimens obtained during microvascular decompression surgery. J Neurosurg 96:532–543.

Devor M, Govrin-Lippmann R, Rappaport ZH, et al (2002b) Cranial root injury in glossopharyngeal neuralgia: electron microscopic observations. Case report. J Neurosurg 96:603–606.

Devor M, Amir R, Rappaport ZH (2002c) Pathophysiology of trigeminal neuralgia: the ignition hypothesis. Clin J Pain 18:4–13.

Dolenc VV (1994) Frontotemporal epidural approach to trigeminal neurinomas. Acta Neurochir (Wien) 130:55–65.

Eldridge PR, Sinha AK, Javadpour M, et al (2003) Microvascular decompression for trigeminal neuralgia in patients with multiple sclerosis. Stereotact Funct Neurosurg 81:57–64.

Forderreuther S, Straube A (1999) The criteria of the International Headache Society for Tolosa-Hunt syndrome need to be revised. J Neurol 246:371–377.

Fraioli B, Esposito V, Guidetti B, et al (1989) Treatment of trigeminal neuralgia by thermocoagulation, glycerolization, and percutaneous compression of the gasserian ganglion and/or retrogasserian rootlets: long-term results and therapeutic protocol. Neurosurgery 24:239–245.

Fukuda H, Ishikawa M, Okumura R (2003) Demonstration of neurovascular compression in trigeminal neuralgia and hemifacial spasm with magnetic resonance imaging: comparison with surgical findings in 60 consecutive cases. Surg Neurol 59:93–99.

Goh BT, Poon CY, Peck RH (2001) The importance of routine magnetic resonance imaging in trigeminal neuralgia diagnosis. Oral Surg Oral Med Oral Pathol Oral Radiol Endod 92:424–429.

Gomori JM, Rappaport ZH (1985) Transovale trigeminal cistern puncture: modified fluoroscopically guided technique. AJNR Am J Neuroradiol 6:93–94.

Gorecki JP, Nashold BS (1995) The Duke experience with the nucleus caudalis DREZ operation. Acta Neurochir Suppl 64:128–131.

Gybels JM, Sweet WH (1989) Neurosurgical Treatment of Persistent Pain. Basel: Karger.

Hassenbusch SJ, Kunkel RS, Kosmorsky GS, et al (1991) Trigeminal cisternal injection of glycerol for treatment of chronic intractable cluster headaches. Neurosurgery 29:504–508.

Henson CF, Goldman HW, Rosenwasser RH, et al (2005) Glycerol rhizotomy versus gamma knife radiosurgery for the treatment of trigeminal neuralgia: an analysis of patients treated at one institution. Int J Radiat Oncol Biol Phys 63:82–90.

Ito M, Sonokawa T, Mishina H, et al (1996) Dural arteriovenous malformation manifesting as tic douloureux. Surg Neurol 45:370–375.

Jannetta PJ (1976) Microsurgical approach to the trigeminal nerve for tic doloreux. Prog Neurol Surg 7:180–200.

Javadpour M, Eldridge PR, Varma TR, et al (2003) Microvascular decompression for trigeminal neuralgia in patients over 70 years of age. Neurology 60:520.

Jho HD, Lunsford LD (1997) Percutaneous retrogasserian glycerol rhizotomy. Current technique and results. Neurosurg Clin N Am 8:63–74.

Kanpolat Y, Savas A, Batay F, et al (1998) Computed tomography-guided trigeminal tractotomy-nucleotomy in the management of vagoglossopharyngeal and geniculate neuralgias. Neurosurgery 43:484–489.

Kanpolat Y, Savas A, Ugur HC, et al (2005) The trigeminal tract and nucleus procedures in treatment of atypical facial pain. Surg Neurol 64(Suppl 2):S96–S100.

Karibe H, Shirane R, Jokura H, et al (2004) Intrinsic arteriovenous malformation of the trigeminal nerve in a patient with trigeminal neuralgia: case report. Neurosurgery 55:1433.

Klun B (1992) Microvascular decompression and partial sensory rhizotomy in the treatment of trigeminal neuralgia: personal experience with 220 patients. Neurosurgery 30:49–52.

Kondo A (1998) Follow-up results of using microvascular decompression for treatment of glossopharyngeal neuralgia. J Neurosurg 88:221–225.

Kondziolka D, Lunsford LD (2005) Percutaneous retrogasserian glycerol rhizotomy for trigeminal neuralgia: technique and expectations. Neurosurg Focus 18:E7.

Kondziolka D, Lunsford LD, Flickinger JC, et al (1996) Stereotactic radiosurgery for trigeminal neuralgia: a multiinstitutional study using the gamma unit. J Neurosurg 84:940–945.

Lee O, Cromwell LD, Weider DJ (2005) Carcinomatous meningitis arising from primary nasopharyngeal carcinoma. Am J Otolaryngol 26:193–197.

Li ST, Pan Q, Liu N, et al (2004) Trigeminal neuralgia: what are the important factors for good operative outcomes with microvascular decompression. Surg Neurol 62:400–404.

Linskey ME, Sekhar LN, Hirsch WL Jr, et al (1990) Aneurysms of the intracavernous carotid artery: natural history and indications for treatment. Neurosurgery 26:933–937.

Lovely TJ, Jannetta PJ (1997a) Microvascular decompression for trigeminal neuralgia. Surgical technique and long-term results. Neurosurg Clin N Am 8:11–29.

Lovely TJ, Jannetta PJ (1997b) Surgical management of geniculate neuralgia. Am J Otol 18:512–517.

Lovely TJ, Kotsiakis X, Jannetta PJ (1998) The surgical management of chronic cluster headache. Headache 38:590–594.

McNatt SA, Yu C, Giannotta SL, et al (2005) Gamma knife radiosurgery for trigeminal neuralgia. Neurosurgery 56:1295–1301.

Mainardi F, Maggioni F, Dainese F, et al (2002) Spontaneous carotid artery dissection with cluster-like headache. Cephalalgia 22:557–559.

Matsuka Y, Fort ET, Merrill RL (2000) Trigeminal neuralgia due to an acoustic neuroma in the cerebellopontine angle. J Orofac Pain 14:147–151.

Meng L, Yuguang L, Feng L, et al (2005) Cerebellopontine angle epidermoids presenting with trigeminal neuralgia. J Clin Neurosci 12:784–786.

Moller AR (1998) Vascular compression of cranial nerves. I. History of the microvascular decompression operation. Neurol Res 20:727–731.

Moller AR (1999) Vascular compression of cranial nerves: II: pathophysiology. Neurol Res 21:439–443.

Moraci A, Buonaiuto C, Punzo A, et al (1992) Trigeminal neuralgia treated by percutaneous thermocoagulation. Comparative analysis of percutaneous thermocoagulation and other surgical procedures. Neurochirurgia (Stuttg) 35:48–53.

Morgenlander JC, Wilkins RH (1990) Surgical treatment of cluster headache. J Neurosurg 72:866–871.

Murali R, Rovit RL (1996) Are peripheral neurectomies of value in the treatment of trigeminal neuralgia? An analysis of new cases and cases involving previous radiofrequency gasserian thermocoagulation. J Neurosurg 85:435–437.

Oturai AB, Jensen K, Eriksen J, et al (1996) Neurosurgery for trigeminal neuralgia: comparison of alcohol block, neurectomy, and radiofrequency coagulation. Clin J Pain 12:311–315.

Pickett GE, Bisnaire D, Ferguson GG (2005) Percutaneous retrogasserian glycerol rhizotomy in the treatment of tic douloureux associated with multiple sclerosis. Neurosurgery 56:537–545.

Pollock BE (2005) Percutaneous retrogasserian glycerol rhizotomy for patients with idiopathic trigeminal neuralgia: a prospective analysis of factors related to pain relief. J Neurosurg 102:223–228.

Pollock BE, Iuliano BA, Foote RL, et al (2000) Stereotactic radiosurgery for tumor-related trigeminal pain. Neurosurgery 46:576–582.

Pulec JL (2002) Geniculate neuralgia: long-term results of surgical treatment. Ear Nose Throat J 81:30–33.

Quinones-Hinojosa A, Chang EF, Khan SA, et al (2003) Isolated trigeminal nerve sarcoid granuloma mimicking trigeminal schwannoma: case report. Neurosurgery 52:700–705.

Rainov NG, Heidecke V (2003) Motor cortex stimulation for neuropathic facial pain. Neurol Res 25:157–161.

Rappaport ZH (1985) Epidermoid tumour of the cerebellopontine angle as a cause of trigeminal neuralgia. *Neurochirurgia (Stuttg)* **28**:211–212.

Rappaport ZH (1996) The choice of therapy in medically intractable trigeminal neuralgia. *Isr J Med Sci* **32**:1232–1234.

Rappaport ZH, Gomori JM (1988) Recurrent trigeminal cistern glycerol injections for tic douloureux. *Acta Neurochir (Wien)* **90**:31–34.

Regis J, Metellus P, Dufour H, *et al* (2001) Long-term outcome after gamma knife surgery for secondary trigeminal neuralgia. *J Neurosurg* **95**:199–205.

Resnick DK, Jannetta PJ, Bissonnette D, *et al* (1995) Microvascular decompression for glossopharyngeal neuralgia. *Neurosurgery* **36**:64–68.

Resnick DK, Jannetta PJ, Lunsford LD, *et al* (1996) Microvascular decompression for trigeminal neuralgia in patients with multiple sclerosis. *Surg Neurol* **46**:358–361.

Rowed DW (1990) Chronic cluster headache managed by nervus intermedius section. *Headache* **30**:401–406.

Saeed AB, Shuaib A, Al-Sulaiti G, *et al* (2000) Vertebral artery dissection: warning symptoms, clinical features and prognosis in 26 patients. *Can J Neurol Sci* **27**:292–296.

Samii M, Carvalho GA, Tatagiba M, *et al* (1997) Surgical management of meningiomas originating in Meckel's cave. *Neurosurgery* **41**:767–774.

Sanders M, Zuurmond WW (1997) Efficacy of sphenopalatine ganglion blockade in 66 patients suffering from cluster headache: a 12- to 70-month follow-up evaluation. *J Neurosurg* **87**:876–880.

Selky AK, Pascuzzi R (1995) Raeder's paratrigeminal syndrome due to spontaneous dissection of the cervical and petrous internal carotid artery. *Headache* **35**:432–434.

Sheehan J, Pan HC, Stroila M, *et al* (2005) Gamma knife surgery for trigeminal neuralgia: outcomes and prognostic factors. *J Neurosurg* **102**:434–441.

Sindou M, Mertens P (1993) Microsurgical vascular decompression (MVD) in trigeminal and glosso-vago-pharyngeal neuralgias. A twenty-year experience. *Acta Neurochir Suppl (Wien)* **58**:168–170.

Sweet WH (1988) Percutaneous methods for the treatment of trigeminal neuralgia and other faciocephalic pain; comparison with microvascular decompression. *Semin Neurol* **8**:272–279.

Taha JM, Tew JM Jr (1995a) Long-term results of surgical treatment of idiopathic neuralgias of the glossopharyngeal and vagal nerves. *Neurosurgery* **36**:926–930.

Taha JM, Tew JM Jr (1995b) Long-term results of radiofrequency rhizotomy in the treatment of cluster headache. *Headache* **35**:193–196.

Taha JM, Tew JM Jr (1996) Comparison of surgical treatments for trigeminal neuralgia: reevaluation of radiofrequency rhizotomy. *Neurosurgery* **38**:865–871.

Tirakotai W, Riegel T, Sure U, *et al* (2004) Image-guided motor cortex stimulation in patients with central pain. *Minim Invasive Neurosurg* **47**:273–277.

Tyler-Kabara EC, Kassam AB, Horowitz MH, *et al* (2002) Predictors of outcome in surgically managed patients with typical and atypical trigeminal neuralgia: comparison of results following microvascular decompression. *J Neurosurg* **96**:527–531.

Voros E, Palko A, Horvath K, *et al* (2001) Three-dimensional time-of-flight MR angiography in trigeminal neuralgia on a 0.5-T system. *Eur Radiol* **11**:642–647.

Yamamoto T, Goto K, Suzuki A, *et al* (2000) Long-term improvement of idiopathic hypertrophic cranial pachymeningitis by lymphocytapheresis. *Ther Apher* **4**:313–316.

Yang J, Simonson TM, Ruprecht A, *et al* (1996) Magnetic resonance imaging used to assess patients with trigeminal neuralgia. *Oral Surg Oral Med Oral Pathol Oral Radiol Endod* **81**:343–350.

Yeh HS, Tew JM Jr (1984) Tic convulsif, the combination of geniculate neuralgia and hemifacial spasm relieved by vascular decompression. *Neurology* **34**:682–683.

Yi HJ, Kim CH, Bak KH, *et al* (2000) Metastatic tumors in the sellar and parasellar regions: clinical review of four cases. *J Korean Med Sci* **15**:363–367.

Young RF (1995) Electrical stimulation of the trigeminal nerve root for the treatment of chronic facial pain. *J Neurosurg* **83**:72–78.

Younger DS (2004) Headaches and vasculitis. *Neurol Clin* **22**:207–228.

Zakrzewska JM, Lopez BC, Kim SE, *et al* (2005) Patient reports of satisfaction after microvascular decompression and partial sensory rhizotomy for trigeminal neuralgia. *Neurosurgery* **56**:1304–1311.

Referred and secondary orofacial pain syndromes

Rafael Benoliel, Yair Sharav and Eli Eliav

This chapter covers post-traumatic headache and a number of entities outside the orofacial region that refer pain to the region.

1. Headache or Facial Pain Secondary to Regional Trauma

Headache or facial pain that occurs *de novo* in close temporal relation to trauma or an existing pain disorder that undergoes significant worsening may be classified as post-traumatic. Post-traumatic headache (PTH) may be subclassified as associated with mild or moderate to severe head injury and may be acute or chronic (Olesen *et al* 2004). Acute PTH occurs within 7 days but resolves within 3 months of injury, whilst chronic PTH is diagnosed if pain persists beyond 3 months (Olesen *et al* 2004).

No comparable criteria to those of the International Headache Society (IHS) have been established for post-traumatic facial pain. Extrapolating from the IHS's criteria would allow the preface 'post-traumatic' to be added to cases where the facial pain began in close temporal proximity to a traumatic event (less than 7 days) and persists beyond 3 months (Benoliel *et al* 1994). The individual distribution of craniofacial post-traumatic pain may dictate the specialist a patient consults but the aetiologic events and mechanisms are probably similar. We therefore refer to post-traumatic headache and/or facial pain as post-traumatic craniofacial pain (PTCFP) throughout the following section.

1.1. Epidemiology

Acute headache that occurs following trauma to the head or face region is relatively common and occurs in 30–90%

of patients (Evans 2004; Nicholson and Martelli 2004; Benoliel *et al* 2005; Walker *et al* 2005; Lew *et al* 2006). The number of patients that continue to suffer pain and develop chronic PTCFP is unclear and often varies across countries (Solomon 2005). About a third of patients with head injury report persistent headache at 3 months, a quarter or more may still report pain 4–5 years following injury and 11% suffer frequent headaches after 22-year follow-up (Edna and Cappelen 1987; Hillier *et al* 1997; Nestvold *et al* 2005; Solomon 2005). Most chronic PTCFP cases are caused by motor vehicle accidents, some by falls or assaults and a minority by sports injuries (Benoliel *et al* 1994; Young *et al* 2001). Most patients are young males and characteristically cases are seen at specialist centres a long time following injury (Benoliel *et al* 1994; Landy 1998), a factor associated with a reduced prognosis (Benoliel *et al* 1994).

1.2. Comorbidity

Chronic PTCFP may form part of a symptom complex termed post-traumatic stress disorder (PTSD) that includes psychological, social and cognitive impairment (Tatrow *et al* 2003; Baandrup and Jensen 2005; De Leeuw *et al* 2005a,b; Sherman *et al* 2005; Branca 2006; Stulemeijer *et al* 2006). Following orofacial injury acute PTSD may be particularly prominent and may persist with significant associated disability (Aghabeigi *et al* 1992; Glynn *et al* 2003). If PTSD becomes established a multidisciplinary approach that involves pain specialists, psychologist/psychiatrists, physiotherapists, social workers, family physician and cooperation from members of the patient's family and co-workers is required. Additionally patients may be involved in litigation and although there is no evidence to suggest that PTCFP is related to ongoing litigation (Evans 2004; Mooney *et al* 2005) careful work up to exclude malingering should be performed (Burgess and Dworkin 1993).

1.3. Assessment and Symptomatology

The assessment of PTCFP is often complicated by the absence of detectable organic pathology or abnormalities in neurophysiologic testing, particularly following mild or blunt craniocervical injury (Olesen *et al* 2004). Indeed the long-term persistence of PTCFP is unrelated to associated physical variables such as trauma severity and the incidence of loss of consciousness (Nestvold *et al* 2005). The factors that significantly increase the persistence of PTCFP 22 years following trauma were found to be female gender, high intensity of the acute PTCFP and psychiatric comorbidity (Nestvold *et al* 2005). The clinical characteristics of chronic PTCFP are usually similar to those of primary headache/facial pain disorders, and more than one disorder may occur together in the same patient (Benoliel *et al* 1994; Haas 1996; Bettucci *et al* 1998; Lane and Arciniegas 2002; Evans 2004; Baandrup and Jensen 2005). About a third of chronic PTCFP patients report symptomatology of tension-type headaches and about 28% of migraine headaches (Lew *et al* 2006). Similarly musculoskeletal pain is most commonly observed in post-traumatic orofacial pain (Benoliel *et al* 1994; De Leeuw *et al* 2005a,b). Migraine-type headaches seem to be more common following acceleration-deceleration injuries to the neck (whiplash) and injuries to the cervical complex (Lew *et al* 2006). Unclassifiable headache disorders are reported in about a fifth to a quarter of cases (Lew *et al* 2006). The importance of accurate diagnosis of all the involved disorders is paramount as it will dictate the prescription of treatment; see Case 13.1.

1.4. Pathophysiology

The pathophysiology of PTCFP is unclear and probably involves a number of mechanisms that interplay with the individual patient's psychosocial capabilities and specific genotype to dictate who will or will not suffer chronic pain. The role of trauma in some craniofacial pain syndromes such as temporomandibular disorders is well established (see Chapters 7 and 8). Direct injury to musculoskeletal structures may initiate changes that in susceptible individuals result in persistent pain. The degree of brain injury is not consistently associated with the incidence or severity of pain. Thus frank injury to brain tissue plays some part but other factors are involved. Shear forces applied to the brain result in a phenomenon termed diffuse axonal injury (see Chapter 11) that may be involved in the initiation of some PTCFP syndromes.

1.5. Treatment

Symptomatic treatment includes the use of drugs relevant to the primary pain disorders (see Chapters 7–11, 15 and 16) and usually requires additional modalities such as physical therapy, trigger point injections and occlusal splints (see Chapters 7 and 8). Cognitive behavioural therapy may be indicated (see Chapter 4) and is very successful in chronic PTCFP (Gurr and Coetzer 2005).

Chronic PTCFP developing after whiplash injury is also classified by the IHS and is discussed in the next section (Olesen *et al* 2004).

2. Headache or Facial Pain of Cervical Origin

Craniofacial pain may originate from the neck in disorders of the cervical vertebrae and associated structures (ligaments, periosteum), the cervical muscles and the cervical nerves. Referred pain from cervical arteries is also discussed below. Rare cervical entities associated with pain and dysfunction involving the head include retropharyngeal tendonitis (Fahlgren 1986, 1988; Ekbom *et al* 1994; Chung *et al* 2005; Kusunoki *et al* 2006) and craniocervical dystonia (Defazio *et al* 1989; Tarsy and First 1999; Ertekin *et al* 2002; Muller *et al* 2002; Ondo *et al* 2005; Bhidayasiri *et al* 2006).

2.1. Head and Neck Pain Associated with Whiplash Injury

Whether whiplash induces temporomandibular disorders is unclear and has been discussed in Chapter 7. Acute pain occurring locally in the neck following whiplash injuries is relatively common (Solomon 2005). Acute headache occurs in a large number of whiplash injuries (Di Stefano and Radanov 1995). Additionally whiplash may lead to chronic cervical pain with disability and may induce headache as described below (Cote *et al* 2000). Whiplash associated disorders have been defined and categorized (Spitzer *et al* 1995); subtype I includes cervical pain and tenderness and type II has additional features of reduced range of motion and point tenderness. Whiplash associated disorders I and II will be referred to in this section as chronic whiplash pain. Types III and IV are associated with fractures and distinct neurological signs and are beyond the scope of this book. Depending on culture and geographical distribution 1–82% of patients continue to suffer from chronic whiplash pain following whiplash injury (Barnsley *et al* 1994; Freeman *et al* 1999; Solomon 2005). The persistence of pain is not consistently related to the degree of trauma or cervical pathology. Similarly there are many patients with structural cervical lesions who suffer no pain (Solomon 2005). Diffuse axonal injury as described earlier (see also

Case 13.1 Chronic Post-traumatic Headache, 22-year-old Male

Present complaint

Pain in left craniofacial area that started immediately after trauma to the area.

History of present complaint

The patient was injured 2 years previously by a stone that hit his head and face on the left side. He had lost consciousness for a brief period only and had been transferred to an emergency department for treatment. There were no fractures but a laceration in the left temporal area was debrided and sutured. He was discharged and healed uneventfully but continued to suffer constant headaches. He complained of disturbed sleep.

Currently he suffered from pain in three locations, associated with different pain characteristics described as follows (see Fig. 13.1):

1. Pain located in all the left side of the head:
   a. Episodic pain appeared a number of times (>8) a month;
   b. Pain lasted up to a number of days;
   c. Pain was moderate (VAS 7.5) and of a throbbing quality; and
   d. Pain was associated with redness of the left eye.
2. Pain specifically around the angle of the mandible and temporomandibular joint:
   a. Pain occurred daily or nearly every day;
   b. Pain lasted for some hours;
   c. Pain was of moderate severity and of a dull, pressing quality (VAS 7); and
   d. Pain was aggravated by chewing or trying to open the mouth widely.
3. Pain in the temporal region:
   a. Episodic pain with no specific pattern;
   b. Paroxysmal, sharp pain that lasted for a number of seconds; and
   c. Pain of extreme severity (VAS 8).

Physical examination

The TMJ and the muscles of mastication on the left side and the cervical muscles bilaterally were tender to palpation. Mouth opening was limited (30 mm interincisal) and increased following vapocoolant (ethyl chloride) spray (35 mm).

A tender scar was palpated in the left temporal area that demonstrated allodynia and increased pain following repeated stimuli (temporal summation).

Relevant medical history

None.

Diagnosis

Since the pain had begun following regional trauma and persisted for 2 years this is a clear case of 'chronic post-traumatic headache'.

Diagnostic and treatment considerations

The pain characteristics outlined above indicated that there were three pain subtypes:

1. Migraine headache (see Chapter 9);
2. Masticatory myofascial pain (see Chapter 7); and
3. Post-traumatic neuropathy (see Chapter 11).

Migraine headache is often associated with regional muscle sensitivity but the particularly unilateral symptomatology, the dysfunction and associated signs suggested that the patient did indeed suffer from myofascial pain.

The patient was initiated on 10 mg amitriptyline, which is an efficacious prophylactic drug for myofascial, neuropathic and migraine-type pains. The dose was to be increased by 10–15 mg every 2 weeks to an initial target of 35 mg daily. At review (including summarizing pain diaries) it was obvious that the pain response was highly specific and although the migraine and myofascial pain responded favourably, the traumatic neuropathy although initially responding was slowly relapsing (see Fig. 13.2). Various antiepileptic drugs were added on to attempt to control the neuropathic pain but the only drug to provide partial relief (VAS reduced to 2) was clonazepam 1.5 mg together with amitriptyline 35 mg at bedtime.

This case demonstrates the importance of isolating individual diagnoses in post-traumatic pain and providing individual therapy.

Chapter 11) may be involved in the initiation of chronic pain following whiplash injury but in the absence of clear proof remains speculative. The role of litigation in persistence of chronic whiplash pain is unclear. However, one study has shown that when compensation for pain and suffering is eliminated there is a decreased incidence and improved prognosis of whiplash injury (Cassidy *et al* 2000).

Structural lesions of the cervical spine should be assessed by an orthopaedic surgeon or neurologist. Similarly, conservative treatment of chronic whiplash pain should be performed in close cooperation with an orthopaedic surgeon or neurologist and involve the use of multimodal therapy—medication, physical therapy, soft collars, trigger point injection and cognitive behavioural therapy.

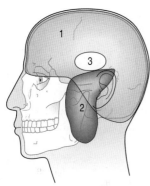

Fig. 13.1 • Pain location for Case 13.1. 1, Migraine headache (grey area): episodic, throbbing pain lasting days. 2, Masticatory myofascial pain (dotted area): chronic, deep, dull pain lasting hours and aggravated by mandibular function. 3, Post-traumatic neuropathy (white area): paroxysmal, severe, sharp pain lasting seconds and associated with an allodynic scar.

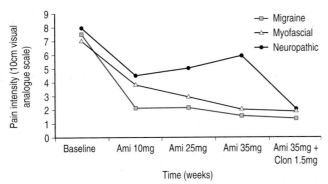

Fig. 13.2 • Response to drug therapy of the different pain disorders. Case 13.1 suffered from chronic post-traumatic head and facial pain. There were three different components diagnosed: migraine headache, masticatory myofascial pain (myofascial) and neuropathic. Migraine and myofascial pain responded well to 35 mg amitriptyline (Ami) whilst the neuropathic pain, although it initially responded reasonably, began to relapse. Addition of 1.5 mg clonazepam (Clon) relieved the neuropathic pain.

2.2. Cervicogenic Headache

Cervicogenic headache (CHA) is clearly defined by the IHS (see Table 13.1), but the reliability of the diagnostic criteria is unclear (Olesen *et al* 2004). The presence of headache associated with cervical spine disease is insufficient to diagnose CHA as virtually all people over the age of 40 will display such changes (Edmeads 1988; Bono *et al* 1998). Sjaastad and colleagues suggest that CHA is a symptom complex or reaction pattern (Sjaastad and Fredriksen 2000). Thus a number of cervical disorders may lead to CHA and its symptomatology may therefore be extremely variable.

2.2.1. Epidemiology

The prevalence of CHA in the general population is 0.4–2.5% and reaches 15–20% in patients with chronic headaches (Haldeman and Dagenais 2001). Mean age is about 43 years and females outnumber males by 4:1 (Haldeman and Dagenais 2001). Mean symptom duration

is about 7 years (Sjaastad and Fredriksen 2000; Antonaci *et al* 2001). However, due to a lack of universal agreement on criteria the exact figures are unclear.

2.2.2. Clinical Features

The clinical features of CHA are nonspecific and often mimic migraines or tension-type headaches. Headaches may be uni- or bilateral with a variable quality. Some suggestive features include a posterior location, triggering by neck movement and a postural component.

Sjastaad and colleagues have outlined several features commonly observed in CHA cases (Sjaastad *et al* 1990, 1992, 1997, 1998a,b; Sjaastad and Bovim 1991; Sjaastad 1999; Sjaastad and Fredriksen 2000). Patients are usually female with a history of neck trauma. Pain is largely unilateral and does not change sides although contralateral spread may occur in severe pain. The pain is located initially in the neck and spreads anteriorly to the oculofrontotemporal regions where it may become the prominent feature. Quality is non-throbbing, is of moderate intensity and may be continuous or intermittent but usually aggravated by neck movements, pressure on the neck or awkward neck postures. There may be reduced cervical range of motion and pain referral to the ipsilateral shoulder and arm. Accompanying signs reported include nausea, vomiting, phono- and photophobia and oedema or flushing around the eye.

The symptom sign complex described above may often be observed in migraine without aura and there has been discussion as to the validity of CHA as a separate entity.

2.2.3. Pathophysiology

Referred pain from cervical disorders to head or facial regions may occur through a number of mechanisms. The greater and lesser occipital branches of the sensory second cervical (C) root may refer pain to the back of the head. The sensory first cervical root may refer pain to the vertex or frontal region, but some consider this unlikely. Connections between C2 branches from the posterior fossa to branches of the ophthalmic nerve would refer pain to the front of the head. The descending spinal tract and upper cervical segments merge into the trigeminocervical complex, providing an anatomical connection for pain referral between trigeminal and cervical structures.

2.2.4. Treatment

Underlying disease processes should be identified and treated if this is possible. Diagnostic blockade of the C2 root may alleviate pain and differentiate CHA from other primary headaches. The use of medications, physical therapy, transcutaneous electrical nerve stimulation, botulinum toxin injections and surgery is largely unvalidated but appears in the literature.

Table 13.1 International Headache Society's (IHS) Criteria for Cervicogenic Headache

	Diagnostic Criteria	Notes
A	Pain, referred from a source in the neck and perceived in one or more regions of the head and/or face, fulfilling criteria C and D	
B	Clinical, laboratory and/or imaging evidence of a disorder or lesion within the cervical spine or soft tissues of the neck known to be, or generally accepted as, a valid cause of headache.	Tumours, fractures, infections and rheumatoid arthritis are not generally validated causes but may be so in individual cases. IHS criteria suggest that cervical myofascial tender areas should be coded as tension-type headache; we suggest simply diagnosing these as cervical myofascial pain.
C	Evidence that the pain can be attributed to the neck disorder or lesion based on at least one of the following: 1. Demonstration of clinical signs that implicate a source of pain in the neck 2. Abolition of headache following diagnostic blockade of a cervical structure or its nerve supply using placebo or other adequate controls	1. The specificity and sensitivity of signs and anamnestic details such as tenderness, reduced range of motion and a history of neck trauma are unclear. These are often observed in other headaches. 2. Reduction of pain by ≥90% is acceptable.
D	Pain resolves within 3 months after successful treatment of the causative disorder or lesion.	Implies complete remission

From Olesen *et al* (2004) with permission

3. Neck Tongue Syndrome (NTS)

NTS consists of the appearance of occipital or upper neck pain associated with an abnormal sensation on the ipsilateral side of the tongue.

3.1. Clinical Features

Pain is initiated by head rotation, usually to one side, and lasts some minutes (Olesen *et al* 2004). Pain is usually sharp and radiates to the occipital, cervical and lingual regions (Lance and Anthony 1980; Elisevich *et al* 1984). In the tongue, paraesthesia, dysaesthesia or anaesthesia may be reported lasting from a few seconds to about 2 minutes (Sjaastad and Bakketeig 2006). This may or may not be preceded by tongue pain (Lance and Anthony 1980; Chedrawi *et al* 2000). Patients may describe radicular symptoms and display restricted neck movements (Sjaastad and Bakketeig 2006).

3.2. Epidemiology

Although considered extremely rare about 59 cases have been reported in the literature and a prevalence of 0.22% has been estimated (Sjaastad and Bakketeig 2006).

3.3. Pathophysiology

Excessive range of movement of the atlantoaxial joint with impaction and stretching of the second cervical root (C2) is thought to underlie NTS (Bogduk 1981). This in turn compresses proprioceptive fibres from the tongue that pass from the ansa hypoglossi to the C2 ventral ramus (Lance and Anthony 1980). Surgical findings confirm C2 nerve compression by the atlantoaxial joint (Elisevich *et al* 1984).

3.4. Treatment

Spinal immobilization (soft collar), atlantoaxial fusion or resection of the C2 spinal nerve may be needed; in uncomplicated cases spinal manipulation may help (Elisevich *et al* 1984; Fortin and Biller 1985; Borody 2004).

4. Medication Overuse Headache

The frequent intake of analgesics has been associated with chronic headache, termed medication overuse headache (MOH). The involvement of the orofacial region in MOH is unreported.

4.1. Clinical Features

The diagnosis of MOH requires the presence for at least 3 months of daily or nearly daily headache (>14 days per month) associated with drug overuse on more than 10–15 days monthly (Olesen *et al* 2004). The change in headache pattern must have occurred or worsened during the onset of drug misuse and will resolve or revert to its original pattern within 2 months of drug control or cessation (Olesen *et al* 2004). Thus MOH can only be reliably diagnosed following a 2-month follow-up period. In some initially diagnosed MOH patients there may be no change or even a worsening of headaches following a 2-month cessation (Zeeberg *et al* 2006).

Patients describe an initial episodic headache that increases in frequency together with increasing intake of anti-headache drugs. The clinical characteristics are variable and partly depend on the underlying primary headache and the drug being abused. Analgesics (including combinations), opioids and ergots induce a mild to moderate, bilateral headache with a pressure-like quality whilst triptans induce a unilateral migraine-like headache (Pageler *et al* 2005). Patients with underlying migraine may report that together with the onset of MOH there was a noticeable waning of accompanying signs such as nausea and vomiting (Smith and Stoneman 2004).

MOH is one of the secondary forms of chronic daily headache (CDH; see Chapter 7) and has been associated with a number of drugs including simple analgesics, opioids and triptans (Meskunas *et al* 2006). Often, however, MOH patients are concomitantly abusing more than one compound and the identification of the responsible drug is difficult (Obermann *et al* 2006). Drugs prominently associated with MOH are the short-acting opioid butalbital, caffeine, aspirin, triptans and aspirin/codeine combinations (Obermann *et al* 2006). Triptans may induce daily migraine-like headaches but have also been associated with an increase in frequency of migraines (Limmroth *et al* 2002). Indeed triptan overuse induces MOH with the least mean latency (1.7 years) and dosages (18/month) whilst analgesics were associated with a latency of 4.8 years and a monthly frequency of 114 doses (Limmroth *et al* 2002).

Because MOH commonly appears in patients with primary headaches it is often overlooked or misdiagnosed as other chronic headache forms such as chronic migraine (see Chapter 9) or chronic tension-type headache (see Chapter 7). In a meta-analysis most MOH patients (65%) reported migraine as their primary headache whilst 27% reported tension-type headache and 8% reported other primary or mixed headaches (Diener and Dahlof 1999). In this series women outnumbered men by 3.5:1, higher than the ratio in migraine and suggesting that women are more prone to develop MOH. The mean duration of the primary headache was about 20 years with CDH/MOH beginning about 6 years previously. Frequent drug use was estimated at a mean of 10 years and indicates a long latency before MOH is induced (Diener and Dahlof 1999). Patients were taking on average 2–6 different medications concomitantly with about 5 tablets or suppositories daily.

4.2. Epidemiology

The abuse of analgesic drugs is a major concern in the management of chronic pain patients. This is due to potential health-related side effects, addiction and more recently the induction of MOH.

Population studies show that about 5% take analgesics daily and about 1% may be taking up to 10 tablets daily (Zwart *et al* 2003; Obermann *et al* 2006). Between 1 and 3% of the population will be taking anti-headache medications daily, putting them at high risk for the development of MOH (Prencipe *et al* 2001; Colas *et al* 2004; Obermann *et al* 2006; Wang *et al* 2006). Overall it has been found that approximately 1% of the population will suffer from MOH that has emerged as the most common headache after migraine and tension-type headaches (Castillo *et al* 1999; Celentano *et al* 1992; Zwart *et al* 2003; Colas *et al* 2004). All age groups are affected including children and adolescents (Hering-Hanit and Gadoth 2003; Dyb *et al* 2006; Wang *et al* 2006). In clinic-based studies MOH has been reported in about 10% of attendees (Granella *et al* 1987; Obermann *et al* 2006). The one-year incidence of MOH in migraine patients was found to be about 9% and two main predictors with individual odds ratios of over 20 emerged: high initial headache frequency (>10 days per month) and expectedly the use of medication on more than 10 days per month (Katsarava *et al* 2004).

4.3. Pathophysiology

Genetic predisposition is suggested by the fact that analgesic abuse in non-headache populations is not associated with comparable incidence rates of MOH (Bahra *et al* 2003; Zwart *et al* 2003, 2004). Further mechanisms include central sensitization secondary to repetitive activation of nociceptive pathways by the frequent primary headaches, central changes in pain inhibitory pathways and receptor dysregulation accompanying the primary headache disorder or secondary to drug use (Smith and Stoneman 2004; Obermann *et al* 2006). A recent study suggests that preceding psychiatric comorbidity with migraine may significantly predispose patients to develop MOH (Radat *et al* 2005); however, the direction of the cause and effect relationship is unclear. Notwithstanding, the study suggested that MOH may be one behavioural result of an addictive problem and this is supported in a further study (Fuh *et al* 2005). In a recent functional imaging study metabolic changes in brain areas involved in the processing of pain were observed and these were reversed following drug withdrawal (Fumal *et al* 2006). These findings are consistent with other imaging studies on chronic pain mechanisms. Moreover persistent metabolic changes were observed in the medial orbitofrontal cortex similar to those observed in substance and alcohol abusers (Fumal *et al* 2006). Whether these latter changes are secondary (drug-induced) or primary genetic factors predisposing to addictive behaviour is unclear.

Patients are often reluctant to cease drug intake due to the positive effects of compounds such as caffeine. Persistent analgesic intake may also be due to the appearance of withdrawal symptoms after cessation, particularly in opioids and caffeine-containing drugs (Obermann *et al* 2006).

4.4. Treatment

Therapy is essentially the management of drug cessation and withdrawal symptoms and these may vary, depending on the substance abused (Dowson et al 2005). In this context it is pertinent to stress the importance of prevention by careful and precise patient information, responsible prescribing and regular follow-up. Treatment may be relatively straightforward and control of drug abuse and symptom resolution easily attained (Hering and Steiner 1991; Warner 2001; Obermann et al 2006). In complex cases cessation and symptom management are best performed by a primary care physician or neurologist with relevant experience, sometimes needing admission to hospital (Obermann et al 2006). Cessation of opioids, ergots and drug combinations may induce nausea, restlessness and anxiety that may last up to 10 days with a mean of 3.5 days (Obermann et al 2006). In contrast patients abusing triptans are reported to be headache- and symptom-free within 4 days of cessation (Obermann et al 2006).

Following the acute phase careful monitoring of the long-term control of drug abuse should be performed and some will need behavioural therapy. Patients need clear instructions on maximum dosages and frequency of intake: triptans <9 dosages per month, opioids or analgesics <50 dosages/month. A pain/drug diary must be carefully managed and reviewed at each follow-up visit. In patients with a high baseline headache frequency a suitable prophylactic drug should be prescribed along with clear instructions on escape medication for breakthrough pain (see Chapters 7, 9 and 17).

Long-term prognosis is relatively good with about 60–70% drug abuse free at 4–6 years (Diener et al 1989; Schnider et al 1996; Fritsche et al 2001; Pini et al 2001; Tribl et al 2001; Grazzi et al 2002). Patients remaining free of drug abuse at 12 months have an excellent prognosis (Tribl et al 2001; Katsarava et al 2003). Negative prognosticators indicating expected relapse include the underlying primary headache disorder (tension-type headache > migraine) and previously abused drug (analgesic > triptans > ergots).

5. Trigeminal Pain and Specific Syndromes Associated with Tumours

5.1. Tolosa Hunt Syndrome (THS)

The trigeminal nerve, internal carotid artery, the third, fourth and sixth cranial nerves and the autonomic nerves of the eye are intimately related in the cavernous sinus. Lesions in this area may therefore cause facial pain associated with a number of ocular signs, depending on which nerves are affected.

THS is characterized by episodes of unilateral orbital pain persisting for weeks. Coinciding with the onset of pain or closely following it is paresis of one or more of the third, fourth and sixth cranial nerves and the demonstration of a granulomatous lesion by magnetic resonance imaging (MRI) or biopsy. As part of the inclusion criteria symptoms should resolve within 72 hours of initiating adequate steroid therapy. Diagnosis is based on the clinical presentation, blood tests and MRI (Cakirer 2003a). An MRI post-treatment showing resolution of the lesion is recommended (Cakirer 2003b).

5.1.1. Clinical Features and Treatment

THS is a painful ophthalmoplegia (PO) caused by granulomatous infiltration of the cavernous sinus (Hunt 1976). Pain is orbital or retro-orbital of severe and fluctuating intensity (Hannerz 1985; Gonzales 1998). Quality is described as pressure, boring, or knife-like pain in the eye (Hannerz 1985). The third nerve is involved in most (90%) and the fourth nerve in under half (40%) of cases (Bogduk 2006). The incidence of identifiable lesions in the cavernous sinus increases with the number of nerves involved (Lin and Tsai 2003). Often there may be a reduced pupillary light reflex and ptosis suggestive of autonomic dysfunction. Periorbital hypoaesthesia and a reduced corneal reflex are secondary to sensory dysfunction of the frontal branch of the ophthalmic nerve. Optic nerve involvement (reduced acuity) and involvement of the maxillary nerve suggests enlargement of the lesion (Bogduk 2006). Treatment is by high-dose steroids (80–100 mg prednisone daily) tapered over 7–14 days. Often, however, there is a need for longer treatment to obtain resolution of symptoms. Biopsy and surgical excision may be necessary.

5.1.2. Diagnostic Issues with THS

Involvement of the facial nerve negates a focal lesion in the cavernous sinus as the aetiological factor (Hannerz 1999; Tessitore and Tessitore 2000; Kang et al 2006). Moreover reports of THS with additional involvement of other cranial nerves suggests that THS may be one presentation of a widespread disorder (Steele and Vasuvat 1970; Hokkanen et al 1978; Hunt and Brightman 1988). The response to steroids is nonspecific and has been observed in other causes of PO such as tumours, lymphoma, nasopharyngeal carcinoma, adenoma and actinomycosis (Dornan et al 1979; Spector and Fiandaca 1986; Thomas et al 1988). Imaging of lesions in the cavernous sinus may not be characteristic and although suggestive of granulomas does not clarify the aetiology (Kwan et al 1988; Goadsby and Lance 1989; Yousem et al 1989; Goto et al 1990; Desai et al 1991; Hannerz 1992, 1999). Findings of actinomyces and aspergillus in granulomas of THS patients have led to the alternative speculation that THS is the result of a fungal infection (Rowed et al 1985; Tobias et al 2002). These issues have led to the proposal that THS be assessed under the differential diagnosis of PO (Bogduk 2006).

5.1.3. Differential Diagnosis

Painful ophthalmoplegia is the prominent symptom in THS, but several other pathologies may also cause orbital pain accompanied by ophthalmoplegia (Gladstone and Dodick 2004; La Mantia *et al* 2005). Careful work up of such cases is therefore indicated. Vascular disorders such as cavernous sinus thrombosis and giant cell arteritis of the temporal artery may mimic these symptoms. Diabetic neuropathy and ophthalmoplegic migraine are possible neurologic causes. Neoplastic and infectious processes in the region and infiltrative disorders such as systemic lupus erythematosus, lymphoma, sarcoid and syphilis have also been associated with orbital pain. Applying current IHS criteria these would not be considered THS. In a recent review of the relevant literature only 21% of published cases met the current IHS criteria for THS (La Mantia *et al* 2006). Cases not defined as THS included those due to tumours or a lack of positive imaging findings.

5.2. Oculosympathetic Syndrome (OSS)

5.2.1. Paratrigeminal OSS (POSS; Previous Term: Raeder's Syndrome)

The syndrome as first described presented patients with trigeminal nerve dysfunction or pain accompanied by ocular sympathetic dysfunction (Merskey and Bogduk 1994). This was proposed to be the result of a lesion in the middle cranial fossa in the paratrigeminal area. The sympathetic nerve supply to the eye (oculosympathetic outflow) arises from the internal carotid plexus in the middle cranial fossa, medial to the trigeminal ganglion. A lesion in this area would induce trigeminal symptoms (paraesthesia, pain) and sympathetic dysfunction of the eye: miosis or ptosis (Horner's syndrome). POSS should appear with no alteration in forehead sweating; sympathetic innervation to the sweat glands is mediated by fibres that exit the carotid plexus prior to the middle cranial fossa and relatively laterally to the oculosympathetic outflow (Goadsby 2002). In some instances, however, the parasympathetic system reinnervates the sweat glands so that intact sweating does not signify a functional sympathetic innervation (Goadsby 2002). Although the original case described had a paratrigeminal neoplasm, later cases presented no organic pathology (Solomon and Lustig 2001). Thus various subgroups that presented with a similar phenotype—a Horner's syndrome with ipsilateral trigeminal pain/dysfunction—were described (Solomon and Lustig 2001).

Patients with oculosympathetic loss, miosis or ptosis, or both, with normal forehead sweating, and evidence of trigeminal involvement, either sensory change or neuralgic pain, are highly likely to have a lesion in the middle cranial fossa medial to the trigeminal ganglion (paratrigeminal). These should be termed POSS and patients thoroughly examined including an MRI at baseline and further studies as needed (Goadsby 2002). In addition to paratrigeminal middle cranial fossa neoplasms the most common differential is pathology of the carotid artery that would affect the sympathetic plexus. Particularly carotid artery dissection may occur with unilateral facial pain and a Horner's syndrome (Mokri 2002).

5.2.2. Cervical Artery Dissection; OSS and Facial Pain

Extracranial dissections of the internal carotid artery (ICA) and vertebral artery (VA) are quite common with an annual combined incidence of 5/100 000 persons; co-occurrences are termed cervical artery dissections (CADs; Mokri 2002). The mean patient age is in the early 40s and approximately 70% of the patients are younger than 50 years (Mokri 2002). Spontaneous dissections occur with no history of trauma whilst some cases report blunt trauma, particularly extension–flexion (whiplash) or rotation injuries to the neck (Mokri 2002). CADs arise from a tear in the intima allowing blood to enter the artery wall under high pressure. The resulting intramural haematoma may compromise the lumen and lead to stenosis or expand outwards as an aneurysmal dilatation (Biousse and Mitsias 2006).

The clinical presentation is varied and may consist of a single or combination of symptoms such as pain, Horner's syndrome and neck tenderness. The most common presentation of CADs is head, face or neck pain with or without other signs: up to 95% in ICA and 70% in VA dissection (Hart and Easton 1983; Biousse *et al* 1998; Solomon and Lustig 2001; Mokri 2002; Biousse and Mitsias 2006). In ICA dissections, a unilateral headache may be the single symptom in 45% and is ipsilateral to dissection with a steady or throbbing quality (Evans and Mokri 2002; Mokri 2002). Frequently pain occurs in the orbital, periorbital and frontal regions and may commonly involve the cheek, angle of the mandible, jaw and the ear. Anterolateral neck pain occurs in 25% of the patients. Other accompanying signs include diplopia, pulsatile tinnitus, tongue paresis and dysgeusia (Biousse and Mitsias 2006).

A Horner's syndrome may be the presenting sign of ICA dissection in about half of cases with or without pain (Hart and Easton 1983; Mokri 1990, 2002; Biousse *et al* 1998). In VA dissections, the headache is unilateral in two-thirds, and ipsilateral to the dissection. Pain is located in the posterior head and is rarely associated with facial pain. Posterior neck pain is noted in almost 50% of patients with VA dissections.

Diagnosis is by angiography, Doppler, MRI or MRA but false-negatives are possible. Treatment may include anticoagulation, surgery or placement of stents and mortality of CAD is low (5%); the prognosis of CADs is considered to be very good in the vast majority of cases (Mokri 2002). Pain resolves within one week but may last up to 5 weeks (Biousse and Mitsias 2006). Recurrence is, however, not uncommon; 6–17% of patients will suffer a dissection in another vessel within 10 years (Mokri 2002).

6. Intracranial and Peripheral Tumours

Intracranial malignancies may give rise to orofacial pain and headache (Bullitt *et al* 1986; Puca *et al* 1993; Bhaya and Har-El 1998; Pfund *et al* 1999; Christiaans *et al* 2002). In large series of patients presenting with facial pain the incidence of intracranial tumours has been found to be 0.8–5.9% (Bullitt *et al* 1986; Cheng *et al* 1993). Even in diagnosed cancer patients with new or changed headache it is difficult to predict intracranial metastases. In one study in cancer patients with headache, factors such as a diagnosis of non-tension-type headache, duration of less than 10 weeks and vomiting were individually highly predictive of metastatic disease (Christiaans *et al* 2002). No information from the neurological examination significantly contributed to diagnosis (Christiaans *et al* 2002). The clinical presentation is therefore often misleading and neurological assessment may be of limited value.

Direct involvement of a branch of the trigeminal nerve by neoplasia may cause numbness and neuralgia-like symptoms. Thus tumours in the maxillary sinus or in the mandible may cause infraorbital or mental nerve symptomatology respectively. In patients that demonstrate paraesthesia with pain, a peripheral neoplastic process with perineural invasion should be ruled out (Ariji *et al* 1994). Neuropathic trigeminal pain associated with systemic disease is discussed in Chapter 14.

7. Giant Cell Arteritis

7.1. Introduction

Giant cell arteritis (GCA), also referred to as temporal arteritis, is a chronic vasculitis of large and medium-sized arteries. GCA is usually accompanied by head, face or neck pain. The diagnosis of GCA relies on the presence of a swollen and tender scalp artery (usually the temporal artery) accompanied by an elevated erythrocyte sedimentation rate (ESR) and a rapid response (<48 hours) to steroid therapy (Olesen *et al* 2004). However, all these factors may not always occur in a particular case and definitive diagnosis is dependent on an artery biopsy demonstrating typical histopathology. Concurrent symptoms commonly include proximal muscle ache, morning stiffness and polymyalgia rheumatica (PMR).

GCA predominantly affects patients over the age of 50 years, typically in the seventh and eighth decades, and women are affected about twice as often as men (Gabriel *et al* 1995; Nordborg *et al* 2000). The incidence is age-related and rises from 2.3/100 000/year in the 60-year-old population to 44.7/100 000/year among 90 year olds

(Machado *et al* 1988; Nordborg and Bengtsson 1990; Baldursson *et al* 1994; Gran and Myklebust 1997; Gonzalez-Gay *et al* 2001). GCA affects mainly patients of Caucasian origin; particularly people of Scandinavian or North European descent, irrespective of their residence (Machado *et al* 1988; Nordborg and Bengtsson 1990; Baldursson *et al* 1994; Gran and Myklebust 1997). Additionally genetic studies suggest an inherited component and most point to an association with the human leucocyte antigen system (Carroll *et al* 2006).

7.2. Clinical Features

GCA is well known for its variable clinical manifestations. The clinical signs are the result of damage to the arterial supply leading to tissue ischaemia and injury. The most common presenting complaints include headache, scalp tenderness, jaw claudication and arthralgia (Hayreh 1998; Smetana and Shmerling 2002; Gonzalez-Gay *et al* 2005a; Carroll *et al* 2006). Jaw claudication may be expressed as tiredness and inefficient chewing leading to clinical similarities with temporomandibular disorders. Uncommonly areas with severe ischaemia may necrose.

Patients with GCA presenting in an orofacial pain clinic complain primarily of pain, most commonly over the muscles of mastication, the temporomandibular joint (TMJ) and the eye. Headache is present in 90% of patients and often localizes to the temple (ipsi- or bilateral) and the forehead but location is highly variable (Schmidt 2006; Wall and Corbett 2006). Pain quality may be throbbing, burning, boring or lancinating and may vary from mild to severe (Wall and Corbett 2006). Head tenderness and allodynia particularly over the temporal regions may be marked. The temporal artery may be prominent, tender or beaded but these findings are inconsistent and in more advanced cases the artery may not be easily located. Ophthalmoscopy may reveal anterior ischaemic optic neuropathy with a pale and swollen optic disc.

Constitutional symptoms may include fever, weight loss, anorexia and malaise. Additionally alterations in mental status including depression, dementia, confusion and delusional thinking have been reported (Carroll *et al* 2006). Many of these symptoms are common in the elderly secondary to infectious, malignant or age-related disease and may therefore be missed as a presenting sign of GCA. Typical clinical manifestations may be totally absent in up to 38% of patients that present with solely visual symptoms, termed silent or occult GCA (Keltner 1982; Carroll *et al* 2006).

Ocular involvement may occur in 14–70% of GCA patients (Carroll *et al* 2006). Transient visual disturbances such as diplopia or ocular pain are reported by 2–30% of cases (Hayreh *et al* 1998). Bilateral blindness has been reported in a third of patients and is usually the result of ischaemic damage to the optic nerve, the retina or choroid.

Associated signs. PMR is very common and affects 1 in every 130 individuals over the age of 50 years and may be the presenting manifestation of GCA in up to 50% of cases (Gonzalez-Gay *et al* 2005a). Clinically PMR is characterized by bilateral severe aching pain and morning stiffness of the neck, shoulder and pelvic girdles. Females are more often affected, incidence increases with age and there are signs of systemic inflammation, suggesting similarities with GCA (Evans and Hunder 2000; Salvarani *et al* 2002). Therefore some consider PMR and GCA to be different phases of the same disease. However, PMR lacks the inflammatory infiltrate and vaso-occlusive ischaemic manifestations of GCA. PMR is often an isolated condition and does not demonstrate the strong HLA association seen in GCA (Dababneh *et al* 1998; Gonzalez-Gay *et al* 1998; Gonzalez-Gay 2001, 2004; Martinez-Taboda *et al* 2004). Debate continues as to the precise nature of the comorbidity of PMR and GCA (Carroll *et al* 2006).

Diagnosis. Overall the clinical signs are not reliable enough to confidently diagnose GCA and special tests, particularly temporal artery biopsy, are relied upon to confirm or refute diagnosis.

In relevant cases, an elevated erythrocyte sedimentation rate is considered indicative of GCA but ESRs of < 40 mm/h occur in up to 22.5% of patients and normal levels do not exclude diagnosis (Salvarani and Hunder 2001; Carroll *et al* 2006). Constitutional symptoms are more common in patients with ESR >100 mm/h, and in cases with elevated ESR disease activity correlates with ESR changes (Gonzalez-Gay *et al* 2005b; Carroll *et al* 2006). ESR is affected by sex, a number of haematological disorders, malignancy, liver dysfunction and the use of anti-inflammatory drugs. Moreover there is some disagreement as to the 'normal' range of ESR. C-reactive protein (CRP) has several advantages over ESR; it is unaffected by gender, age, plasma composition and red cell morphology and has an accurately defined and accepted normal range. CRP is commonly used in conjunction with ESR for the diagnosis of GCA and significantly improves specificity (Hayreh *et al* 1997). Elevated platelet counts are commonly observed in GCA and promptly return to normal following steroid therapy. A number of other tests are more rarely used for the diagnosis and/or monitoring of GCA including plasma viscosity, interleukin-6, fibrinogen and liver function tests (Salvarani *et al* 2003).

Significantly increased likelihood ratios (LR) have been associated with signs and symptoms such as jaw claudication (LR 4–4.2), diplopia (LR 3.4), thrombocytosis (5.9) and a painful or abnormal temporal artery (LR 2.3, 3.1 respectively) and an ESR >100 mm/h (Smetana and Shmerling 2002; Niederkohr and Levin 2005). It is important, however, to realize that in patients with positive biopsy, jaw claudication and diplopia were present in only 34 and 14% of patients, respectively (Smetana and Shmerling 2002).

Imaging techniques that may be useful include duplex ultrasonography (US), angiography, positron emission tomography, MRI and computerized tomography (Schmidt 2006). However, most of these techniques are suitable for the assessment of large vessels and are of limited value in the small cranial vessels. In expert hands with state-of-the-art equipment US is very reliable (sensitivity 88%, specificity 99.5%) for the diagnosis of GCA even in small vessels (Schmidt 2006). MRI has recently been shown to accurately detect areas of mural inflammation, even in the relatively small temporal artery (Bley *et al* 2005a,b, 2007). MRI may therefore be a future possibility for diagnosis or to guide biopsy site selection.

The diagnosis of GCA is dependent on temporal artery (TA) biopsy and should be performed in all cases but up to 15% of patients may have a negative biopsy (Smetana and Shmerling 2002; Schmidt and Gromnica-Ihle 2005; Carroll *et al* 2006). The threat of blindness mandates that corticosteroid therapy not be delayed but TA biopsy should be performed within a week (Ray-Chaudhuri *et al* 2002; Nordborg and Nordborg 2004; Schmidt 2006). Because of the presence of 'skip lesions' (see below) biopsy should include a length of at least 2–2.5 cm of artery and serially sectioned every 1 mm. Sections should be stained with haematoxylin and eosin and with an elastin specific stain. A negative biopsy in a clinically suspect patient may be an indication for a further, contralateral, biopsy. Contralateral biopsy may be positive in up to 15% of cases following an initially negative ipsilateral result (Ponge *et al* 1988; Danesh-Meyer *et al* 2000).

7.3. Pathophysiology

The initial event that triggers the cascade of immune and inflammatory reactions underlying GCA has been suggested to be infective but remains unclear (Carroll *et al* 2006). Current theory points to the activation of immature dendritic cells residing in the arterial wall. Activated dendritic cells then produce inflammatory cytokines and chemokines, ultimately attracting T cells and macrophages (Weyand and Goronzy 2003; Ma-Krupa *et al* 2004). Many GCA patients demonstrate signs of systemic inflammation. Interleukins-1 and -6 are considered to play a key role in the pathophysiology of GCA and induce the production of acute-phase proteins by the liver, fever and myalgia (Carroll *et al* 2006).

The aorta and its extracranial branches are specifically but not solely affected. In particular the superficial temporal, ophthalmic, posterior ciliary and vertebral arteries are commonly involved (Carroll *et al* 2006). The central retinal and other branches of the external carotid artery are less commonly affected whilst the intracranial arteries are spared.

In active disease there are nodular inflammatory granulomatous reactions affecting arteries with an elastic lamina; the distribution of disease correlates with the distribution of elastin (Nordborg and Nordborg 1998). Often disease activity is variable within the same artery, leading to skip lesions — segments of inflamed regions adjacent to unaffected areas (Lie 1996; Poller *et al* 2000; Taylor-Gjevre *et al* 2005). This is the rationale for long sections of artery being obtained as biopsy specimens.

Histopathology of affected arteries shows inflammation of the adventitia, media and intima. There is predominant aggregation of CD4+ (T-helper/inducer) cells and a select group of T cells within the adventitial layer produces interferon gamma (IFN-γ) thought to be the key regulating cytokine in GCA (Wagner *et al* 1996). Macrophages are present in distinct functional groups throughout the arterial wall and induce a proinflammatory response in the adventitia and destruction of the media. Ischaemic symptoms are probably secondary to narrowing of the lumen, but often thrombosis is present. Intimal thickening observed in GCA correlates with circulating levels of IFN-γ and is probably a healing response (Kaiser *et al* 1998, 1999; Weyand and Goronzy 2003).

Treatment. GCA may run a self-limiting course lasting 2–4 years but many patients require long-term therapy (Kyle 1991; Kyle and Hazleman 1993; Swannell 1997; Schmidt 2006). Because of the potentially severe effects rapid and efficient treatment with corticosteroids is indicated (Carroll *et al* 2006; Schmidt 2006). Patients with suspected GCA should be rapidly assessed and referred for ophthalmological examination and biopsy; steroid therapy should not, however, be withheld (Nordborg and Nordborg 2004; Schmidt 2006). Onset of visual loss following initial symptoms may be rapid and varies from weeks to months. The loss of vision in one eye usually indicates loss of vision in the second eye within 1–2 months (Carroll *et al* 2006; Wall and Corbett 2006).

Recent recommendations suggest beginning with 60–80mg prednisone daily (Carroll *et al* 2006; Schmidt 2006). Patients with ocular involvement at presentation commonly receive very high initial doses (1000mg/d for 3 days). Resolution of systemic symptoms occurs within 24–72 hours and the dose should be increased if necessary to attain symptomatic relief; the ESR normalizes only after several weeks. The effective dose should be maintained for 4–6 weeks and then tapered whilst closely monitoring clinical signs, ESR and CRP. The dose is reduced by 10mg per month, 5mg per month, then 1mg/month once a daily dose of 10–15mg/d is attained (Carroll *et al* 2006). Total treatment may span 1–2 years and all dose adjustments should be accompanied by clinical and laboratory testing. Relapses are common particularly in the first 18 months and may be accurately predicted by changes in CRP levels (Proven *et al* 2003; Carroll *et al* 2006).

Patients on corticosteroids require expert medical management of side effects including osteoporosis, depression and gastrointestinal (GI) problems (Schmidt 2006). The incidence of serious effects associated with corticosteroid therapy is >50% (Proven *et al* 2003). For this reason steroid sparing drugs have been tested but there is no consensus concerning their use. Patients taking aspirin

before or at diagnosis demonstrate lower risk for visual loss (Nesher *et al* 2004) and adjuvant aspirin (20–100 mg/day) therapy may antagonize IFN-γ. However, aspirin may further increase GI morbidity and a proton pump inhibitor should therefore be prescribed.

8. Facial Pain of Cardiac Origin

Ischaemic heart disease (IHD) may lead to the onset of painful symptoms usually located retrosternally or precordially with radiation to the left arm, left shoulder and neck (Eslick 2005). This symptom is termed angina pectoris (AP) and may be more rarely accompanied by referred pain to the back, the right arm, epigastrium, head and orofacial region (Edmondstone 1995; Culic *et al* 2001; Theroux 2004; Kosuge *et al* 2006).

Stable AP is precipitated by effort, relieved by rest and associated with coronary artery disease whilst unstable AP is characterized by increasing pain frequency and/or duration and novel onset at rest or with minimal effort (Theroux 2004). Atypical forms of AP may occur during sleep or at rest (e.g. Prinzmetal's angina) or not be associated with detectable coronary artery disease (e.g. microvascular angina). Acute coronary syndrome describes the continuum from unstable AP at one end of the spectrum to myocardial infarction (MI) at the other end (Theroux 2004).

Ischaemic cardiac pain is usually described as variations of pressure-like descriptors (heavy, pressing, tight, squeezing) but may also be aching, sharp, burning/searing or a burst open feeling (Culic *et al* 2001; Kosuge *et al* 2006). Accompanying manifestations will vary depending on whether the symptoms reflect stable/unstable AP or MI. Commonly patients report accompanying sweating, weakness, nausea, dyspnoea and vomiting but may not report any manifestation other than pain (Culic *et al* 2001; Kosuge *et al* 2006).

Pain referral to the orofacial region in AP or MI has been variably reported from 4 to 18% of cases (Edmondstone 1995; Culic *et al* 2001; Kosuge *et al* 2006). Headache associated with ischaemic chest pain (cardiac cephalgia) is defined by the IHS and requires the presence of head pain aggravated by exercise and accompanied by nausea. There must be evidence for concomitant acute myocardial ischaemia, and resolution of symptoms with effective cardiac therapy. Cardiac cephalgia has been reported in 5.2% of one series of MI patients and usually accompanies chest symptoms (Culic *et al* 2001). In rarer instances MI pain may be primarily felt as headache (3.4%), jaw pain (3.6%) or neck pain (8.4%) (Culic *et al* 2001). Orofacial pain (8.3%) is more common in inferior MI and cardiac cephalgia is more frequently reported (7.3%) in anterior MI (Culic *et al* 2001), suggesting that anatomic factors influence the prevalence of pain referral. However, other studies have shown that women report a higher frequency of jaw pain associated with AP than do men, even after controlling for MI severity and location (Granot *et al* 2004; Kosuge *et al* 2006; Lovlien *et al* 2006).

Reports of patients with orofacial pain as the cardinal manifestation of IHD have appeared in the literature (Natkin *et al* 1975; Tzukert *et al* 1981; Graham and Schinbeckler 1982; Batchelder *et al* 1987; Sandler *et al* 1995; Kreiner and Okeson 1999; Stollberger *et al* 2001; Durso *et al* 2003; de Oliveira Franco *et al* 2005). Diagnosis is often dependent on the temporal profile that may be suggestive of cardiac cephalgia/orofacial pain. Typically, onset is in close proximity to exercise and subsides with rest or antianginal therapy. Rarely, as in unstable AP, pain may be felt at rest (Gutierrez-Morlote and Pascual 2002). Pain may be moderate to severe and located in the neck and lower jaw (may involve teeth and gums), unilaterally in the head or even at the vertex. At-risk groups are patients over 50 with new onset headache and risk factors for heart disease.

The mechanisms of referred pain in IHD are unclear and may be multiple (Foreman 1999; Kreiner and Okeson 1999). Convergence of sympathetic or vagal fibres that transduce cardiac pain with trigeminocervical pathways has been shown and indeed sympathectomy relieves AP in a subset of patients. Compromised cardiac function with impaired venous return may lead to increased intracranial pressure and subsequent pain. Cardiac ischaemia may induce the release of a number of mediators that can cause distant pain.

References

Aghabeigi B, Feinmann C, Harris M (1992) Prevalence of post-traumatic stress disorder in patients with chronic idiopathic facial pain. *Br J Oral Maxillofac Surg* 30(6):360–364.

Antonaci F, Fredriksen TA, Sjaastad O (2001) Cervicogenic headache: clinical presentation, diagnostic criteria, and differential diagnosis. *Curr Pain Headache Rep* 5(4):387–392.

Ariji E, Ozeki S, Yonetsu K, *et al* (1994) Central squamous cell carcinoma of the mandible. Computed tomographic findings. *Oral Surg Oral Med Oral Pathol* 77(5):541–548.

Baandrup L, Jensen R (2005) Chronic post-traumatic headache—a clinical analysis in relation to the International Headache Classification 2nd Edition. *Cephalalgia* 25(2):132–138.

Bahra A, Walsh M, Menon S, *et al* (2003) Does chronic daily headache arise de novo in association with regular use of analgesics? *Headache* 43(3):179–190.

Baldursson O, Steinsson K, Bjornsson J, *et al* (1994) Giant cell arteritis in Iceland. An epidemiologic and histopathologic analysis. *Arthritis Rheum* 37(7):1007–1012.

Barnsley L, Lord S, Bogduk N (1994) Whiplash injury. *Pain* 58(3):283–307.

Batchelder BJ, Krutchkoff DJ, Amara J (1987) Mandibular pain as the initial and sole clinical manifestation of coronary insufficiency: report of case. *J Am Dent Assoc* 115(5):710–712.

Benoliel R, Eliav E, Elishoov H, *et al* (1994) Diagnosis and treatment of persistent pain after trauma to the head and neck. *J Oral Maxillofac Surg* 52(11):1138–1147; discussion 1147–1148.

Benoliel R, Birenboim R, Regev E, *et al* (2005) Neurosensory changes in the infraorbital nerve following zygomatic fractures. *Oral Surg Oral Med Oral Pathol Oral Radiol Endod* 99(6):657–665.

Bettucci D, Aguggia M, Bolamperti L, *et al* (1998) Chronic post-traumatic headache associated with minor cranial trauma: a description of cephalalgic patterns. *Ital J Neurol Sci* 19(1):20–24.

Bhaya MH, Har-El G (1998) Referred facial pain from intracranial tumors: a diagnostic dilemma. *Am J Otolaryngol* 19(6):383–386.

Bhidayasiri R, Cardoso F, Truong DD (2006) Botulinum toxin in blepharospasm and oromandibular dystonia: comparing different botulinum toxin preparations. *Eur J Neurol* 13(Suppl 1):21–29.

Biousse V, Mitsias P (2006) Carotid or vertebral artery disease. In: Olesen J, Goadsby PJ, Ramadan NM, *et al* (eds) *The Headaches*, 3rd edn. Philadelphia: Lippincott Williams and Wilkins, pp 911–918.

Biousse V, Touboul PJ, D'Anglejan-Chatillon J, *et al* (1998) Ophthalmologic manifestations of internal carotid artery dissection. *Am J Ophthalmol* 126(4):565–577.

Bley TA, Weiben O, Uhl M, *et al* (2005a) Assessment of the cranial involvement pattern of giant cell arteritis with 3T magnetic resonance imaging. *Arthritis Rheum* 52(8):2470–2477.

Bley TA, Wieben O, Uhl M, *et al* (2005b) High-resolution MRI in giant cell arteritis: imaging of the wall of the superficial temporal artery. *AJR Am J Roentgenol* 184(1):283–287.

Bley TA, Uhl M, Venhoff N, *et al* (2007) 3-T MRI reveals cranial and thoracic inflammatory changes in giant cell arteritis. *Clin Rheumatol*. 26(3):448–450.

Bogduk N (1981) An anatomical basis for the neck-tongue syndrome. *J Neurol Neurosurg Psychiatry* 44(3):202–208.

Bogduk N (2006) Pain of cranial nerve and cervical nerve origin other than primary neuralgias. In: Olesen J, Goadsby PJ, Ramadan NM, *et al* (eds) *The Headaches*, 3rd edn. Philadelphia: Lippincott Williams and Wilkins, pp 1043–1051.

Bono G, Antonaci F, Ghirmai S, *et al* (1998) The clinical profile of cervicogenic headache as it emerges from a study based on the early diagnostic criteria (Sjaastad *et al* 1990). *Funct Neurol* 13(1):75–77.

Borody C (2004) Neck-tongue syndrome. *J Manipulative Physiol Ther* 27(5):e8.

Branca B (2006) Neuropsychologic aspects of post-traumatic headache and chronic daily headache. *Curr Pain Headache Rep* 10(1):54–66.

Bullitt E, Tew JM, Boyd J (1986) Intracranial tumors in patients with facial pain. *J Neurosurg* 64(6):865–871.

Burgess JA, Dworkin SF (1993) Litigation and post-traumatic TMD: how patients report treatment outcome. *J Am Dent Assoc* 124(6):105–110.

Cakirer S (2003a) MRI findings in the patients with the presumptive clinical diagnosis of Tolosa-Hunt syndrome. *Eur Radiol* 13(1):17–28.

Cakirer S (2003b) MRI findings in Tolosa-Hunt syndrome before and after systemic corticosteroid therapy. *Eur J Radiol* 45(2):83–90.

Carroll SC, Gaskin BJ, Danesh-Meyer HV (2006) Giant cell arteritis. *Clin Experiment Ophthalmol* 34(2):159–173.

Cassidy JD, Carroll LJ, Cote P, *et al* (2000) Effect of eliminating compensation for pain and suffering on the outcome of insurance claims for whiplash injury. *N Engl J Med* 342(16):1179–1186.

Castillo J, Munoz P, Guitera V, *et al* (1999) Epidemiology of chronic daily headache in the general population. *Headache* 39(3):190–196.

Celentano DD, Stewart WF, Lipton RB, *et al* (1992) Medication use and disability among migraineurs: a national probability sample survey. *Headache* 32(5):223–228.

Chedrawi AK, Fishman MA, Miller G (2000) Neck-tongue syndrome. *Pediatr Neurol* 22(5):397–399.

Cheng TM, Cascino TL, Onofrio BM (1993) Comprehensive study of diagnosis and treatment of trigeminal neuralgia secondary to tumors. *Neurology* 43(11):2298–2302.

Christiaans MH, Kelder JC, Arnoldus EP, *et al* (2002) Prediction of intracranial metastases in cancer patients with headache. *Cancer* 94(7):2063–2068.

Chung T, Rebello R, Gooden EA (2005) Retropharyngeal calcific tendinitis: case report and review of literature. *Emerg Radiol* **11**(6):375–380.

Colas R, Munoz P, Temprano R, *et al* (2004) Chronic daily headache with analgesic overuse: epidemiology and impact on quality of life. *Neurology* **62**(8):1338–1342.

Cote P, Cassidy JD, Carroll L (2000) Is a lifetime history of neck injury in a traffic collision associated with prevalent neck pain, headache and depressive symptomatology? *Accid Anal Prev* **32**(2):151–159.

Culic V, Miric D, Eterovic D (2001) Correlation between symptomatology and site of acute myocardial infarction. *Int J Cardiol* **77**(2–3):163–168.

Dababneh A, Gonzalez-Gay MA, Garcia-Porrua C, *et al* (1998) Giant cell arteritis and polymyalgia rheumatica can be differentiated by distinct patterns of HLA class II association. *J Rheumatol* **25**(11):2140–2145.

Danesh-Meyer HV, Savino PJ, Eagle RC Jr, *et al* (2000) Low diagnostic yield with second biopsies in suspected giant cell arteritis. *J Neuroophthalmol* **20**(3):213–215.

Defazio G, Lamberti P, Lepore V, *et al* (1989) Facial dystonia: clinical features, prognosis and pharmacology in 31 patients. *Ital J Neurol Sci* **10**(6):553–560.

De Leeuw R, Bertoli E, Schmidt JE, *et al* (2005a) Prevalence of post-traumatic stress disorder symptoms in orofacial pain patients. *Oral Surg Oral Med Oral Pathol Oral Radiol Endod* **99**(5):558–568.

De Leeuw R, Bertoli E, Schmidt JE, *et al* (2005b) Prevalence of traumatic stressors in patients with temporomandibular disorders. *J Oral Maxillofac Surg* **63**(1):42–50.

de Oliveira Franco AC, de Siqueira JT, Mansur AJ (2005) Bilateral facial pain from cardiac origin. A case report. *Br Dent J* **198**(11):679–680.

Desai SP, Carter J, Jinkins JR (1991) Contrast-enhanced MR imaging of Tolosa-Hunt syndrome: a case report. AJNR *Am J Neuroradiol* **12**(1):182–183.

Diener HC, Dahlof C (1999) Headache associated with chronic use of substances. In: Olesen J, Tfelt-Hansen P, Welch KMA (eds) *The Headaches*, 2nd edn. Philadelphia: Lippincot Williams and Wilkins, pp 871–878.

Diener HC, Dichgans J, Scholz E, *et al* (1989) Analgesic-induced chronic headache: long-term results of withdrawal therapy. *J Neurol* **236**(1):9–14.

Di Stefano G, Radanov BP (1995) Course of attention and memory after common whiplash: a two-years prospective study with age, education and gender pair-matched patients. *Acta Neurol Scand* **91**(5):346–352.

Dornan TL, Espir ML, Gale EA, *et al* (1979) Remittent painful ophthalmoplegia: the Tolosa-Hunt syndrome? A report of seven cases and review of the literature. *J Neurol Neurosurg Psychiatry* **42**(3):270–275.

Dowson AJ, Dodick DW, Limmroth V (2005) Medication overuse headache in patients with primary headache disorders: epidemiology, management and pathogenesis. *CNS Drugs* **19**(6):483–497.

Durso BC, Israel MS, Janini ME, *et al* (2003) Orofacial pain of cardiac origin: a case report. *Cranio* **21**(2):152–153.

Dyb G, Holmen TL, Zwart JA (2006) Analgesic overuse among adolescents with headache: the Head-HUNT-Youth Study. *Neurology* **66**(2):198–201.

Edmeads J (1988) The cervical spine and headache. *Neurology* **38**(12):1874–1878.

Edmondstone WM (1995) Cardiac chest pain: does body language help the diagnosis? *Bmj* **311**(7021):1660–1661.

Edna TH, Cappelen J (1987) Late post-concussional symptoms in traumatic head injury. An analysis of frequency and risk factors. *Acta Neurochir (Wien)* **86**(1–2):12–17.

Ekbom K, Torhall J, Annell K, *et al* (1994) Magnetic resonance imaging in retropharyngeal tendinitis. *Cephalalgia* **14**(4): 266–269; discussion 257.

Elisevich K, Stratford J, Bray G, *et al* (1984) Neck tongue syndrome: operative management. *J Neurol Neurosurg Psychiatry* **47**(4):407–409.

Ertekin C, Aydogdu I, Secil Y, *et al* (2002) Oropharyngeal swallowing in craniocervical dystonia. *J Neurol Neurosurg Psychiatry* **73**(4):406–411.

Eslick GD (2005) Usefulness of chest pain character and location as diagnostic indicators of an acute coronary syndrome. *Am J Cardiol* **95**(10):1228–1231.

Evans JM, Hunder GG (2000) Polymyalgia rheumatica and giant cell arteritis. *Rheum Dis Clin North Am* **26**(3):493–515.

Evans RW (2004) Post-traumatic headaches. *Neurol Clin* **22**(1): 237–249, viii.

Evans RW, Mokri B (2002) Headache in cervical artery dissections. *Headache* **42**(10):1061–1063.

Fahlgren H (1986) Retropharyngeal tendinitis. *Cephalalgia* **6**(3): 169–174.

Fahlgren H (1988) Retropharyngeal tendinitis: three probable cases with an unusually low epicentre. *Cephalalgia* **8**(2):105–110.

Foreman RD (1999) Mechanisms of cardiac pain. *Annu Rev Physiol* **61**:143–167.

Fortin CJ, Biller J (1985) Neck tongue syndrome. *Headache* **25**(5): 255–258.

Freeman MD, Croft AC, Rossignol AM, *et al* (1999) A review and methodologic critique of the literature refuting whiplash syndrome. *Spine* **24**(1):86–96.

Fritsche G, Eberl A, Katsarava Z, *et al* (2001) Drug-induced headache: long-term follow-up of withdrawal therapy and persistence of drug misuse. *Eur Neurol* **45**(4):229–235.

Fuh JL, Wang SJ, Lu SR, *et al* (2005) Does medication overuse headache represent a behavior of dependence? *Pain* **119**(1–3):49–55.

Fumal A, Laureys S, Di Clemente L, *et al* (2006) Orbitofrontal cortex involvement in chronic analgesic-overuse headache evolving from episodic migraine. *Brain* **129**(Pt 2):543–550.

Gabriel SE, O'Fallon WM, Achkar AA, *et al* (1995) The use of clinical characteristics to predict the results of temporal artery biopsy among patients with suspected giant cell arteritis. *J Rheumatol* **22**(1):93–96.

Gladstone JP, Dodick DW (2004) Painful ophthalmoplegia: overview with a focus on Tolosa-Hunt syndrome. *Curr Pain Headache Rep* **8**(4):321–329.

Glynn SM, Asarnow JR, Asarnow R, *et al* (2003) The development of acute post-traumatic stress disorder after orofacial injury: a prospective study in a large urban hospital. *J Oral Maxillofac Surg* **61**(7):785–792.

Goadsby PJ (2002) Raeder's syndrome [corrected]: paratrigeminal paralysis of the oculopupillary sympathetic system. *J Neurol Neurosurg Psychiatry* **72**(3):297–299.

Goadsby PJ, Lance JW (1989) Clinicopathological correlation in a case of painful ophthalmoplegia: Tolosa-Hunt syndrome. *J Neurol Neurosurg Psychiatry* **52**(11):1290–1293.

Gonzales GR (1998) Pain in Tolosa-Hunt syndrome. *J Pain Symptom Manage* **16**(3):199–204.

Gonzalez-Gay MA (2001) Genetic epidemiology. Giant cell arteritis and polymyalgia rheumatica. *Arthritis Res* **3**(3): 154–157.

Gonzalez-Gay MA (2004) Giant cell arteritis and polymyalgia rheumatica: two different but often overlapping conditions. *Semin Arthritis Rheum* **33**(5):289–293.

Gonzalez-Gay MA, Garcia-Porrua C, Vazquez-Caruncho M (1998) Polymyalgia rheumatica in biopsy proven giant cell arteritis does not constitute a different subset but differs from isolated polymyalgia rheumatica. *J Rheumatol* **25**(9):1750–1755.

Gonzalez-Gay MA, Garcia-Porrua C, Rivas MJ, *et al* (2001) Epidemiology of biopsy proven giant cell arteritis in northwestern Spain: trend over an 18 year period. *Ann Rheum Dis* **60**(4):367–371.

Gonzalez-Gay MA, Barros S, Lopez-Diaz MJ, *et al* (2005a) Giant cell arteritis: disease patterns of clinical presentation in a series of 240 patients. *Medicine (Baltimore)* **84**(5):269–276.

Gonzalez-Gay MA, Lopez-Diaz MJ, Barros S, *et al* (2005b) Giant cell arteritis: laboratory tests at the time of diagnosis in a series of 240 patients. *Medicine (Baltimore)* **84**(5):277–290.

Goto Y, Hosokawa S, Goto I, et al (1990) Abnormality in the cavernous sinus in three patients with Tolosa-Hunt syndrome: MRI and CT findings. *J Neurol Neurosurg Psychiatry* **53**(3):231–234.

Graham LL, Schinbeckler GA (1982) Orofacial pain of cardiac origin. *J Am Dent Assoc* **104**(1):47–48.

Gran JT, Myklebust G (1997) The incidence of polymyalgia rheumatica and temporal arteritis in the county of Aust Agder, south Norway: a prospective study 1987-94. *J Rheumatol* **24**(9):1739–1743.

Granella F, Farina S, Malferrari G, et al (1987) Drug abuse in chronic headache: a clinico-epidemiologic study. *Cephalalgia* **7**(1):15–19.

Granot M, Goldstein-Ferber S, Azzam ZS (2004) Gender differences in the perception of chest pain. *J Pain Symptom Manage* **27**(2):149–155.

Grazzi L, Andrasik F, D'Amico D, et al (2002) Behavioral and pharmacologic treatment of transformed migraine with analgesic overuse: outcome at 3 years. *Headache* **42**(6):483–490.

Gurr B, Coetzer BR (2005) The effectiveness of cognitive-behavioural therapy for post-traumatic headaches. *Brain Inj* **19**(7):481–491.

Gutierrez-Morlote J, Pascual J (2002) Cardiac cephalgia is not necessarily an exertional headache: case report. *Cephalalgia* **22**(9):765–766.

Haas DC (1996) Chronic post-traumatic headaches classified and compared with natural headaches. *Cephalalgia* **16**(7):486–493.

Haldeman S, Dagenais S (2001) Cervicogenic headaches: a critical review. *Spine J* **1**(1):31–46.

Hannerz J (1985) Pain characteristics of painful ophthalmoplegia (the Tolosa-Hunt syndrome). *Cephalalgia* **5**(2):103–106.

Hannerz J (1992) Recurrent Tolosa-Hunt syndrome. *Cephalalgia* **12**(1):45–51.

Hannerz J (1999) Recurrent Tolosa-Hunt syndrome: a report of ten new cases. *Cephalalgia* **19**(Suppl 25):33–35.

Hart RG, Easton JD (1983) Dissections of cervical and cerebral arteries. *Neurol Clin* **1**(1):155–182.

Hayreh SS (1998) Masticatory muscle pain: an important indicator of giant cell arteritis. *Spec Care Dentist* **18**(2):60–65.

Hayreh SS, Podhajsky PA, Raman R, et al (1997) Giant cell arteritis: validity and reliability of various diagnostic criteria. *Am J Ophthalmol* **123**(3):285–296.

Hayreh SS, Podhajsky PA, Zimmerman B (1998) Ocular manifestations of giant cell arteritis. *Am J Ophthalmol* **125**(4):509–520.

Hering R, Steiner TJ (1991) Abrupt outpatient withdrawal of medication in analgesic-abusing migraineurs. *Lancet* **337**(8755):1442–1443.

Hering-Hanit R, Gadoth N (2003) Caffeine-induced headache in children and adolescents. *Cephalalgia* **23**(5):332–335.

Hillier SL, Sharpe MH, Metzer J (1997) Outcomes 5 years post-traumatic brain injury (with further reference to neurophysical impairment and disability). *Brain Inj* **11**(9):661–675.

Hokkanen E, Haltia T, Myllyla VV (1978) Recurrent multiple cranial neuropathies. *Eur Neurol* **17**(1):32–37.

Hunt WE (1976) Tolosa-Hunt syndrome: one cause of painful ophthalmoplegia. *J Neurosurg* **44**(5):544–549.

Hunt WE, Brightman RP (1988) The Tolosa-Hunt syndrome: a problem in differential diagnosis. *Acta Neurochir Suppl (Wien)* **42**:248–252.

Kaiser M, Weyand CM, Bjornsson J, et al (1998) Platelet-derived growth factor, intimal hyperplasia, and ischemic complications in giant cell arteritis. *Arthritis Rheum* **41**(4):623–633.

Kaiser M, Younge B, Bjornsson J, et al (1999) Formation of new vasa vasorum in vasculitis. Production of angiogenic cytokines by multinucleated giant cells. *Am J Pathol* **155**(3):765–774.

Kang H, Park KJ, Son S, et al (2006) MRI in Tolosa-Hunt syndrome associated with facial nerve palsy. *Headache* **46**(2):336–339.

Katsarava Z, Limmroth V, Finke M, et al (2003) Rates and predictors for relapse in medication overuse headache: a 1-year prospective study. *Neurology* **60**(10):1682–1683.

Katsarava Z, Schneeweiss S, Kurth T, et al (2004) Incidence and predictors for chronicity of headache in patients with episodic migraine. *Neurology* **62**(5):788–790.

Keltner JL (1982) Giant-cell arteritis. Signs and symptoms. *Ophthalmology* **89**(10):1101–1110.

Kosuge M, Kimura K, Ishikawa T, et al (2006) Differences between men and women in terms of clinical features of ST-segment elevation acute myocardial infarction. *Circ J* **70**(3):222–226.

Kreiner M, Okeson JP (1999) Toothache of cardiac origin. *J Orofac Pain* **13**(3):201–207.

Kusunoki T, Muramoto D, Murata K (2006) A case of calcific retropharyngeal tendinitis suspected to be a retropharyngeal abscess upon the first medical examination. *Auris Nasus Larynx* **33**(3):329–331.

Kwan ES, Wolpert SM, Hedges TR 3rd, et al (1988) Tolosa-Hunt syndrome revisited: not necessarily a diagnosis of exclusion. *AJR Am J Roentgenol* **150**(2):413–418.

Kyle V (1991) Treatment of polymyalgia rheumatica/giant cell arteritis. *Baillieres Clin Rheumatol* **5**(3):485–491.

Kyle V, Hazleman BL (1993) The clinical and laboratory course of polymyalgia rheumatica/giant cell arteritis after the first two months of treatment. *Ann Rheum Dis* **52**(12):847–850.

La Mantia L, Erbetta A, Bussone G (2005) Painful ophthalmoplegia: an unresolved clinical problem. *Neurol Sci* **26**(Suppl 2):S79–S82.

La Mantia L, Curone M, Rapoport AM, et al (2006) Tolosa-Hunt syndrome: critical literature review based on IHS 2004 criteria. *Cephalalgia* **26**(7):772–781.

Lance JW, Anthony M (1980) Neck-tongue syndrome on sudden turning of the head. *J Neurol Neurosurg Psychiatry* **43**(2):97–101.

Landy PJ (1998) Neurological sequelae of minor head and neck injuries. *Injury* **29**(3):199–206.

Lane JC, Arciniegas DB (2002) Post-traumatic headache. *Curr Treat Options Neurol* **4**(1):89–104.

Lew HL, Lin PH, Fuh JL, et al (2006) Characteristics and treatment of headache after traumatic brain injury: a focused review. *Am J Phys Med Rehabil* **85**(7):619–627.

Lie JT (1996) Temporal artery biopsy diagnosis of giant cell arteritis: lessons from 1109 biopsies. *Anat Pathol* **1**:69–97.

Limmroth V, Katsarava Z, Fritsche G, et al (2002) Features of medication overuse headache following overuse of different acute headache drugs. *Neurology* **59**(7):1011–1014.

Lin CC, Tsai JJ (2003) Relationship between the number of involved cranial nerves and the percentage of lesions located in the cavernous sinus. *Eur Neurol* **49**(2):98–102.

Lovlien M, Schei B, Gjengedal E (2006) Are there gender differences related to symptoms of acute myocardial infarction? A Norwegian perspective. *Prog Cardiovasc Nurs* **21**(1):14–19.

Machado EB, Michet CJ, Ballard DJ, et al (1988) Trends in incidence and clinical presentation of temporal arteritis in Olmsted County, Minnesota, 1950-1985. *Arthritis Rheum* **31**(6):745–749.

Ma-Krupa W, Jeon MS, Spoerl S, et al (2004) Activation of arterial wall dendritic cells and breakdown of self-tolerance in giant cell arteritis. *J Exp Med* **199**(2):173–183.

Martinez-Taboda VM, Bartolome MJ, Lopez-Hoyos M, et al (2004) HLA-DRB1 allele distribution in polymyalgia rheumatica and giant cell arteritis: influence on clinical subgroups and prognosis. *Semin Arthritis Rheum* **34**(1):454–464.

Merskey H, Bogduk N (1994). *Classification of Chronic Pain: Descriptions of Chronic Pain Syndromes and Definition of Pain Terms*, 2nd edn. IASP Press: Seattle.

Meskunas CA, Tepper SJ, Rapoport AM, et al (2006) Medications associated with probable medication overuse headache reported in a tertiary care headache center over a 15-year period. *Headache* **46**(5):766–772.

Mokri B (1990) Traumatic and spontaneous extracranial internal carotid artery dissections. *J Neurol* **237**(6):356–361.

Mokri B (2002) Headaches in cervical artery dissections. *Curr Pain Headache Rep* **6**(3):209–216.

Mooney G, Speed J, Sheppard S (2005) Factors related to recovery after mild traumatic brain injury. *Brain Inj* **19**(12):975–987.

Muller J, Kemmler G, Wissel J, et al (2002) The impact of blepharospasm and cervical dystonia on health-related quality of life and depression. *J Neurol* **249**(7):842–846.

Natkin E, Harrington GW, Mandel MA (1975) Anginal pain referred to the teeth. Report of a case. *Oral Surg Oral Med Oral Pathol* **40**(5):678–680.

Nesher G, Berkun Y, Mates M, et al (2004) Low-dose aspirin and prevention of cranial ischemic complications in giant cell arteritis. *Arthritis Rheum* **50**(4):1332–1337.

Nestvold K, Lundar T, Mowinckel P, et al (2005) Predictors of headache 22 years after hospitalization for head injury. *Acta Neurol Scand* **112**(1):13–18.

Nicholson K, Martelli MF (2004) The problem of pain. *J Head Trauma Rehabil* **19**(1):2–9.

Niederkohr RD, Levin LA (2005) Management of the patient with suspected temporal arteritis a decision-analytic approach. *Ophthalmology* **112**(5):744–756.

Nordborg C, Nordborg E, Petursdottir V (2000) Giant cell arteritis. Epidemiology, etiology and pathogenesis. *Apmis* **108**(11):713–724.

Nordborg E, Bengtsson BA (1990) Epidemiology of biopsy-proven giant cell arteritis (GCA). *J Intern Med* **227**(4):233–236.

Nordborg E, Nordborg C (1998) The inflammatory reaction in giant cell arteritis: an immunohistochemical investigation. *Clin Exp Rheumatol* **16**(2):165–168.

Nordborg E, Nordborg C (2004) Giant cell arteritis: strategies in diagnosis and treatment. *Curr Opin Rheumatol* **16**(1):25–30.

Obermann M, Bartsch T, Katsarava Z (2006) Medication overuse headache. *Expert Opin Drug Saf* **5**(1):49–56.

Olesen J, Bousser M-G, Diener HC, et al (2004) The International Classification of Headache Disorders, 2nd Edition. *Cephalalgia* **24** (suppl 1):24–150.

Ondo WG, Gollomp S, Galvez-Jimenez N (2005) A pilot study of botulinum toxin A for headache in cervical dystonia. *Headache* **45**(8):1073–1077.

Pageler L, Savidou I, Limmroth V (2005) Medication-overuse headache. *Curr Pain Headache Rep* **9**(6):430–435.

Pfund Z, Szapary L, Jaszberenyi O, et al (1999) Headache in intracranial tumors. *Cephalalgia* **19**(9):787–790; discussion 765.

Pini LA, Cicero AF, Sandrini M (2001) Long-term follow-up of patients treated for chronic headache with analgesic overuse. *Cephalalgia* **21**(9):878–883.

Poller DN, van Wyk Q, Jeffrey MJ (2000) The importance of skip lesions in temporal arteritis. *J Clin Pathol* **53**(2):137–139.

Ponge T, Barrier JH, Grolleau JY, et al (1988) The efficacy of selective unilateral temporal artery biopsy versus bilateral biopsies for diagnosis of giant cell arteritis. *J Rheumatol* **15**(6):997–1000.

Prencipe M, Casini AR, Ferretti C, et al (2001) Prevalence of headache in an elderly population: attack frequency, disability, and use of medication. *J Neurol Neurosurg Psychiatry* **70**(3):377–381.

Proven A, Gabriel SE, Orces C, et al (2003) Glucocorticoid therapy in giant cell arteritis: duration and adverse outcomes. *Arthritis Rheum* **49**(5):703–708.

Puca A, Meglio M, Tamburrini G, et al (1993) Trigeminal involvement in intracranial tumours. Anatomical and clinical observations on 73 patients. *Acta Neurochir (Wien)* **125**(1–4):47–51.

Radat F, Creac'h C, Swendsen JD, et al (2005) Psychiatric comorbidity in the evolution from migraine to medication overuse headache. *Cephalalgia* **25**(7):519–522.

Ray-Chaudhuri N, Kine DA, Tijani SO, et al (2002) Effect of prior steroid treatment on temporal artery biopsy findings in giant cell arteritis. *Br J Ophthalmol* **86**(5):530–532.

Rowed DW, Kassel EE, Lewis AJ (1985) Transorbital intracavernous needle biopsy in painful ophthalmoplegia. Case report. *J Neurosurg* **62**(5):776–780.

Salvarani C, Hunder GG (2001) Giant cell arteritis with low erythrocyte sedimentation rate: frequency of occurence in a population-based study. *Arthritis Rheum* **45**(2):140–145.

Salvarani C, Cantini F, Boiardi L, et al (2002) Polymyalgia rheumatica and giant-cell arteritis. *N Engl J Med* **347**(4):261–271.

Salvarani C, Cantini F, Boiardi L, et al (2003) Laboratory investigations useful in giant cell arteritis and Takayasu's arteritis. *Clin Exp Rheumatol* **21**(6 Suppl 32):S23–S28.

Sandler NA, Ziccardi V, Ochs M (1995) Differential diagnosis of jaw pain in the elderly. *J Am Dent Assoc* **126**(9):1263–1272.

Schmidt WA (2006) Current diagnosis and treatment of temporal arteritis. *Curr Treat Options Cardiovasc Med* **8**(2):145–151.

Schmidt WA, Gromnica-Ihle E (2005) What is the best approach to diagnosing large-vessel vasculitis? *Best Pract Res Clin Rheumatol* **19**(2):223–242.

Schnider P, Aull S, Baumgartner C, et al (1996) Long-term outcome of patients with headache and drug abuse after inpatient withdrawal: five-year follow-up. *Cephalalgia* **16**(7):481–485; discussion 461.

Sherman JJ, Carlson CR, Wilson JF, et al (2005) Post-traumatic stress disorder among patients with orofacial pain. *J Orofac Pain* **19**(4):309–317.

Sjaastad O (1999) Reliability of cervicogenic headache diagnosis. *Cephalalgia* **19**(9):767–768.

Sjaastad O, Bakketeig L (2006) Neck-tongue syndrome and related conditions. *Cephalalgia* **26**(3):233–240.

Sjaastad O, Bovim G (1991) Cervicogenic headache. The differentiation from common migraine. An overview. *Funct Neurol* **6**(2):93–100.

Sjaastad O, Fredriksen TA (2000) Cervicogenic headache: criteria, classification and epidemiology. *Clin Exp Rheumatol* **18** (2 Suppl 19):S3–S6.

Sjaastad O, Fredriksen TA, Pfaffenrath V (1990) Cervicogenic headache: diagnostic criteria. *Headache* **30**(11):725–726.

Sjaastad O, Bovim G, Stovner LJ (1992) Laterality of pain and other migraine criteria in common migraine. A comparison with cervicogenic headache. *Funct Neurol* **7**(4):289–294.

Sjaastad O, Fredriksen TA, Stolt-Nielsen A, et al (1997) Cervicogenic headache: a clinical review with special emphasis on therapy. *Funct Neurol* **12**(6):305–317.

Sjaastad O, Fredriksen TA, Pfaffenrath V (1998a) Cervicogenic headache: diagnostic criteria. The Cervicogenic Headache International Study Group. *Headache* **38**(6):442–445.

Sjaastad O, Salvesen R, Jansen J, et al (1998b) Cervicogenic headache a critical view on pathogenesis. *Funct Neurol* **13**(1):71–74.

Smetana GW, Shmerling RH (2002) Does this patient have temporal arteritis? *Jama* **287**(1):92–101.

Smith TR, Stoneman J (2004) Medication overuse headache from antimigraine therapy: clinical features, pathogenesis and management. *Drugs* **64**(22):2503–2514.

Solomon S (2005) Chronic post-traumatic neck and head pain. *Headache* **45**(1):53–67.

Solomon S, Lustig JP (2001) Benign Raeder's syndrome is probably a manifestation of carotid artery disease. *Cephalalgia* **21**(1):1–11.

Spector RH, Fiandaca MS (1986) The "sinister" Tolosa-Hunt syndrome. *Neurology* **36**(2):198–203.

Spitzer WO, Skovron ML, Salmi LR, et al (1995) Scientific monograph of the Quebec Task Force on Whiplash-Associated Disorders: redefining "whiplash" and its management. *Spine* **20**(8 Suppl):1S–73S.

Steele JC, Vasuvat A (1970) Recurrent multiple cranial nerve palsies: a distinctive syndrome of cranial polyneuropathy. *J Neurol Neurosurg Psychiatry* **33**(6):828–832.

Stollberger C, Finsterer J, Habitzl W, et al (2001) Toothache leading to emergency cardiac surgery. *Intensive Care Med* **27**(6):1100–1101.

Stulemeijer M, van der Werf S, Bleijenberg G, et al (2006) Recovery from mild traumatic brain injury: a focus on fatigue. *J Neurol* **253**(8):1041–1047.

Swannell AJ (1997) Polymyalgia rheumatica and temporal arteritis: diagnosis and management. *Bmj* **314**(7090):1329–1332.

Tarsy D, First ER (1999) Painful cervical dystonia: clinical features and response to treatment with botulinum toxin. *Mov Disord* **14**(6):1043–1045.

Tatrow K, Blanchard EB, Hickling EJ, *et al* (2003) Posttraumatic headache: biopsychosocial comparisons with multiple control groups. *Headache* **43**(7):755–766.

Taylor-Gjevre R, Vo M, Shukla D, *et al* (2005) Temporal artery biopsy for giant cell arteritis. *J Rheumatol* **32**(7):1279–1282.

Tessitore E, Tessitore A (2000) Tolosa-Hunt syndrome preceded by facial palsy. *Headache* **40**(5):393–396.

Theroux P (2004) Angina pectoris. In: Goldman L, Ausiello D (eds) *Cecil Textbook of Medicine*, 22nd edn. Saunders: Philadelphia, pp 389–400.

Thomas DJ, Charlesworth MC, Afshar F, *et al* (1988) Computerised axial tomography and magnetic resonance scanning in the Tolosa-Hunt syndrome. *Br J Ophthalmol* **72**(4):299–302.

Tobias S, Lee JH, Tomford JW (2002) Rare Actinobacillus infection of the cavernous sinus causing painful ophthalmoplegia: case report. *Neurosurgery* **51**(3):807–809; discussion 809–810.

Tribl GG, Schnider P, Wober C, *et al* (2001) Are there predictive factors for long-term outcome after withdrawal in drug-induced chronic daily headache? *Cephalalgia* **21**(6):691–696.

Tzukert A, Hasin Y, Sharav Y (1981) Orofacial pain of cardiac origin. *Oral Surg Oral Med Oral Pathol* **51**(5):484–486.

Wagner AD, Bjornsson J, Bartley GB, *et al* (1996) Interferon-gamma-producing T cells in giant cell vasculitis represent a minority of tissue-infiltrating cells and are located distant from the site of pathology. *Am J Pathol* **148**(6):1925–1933.

Walker WC, Seel RT, Curtiss G, *et al* (2005) Headache after moderate and severe traumatic brain injury: a longitudinal analysis. *Arch Phys Med Rehabil* **86**(9):1793–1800.

Wall M, Corbett JJ (2006) Arteritis. In: Olesen J, Goadsby PJ, Ramadan NM, *et al* (eds) *The Headaches*, 3rd edn. Philadelphia: Lippincott Williams and Wilkins, pp 901–910.

Wang SJ, Fuh JL, Lu SR, *et al* (2006) Chronic daily headache in adolescents: prevalence, impact, and medication overuse. *Neurology* **66**(2):193–197.

Warner JS (2001) The outcome of treating patients with suspected rebound headache. *Headache* **41**(7):685–692.

Weyand CM, Goronzy JJ (2003) Medium- and large-vessel vasculitis. *N Engl J Med* **349**(2):160–169.

Young W, Packard RC, Ramadan N (2001) Headaches associated with head trauma. In: Silberstein S, Lipton RB, Dalesio DJ (eds) *Wolf's Headache and Other Head Pain*, 7th edn. New York: Oxford University Press, pp 325–348.

Yousem DM, Atlas SW, Grossman RI, *et al* (1989) MR imaging of Tolosa-Hunt syndrome. *AJNR Am J Neuroradiol* **10**(6):1181–1184.

Zeeberg P, Olesen J, Jensen R (2006) Probable medication-overuse headache. *Neurology* **66**(12):1894–1898.

Zwart JA, Dyb G, Hagen K, *et al* (2003) Analgesic use: a predictor of chronic pain and medication overuse headache: the Head-HUNT Study. *Neurology* **61**(2):160–164.

Zwart JA, Dyb G, Hagen K, *et al* (2004) Analgesic overuse among subjects with headache, neck, and low-back pain. *Neurology* **62**(9):1540–1544.

CHAPTER 14

Orofacial pain in the medically complex patient

Sharon Elad, Joel Epstein, Gary Klasser and Herve Sroussi

1. Introduction

This chapter presents an overview of systemic diseases that may induce orofacial pain or headache. This approach is useful when dealing with pain patients who report comorbid systemic disease. As clinicians it is important to differentiate pain that may be secondary to remote disease processes and therefore amenable to therapy of the primary condition. These conditions include relatively common entities such as hypertension, whereas others such as dialysis-induced headaches are rare. The mechanisms involved in the pathogenesis of systemically induced pain are highly variable but may include inflammatory (see Chapter 15) and neuropathic processes Chapters 2 and 11. Neuronal injury may be induced by ischaemia or demyelinating or metabolic processes.

2. Orofacial Pain in Metabolic and Endocrine Disorders

The clinician must be cognizant of the possibility that certain systemic metabolic disorders may present as facial pain. Because the metabolic condition is systemic, the effects are usually noticeable in multiple sites appearing secondary to the underlying condition. The more common pain-inducing metabolic disorders that the clinician should be aware of are diabetic, alcoholic and nutritional neuropathies. The common hallmark of these diseases is involvement of peripheral nerves by alteration of the structure or function of myelin and axons due to metabolic pathway dysregulation. However, the exact mechanism by which a systemic condition can induce pain is still controversial (see also neuropathic pain Chapter 11). In the majority of these conditions, the pain associated with these metabolic polyneuropathies is customarily found in the extremities and not in the orofacial structures. However, even though pain in the facial region is rare, the clinician must appreciate the possibility that such neuropathies exist in order to direct therapy to the actual source of the condition.

2.1. Diabetic Neuropathy

Demyelination of peripheral nerves that occurs in diabetes leads to neuropathic changes in the motor, autonomic and sensory nervous systems. Up to 48% of diabetics suffer from neuropathy (Dyck *et al* 1999). The incidence of cranial nerve involvement ranges from 3 to 14%, but most of these are motor neuropathies (Irkec *et al* 2001).

Diabetic polyneuropathy is multifactorial in aetiology. The results from the Diabetes Control and Complications Trial demonstrated that hyperglycaemia and insulin deficiency contribute to the development of diabetic neuropathy and that glycaemic control lowers the risk of neuropathy by 60% over 5 years (Tamborlane and Ahern 1997). It is hypothesized that decreased bioavailability of systemic insulin in diabetes may contribute to more severe axonal atrophy or loss. Additionally hyperglycaemia may cause a microvasculitis leading to an ischaemic injury, resulting in demyelination and axonal dystrophy (Dyck and Norell 1999). Elevated endoneurial glucose, fructose and sorbitol levels in diabetes are associated with fibre degeneration and the severity of neuropathy (Dyck *et al* 1988).

Involvement of the third, fourth, sixth and seventh cranial nerves in diabetic neuropathies have been well documented (Thomas and Tomlinson 1993; Eshbaugh *et al* 1995). The trigeminal (fifth cranial) nerve rarely appears to be involved in diabetes, although there are case reports

(Cruccu *et al* 1998; Urban *et al* 1999). Patients with diabetic neuropathy often complain of a sharp, shooting pain in the mandible and tongue with occasional involvement of the mucosa. Additionally, it has been found that peripheral polyneuropathies often cause subclinical damage to the trigeminal nerve (thus leading to an underreporting of such events). The mandibular branch is often affected and patients complain of unilateral facial paraesthesia or hypoaesthesia in the mental nerve territory, mandibular pain and abnormal motor responses in facial or masseter muscles (Cruccu *et al* 1998). The cramped anatomical route of nerves in the mandibular canal or below the internal pterygoid muscle and fascia may expose them to an increased risk of damage (Cruccu *et al* 1998). Primary treatment should be directed at the underlying metabolic condition by appropriate referral to the medical specialist to manage the systemic condition. Symptoms of polyneuropathy may be treated with an approach similar to that of other neuropathic pains; see Chapters 11 and 16.

2.2. Alcohol and Nutritional Neuropathy

Alcoholism, or addiction to alcohol, is a worldwide problem with enormous medical, social and economic costs to the individual and to society. Individuals who engage in chronic alcohol consumption have a number of serious medical complications including neurological disorders. Alcoholic polyneuropathy can be purely motor or purely sensory in its effects, although the most common clinical presentation is mixed. Alcoholics frequently suffer from entrapment or pressure neuropathies especially in the ulnar and peroneal nerves. Paraesthesias, pain and weakness mainly in the extremities are common. Several reports of alcoholics with hearing loss, balance disturbances and facial weakness related to degeneration of the eighth cranial nerve appear in the literature. Distal muscle weakness and atrophy are also common findings in the extremities, but have not been reported from the orofacial region (Preedy *et al* 2003).

The pathogenesis of alcoholic polyneuropathy is not fully understood. Some believe that the majority of associated medical disorders may be due to ethanol neurotoxicity (Charness *et al* 1989). There are also reports that malnutrition is the cause of most alcohol-related neurologic disorders as alcoholics often obtain as much as 50% of their calories from ethanol, allowing serious nutritional deficiencies to develop, particularly for protein, thiamine, folate and niacin (Diamond and Messing 1994). Another possibility may be that alcohol consumption has direct negative effects on the gastrointestinal mucosa and pancreas. A consequence of these actions may be malabsorption of essential nutrients (Stickel *et al* 2003). Neuropathy is characterized by axonal degeneration and demyelination with evidence suggesting a direct neurotoxic effect of ethanol on the peripheral nerves.

2.3. Hypothyroidism

Hypofunction of the thyroid gland is one of the most common endocrine disorders in older women and may be associated with headaches. Thirty percent of 102 adult patients with hypothyroidism reported headaches 1–2 months following initial symptoms of hypothyroidism (Moreau *et al* 1998). Headaches are usually bilateral, mild, nonpulsatile and continuous. There is a good response to abortive salicylates and administration of thyroid hormone usually leads to headache resolution. The pathophysiology of hypothyroidism-related headache may be due to an underlying metabolic or vascular process (Moreau *et al* 1998).

2.4. Fabry's Disease

This is an X-linked metabolic disease caused by the deficiency of the lysosomal enzyme alpha-galactosidase A, which induces a progressive accumulation of galactosyl containing glycosphingolipid residues in multiple organs. One of the predominant signs of Fabry's disease found in a cohort of young patients was acroparaesthesia (paraesthesia of limbs and tips of other extremities due to nerve compression or polyneuritis) (Ries *et al* 2003). Cranial nerve dysfunction resulting in facial paraesthesia, odontogenic-like pain, trigeminal neuralgia, taste and smell impairment, or glossomotor dysfunction, has been described (Cable *et al* 1982). Neurological and psychological changes, such as headache, recurrent vertigo, tinnitus, diminished level of activity, fatigue and depression, have also been reported in patients with Fabry's disease (Ries *et al* 2003). It is noteworthy that there is an increased prevalence of cutaneous and mucosal angiokeratomas and telangiectasia as well as cysts or pseudocysts of the maxillary sinuses in patients with Fabry's disease (Baccaglini *et al* 2001).

2.5. Amyloidosis

Amyloid is an eosinophilic hyaline protein which pathologically accumulates within tissues in a number of diseases and is thus nonspecific. It has a characteristic fibrillar structure on electron microscopy which varies in different forms of amyloidosis, but is in all cases associated with a non-fibrillar component termed amyloid-P.

The widespread lesions in amyloid disease and the possible involvement of virtually any system make this disorder protean in its manifestations. However, amyloid is deposited mainly in the heart, skeletal muscle and gastrointestinal tract so that normal function of these organs is severely compromised. Orofacial manifestations may occur by amyloid deposits developing in the temporal arteries mimicking the symptoms of temporal arteritis (Chapter 13) (Ing *et al* 1997). Other complaints include burning pain in the oral cavity, especially on the tongue. Additionally, the development of papules and xerostomia has been reported (Koloktronis *et al* 2003).

3. Orofacial Pain in Joint Disorders

Polyarthritides are a group of disorders in which the articular surfaces become inflamed, sometimes involving the temporomandibular joint (TMJ). The signs and symptoms in polyarthritides may be similar to those found in degenerative joint disease (osteoarthritis); however, the causative factors are different (see Chapter 8). The polyarthritides include rheumatoid arthritis, psoriatic arthritis, ankylosing spondylitis, infectious arthritis, hyperuricaemia, traumatic arthritis and Reiter's syndrome. It is important for the clinician to differentiate amongst these various conditions as treatment modalities differ. As a general rule systemic polyarthritides rarely involve the TMJ. Primary osteoarthritis of the TMJ is covered in Chapter 8.

3.1. Rheumatoid Arthritis

Rheumatoid arthritis (RA) is a systemic, chronic, inflammatory disease of unknown aetiology. Factors associated with RA include the possibility of infectious triggers, genetic predisposition and autoimmune response in that CD4+ T cells stimulate the immune cascade leading to cytokine production such as tumour necrosis factor alpha and interleukin-1 (Dodeller and Schulze-Koops 2006; Dombrecht et al 2006). The disease affects the articular surfaces including the synovial tissues, capsule, tendons and ligaments. The inflammatory process leads to the secondary destruction of the articular cartilage and subchondral bone (Bayar et al 2002; Helenius et al 2005). RA has an insidious onset with periods of exacerbation and remission. The prevalence in Western populations is 0.5–1% with a female-to-male ratio of approximately 3:1 (Symmons et al 1994). The disease can occur at any age with onset usually between 25 and 50 years, and the incidence peaks in the fourth and fifth decades of life (Yelin 1992). Characteristically RA affects small peripheral joints such as in the hands, wrists and feet. Joint involvement in RA tends to be symmetrical and more generalized in its clinical presentation as compared to degenerative joint disease (Laskin 1995).

The prevalence of TMJ involvement in patients with rheumatic disease varies greatly, depending on the diagnostic criteria, the population studied and the measures of assessment. Clinical involvement of the TMJ is present in approximately 50% of patients with RA and seems to correlate with disease duration and severity (Tabeling and Dolwick 1985; Gleissner et al 2003). The most common clinical signs and symptoms in the orofacial region are bilateral deep, dull, aching pain (exacerbated during function); tenderness and swelling in the preauricular regions; limitation of mandibular range of movement; stiffness in the TMJ upon awakening; intracapsular joint sounds (crepitus/clicking); and tenderness of the masticatory muscles (Kononen et al 1992; Laskin 1995; Helenius

et al 2005). As the disease progresses, limitation in opening may be worsened due to fibrous or bony ankylosis (Kobayashi et al 2001). If greater destruction of the condyles occurs, the patient may develop a progressive Class II malocclusion with heavy posterior occlusal contacts and an anterior open bite caused by loss of ramus height (Laskin 1995; Marini et al 1999).

Approximately 50–80% of RA patients have radiographic evidence of TMJ abnormalities (Larheim et al 1990; Wenneberg et al 1990). The radiographic findings of the TMJ, although not evident in the early stages of the disease process, become more apparent with disease progression. Use of magnetic resonance imaging (MRI) and computed tomography (CT) show joint effusions, disc displacements and condylar abnormalities including erosions, flattening, sclerosis, subchondral cysts and osteophytes (Bayar et al 2002; Voog et al 2003; Manfredini et al 2005).

Symptomatic TMJs in RA patients demonstrate a high frequency of synovial inflammation and connective tissue degeneration, similar to patients with osteoarthritis but different from matched-controls. Additionally, pronounced inflammatory and degenerative changes develop faster in RA than in osteoarthritis (Gynther et al 1997).

A paediatric form termed juvenile RA occurs in patients under the age of 16 years. Prevalence estimates in the United States range from 0.2 to 0.5 cases per 1000 children (Gewanter et al 1983) with a predominance in females (female:male ratio of 2–3:1). Juvenile RA is characterized by two peaks of onset, one between the ages of 1 and 3 years and the other between the ages of 8 and 12 years (Katz 1988). The prevalence of TMJ involvement in patients with juvenile RA is variable because different methods are utilized in assessment (Pedersen et al 2001; Twilt et al 2004) and when present may lead to adverse effects on occlusion and facial growth (Walton et al 1999).

Juvenile RA is subclassified into three categories: polyarticular (i.e. multiple joints affected), pauciarticular (i.e. fewer than 4 joints affected) and systemic with high fever, rash and multiple organ involvement (Katz 1988). Although the TMJ may be involved in any of these categories, it is most often affected by the polyarticular form (Pedersen et al 2001). The clinical and radiographic features are similar to those observed in the adult form of the disease. A characteristic feature of advanced juvenile RA is a significant reduction in the dimensions of the lower third of the face caused by a combination of micrognathia and a Class II skeletal distortion termed 'birdface' deformity. This is the result of destruction of the condylar growth site by the disease process.

3.2. Psoriatic Arthritis

Psoriatic arthritis is an inflammatory condition associated with psoriasis, which is a chronic, often pruritic dermatologic disease with a genetic component affecting 1–2% of the population. Associated arthritis affects approximately 6% of this population, making this a relatively uncommon condition (Wilson *et al* 1990; Koorbusch *et al* 1991; Zhu *et al* 1996). Indeed, there have been only 35 reported cases of psoriatic arthritis affecting the TMJ (Dervis 2005). However, clinical and radiographic findings associated with temporomandibular disorders in patients with generalized psoriatic arthritis seem to be more common than these case reports suggest (Kononen 1986).

Psoriatic arthritis of the TMJ is often unilateral, of sudden onset and episodic. Patients commonly complain of tenderness and pain in the preauricular region and the muscles of mastication, morning stiffness, fatigue and tiredness in the jaws. Signs include joint crepitation, painful mandibular function and a progressive decrease in interincisal opening (Kononen 1987; Koorbusch *et al* 1991; Dervis 2005). Ankylosis of the joint has been reported in severe cases (Miles and Kaugars 1991). There are, however, reports of spontaneous remission.

Radiographic changes of the TMJs associated with psoriatic arthritis are quite common and include the following nonspecific findings: erosion, flattening, osteoporosis, limited range of motion, joint space narrowing, subchondral cysts and ankylosis (Kononen and Kilpinen 1990; Melchiorre *et al* 2003).

3.3. Ankylosing Spondylitis

Ankylosing spondylitis (Bechterew's disease) is a chronic inflammatory disease of unknown aetiology, is usually progressive and most often affects the sacroiliac joints and vertebral column. The main locus of pathology is the site where the ligaments and capsule insert into the bone and not the synovium (McGonagle *et al* 1998). This condition affects 1–2% of the Caucasian population with a male-to-female prevalence ratio ranging from 6:1 (Locher *et al* 1996) to 2:1 (Helenius *et al* 2005). The affected male population demonstrates more involved joints and increased disease severity than the female population. Onset of the disease is usually between ages 16 and 40 (Locher *et al* 1996). The prevalence of TMJ involvement is quite rare and ranges from 4 to 35%, depending on the diagnostic criteria used, the population studied and the methods used to assess TMJ involvement (Kononen *et al* 1992; Ramos-Remus *et al* 1997).

The clinical findings are similar to those of other arthritic conditions and include tenderness and/or pain in the masticatory muscles and TMJ, morning stiffness/fatigue in the jaws, limitation in mouth opening and joint sounds (Kononen *et al* 1992; Locher *et al* 1996; Ramos-Remus *et al* 1997). Common radiographic signs consist of condylar erosions, flattening and sclerosis, flattening of the temporal bone and joint space narrowing (Ramos-Remus *et al* 1997; Major *et al* 1999; Helenius *et al* 2005).

3.4. Infectious Arthritis

Infectious (septic) arthritis of the TMJ is a rare disease, not frequently documented in the literature. It is an inflammatory reaction of the articular surfaces resulting from bacterial invasion caused by a penetrating external injury, spreading infection from adjacent structures (dental, parotid gland or otic origins) or from bacteraemia associated with systemic infection such as tuberculosis, syphilis and gonorrhea (Moses *et al* 1998; Henry *et al* 1999; Okeson 2003). The most common bacteria involved with infectious arthritis are *Staphylococcus aureus*, *Neisseria gonorrhea* and *Haemophilus influenzae* (Hincapie *et al* 1999). Risk factors include diabetes mellitus, systemic lupus erythematosus, rheumatoid arthritis, other immunosuppressive diseases or previous joint disease. Patients often complain of limited and painful mouth opening with a warm, erythematous preauricular mass. Mandibular deviation at rest to the contralateral side is due to joint effusion, and is often associated with a malocclusion (Hekkenberg *et al* 1999). Radiographically, the TMJ may appear normal; however, with disease progression, there may be signs of erosion of the articular surfaces and bone destruction (Thomson 1989; Leighty *et al* 1993). Bone scanning utilizing technetium-99 phosphate has been employed to detect physiologic bone changes earlier than radiographic anatomic changes; specificity is low but sensitivity is high so a negative result strongly argues against an infectious arthritis (Goldschmidt *et al* 2002). TMJ fibrosis and ankylosis resulting in impaired joint mobility and function are potential complications that usually occur in the later stages of the disease process (Leighty *et al* 1993).

3.5. Hyperuricaemia

Hyperuricaemia (gout) comprises a heterogenous group of arthritic disorders characterized by the deposition or concentration of monosodium urate monohydrate crystals in joints and tendons (crystal arthritis). The metatarsophalangeal joint (big toe) is involved in 90% of cases (Terkeltaub 2003; Saag and Mikuls 2005). Gout progresses through four clinical phases: asymptomatic hyperuricaemia, acute gouty arthritis, intercritical gout (intervals between acute attacks) and chronic tophaceous gout characterized by radiographically evident chalky deposits of sodium urate (Harris *et al* 1999). Pseudogout, another form of crystal arthritis, is due to the deposition of calcium pyrophosphate dihydrate crystals. Gout is rare and affects at least 1% of the population in Western countries with a peak incidence occurring in male patients 30 to 50 years old (Terkeltaub 2003; Saag and Mikuls 2005).

Uric acid is the end product of purine metabolism and has no physiologic role. Humans genetically lack the enzyme uricase, which allows for the degradation of uric acid to the water soluble and easily excreted product known as allantoin, thereby preventing uric acid accumulation. Elevated serum levels are a result of an overproduction and/or an underexcretion of uric acid. These mechanisms predispose the individual for developing microcrystals that may precipitate in the synovium. Additionally, it may be caused by haematologic disorders or by the use of certain medications (Halabe and Sperling 1994; Pittman and Bross 1999).

Hyperuricaemia seldom affects the TMJ and if so, rarely alone. If the TMJ is involved, the disease is usually confined to the joint space, which leads to pain and limitation of mouth opening (Gross *et al* 1987; Barthelemy *et al* 2001). However, a case where the disease process extended beyond the joint capsule into the pterygoid muscle with concomitant destruction of the head of the condyle, the temporal bone and the greater wing of the sphenoid bone has been described (Barthelemy *et al* 2001).

3.6. Reiter's Syndrome

Reiter's syndrome, also known as reactive arthritis, was described in 1916 by Hans Reiter as a triad of arthritis, nongonococcal urethritis and conjunctivitis, occurring concurrently or sequentially. More recently, Reiter's syndrome has also been defined as a peripheral arthritis lasting longer than 1 month, associated with urethritis, cervicitis or diarrhoea with additional features including mucocutaneous lesions, cardiac involvement and central or peripheral nerve involvement (Amor 1998; Kataria and Brent 2004). Reactive arthritis refers to an acute nonpurulent (aseptic) arthritis initiated by a remote infection. Reiter's syndrome is triggered by enteric or urogenital (venereal) infections. The bacteria implicated in the enteric form include *Shigella*, *Salmonella* and *Yersinia* spp. whilst *Chlamydia*, *Mycoplasma* and *Yersinia* spp. are associated with the urogenital type (Hughes and Keat 1994; Dworkin *et al* 2001).

Reiter's syndrome is associated with human leukocyte antigen HLA-B27, although HLA-B27 is not always present in an affected individual, particularly in the presence of HIV. The arthritis involved with this syndrome is usually in multiple joints with the lower extremities affected most often. The syndrome occurs mostly in males between the ages of 20 and 30 years.

Signs and symptoms of muscle and joint dysfunction in 52 males with Reiter's syndrome were more frequent and severe than those in 52 matched controls with no general joint disease (Kononen 1992). One-quarter of the Reiter's syndrome group reported TMJ signs or symptoms with the most characteristic being pain on function, tenderness to palpation and pain when opening wide (15%). Tenderness to palpation of the masticatory muscles (19%) and stiffness/tiredness of the jaws in the morning were also reported.

Patients with Reiter's syndrome more frequently display radiographic findings in the condyle (33%), with the most common finding being unilateral erosion (12%) (Kononen *et al* 2002).

4. Orofacial Pain in Bone Disorders

Osteoporosis is the most common bone disease in humans and affects both men and women (Mauck and Clarke 2006). Osteoporosis may be diagnosed following a low-impact or fragility fracture. Alternatively low bone mineral density, which is best assessed by central dual-energy X-ray absorptiometry, accurately identifies patients. Both nonpharmacological therapy (calcium and vitamin D supplementation, weight-bearing exercise and fall prevention) and pharmacological treatments (antiresorptive and anabolic agents) may be helpful in the prevention and treatment of osteoporosis.

There is a suggestion in the literature that osteoporosis is linked to temporomandibular disorders (Klemetti *et al* 1995) and atypical facial pain (Woda and Pionchon 2000) with female hormones being implicated as a common risk factor. This is based on the strong female prevalence in atypical facial pain and the physiologic and therapeutic modification of oestrogen levels in patients with these pain conditions as well as in patients with osteoporosis (Graff-Radford and Solberg 1992; Pfaffenrath *et al* 1993). The connection remains, however, speculative (see also Chapter 11; atypical facial pain).

Paget's disease of bone is characterized by bone resorption in focal areas followed by excessive new bone formation, with eventual replacement of the normal bone marrow by vascular and fibrous tissue. The aetiology of Paget's disease is not well understood; however, one Paget-disease-linked gene and several other susceptibility loci have been identified, and paramyxoviral gene products have been detected in Pagetic osteoclasts (Roodman and Windle 2005). Because of the excessive bone formation in the craniofacial complex, neurological deficits are common and include hearing, sight and smell changes (Wheeler *et al* 1995). Comparison of oral status between Paget's patients and healthy controls demonstrated that Paget's subjects were more likely to report pain when opening the mouth (Wheeler *et al* 1995).

5. Orofacial Pain in Immunologically Mediated Diseases

Immunologically mediated diseases are those with a prominent involvement of immunocytes and/or their products. We review the presentation of orofacial pain in autoimmune diseases, allergy and granulomatous and immune complex diseases.

5.1. Autoimmune Diseases

Autoimmune diseases encompass a large group of disorders which often present with overlapping and mixed clinical and laboratory features. Most often these disorders affect multisystems and although they appear to be related to a systemic autoimmune dysfunction the exact aetiology remains unclear. There are a variety of autoimmune diseases related to orofacial pain and dysfunction.

5.1.1. Systemic Lupus Erythematosus

Systemic lupus erythematosus (SLE) is a chronic autoimmune disease involving multiple organ systems. Characteristically there is a state of immune hyperactivity and antibodies directed against cell nuclei. Autoantibodies, circulating immune complexes and T lymphocytes all contribute to the expression of disease. Multisystem involvement appears as dermatologic, renal, central and peripheral nervous systems, haematologic, musculoskeletal, cardiovascular, pulmonary, vascular endothelium and gastrointestinal manifestations. Ninety percent of cases are women with the majority (80%) in their childbearing years. This has led to the hypothesis that women who are exposed to oestrogen-containing oral contraceptives or hormone replacement therapy have an increased risk of developing or exacerbating SLE (Julkunen 1991; Skaer 1992; Sanchez-Guerrero et al 1997); however, other studies do not support this finding (Mok et al 2001; Cooper et al 2002).

TMJ involvement has been reported in SLE; one-third of patients had current complaints and two-thirds had a history of severe symptoms from the TMJ (Jonsson et al 1983). Objective findings included locking or dislocation, tenderness to palpation and pain on movement of the mandible in 22% of cases. Additionally, radiographic changes of the condyles, including flattening, erosions, osteophytes and sclerosis, were observed in 30% of these patients.

Trigeminal sensory neuropathy has been associated with SLE, commonly with facial numbness, paraesthesia, dysaesthesia and pain; however, other cranial nerves may be involved (Hagen et al 1990). Trigeminal neuropathy may be the initial feature of SLE or it may follow disease onset and usually develops slowly (Hagen et al 1990; Shotts et al 1999). Oral ulcerations have also been associated with SLE and may induce acute pain (Jorizzo et al 1992).

Intractable headaches, the so-called 'lupus headaches', have long been thought of as a common and characteristic manifestation of SLE. However, a controlled study showed that headache is not specifically related to SLE expression or severity (Sfikakis et al 1998). Accepting the presence of headaches, even severe, as a neurological manifestation of SLE in the absence of seizures or overt psychosis may result in overestimation of the disease status (Sfikakis et al 1998). This approach was further supported by a recent meta-analysis (Mitsikostas et al 2004).

5.1.2. Sjögren Syndrome

Sjögren syndrome (SS) is a chronic, systemic autoimmune disorder of unknown aetiology which affects the exocrine glands; histologically characterized by a lymphocytic infiltrate of the affected glands (Fox 2005). The hallmark manifestations of SS are dryness of the mouth and eyes due to involvement of the salivary and lacrimal glands. SS is also associated with other disorders such as rheumatoid arthritis, systemic lupus erythematosus and scleroderma. In addition, SS may cause skin, nose and vaginal dryness, and may affect other organs of the body including the kidneys, blood vessels, lungs, liver, pancreas and brain. SS affects 1–4 million people in the United States, usually over the age of 40 at diagnosis. Women are nine times more likely to have SS than men. 'Primary' SS occurs in people with no other rheumatologic disease. 'Secondary' SS occurs in people who do have another rheumatologic disease, most often SLE or RA.

The presence of dry mouth increases the risk for mucosal sensitivity and, due to impaired lubrication, often leads to secondary infection, mostly candidiasis (Guggenheimer and Moore 2003). When interductal salivary flow rate is reduced, the cleansing effect of saliva is minimized and retrograde infection with acute sialoadenitis may be associated with pain.

Distal, symmetrical sensory neuropathy is present in 10–20% of cases with primary SS (Olney 1998), but there are reports of asymmetric neuropathies (Denislic and Meh 1997). Isolated cranial nerve sensory neuropathy has been reported in a number of patients with SS (Urban et al 2001; Mori et al 2005), including the trigeminal nerve (Font et al 2003). Trigeminal sensory neuropathy in SS is characterized by a slowly progressing, unilateral or bilateral facial numbness or paraesthesia, occasionally associated with pain (Urban et al 1999).

5.1.3. Scleroderma

Scleroderma, also known as systemic sclerosis, is a multisystem connective tissue disorder of unknown aetiology. It is characterized by inflammation and vascular and fibrotic alterations in the skin, which becomes indurated and fixed to the underlying connective tissue (Spackman 1999). It also involves various other internal organs, the gastrointestinal tract, heart, lungs and kidneys, causing fibrosis by the deposition of too much collagen. Scleroderma is a rather generic term used to describe a systemic as well as a localized cutaneous variant. The systemic form of scleroderma is classified as CREST syndrome, which is an acronym for the clinical manifestations: calcinosis, Raynaud's phenomenon, esophageal dysmotility, sclerodactyly and telangiectasia. This can be further subdivided into morphea scleroderma (a localized form of the disease) and linear scleroderma (a specific type of localized scleroderma). Diffuse systemic sclerosis, or progressive systemic sclerosis, is rare and carries a poor prognosis (Scardina and Messina 2004). Females are affected more often than males with a ratio of 3:1 and this tends to increase to 4:1 during the childbearing years (Spackman 1999) with the highest onset of symptoms being between the ages of 30 and 50 years.

The most characteristic orofacial manifestations are microstomia, resulting in limited mouth opening, mucogingival problems, fibrosis of the hard and soft palate, telangiectasis and chromatosis of the face and oral mucosa, xerostomia, dry eyes, widening of the periodontal ligament space, TMJ dysfunction and trigeminal neuropathy (Nagy *et al* 1994; Chaffee 1998). These manifestations are either a direct result of the substitutions of normal tissues with collagen or the deposition of collagen around nerves or endothelial tissues (Wood and Lee 1988).

TMJ dysfunction is most often related to gross changes to the mandible which include osteolytic activity resulting in bone resorption of the coronoid process, condyles, angle of the mandible and ramus (Chaffee 1998; Scardina and Messina 2004). These changes result in articular pain and swelling due to tendonitis and synovitis with accompanying radiographic changes described earlier (Ramon *et al* 1987).

Trigeminal sensory neuropathy may involve all three branches and appears to be the most frequent orofacial phenomenon to precede this disorder (Hagen *et al* 1990). Of 22 patients with scleroderma, 9 displayed trigeminal neuropathy as the first symptom (Lecky *et al* 1987). The symptomatology consists of paraesthesia, burning and/or an intense sharp/stabbing pain that may be provoked by jaw use or movement, thus mimicking the presentation of trigeminal neuralgia (Spackman 1999; Fischoff and Sirois 2000).

5.1.4. Mixed Connective Tissue Disorder

The clinical findings in mixed connective tissue disorder (MCTD) often include Raynaud's phenomenon, polyarthralgia or arthritis, lymphadenitis, cutaneous and mucosal lesions and serositis in the form of pulmonary involvement. These features are commonly found in a number of different connective tissue diseases including systemic lupus erythematosus, scleroderma, rheumatoid arthritis and polymyositis. Thus MCTD is characterized by overlapping, nonspecific clinical features that may occur simultaneously or sequentially (Alfaro-Giner *et al* 1992).

The orofacial manifestations of these connective tissue disorders, although uncommon, appear as trigeminal sensory neuropathy and arthritis of the TMJ. The presence of trigeminal neuropathy has also been reported to include both pain and numbness, and it appears that neurovascular headaches of mild to moderate severity are relatively common in this disorder (Hagen *et al* 1990; Alfaro-Giner *et al* 1992).

Patients with MCTD demonstrate signs and symptoms of dysfunction of the masticatory system (Konttinen *et al* 1990). Masticatory muscle and TMJ tenderness, with associated clicking or crepitation, are common (Helenius *et al* 2005). Radiographic changes of the temporomandibular joints were observed in 7 of 10 patients examined (Konttinen *et al* 1990). Moreover, in 5 of 6 patients with

normal-appearing mucosa, histological examination revealed chronic inflammation. Three of the 10 patients had clinically atrophic and erythematous oral mucosa; histological examination again revealed chronic inflammation.

MCTD is often associated with secondary Sjögren syndrome (Alarcon-Segovia 1984), although this association does not influence the clinical course of MCTD (Ohtsuka *et al* 1992). Suspicious cases of Sjögren-like symptoms that are undiagnosed should be referred for medical assessment.

5.1.5. Antiphospholipid Syndrome

The antiphospholipid syndrome (APS, Hughes syndrome), first described in 1983, is a prothrombotic disease in which neurological events feature prominently. Cerebrovascular accidents (CVA), transient ischaemic attacks (TIA) and headaches are important complications. Other neurological symptoms, including diplopia, memory loss, ataxia and 'multiple sclerosis-like' features are common (Hughes 2003). APS is characterized by serum autoantibodies to phospholipids, which are deposited in small vessels, leading to intimal hyperplasia and acute thromboses, especially in cerebral, renal, pulmonary, cutaneous and cardiac arteries. APS may be seen in isolation or associated with SLE or other connective tissue diseases including Sjögren's syndrome.

Headache in APS can vary from typical episodic migraine to an almost continuous incapacitating headache. The patient history is often remarkably similar with teenage headaches, frequently migrainous in character and temporally associated with premenstrual days. These headaches may subsequently disappear for 10–20 years only to return when the patient reaches the age of 30–40 years. Significantly, there is a strong family history of headaches or of migraine in many of these patients, suggesting common genetic influences. Moreover as in migraine with aura, some patients report headaches accompanied by visual or speech disturbance, or by transient ischaemic attacks (Hughes 2003).

The association of migraine and anti-phospholipid antibodies (aPL) is controversial, with widely varying results. Some have reported association with lupus anticoagulant (LA) or anti-cardiolipin (aCL) (Levine *et al* 1987; Hogan *et al* 1988), but others report no associations (Alarcon-Segovia *et al* 1989). The difficulty in demonstrating a true association between aCL positivity and migraine stems in part from the high prevalence of migraine in the normal population and the relatively low prevalence of aCL positivity in otherwise healthy individuals (see Chapter 9 for migraine description). One of the major problems is that headaches, often nonmigrainous, have been loosely termed 'migraine', and these headaches may precede or accompany TIAs or CVA (Tzourio *et al* 2000). Anti-phospholipid antibodies have also been detected in patients with transient neurological symptoms including migraine aura. Therefore, the controversy may be in part due to the inherent difficulty in distinguishing the transient focal neurological events of migraine from TIA (Sanna *et al* 2003). The available data suggest an association between the migraine-like *phenomena* and aPL but not between migraine headache and aPL (Shuaib *et al* 1989; Montalban *et al* 1992; Tietjen 1992; Tietjen *et al* 1998; Verrotti *et al* 2000).

Anecdotal reports show that anticoagulation treatment is sometimes effective in reducing the number and intensity of headache attacks in selected APS patients (Cuadrado *et al* 2000). Similarly, memory loss often improves dramatically with appropriate warfarin dosage (Cuadrado *et al* 2001; Hughes 2003).

5.2. Allergy

Orofacial allergic reactions may have a protean presentation in regard to acuity and spectrum of symptoms. The acute form of oral allergy, also known as oral allergy syndrome, is an uncommon variant of allergic reactions. It refers to the combination of irritation, pruritus and swelling of the lips, tongue, palate and throat, sometimes associated with other allergic features such as rhinoconjunctivitis, asthma, urticaria-angioedema and even anaphylactic shock. Symptoms usually develop within minutes but occasionally are delayed for over an hour. They may include itching and burning of the lips, mouth and throat, watery itchy eyes, runny nose and sneezing.

Most chronic forms of oral allergy are attributed to dental restorative materials. Gold is reported to cause itching, a burning pain sensation and, at times, ulceration of the oral tissues adjacent to the gold restoration (van Loon *et al* 1992). Immunologic-mediated lichenoid reactions have also been attributed to dental restorative materials and drugs (Scully and Bagan 2004; Issa *et al* 2005).

In the context of allergy and headache, an interdisciplinary consensus committee of the International Headache Society (IHS) and the American Academy of Otolaryngology-Head and Neck Surgery suggested that in patients with allergies and headaches, management of the allergies may reduce the frequency of the headaches. The mechanism for this may be related to reducing a trigger for the headache (i.e. allergies) or by decreasing mucosal inflammation which may be responsible for precipitating the headache. Patients with typical itchy eyes, itchy nose and nasal congestion may benefit from an allergy evaluation (Cady *et al* 2005). This consensus meeting was part of an attempt to define conditions that lead to headaches of rhinogenic origin (see also Chapter 6). This conclusion is supported by a previous study (Gazerani *et al* 2003) which showed that the relationship between allergy and migraine can be based, in part, on an IgE-mediated mechanism with histamine release playing an important role.

5.3. Granulomatous Diseases

5.3.1. Wegener's Granulomatosis

Wegener's granulomatosis (WG) is an autoimmune disease which has a clinical predilection for the upper airways, lungs and kidneys. WG is a necrotizing granulomatous vasculitis characterized by the presence of antineutrophil cytoplasmic antibody (ANCA). Neurological involvement in this autoimmune disease is rare at onset. However, a case where headache was the initial, dominant presentation was reported (Lim *et al* 2002). The headache was migratory, throbbing and accentuated by head movement and symptoms disappeared when the treatment was directed at the underlying WG. Two further cases where the headache in WG was described as a severe lancinating left-sided facial pain with green nasal discharge, postnasal drip, nasal obstruction and photophobia with the eventual development of hyperalgesia and allodynia have been published (Makura and Robson 1996). The described pain was localized to the frontoethmoid area and extended retro-orbitally and kept the patient awake at night. In the second case, hearing loss was also present.

5.3.2. Neurosarcoidosis

Neurosarcoidosis (NS) is a multisystem granulomatous disease of unknown cause, most commonly affecting young adults. Sarcoid lesions are non-caseating epithelioid granulomas. Involvement of the CNS is clinically evident in 5% and silent in 10% of the cases with systemic sarcoidosis: it may occur at presentation in 10–30% of patients and more rarely is strictly confined to the central nervous system (CNS). Intracranial lesions are detectable by magnetic resonance imaging (MRI) (La Mantia and Erbetta 2004).

Headaches are frequently reported in patients with neurosarcoidosis (30%). Headache character varies in relation to neuropathologic involvement—focal lesions, meningitis, cranial nerve palsies—so no typical characteristics of headache are known. Intractable headaches located occipitally and radiating frontally, with associated nausea and visual disturbances, have been reported in patients with isolated supratentorial tumour-like lesions (Vannemreddy *et al* 2002). Diffuse or bifrontal pain is a more typical symptom of leptomeningeal involvement which may be associated with papilloedema (Katz *et al* 2003). Other forms of cranial pain may be related to trigeminal or optic nerve involvement and migraine has also been reported (Dizdarevic *et al* 1998).

5.3.3. Melkersson Rosenthal Syndrome

Melkersson Rosenthal syndrome is an uncommon condition of uncertain pathogenesis and course. The classic triad of signs includes recurrent orofacial oedema, recurrent facial nerve palsy and lingua plica (fissured tongue). The condition produces non-tender, persistent swelling of one or both lips and affects primarily young adults. Histologically, non-necrotizing granulomatous inflammation is seen (Allen *et al* 1990). Therefore, facial neuropathy involving facial palsy or symptomatic lip swelling should include Melkersson Rosenthal syndrome as a differential diagnosis. Some authors suggest that Melkerson Rosenthal syndrome is a variant of Crohn's disease (Scully 2005).

5.4. Immune Complex Diseases

5.4.1. Behçet's Disease

Behçet's disease is a clinical triad of oral and genital ulceration and uveitis that affects young adult males, particularly in Turkey and Japan, with an association to HLA-B5 and HLA-B51. Clinical features such as arthralgia and vasculitis suggest an immune complex-mediated basis, which is supported by finding of circulating immune complexes, but the antigen responsible has not been identified. There are immunological changes in Behçet's disease such as T-lymphocyte abnormalities, changes in serum complement and increased polymorphonuclear motility. Mononuclear cells and natural killer cells may also be involved (Yamashita 1997; Zierhut *et al* 2003).

Recurrent headache has been reported in over 80% of Behçet's patients (Monastero *et al* 2003; Kidd 2006). The majority fulfil the IHS criteria for migraine (Chapter 9), with a higher than normal prevalence of visual sensory aura (52%). Sixty-two percent of patients showed moderate or severe disability using the Migraine Disability Assessment Score (Kidd 2006). Since the nervous system is involved in 5% of Behçet's patients, headache appears to occur independently (Saip *et al* 2005). A much lower incidence of headache in Behçet's patients (58%) has been reported (Saip *et al* 2005); however, migrainous headache was commonly associated with exacerbations of some of the systemic symptoms of the syndrome. Therefore, this form of headache is not specific to Behçet's disease, but may be explained by a vascular headache triggered by the immuno-mediated disease activity in susceptible individuals.

6. Orofacial Pain in Neurologic Disorders

Headaches associated with neurologic disorders are mainly observed in cerebrovascular accident (CVA), multiple sclerosis (MS) and changes in intracranial pressure; see also Chapters 11 and 13.

CVA is a syndrome of rapidly developing clinical signs and symptoms of focal, and at times, global disturbances of cerebral function lasting greater than 24 hours or resulting in death within that time. When blood flow to the brain is interrupted for more than a few seconds, brain cells can die, causing infarction. The most common cause of CVA or stroke is cerebral atherosclerosis that may lead to the

main types of CVA: haemorrhagic (intracerebral or subarachnoid), thrombotic or embolic. Rarely strokes are secondary to other pathologies, such as carotid dissection (Chapter 13), carotid stenosis, cocaine use and syphilis.

In a prospective study involving 240 patients experiencing an acute CVA, it was found that headache occurred in 38% of this population. Headache patients were younger with a history of tension-type headache being more significant in the headache group than in the non-headache group. In patients with ischaemic stroke, the incidence of headache was lower, with shorter, more localized less intense pain compared to patients with haemorrhagic CVA (Arboix *et al* 1994).

The association between migraine and stroke remains controversial (Agostoni *et al* 2004; Rothrock 2004). Epidemiological studies suggest that migraine may be an independent risk factor for ischaemic stroke in women under 45 years of age, with additional risk factors being cigarette smoking and oral contraceptive use (Tzourio *et al* 1995). The pathogenesis is not well understood, but is thought to be related to common biochemical mechanisms between migraine and stroke. A classification of migraine-related stroke has been proposed which includes three major entities: coexisting stroke and migraine, stroke with clinical features of migraine and migraine-induced stroke (Agostoni *et al* 2004). Coexisting stroke and migraine was proposed as an explanation for the relationship between stroke and migraine in patients affected by cardiac disease. In such a condition, a possible cause of ischaemic stroke may be an increased propensity towards paradoxical cerebral emboli during migraine attacks, when there is a condition of platelet hyperaggregation.

Stroke with clinical features of migraine stems from the hypothesis that in some arteriovenous malformations or neurological diseases, the circulation in the central nervous system may be affected by multiple minor infarcts, and the patient may present with migraine as a symptom of a minor infarct.

The concept of migraine-induced stroke is well represented by migrainous infarction. It is described in the most recent classification of headaches (IHS 2004) and represents the strongest evidence for the relationship between ischaemic stroke and migraine (Chapter 9).

An association between MS and headaches has been suggested (Rolak and Brown 1990). In 137 MS patients, 88 reported headache, 21 of whom developed headache after initiation of interferon treatment (D'Amico *et al* 2004). The prevalence of all headaches not due to interferon was 57.7%. Migraine was found in 25%, tension-type headache in 31.9% and cluster headache in one patient. A significant correlation between migraine and relapsing–remitting MS also was found. Some authors suggest that the mechanism for this is a serotoninergic link between MS and migraine headache (Sandyk and Awerbuch 1994).

Headache may be caused by both raised intracranial pressure and intracranial hypotension (Ramadan 1996;

Mokri 2003). Extremely high intracranial pressure commonly causes headache. Benign intracranial hypertension is a rare syndrome of increased intracranial pressure manifesting as headache, transient visual obscuration and palsy of the sixth cranial nerve. The majority of patients with benign intracranial hypertension are idiopathic but possible causes include tetracycline use, endocrine disorders such as obesity, hypoparathyroidism, hypervitaminosis A and thyroid replacement therapy. Cerebral oedema, high cerebrospinal fluid outflow resistance, high cerebral venous pressure or a combination of the three is thought to underlie benign intracranial hypertension. The management of benign intracranial hypertension includes symptomatic headache relief, removal of offending risk factors and medical or surgical reduction of intracranial pressure. Spontaneous intracranial hypotension, characterized by postural headache, is rarer than benign intracranial hypertension. Diminished cerebrospinal fluid production, hyperabsorption and cerebrospinal fluid (CSF) leak are postulated mechanisms of spontaneous intracranial hypotension; CSF pressure is typically less than 60 mmH$_2$O. Empirical treatment includes bed rest, administration of caffeine, corticosteroids or mineralocorticoids, epidural blood patch and epidural saline infusion.

In summary, the IHS has recently recognized that secondary headaches may occur in patients affected by inflammatory diseases of the central nervous system, classified as headaches attributed to non-vascular intracranial disorders. Headaches are frequently reported in patients with neurosarcoidosis (30%), Behçet's syndrome (55%) and acute disseminated encephalomyelitis (45–58%) (La Mantia and Erbetta 2004).

7. Orofacial Pain in Hypertension

Headache is generally regarded as a symptom of high blood pressure, despite conflicting opinions on their precise association. Most studies have shown that mild, chronic hypertension and headache are not associated (Cortelli et al 2004). Whether moderate hypertension predisposes an individual to headache remains controversial, but there is little evidence. However, headaches caused by significant disturbances in arterial pressure are included in the IHS classification. The headaches associated with severe disturbance in arterial pressure were attributed to phaeochromocytoma, malignant hypertension, preeclampsia and eclampsia and acute pressor response to an exogenous agent.

The most common symptom of phaeochromocytoma is a rapid-onset headache, which has been reported by up to 92% of these patients (Mannelli et al 1999). The headache, which lasts less than an hour in most patients, is bilateral, severe and throbbing, and may be associated with nausea in 50% of cases. Paroxysms can begin spontaneously or be triggered by physical exertion, certain medications,

emotional stress and changes in posture and increases in intraabdominal pressure (Cortelli et al 2004).

In malignant hypertension, the rate and extent of the rise in blood pressure are the most important factors in the development of acute cerebral syndrome. The presenting symptoms can be headache, nausea and vomiting. Additional signs and symptoms include blurred vision, scintillating scotoma or visual loss, anxiety and then decreased levels of consciousness until seizures begin (Cortelli et al 2004).

Preeclampsia occurs in up to 7% of pregnancies and eclampsia is found in up to 0.3%. It was suggested that headache in women with preeclampsia is strongly associated with the presence of abnormal cerebral perfusion pressure (Belfort et al 1999). A strong association between migraine history and preeclampsia development, specifically with the severe form of preeclampsia, has been shown (Facchinetti et al 2005).

A sudden severe headache, due to a rapid increase in blood pressure, may occur in individuals taking monoamine oxidase inhibitors (MAOI) concomitantly with the drinking of red wine, eating foods with high tyramine content (cheese, chicken livers or pickled herring) or taking sympathomimetic medications such as pseudoephedrine (Cortelli et al 2004). However MAOIs are rarely employed.

8. Orofacial Pain in Blood Disorders

Disorders of the red blood cells can cause headaches. Anaemia, defined as a reduction in the oxygen-carrying capacity of the blood, is usually related to a decrease in the number of circulating red blood cells or to an abnormality in their haemoglobin content. In some forms of haemoglobinopathies—thalassaemia and sickle cell anaemia—facial pain or headache may be present as part of compensative changes in the jaws.

Thalassaemias are autosomally dominant inherited disorders in which either alpha- or beta-globin chains are synthesized at a low rate, thereby lessening the production of haemoglobin. The unaffected chains are produced in excess and precipitate within the erythrocytes to cause excessive erythrocyte fragility and haemolysis. Thalassaemias are characterized by a hypochromic microcytic anaemia and may be severe (major, homozygous) or mild (minor, heterozygous) and may affect beta- (beta-thalassaemia) or alpha-chains (alpha thalassaemia).

In beta-thalassaemia, neurological complications have been attributed to various factors such as chronic hypoxia, bone marrow expansion, iron overload and desferrioxamine neurotoxicity (Zafeiriou et al 2006). Cranial nerve palsies have been described in thalassaemia due to the extramedullary haematopoiesis resulting in pressure on the nerves (To and Nadel 1991; Aarabi et al 1998). Thromboembolic events have been frequently reported in beta-thalassaemic patients in association with risk factors such as diabetes, complex cardiopulmonary abnormalities, hypothyroidisim, liver function anomalies and postsplenectomy thrombocytosis. A multicentral Italian study identified 32 patients with thromboembolic episodes in a total of 735 thalassaemic subjects. There was great variation in localization of the thromboemboli, mainly the CNS (16/32), with a clinical picture of headache, seizures and haemiparesis (Borgna Pignatti et al 1998). Anecdotally, thalassaemic patients may experience painful swelling of the parotid glands with xerostomia caused by iron deposition, and a sore or burning tongue related to folate deficiency (Goldfarb et al 1983).

In sickle-cell anaemia, amino-acid substitution in the globin chain results in haemoglobin with a propensity to polymerize or precipitate, causing gross distortions in the shape of erythrocytes and membrane damage. The erythrocytes stiffen and cause microvascular occlusions. Painful crises usually due to infarction as a result of sickling are brought on by infection, dehydration, hypoxia, acidosis or cold, and cause severe pain and pyrexia. Cases of mental nerve paraesthesia in sickle cell crisis, probably due to the intensive extramedullary haematopoiesis in the jaws, have been described.

Painful infarcts in the jaws may be mistaken for toothache or osteomyelitis. Pulpal symptoms are common in the absence of any obvious dental disease and sometimes pulpal necrosis has resulted (O'Rourke and Mitropoulos 1990; Demirbas Kaya et al 2004). Skull infarction should be considered as a cause of new onset headache located at the vertex in patients with sickle cell disease, especially if scalp oedema is present (Pari and Schipper 1996).

A study on the characteristics of headaches in children with sickle cell disease showed an incidence of 31.2% of frequent headaches (greater than once a week) with moderate average pain severity (5.8 on a 0–10 scale). Duration of headaches ranged from 30 minutes to several days, with a mean of 5 hours. Based on IHS criteria, 43.8% of children had headache symptoms consistent with migraines, 6.2% with migraine with aura and 50% with tension-type headaches. Children with symptoms of migraine had functional disability significantly greater than that in children with symptoms of tension-type headaches.

The use of cytokines and growth factors, some with known toxicities, has become common in the treatment of haematological disorders (Vial and Descotes 1995). Granulocyte macrophage colony stimulating factor (GM-CSF) is administered to prevent myelotoxicity or accelerate haematopoietic recovery after chemotherapy and has been reported to cause headache (Hovgaard and Nissen 1992). A common adverse event due to the ability of GM-CSF to increase haematopoiesis in bone marrow is bone pain with the potential involvement of the jaw. GM-CSF is increasingly used to mobilize haematopoietic stem cells to the peripheral blood in the healthy donor population, thereby exposing this group to potential adverse events presenting in the orofacial complex.

9. Orofacial Pain in Dialysis and Renal Disorders

Dialysis may induce severe headache as a result of overhydration and electrolyte shifts. About 70% of haemodialysis patients complain of headache and about 57% of patients experience headache during haemodialysis sessions (Antoniazzi et al 2003). The most prevalent features of dialysis headache include frontotemporal location, moderate severity, throbbing quality and a duration of less than 4 hours (Goksan et al 2004).

The IHS criteria for headache related to haemodialysis consider that the headaches must begin during haemodialysis and terminate within 24 hours. However, there are variations of headache related to haemodialysis that may not follow these specific criteria (Antoniazzi et al 2003). The literature suggests that the dialysis protocol may also affect the frequency of headache (Heidenheim et al 2003).

There are also sporadic reports regarding a complication of nephrotic syndrome causing headache, specifically cerebral venous thrombosis (Pillekamp et al 1997; Chan 2004).

Alport's syndrome is an unusual genetic disease that ultimately results in renal failure and has an associated high incidence of sensorineural hearing loss. A case of a patient with Alport's syndrome and TMJ involvement is described in the literature (Gingrass 1993). The patient had complaints of facial and joint pain that resembled temporomandibular disorder with headache, tinnitus, joint pain and temporal swelling.

10. Orofacial Pain in Pulmonary Diseases

Chronic obstructive pulmonary disease (COPD) is a chronic, slowly progressive irreversible disease characterized by breathlessness, wheezing, cough and sputum production. About 30% of patients with moderate or severe, stable COPD complain of headache and 45.5% report sleep disorders. Significant risk factors include a family history of COPD, having other systemic or sleep disorders (snoring, bruxism) and laboratory data of chronic hypoxaemia and airway obstruction (Ozge et al 2006). This suggests a relationship between chronic hypoxaemia and headache.

Asthma is a state of bronchial hyper-reactivity causing paroxysmal expiratory wheezing, dyspnoea and cough. Generalized reversible bronchial narrowing is caused by excessive bronchial smooth muscle tone, mucosal oedema and congestion, and mucus hypersecretion with diminished ciliary clearance. Evidence for an association between migraine and asthma is based on a matched case-control study including a patient population of over 5 million subjects (Davey et al 2002). However, the mechanism shared by migraine and asthma is unclear.

11. Orofacial Pain in Cancer Patients

Regional pain may occur with oropharyngeal and head and neck cancers, systemic cancers, cancer metastatic to the head and neck and cancers distant to the site of pain. Cancer surgery, radiation and chemotherapy inevitably lead to pain (Table 14.1). Pain in oropharyngeal and head and neck cancer patients is extremely common and is associated with significant suffering markedly affecting quality of life. Treatment and prevention of pain in cancer requires knowledge of the multifactorial processes and mechanisms involved.

Classification of orofacial pain in cancer patients may be based upon the underlying pathophysiology (e.g. nociceptive, inflammatory, infectious, neuropathic), the location of the tumour (local vs distant) or the primary initiating agent (cancer or cancer therapy). It is convenient to examine cancer-related pain according to the timing of its appearance (e.g. presenting sign, or during and following therapy).

Patients with advanced cancer experience significant pain, see Table 14.2 (Portenoy and Lesage 1999). In patients with head and neck (H&N) cancers, pain is reported in up to 85% of cases at diagnosis (Foley and Inturrisi 1987; Epstein and Stewart 1993). The majority (approximately three-quarters) will suffer from pain secondary to bone destruction and nerve injury (Coleman 1998; Foley 1999) that involves inflammatory and neuropathic mechanisms (Caraceni and Portenoy 1999; Kanner 2001). In large surveys of H&N cancer patients (Grond et al 1996; Caraceni and Portenoy 1999), pain was frequently associated with the tumour (87–92.5%), while in 17–20.8% pain was secondary to therapy, and many patients reported pain from both disease and treatment. Following treatment of H&N cancer, 78% of patients reported pain in the head, face or mouth and 54% in the cervical region or shoulder and some reported pain in distant sites (thoracic region (7%), lower back (7%), and limbs (5%)) (Grond et al 1996).

It is estimated that between 45 and 60% of all cancer patients may not have adequate pain control (de Wit et al 2001; Meuser et al 2001). Barriers to achieving adequate pain management include the patient's reluctance to report pain, practices of healthcare providers and patient's preconceived fears of addiction and regulatory barriers to the use of opioids. Cancer pain causes significant negative impact on quality of life (QoL) and increases anxiety and depression (Caraceni and Portenoy 1999; Portenoy et al 1999; Epstein and Schubert 2003; Sonis 2004a).

Orofacial pain may be aggravated by motor functions of the H&N and oropharynx. The oral mucosa is highly sensitive to the effects of systemic chemotherapy and regional radiotherapy, whereby oral function and QoL can be affected and therapy is limited due to painful mucositis. Pain associated with oropharyngeal mucositis may prevent oral intake of food and medications and affect speech and respiration, frequently requiring the use of opioid analgesics. Oral microbial flora are a potential source of opportunistic infection, particularly in cases of mucosal damage and myelosuppression with attendant pain and morbidity affecting communication, oral nutrition and medication.

The economic cost of treatment-associated side effects is demonstrated by chemotherapy- and radiotherapy-induced mucositis (Sonis et al 2001; Elting et al 2003; Oster et al 2005). Severe and painful mucositis is associated with enteral/parenteral nutrition, analgesic requirements, additional admissions and prolonged stay in hospital, leading to increased cost of care and potentially to delayed, interrupted or altered cancer therapy affecting prognosis.

Graft-versus-host disease (GVHD) is a major painful complication of allogeneic haematopoietic stem cell transplant (HSCT), occurring in 25–70% of patients (Woo et al 1997).

Pain in cancer patients may also occur coincidentally due to other conditions unrelated to cancer, but may be interpreted by the patient as progression or recurrence of the cancer.

11.1. Orofacial Pain due to Cancer

11.1.1. Pain in Regional Malignancy

Local-regional cancers commonly causing pain in the H&N include oropharyngeal, sinus, nasopharyngeal, salivary glands, intracranial and extracranial primary and metastatic tumours. In a retrospective study, pain as the initial complaint of oral cancer was found in 19.2% of 1412 patients and was more prevalent in men (Cuffari et al 2006). Pain complaints were nonspecific and included descriptions such as sore throat, pain on function (swallowing, chewing) and pain in the region of the tongue, mouth, teeth and ear. Pain was found to be associated with advanced disease and tongue location (Cuffari et al 2006). In another study primary squamous cell carcinomas of the oral mucosa presented with pain in up to 85% of patients presenting for diagnosis of oral cancer (Epstein and Stewart 1993). The most common presenting symptom of osteosarcoma of the jaw is a mass (85–95.5%) (Bennett et al 2000; Gorsky and Epstein 2000) with pain associated with the mass in approximately half of cases (Mardinger et al 2001).

Manifestations of systemic cancers such as leukaemia may affect the H&N and cause pain and loss of function (Epstein and Stewart 1993; McGuire et al 1998). Haematologic cancers and cancer therapies for solid tumours increase the risk of secondary infections (fungal, bacterial, viral) due to damage to mucosal barriers and possible myelosuppression. Pain may be induced by infection due to reactivation of latent or exacerbation of prior chronic infection or a new infection, including secondary to nosocomial flora and acquired pathogens (Bergmann and Andersen 1990; Bergmann et al 1990; Epstein and Polsky 1998).

Lymphoma is a common neoplasm occurring in the oral region accounting for 3.5% of oral malignancies (Hoffman *et al* 1998; Epstein *et al* 2001a). Lymphoma presents as a firm rubbery mass associated with discomfort in approximately one-half of patients. Lymphomas and leukaemias may induce pain by infiltration of pain-sensitive structures such as periosteum and gingivae.

Multiple myeloma frequently presents with pain that may be associated with the teeth and may cause radiolucent periapical lesions without bony margins resulting in a diagnostic challenge (Epstein 1997; Witt *et al* 1997). Other orofacial malignancies such as malignant melanoma and intraoral sarcomas are rare, but may present as a mass with or without ulceration that may be accompanied by discomfort (Gorsky and Epstein 1998a,b). Primary or metastatic tumours of the jaw and of the infratemporal fossa may cause numbness or pain that may precede tumour diagnosis (Schreiber *et al* 1991; Cohen and Rosenheck 1998).

Orofacial pain or headache is reported with intracranial tumours in up to 6% of cases; see also Chapters 11 and 13 (Bullitt *et al* 1986; Luyk *et al* 1991; Puca *et al* 1993; Bhaya and Har-El 1998; Pfund *et al* 1999; Christiaans *et al* 2002).

Metastases to bone may present with neurologic symptoms, such as pain and numbness, or a mass and commonly arise from the breast, colon, prostate, thyroid, lung and kidney (Coleman 1997). Bone pain results from structural damage, periosteal irritation and nerve entrapment. Metastases to the jaw rarely involve soft tissue and most commonly occur in the posterior mandible, angle of the jaw and ramus (Hirshberg and Buchner 1995). Of tumours metastasizing to the jaws, lung is the most common source in men and breast cancer is the most common primary cancer in women (Sanchez Aniceto *et al* 1990; Hirshberg *et al* 1993, 1994; Hirshberg and Buchner 1995). In up to 30% of cases, oral metastases are the first indication of a distant undiscovered cancer (Hirshberg and Buchner 1995). Patients with nasopharyngeal cancer often report pain that is referred to the TMJ region and may be misdiagnosed as temporomandibular disorder (TMD) (Epstein and Jones 1993; Su and Lui 1996; Wang and Howng 2001). In one study, approximately 10% of patients with nasopharyngeal carcinoma presented with common TMD signs and symptoms. About 40% described dull, aching pain resulting in headache, earache, jaw, midface or neck pain (Epstein and Jones 1993).

Pain is therefore an unreliable predictor of orofacial malignancy as pain quality and intensity are highly variable and in most studies pain occurs in from 20 to 85% of cancer patients at diagnosis. However, the combination of numbness, pain and swelling together is highly predictive of malignancy, particularly in the presence of systemic signs (weight loss, fatigue, anaemia). Patients with pain before treatment develop significantly greater impairment due to pain during and after treatment

Table 14.1 Distribution of pain during various stages of cancer and it therapy

Timing	Aetiology of pain
At clinical presentation	Space occupying lesion (oral)
	Space occupying lesion (infratemporal fossa, intra-cranial)
	Leukaemic infiltration
	Secondary syndromes such as anaemia
Early in the treatment course	Nerve damage due to cytotoxics (vinca alkaloids)/radiation
	Mucosal damage due to cytotoxics/radiation
	Acute GVHD
	Infection
	Post surgery
Late in the treatment course	Chronic GVHD
	Post-mucositis pain
	Osteoradionecrosis
	Osteonecrosis (bisphosphonates)
	Post surgery
In terminal stage	Same aetiologies
In recurrence	Same as 'at clinical presentation'

GVHD, graft versus host disease.

(Gellrich *et al* 2002a), suggesting sensitization has occurred. Mechanisms of pain are outlined in Table 14.1; see also Chapters 2 (neuroanatomy and mechanisms), 11 (neuropathies) and 15 (inflammation).

11.1.2. Pain Secondary to Malignancy at a Distant Site

Orofacial pain may arise from a distant and non-metastasized cancer, most commonly from the lungs (Abraham *et al* 2003; Eross *et al* 2003; Sarlani *et al* 2003), due to activation of nociceptive pathways in mediastinal or H&N structures (Sarlani *et al* 2003). Pain may also be due to invasion or compression of the vagus nerve (Bindoff and Heseltine 1988); referred facial pain may be mediated by termination of vagal afferents in the spinal trigeminal nucleus (Contreras *et al* 1982; Gwyn *et al* 1985). In addition, the phrenic nerve may refer pain from the pleura and subdiaphragmatic areas to the H&N (Goldberg 1997). Paraneoplastic processes resulting in peripheral neuropathies and cytokine production are common, particularly in lung cancer (Amato and Collins 1998; Antoine *et al* 1999; Mallecourt and Delattre 2000). Typical presentations include unilateral dull aching pain (ipsilateral to the lung tumour), often located around the ear, jaw and temporal regions, weight loss, haemoptysis, persistent cough and chest wall pain (Sarlani *et al* 2003). Similar mechanisms may be associated with gastrointestinal and pancreatic cancer that present with orofacial pain (Daggett and Nabarro 1984; Littlewood and Mandelli 2002).

In patients with lung cancer, peripheral neuropathy was found in 48% prior to chemotherapy (Teravainen and Larsen 1977). Neuromuscular dysfunction occurs in 30% of patients with diverse tumours, most commonly in ovarian, testicular and bronchogenic cancers (Paul *et al* 1978). Often these neuropathies are accompanied by detectable autoantibodies that may aid in diagnosis.

11.2. Orofacial Pain due to Cancer Therapy

Treatment-related orofacial pain is almost universal in chemotherapy and H&N cancer patients. Pain may be acute during active therapy, or delayed due to late complications of therapy such as dysfunction of the masticatory system, soft tissue and bone necrosis, secondary infection, dental pain due to dentinal sensitivity and caries, mucosal atrophy, neuropathy and oral GVHD.

11.2.1. Pain due to Chemo- and Radiotherapy

The most common acute oral side effect of cancer chemotherapy or radiotherapy is oral mucositis (Table 14.2). In chemotherapy-induced mucositis, the sites most commonly involved are nonkeratinized tissue (buccal and labial mucosa, ventral and lateral aspects of the tongue, soft palate and floor of the mouth). Signs of mucositis appear approximately 6–10 days after treatment, although the biological changes begin immediately (Sonis 2004a). Pain associated with mucositis is the most distressing symptom in patients receiving aggressive neutropenia-inducing chemotherapy regimens (Epstein *et al* 2002a; Rubenstein *et al* 2004; Duncan *et al* 2005). Mucositis is well documented in HSCT patients and is the most frequent serious side effect of therapy in the first 100 days (Bellm *et al* 2000; Stiff 2001; Oster *et al* 2005). Patients treated with high-dose cancer chemotherapy for solid malignancies particularly of epithelial origin (e.g. GI and breast) suffer painful oral mucositis due to mucosal toxicity of chemotherapy more frequently than generally recognized, and prevalence and severity increase throughout successive courses of chemotherapy (Stiff 2001; Elting *et al* 2003).

In radiation therapy, mucositis typically affects non-keratinized mucosa in the radiation field beginning in week 3 and peaking at weeks 5–6 of therapy, then remitting 4–8 weeks after therapy (Epstein *et al* 2001b,c).

Table 14.2 Incidence of Severe Oropharyngeal Mucositis

Disease	Therapy	Incidence (%)
Oropharyngeal cancer	RT, RT/CT	55–86
Haematological malignancies and multiple myeloma	HSCT	31–64
Breast cancer and NHL	CT	2.3–13.64
Colon cancer	CT	1.35–4.43

RT, radiotherapy; CT, chemo-therapy; RT/CT, chemoradiotherapy; HSCT, haematopoietic stem cell transplantation; NHL, non-Hodgkin's lymphoma. (Epstein *et al* 2007).

Mucositis pain is common (58–75%) and interferes with daily activities in approximately 33–60% of patients (McGuire *et al* 1993; Trotti *et al* 2003; Bernier *et al* 2004; Cooper *et al* 2004; Sonis *et al* 2004a). The incidence, severity and duration of mucositis increase with use of combined chemoradiotherapy of H&N cancer (List *et al* 1999; Bernier *et al* 2004; Cooper *et al* 2004). Mucosal symptoms continue for 6–12 months in up to a third of the patients, even after clinical resolution of the mucosal lesion (List *et al* 1999; Huang *et al* 2003; Bernier *et al* 2004; Cooper *et al* 2004), suggesting epithelial atrophy and/or neuropathy. Patients with mucosal pain prior to cancer therapy may experience more severe mucositis-associated pain during treatment, suggesting the establishment of sensitization.

Pain due to oral mucositis has a dramatic impact on QoL, and frequently requires opioid analgesics, tube feeding, extended hospitalization and unanticipated re-hospitalization, and may lead to modification or interruption of cancer therapy (Epstein *et al* 2001c; Sonis *et al* 2001; Elting *et al* 2003). Mucositis pain can be severe, preventing oral intake of food and medications, and limits verbal communication, causing psychosocial distress. Oral mucosal pain can be aggravated by comorbidities such as dry mouth and secondary mucosal infection (e.g. candidiasis) (Epstein *et al* 2002b). The breakdown of the epithelial barrier in mucositis is a potential portal for systemic infection (Sonis *et al* 2001; Elting *et al* 2003; Giles *et al* 2003). Dry mouth secondary to dehydration or the effects of radiation therapy on salivary glands may aggravate mucosal pain.

Some neurotoxic cytotoxic agents (e.g. vincristine, vinblastine, platinum derivatives, taxanes, thalidomide) may cause jaw pain and neuropathy (McCarthy and Skillings 1992; Hilkens *et al* 1997; Cella *et al* 2003; Forman 2004).

11.2.2. Pain due to Surgical Procedures

Surgical procedures result in acute orofacial pain and may ultimately lead to chronic pain, involving inflammatory and neuropathic mechanisms. Adjuvant therapies may affect the severity and frequency of pain; neck dissection may increase musculoskeletal dysfunction and neuropathic pain (Terrell *et al* 2000). Radiation therapy may increase postsurgical fibrosis and dysfunction, and pain in post-traumatic neuropathy.

Orofacial pain following H&N cancer therapy can develop due to secondary musculoskeletal (TMDs) or neuropathic syndromes. The impact may be severe if discontinuity of the jaw or fibrosis of muscles and soft tissue occurs. Resection of the mandible for tumour excision will inevitably lead to sensory impairment, with 50% experiencing regional hyperalgesia or allodynia (Chow and Teh 2000). At 2–5 years post-maxillectomy approximately 90% of patients reported persistent pain (Rogers *et al* 2003). Functional consequences are often secondary to pain and post-surgical fibrosis (Gellrich *et al* 2002b).

Pain scores following H&N cancer surgery were highest for oral cavity cancer followed by the larynx, oropharynx and nasopharynx (Terrell *et al* 1999), and postoperative functional problems were present in more than 50% of patients (Gellrich *et al* 2002a). Persistent impairment due to moderate to severe pain was found in 34.3% of cases more than 6 months postoperatively (Gellrich *et al* 2002a). The most frequent sites of pain were the shoulder (31–38.5%), the neck (4.9–34.9%), the TMJ (4.9–20.1%), the oral cavity (4.2–18.7%) and other sites of the head and face (4.2–15.6%) (Gellrich *et al* 2002a,b), reflecting morbidity secondary to tumour and regional lymph node resection (Terrell *et al* 2000; Taylor *et al* 2004). While more than 60% of patients reported pain, of which the majority was rated as severe, 75% of these patients were not taking analgesics (Gellrich *et al* 2002a). In any event, analgesics and physiotherapy were largely ineffective in the treatment of chronic pain in these patients (Gellrich *et al* 2002b). At 54–60 months post surgery, a smaller proportion of reviewed patients (14.9%) had persistent pain (Gellrich *et al* 2002b), suggesting spontaneous resolution over time. In postsurgical cancer patients, pain is characterized by acute pain lasting 1–2 months with a gradual time-related improvement (Bjordal *et al* 2001; Hammerlid *et al* 2001; Hammerlid and Taft 2001). However, H&N cancer survivors (>3 years) suffer significantly more pain and functional problems than matched control subjects (Hammerlid *et al* 2001). Chronic pain in cancer patients is therefore often underestimated and undertreated.

11.3. Orofacial Pain due to other Aetiology in Cancer Patients

Orofacial pain of any cause, related or unrelated to cancer, may occur during cancer treatment. Pain may be due to local dental infection (Chapter 5) which may be of increased importance in myelosuppressed patients (Schubert 1991; Jones *et al* 1993). Postherpetic neuralgia may result in chronic pain in approximately 10% of cases and pain may persist for years (see Chapter 11). Pain of any cause arising in cancer patients is likely to be associated with heightened anxiety which impacts pain perception and pain behaviour.

Post-radiation soft tissue necrosis and osteonecrosis are well-recognized chronic complications that may be associated with pain (Marx and Johnson 1987; Epstein *et al* 1997). The onset of symptoms is variable and may appear decades post radiotherapy (McKenzie *et al* 1993; Epstein *et al* 1997; Cramer *et al* 2002; Reuther *et al* 2003).

Bisphosphonate-related osteonecrosis and osteomyelitis of the jaws are frequently first recongnized due to pain (Ruggiero and Mehrotra 2004; Marx *et al* 2005). The cumulative incidence of bisphosphonate-related osteonecrosis is rising, and is reported to be 10% after 3 years of intravenous bisphosphonate use, with lower risk in oral bisphosphonate use (Durie *et al* 2005). As research data accumulate we may gain insight to the pathophysiology of bisphosphonate-related osteonecrosis and may thus be able to offer improved preventative and therapeutic strategies.

Pain due to oral GVHD represents a local manifestation of a systemic disease, secondary to allogeneic HSCT. Oral GVHD mimics a number of autoimmune disorders, including lichen planus, lupus and scleroderma (systemic sclerosis) (Woo *et al* 1997). The clinical presentation includes mucosal erythema, atrophy, pseudomembranous ulceration and hyperkeratotic striae, plaques and papules, similar to oral lichen planus and, less commonly, systemic lupus erythematosus (Woo *et al* 1997).

11.4. Treatment of Orofacial Pain in Cancer

Effective management of orofacial pain in cancer patients requires comprehensive assessment and diagnosis of potentially multifactorial aetiologies and treatment directed at the various factors involved in the pain experience. Treatment of cancer-related pain is attained by effective treatment of the malignant disease. Treatment of H&N cancer is beyond the scope of this textbook; for recent review see Modi *et al* (2005). Palliative treatment with radiation or chemotherapy may provide control of pain when used for cure or palliation.

11.4.1. Pain due to Oral Mucositis

Oral mucositis pain results from injury to tissues that causes release of reactive oxygen species, proinflammatory cytokines and neurotransmitters that activate nociceptive receptors. Pain experienced is related to the degree of tissue damage and is modified by the emotional and sociocultural background of the patient (Pederson et al 2000; Borbasi et al 2002; Schulz-Kindermann et al 2002). Mucotoxic chemotherapy, combined chemoradiotherapy and dose dense chemotherapy increase the risk of mucositis. If patients have received prior courses of chemotherapy, risk can be estimated based upon whether the person experienced mucositis in prior courses of treatment. Other factors that may influence severity of mucositis include age, mucosal infection and oral hygiene (Dodd et al 2001; Epstein and Schubert 2001; Borbasi et al 2002).

11.4.2. Prevention of Mucosal Damage

Treating malignancies with reduced toxicity regimens is a continuing goal. However, due to poor cure rates in H&N cancer, particularly of advanced disease, more intensive radiation protocols that include hyperfractionation, combined chemoradiotherapy, and reirradiation for recurrence increase the intensity, severity and duration of mucositis. Patients receiving intensive regimens and dose dense chemotherapy regimens are at increased risk of mucositis, which continues to limit therapy (Elting et al 2003). Considerable effort is invested to reduce mucositis, including radiation treatment planning (3D-sparing radiotherapy and intensive modulated radiotherapy (IMRT)), changes in chemotherapy drugs, doses, or schedule of delivery and effective prophylaxis and early treatment of emerging mucositis.

11.4.3. Basic Oral Care

The goal of basic oral care is to maintain oral health, reduce tissue irritation and control dental plaque levels. Reduction of oral microbial load and local infectious/inflammatory disease may minimize gingivitis and reduce the risk of mucositis and pain. While there are no controlled studies showing effectiveness of basic oral care, they remain standard treatment. There is evidence, however, that good oral hygiene may reduce the frequency and severity of oral mucositis and, therefore, of associated pain (Borowski et al 1994). Good oral hygiene does not increase the risk of bacteraemia even in neutropenic patients.

11.4.4. Topical Approaches for Mucosal Pain Relief

The oral mucosa is accessible for topical interventions although the adverse taste of drugs, induced nausea and diluting effects of saliva may limit compliance and effect (see Chapter 15). Topical anaesthetics are used for mucositis pain, despite a lack of controlled trials. Topical

anaesthetics also have a limited duration of effect (15–30 minutes), have a potential stinging with initial application on damaged mucosa and suppress taste and the gag reflex. One study demonstrated limited systemic absorption across compromised mucosal surfaces (Elad et al 1999). Topical anaesthetics are often mixed with coating and antimicrobial agents such as milk of magnesia, diphenhydramine or nystatin (e.g. 'magic mouthwash' or 'oncology mouthwash').

Topical benzydamine, an anti-inflammatory and anaesthetic agent, has been shown in randomized, controlled studies to reduce pain in oral mucositis and reduce the need for systemic analgesics (Pederson et al 2000; Epstein et al 2001c). Topical doxepin, a tricyclic antidepressant, produces analgesia for 4 hours or longer following a single application in cancer patients (Epstein et al 2006). Topical morphine has been shown to be effective for relieving pain (Cerchietti et al 2002), but there is concern about dispensing large volumes of the medication. Topical fentanyl prepared as lozenges induced relief of oral mucositis pain in a randomized placebo-controlled study, although its analgesic potential was not shown to be superior to placebo (Shaiova et al 2004). Other miscellaneous agents including topical ketamine, a general anaesthetic agent, have been assessed (Slatkin and Rhiner 2003). Topical capsaicin has been studied for the control of oral mucositis pain (Berger et al 1995), but it is poorly tolerated by patients.

Coating agents have been promoted for use in managing pain of mucositis. Sucralfate may have a role to play in pain management, although it has not been shown to reduce oral mucositis (Epstein and Wong 1994). Other coating agents such as antacids and milk of magnesia, often mixed as discussed earlier, have not been shown to significantly reduce pain.

A non-pharmacologic local approach for pain relief in cancer patients by using laser treatment is effective (Whelan et al 2001; Elad et al 2003; Genot and Klastersky 2005).

11.4.5. Systemic Medications

The World Health Organization (WHO) Pain Management Ladder has been recommended for managing pain in cancer patients (Meuser et al 2001). Pain is reduced by following the WHO ladder to one-third of pretreatment intensity in 70–90% of cases (Zech et al 1995; Ripamonti and Dickerson 2001). Thus, 10–30% of cancer patients do not achieve adequate pain control using the three-step ladder (Larue et al 1995). The WHO analgesic ladder assumes gradual progression of pain; however, pain management must be directed at the severity of pain at the time and a stepwise gradual approach may not be logical. Furthermore, a meta-analysis has challenged the effectiveness of 'weak' opioids (Step II medications); no difference was seen between effectiveness of nonsteroidal anti-inflammatory drugs (NSAIDs) (Step I) and that of weak opioids (Step II) with increased side effects when using weak opioids (Eisenberg *et al* 1994; McNicol *et al* 2004). A change from Step I to Step II medications does not improve pain management and patients begun on 'strong' opioids (Step III) enjoy better pain control (Benedetti *et al* 2000). Therefore, a change in the WHO ladder has been discussed, where Step I medications are used for mild pain, whilst for more severe pain, the lowest effective dose of strong opioids is individually titrated to provide pain control (Fig. 14.1, Table 14.3) (Eisenberg *et al* 2005). Medications are provided on a time-contingent basis. Opioids should be prescribed at appropriate doses and routes and at a frequency based upon the pharmacokinetics and report of adequate pain relief. Patient-controlled analgesia (PCA) has been shown to result in improved mucositis pain management for HSCT patients, with lower total doses of opioid analgesics and fewer side effects (Dunbar *et al* 1996; Coda *et al* 1997; Pillitteri and Clark 1998). Transdermal fentanyl has become widely utilized in management of oropharyngeal pain in cancer patients (Sloan *et al* 1998; Mystakidou *et al* 2002; Menahem and Shvartzman 2004). A steady state of analgesia should be maintained with additional analgesics for breakthrough pain (Coluzzi *et al* 2001; Payne *et al* 2001; Lucas and Lipman

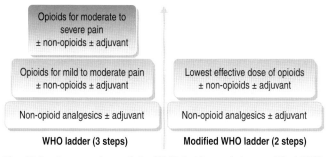

Fig. 14.1 • A comparison of the WHO ladder and the modified WHO ladder.

Table 14.3	Management of Orofacial Pain in Cancer Patients
Step 1	Diagnose/treat cause
Step 2	Topical therapy for mucosal pain
Step 3	Non-opioid analgesics
Step 4	Strong opioids
	Adjunctive medications: centrally acting analgesics[a]
	Adjunctive/complementary management[b]
Step 5	Repeated assessment of effect and side effects

Based on the Modified WHO's Pain ladder.
[a] For example, tricyclic antidepressants, gabapentin, antiseizure medications, antianxiety agents, muscle relaxants, sleep-promoting medications.
[b] Physical therapy, acupuncture, psychological management.

2002). Daily assessment of pain levels and modification of pain medications following the WHO ladder has been shown to improve pain control in H&N cancer patients receiving radiotherapy (Menzies *et al* 2000).

Addiction to opioids is not a concern for cancer patients. The focus should be on escalating to stronger opioids as needed and to employ adjuvant approaches in order to provide adequate pain relief. Tolerance and physical side effects such as constipation, nausea, vomiting and mental clouding may occur with opioid use and should be anticipated and managed prophylactically if possible. Bowel management should be implemented with the initial opioid prescription, and adequacy of the approach should be assessed on a regular basis.

Improved pain control may be achieved with opioid substitution and opioid rotation (Coluzzi *et al* 2001; Lucas and Lipman 2002; Drake *et al* 2004). Parenteral opioids have been shown to provide improved analgesia for cancer pain patients who have not responded to oral opioids, suggesting a change in route of administration may be effective in some cases. Administration of more than one opioid may offer increased pain relief, for example oxycodone when used in addition to morphine and methadone (Ripamonti and Dickerson 2001).

Cyclo-oxygenase (COX)-2 is upregulated in mucositis, and levels correlate with developing mucositis (Mohan and Epstein 2003; Sonis *et al* 2004b). Therefore, COX-2 inhibitors represent potential agents that may affect pain and the evolution of mucositis (see Chapters 15 and 16). Selective COX-2 inhibition (leaving COX-1 activity) will not affect platelet aggregation and will not increase the risk of bleeding. In addition to the pain and opioid sparing effects, COX-2 inhibitors may provide benefits including possible chemoprevention and effect on angiogenesis (Vickers and Cassileth 2001; Lucas and Lipman 2002; Mohan and Epstein 2003; Ruoff and Lema 2003). NSAIDs for cancer patients reduce the need for opioids, although they may lead to gastrointestinal discomfort (Enting *et al* 2002). Additional concerns with COX-2 inhibitors are increased risk for cardiovascular and renal complications, particularly in specific patient groups (Chapter 15). For oral mucosal pain, treatment should begin with topicals to which, following the analgesic ladder, systemic analgesics are added if pain continues (Table 14.3). Topical agents should be continued even after systemic medications have been started.

Adjuvant medications such as centrally acting pain medications (tricyclic antidepressants, gabapentin) should be employed (Devulder *et al* 2001; Ripamonti and Dickerson 2001); see Chapters 15 and 16. Amitriptyline has been studied in a placebo-controlled trial in addition to morphine in neuropathic cancer pain. While limited additional analgesic effect was seen, improved sleep was reported. However, increased side effects including drowsiness, confusion and dry mouth were seen (Coluzzi *et al* 2001; Lucas and Lipman 2002).

Gabapentin can provide improved pain control when used in addition to morphine in cancer patients as assessed during wound dressing changes (Devulder *et al* 2001) and may affect the neuropathic component of pain (Ripamonti and Dickerson 2001).

Quality and quantity of sleep must be assessed. Good sleep is critical in pain management and inadequate pain control may result in nonrestorative sleep; see Chapter 1. Attention must be paid to sleep hygiene and medication use may be indicated. Tricyclic antidepressants, some of the benzodiazepines and non-benzodiazepine anxiolytic/hypnotics, can be useful in these situations.

Physical therapy including treatment of myofascial pain and TMDs in cancer patients may include use of oral appliances, physiotherapy, exercises, heat and cold application, medications and complementary pain management strategies (see Chapters 7, 8, 17).

11.4.6. Complementary Pain Management Strategies

Complementary pain management techniques are presented in Table 14.4; see also Chapter 17. Hypnosis has been studied in randomized trials as a 'complementary method' of pain control in cancer patients. A variety of hypnotic techniques including vocal techniques, listening and instrumental techniques have been discussed, and controlled studies on the impact on cancer pain have been identified (Syrjala *et al* 1992; Magill 2001; Ripamonti and Dickerson 2001; Bardia 2006). Additional complementary and alternative medicine (CAM) techniques including counselling, distraction, relaxation techniques and other

Table 14.4	Additional and Complementary Pain Management Techniques in Oncology

Palliative radiation therapy
Cold/moist heat applications
Hypnosis
Acupuncture
Psychological: Distraction techniques Relaxation/ imagery techniques
Music therapy; drama therapy
Counselling
Cognitive/behavioural therapy
Topical anesthetics/analgesics
Adjunctive medications: Anxiolytics Co-analgesics/centrally acting agents: Anticonvulsants Antidepressants

cognitive and behavioural training programs have been discussed. Physical management of orofacial pain may include ice chips for oral cooling and cold compresses.

CAM techniques, such as acupuncture, transcutaneous nerve stimulation, group therapy, self-hypnosis, relaxation, imagery, cognitive behavioural training and massage therapy have also been assessed for pain management in cancer patients (Pan *et al* 2000). Relaxation and imagery have been shown in one controlled trial to affect pain in oral mucositis (Syrjala *et al* 1995).

12. Orofacial Pain in HIV Positive Patients

12.1. Human Immunodeficiency Virus (HIV)-Related Headache

Headache is a common symptom in patients with HIV infection. Primary or secondary headache may be seen in 42–50% of patients (Lipton *et al* 1991; Berger *et al* 1996; Norval 2004). There is great variability in the reported incidence of primary headache in HIV-infected patients. Primary headache was found to occur in 2.8% of HIV-infected patients admitted to an HIV service over a 1-year period. This incidence was much higher than the incidence of patients complaining about headache among HIV-negative patients admitted to the neurology service (0.8%) (Brew and Miller 1993). However, the incidence of primary headache in HIV-positive patients reported by others has been as high as 38% (Lipton *et al* 1991; Mirsattari *et al* 1999). The most prevalent types of primary headaches are tension-type headache and migraine (14–45.8% and 16–76%, respectively). Cluster headache is much less common (10%) (Mirsattari *et al* 1999; Evers *et al* 2000). Identifiable, serious causes of headache are found in up to 82% of HIV-infected patients who presented with headache (Lipton *et al* 1991; Mirsattari *et al* 1999).

HIV is neurotropic so neurologic complications in acquired immunodeficiency syndrome (AIDS) are common (Goldstein 1990; Graham and Wippold 2001). HIV crosses the blood–brain barrier (Graham and Wippold 2001), infects macrophages and microglia in the CNS and frequently causes neurocognitive impairment (Dunfee *et al* 2006). The release of inflammatory mediators by HIV-infected microglia and macrophages and the concurrent neuronal damage play central roles in the conceptualization of HIV-related neuropathology (Power and Johnson 2001).

There are numerous causes for secondary headaches in HIV patients, such as acute HIV meningitis. A chronic form of headache also thought to be caused by HIV itself may or may not be associated with cerebrospinal pleocytosis. Headaches may be caused by neoplasms and opportunistic infections resulting in meningitis (cryptococcal, tuberculous, or syphilitic), focal brain lesions (lymphoma, toxoplasmosis) or diffuse brain disease (cytomegalovirus, herpes simplex, progressive multifocal leukoencephalopathy) (Goldstein 1990; Holloway and Kieburtz 1995). Cryptococcal meningitis (39%) and CNS toxoplasmosis (16%) were the leading infectious aetiologies for HIV headache (Lipton *et al* 1991).

Facial pain may be caused by sinusitis, ocular pathology, systemic infection and even intracranial hypotension from diagnostic lumbar puncture (LP) (so-called 'post-LP-headache') (Goldstein 1990; Holloway and Kieburtz 1995; Rinaldi *et al* 1997).

The affected patients usually have advanced HIV infection (Brew and Miller 1993). A correlation between the presence of headache and the degree of immunosuppression has been observed (Berger and Nath 2000). Nevertheless, HIV-related headaches can occur at any time during infection: at seroconversion, during the incubation period, in patients with symptomatic HIV infection or after an AIDS-defining illness (Holloway and Kieburtz 1995). It was suggested that progression of immunological deficiency is related to a decrease in the frequency of migraine and to an increase in the frequency of tension-type headache (Evers *et al* 2000).

The stage of disease also has a practical implication as the value of CT scan was shown to be highest for patients with CD4 counts less than 200 cells/μL (Gifford and Hecht 2001; Graham and Wippold 2001). The highest prevalence of positive scans was found in patients with advanced disease. This is in accordance with the fact that CD4 counts predict the relative risk of developing opportunistic infections and neoplasms in the CNS. Thus, in the absence of significant immunosuppression, CT or MRI is not suggested unless focal findings are present on neurologic examination. The headache frequency and characteristics, however, bear no relation to CD4 counts, cerebrospinal fluid parameters, cranial MRI abnormalities, the presence of sinusitis or the use of zidovudine.

Treatment of head or facial pain is directed at the aetiology when this is possible. Unfortunately, headaches in HIV patients frequently do not respond to conventional management and carry a poor prognosis (Mirsattari *et al* 1999).

12.2. HIV-Related Oral Painful Mucosal Lesions

The oral cavity is a common site for the occurrence of lesions in patients who are seropositive for HIV (Gillespie and Marino 1993; Patton *et al* 2002). In HIV patients, the oral cavity is one of the most common sites of pain in the whole body (Norval 2004).

Oral candidiasis is the most common oral lesion identified, and may be associated with a burning sensation. Other oral infections—fungal, viral or bacterial—are well recognized and often result in local pain with possible systemic febrile episodes.

HIV patients may suffer from the major form of oral recurrent aphthous ulcers (RAU). Although RAU is not aetiologically related to a specific pathogen, secondary infection can occur at the lesion's site (Kerr and Ship 2003).

Necrotizing gingivitis and necrotizing periodontitis can progress rapidly and be extremely painful (Barr 1995). A more extensive form, necrotizing stomatitis, has also been reported (Barr 1995; Barasch *et al* 2003).

12.3. HIV-Related Neuropathy

Neurological manifestations of HIV in the head and neck have been reported (Milam *et al* 1986), but are rare (Schiodt 1997). There are some cases of facial nerve dysfunction (Belec *et al* 1991; Durham *et al* 1993) as well as cases of recalcitrant headaches (Penfold and Clark 1992). Peripheral neurological symptoms have been recognized early in primary HIV infection (Denning 1988; Ackerman *et al* 1989) and later in the disease progression, mainly as a potential side effect of HIV antiviral medications (Moyle *et al* 1997; Nieuwkerk *et al* 2000; Kilbourne *et al* 2001). One case of H&N neuropathy has been reported with thalidomide (Elad *et al* 1997). Strong associations between neuropathies and opportunistic viral herpetic infections (Chopra *et al* 1999) or thalidomide (Paterson *et al* 1995) have been documented.

Clinical management of neuropathic pain should be aggressive with a multidisciplinary, comprehensive approach similar to that to cancer-related pain (Penfold and Clark 1992; Katz 2000). Clinicians should address the aetiology of the pain, especially in cases of viral-related pain still commonly observed in HIV disease (Gebo *et al* 2005).

References

Aarabi B, Haghshenas M, Rakeii V (1998) Visual failure caused by suprasellar extramedullary hematopoiesis in beta thalassemia: case report. *Neurosurgery* **42**(4):922–925; discussion 925–926.

Abraham PJ, Capobianco DJ, Cheshire WP (2003) Facial pain as the presenting symptom of lung carcinoma with normal chest radiograph. *Headache* **43**(5):499–504.

Ackerman Z, Zeltser R, Maayan S (1989) AIDS and oropharyngeal candidiasis. *Isr J Dent Sci* **2**(3):162–166.

Agostoni E, Fumagalli L, Santoro P, *et al* (2004) Migraine and stroke. *Neurol Sci* **25**(Suppl 3):S123–S125.

Alarcon-Segovia D (1984) Symptomatic Sjögren's syndrome in mixed connective tissue disease. *J Rheumatol* **11**(5):582–583.

Alarcon-Segovia D, Deleze M, Oria CV, *et al* (1989) Antiphospholipid antibodies and the antiphospholipid syndrome in systemic lupus erythematosus. A prospective analysis of 500 consecutive patients. *Medicine (Baltimore)* **68**(6):353–365.

Alfaro-Giner A, Penarrocha-Diago M, Bagan-Sebastian JV (1992) Orofacial manifestations of mixed connective tissue disease with an uncommon serologic evolution. *Oral Surg Oral Med Oral Pathol* **73**(4):441–444.

Allen CM, Camisa C, Hamzeh S, *et al* (1990) Cheilitis granulomatosa: report of six cases and review of the literature. *J Am Acad Dermatol* **23**(3 Pt 1):444–450.

Amato AA, Collins MP (1998) Neuropathies associated with malignancy. *Semin Neurol* **18**(1):125–144.

Amor B (1998) Reiter's syndrome. Diagnosis and clinical features. *Rheum Dis Clin North Am* **24**(4):677–695, vii.

Antoine JC, Mosnier JF, Absi L, *et al* (1999) Carcinoma associated paraneoplastic peripheral neuropathies in patients with and without anti-onconeural antibodies. *J Neurol Neurosurg Psychiatry* **67**(1):7–14.

Antoniazzi AL, Bigal ME, Bordini CA, *et al* (2003) Headache and hemodialysis: a prospective study. *Headache* **43**(2):99–102.

Arboix A, Massons J, Oliveres M, *et al* (1994) Headache in acute cerebrovascular disease: a prospective clinical study in 240 patients. *Cephalalgia* **14**(1):37–40.

Baccaglini L, Schiffmann R, Brennan MT, *et al* (2001) Oral and craniofacial findings in Fabry's disease: a report of 13 patients. *Oral Surg Oral Med Oral Pathol Oral Radiol Endod* **92**(4):415–419.

Barasch A, Gordon S, Geist RY, *et al* (2003) Necrotizing stomatitis: report of 3 Pseudomonas aeruginosa-positive patients. *Oral Surg Oral Med Oral Pathol Oral Radiol Endod* **96**(2):136–140.

Bardia A, Barton DL, Prokop LJ, *et al* (2006) Efficacy of complementary and alternative medicine therapies in relieving cancer pain: a systematic review. *J Clin Oncol* **24**:5457–5464.

Barr CE (1995) Periodontal problems related to HIV-1 infection. *Adv Dent Res* **9**(2):147–151.

Barthelemy I, Karanas Y, Sannajust JP, *et al* (2001) Gout of the temporomandibular joint: pitfalls in diagnosis. *J Craniomaxillofac Surg* **29**(5):307–310.

Bayar N, Kara SA, Keles I, *et al* (2002) Temporomandibular joint involvement in rheumatoid arthritis: a radiological and clinical study. *Cranio* **20**(2):105–110.

Belec L, Georges AJ, Bouree P, *et al* (1991) Peripheral facial nerve palsy related to HIV infection: relationship with the immunological status and the HIV staging in Central Africa. *Cent Afr J Med.* **37**(3):88–93.

Belfort MA, Saade GR, Grunewald C, *et al* (1999) Association of cerebral perfusion pressure with headache in women with pre-eclampsia. *Br J Obstet Gynaecol* **106**(8):814–821.

Bellm LA, Epstein JB, Rose-Ped A, *et al* (2000) Patient reports of complications of bone marrow transplantation. *Support Care Cancer* **8**(1):33–39.

Benedetti C, Brock C, Cleeland C, *et al* (2000) NCCN Practice Guidelines for Cancer Pain. *Oncology (Williston Park)* **14**(11A):135–150.

Bennett JH, Thomas G, Evans AW, *et al* (2000) Osteosarcoma of the jaws: a 30-year retrospective review. *Oral Surg Oral Med Oral Pathol Oral Radiol Endod* **90**(3):323–332.

Berger A, Henderson M, Nadoolman W, *et al* (1995) Oral capsaicin provides temporary relief for oral mucositis pain secondary to chemotherapy/radiation therapy. *J Pain Symptom Manage* **10**(3):243–248.

Berger JR, Nath A (2000) A careful neurologic examination should precede neuroimaging studies in HIV-infected patients with headache. *AJNR Am J Neuroradiol* **21**(3):441–442.

Berger JR, Stein N, Pall L (1996) Headache and human immunodeficiency virus infection: a case control study. *Eur Neurol* **36**(4):229–233.

Bergmann OJ, Andersen PL (1990) Acute oral candidiasis during febrile episodes in immunocompromised patients with haematologic malignancies. *Scand J Infect Dis* **22**(3):353–358.

Bergmann OJ, Mogensen SC, Ellegaard J (1990) Herpes simplex virus and intraoral ulcers in immunocompromised patients with haematologic malignancies. *Eur J Clin Microbiol Infect Dis* **9**(3):184–190.

Bernier J, Domenge C, Ozsahin M, *et al* (2004) Postoperative irradiation with or without concomitant chemotherapy for locally advanced head and neck cancer. *N Engl J Med* **350**(19):1945–1952.

Bhaya MH, Har-El G (1998) Referred facial pain from intracranial tumors: a diagnostic dilemma. *Am J Otolaryngol* **19**(6):383–386.

Bindoff LA, Heseltine D (1988) Unilateral facial pain in patients with lung cancer: a referred pain via the vagus? *Lancet* **1**(8589):812–815.

Bjordal K, Ahlner-Elmqvist M, Hammerlid E, *et al* (2001) A prospective study of quality of life in head and neck cancer patients. Part II: Longitudinal data. *Laryngoscope* **111**(8):1440–1452.

Borbasi S, Cameron K, Quested B, *et al* (2002) More than a sore mouth: patients' experience of oral mucositis. *Oncol Nurs Forum* **29**(7):1051–1057.

Borgna Pignatti C, Carnelli V, Caruso V, *et al* (1998) Thromboembolic events in beta thalassemia major: an Italian multicenter study. *Acta Haematol* **99**(2):76–79.

Borowski B, Benhamou E, Pico JL, *et al* (1994) Prevention of oral mucositis in patients treated with high-dose chemotherapy and bone marrow transplantation: a randomised controlled trial comparing two protocols of dental care. *Eur J Cancer B Oral Oncol* **30B**(2):93–97.

Brew BJ, Miller J (1993) Human immunodeficiency virus-related headache. *Neurology* **43**(6):1098–1100.

Bullitt E, Tew JM, Boyd J (1986) Intracranial tumors in patients with facial pain. *J Neurosurg* **64**(6):865–871.

Cable WJ, Kolodny EH, Adams RD (1982) Fabry disease: impaired autonomic function. *Neurology* **32**(5):498–502.

Cady RK, Dodick DW, Levine HL, *et al* (2005) Sinus headache: a neurology, otolaryngology, allergy, and primary care consensus on diagnosis and treatment. *Mayo Clin Proc* **80**(7):908–916.

Caraceni A, Portenoy RK (1999) An international survey of cancer pain characteristics and syndromes. IASP Task Force on Cancer Pain. International Association for the Study of Pain. *Pain* **82**(3):263–274.

Cella D, Peterman A, Hudgens S, *et al* (2003) Measuring the side effects of taxane therapy in oncology: the functional assesment of cancer therapy-taxane (FACT-taxane). *Cancer* **98**(4):822–831.

Cerchietti LC, Navigante AH, Bonomi MR, *et al* (2002) Effect of topical morphine for mucositis-associated pain following concomitant chemoradiotherapy for head and neck carcinoma. *Cancer* **95**(10):2230–2236.

Chaffee NR (1998) CREST syndrome: clinical manifestations and dental management. *J Prosthodont* **7**(3):155–160.

Chan KH, Cheung RT, Mak W, Au-Yeung KM, Ho SL (2004) Cerebral venous thrombosis presenting as unilateral headache and visual blurring in a man with nephrotic syndrome. *Hosp Med* **65**(1):54–55.

Charness ME, Simon RP, Greenberg DA (1989) Ethanol and the nervous system. *N Engl J Med* **321**(7):442–454.

Chopra KF, Evans T, Severson J, *et al* (1999) Acute varicella zoster with postherpetic hyperhidrosis as the initial presentation of HIV infection. *J Am Acad Dermatol* **41**(1):119–121.

Chow HT, Teh LY (2000) Sensory impairment after resection of the mandible: a case report of 10 cases. *J Oral Maxillofac Surg* **58**(6):629–635.

Christiaans MH, Kelder JC, Arnoldus EP, *et al* (2002) Prediction of intracranial metastases in cancer patients with headache. *Cancer* **94**(7):2063–2068.

Coda BA, O'Sullivan B, Donaldson G, *et al* (1997) Comparative efficacy of patient-controlled administration of morphine, hydromorphone, or sufentanil for the treatment of oral mucositis pain following bone marrow transplantation. *Pain* **72**(3):333–346.

Cohen HV, Rosenheck AH (1998) Metastatic cancer presenting as TMD. A case report. *J N J Dent Assoc* **69**(3):17–19.

Coleman RE (1997) Skeletal complications of malignancy. *Cancer* **80**(8 Suppl):1588–1594.

Coleman RE (1998) How can we improve the treatment of bone metastases further? *Curr Opin Oncol* **10**(Suppl 1):S7–S13.

Coluzzi PH, Schwartzberg L, Conroy JD, *et al* (2001) Breakthrough cancer pain: a randomized trial comparing oral transmucosal fentanyl citrate (OTFC) and morphine sulfate immediate release (MSIR). *Pain* **91**(1–2):123–130.

Contreras RJ, Beckstead RM, Norgren R (1982) The central projections of the trigeminal, facial, glossopharyngeal and vagus nerves: an autoradiographic study in the rat. *J Auton Nerv Syst* **6**(3):303–322.

Cooper GS, Dooley MA, Treadwell EL, *et al* (2002) Hormonal and reproductive risk factors for development of systemic lupus erythematosus: results of a population-based, case-control study. *Arthritis Rheum* **46**(7):1830–1839.

Cooper JS, Pajak TF, Forastiere AA, *et al* (2004) Postoperative concurrent radiotherapy and chemotherapy for high-risk squamous-cell carcinoma of the head and neck. *N Engl J Med* **350**(19):1937–1944.

Cortelli P, Grimaldi D, Guaraldi P, *et al* (2004) Headache and hypertension. *Neurol Sci* **25** (Suppl 3):S132–S134.

Cramer CK, Epstein JB, Sheps SB, *et al* (2002) Modified Delphi survey for decision analysis for prophylaxis of post-radiation osteonecrosis. *Oral Oncol* **38**(6):574–583.

Cruccu G, Agostino R, Inghilleri M, *et al* (1998) Mandibular nerve involvement in diabetic polyneuropathy and chronic inflammatory demyelinating polyneuropathy. *Muscle Nerve* **21**(12):1673–1679.

Cuadrado MJ, Khamashta MA, Hughes GR (2000) Migraine and stroke in young women. *Qjm* **93**(5):317–318.

Cuadrado MJ, Khamashta MA, D'Cruz D, *et al* (2001) Migraine in Hughes syndrome–heparin as a therapeutic trial? *Qjm* **94**(2): 114–115.

Cuffari L, Tesseroli de Siqueira JT, Nemr K, *et al* (2006) Pain complaint as the first symptom of oral cancer: a descriptive study. *Oral Surg Oral Med Oral Pathol Oral Radiol Endod* **102**(1):56–61.

Daggett P, Nabarro J (1984) Neurological aspects of insulinomas. *Postgrad Med J* **60**(707):577–581.

D'Amico D, La Mantia L, Rigamonti A, *et al* (2004) Prevalence of primary headaches in people with multiple sclerosis. *Cephalalgia* **24**(11):980–984.

Davey G, Sedgwick P, Maier W, *et al* (2002) Association between migraine and asthma: matched case-control study. *Br J Gen Pract* **52**(482):723–727.

Demirbas Kaya A, Aktener BO, Unsal C (2004) Pulpal necrosis with sickle cell anaemia. *Int Endod J* **37**(9):602–606.

Denislic M, Meh D (1997) Early asymmetric neuropathy in primary Sjögren's syndrome. *J Neurol* **244**(6):383–387.

Denning DW (1988) The neurological features of acute HIV infection. *Biomed Pharmacother* **42**(1):11–14.

Dervis E (2005) The prevalence of temporomandibular disorders in patients with psoriasis with or without psoriatic arthritis. *J Oral Rehabil* **32**(11):786–793.

Devulder J, Lambert J, Naeyaert JM (2001) Gabapentin for pain control in cancer patients' wound dressing care. *J Pain Symptom Manage* **22**(1):622–626.

de Wit R, van Dam F, Loonstra S, *et al* (2001) The Amsterdam Pain Management Index compared to eight frequently used outcome measures to evaluate the adequacy of pain treatment in cancer patients with chronic pain. *Pain* **91**(3):339–349.

Diamond I, Messing RO (1994) Neurologic effects of alcoholism. *West J Med* **161**(3):279–287.

Dizdarevic K, Dizdarevic S, Dizdarevic Z (1998) [Neurosarcoidosis presenting with transitory neurodeficit and generalized epileptic seizures associated with migraine]. *Med Arh* **52**(3):159–162.

Dodd MJ, Dibble S, Miaskowski C, *et al* (2001) A comparison of the affective state and quality of life of chemotherapy patients who do and do not develop chemotherapy-induced oral mucositis. *J Pain Symptom Manage* **21**(6):498–505.

Dodeller F, Schulze-Koops H (2006) The p38 mitogen-activated protein kinase signaling cascade in CD4 T cells. *Arthritis Res Ther* **8**(2):205.

Dombrecht EJ, Aerts NE, Schuerwegh AJ, *et al* (2006) Influence of anti-tumor necrosis factor therapy (Adalimumab) on regulatory T cells and dendritic cells in rheumatoid arthritis. *Clin Exp Rheumatol* **24**(1):31–37.

Drake R, Longworth J, Collins JJ (2004) Opioid rotation in children with cancer. *J Palliat Med* **7**(3):419–422.

Dunbar PJ, Chapman CR, Buckley FP, *et al* (1996) Clinical analgesic equivalence for morphine and hydromorphone with prolonged PCA. *Pain* **68**(2–3): 265–270.

Duncan GG, Epstein JB, Tu D, *et al* (2005) Quality of life, mucositis, and xerostomia from radiotherapy for head and neck cancers: a report from the NCIC CTG HN2 randomized trial of an antimicrobial lozenge to prevent mucositis. *Head Neck* **27**(5):421–428.

Dunfee R, Thomas ER, Gorry PR, *et al* (2006) Mechanisms of HIV-1 neurotropism. *Curr HIV Res* **4**(3):267–278.

Durham TM, Hodges ED, Swindels S, *et al* (1993) Facial nerve paralysis related to HIV disease. Case report and dental considerations. *Oral Surg Oral Med Oral Pathol.* **75**(1):37–40.

Durie BG, Katz M, Crowley J (2005) Osteonecrosis of the jaw and bisphosphonates. *N Engl J Med* **353**(1):99–102; discussion 99–102.

Dworkin MS, Shoemaker PC, Goldoft MJ, *et al* (2001) Reactive arthritis and Reiter's syndrome following an outbreak of gastroenteritis caused by Salmonella enteritidis. *Clin Infect Dis* **33**(7): 1010–1014.

Dyck PJ, Norell JE (1999) Microvasculitis and ischemia in diabetic lumbosacral radiculoplexus neuropathy. *Neurology* **53**(9): 2113–2121.

Dyck PJ, Zimmerman BR, Vilen TH, *et al* (1988) Nerve glucose, fructose, sorbitol, myo-inositol, and fiber degeneration and regeneration in diabetic neuropathy. *N Engl J Med* **319**(9):542–548.

Dyck PJ, Davies JL, Wilson DM, *et al* (1999) Risk factors for severity of diabetic polyneuropathy: intensive longitudinal assessment of the Rochester Diabetic Neuropathy Study cohort. *Diabetes Care* **22**(9):1479–1486.

Eisenberg E, Berkey CS, Carr DB, *et al* (1994) Efficacy and safety of nonsteroidal antiinflammatory drugs for cancer pain: a meta-analysis. *J Clin Oncol* **12**(12):2756–2765.

Eisenberg E, Marinangeli F, Birkhahn J, *et al* (2005) Time to modify the WHO analgesic ladder? *Pain: Clinical Updates* **13**(5): 1–4.

Elad S, Galili D, Garfunkel AA, *et al* (1997) Thalidomide-induced perioral neuropathy. *Oral Surg Oral Med Oral Pathol Oral Radiol Endod* **84**(4):362–364.

Elad S, Cohen G, Zylber-Katz E, *et al* (1999) Systemic absorption of lidocaine after topical application for the treatment of oral mucositis in bone marrow transplantation patients. *J Oral Pathol Med* **28**(4):170–172.

Elad S, Or R, Shapira MY, *et al* (2003) CO2 laser in oral graft-versus-host disease: a pilot study. *Bone Marrow Transplant* **32**(10):1031–1034.

Elting LS, Cooksley C, Chambers M, *et al* (2003) The burdens of cancer therapy. Clinical and economic outcomes of chemotherapy-induced mucositis. *Cancer* **98**(7):1531–1539.

Enting RH, Oldenmenger WH, van der Rijt CC, *et al* (2002) A prospective study evaluating the response of patients with unrelieved cancer pain to parenteral opioids. *Cancer* **94**(11):3049–3056.

Epstein J, van der Meij E, McKenzie M, *et al* (1997) Postradiation osteonecrosis of the mandible: a long-term follow-up study. *Oral Surg Oral Med Oral Pathol Oral Radiol Endod* **83**(6):657–662.

Epstein JB (1997) Radiographic manifestations of multiple myeloma in the mandible: A retrospective study of 77 patients. *J Oral Maxillofac Surg* **55**:454–455.

Epstein JB, Jones CK (1993) Presenting signs and symptoms of nasopharyngeal carcinoma. *Oral Surg Oral Med Oral Pathol* **75**(1): 32–36.

Epstein JB, Polsky B (1998) Oropharyngeal candidiasis: a review of its clinical spectrum and current therapies. *Clin Ther* **20**(1):40–57.

Epstein JB, Schubert MM (2001) Oral mucositis in cancer patients. In: Loeser JD, Butler SH, Chapman CR *et al* (eds) *Bonica's Management of Pain*. Philadephia: Lippincott Williams and Wilkins, pp 730–738.

Epstein JB, Schubert MM (2003) Oropharyngeal mucositis in cancer therapy. Review of pathogenesis, diagnosis, and management. *Oncology (Huntingt)* **17**(12):1767–1779; discussion 1779–1782, 1791–1792.

Epstein JB, Stewart KH (1993) Radiation therapy and pain in patients with head and neck cancer. *Eur J Cancer B Oral Oncol* **29B**(3):191–199.

Epstein JB, Wong FL (1994) The efficacy of sucralfate suspension in the prevention of oral mucositis due to radiation therapy. *Int J Radiat Oncol Biol Phys* **28**(3):693–698.

Epstein JB, Epstein JD, Le ND, *et al* (2001a) Characteristics of oral and paraoral malignant lymphoma: a population-based review of 361 cases. *Oral Surg Oral Med Oral Pathol Oral Radiol Endod* **92**(5):519–525.

Epstein JB, Robertson M, Emerton S, *et al* (2001b) Quality of life and oral function in patients treated with radiation therapy for head and neck cancer. *Head Neck* **23**(5):389–398.

Epstein JB, Silverman S Jr, Paggiarino DA, *et al* (2001c) Benzydamine HCl for prophylaxis of radiation-induced oral mucositis: results from a multicenter, randomized, double-blind, placebo-controlled clinical trial. *Cancer* **92**(4):875–885.

Epstein JB, Phillips N, Parry J, *et al* (2002a) Quality of life, taste, olfactory and oral function following high-dose chemotherapy and allogeneic hematopoietic cell transplantation. *Bone Marrow Transplant* **30**(11):785–792.

Epstein JB, Tsang AH, Warkentin D, *et al* (2002b) The role of salivary function in modulating chemotherapy-induced oropharyngeal mucositis: a review of the literature. *Oral Surg Oral Med Oral Pathol Oral Radiol Endod* **94**(1):39–44.

Epstein JB, Epstein JD, Epstein MS, *et al* (2006) Oral doxepin rinse: the analgesic effect and duration of pain reduction in patients with oral mucositis due to cancer therapy. *Anesth Analg* **103** (2):465–470, table of contents.

Epstein JB, Elad S, Eliav E, *et al* (2007) Orofacial pain in cancer part II: clinical perspectives and management. *J Dent Res* **86**(6):506–518.

Eross EJ, Dodick DW, Swanson JW, *et al* (2003) A review of intractable facial pain secondary to underlying lung neoplasms. *Cephalalgia* **23**(1):2–5.

Eshbaugh CG, Siatkowski RM, Smith JL, *et al* (1995) Simultaneous, multiple cranial neuropathies in diabetes mellitus. *J Neuroophthalmol* **15**(4):219–224.

Evers S, Wibbeke B, Reichelt D, *et al* (2000) The impact of HIV infection on primary headache. Unexpected findings from retrospective, cross-sectional, and prospective analyses. *Pain* **85**(1–2):191–200.

Facchinetti F, Allais G, D'Amico R, *et al* (2005) The relationship between headache and preeclampsia: a case-control study. *Eur J Obstet Gynecol Reprod Biol* **121**(2):143–148.

Fischoff DK, Sirois D (2000) Painful trigeminal neuropathy caused by severe mandibular resorption and nerve compression in a patient with systemic sclerosis: case report and literature review. *Oral Surg Oral Med Oral Pathol Oral Radiol Endod* **90**(4):456–459.

Foley KM (1999) Advances in cancer pain. *Arch Neurol* **56**(4):413–417.

Foley KM, Inturrisi CE (1987) Analgesic drug therapy in cancer pain: principles and practice. *Med Clin North Am* **71**(2):207–232.

Font J, Ramos-Casals M, de la Red G, *et al* (2003) Pure sensory neuropathy in primary Sjögren's syndrome. Longterm prospective followup and review of the literature. *J Rheumatol* **30**(7):1552–1557.

Forman AD (2004) Peripheral neuropathy and cancer. *Curr Oncol Rep* **6**(1):20–25.

Fox RI (2005) Sjögren's syndrome. *Lancet* **366**(9482):321–331.

Gazerani P, Pourpak Z, Ahmadiani A, *et al* (2003) A correlation between migraine, histamine and immunoglobulin E. *Scand J Immunol* **57**(3):286–290.

Gebo KA, Kalyani R, Moore RD, *et al* (2005) The incidence of, risk factors for, and sequelae of herpes zoster among HIV patients in the highly active antiretroviral therapy era. *J Acquir Immune Defic Syndr* **40**(2):169–174.

Gellrich NC, Schimming R, Schramm A, *et al* (2002a) Pain, function, and psychologic outcome before, during, and after intraoral tumor resection. *J Oral Maxillofac Surg* **60**(7):772–777.

Gellrich NC, Schramm A, Bockmann R, *et al* (2002b) Follow-up in patients with oral cancer. *J Oral Maxillofac Surg* **60**(4):380–386; discussion 387–388.

Genot MT, Klastersky J (2005) Low-level laser for prevention and therapy of oral mucositis induced by chemotherapy or radiotherapy. *Curr Opin Oncol* **17**(3):236–240.

Gewanter HL, Roghmann KJ, Baum J (1983) The prevalence of juvenile arthritis. *Arthritis Rheum* **26**(5):599–603.

Gifford AL, Hecht FM (2001) Evaluating HIV-infected patients with headache: who needs computed tomography? *Headache* **41**(5):441–448.

Giles FJ, Miller CB, Hurd DD, *et al* (2003) A phase III, randomized, double-blind, placebo-controlled, multinational trial of iseganan for the prevention of oral mucositis in patients receiving stomatotoxic chemotherapy (PROMPT-CT trial). *Leuk Lymphoma* **44**(7):1165–1172.

Gillespie GM, Marino R (1993) Oral manifestations of HIV infection: a Panamerican perspective. *J Oral Pathol Med* **22**(1):2–7.

Gingrass D (1993) Temporomandibular joint degeneration in Alport's syndrome: review of literature and case report. *J Orofac Pain* **7**(3):307–310.

Gleissner C, Kaesser U, Dehne F, *et al* (2003) Temporomandibular joint function in patients with longstanding rheumatoid arthritis - I. Role of periodontal status and prosthetic care - a clinical study. *Eur J Med Res* **8**(3):98–108.

Goksan B, Karaali-Savrun F, Ertan S, *et al* (2004) Haemodialysis-related headache. *Cephalalgia* **24**(4):284–287.

Goldberg HL (1997) Chest cancer refers pain to face and jaw: a case review. *Cranio* **15**(2):167–169.

Goldfarb A, Nitzan DW, Marmary Y (1983) Changes in the parotid salivary gland of beta-thalassemia patients due to hemosiderin deposits. *Int J Oral Surg* **12**(2):115–119.

Goldschmidt MJ, Butterfield KJ, Goracy ES, *et al* (2002) Streptococcal infection of the temporomandibular joint of hematogenous origin: a case report and contemporary therapy. *J Oral Maxillofac Surg* **60**(11):1347–1353.

Goldstein J (1990) Headache and acquired immunodeficiency syndrome. *Neurol Clin* **8**(4):947–960.

Gorsky M, Epstein JB (1998a) Melanoma arising from the mucosal surfaces of the head and neck. *Oral Surg Oral Med Oral Pathol Oral Radiol Endod* **86**(6):715–719.

Gorsky M, Epstein JB (1998b) Head and neck and intra-oral soft tissue sarcomas. *Oral Oncol* **34**(4):292–296.

Gorsky M, Epstein JB (2000) Craniofacial osseous and chondromatous sarcomas in British Columbia–a review of 34 cases. *Oral Oncol* **36**(1):27–31.

Graff-Radford SB, Solberg WK (1992) Atypical odontalgia. *J Craniomandib Disord* **6**(4):260–265.

Graham CB 3rd, Wippold FJ 3rd (2001) Headache in the HIV patient: a review with special attention to the role of imaging. *Cephalalgia* **21**(3):169–174.

Grond S, Zech D, Diefenbach C, *et al* (1996) Assessment of cancer pain: a prospective evaluation in 2266 cancer patients referred to a pain service. *Pain* **64**(1):107–114.

Gross BD, Williams RB, DiCosimo CJ, *et al* (1987) Gout and pseudogout of the temporomandibular joint. *Oral Surg Oral Med Oral Pathol* **63**(5):551–554.

Guggenheimer J, Moore PA (2003) Xerostomia: etiology, recognition and treatment. *J Am Dent Assoc* **134**(1):61–69; quiz 118–119.

Gwyn DG, Leslie RA, Hopkins DA (1985) Observations on the afferent and efferent organization of the vagus nerve and the innervation of the stomach in the squirrel monkey. *J Comp Neurol* **239**(2):163–175.

Gynther GW, Holmlund AB, Reinholt FP, *et al* (1997) Temporomandibular joint involvement in generalized osteoarthritis and rheumatoid arthritis: a clinical, arthroscopic, histologic, and immunohistochemical study. *Int J Oral Maxillofac Surg* **26**(1):10–16.

Hagen NA, Stevens JC, Michet CJ Jr (1990) Trigeminal sensory neuropathy associated with connective tissue diseases. *Neurology* **40**(6):891–896.

Halabe A, Sperling O (1994) Uric acid nephrolithiasis. *Miner Electrolyte Metab* **20**(6):424–431.

Hammerlid E, Taft C (2001) Health-related quality of life in long-term head and neck cancer survivors: a comparison with general population norms. *Br J Cancer* **84**(2):149–156.

Hammerlid E, Silander E, Hornestam L, *et al* (2001) Health-related quality of life three years after diagnosis of head and neck cancer–a longitudinal study. *Head Neck* **23**(2):113–125.

Harris MD, Siegel LB, Alloway JA (1999) Gout and hyperuricemia. *Am Fam Physician* **59**(4):925–934.

Heidenheim AP, Leitch R, Kortas C, *et al* (2003) Patient monitoring in the London Daily/Nocturnal Hemodialysis Study. *Am J Kidney Dis* **42**(1 Suppl):61–65.

Hekkenberg RJ, Piedade L, Mock D, *et al* (1999) Septic arthritis of the temporomandibular joint. *Otolaryngol Head Neck Surg* **120**(5):780–782.

Helenius LM, Hallikainen D, Helenius I, *et al* (2005) Clinical and radiographic findings of the temporomandibular joint in patients with various rheumatic diseases. A case-control study. *Oral Surg Oral Med Oral Pathol Oral Radiol Endod* **99**(4):455–463.

Henry CH, Hudson AP, Gerard HC, *et al* (1999) Identification of Chlamydia trachomatis in the human temporomandibular joint. *J Oral Maxillofac Surg* **57**(6):683–688; discussion 689.

Hilkens PH, Pronk LC, Verweij J, *et al* (1997) Peripheral neuropathy induced by combination chemotherapy of docetaxel and cisplatin. *Br J Cancer* **75**(3):417–422.

Hincapie JW, Tobon D, Diaz-Reyes GA (1999) Septic arthritis of the temporomandibular joint. *Otolaryngol Head Neck Surg* **121**(6):836–837.

Hirshberg A, Buchner A (1995) Metastatic tumours to the oral region. An overview. *Eur J Cancer B Oral Oncol* **31B**(6):355–360.

Hirshberg A, Leibovich P, Buchner A (1993) Metastases to the oral mucosa: analysis of 157 cases. *J Oral Pathol Med* **22**(9):385–390.

Hirshberg A, Leibovich P, Buchner A (1994) Metastatic tumors to the jawbones: analysis of 390 cases. *J Oral Pathol Med* **23**(8):337–341.

Hoffman HT, Karnell LH, Funk GF, *et al* (1998) The National Cancer Data Base report on cancer of the head and neck. *Arch Otolaryngol Head Neck Surg* **124**(9):951–962.

Hogan MJ, Brunet DG, Ford PM, *et al* (1988) Lupus anticoagulant, antiphospholipid antibodies and migraine. *Can J Neurol Sci* **15**(4):420–425.

Holloway RG, Kieburtz KD (1995) Headache and the human immunodeficiency virus type 1 infection. *Headache* **35**(5):245–255.

Hovgaard DJ, Nissen NI (1992) Effect of recombinant human granulocyte-macrophage colony-stimulating factor in patients with Hodgkin's disease: a phase I/II study. *J Clin Oncol* **10**(3):390–397.

Huang HY, Wilkie DJ, Chapman CR, *et al* (2003) Pain trajectory of Taiwanese with nasopharyngeal carcinoma over the course of radiation therapy. *J Pain Symptom Manage* **25**(3):247–255.

Hughes GR (2003) Migraine, memory loss, and 'multiple sclerosis'. Neurological features of the antiphospholipid (Hughes') syndrome. *Postgrad Med J* **79**(928):81–83.

Hughes RA, Keat AC (1994) Reiter's syndrome and reactive arthritis: a current view. *Semin Arthritis Rheum* **24**(3):190–210.

Ing EB, Woolf IZ, Younge BR, *et al* (1997) Systemic amyloidosis with temporal artery involvement mimicking temporal arteritis. *Ophthalmic Surg Lasers* **28**(4):328–331.

International Headache Society (IHS) (2004) Classification and diagnostic criteria for headache disorders cranial neuralgias and facial pain of the Headache Classification Committee of the IHS. *Cephalalgia* **24**(Suppl 1):32–33.

Irkec C, Nazliel B, Yetkin I, *et al* (2001) Facial nerve conduction in diabetic neuropathy. *Acta Neurol Belg* **101**(3):177–179.

Issa Y, Duxbury AJ, Macfarlane TV, *et al* (2005) Oral lichenoid lesions related to dental restorative materials. *Br Dent J* **198**(6):361–366; disussion 549; quiz 372.

Jones AC, Freedman PD, Phelan JA, *et al* (1993) Cytomegalovirus infections of the oral cavity. A report of six cases and review of the literature. *Oral Surg Oral Med Oral Pathol* **75**(1):76–85.

Jonsson R, Lindvall AM, Nyberg G (1983) Temporomandibular joint involvement in systemic lupus erythematosus. *Arthritis Rheum* **26**(12):1506–1510.

Jorizzo JL, Salisbury PL, Rogers RS 3rd, *et al* (1992) Oral lesions in systemic lupus erythematosus. Do ulcerative lesions represent a necrotizing vasculitis? *J Am Acad Dermatol* **27**(3):389–394.

Julkunen HA (1991) Oral contraceptives in systemic lupus erythematosus: side-effects and influence on the activity of SLE. *Scand J Rheumatol* **20**(6):427–433.

Kanner R (2001) Diagnosis and management of neuropathic pain in patients with cancer. *Cancer Invest* **19**(3):324–333.

Kataria RK, Brent LH (2004) Spondyloarthropathies. *Am Fam Physician* **69**(12):2853–2860.

Katz JM, Bruno MK, Winterkorn JM, *et al* (2003) The pathogenesis and treatment of optic disc swelling in neurosarcoidosis: a unique therapeutic response to infliximab. *Arch Neurol* **60**(3):426–430.

Katz N (2000) Neuropathic pain in cancer and AIDS. *Clin J Pain* **16**(2 Suppl):S41–S48.

Katz W (1988) *Diagnosis and Management of Rheumatic Diseases*, 2nd edn. Philadelphia: Lippincott.

Kerr AR, Ship JA (2003) Management strategies for HIV-associated aphthous stomatitis. *Am J Clin Dermatol* **4**(10):669–680.

Kidd D (2006) The prevalence of headache in Behcet's syndrome. *Rheumatology (Oxford)* **45**(5):621–623.

Kilbourne AM, Justice AC, Rabeneck L, *et al* (2001) General medical and psychiatric comorbidity among HIV-infected veterans in the post-HAART era. *J Clin Epidemiol* **54**(Suppl 1):S22–S28.

Klemetti E, Vainio P, Kroger H (1995) Craniomandibular disorders and skeletal mineral status. *Cranio* **13**(2):89–92.

Kobayashi R, Utsunomiya T, Yamamoto H, *et al* (2001) Ankylosis of the temporomandibular joint caused by rheumatoid arthritis: a pathological study and review. *J Oral Sci* **43**(2):97–101.

Koloktronis A, Chatzigiannis I, Paloukidou N (2003) Oral involvement in a case of AA amyloidosis. *Oral Dis* **9**(5):269–272.

Kononen M (1986) Craniomandibular disorders in psoriatic arthritis. Correlations between subjective symptoms, clinical signs, and radiographic changes. *Acta Odontol Scand* **44**(6):369–375.

Kononen M (1987) Clinical signs of craniomandibular disorders in patients with psoriatic arthritis. *Scand J Dent Res* **95**(4):340–346.

Kononen M (1992) Signs and symptoms of craniomandibular disorders in men with Reiter's disease. *J Craniomandib Disord* **6**(4):247–253.

Kononen M, Kilpinen E (1990) Comparison of three radiographic methods in screening of temporomandibular joint involvement in patients with psoriatic arthritis. *Acta Odontol Scand* **48**(4):271–277.

Kononen M, Wenneberg B, Kallenberg A (1992) Craniomandibular disorders in rheumatoid arthritis, psoriatic arthritis, and ankylosing spondylitis. A clinical study. *Acta Odontol Scand* **50**(5):281–287.

Kononen M, Kovero O, Wenneberg B, *et al* (2002) Radiographic signs in the temporomandibular joint in Reiter's disease. *J Orofac Pain* **16**(2):143–147.

Konttinen YT, Tuominen TS, Piirainen HI, *et al* (1990) Signs and symptoms in the masticatory system in ten patients with mixed connective tissue disease. *Scand J Rheumatol* **19**(5):363–373.

Koorbusch GF, Zeitler DL, Fotos PG, *et al* (1991) Psoriatic arthritis of the temporomandibular joints with ankylosis. Literature review and case reports. *Oral Surg Oral Med Oral Pathol* **71**(3):267–274.

La Mantia L, Erbetta A (2004) Headache and inflammatory disorders of the central nervous system. *Neurol Sci* **25** (Suppl 3):S148–S153.

Larheim TA, Smith HJ, Aspestrand F (1990) Rheumatic disease of the temporomandibular joint: MR imaging and tomographic manifestations. *Radiology* **175**(2):527–531.

Larue F, Colleau SM, Brasseur L, et al (1995) Multicentre study of cancer pain and its treatment in France. *Bmj* **310**(6986): 1034–1037.

Laskin D (1995) The clinical diagnosis of temporomandibular disorders in the orthodontic patient. *Seminars in Orthodontics* **1**(4):197–206.

Lecky BR, Hughes RA, Murray NM (1987) Trigeminal sensory neuropathy. A study of 22 cases. *Brain* **110**(Pt 6):1463–1485.

Leighty SM, Spach DH, Myall RW, et al (1993) Septic arthritis of the temporomandibular joint: review of the literature and report of two cases in children. *Int J Oral Maxillofac Surg* **22**(5):292–297.

Levine SR, Joseph R, D'Andrea G, et al (1987) Migraine and the lupus anticoagulant. Case reports and review of the literature. *Cephalalgia* **7**(2):93–99.

Lim IG, Spira PJ, McNeil HP (2002) Headache as the initial presentation of Wegener's granulomatosis. *Ann Rheum Dis* **61**(6):571–572.

Lipton RB, Feraru ER, Weiss G, et al (1991) Headache in HIV-1-related disorders. *Headache* **31**(8):518–522.

List MA, Siston A, Haraf D, et al (1999) Quality of life and performance in advanced head and neck cancer patients on concomitant chemoradiotherapy: a prospective examination. *J Clin Oncol* **17**(3): 1020–1028.

Littlewood T, Mandelli F (2002) The effects of anemia in hematologic malignancies: more than a symptom. *Semin Oncol* **29**(3 Suppl 8):40–44.

Locher MC, Felder M, Sailer HF (1996) Involvement of the temporomandibular joints in ankylosing spondylitis (Bechterew's disease). *J Craniomaxillofac Surg* **24**(4):205–213.

Lucas LK, Lipman AG (2002) Recent advances in pharmacotherapy for cancer pain management. *Cancer Pract* **10**(Suppl 1):S14–S20.

Luyk NH, Hammond-Tooke G, Bishara SN, et al (1991) Facial pain and muscle atrophy secondary to an intracranial tumour. *Br J Oral Maxillofac Surg* **29**(3):204–207.

McCarthy GM, Skillings JR (1992) Jaw and other orofacial pain in patients receiving vincristine for the treatment of cancer. *Oral Surg Oral Med Oral Pathol* **74**(3):299–304.

McGonagle D, Gibbon W, Emery P (1998) Classification of inflammatory arthritis by enthesitis. *Lancet* **352** (9134):1137–1140.

McGuire DB, Altomonte V, Peterson DE, et al (1993) Patterns of mucositis and pain in patients receiving preparative chemotherapy and bone marrow transplantation. *Oncol Nurs Forum* **20**(10):1493–1502.

McGuire DB, Yeager KA, Dudley WN, et al (1998) Acute oral pain and mucositis in bone marrow transplant and leukemia patients: data from a pilot study. *Cancer Nurs* **21**(6):385–393.

McKenzie MR, Wong FL, Epstein JB, et al (1993) Hyperbaric oxygen and postradiation osteonecrosis of the mandible. *Eur J Cancer B Oral Oncol* **29B**(3):201–207.

McNicol E, Strassels S, Goudas L, et al (2004) Nonsteroidal anti-inflammatory drugs, alone or combined with opioids, for cancer pain: a systematic review. *J Clin Oncol* **22**(10): 1975–1992.

Magill L (2001) The use of music therapy to address the suffering in advanced cancer pain. *J Palliat Care* **17**(3):167–172.

Major P, Ramos-Remus C, Suarez-Almazor ME, et al (1999) Magnetic resonance imaging and clinical assessment of temporomandibular joint pathology in ankylosing spondylitis. *J Rheumatol* **26**(3):616–621.

Makura ZG, Robson AK (1996) Wegener's granulomatosis presenting as a temporal headache. *J Laryngol Otol* **110**(8): 802–804.

Mallecourt C, Delattre JY (2000) [Paraneoplastic neuropathies]. *Presse Med* **29**(8):447–452.

Manfredini D, Tognini F, Melchiorre D, et al (2005) Ultrasonography of the temporomandibular joint: comparison of findings in patients with rheumatic diseases and temporomandibular disorders. A preliminary report. *Oral Surg Oral Med Oral Pathol Oral Radiol Endod* **100**(4):481–485.

Mannelli M, Ianni L, Cilotti A, et al (1999) Pheochromocytoma in Italy: a multicentric retrospective study. *Eur J Endocrinol* **141**(6): 619–624.

Mardinger O, Givol N, Talmi YP, et al (2001) Osteosarcoma of the jaw. The Chaim Sheba Medical Center experience. *Oral Surg Oral Med Oral Pathol Oral Radiol Endod* **91**(4):445–451.

Marini I, Vecchiet F, Spiazzi L, et al (1999) Stomatognathic function in juvenile rheumatoid arthritis and in developmental open-bite subjects. *ASDC J Dent Child* **66**(1):30–35, 12.

Marx RE, Johnson RP (1987) Studies in the radiobiology of osteoradionecrosis and their clinical significance. *Oral Surg Oral Med Oral Pathol* **64**(4):379–390.

Marx RE, Sawatari Y, Fortin M, et al (2005) Bisphosphonate-induced exposed bone (osteonecrosis/osteopetrosis) of the jaws: risk factors, recognition, prevention, and treatment. *J Oral Maxillofac Surg* **63**(11):1567–1575.

Mauck KF, Clarke BL (2006) Diagnosis, screening, prevention, and treatment of osteoporosis. *Mayo Clin Proc* **81**(5):662–672.

Melchiorre D, Calderazzi A, Maddali Bongi S, et al (2003) A comparison of ultrasonography and magnetic resonance imaging in the evaluation of temporomandibular joint involvement in rheumatoid arthritis and psoriatic arthritis. *Rheumatology (Oxford)* **42**(5):673–676.

Menahem S, Shvartzman P (2004) High-dose fentanyl patch for cancer pain. *J Am Board Fam Pract* **17**(5):388–390.

Menzies K, Murray J, Wilcock A (2000) Audit of cancer pain management in a cancer centre. *Int J Palliat Nurs* **6**(9):443–447.

Meuser T, Pietruck C, Radbruch L, et al (2001) Symptoms during cancer pain treatment following WHO-guidelines: a longitudinal follow-up study of symptom prevalence, severity and etiology. *Pain* **93**(3):247–257.

Milam SB, Rees TD, Leiman HI (1986) An unusual cause of bilateral mental neuropathy in an AIDS patient. Report of a case. *J Periodontol* **57**(12):753–755.

Miles DA, Kaugars GA (1991) Psoriatic involvement of the temporomandibular joint. Literature review and report of two cases. *Oral Surg Oral Med Oral Pathol* **71**(6):770–774.

Mirsattari SM, Power C, Nath A (1999) Primary headaches in HIV-infected patients. *Headache* **39**(1):3–10.

Mitsikostas DD, Sfikakis PP, Goadsby PJ (2004) A meta-analysis for headache in systemic lupus erythematosus: the evidence and the myth. *Brain* **127**(Pt 5):1200–1209.

Modi BJ, Knab B, Feldman LE, et al (2005) Review of current treatment practices for carcinoma of the head and neck. *Expert Opin Pharmacother* **6**(7):1143–1155.

Mohan S, Epstein JB (2003) Carcinogenesis and cyclooxygenase: the potential role of COX-2 inhibition in upper aerodigestive tract cancer. *Oral Oncol* **39**(6):537–546.

Mok CC, Lau CS, Wong RW (2001) Use of exogenous estrogens in systemic lupus erythematosus. *Semin Arthritis Rheum* **30**(6): 426–435.

Mokri B (2003) Headaches caused by decreased intracranial pressure: diagnosis and management. *Curr Opin Neurol* **16**(3):319–326.

Monastero R, Mannino M, Lopez G, et al (2003) Prevalence of headache in patients with Behcet's disease without overt neurological involvement. *Cephalalgia* **23**(2):105–108.

Montalban J, Cervera R, Font J, et al (1992) Lack of association between anticardiolipin antibodies and migraine in systemic lupus erythematosus. *Neurology* **42**(3 Pt 1):681–682.

Moreau T, Manceau E, Giroud-Baleydier F, et al (1998) Headache in hypothyroidism. Prevalence and outcome under thyroid hormone therapy. *Cephalalgia* **18**(10):687–689.

Mori K, Iijima M, Koike H, et al (2005) The wide spectrum of clinical manifestations in Sjögren's syndrome-associated neuropathy. *Brain* **128**(Pt 11):2518–2534.

Moses JJ, Lange CR, Arredondo A (1998) Septic arthritis of the temporomandibular joint after the removal of third molars. *J Oral Maxillofac Surg* **56**(4):510–512.

Moyle GJ, Bouza E, Antunes F, et al (1997) Zidovudine monotherapy versus zidovudine plus zalcitabine combination therapy in HIV-positive persons with CD4 cell counts 300–500 cells/mm3: a double-blind controlled trial. The M50003 Study

Group Coordinating and Writing Committee. *Antivir Ther* **2**(4):229–236.

Mystakidou K, Befon S, Tsilika E, et al (2002) Use of TTS fentanyl as a single opioid for cancer pain relief: a safety and efficacy clinical trial in patients naive to mild or strong opioids. *Oncology* **62**(1):9–16.

Nagy G, Kovacs J, Zeher M, et al (1994) Analysis of the oral manifestations of systemic sclerosis. *Oral Surg Oral Med Oral Pathol* **77**(2):141–146.

Nieuwkerk PT, Gisolf EH, Colebunders R, et al (2000) Quality of life in asymptomatic- and symptomatic HIV infected patients in a trial of ritonavir/saquinavir therapy. The Prometheus Study Group. *Aids.* **14**(2):181–187.

Norval DA (2004) Symptoms and sites of pain experienced by AIDS patients. *S Afr Med J* **94**(6):450–454.

Ohtsuka E, Nonaka S, Shingu M, et al (1992) Sjögren's syndrome and mixed connective tissue disease. *Clin Exp Rheumatol* **10**(4):339–344.

Okeson J (2003) Diagnosis of temporomandibular disorders. In: Okeson J (ed) *Management of Temporomandibular Disorders and Occlusion*, 5th edn. St Louis: Mosby, p 356.

Olney RK (1998) Neuropathies associated with connective tissue disease. *Semin Neurol* **18**(1):63–72.

O'Rourke C, Mitropoulos C (1990) Orofacial pain in patients with sickle cell disease. *Br Dent J* **169**(5):130–132.

Oster G, Vera-Llonch M, Ford C, et al (2005) Oral mucositis (OM) and outcomes of allogeneic (AL) hematopoietic stem cell transplantation (HSCT). *Support Care Cancer* **13**(6):447.

Ozge A, Ozge C, Kaleagasi H, et al (2006) Headache in patients with chronic obstructive pulmonary disease: effects of chronic hypoxaemia. *J Headache Pain* **7**(1):37–43.

Pan CX, Morrison RS, Ness J, et al (2000) Complementary and alternative medicine in the management of pain, dyspnea, and nausea and vomiting near the end of life. A systematic review. *J Pain Symptom Manage* **20**(5):374–387.

Pari G, Schipper HM (1996) Headache and scalp edema in sickle cell disease. *Can J Neurol Sci* **23**(3):224–226.

Paterson DL, Georghiou PR, Allworth AM, et al (1995) Thalidomide as treatment of refractory aphthous ulceration related to human immunodeficiency virus infection. *Clin Infect Dis.* **20**(2):250–254.

Patton LL, Phelan JA, Ramos-Gomez FJ, et al (2002) Prevalence and classification of HIV-associated oral lesions. *Oral Dis* **8**(Suppl 2):98–109.

Paul T, Katiyar BC, Misra S, et al (1978) Carcinomatous neuromuscular syndromes. A clinical and quantitative electrophysiological study. *Brain* **101**(1):53–63.

Payne R, Coluzzi P, Hart L, et al (2001) Long-term safety of oral transmucosal fentanyl citrate for breakthrough cancer pain. *J Pain Symptom Manage* **22**(1):575–583.

Pederson C, Parran L, Harbaugh B (2000) Children's perceptions of pain during 3 weeks of bone marrow transplant experience. *J Pediatr Oncol Nurs* **17**(1):22–32.

Pedersen TK, Jensen JJ, Melsen B, et al (2001) Resorption of the temporomandibular condylar bone according to subtypes of juvenile chronic arthritis. *J Rheumatol* **28**(9):2109–2115.

Penfold J, Clark AJ (1992) Pain syndromes in HIV infection. *Can J Anaesth* **39**(7):724–730.

Pfaffenrath V, Rath M, Pollmann W, et al (1993) Atypical facial pain–application of the IHS criteria in a clinical sample. *Cephalalgia* **13**(Suppl 12):84–88.

Pfund Z, Szapary L, Jaszberenyi O, et al (1999) Headache in intracranial tumors. *Cephalalgia* **19**(9):787–790; discussion 765.

Pillekamp F, Hoppe B, Roth B, et al (1997) Vomiting, headache and seizures in a child with idiopathic nephrotic syndrome. *Nephrol Dial Transplant* **12**(6): 1280–1281.

Pillitteri LC, Clark RE (1998) Comparison of a patient-controlled analgesia system with continuous infusion for administration of diamorphine for mucositis. *Bone Marrow Transplant* **22**(5): 495–498.

Pittman JR, Bross MH (1999) Diagnosis and management of gout. *Am Fam Physician* **59**(7):1799–1806, 1810.

Portenoy RK, Lesage P (1999) Management of cancer pain. *Lancet* **353**(9165): 1695–1700.

Portenoy RK, Payne D, Jacobsen P (1999) Breakthrough pain: characteristics and impact in patients with cancer pain. *Pain* **81**(1–2):129–134.

Power C, Johnson RT (2001) Neuroimmune and neurovirological aspects of human immunodeficiency virus infection. *Adv Virus Res* **56**:389–433.

Preedy VR, Ohlendieck K, Adachi J, et al (2003) The importance of alcohol-induced muscle disease. *J Muscle Res Cell Motil* **24**(1): 55–63.

Puca A, Meglio M, Tamburrini G, et al (1993) Trigeminal involvement in intracranial tumours. Anatomical and clinical observations on 73 patients. *Acta Neurochir (Wien)* **125** (1–4):47–51.

Ramadan NM (1996) Headache caused by raised intracranial pressure and intracranial hypotension. *Curr Opin Neurol* **9**(3):214–218.

Ramon Y, Samra H, Oberman M (1987) Mandibular condylosis and apertognathia as presenting symptoms in progressive systemic sclerosis (scleroderma). Pattern of mandibular bony lesions and atrophy of masticatory muscles in PSS, presumably caused by affected muscular arteries. *Oral Surg Oral Med Oral Pathol* **63**(3):269–274.

Ramos-Remus C, Major P, Gomez-Vargas A, et al (1997) Temporomandibular joint osseous morphology in a consecutive sample of ankylosing spondylitis patients. *Ann Rheum Dis* **56**(2):103–107.

Reuther T, Schuster T, Mende U, et al (2003) Osteoradionecrosis of the jaws as a side effect of radiotherapy of head and neck tumour patients–a report of a thirty year retrospective review. *Int J Oral Maxillofac Surg* **32**(3):289–295.

Ries M, Ramaswami U, Parini R, et al (2003) The early clinical phenotype of Fabry disease: a study on 35 European children and adolescents. *Eur J Pediatr* **162**(11):767–772.

Rinaldi R, Manfredi R, Azzimondi G, et al (1997) Recurrent 'migrainelike' episodes in patients with HIV disease. *Headache* **37**(7):443–448.

Ripamonti C, Dickerson ED (2001) Strategies for the treatment of cancer pain in the new millennium. *Drugs* **61**(7):955–977.

Rogers SN, Lowe D, McNally D, et al (2003) Health-related quality of life after maxillectomy: a comparison between prosthetic obturation and free flap. *J Oral Maxillofac Surg* **61**(2): 174–181.

Rolak LA, Brown S (1990) Headaches and multiple sclerosis: a clinical study and review of the literature. *J Neurol* **237**(5): 300–302.

Roodman GD, Windle JJ (2005) Paget disease of bone. *J Clin Invest* **115**(2):200–208.

Rothrock JF (2004) Headaches due to vascular disorders. *Neurol Clin* **22**(1):21–37, v.

Rubenstein EB, Peterson DE, Schubert M, et al (2004) Clinical practice guidelines for the prevention and treatment of cancer therapy-induced oral and gastrointestinal mucositis. *Cancer* **100** (9 Suppl):2026–2046.

Ruggiero SL, Mehrotra B (2004) Ten years of alendronate treatment for osteoporosis in postmenopausal women. *N Engl J Med* **351**(2):190–192; author reply 190–192.

Ruoff G, Lema M (2003) Strategies in pain management: new and potential indications for COX-2 specific inhibitors. *J Pain Symptom Manage* **25**(2 Suppl):S21–S31.

Saag KG, Mikuls TR (2005) Recent advances in the epidemiology of gout. *Curr Rheumatol Rep* **7**(3):235–241.

Saip S, Siva A, Altintas A, et al (2005) Headache in Behcet's syndrome. *Headache* **45**(7):911–919.

Sanchez Aniceto G, Garcia Penin A, de la Mata Pages R, et al (1990) Tumors metastatic to the mandible: analysis of nine cases and review of the literature. *J Oral Maxillofac Surg* **48**(3): 246–251.

Sanchez-Guerrero J, Karlson EW, Liang MH, et al (1997) Past use of oral contraceptives and the risk of developing systemic lupus erythematosus. *Arthritis Rheum* **40**(5):804–808.

Sandyk R, Awerbuch GI (1994) The co-occurrence of multiple sclerosis and migraine headache: the serotoninergic link. *Int J Neurosci* 76(3–4):249–257.

Sanna G, Bertolaccini ML, Cuadrado MJ, *et al* (2003) Central nervous system involvement in the antiphospholipid (Hughes) syndrome. *Rheumatology (Oxford)* 42(2):200–213.

Sarlani E, Schwartz AH, Greenspan JD, *et al* (2003) Facial pain as first manifestation of lung cancer: a case of lung cancer-related cluster headache and a review of the literature. *J Orofac Pain* 17(3):262–267.

Scardina GA, Messina P (2004) Systemic sclerosis: description and diagnostic role of the oral phenomena. *Gen Dent* 52(1):42–47.

Schiodt M (1997) Less common oral lesions associated with HIV infection: prevalence and classification. *Oral Dis* 3(Suppl 1):S208–S213.

Schreiber A, Kinney LA, Salman R (1991) Large-cell lymphoma of the infratemporal fossa presenting as myofascial pain. *J Craniomandib Disord* 5(4):286–289.

Schubert MM (1991) Oral manifestations of viral infections in immunocompromised patients. *Curr Opin Dent* 1(4):384–397.

Schulz-Kindermann F, Hennings U, Ramm G, *et al* (2002) The role of biomedical and psychosocial factors for the prediction of pain and distress in patients undergoing high-dose therapy and BMT/PBSCT. *Bone Marrow Transplant* 29(4):341–351.

Scully C (2005) *Medical problems in dentistry*. Elsevier: Edinburgh.

Scully C, Bagan JV (2004) Adverse drug reactions in the orofacial region. *Crit Rev Oral Biol Med* 15(4):221–239.

Sfikakis PP, Mitsikostas DD, Manoussakis MN, *et al* (1998) Headache in systemic lupus erythematosus: a controlled study. *Br J Rheumatol* 37(3):300–303.

Shaiova L, Lapin J, Manco LS, *et al* (2004) Tolerability and effects of two formulations of oral transmucosal fentanyl citrate (OTFC; ACTIQ) in patients with radiation-induced oral mucositis. *Support Care Cancer* 12(4):268–273.

Shotts RH, Porter SR, Kumar N, *et al* (1999) Longstanding trigeminal sensory neuropathy of nontraumatic cause. *Oral Surg Oral Med Oral Pathol Oral Radiol Endod* 87(5):572–576.

Shuaib A, Barklay L, Lee MA, *et al* (1989) Migraine and anti-phospholipid antibodies. *Headache* 29(1):42–45.

Skaer TL (1992) Medication-induced systemic lupus erythematosus. *Clin Ther* 14(4):496–506, discussion 495.

Slatkin NE, Rhiner M (2003) Topical ketamine in the treatment of mucositis pain. *Pain Med* 4(3):298–303.

Sloan PA, Moulin DE, Hays H (1998) A clinical evaluation of transdermal therapeutic system fentanyl for the treatment of cancer pain. *J Pain Symptom Manage* 16(2):102–111.

Sonis ST (2004a) The pathobiology of mucositis. *Nat Rev Cancer* 4(4):277–284.

Sonis ST (2004b) Oral mucositis in cancer therapy. *J Support Oncol* 2(6 Suppl 3):3–8.

Sonis ST, Oster G, Fuchs H, *et al* (2001) Oral mucositis and the clinical and economic outcomes of hematopoietic stem-cell transplantation. *J Clin Oncol* 19(8):2201–2205.

Sonis ST, Elting LS, Keefe D, *et al* (2004a) Perspectives on cancer therapy-induced mucosal injury: pathogenesis, measurement, epidemiology, and consequences for patients. *Cancer* 100(9 Suppl):1995–2025.

Sonis ST, O'Donnell KE, Popat R, *et al* (2004b) The relationship between mucosal cyclooxygenase-2 (COX-2) expression and experimental radiation-induced mucositis. *Oral Oncol* 40(2):170–176.

Spackman GK (1999) Scleroderma: what the general dentist should know. *Gen Dent* 47(6):576–579.

Stickel F, Hoehn B, Schuppan D, *et al* (2003) Review article: Nutritional therapy in alcoholic liver disease. *Aliment Pharmacol Ther* 18(4):357–373.

Stiff P (2001) Mucositis associated with stem cell transplantation: current status and innovative approaches to management. *Bone Marrow Transplant* 27(Suppl 2):S3–S11.

Su CY, Lui CC (1996) Perineural invasion of the trigeminal nerve in patients with nasopharyngeal carcinoma. Imaging and clinical correlations. *Cancer* 78(10):2063–2069.

Symmons DP, Barrett EM, Bankhead CR, *et al* (1994) The incidence of rheumatoid arthritis in the United Kingdom: results from the Norfolk Arthritis Register. *Br J Rheumatol* 33(8):735–739.

Syrjala KL, Cummings C, Donaldson GW (1992) Hypnosis or cognitive behavioural training for the reduction of pain and nausea during cancer treatment: a controlled clinical trial. *Pain* 48:137–146.

Syrjala KL, Donaldson GW, Davis MW, *et al* (1995) Relaxation and imagery and cognitive-behavioral training reduce pain during cancer treatment: a controlled clinical trial. *Pain* 63(2):189–198.

Tabeling HJ, Dolwick MF (1985) Rheumatoid arthritis: diagnosis and treatment. *Fla Dent J* 56(1):16–18.

Tamborlane WV, Ahern J (1997) Implications and results of the Diabetes Control and Complications Trial. *Pediatr Clin North Am* 44(2):285–300.

Taylor JC, Terrell JE, Ronis DL, *et al* (2004) Disability in patients with head and neck cancer. *Arch Otolaryngol Head Neck Surg* 130(6):764–769.

Teravainen H, Larsen A (1977) Some features of the neuromuscular complications of pulmonary carcinoma. *Ann Neurol* 2(6):495–502.

Terkeltaub RA (2003) Clinical practice. Gout. *N Engl J Med* 349(17):1647–1655.

Terrell JE, Nanavati K, Esclamado RM, *et al* (1999) Health impact of head and neck cancer. *Otolaryngol Head Neck Surg* 120(6):852–859.

Terrell JE, Welsh DE, Bradford CR, *et al* (2000) Pain, quality of life, and spinal accessory nerve status after neck dissection. *Laryngoscope* 110(4):620–626.

Thomas PK, Tomlinson DR (1993). Diabetic and hypoglycemic neuropathy. In: Dyck PJ, Griffin J, Low P, Poduslo JF. *Peripheral neuropathy*, 3rd edn. Philadelphia: Saunders, pp 1219–1250.

Thomson HG (1989) Septic arthritis of the temporomandibular joint complicating otitis externa. *J Laryngol Otol* 103(3):319–321.

Tietjen GE (1992) Migraine and antiphospholipid antibodies. *Cephalalgia* 12(2):69–74.

Tietjen GE, Day M, Norris L, *et al* (1998) Role of anticardiolipin antibodies in young persons with migraine and transient focal neurologic events: a prospective study. *Neurology* 50(5):1433–1440.

To KW, Nadel AJ (1991) Ophthalmologic complications in hemoglobinopathies. *Hematol Oncol Clin North Am* 5(3):535–548.

Trotti A, Bellm LA, Epstein JB, *et al* (2003) Mucositis incidence, severity and associated outcomes in patients with head and neck cancer receiving radiotherapy with or without chemotherapy: a systematic literature review. *Radiother Oncol* 66(3):253–262.

Twilt M, Mobers SM, Arends LR, *et al* (2004) Temporomandibular involvement in juvenile idiopathic arthritis. *J Rheumatol* 31(7):1418–1422.

Tzourio C, Tehindrazanarivelo A, Iglesias S, *et al* (1995) Case-control study of migraine and risk of ischaemic stroke in young women. *Bmj* 310(6983):830–833.

Tzourio C, Kittner SJ, Bousser MG, *et al* (2000) Migraine and stroke in young women. *Cephalalgia* 20(3):190–199.

Urban PP, Forst T, Lenfers M, *et al* (1999) Incidence of subclinical trigeminal and facial nerve involvement in diabetes mellitus. *Electromyogr Clin Neurophysiol* 39(5):267–272.

Urban PP, Keilmann A, Teichmann EM, *et al* (2001) Sensory neuropathy of the trigeminal, glossopharyngeal, and vagal nerves in Sjögren's syndrome. *J Neurol Sci* 186(1–2):59–63.

van Loon LA, Bos JD, Davidson CL (1992) Clinical evaluation of fifty-six patients referred with symptoms tentatively related to allergic contact stomatitis. *Oral Surg Oral Med Oral Pathol* 74(5):572–575.

Vannemreddy PS, Nanda A, Reddy PK, *et al* (2002) Primary cerebral sarcoid granuloma: the importance of definitive diagnosis in the high-risk patient population. *Clin Neurol Neurosurg* 104(4):289–292.

Verrotti A, Cieri F, Pelliccia P, *et al* (2000) Lack of association between antiphospholipid antibodies and migraine in children. *Int J Clin Lab Res* **30**(2):109–111.

Vial T, Descotes J (1995) Clinical toxicity of cytokines used as haemopoietic growth factors. *Drug Saf* **13**(6):371–406.

Vickers AJ, Cassileth BR (2001) Unconventional therapies for cancer and cancer-related symptoms. *Lancet Oncol* **2**(4):226–232.

Voog U, Alstergren P, Eliasson S, *et al* (2003) Inflammatory mediators and radiographic changes in temporomandibular joints of patients with rheumatoid arthritis. *Acta Odontol Scand* **61**(1):57–64.

Walton AG, Welbury RR, Foster HE, *et al* (1999) Juvenile chronic arthritis: a dental review. *Oral Dis* **5**(1):68–75.

Wang CJ, Howng SL (2001) Trigeminal neuralgia caused by nasopharyngeal carcinoma with skull base invasion–a case report. *Kaohsiung J Med Sci* **17**(12):630–632.

Wenneberg B, Kononen M, Kallenberg A (1990) Radiographic changes in the temporomandibular joint of patients with rheumatoid arthritis, psoriatic arthritis, and ankylosing spondylitis. *J Craniomandib Disord* **4**(1):35–39.

Wheeler TT, Alberts MA, Dolan TA, *et al* (1995) Dental, visual, auditory and olfactory complications in Paget's disease of bone. *J Am Geriatr Soc* **43**(12):1384–1391.

Whelan HT, Smits RL Jr, Buchman EV, *et al* (2001) Effect of NASA light-emitting diode irradiation on wound healing. *J Clin Laser Med Surg* **19**(6):305–314.

Wilson AW, Brown JS, Ord RA (1990) Psoriatic arthropathy of the temporomandibular joint. *Oral Surg Oral Med Oral Pathol* **70**(5):555–558.

Witt C, Borges AC, Klein K, *et al* (1997) Radiographic manifestations of multiple myeloma in the mandible: a retrospective study of 77 patients. *J Oral Maxillofac Surg* **55**(5):450–453; discussion 454–455.

Woda A, Pionchon P (2000) A unified concept of idiopathic orofacial pain: pathophysiologic features. *J Orofac Pain* **14**(3): 196–212.

Woo SB, Lee SJ, Schubert MM (1997) Graft-vs.-host disease. *Crit Rev Oral Biol Med* **8**(2):201–216.

Wood RE, Lee P (1988) Analysis of the oral manifestations of systemic sclerosis (scleroderma). *Oral Surg Oral Med Oral Pathol* **65**(2):172–178.

Yamashita N (1997) Hyperreactivity of neutrophils and abnormal T cell homeostasis: a new insight for pathogenesis of Behcet's disease. *Int Rev Immunol* **14**(1):11–19.

Yelin E (1992) Arthritis. The cumulative impact of a common chronic condition. *Arthritis Rheum* **35**(5):489–497.

Zafeiriou DI, Economou M, Athanasiou-Metaxa M (2006) Neurological complications in beta-thalassemia. *Brain Dev* **28**(8):477–481.

Zech DF, Grond S, Lynch J, *et al* (1995) Validation of World Health Organization Guidelines for cancer pain relief: a 10-year prospective study. *Pain* **63**(1):65–76.

Zhu JF, Kaminski MJ, Pulitzer DR, *et al* (1996) Psoriasis: pathophysiology and oral manifestations. *Oral Dis* **2**(2): 135–144.

Zierhut M, Mizuki N, Ohno S, *et al* (2003) Immunology and functional genomics of Behcet's disease. *Cell Mol Life Sci* **60**(9):1903–1922.

CHAPTER 15

Pharmacotherapy of acute orofacial pain

Yair Sharav and Rafael Benoliel

1. Introduction

The aim of drug therapy for acute orofacial pain is to relieve pain with maximum efficacy and minimum side effects. Ideally an analgesic drug provides significant relief across all pain severities, has minimal side effects, has few drug interactions and is convenient to administer (e.g. single daily oral dose, pleasant tasting and rapid absorption). However, ideal drugs do not exist and when administering an analgesic consideration should be given to pain severity, the patient's medical background, susceptibility to the various side effects (e.g. gastrointestinal, cardiac, renal) and the fact that patients may differ genetically in their response to analgesics (Lotsch and Geisslinger 2006). The orofacial pain practitioner needs to thoroughly understand the different classes of analgesics and their mechanisms of actions and appreciate that drug actions and interactions change with the patient's age and medical status (Kim *et al* 2004). Analgesics also have gender-specific adverse events and complex pharmacological interactions with other medications that the patient may be taking. This chapter reviews the clinical pharmacology of drugs usually employed in the treatment of acute orofacial pain. Since long-term nonsteroidal anti-inflammatory drugs (NSAIDs) and opioids are sometimes employed in the management of persistent or recurring orofacial pain conditions, relevant 'chronic' adverse effects are also discussed.

The pathogenesis of acute and chronic pain involves peripheral as well as central mechanisms of sensitization that are associated with plasticity in primary sensory and dorsal horn neurons (Woolf and Salter 2000). The local inflammatory response leads to heightened sensitivity and activity of local nociceptors and to distant effects at the level of the central nervous system (CNS). A mechanism-based strategy for pain control with analgesics should have, at least, three major aims (Camu *et al* 2003):

a. Prevention of sensitization of peripheral nociceptors;
b. Interruption of the neuronal transmission of nociceptive signals; and
c. Attenuation of the nociceptive message in the spinal cord and other parts of the CNS.

Acute pain is usually activated by an inflammatory process, so the initial strategy to attain analgesia normally involves the use of anti-inflammatory drugs. However, the sole inhibition of inflammation may not be sufficient to obtain adequate analgesia. NSAIDs, including selective cyclo-oxygenase enzyme (COX)-2 inhibitors, combine anti-inflammatory effects with analgesic actions on peripheral and central neural targets (Cashman 1996). The clinical success of NSAIDs has resulted in their widespread use, and it is estimated that over 30 million patients ingest these for the treatment of pain and inflammation on a daily basis (Singh and Triadafilopoulos 1999).

1.1. The Inflammatory 'Soup'

The 'inflammatory soup' is a mixture of bioactive molecules (bradykinin, histamine, prostaglandins, neurotrophins and interleukins) produced in response to a variety of stimuli and tissue injury. These molecules may act peripherally on primary afferents by direct and/or indirect effects. Direct effects include activation of primary afferent nociceptors and sensitization of nociceptors that result in increasing responses to various stimuli. Indirect effects are mediated by leukocytes and the sympathetic nervous system. These effects may involve increased excitability of dorsal horn neurons (DHNs), leading to altered descending pain control mechanisms and adaptive changes in the thalamus, cortex and higher centres (Millan 1999).

The concomitant presence of mediators such as nerve growth factor (NGF), 5HT, interleukin (IL)-1 and bradykinin at sites of inflammation has led to the collective term inflammatory soup (Mamet *et al* 2002). This soup synergistically activates peripheral nociceptors (Kessler *et al* 1992). An important characteristic of inflammation is acidosis, and protons will directly and indirectly cause pain and hyperalgesia (Steen *et al* 1995). Protons directly activate sensory neurons, mainly through acid-sensing ion channels (ASICs) (Sutherland *et al* 2000; Julius and Basbaum 2001; Ichikawa and Sugimoto 2002; Kido *et al* 2003). The inflammatory soup also induces ASIC upregulation, increases ASIC-expressing neurons and activates sensory neurons leading to increased excitability (Mamet *et al* 2002, 2003). An additional receptor, the dorsal-root ASIC (DRASIC or ASIC3), is both proton and mechanosensitive (Price *et al* 2001). Further synergism is observed via an interaction between mediators in the inflammatory soup and an acidic pH; enhanced effects are mutual and a two-way intensification of experimental human pain has been reported (Steen *et al* 1996). Protons also induce a decrease in the activation threshold for other receptors and therefore increase pain.

1.2. Prostaglandins

Prostaglandins (PG) are synthesized by the constitutive enzyme COX-1 and its inducible isoform COX-2, which is induced in peripheral tissues by a number of inflammatory mediators including cytokines and growth factors (Ballou *et al* 2000). Neuronal effects of PG are mediated by a direct action on the nociceptor (Taiwo and Levine 1989; Noda *et al* 1997) and are not under the control of NGF (Southall and Vasko 2000). PGs are prime examples of sensitizing agents, and specific subtypes (PGE$_2$ and PGI$_2$) have been found to mediate the hyperalgesia induced by bradykinin and noradrenaline (Taiwo *et al* 1990). Experimentally, PGE$_2$ will induce sensitization of multiple classes of cutaneous afferents including C-polymodal nociceptors and Aδ high-threshold mechanonociceptors (Martin *et al* 1987).

COX-2 is upregulated in the spinal cord during peripheral inflammation and COX-2 products contribute to the increased excitability of spinal cord neurons during persistent peripheral inflammation (Samad *et al* 2001; Seybold *et al* 2003). This suggests that PGs are involved at various sites and anatomical levels of the inflammatory-nociceptive pathway (Rueff and Dray 1993). It is not surprising therefore that drugs acting on PGs such as nonselective NSAIDs and selective COX-2 inhibitors are effective analgesic and anti-inflammatory drugs.

The diagram presented in Fig. 15.1 is a highly simplified version of the metabolic pathway from arachidonic acid to PGs, thromboxanes (TX) and leukotrienes (LT) (Funk 2001). Arachidonic acid is a product of cell membrane phospholipids, and its formation may be enhanced by tissue injury. After the release of arachidonic acid (AA), COX catalyzes a complex reaction that converts

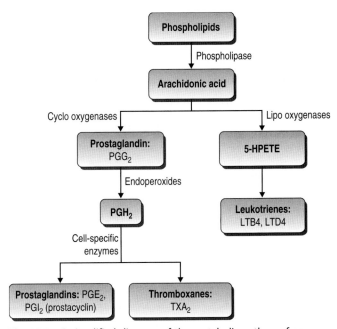

Fig. 15.1 • A simplified diagram of the metabolic pathway from arachidonic acid to prostaglandins, thromboxanes, and leukotrienes. The mechanisms of analgesia-associated adverse effects occur through the regulation of prostaglandin synthesis by anti-inflammatory drugs. Blocking the effect of cyclooxygenases (COX1 and COX-2), by aspirin or traditional NSAIDs, inhibits the production of prostaglandins, in particular PGE$_2$, and causes analgesia. However, prostaglandins are needed for protection of the gastric mucosa, and kidney blood perfusion, hence the deleterious effect on these organs as a possible side effect of NSAID administration. Blocking COX-1 activity also inhibits production of thromboxanes, needed for platelet aggregation and normal blood clotting. By blocking the COX pathway more arachidonic acid is available for the lipo-oxygenase pathway and more leukotrienes such as leukotriene B$_4$ (LTB4) and LTD4 are produced. LTB4 induces neutrophil-dependent hyperalgesia; LTD$_4$ is associated with sensitivity reactions. Selective inhibition of COX-2 minimally blocks the production of PGE$_2$, but selectively suppresses prostacyclin (PGI$_2$) production (that has antithrombotic and antihypertensive effects) without affecting TXA$_2$, and could therefore predispose the patient (especially the elderly, or with other CV risk factors) to thromboembolic adverse effects and hypertension. Additionally some leukotrienes increase gastric acid production that is unbalanced by the protective prostaglandins, leading to increased GI side effects.

AA to PGG$_2$. In a second step a peroxidase-catalyzed reaction converts PGG$_2$ to PGH$_2$ (Funk 2001), which then reacts with other enzymes, determined by the host tissue/cell, into different PGs or TX. For example, PGH$_2$ in platelets is converted into TXA$_2$, whilst in endothelial cells it will be converted into PGE$_2$ and PGI$_2$ (Smith and Marnett 1991; Smith *et al* 1994). TXA$_2$ is a powerful vasoconstrictor that stimulates platelet aggregation. PGE$_2$ and PGI$_2$ are vasodilators that affect renal glomerular filtration rate and possess gastroprotective properties (Brune 2004). Specific leukotrienes lead to vasoconstriction and increased acid secretion in gastric mucosa whilst others lead to hypersensitivity reactions such as oedema and bronchospasm (Brune 2004). Additionally, leukotriene B4 is known to induce a number of proinflammatory effects and has been implicated in chronic inflammation and tissue destruction in inflammatory joint disease (Bertolini *et al* 2001).

2. Modes of Action of NSAIDs

The blockade of the enzymatic effects of COX by aspirin or other NSAIDs inhibits the production of PGs associated with nociception (in particular PGE_2), hence the analgesic effect of these drugs (Vane 1971). However, as we later describe in detail, prostaglandins are essential for the normal function of many organs (e.g. gastrointestinal, kidney) and their disruption is associated with serious side effects. Additionally, the production of TXs is also blocked. TXA_2 is associated with platelet aggregation, and blocking the production of TXA_2 interferes with normal blood clotting. In addition, the blockade of the COX pathway increases the amount of AA substrate available for the lipo-oxygenase pathway, thereby enhancing the production of LTs. An excess of LT is associated with asthmatic attacks, urticaria and other sensitivity reactions (see Fig. 15.1) (Israel et al 1993). There is evidence that some NSAIDs such as ibuprofen and indomethacin exert part of their effect by COX-independent mechanisms (Tegeder et al 2001). These mechanisms probably involve inhibition of transcription factors mediated by alterations in the activity of cellular kinases.

2.1. COX Isoforms

An important advance in prostaglandin research was the discovery that COX exists in various isoforms: primarily COX-1 and COX-2 (Fu et al 1990), and recent evidence points to the existence of COX-3. The level of COX-1 in cells varies relatively over a narrow range (two- to four-fold), and is considered a constitutive or housekeeping enzyme, largely unrelated to inflammation. COX-1 maintains PG and TX synthesis in the stomach, the kidney, endothelial cells, blood platelets and other tissues. COX-2, however, is mostly an inducible enzyme and is considered part of the inflammatory process (Robinson 1997). COX-2 is produced in monocytes, synovial cells and fibroblasts after stimulation by cytokines and growth factors, and its expression is augmented 10- to 80-fold when cells are activated (Smith et al 1994). Less is known about COX-3, which is found in the cerebral cortex and cardiac tissue and appears to be involved in centrally mediated pain. The kinetics of COX-2 inhibition is different from that of COX-1. COX-1 inhibition is instantaneous and competitively reversible. COX-2 inhibition is time-dependent, with selectivity developing over 15–30 minutes, and is thereafter essentially irreversible (Hawkey 1999). Different genes encode these two enzymes, and separate experiments in mice have used stem cell technology to knock out the genes for COX-1 and COX-2 to provide evidence of each of these enzymes' role (Dinchuk et al 1995; Langenbach et al 1995). However, some of the results were quite unexpected, stressing a possible constitutive role for COX-2. Thus, deletion of the COX-2 gene was associated with a shortened life span, infertility due to failure of ovarian development and incomplete maturation of nephrons resulting in renal failure (Dinchuk et al 1995). Also the results of experimental inflammation were similar in mice lacking the COX-2 gene and control mice, stressing the important role of COX-1 in inflammation (Dinchuk et al 1995). Another surprising find was that even though mice lacking COX-1 had gastric PGE levels that were only 1% of controls, they had no gastric pathology, and were less susceptible to indomethacin-induced gastropathy than controls (Langenbach et al 1995).

Indeed, it was first assumed that drugs with COX-2 selectivity would spare physiological PG synthesis, and possess anti-inflammatory action with fewer or none of the typical adverse effects of NSAIDs on the gastrointestinal tract, kidneys, platelets and lungs (Vane 1994). However, it became obvious that COX-1 has an important role in the inflammatory response whilst COX-2 has fundamental constitutive roles. Animal experiments and clinical trials with specific COX-2 inhibitors have revealed that COX-2 is important for the normal function of many systems (Crofford et al 2000; Katori and Majima 2000). This is particularly true for the kidney, central nervous, cardiovascular and reproductive systems.

Novel coxibs (e.g. etoricoxib, valdecoxib, parecoxib, lumiracoxib) have been recently developed with enhanced biochemical COX-2 selectivity over that of older ones such as rofecoxib and celecoxib. They have the potential advantage to spare COX-1 activity, thus reducing gastrointestinal toxicity, even when administered at high doses to improve efficacy. However, several randomized clinical studies suggest that the novel coxibs have comparable efficacy to nonselective NSAIDs in the treatment of osteoarthritis, rheumatoid arthritis and acute pain, but they share similar renal side effects.

3. Adverse Effects of NSAIDs

NSAIDs interfere with the production of prostaglandins and thromboxanes, and enhance the amount of leukotrienes. The main adverse effects of NSAID administration associated with inhibition of PG are gastrointestinal toxicity and renal failure. Inhibition of TX is associated with coagulation problems, and the surplus production of LT is mainly associated with hypersensitive reactions such as asthma and urticaria. The selective COX-2 inhibitors gained widespread popularity, having equivalent analgesic and anti-inflammatory effects as the conventional NSAIDs, yet with reduced gastrointestinal (GI) side effects (Bombardier et al 2000; Silverstein et al 2000; Schnitzer et al 2004). A recent review discusses the clinical implications of COX-2 inhibitors for acute dental pain management and its benefits and risks (Spink et al 2005).

Recently COX-2 inhibitors have been shown to increase the risk of cardiovascular (CV) events such as myocardial infarction and ischaemic stroke (Wong et al 2005). They are also intimately involved in prostaglandin-dependent renal homeostatic processes, and therefore do not offer renal safety over that of NSAIDs (Brater *et al* 2001). In a very short time, COX-2 inhibitors have gone from the darlings to the pariahs of the pharmaceutical industry (Brophy 2005). The risks and adverse effects of traditional NSAIDs and of the newer more selective COX-2 inhibitors are detailed below.

3.1. Gastrointestinal

3.1.1. Pathophysiology

Gastroduodenal mucosal injury develops when the deleterious effect of gastric acid overwhelms the normal defensive properties of the mucosa. Concepts about NSAID-induced gastroduodenal mucosal injury have evolved from a simple notion of topical injury to theories involving multiple mechanisms with both local and systemic effects. Topical injury caused by NSAIDs contributes to the development of gastroduodenal mucosal injury but the systemic effects of these agents appear to have the predominant role (Schoen and Vender 1989), largely through the decreased synthesis of mucosal prostaglandins (Lanza *et al* 1980). Aspirin, at a dose as low as 30mg, is sufficient to suppress prostaglandin synthesis in the gastric mucosa (Lee *et al* 1994). Prostaglandin inhibition, in turn, leads to decreases in epithelial mucus production, secretion of bicarbonate, mucosal blood flow, epithelial proliferation and mucosal resistance to injury (Wolfe and Soll 1988). The impairment in mucosal resistance permits injury by endogenous factors, including acid, pepsin and bile salts, as well as by exogenous noxious agents.

Selective COX-2 inhibitors hold the promise of fewer adverse effects as far as the gastrointestinal tract and platelets are concerned (Silverstein *et al* 2000; FitzGerald and Patrono 2001; Schnitzer *et al* 2004). However, despite the 50% reduction of symptomatic ulcers, perforations and bleeding observed for rofecoxib (Bombardier *et al* 2000), the risk for serious GI toxicity by selective COX-2 inhibitors is still within the 2–4% range for COX-nonselective NSAIDs. Furthermore, there is increasing evidence of the importance of COX-2 in resolution of mucosal inflammation and in ulcer healing (Wallace and Devchand 2005). COX-2 inhibitors are therefore contraindicated for use in patients with diagnosed and actively treated GI ulcers (Stichtenoth and Frolich 2003).

3.1.2. Epidemiology

According to prospective data 13 of every 1000 patients with rheumatoid arthritis who take NSAIDs for one year have a serious GI complication. The risk in patients with osteoarthritis is somewhat lower (7.3 per 1000 patients per year) (Singh and Triadafilopoulos 1999). Mortality attributed to NSAID-related GI toxic effects is 0.22% per

year, with an annual relative risk of 4.21 as compared with the risk for persons not using NSAIDs (Singh and Triadafilopoulos 1999). However, these figures are true for 1999, before the wide introduction of COX-2 inhibitors such as celecoxib or rofecoxib. The severity of the NSAID-associated GI injury is not to be underestimated; on average 1 in 1200 patients taking NSAIDs for at least 2 months, who would not have died had they not taken NSAIDs, will die from gastroduodenal complications. This extrapolates to about 2000 deaths each year in the UK alone (Tramer *et al* 2000).

3.1.3. Risk Factors

The risk for adverse GI events increases linearly with age (Longstreth 1995). Other risk factors that have been identified in multiple studies are higher doses of NSAIDs (including the use of two or more NSAIDs), a history of gastroduodenal ulcer or gastrointestinal bleeding, concomitant use of corticosteroids, serious coexisting conditions, alcohol abuse and concomitant use of anticoagulants (Hernandez-Diaz and Garcia-Rodriguez 2001). However, many of these studies are based on univariate analysis and do not consider the interactions among multiple factors and coexisting conditions so for medically complex patients the risk may be even higher (Wolfe *et al* 1999).

3.1.4. Clinical Spectrum of Injury

In the majority of patients, NSAID-induced gastroduodenal mucosal injury is superficial and self-limiting. However, peptic ulcers develop in some patients, and they may lead to gastroduodenal haemorrhage, perforation, and death. After ingestion of an NSAID, ultrastructural damage to the gastric surface epithelium occurs within minutes, and gross, endoscopically detectable haemorrhages and erosions in the gastroduodenal epithelium occur within several hours (Graham and Smith 1986).

3.1.5. Prevention and Management

At least 10–20% of patients have dyspeptic symptoms during NSAID therapy (Singh *et al* 1996). However, such symptoms are poorly correlated with the endoscopic appearance and severity of mucosal injury. Up to 40% of persons with endoscopic evidence of erosive gastritis are asymptomatic (Larkai *et al* 1987; Pounder 1989) and as many as 50% of patients with dyspepsia have normal-appearing mucosa (Larkai *et al* 1987). Histamine H_2-receptor antagonists improve dyspeptic symptoms, but still permit a high risk of GI complications (Wolfe *et al* 1999).

The concomitant use of antacid medication in susceptible individuals or for long-term therapy is common practice. The proton-pump inhibitor omeprazole and misoprostol, a prostaglandin E_1 analogue, are commonly used for the treatment and prevention of NSAID-related gastroduodenal ulcers. However, omeprazole provided greater symptomatic relief, and also better healing of gastroduodenal ulcers in patients receiving ongoing NSAIDs (Hawkey *et al* 1998). A quality-of-life evaluation showed that patients receiving omeprazole had significantly greater improvement in scores on the Gastrointestinal Symptom Rating Scale than the patients receiving misoprostol (Hawkey *et al* 1998). Additionally, based on a cost-effectiveness analysis omeprazole is preferable to misoprostol (Eccles *et al* 1998). Proton-pump inhibitors represent a suitable means of preventing the development of gastroduodenal ulcers associated with the use of NSAIDs; they appear to provide a safe and effective form of therapy for NSAID-associated dyspepsia (Lanza 1998; Morgner *et al* 2007).

3.2. Renal

The kidney is the second most frequent target of serious adverse effects of NSAIDs related to inhibition of COX and is estimated to affect 2 million patients annually in the USA alone (Sandhu and Heyneman 2004). The renal side effects of NSAIDs comprise reduction in renal blood flow (RBF) and glomerular filtration rate (GFR), sodium/water retention and hyperkalaemia (Sandhu and Heyneman 2004). Animal experiments and clinical trials with preferential and specific COX-2 inhibitors revealed that COX-2 is the critical enzyme for sodium excretion and renin release and likely antagonism of antidiuretic hormone—a prime example of a constitutive role for COX-2. Additionally, a significant role of COX-2 in nephrogenesis is suggested. For renal haemodynamics the available evidence points to COX-1 as the predominant enzyme, but further investigations are required (Stichtenoth and Frolich 2000).

Furthermore, PGI_2 significantly influences the renal system of medically compromised patients, especially with diabetes, peripheral vascular disease or other causes of renal insufficiency. COX-2 inhibition decreases PGE_2 and PGI_2, modifiers of glomerular filtration in compromised kidneys, and causes sodium retention, promoting peripheral oedema and hypertension, lower renal perfusion with renal ischaemia (Khan *et al* 2001). The dose-dependent consequences of standard NSAIDs and COX-2 inhibitors on the kidney include elevated blood pressure, oedema and congestive heart failure in some compromised patients and in patients taking beta-adrenergic blocker drugs or angiotensin-converting enzyme (ACE) inhibitors (Whelton *et al* 2002).

The second generation of COX-2 inhibitors with higher COX-2 selectivity (valdecoxib, parecoxib, and especially etoricoxib and lumaricoxib) possesses marginal, if any, gain in safety compared with the first generation (Sandhu and Heyneman 2004). The apparent dose dependence of renal toxicity also limits the use of higher dosages. It can be concluded at this stage that with regards to renal adverse events, selective COX-2 inhibitors do not offer a clinically relevant advantage over conventional NSAIDs

(Stichtenoth and Frolich 2003; Sandhu and Heyneman 2004). It seems, however, that renal effects are related to individual COX-2 inhibitors and are not a 'class effect' (Sandhu and Heyneman 2004; Zhang *et al* 2006).

The epidemiological impact is substantial and current users of NSAIDs are estimated to be 2–4 times more at risk for acute renal failure (Evans *et al* 1995; Perez Gutthann *et al* 1996; Henry *et al* 1997). This risk is dose dependent and is highest (relative risk >8) during the first month of therapy (Perez Gutthann *et al* 1996; Henry *et al* 1997). Other risk factors for acute renal failure are long drug half-life, male gender, increasing age, cardiovascular comorbidity, renal diseases, concomitant use of other nephrotoxic drugs and any recent hospitalization (Perez Gutthann *et al* 1996; Henry *et al* 1997). Of the specific COX-2 inhibitors rofecoxib has been found to significantly increase the risk for peripheral oedema, hypertension, renal dysfunction and arrhythmias (Zhang *et al* 2006). Increased risk was associated with increased dose and duration of rofecoxib use (Zhang *et al* 2006). The NSAID effect on acute renal failure is stronger among subjects with a previous history of renal disease and in those with a history of gout or hyperuricaemia. Among these patients, NSAID exposure increases the risk of acute renal failure by a factor of 7 (Whelton *et al* 1990; Henry *et al* 1997). Only indomethacin presented a higher relative risk for acute renal failure than the other conventional NSAIDs (Perez Gutthann *et al* 1996).

3.3. Cardiovascular

Current users of any NSAIDs are estimated to have up to a twofold increase in risk of hospitalization for congestive heart failure, even greater in patients with pre-existing heart disease (Hernandez-Diaz and Garcia-Rodriguez 2001; Kearney *et al* 2006). The risk is dose dependent, and higher during the first month of therapy (Heerdink *et al* 1998; Page and Henry 2000; Kearney *et al* 2006).

While COX-2 inhibitors gained widespread popularity as effective anti-inflammatory and analgesic agents with reduced GI side effects (Bombardier *et al* 2000; Silverstein *et al* 2000; Schnitzer *et al* 2004), concerns over cardiovascular risk of selective COX-2 inhibitors have been raised, which may outweigh any gain in GI safety (FitzGerald and Patrono 2001). Increased risk was shown for certain vascular events: myocardial infarction (MI) and ischaemic stroke (Bresalier *et al* 2005; Kearney *et al* 2006). The cardiovascular harm associated with COX-2 inhibitors became apparent in trials conducted for other indications. Therefore, even with the evidence from these trials, we lack information to make confident statements about the exact levels of risk for each drug, the time course of the risk and the populations of patients (if any) in whom the benefits might exceed the known risks (Psaty and Furberg 2005). Cardiovascular safety of all COX-2 inhibitors and traditional NSAIDs has since been under intense investigation.

Rofecoxib was withdrawn from the market following the findings of a doubling of risk of vascular events in the rofecoxib group compared to placebo (relative risk, 1.92; 95% CI: 1.19–3.11) (Bresalier et al 2005). Meta-analysis of controlled studies using rofecoxib had previously shown that the risk of MI was increased after a few months of treatment (Juni et al 2004; Solomon et al 2004). Rofecoxib at all doses increases the risk by a factor of 1.59 (95% CI: 1.1–2.3) and for rofecoxib >25mg/d by a factor of 3.58 (CI: 1.3–10.1). Rofecoxib is also associated with higher incidences of hypertension, peripheral oedema and congestive heart failure compared with celecoxib and other NSAIDs (Bombardier et al 2000; Mamdani et al 2004; Solomon et al 2004). A significant elevation in the cardiovascular event rate for rofecoxib has been confirmed in recent studies (Solomon et al 2006). The increase rate for rofecoxib was seen in the first 60 days of use and thereafter.

Death from CV causes, MI, stroke, or heart failure was higher in a group taking celecoxib 200mg twice per day and 400mg twice per day than in the placebo group (relative risk 2.8; 95% CI: 1.3–6.3) (Solomon et al 2005). CV risk with celecoxib became apparent only after 12 months of treatment and increased with higher doses but this has not been a consistent finding (ADAPT 2006).

MI, cardiac arrest, stroke and pulmonary embolism were more frequent among the patients given the newer coxibs, valdecoxib and its prodrug parecoxib, than among those given placebo (2.0 vs. 0.5%; relative risk 3.7) (Ott et al 2003; Nussmeier et al 2005). In one study the risks of using COX-2 inhibitors in high CV risk patients, who were excluded from previous randomized controlled studies, were noted (Nussmeier et al 2005). A pooled analysis of these studies suggests that parecoxib/valdecoxib elevate the combined incidence of MI and stroke by threefold in these populations (Furberg et al 2005).

Traditional NSAIDs, such as diclofenac and ibuprofen, have also been implicated in increased MI risk (Hippisley-Cox and Coupland 2005; Kearney et al 2006; McGettigan and Henry 2006). These findings have not, however, been universally duplicated (Solomon et al 2006). For naproxen versus any NSAID, taken at least 60 days previously, the adjusted odds ratio was not significant (1.14, CI: 1–1.3) (Graham et al 2005). A significant reduction in CV events was noted for naproxen in one study (RR 0.75, CI: 0.62–0.92) (Solomon et al 2006), whilst in another naproxen significantly increased CV risk (ADAPT 2006). It may be concluded that naproxen may not significantly protect against serious coronary heart disease; however, it is not consistently associated with any increased risk (Graham et al 2005; Kearney et al 2006; McGettigan and Henry 2006). Hypertensive patients on NSAIDs are more susceptible to blood pressure increases than normotensives (Johnson et al 1994) and demonstrate significantly increased rates of MI or CVA relative to normotensive patients (Spalding et al 2007).

Concomitant NSAID and antihypertensive treatment may induce clinically significant drug interactions. Indomethacin and piroxicam induce a hypertensive effect greater than that of alternative NSAIDs. There is also relatively greater antagonism between NSAIDs and beta-blockers compared with other antihypertensives (Johnson 1998). Fortunately, the CV risk of short-term use of most NSAIDs is minimal and most serious side effects occur only after long-term use. There are, however, three classes of antihypertensive agents that can interact with NSAIDs: ACE inhibitors, beta-blockers and diuretics. The action of all these drugs is aided by renal prostaglandins. With the principal effect of NSAIDs being PG inhibition, the effectiveness of these agents may be diminished. This interaction usually takes approximately 7–8 days to occur. Therefore, NSAID use in a hypertensive patient on these medications should be limited to 4–6 days (Haas 1999).

The American Heart Association released a scientific statement to aid clinicians in selection of analgesics for patients with increased CV risk (Antman et al 2007). Their recommendations reiterate our conclusions summarized in detail at the end of this chapter. In brief, for patients with increased CV risk acetaminophen or aspirin should initially be tried. Naproxen remains the NSAID with the most data indicating no increased risk for CV events and is therefore a logical second option; the use of gastroprotective agents should be considered in at-risk individuals. COX-2 inhibitors are contraindicated in patients with recent bypass surgery, unstable angina, previous MI, ischaemic cerebrovascular events or any other active atherosclerotic process as they are associated with significantly increased risk for adverse CV events (Antman et al 2007). Additionally COX-2 inhibitors may lead to impaired renal perfusion, sodium retention and increased blood pressure which contribute to increased CV risk. When NSAIDs, particularly COX-2 inhibitors, are indicated they should be used at the lowest dose for the shortest time (Antman et al 2007).

3.4. Platelet Effects and Concomitant Aspirin Use

Human platelets and vascular endothelial cells process PGH_2 to produce TXA_2 and prostacyclin (PGI_2), respectively (Majerus 1983). COX-1 converts arachidonic acid to TXA_2 (mostly from platelets), which induces platelet aggregation and vasoconstriction. COX-2 is responsible for the conversion of AA to PGI_2, which inhibits platelet aggregation and induces vasodilatation. Selective inhibition of COX-2 causes suppression of PGI_2 production without affecting TXA_2, and predisposes to hypertension and increased thromboembolic risks (Fitzgerald 2004; Grosser et al 2006).

The best characterized mechanism of action of aspirin is related to its capacity to irreversibly inactivate COX-1 and COX-2. Since aspirin probably also inactivates COX-1 in relatively mature megakaryocytes, and only 10% of the platelet pool is replenished each day, once-a-day dosing of aspirin is able to maintain virtually complete inhibition of platelet TXA_2 production (Patrono *et al* 2001). Vascular PGI_2 can be derived from both COX-1 and COX-2 (McAdam *et al* 1999) and there is substantial residual COX-2-dependent PGI_2 biosynthesis *in vivo* at daily doses of aspirin in the range of 30 to 100mg to maintain vascular homeostasis (Clarke *et al* 1991). Experimental studies support the importance of PGI_2 in the prevention of arterial thrombosis (Murata *et al* 1997). It has not been established that more profound suppression of PGI_2 formation by higher doses of aspirin is sufficient to initiate or to predispose to thrombosis. However, one trial showed a significantly lower rate of vascular events in patients receiving 80 or 325mg aspirin than in patients receiving 650 or 1300mg daily, consistent with an important role for PGI_2 in preventing thrombosis (Taylor *et al* 1999).

In contrast to the irreversible effects of aspirin, traditional NSAIDs reversibly inhibit platelet aggregation and prolong bleeding time (Schafer 1999). The regular administration of naproxen 500mg BID can mimic the antiplatelet COX-1 effect of low-dose aspirin but does not decrease prostacyclin biosynthesis *in vivo* (Capone *et al* 2004). Rofecoxib and valdecoxib do not impair platelet aggregation, and rofecoxib does not alter the antiplatelet effect of aspirin (Ouellet *et al* 2001; Leese *et al* 2002). Thus, in terms of bleeding COX-2 inhibitors may be given more safely than traditional NSAIDs in the dental perioperative setting.

Aspirin is taken on a daily basis by a large number of patients, especially for cardioprotection (Gaziano and Gibson 2006). Choosing an analgesic that does not interfere with aspirin's action or increase adverse events is important. For example, the use of NSAIDs in conjunction with aspirin may increase the risk of GI complications. Moreover, ibuprofen and naproxen interfere with aspirin's ability to irreversibly acetylate platelet COX-1, and theoretically may reduce aspirin's protective antithrombotic effect (Catella-Lawson *et al* 2001; Capone *et al* 2005). Data from epidemiological studies suggest that taking any NSAID may cancel aspirin's cardioprotective effects (Gaziano and Gibson 2006). Treatment with NSAIDs, particularly ibuprofen or naproxen, should be avoided in patients taking concomitant low-dose aspirin (Antman *et al* 2007). Taking aspirin prior to ibuprofen or naproxen ingestion does not seem to resolve this interaction (Capone *et al* 2005; Antman *et al* 2007). However, concomitant administration of rofecoxib, acetaminophen or diclofenac did not affect the pharmacodynamics of aspirin (Catella-Lawson *et al* 2001). The use of COX-2 inhibitors in patients taking aspirin a priori defeats the very reason for prescribing COX-2 inhibitors: GI safety. It would therefore seem prudent to preferentially use acetaminophen for these patients (Gaziano and Gibson 2006).

3.5. Hypersensitivity Reaction

It is well known that aspirin and other NSAIDs can exacerbate various forms of urticaria and asthma (Szczeklik and Stevenson 1999; Stevenson *et al* 2001). Aspirin sensitivity can be confirmed by drug challenge tests in 20–41% of patients with urticaria (Juhlin 1981). In contrast, the rate of aspirin sensitivity in the normal population is about 1% (Bigby 2001). Susceptible individuals have cross-sensitivity to the entire class of drugs regardless of their chemical structure.

The most common clinical presentation is urticaria and angioedema. Current theories regarding the mechanisms of NSAID sensitivity in chronic idiopathic urticaria (CIU) are largely inferred from studies of an analogous, well-defined clinical syndrome of aspirin-induced asthma (AIA), which affects about 10% of adult asthmatic patients (Szczeklik and Stevenson 1999). Both syndromes affect middle-aged individuals, with a female preponderance. Sensitivity to NSAIDs is present in only a subset of patients with asthma and CIU. Although some NSAID-induced cutaneous eruptions are immunologic, in most cases the mechanism involves inhibition of COX. It is well established that in AIA the mechanism of sensitivity involves inhibition of COX-1 (Szczeklik 1990). At the biochemical level, AIA is characterized by overproduction of leukotrienes and increased urinary excretion of leukotriene E_4 (LTE_4) (Christie *et al* 1991). The mechanism of sensitivity to NSAIDs in CIU is also associated with overproduction of leukotrienes and mast cell activation and most likely depends on inhibition of COX-1 (Zembowicz *et al* 2003). COX-2 inhibitors (rofecoxib, up to 37.5mg, and celecoxib, up to 300mg) do not induce urticaria in patients with CIU sensitive to NSAIDs. Etoricoxib, a second-generation COX-2 inhibitor, at 120mg dosage was also found safe in patients with NSAID-induced urticaria and angioedema (Sanchez-Borges *et al* 2005). The COX-2 inhibitor rofecoxib, up to 25mg, was also safe in AIA patients also sensitive to other NSAIDs (Martin-Garcia *et al* 2002; Perrone *et al* 2003; Nettis *et al* 2005; Micheletto *et al* 2006). Celecoxib 200mg was also safe in AIA patients (Martin-Garcia *et al* 2003; Celik *et al* 2005). However, valdecoxib, one of the newer COX-2 inhibitors, is not recommended in patients with a history of asthma or urticaria. Valdecoxib is a benzene-sulphonamide and could also have cross reactivity in patients who are allergic to sulpha-type drugs (Glasser and Burroughs 2003).

About 7% of AIA patients who had no adverse reaction to rofecoxib had experienced asthma induced by acetaminophen (Martin-Garcia *et al* 2002). Cross reactivity of patients with AIA to acetaminophen is fairy prevalent, especially in doses >1000mg. Thus, 34% of AIA patients reacted to acetaminophen in doses of 1000–1500mg (95% CI: 20–49%). By contrast, none of the non-AIA patients reacted to acetaminophen (95% CI: 0–14%). This difference was highly significant, supporting the hypothesis that cross sensitivity between aspirin and acetaminophen is unique in AIA patients. Daily paracetamol use increases the risk of asthma by a factor of 2.38 (CI: 1.22–4.64). It is recommended that frequent (daily) or high doses of acetaminophen (1000mg or greater) should be avoided in aspirin-sensitive asthmatic patients (Settipane *et al* 1995).

Anaphylactic shock and urticaria/angio-oedema after a single dose of dipyrone has been reported (Szczeklik *et al* 1977). All patients had positive skin tests to these drugs but no cross reactivity with NSAIDs. Dipyrone-induced hypersensitivity reactions include skin rash with an intriguing geographical difference in frequency (Levy 2000). Respiratory asthma-like reactions with cross reactivity in patients sensitive to aspirin have been more rarely reported (Levy 2000). Dipyrone has been clearly shown to cause agranulocytosis, but there is insufficient useful information to adequately quantify the risk. Most studies are old, methodologically weak and small, and use different definitions of agranulocytosis (Edwards and McQuay 2002). It is absolute risks that are important when determining harm. Absolute risks of rare events following some drug treatments have been determined but it is not possible to determine the risk of agranulocytosis with dipyrone and uncertainty is likely to remain (Tramer *et al* 2000; Edwards and McQuay 2002).

The pathogenesis of agranulocytosis following the use of dipyrone (and other pyrazolones) is considered immunological (Levy 2000). Conflicting data and regulations prevail worldwide as to the incidence of agranulocytosis following the use of pyrazolones in general, and dipyrone in particular (Levy 2000). A multinational study found significant regional variability in the risk ratio for agranulocytosis following the use of dipyrone (International Agranulocytosis and Aplastic Anemia Study 1986). In Ulm, Berlin and Barcelona the risk ratio was 23.7 and the excess risk estimate connected with hospital admission for agranulocytosis from any dipyrone use in a seven-day period amounted to 1.1 cases per million users. In Israel and Budapest there was no evidence of increased risk associated with dipyrone use (International Agranulocytosis and Aplastic Anemia Study 1986). The reason for the geographical variation in the risk of dipyrone-induced agranulocytosis and rash is unclear (Levy 2000).

3.6. Effects on Bone Healing

Studies suggest that nonspecific NSAIDs, which inhibit both COX-1 and COX-2 isoforms, delay bone healing. Recent studies investigating the effects of COX-2-selective inhibitors on bone healing have yielded similar results (Harder and An 2003). A recent animal study demonstrated that ketorolac significantly delays fracture healing (Gerstenfeld *et al* 2003). It was further demonstrated that a COX-2-selective NSAID, such as parecoxib (valdecoxib), has only a small effect on delaying fracture healing even at doses known to fully inhibit prostaglandin production (Gerstenfeld *et al* 2003). Despite the understanding of the potential mechanism through which NSAIDs and COX-2

inhibitors hamper bone healing in a laboratory setting, few studies exist that show whether these inhibitory effects are also evident clinically (Harder and An 2003).

3.7. Reproductive System and Pregnancy Risk

COX-2 plays a prominent role at all stages of reproduction (Chan 2004). Thus prolonged use of COX-2 inhibitors in women may lead to pregnancy risks and infertility (Silverstein *et al* 2000; Nielsen *et al* 2001; Li *et al* 2003; Norman and Wu 2004). Both oestrogen and progesterone are involved in the regulation of COX production in tissues of the reproductive tract (Chan 2004). Therefore changes in oestrogen and progesterone levels during pregnancy contribute to the dramatic increase in COX-2 expression although this effect seems to vary at different stages of pregnancy. This further strengthens the earlier findings that COX-2 activities are necessary to support pregnancy.

Use of NSAIDs during the first 20 weeks of pregnancy has been associated with an 80% increased risk of miscarriage over non-use (risk ratio 1.8, CI: 1–3.2). Risk of miscarriage was highest when the drug was taken around the time of conception (risk ratio 5.6, CI: 2.3–13.7) or used for more than a week (risk ratio 8.1, CI: 2.8–23.4). Absolute risk of NSAID-associated miscarriage was 10% for any use, 35% for use around time of conception and 52% for use longer than one week (Li *et al* 2003). However, prenatal use of paracetamol, pharmacologically different from NSAIDs and aspirin, was not associated with increased risk of miscarriage regardless of timing and duration of use (Li *et al* 2003). In view of the above, warnings of drug effects on reproduction have been included in the product labelling of marketed NSAIDs and COX-2-specific inhibitors (Chan 2004).

Paracetamol is generally considered to be the analgesic of choice in pregnant patients. However, the use of paracetamol, but not aspirin, was positively associated with asthma and persistent wheezing in infants of mothers who took paracetamol frequently (defined as most days or daily use) in late pregnancy (Shaheen *et al* 2005). No association was found with hay fever, eczema or skin test positivity. The proportion of asthma attributable to paracetamol use in late pregnancy, assuming a causal relation, was 7% (Shaheen *et al* 2005). The number of pregnant women taking frequent doses was very small so the authors recommend that infrequent paracetamol remain the analgesic of choice in pregnancy (Shaheen *et al* 2005).

4. Efficacy of NSAIDs

Prostaglandins represent one of the key chemicals involved in the sensitization of peripheral nociceptors, thereby contributing to the development of both primary and subsequent secondary hyperalgesia. PGs are synthesized rather rapidly following tissue injury and appear in significant concentrations just one hour after trauma (Henman *et al* 1979). The PGE$_2$ prostanoid is especially important in inflammatory pain and levels of PGE$_2$ correlate with pain intensity levels following the extraction of impacted wisdom teeth (Roszkowski *et al* 1997). The dental model for analgesic efficacy examines the effect of analgesics after surgical extraction of the third mandibular molar. This is a widely established model for inducing postsurgical inflammation-based moderate to severe pain and a useful tool for examining the efficacy of analgesics (Norholt 1998). This model is particularly relevant to our discussion on analgesic efficacy for acute orofacial pain, since there is evidence that NSAIDs may be more effective in dental surgery than in, for example, orthopaedic surgery (Hyllested *et al* 2002).

Measuring analgesic efficacy. The number needed to treat (NNT) represents the number of patients treated to achieve one patient with at least 50% pain relief; it describes the differences between active treatment and control and provides a useful way of comparing the relative efficacy of analgesics. The relative efficacy of non-opioid analgesics is presented in Fig. 15.2. Information on dosing and side effects are shown in Table 15.1.

4.1. Conventional NSAIDs

The use of NSAIDs is advocated for the management of postoperative pain, and these drugs have been widely used for pain relief in dentistry (Gobetti 1992). Conventional NSAIDs typically inhibit prostaglandin production by both COX-1 and COX-2 enzyme systems. Even though significant advances in the understanding of cyclooxygenases and prostaglandins and their involvement in pain production have led to the development of the specific COX-2 inhibitors, the nonselective NSAIDs have retained their position as analgesics of choice for the general population (Gotzsche 2005). Important differences in adverse effects exist between different NSAIDs; in contrast their beneficial effects seem similar (Gotzsche 2005). The differences in side effects are most important in considering which NSAID to choose, such as the relative risks of GI ulceration compared with the potential increase in CV risk (Juni *et al* 2005). The evidence suggests that if one NSAID is unsatisfactory, then switching to another NSAID will not provide better analgesia. Likewise doubling the therapeutic dose of an NSAID leads to only a small increase in effect, which may not be clinically relevant (Huskisson *et al* 1976). The dose–response curve saturates at high doses, and recommended dosages are close to providing a ceiling effect (Eisenberg *et al* 1994). However, the incidence of adverse effects increases in an approximately linear fashion with the dose (Henry *et al* 1996; Henry and McGettigan 2003). Thus, there is a ceiling effect on the analgesic efficacy but not on the adverse effects. Therefore, general principles of NSAID use include:

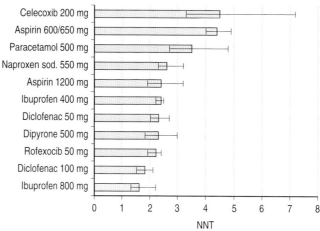

Fig. 15.2 • Number needed to treat (NNT) for one patient to achieve at least 50% pain relief, ±95% confidence interval (CI), for non-opioid analgesics at usual recommended doses.

Data from Collins *et al* (2000b), Barden *et al* (2003, 2004, 2005) and Mason *et al* (2004).

- Use the lowest effective dose for the shortest possible duration; and
- After observing initial response and side effects, titrate the dose and frequency so as to meet the needs of the individual patient.

4.1.1. Ibuprofen

Ibuprofen is a prototypical NSAID and represents the gold standard against which new analgesic agents are evaluated for efficacy in acute orofacial pain (Dionne and Berthold 2001; Zelenakas *et al* 2004). Ibuprofen is one of the most commonly prescribed NSAIDs for dental pain and this drug is widely available over the counter (OTC, i.e. without prescription) around the world. It has been shown that ibuprofen is an effective analgesic in the control of postoperative dental pain in a number of clinical trials (Winter *et al* 1978; Seymour *et al* 1996; Hersh *et al* 2000). Ibuprofen 400mg is apparently the most suitable dose after third molar surgery; 200mg did not differ from placebo and there is little analgesic advantage in increasing the dose to 600mg (Seymour *et al* 1996). Ibuprofen 800mg is, however, extremely effective in acute pain and may be indicated in moderate to severe cases (Fig. 15.2). Analgesic efficacy relative to placebo is similar for ibuprofen 400mg (NNT 2.4, CI: 2.3–2.6), diclofenac 50mg (NNT 2.3, CI: 2.0–2.7) and naproxen sodium 550 mg (NNT 2.6, CI: 2.2–3.2) (Collins *et al* 2000a). Ibuprofen 400mg is, however, superior to paracetamol 500mg (NNT 3.5, CI: 2.7–4.8) and aspirin 600/650mg (NNT 4.4, CI: 4.0–4.9) (Collins *et al* 2000a; Barden *et al* 2004; Mason *et al* 2004). Overall, ibuprofen was associated with the lowest relative GI risk, followed by diclofenac. Indeed, ibuprofen in dosages of 800–1200mg per day over 1–10 days duration has an excellent GI safety profile not significantly different from placebo (Kellstein *et al* 1999). Other NSAIDs such as ketoprofen and piroxicam ranked

Table 15.1 Doses and Medical Considerations of Common Analgesics

Drug	Dose (mg)[a]	Maintenance Dose (In mg × Dosages per day)[b]	Medical Considerations[c]	Pregnancy[d] Category	Pregnancy[d] Comment	Breast Feeding	Common Side Effects[e]
Ibuprofen	400	400 × 4	RI, AIA, CIU GI, Asthma	D	DA 3rd	Minimal	CSE, stomatitis
Naproxen Na	275–550	a. 275 × 3 b. 550 × 2	RI, Hep GI, Asthma	B	DA 3rd	Minimal	
Naproxen	250–500	a. 250 × 3 b. 500 × 2					
Etodolac	200 400	a. 200 × 3 b. 400 × 3	CV, GI, Neu, Asthma	C	DA	Unclear	CSE, malaise, flatulence
Etodolac ER[f]	400–1000	once daily					
Indomethacin	25–50	a. 25 × 3 b. 50 × 3	CV, GI, Asthma, AIA	B	DA 3rd	Minimal	CSE, fatigue, depression
Diclofenac[g]	25–50	a. 25 × 3 or 4 b. 50 × 2 or 3	CV, GI, Asthma, AIA	C	DA 3rd	Unclear	CSE, flatulence
Diclofenac SR[f]	100	1 daily					
Celecoxib	400	200 × 2	AIA, CIU, Sulfa	C	CI	CI	CSE, pharyngitis
Etoricoxib	120	a. 60 × 1 b. 120 × 1	Asthma, AIA, CIU, CV, GI, Prothrombotic	NS	CI	CI	CSE, taste disturbance, flatulence, fatigue
Lumiracoxib	400	a. 200 × 1 b. 400 × 1	GI, AIA, CIU, CV, Prothrombotic	NS		Unknown	CSE
Acetaminophen[h]	500 1000	a. 500 × 4 b. 1000 × 4	RI, Derm, alcohol, Hypothermia	A	Avoid frequent use in third trimester	Minimal	Rash, hypothermia
Dipyrone	500 1000	a. 500 × 4 b. 1000 × 4	Haem, G6PD, Hep	NS		Unclear	Rash, GI, AGRAN, AN

[a] For moderate to severe pain.

[b] Alternative regimens, when available, are shown as a, b.

[c] RI, renal insufficiency; AIA, aspirin-induced asthma; CIU, chronic idiopathic urticaria; GI, gastrointestinal; Hep, liver disease; CV, cardiovascular; Neu, neurological; Derm, dermatologic; Haem, haematologic; G6PD, glucose-6-phosphate dehydrogenase deficiency; alcohol, abusers (>3 drinks daily).

[d] According to the American or Australian food and drug administrations and United Kingdom product labelling. DA, use in late pregnancy may induce premature closure of the ductus arteriosus. 3rd, use in third trimester may delay birth.

[e] CSE: Common side effects of all NSAIDs include oedema, gastrointestinal complaints (abdominal pain, diarrhoea, constipation, dyspepsia, heartburn, nausea, vomiting), rashes or pruritus, tinnitus, dizziness, somnolence, headache and increased liver function tests. AGRAN, agranulocytosis; AN, anaemia.

[f] Extended or modified release formulation.

[g] Diclofenac is also available in 50 and 75 mg with 200 μg misoprostol—this formulation is contraindicated during pregnancy.

[h] Contraindicated in first and second trimesters unless the potential benefit to the patient outweighs the potential risk to the foetus.

highest for risk and indomethacin, naproxen, sulindac and aspirin occupied intermediate positions. Higher doses of ibuprofen (>1200 mg/d) were associated with relative risks similar to those with naproxen and indomethacin (Henry et al 1996). In summary, extensive epidemiological data on efficacy and safety support the use of 400 mg of ibuprofen first when choosing an NSAID (Henry et al 1996). Recent evidence points to an increased risk for serious CV events with ibuprofen particularly at

high doses (Juni et al 2005; Kearney et al 2006; McGettigan and Henry 2006).

Clinical considerations. For mild to moderate pain 400 mg as an initial dose followed by 400 mg orally every 4 hours or as needed is effective. Strong pain may be treated with an 800 mg initial dose. Analgesic onset occurs within 30 minutes (Malmstrom et al 2004a).

Common side effects of ibuprofen include oedema, GI complaints (abdominal pain, diarrhoea, constipation, dyspepsia, heartburn, nausea, vomiting), rashes or pruritus, tinnitus, dizziness, somnolence, headache and increased liver function tests. Rarer but serious side effects include CV events, GI ulceration, anaemia, agranulocytosis, leukopenia, hepatitis and depression. Erythema multiforme or Stevens-Johnson syndrome has also been reported. Severe, even fatal, anaphylactic-like reactions have been reported in patients who have experienced asthma, urticaria or allergic-type reactions after taking aspirin or other nonsteroidal anti-inflammatory agents. Treatment of patients with renal impairment should be coordinated with the treating physician and initiated at the lowest recommended dosage. The patient must be monitored closely and dosage reduced if necessary. Ibuprofen should be avoided in late pregnancy particularly as it may cause premature closure of the ductus arteriosus (Pregnancy Category: D). As for all NSAIDS, ibuprofen may delay the onset of childbirth. The danger for breastfeeding infants is minimal.

4.1.2. Naproxen

Meta-analysis of six trials that compared naproxen sodium 550 mg with placebo gave an NNT of 2.6 (95% CI: 2.2–3.2) (Mason *et al* 2003, 2004). Naproxen sodium is more suitable for treatment of acute pain than naproxen due to an earlier onset of analgesia (30 minutes versus 1 hour, respectively). The analgesic efficacy and onset are similar to that of ibuprofen 400 mg (Fig. 15.2) but naproxen produces a longer duration of analgesia. Weighted mean time to re-medication for naproxen sodium 550 mg was 7.6 hours compared with 2.6 hours for placebo, and the effects of one dose last, on average, up to 7 hours (Mason *et al* 2003, 2004). It was concluded that naproxen sodium 440–550 mg and naproxen 400 mg administered orally are effective analgesics for the treatment of acute postoperative pain in adults. A low incidence of adverse events was found with no significant difference between treatment and placebo, but reporting was inconsistent (Mason *et al* 2003).

Clinical considerations. For mild to moderate pain an initial dose of naproxen sodium 550 mg will provide efficient and rapid analgesia. Maintenance of relief may be obtained with 275 mg of naproxen sodium orally every 6–8 hours or 550 mg every 12 hours as needed. Its long half-life may offer some advantages. There is evidence that naproxen may also possess fewer CV complications for both short- and long-term therapy (Juni *et al* 2005; Kearney *et al* 2006; McGettigan and Henry 2006). This may therefore lead to naproxen becoming the NSAID of choice, particularly in at-risk individuals (Antman *et al* 2007), but the evidence must be regularly reviewed by clinicians. Doses should not exceed 1350 mg/d initially, then 1100 mg/d. Alternatively, in order to reduce sodium consumption, maintenance may be performed with naproxen 250 mg orally every 6–8 hours or 500 mg every 12 hours as needed.

Common side effects of naproxen include oedema, GI complaints (abdominal pain, diarrhoea, constipation, dyspepsia, heartburn, nausea, vomiting), stomatitis, rashes or pruritus, tinnitus, dizziness, somnolence, headache and increased liver function tests. Rarer but serious side effects include CV events, GI ulceration, anaemia, agranulocytosis, leukopenia, hepatitis and depression. Stevens-Johnson syndrome as well as severe, even fatal, anaphylactic-like reactions have been reported in patients who had experienced asthma, urticaria or allergic-type reactions after taking aspirin or other nonsteroidal anti-inflammatory agents. Naproxen should be used only if absolutely necessary and with caution in patients with a history of asthma. Geriatric patients should not exceed 200 mg every 12 hours. Patients with liver disease or renal impairment may require dosage reduction and need to be monitored closely; such cases should be treated in conjunction with the treating physician. Naproxen should be avoided in late pregnancy particularly as it may cause premature closure of the ductus arteriosus (Pregnancy Category: B). As for all NSAIDs, naproxen may delay the onset of childbirth. The danger for breastfeeding infants is minimal.

4.1.3. Etodolac

Etodolac, a pyrano-indoleacetic acid derivative, is a member of a new class of NSAIDs that preferentially inhibit COX-2 (Riendeau *et al* 2001). Etodolac is approved by the US Food and Drug Administration (FDA) for treating acute pain, in adults but not children. Some studies have indicated a more rapid onset of analgesic action with etodolac 200 mg and significantly better analgesic efficacy compared to aspirin 650 mg (Gaston *et al* 1986); however, other studies have not confirmed these findings (Hutton 1983). The analgesic efficacy of etodolac 200 mg is comparable to paracetamol 600 mg plus codeine 60 mg, and etodolac 400 mg is significantly superior to the latter combination (Mizraji 1990). Etodolac possesses a more favourable therapeutic index between anti-inflammatory effects and gastric irritation than other NSAIDs (Martel and Klicius 1982).

Clinical considerations. Etodolac is also available in an extended (modified) release formulation. For mild to moderate acute pain it is advisable to use the immediate release formulation: 200–400 mg orally every 6–8 hours as needed up to a maximum of 1200 mg/d. Maintenance can also be performed with the extended release formulation: for adults over 50 kg in weight 800–1200 mg every 24 hours.

Common side effects of etodolac include GI complaints (abdominal pain, diarrhoea, dyspepsia, flatulence, nausea) and malaise. Oedema has been reported with the use of etodolac so it should be avoided in patients with CV disease. Rarer but serious side effects include bronchospasm, CV events, GI ulceration, anaemia, agranulocytosis, leukopenia, hepatitis and depression.

Stevens-Johnson syndrome and toxic epidermal necrolysis have also been reported. As for other NSAIDs etodolac is to be avoided in late pregnancy since it may cause premature closure of the ductus arteriosus (Pregnancy Category: C). The danger for breastfeeding infants is minimal.

4.1.4. Diclofenac

Diclofenac is a preferential COX-2 inhibitor that has been extensively used for the treatment of acute and chronic inflammatory pain. Diclofenac is FDA approved for rheumatoid and osteoarthritis, ankylosing spondylitis, inflammatory disorder of the eye and refractive keratoplasty. In addition to standard (12.5, 25, 50, 75 mg) and slow release (100 mg) formulations, diclofenac is available as suppositories and a 1% topical gel (see Chapter 16). For patients with GI discomfort diclofenac is available as 50 or 75 mg with 200 µg of misoprostol, a gastroprotective prostaglandin analogue.

Clinical considerations. Diclofenac is efficacious in acute pain; the analgesic efficacy of diclofenac 50 mg (NNT 2.3, CI: 2.0–2.7) is similar to that of ibuprofen 400 mg or naproxen sodium 550 mg (Collins *et al* 2000a). It may be prescribed as 25–50 mg three times daily or as once-daily dosage of 100 mg of its slow release formulation.

Diclofenac is usually well tolerated with relatively few GI side effects but may cause dyspepsia, nausea, abdominal pain and constipation. However, GI bleeding and perforation have been reported. Headache, dizziness and drowsiness are common side effects. It is contraindicated in patients who have experienced asthma, urticaria or allergic-type reactions after taking aspirin or other nonsteroidal anti-inflammatory agents; severe, even fatal, anaphylactic-like reactions have been reported. Recently diclofenac has been shown to significantly increase the risk of serious CV events (Andersohn *et al* 2006; Helin-Salmivaara *et al* 2006; Kearney *et al* 2006; McGettigan and Henry 2006) and has also been associated with fluid retention and oedema. Increased liver function tests are commonly observed but hepatitis is relatively uncommon. Stevens-Johnson syndrome and toxic epidermal necrolysis have also been reported.

Diclofenac should be avoided in late pregnancy particularly as it may cause premature closure of the ductus arteriosus (Pregnancy Category: B). As for all NSAIDs, it may delay the onset of childbirth. The diclofenac/misoprostol combination is contraindicated in pregnancy. The risks of diclofenac for lactating infants are unclear.

4.1.5. Indomethacin

Currently indomethacin is largely unused in routine dentistry or indeed for the control of any acute pain due to commonly occurring and significant side effects. However, its important diagnostic and therapeutic role in paroxysmal hemicrania and hemicrania continua mandates a brief review. Indomethacin is FDA-approved for rheumatoid and osteoarthritis, gout, ankylosing spondylitis, patent ductus arteriosus and acute shoulder pain.

Indomethacin has been shown to experimentally block neurogenic inflammation (Buzzi *et al* 1989). Data from animal and human experiments have shown that IV indomethacin produces rapid, significant reductions (26–40%) in cerebral blood flow (Wennmalm *et al* 1984; Slavik and Rhoney 1999; Speziale *et al* 1999). Indomethacin also possesses non-cyclooxygenase-based modes of action that may differentially modulate blood vessels (Feigen *et al* 1981; Quintana *et al* 1983, 1988). An interaction between indomethacin and nitric oxide (NO), involved in headache pathogenesis, has been proposed (Castellano *et al* 1998). Findings from an experimental pain model suggest that an interaction between indomethacin and local NO synthesis is involved in the antinociceptive effects of indomethacin (Ventura-Martinez *et al* 2004).

Clinical considerations. Indomethacin is available in standard and slow release formulations (75 mg) and additionally as suppositories. Standard dosages are 25–50 mg twice or three times daily. In paroxysmal hemicrania (see Chapter 10) most cases will respond to 25 mg three times daily within 24 hours; however, therapy should be continued for 3 days at 75 mg followed, if needed, by 150 mg for a further 3 days (Pareja and Sjaastad 1996).

Adverse effects are probably more frequent with indomethacin than with most other NSAIDs. The most common are GI disturbances (abdominal pain, constipation, diarrhoea, dyspepsia, nausea, vomiting), headache, vertigo, dizziness and lightheadedness. More serious but rarer events include GI perforation, ulceration and bleeding. Rectal irritation and bleeding have been reported occasionally in patients who have received indomethacin suppositories. Other adverse effects include depression, drowsiness, tinnitus, confusion, insomnia, oedema and weight gain, hypertension, haematuria and stomatitis. Indomethacin may increase the risk of serious CV events and is to be avoided in at-risk patients (Helin-Salmivaara *et al* 2006; McGettigan and Henry 2006). Indomethacin is contraindicated in patients who have experienced asthma, urticaria or allergic-type reactions after taking aspirin or other nonsteroidal anti-inflammatory agents; severe, even fatal, anaphylactic-like reactions have been reported. Serious skin reactions such as Stevens-Johnson syndrome and toxic epidermal necrolysis are rare. No dose adjustment is needed in renal disease but indomethacin should be used with caution in hepatic disease; the elderly require a 25% dose reduction. A complaint of blurred vision may be an early symptom of indomethacin-related corneal deposits and warrants evaluation by an ophthalmologist; these effects are reversible.

Indomethacin should be avoided in late pregnancy particularly as it may cause premature closure of the ductus arteriosus (Pregnancy Category: B). As for all NSAIDs, indomethacin may delay the onset of childbirth.

Maternal indomethacin is considered compatible with breastfeeding.

4.2. Selective COX-2 Inhibitors (Coxibs)

The documentation of significantly increased cardiovascular and renal risks with COX-2 inhibitors has raised important issues relating to their continued use, particularly for chronic pain (McGettigan and Henry 2006; Zhang et al 2006). Moreover the lack of any significant increase in analgesic efficacy of COX-2 inhibitors over the classical NSAIDs suggests that we should probably stay with the well-researched older NSAIDs such as ibuprofen and naproxen. Recent meta-analyses also show that adverse CV events associated with COX-2 inhibitors actually occur quite quickly after initiation of therapy and not months afterwards as was initially claimed (McGettigan and Henry 2006). This raises the important question whether COX-2 inhibitors should be used at all for pain control (Graham 2006). Our approach has been to first employ conventional NSAIDs particularly ibuprofen and naproxen. Emerging evidence of CV safety would suggest that naproxen is presently the drug of choice. However, the COX-2 inhibitors are still widely available and are extensively used particularly in patients with GI problems.

4.2.1. Rofecoxib

Rofecoxib was voluntarily withdrawn by the manufacturer in 2004 due to safety concerns of an increased risk for CV events, including heart attack and stroke. However, rofecoxib's effectiveness for acute pain is excellent and as one of the first selective COX-2 inhibitors it deserves brief review.

The NNT for rofecoxib 50 mg versus placebo was found to be 2.2 (95% CI: 1.9–2.4) (Barden et al 2005) with a median time to onset of analgesia of 34 minutes (Desjardins et al 2005). After surgical extraction of third molars rofecoxib 50 mg demonstrated significantly better analgesic efficacy and duration than celecoxib 400 mg (Malmstrom et al 2002), enteric-coated diclofenac sodium (as a single 50-mg dose and 3×50 mg doses) (Chang et al 2002) and codeine/acetaminophen 60/600 mg (Chang et al 2005). The overall analgesic efficacy of rofecoxib 50 mg was similar to that of ibuprofen 400 mg but lasted significantly longer (up to 24 hours). A further study showed that 50 mg rofecoxib was the lowest dose that reproducibly demonstrated an analgesic effect comparable to that of naproxen sodium 550 mg or ibuprofen 400 mg (Morrison et al 2000).

4.2.2. Celecoxib

Ibuprofen 1200 mg per day ('liquigel') was compared to a single dose of celecoxib (200 mg) and placebo in patients with moderate or severe pain following surgical extraction of impacted third molars (Doyle et al 2002). Time to meaningful relief was significantly shorter, and the mean 4-, 8-, and 12-hour summed pain relief combined with pain intensity difference scores were significantly higher for ibuprofen liquigel than for celecoxib. Both active treatments were significantly more effective than placebo, well tolerated with no differences in incidence or severity of adverse events. Ibuprofen 400–600 mg has been shown superior to celecoxib 200–400 mg, respectively (Khan et al 2002; Malmstrom et al 2002). Similarly, rofecoxib 50 mg has greater overall analgesic efficacy than celecoxib 400 mg, as well as a significantly longer duration of analgesic effect (Malmstrom et al 2002).

A recent systematic review concluded that celecoxib 200 mg is an effective means of postoperative pain relief, similar in efficacy to aspirin 600/650 mg, and paracetamol 1000 mg. The NNT for celecoxib 200 mg was 4.5 (CI: 3.3–7.2). However, the trials included used celecoxib 200 mg, half the recommended dose for acute pain. More trials are needed to estimate efficacy for 400 mg and provide data for pooled quantitative estimates of adverse effects (Barden et al 2003). Importantly it seems that although 200 mg celecoxib is safe in terms of CV events, 400 mg significantly increases the risk for serious CV events (McGettigan and Henry 2006). Celecoxib is therefore inferior to first-line NSAIDs, such as naproxen or ibuprofen, both in analgesic efficacy and safety profile so it is rarely employed for pain control.

Clinical considerations. For mild to moderate acute pain an initial dose of 400 mg orally once plus 1 additional 200 mg dose as needed on the first day is recommended. Maintenance may be achieved by 200 mg twice a day as needed.

Common side effects of celecoxib include oedema, GI complaints (abdominal pain, diarrhoea, dyspepsia, flatulence, nausea), rash, dizziness, headache, insomnia and respiratory problems (pharyngitis, sinusitis, rhinitis). Rarer but serious side effects include CV events, GI ulceration, anaemia, increased liver function tests and hepatitis. Severe, even fatal, anaphylactic-like reactions have been reported in patients who have experienced asthma, urticaria or allergic-type reactions after taking aspirin or other nonsteroidal anti-inflammatory agents. Erythema multiforme or Stevens-Johnson syndrome has also been reported. Celecoxib is contraindicated in patients with hypersensitivity to sulphonamides and in asthmatics. Patients with a history of urticaria or allergic-type reactions after taking aspirin or other nonsteroidal anti-inflammatory agents are at risk of severe, even fatal, anaphylactic-like reactions. Celecoxib is in pregnancy category C but many consider all COX-2 contraindicated during pregnancy. Use during breastfeeding is contraindicated.

4.2.3. Valdecoxib

Valdecoxib was voluntarily withdrawn in 2005 due to safety concerns of increased risk of CV events, and reports of serious and potentially life-threatening skin reactions, including death. Valdecoxib is a new highly selective COX-2 inhibitor with a rapid onset of action and significant analgesic properties. In patients with rheumatoid arthritis, valdecoxib 10, 20 or 40 mg/d was significantly more effective than placebo, and similar in efficacy to naproxen 500 mg twice daily; there were no significant differences in efficacy between the three dosages of valdecoxib (Ormrod *et al* 2002).

Patients undergoing oral surgery and receiving valdecoxib 40 mg experienced a significantly quicker onset of analgesia, significantly improved pain relief and lower pain intensity than did patients receiving rofecoxib 50 mg (Fricke *et al* 2002). Valdecoxib, rofecoxib and placebo were equally well tolerated.

Following oral surgery, subjects receiving valdecoxib (20 or 40 mg) experienced a rapid onset of analgesia and, at valdecoxib 40 mg, a level of pain relief comparable with that of those who received oxycodone/acetaminophen (10 mg/1000 mg) (Daniels *et al* 2002). Both valdecoxib doses had a significantly longer duration of analgesic effect than did oxycodone/acetaminophen. Pooled safety data demonstrated that each valdecoxib dose had a tolerability profile superior to that of oxycodone/acetaminophen and similar to that of placebo.

4.2.4. Etoricoxib

Etoricoxib is a novel COX-2 inhibitor with high selectivity for COX-2 (106 COX-2/COX-1 ratio, as compared to 35 for rofecoxib or 1.78 for ibuprofen), and is as effective as ibuprofen and naproxen and more effective than acetaminophen for arthritic pain (Cochrane *et al* 2002).

In patients, after extraction of two or more third molars etoricoxib 120 mg and oxycodone/acetaminophen 10/650 mg achieved significant analgesia with a rapid onset, although the time was slightly faster for oxycodone/acetaminophen (Chang *et al* 2004). The peak effect was similar for both drugs. Oxycodone/acetaminophen treatment resulted in more frequent drug-related nausea and vomiting compared with etoricoxib treatment (Chang *et al* 2004).

The duration of analgesic effect after third molar extractions, defined as median time to rescue medication use, was >24 hours for etoricoxib 120 mg, 20.8 hours for naproxen sodium 550 mg, 3.6 hours for acetaminophen/codeine 600/60 mg and 1.6 hours for placebo. All three active treatments had rapid onset of analgesia (Malmstrom *et al* 2004a). The median time to onset of analgesia for etoricoxib 120–240 mg is about 25–30 minutes (Malmstrom *et al* 2004a,b). There were no significant differences in the onset of analgesia between etoricoxib and ibuprofen. The duration of analgesic effect was >24 hours for etoricoxib 120–240 mg, and 12.1 hours for etoricoxib 60 mg. The duration of effect was significantly longer with all four etoricoxib doses than with ibuprofen (Malmstrom *et al* 2004b). Etoricoxib 120 mg provided superior overall analgesic effect with a smaller percentage of patients experiencing nausea compared to both oxycodone/

acetaminophen 10/650 mg and codeine/acetaminophen 60/600 mg (Malmstrom *et al* 2005). Based on these placebo-controlled studies we calculated a mean NNT of 1.6 for good to excellent pain relief at 8 hours using 120 mg etoricoxib and an NNT of 1.4 using 180 mg etoricoxib (Malmstrom *et al* 2004a,b, 2005). These attractive NNTs must, however, be taken together with NNTs for the active controls in these studies that were similarly low: 1.4 for 550 mg naproxen sodium, 1.7 for 400 mg ibuprofen and 1.6 for an oxycodone/paracetamol 10/650 mg combination.

Clinical considerations. The optimal doses of etoricoxib have not been clearly established. An oral dose of 120 mg has been effective in acute post-dental surgery with a rapid onset (25–30 minutes) with no significant benefit obtained at higher doses (180 or 240 mg). Its long half-life offers the possibility of once-daily dosing.

GI effects (nausea, vomiting, diarrhoea, flatulence, taste disturbances, decreased appetite), headache, dizziness and fatigue have been reported but are relatively rare. Whether etoricoxib is as problematic in terms of CV safety as the earlier COX-2 drugs is unclear. Early data suggest that etoricoxib is indeed associated with thromboembolic events and an increased CV risk and we advise great caution until further data accumulate (Andersohn *et al* 2006; Helin-Salmivaara *et al* 2006). Etoricoxib is contraindicated in patients with a history of bronchospasm, rhinoconjunctivitis or urticaria/angioedema associated with aspirin or other NSAIDs due to a risk of anaphylactic-like reactions. A history of adult-onset asthma, chronic rhinitis, nasal polyps and chronic urticaria/angioedema predispose to these reactions. It is also contraindicated in patients with hypertension, recent MI, angina or other CV disease due to a potential for fluid retention and the possibility of prothrombotic activity. Etoricoxib has not been categorized for use in pregnancy; however, many consider all COX-2 contraindicated during pregnancy. Similarly, use during breastfeeding is contraindicated.

4.2.5. Lumiracoxib

Lumiracoxib is a new coxib with even higher COX-2 selectivity (COX-2/COX-1 ratio=700) (Stichtenoth and Frolich 2003). In patients with postoperative dental pain lumiracoxib 100 mg was comparable to ibuprofen 400 mg but lumiracoxib 400 mg was superior to both (Zelenakas *et al* 2004). Lumiracoxib 400 mg demonstrated the fastest time to analgesic onset (37.4 min) followed by ibuprofen then lumiracoxib 100 mg (Zelenakas *et al* 2004).

Following third molar extraction a single oral dose of lumiracoxib 400 mg was superior to rofecoxib 50 mg, celecoxib 200 mg or placebo at 8 hours post dose (Kellstein *et al* 2004). Lumiracoxib demonstrated the fastest onset of analgesia and the longest time to rescue medication use. Patient global evaluation of lumiracoxib was comparable to rofecoxib and superior to celecoxib and placebo.

All treatments were well tolerated. A recent review (Bannwarth and Berenbaum 2005) found that in patients with acute pain related to primary dysmenorrhoea or dental or orthopaedic surgery, lumiracoxib 400mg/d was at least as effective as standard doses of traditional NSAIDs and other coxibs.

Endoscopic studies have indicated that lumiracoxib is associated with a rate of gastroduodenal ulcer formation significantly lower than that with ibuprofen and does not differ from celecoxib. The cumulative 1-year incidence of ulcer complications (primary endpoint) was significantly reduced by approximately threefold on lumiracoxib 400mg/d compared with naproxen 1000 mg/d or ibuprofen 2400mg/d. Regarding CV events there was no significant difference between lumiracoxib and combined NSAIDs.

Clinical considerations. A single dose of lumiracoxib 400mg is an effective analgesic for mild to moderate pain (extraction of impacted third molars). Analgesic onset occurs in about 35 minutes with about 12 hours duration. If needed, maintenance may be obtained with 200–400mg daily. Lumiracoxib is contraindicated in acute peptic ulcer or GI bleeding as it may delay healing. As with other NSAIDs a history of bronchospasm with rhinoconjunctivitis or urticaria/angioedema associated with aspirin or other nonsteroidal anti-inflammatory agents carries a high risk of anaphylactic-like reactions.

Side effects of lumiracoxib include abdominal pain that may rarely reflect GI ulceration. Because of its potential to induce fluid retention and prothrombotic activity lumiracoxib is contraindicated in patients with hypertension, recent MI, angina or other CV disease. There is no available data on the use of lumiracoxib in pregnancy and breastfeeding. However, in view of the contraindications to other selective COX-2 inhibitors we suggest not to use these drugs in pregnant or lactating mothers till further data are collected. It should be noted that the last two drugs (etoricoxib and lumiracoxib) have yet to be approved by the US FDA (Huber and Terezhalmy 2006).

4.3. Dual-Acting NSAIDs

As discussed earlier the standard NSAIDs and the newer selective COX-2 inhibitors are associated with a number of severe GI, CV and renal side effects. This is due to the inhibition of protective prostaglandins and the unchecked effects of specific leukotrienes on the gastric mucosa. Additionally the proalgesic and proinflammatory effects of the leukotrienes are largely unaffected by these drugs. Drugs acting on both COX and lipo-oxygenase enzymes are an attractive option and are collectively referred to as dual-acting NSAIDs (Bertolini *et al* 2001; Charlier and Michaux 2003). The dual-acting NSAIDs are still in the experimental stage but show promising results in animal models of pain and osteoarthritis (Hinz and Brune 2004; Moreau *et al* 2006; Singh *et al* 2006).

4.4. Conclusions

Significant advances in the understanding of COXs and prostaglandins have led to the development of the specific COX-2 inhibitors. Yet the nonselective NSAIDs remain a reliable class of analgesics due to their predictability and tolerability (Gotzsche 2005). Important differences in adverse effects exist between different NSAIDs and depend amongst other factors on their selectivity for the different COXs. As reviewed earlier, however, the analgesic efficacy of NSAIDs and the newer COX-2 inhibitors seems similar. These differences have a major effect on our considerations; for example, reduction in ulcers with COX-2 inhibitors should be weighed against their potential increase in CV risk compared with the older NSAIDs (Juni *et al* 2005). The medical history of the patient is therefore mandatory, and provides the most important consideration for selection of the proper analgesic (Antman *et al* 2007).

Ibuprofen remains the gold 'analgesic' standard against which new pain relieving drugs are evaluated (Dionne and Berthold 2001; Zelenakas *et al* 2004). However, naproxen has been shown in most studies not to increase CV risk and is thus the NSAID of choice, particularly in at-risk individuals (Graham *et al* 2005; Kearney *et al* 2006; McGettigan and Henry 2006). Unless there is a specific contraindication to their use, short-term NSAIDs are effective for treating acute dental pain in ambulatory patients who generally experience a higher incidence of adverse effects after ingesting an opioid analgesic (Dionne and Berthold 2001; Savage and Henry 2004). COX-2 inhibitors do not posses any additional efficacy over traditional NSAIDs, except for a longer duration of analgesia in single-dose studies (Romsing and Moiniche 2004). Ibuprofen 400mg is considered the first-line NSAID based on its good safety profile, high efficacy and low cost (Sachs 2005). The evidence to date fails to demonstrate any therapeutic advantage of COX-2 inhibitors over ibuprofen in the treatment of acute dental pain (Huber and Terezhalmy 2006). Accumulating evidence continues to support that naproxen is not cardioprotective as once thought. In most studies naproxen does not increase the risk for serious CV events, suggesting that it may be safer than other NSAIDs (Graham 2006). However, recent data indicate that naproxen does have potentially serious CV complications (ADAPT 2006).

5. Paracetamol (Acetaminophen)

Single doses of paracetamol are effective analgesics for acute postoperative pain and with few adverse effects. Paracetamol is generally considered to be a weak inhibitor of the synthesis of prostaglandins. Indeed, paracetamol fails to inhibit the formation of PGs in peripheral tissues and does not suppress the inflammation of rheumatoid arthritis (Flower *et al* 1972). It does, however, decrease postoperative swelling in humans and suppresses inflammation in rats and mice (Graham and Scott 2005). Paracetamol depresses nociceptive activity evoked in thalamic neurons by electrical stimulation of nociceptive afferents, and presents evidence for a central analgesic effect independent of endogenous opioids (Carlsson and Jurna 1987). COX-3, a splice variant of COX-1, has been suggested to be the target of paracetamol's action (Chandrasekharan et al 2002), but genomic and kinetic analysis indicates that this selective interaction is unlikely to be clinically relevant (Graham and Scott 2005). There is considerable evidence that the analgesic effect of paracetamol is central and is due to activation of descending serotonergic pathways, but its primary site of action may still be inhibition of PG synthesis (Libert et al 2004; Graham and Scott 2005).

Forty-seven reports were included in a recent systematic review of paracetamol (Barden et al 2004). The NNT over 4–6 hours following a single dose of paracetamol 500 mg was 3.5 (2.7–4.8) and increasing doses up to 1500 mg did not result in better NNTs. Studies report a variable incidence of adverse effects that are generally mild and transient and there were no statistically significant differences between paracetamol 975/1000 mg and placebo. Other reviews demonstrate similar ranges of efficacy with NNTs of 3.5–5.0 for 600–1000 mg of paracetamol (Moore et al 1997, 2000).

Paracetamol 975/1000 mg is as effective as aspirin 600/650 mg (NNT 4.4, CI: 4.0–4.9), but less effective than ibuprofen 400 mg (NNT 2.4, CI: 2.3–2.6), and diclofenac 50 mg (NNT 2.3, CI: 2.0–2.7); see Fig. 15.2 (Barden et al 2004). Paracetamol is known to have fewer long-term GI adverse effects than other NSAID treatment options, though long-term use is associated with renal and hepatic problems. Ibuprofen liquigel 200/400 mg provided greater overall and peak analgesic effects with a more rapid onset to

analgesia than did acetaminophen 1000 mg following surgical removal of impacted third molars (Hersh et al 2000).

A recent qualitative review of head-to-head comparisons of paracetamol with NSAIDs found that of 16 dental studies, 8 showed that NSAIDs were superior to paracetamol, 5 showed equal results and 2 showed paracetamol was superior to NSAIDs (Hyllested et al 2002). NSAIDs therefore seem to be superior to paracetamol in dental surgery, regarding both pain scores and re-medication (Hyllested et al 2002). On the other hand, a recent crossover study of 36 patients subjected to surgical removal of bilateral third molars, and acting as their own controls, compared the effects of ibuprofen $600 \text{ mg} \times 4/\text{d}$ with those of paracetamol $1000 \text{ mg} \times 4/\text{d}$, and found no significant differences in pain scores or swelling between the two drugs (Bjornsson et al 2003).

Paracetamol is therefore a viable alternative to the NSAIDs, especially because of the low incidence of adverse effects, and should be the preferred choice in high-risk patients (Hyllested et al 2002); see also Table 15.2. For example, the sustained use of paracetamol during oral anticoagulant therapy in itself does not provoke clinically relevant INR changes (Gadisseur et al 2003). Furthermore, based on the data available to date, it still seems prudent to use NSAIDs only in those patients in whom there is good evidence of improved efficacy over paracetamol (Nikles et al 2005). The use of high-dose paracetamol (4 g daily) for 4 or more days is, however, associated with increased levels of alanine aminotransferase, suggesting significant liver toxicity (Watkins et al 2006).

The available evidence supports the use of acetaminophen in doses up to 1000 mg as the initial choice for mild to moderate acute pain. In some cases, modest improvements in analgesic efficacy can be achieved by adding or changing to an NSAID.

Table 15.2 Pharmacotherapeutic Strategy for the Management of Acute Orofacial Pain

Pain Intensity	Options	Healthy Patient	Gastrointestinal Limitations	Cardiovascular Limitations	Anticoagulants	Asthma, Urticaria or Angioedema
Mild to moderate	1st 2nd 3rd	Paracetamol 500 mg Ibuprofen 400 mg Naproxen 500 mg	Paracetamol 500 mg COX-2 inhibitor Naproxen/ibuprofen with proton pump inhibitor	Paracetamol 500 mg Naproxen 500 mg	Paracetamol 500 mg COX-2 inhibitor	COX-2 inhibitor[a] Paracetamol 500 mg[b]
Moderate to severe	1st 2nd	Ibuprofen 800 mg Oxycodone 5 mg paracetamol 500 mg	Oxycodone 5 mg paracetamol 500 g Dipyrone 500–1000 mg	Oxycodone 5 mg paracetamol 500 mg Dipyrone 500–1000 mg	Oxycodone 5 mg paracetamol 500 mg COX-2 inhibitor	COX-2 inhibitor[a] Oxycodone 5 mg paracetamol 500 mg[b]

[a] There is a standard warning against use of COX-2 inhibitors in cases of asthma and urticaria. However, this warning could not be validated by several controlled studies that found rofecoxib, celecoxib and etoricoxib safe in these cases (Martin-Garcia et al 2002; Martin-Garcia et al 2003; Celik et al 2005; Sanchez-Borges et al 2005).

[b] Paracetamol demonstrates cross reactivity in aspirin-induced asthma but usually at doses higher than 500 mg (Settipane et al 1995).

Clinical considerations. For mild to moderate pain 500–1000 mg orally every 4 hours as needed to a maximum of 4 g/d. Common adverse effects include rash and hypothermia. The use of paracetamol in alcohol abusers (>3 alcoholic drinks per day) is contraindicated. Moreover the observation of elevated liver enzymes during high-dose therapy (4 g daily) is a significant concern in patients with liver disease (Watkins *et al* 2006). Paracetamol is the analgesic of choice during pregnancy or breast-feeding (Pregnancy Category: A). However, frequent use of paracetamol during the last trimester of pregnancy is contraindicated.

6. Dipyrone

Dipyrone, the most widely used pyrazolone derivative, is a rapidly reversible inhibitor of cyclooxygenase (Brogden 1986). Dipyrone possesses analgesic, antipyretic, anti-inflammatory and spasmolytic properties, and is often classified as peripherally acting. For example, it was found that dipyrone inhibited platelet aggregation and markedly decreased TXA_2 synthesis, which is consistent with a competitive inhibitory effect of dipyrone on PG synthetase activity (Eldor *et al* 1984). It has been suggested that a central action is also involved in the analgesic effect of dipyrone, and that this central action manifests itself by an activation of inhibition originating in the periaqueductal grey (Carlsson *et al* 1986). Dipyrone depresses pain-evoked potentials in thalamic neurons but less effectively than morphine (Carlsson *et al* 1988). Naloxone abolishes the depressant effects of morphine but not of dipyrone (Carlsson *et al* 1988). Thus it appears that several mechanisms contribute to the analgesic effect of dipyrone, including the possibility that the effects of dipyrone result from antagonism of the pharmacological effects of PGs rather than from inhibition of their synthesis (Brogden 1986).

Dipyrone is relatively safe for the GI tract. Thus, administered for 2 weeks, dipyrone has effects on the gastric and duodenal mucosa comparable to those of paracetamol and placebo, though noticeable damage is detectable at a dosage of 3 g/d (Bianchi Porro *et al* 1996). Dipyrone is comparable in this respect to paracetamol and much safer than diclofenac (Sanchez *et al* 2002). Dipyrone inhibits platelet aggregation and markedly decreases TXA_2 synthesis (Eldor *et al* 1984).

Pyrazolone hypersensitivity associated with chronic asthma is similar to aspirin-induced asthma and probably involves PG inhibition and overproduction of cysteinyl leukotrienes. Other patients may develop anaphylaxis, urticaria and other forms of rash and the hypersensitivity is due to immunological mechanisms (Czerniawska-Mysik and Szczeklik 1981). However, a mixed form is probably more common. Thus, of patients with dipyrone intolerance with and without asthma, 76% of asthmatics and 9% of non-asthmatics reacted with bronchospasm after ingestion of dipyrone, while urticaria developed in 26% of asthmatics and 65% of non-asthmatics (Karakaya and Kalyoncu 2002).

The use of dipyrone as an analgesic is controversial. It is used most commonly to treat postoperative pain, colic pain, cancer pain and migraine, and in many countries, e.g. Russia, Spain, Brazil, and in many parts of South-America and Africa, it is the most popular non-opioid first-line analgesic. In others it has been banned (e.g. USA, UK) because of its association with potentially life-threatening blood dyscrasias such as agranulocytosis. This side effect is discussed in the section that deals with NSAID-related hypersensitivity reactions. Dipyrone is currently available in Austria, Belgium, France, Germany, Italy, The Netherlands, Spain, Switzerland, South Africa, Latin America, Russia, Israel and India (Edwards *et al* 2001).

Clinical considerations. Dipyrone is effective for adults with moderate to severe postoperative pain, and single-dose oral dipyrone 500 mg was found to be of similar efficacy to ibuprofen 400 mg. Adverse effects were poorly reported but the commonest were drowsiness, gastric discomfort and nausea. For a single oral dose of oral dipyrone 500 mg, the NNT was 2.3 (95% CI: 1.8–3.0) (Edwards *et al* 2001). The risk in pregnant or lactating mothers is unclear.

7. Omega-3 Fatty Acids

Recently, the effect of omega-3 fatty acids as an anti-inflammatory agent has emerged, with the possibility that they may serve as an alternative to NSAIDs for long-term use (Cleland and James 2006; Maroon and Bost 2006). They are not suitable for treatment of acute pain, but their use for chronic pain is further discussed in Chapter 17 on complementary medicine.

8. Opioids

Opiates are drugs derived from opium and include morphine, codeine and a wide variety of semisynthetic congeners derived from them and from thebaine, another component of opium. The term *opioid* is more inclusive, applying to all agonists and antagonists with morphine-like activity as well as to naturally occurring and synthetic opioid peptides. *Endorphin* is a generic term referring to the three families of endogenous opioid peptides: the enkephalins, dynorphins and beta-endorphins.

Multiple opioid receptors. There is convincing evidence for three major classes of opioid receptors in the CNS, designated mu, kappa and delta, as well as indications of subtypes within each class. While the commonly prescribed opioids bind preferentially to the mu receptor, they do associate with all three receptor types (Gourlay 2002). Morphine shows the greatest relative preference for the mu receptor. Codeine displays exceedingly poor binding to opioid receptors, which raises the possibility that it is a prodrug where the pharmacologically active species is morphine (Sindrup and Brosen 1995). A similar situation probably applies to oxycodone, where the metabolite oxymorphone may be responsible for the pharmacological effect. Alternatively, the intrinsic anti-nociceptive effect of oxycodone may be mediated via kappa receptors (Ross and Smith 1997).

Mechanisms and sites of opioid-induced analgesia. Opioid-induced analgesia is due to action at several sites within the CNS; both spinal and multiple supraspinal sites have been identified. Peripherally, opioid receptors on the terminals of primary afferent nerves mediate inhibition of the release of neurotransmitters, including substance P. Morphine also antagonizes the effects of exogenously administered substance P by exerting postsynaptic inhibitory action on interneurons and on the output neurons of the spinothalamic tract that conveys nociceptive information to higher centres in the brain. Morphine selectively inhibits various nociceptive reflexes and induces profound analgesia without affecting other sensory modalities. Intrathecal administration of opioids can produce profound segmental analgesia without causing significant alteration of motor or sensory functions (Yaksh and Rudy 1978).

Tramadol is a synthetic, centrally acting opioid analgesic. However, it only binds weakly to mu opioid receptors and with weak affinity to delta and kappa receptors. Tramadol-induced anti-nociception is mediated by the opioid mu receptor and additionally by non-opioid mechanisms (Raffa 2001). Non-opioid mechanisms include the inhibition of norepinephrine and serotonin pathways within the CNS (Scott and Perry 2000).

8.1. Efficacy for Acute Pain

Traditionally, opioids have been classified as weak and strong opioids. Weak opioids include codeine, dihydrocodeine, dextropropoxyphene and tramadol. Morphine, fentanyl, methadone, oxycodone and buprenorphine are considered strong opioids (Schug and Gandham 2006). The weak opioids are relatively poor analgesics on their own, e.g. codeine 30mg NNT 16.7; tramadol 75mg NNT 9.9; dextropropoxyphene 65mg NNT 7.7 (Collins *et al* 2000b; Edwards *et al* 2002). In addition, codeine, a prodrug for morphine, is converted to morphine in the liver but 8–10% of the population lacks the enzyme for this conversion, a further limitation of the analgesic activity of codeine.

Morphine is the gold standard for opioid therapy and only lately was replaced by oxycodone as the most utilized opioid worldwide (Schug and Gandham 2006). While oral morphine is fully absorbed, it has a limited and very variable oral bioavailability of between 10 and 45% due to extensive first-pass metabolism (Gourlay *et al* 1986). Oxycodone, a synthetic derivative of thebaine, has a bioavailability higher than that of morphine (approx. 60%) and is available in a wide range of oral (including controlled release preparations) and parenteral preparations. Oxycodone analgesic efficacy is comparable with that of morphine, with a median oxycodone:morphine dose ratio of 1:1.5, and controlled release oxycodone is as safe and as effective as controlled release morphine (Bruera *et al* 1998). The data also suggest that oxycodone has a reduced rate of hallucinations and itch compared with morphine (Bruera *et al* 1998).

Although there was no benefit for oxycodone 5mg, a significant effect for oxycodone 15mg relative to placebo was shown with an NNT of 2.4 (1.5–4.9) for moderate to severe postoperative pain (Edwards *et al* 2000).

8.2. Adverse Effects

8.2.1. Administration for Acute Pain

For a patient to report an adverse effect with a single dose of oxycodone 15mg compared with placebo the NNH was 3.1 (1.8–11), but no increased adverse effects were shown for oxycodone 5mg over placebo (Edwards *et al* 2000). Use of any oral opioid produced higher rates of adverse events than did placebo. Dry mouth (25%), nausea (21%) and constipation (15%) were the most commonly reported. A substantial proportion of patients on opioids (22%) withdrew because of adverse events (Moore and McQuay 2005). As most side effects are reported at the initial stage of opioid use, and since the above figures refer mostly to trials of opioids in chronic non-malignant pain, it is assumed that even more side effects prevail in patients starting on opioids for acute pain (Moore and McQuay 2005).

8.2.2. Administration for Chronic Pain

Opinions are divided about the chronic use of opioids. The development of the Analgesic Ladder by the World Health Organization (WHO) in 1984 paved the way for a rational approach to the management of chronic cancer pain, and 'legitimized' the regular administration of oral opioids for these patients. However, opinions are even more divided about the use of opioids in non-cancer pain patients that have a normal expected life span (O'Callaghan 2001). The potential complications of chronic opioids use may include organ toxicity, cognitive impairment, tolerance and physical and psychological dependence. These views have been balanced against the reports of improved pain relief in patients resistant to other therapies (Portenoy and Foley 1986), and improvement in function (Zenz *et al* 1992). Moreover, studies on chronic non-cancer pain patients showed a reduction in pain and disability and little effect on cognitive state (Arkinstall *et al* 1995; Moulin *et al* 1996). A controlled study in patients on stable doses of oral morphine (mean daily dose 209mg) considered them non-hazardous with regard to driving ability (Vainio *et al*

1995). Many patients with postherpetic neuralgia report that they prefer opioids to other standard pharmacotherapies (Raja *et al* 2002; Hempenstall *et al* 2005). A survey of analgesic use in the US burn units did not reveal any case of iatrogenic dependence in more than 10000 patients given opioid analgesics (Perry and Heidrich 1982). Tolerance to analgesic effects seems to be irrelevant in clinical practice (Collett 1998). Therefore when the dose needs increasing tolerance should not be considered automatically, and the following factors should be evaluated: deterioration of the underlying condition, new pathology, increased physical activity (e.g. walking, chewing) and poor compliance. A 10-year follow-up study on opioids in chronic pain revealed that dose escalation occurred in only a few patients, suggesting that pain-related tolerance is rare (Jensen *et al* 2006). However, tolerance to respiratory depression develops rapidly and is rapidly reversible. Tolerance to sedation, cognitive effects, nausea and vomiting develops more slowly. Unfortunately, constipation and miosis are the two receptor-mediated effects to which no tolerance develops (Schug *et al* 1992). Physical dependence can be easily avoided by gradual reduction in dosage, and is not to be confused with psychological dependency. The risk of psychological dependence on opioids when used in the management of chronic pain is low, unless there is a prior history of substance abuse, major personality disorder or social disruption (Moulin 1999). Unfortunately, a significant number of patients attending multidisciplinary pain clinics do suffer these psychological factors, thereby making detailed clinical assessment prior to the commencement of opioid therapy essential (O'Callaghan 2001).

Guidelines for the use of opioids in chronic pain. The appropriate use of potent opioids is accepted medical practice for chronic recalcitrant pain in patients with normal life expectancy (Breivik 2003). Following initial diagnosis evidence-based pain therapies will reduce the need for opioids and only a minority of patients referred to a pain clinic will qualify for long-term treatment with potent opioids (Maier *et al* 2002). When indicated opioids should be used according to published guidelines on the use of opioids in chronic pain (Savage 1996; Kalso *et al* 2003).

Ideally one physician should take responsibility for the treatment and follow-up of patients. Strong opioids are not recommended as monotherapy and should be incorporated into a comprehensive rehabilitation programme that includes the attainment of improved physical and social function. Other pharmacological treatments for pain or comorbid conditions (such as antidepressants) and non-pharmacological treatments such as cognitive behavioural therapy and physiotherapy may be indicated. These should be carefully coordinated with the family physician. A written agreement with the patient that outlines therapeutic aims, prescribing legislation, dosages, side effects, risks of dependence and indications for cessation of therapy is recommended (Breivik

2003). Baseline recordings of pain severity and frequency, quality of life and functional status must precede the initiation of treatment. Only sustained-release strong opioids are recommended and these should be titrated over a trial period of 3–4 months. No rapidly acting opioids should be prescribed for breakthrough pain as they are very difficult to control and may rapidly induce dependence. The maximum length of the trial period must be clearly defined for the patient. Additionally patients must understand that opioids are not considered lifelong treatments.

Conclusions. It seems that for moderate to strong acute orofacial pain when the use of opioids is indicated, especially when NSAIDs are not recommended, the oral administration of a combination of oxycodone plus paracetamol is a good choice (see below). Opioid administration for chronic pain is largely reserved for resistant neuropathic pain syndromes as discussed in Chapter 11 (Eisenberg *et al* 2005; Finnerup *et al* 2005). Meta-analysis of published intermediate term trials (weeks–months) showed consistent and significant opioid analgesic efficacy in reducing spontaneous neuropathic pain (Eisenberg *et al* 2005). These trials are more clinically relevant than shorter ones because they assess the benefits and risks associated with opioid treatment for weeks to months.

9. Analgesic Drug Combinations

Combination pharmacotherapy is not new in medicine and is commonly used in the management of hypertension and other CV diseases. Clinical outcomes might be improved under certain conditions with the use of a combination of analgesics, rather than reliance on a single agent. Combination analgesic formulations are an important and effective means of pain relief, and could prove useful in treating elderly and other groups of patients who often cannot tolerate NSAIDs, including the newer COX-2 inhibitors (McQuay and Edwards 2003). A combination of systemic analgesics is most effective when the individual agents act through different mechanisms and result in synergistic pain control (Raffa 2001). Combinations aim at taking advantage of such complementary modes and sites of action and additionally at providing reduced side effects. The combination of an NSAID with paracetamol is a good example (Miranda *et al* 2006). Moreover drug combinations may not necessarily be synergistic in order to provide an improved risk–benefit ratio; additive or even subadditive analgesic effects but with reduced side effects may offer clinical benefits. NSAIDs clearly have an analgesic 'ceiling' (Forbes *et al* 1992; Eisenberg *et al* 1994), but the combination of two NSAIDs with different toxicity profiles would be advantageous in terms of side effects without a significant increase in analgesic potency. The combination of 75mg tramadol with 500mg paracetamol (described below) provides equivalent analgesia to tramadol 150 mg but with reduced side effects. Future work may analyze the combinations of more than two analgesics with complementary modes of action.

9.1. Paracetamol in Combination with Opioids

Paracetamol has been combined with several drugs, particularly of the opioid family (e.g. codeine, oxycodone, tramadol) as well as with other drugs, e.g. NSAIDs.

The weak opioids are relatively poor analgesics on their own (Collins *et al* 2000b; Edwards *et al* 2002). All are more effective when combined with paracetamol

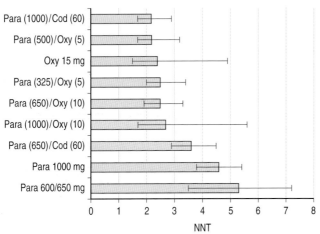

Fig. 15.3 • Number needed to treat (NNT), for one patient to achieve at least 50% pain relief, ±95% confidence interval (CI), for paracetamol (Para) and for paracetamol combined with codeine (Cod) or with oxycodone (Oxy).

Data from Edwards *et al* (2000) and Moore *et al* (1997, 2000).

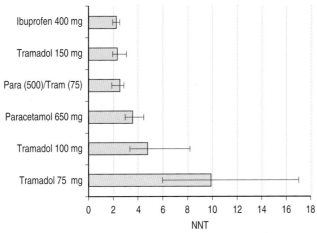

Fig. 15.4 • Number needed to treat (NNT), for one patient to achieve at least 50% pain relief, ±95% confidence interval (CI), for paracetamol (Para), tramadol (Tram) and paracetamol combined with tramadol compared to ibuprofen.

Data from Moore and McQuay (1997) and Edwards *et al* (2002).

(see Figs. 15.3, 15.4) and show synergistic efficacy; with lower opioid dosage there are significantly fewer side effects.

9.1.1. Codeine and Paracetamol

The analgesic efficacy of paracetamol 1000 mg was compared to that of paracetamol 1000 mg plus codeine 30 mg in patients after extractions of impacted third molars. The average increase in pain intensity over 12 hours was significantly less in patients receiving paracetamol plus codeine and there was no difference in adverse events between the two groups (Macleod *et al* 2002). In two systematic reviews on postoperative pain, paracetamol 1000 mg had an NNT of 4.6 (3.8–5.4) when compared with placebo, and paracetamol 600/650 mg had an NNT of 5.3 (4.1–7.2). Paracetamol 600/650 mg plus codeine 60 mg had an NNT of 3.6 (2.9–4.5). The combination of 1000 mg paracetamol with 60 mg codeine improves the NNT to 2.2 (1.7–2.9) with no significant increase in side effect profile relative to lower paracetamol containing combinations (Fig. 15.3).

Relative risk estimates for paracetamol 600/650 mg plus codeine 60 mg versus placebo showed a significant difference for 'drowsiness'/somnolence (NNH 11 (7.5–20)) and dizziness (NNH 27 (15–164)) but no significant difference for nausea/vomiting (Moore *et al* 1997, 2000).

Clinical considerations. For mild to moderate pain paracetamol 300–1000 mg (=4000 mg/d) with codeine 15–60 mg (=360 mg/d) orally every 4 hours as needed is very effective. Common adverse effects of these combinations include lightheadedness, nausea, vomiting, dizziness, sedation and dyspnea that may be severe. Codeine is in pregnancy category A and is considered compatible with breastfeeding although infant risk cannot be completely ruled out.

9.1.2. Oxycodone and Paracetamol

Oxycodone is a strong opioid and is similar to morphine in its effects, with the exception of hallucinations which occur rarely with morphine. The efficacies of oxycodone 15 mg, oxycodone 5 mg plus paracetamol 325 mg and oxycodone 10 mg plus paracetamol 650 mg were similar; the relative benefit estimates and NNTs were about 2.5 for each. This indicates that the dose of oxycodone may be lowered when it is combined with paracetamol, with no loss of efficacy (Edwards *et al* 2000). The combination of other NSAIDs with opioids seems less successful. Trials of combinations of an NSAID with an opioid have disclosed no difference (4 out of 14 papers), a statistically insignificant trend towards superiority (1 out of 14 papers) or at most a slight but statistically significant advantage (9 out of 14 papers), compared with either single entity (McNicol *et al* 2005).

Oxycodone 5 mg plus paracetamol (325, 500 and 1000 mg) was significantly more effective than placebo; with

NNTs of 2.5 (2.0–3.4), 2.2 (1.7–3.2) and 3.9 (2.1–20) respectively for moderate to severe postoperative pain over 4–6 hours (Edwards *et al* 2000). For single-dose oxycodone 10 mg plus paracetamol (650 or 1000 mg) NNTs were 2.5 (2.0–3.3) and 2.7 (1.7–5.6) for moderate to severe postoperative pain over 4–6 hours (Fig. 15.3). Since the combination of oxycodone 10 mg with paracetamol did not show a better NNT than oxycodone 5 mg plus paracetamol (Fig. 15.3), and oxycodone 10 mg exhibited more adverse effects than 5 mg (whether on its own or combined with paracetamol) (Edwards *et al* 2000), it seems prudent to use the oxycodone 5 mg/paracetamol 500 mg combination as first choice.

Clinical considerations. This combination is indicated for moderate to severe pain. Dosing is every 6 hours and the total daily dosage of paracetamol/oxycodone should not exceed 4000/60 mg. Common adverse effects include lightheadedness, pruritus, rash, constipation, nausea and vomiting. Dizziness, sedation and a dysphoric mood have also been reported. Headache and vomiting were also reported with oxycodone 10 mg plus paracetamol 650 mg, but no adverse effects were severe in nature (Edwards *et al* 2000). Oxycodone is in pregnancy category B but is associated with infant risk during breastfeeding and therefore contraindicated for lactating mothers.

9.1.3. Tramadol and Paracetamol

Tramadol is a synthetic, centrally acting analgesic that binds weakly to mu opioid receptors and also inhibits norepinephrine and serotonin pathways within the CNS (Scott and Perry 2000). After third molar extraction a single oral dose of tramadol 75 mg plus acetaminophen 650 mg produces effective analgesia in moderate to severe pain, NNT 2.6 (2.3–3.0) (Edwards *et al* 2002). For tramadol 75 mg on its own, the equivalent NNT was 9.9 (6.0–17), and for acetaminophen 650 mg 3.6 (3.0–4.5) (Fig. 15.4; Edwards *et al* 2002).

In a meta-analysis of postsurgical pain tramadol 50, 100 and 150 mg had NNTs of 7.1 (4.6–18), 4.8 (3.4–8.2) and 2.4 (2.0–3.1), comparable with aspirin 650 mg plus codeine 60 mg NNT 3.6 (2.5–6.3) and acetaminophen 650 mg plus propoxyphene 100 mg NNT 4.0 (3.0–5.7). However, with the same doses of drug postsurgical patients at large had more pain relief than those having dental surgery (Moore and McQuay 1997). Moore and McQuay concluded that absolute ranking of analgesic performance should be done separately for dental pain. Such a study recently examined the tramadol/paracetamol combination specifically for dental pain in 456 patients after third molar extraction (Fricke *et al* 2004). This study established the superiority of tramadol/paracetamol 75/650 mg over tramadol 100 mg in the treatment of acute pain following oral surgery. Adverse events occurred more frequently in the tramadol group than in the tramadol/paracetamol group. Significantly more patients reported adverse effects with tramadol 75 mg or

tramadol 75 mg plus acetaminophen 650 mg than with placebo; the NNH for a patient to report any adverse effects was 5.0 (3.7–7.3) and 5.4 (4.0–8.2) respectively. No significant difference in reported incidence of adverse effects was shown for acetaminophen 650 mg or ibuprofen 400 mg compared with placebo. Almost all reported adverse effects were of mild or moderate severity and all resolved (Edwards *et al* 2002).

Clinical considerations. For acute pain paracetamol (500–650 mg)/tramadol (75 mg) orally every 4–6 hours as needed for 5 days or less is moderately effective. Maximum daily doses should not exceed 3000 mg of paracetamol and 300 mg of tramadol. In patients with pulmonary disease, on higher doses or prolonged treatment, regular monitoring of vital signs is indicated. Common adverse effects include nausea, dizziness, vomiting, excessive sweating, pruritus, rash and slight weight loss. Confusion, headache, somnolence, tremor, anxiety and fatigue are also commonly reported.

Withdrawal of tramadol, particularly if this is abrupt, may induce anxiety, insomnia, nausea, tremors, diaphoresis and hallucinations; slow tapering will minimize or alleviate these withdrawal symptoms. Tramadol is in pregnancy category C and the risk to breastfeeding is unclear.

9.2. NSAIDs and Paracetamol

Several controlled clinical studies among patients with musculoskeletal conditions, dental pain or postoperative pain have shown that combinations of acetaminophen and NSAIDs provide additive pain-relieving activity, thereby leading to dose-sparing effects and improved safety (Altman 2004).

Patients with moderate to strong pain after surgical removal of wisdom teeth were given the following in single oral doses: 100 mg diclofenac; 1 g paracetamol; 1 g paracetamol/60 mg codeine; 100 mg diclofenac/1 g paracetamol; or 100 mg diclofenac/1 g paracetamol/60 mg codeine. Diclofenac plus paracetamol with and without codeine had superior analgesic effect compared with diclofenac, paracetamol, or paracetamol plus codeine. However, the addition of 60 mg codeine increased the degree of side effects. These results support the clinical practice of combining diclofenac with paracetamol for acute pain. Of clinical importance is superior and prolonged analgesia with fewer side effects after enteric-coated diclofenac tablets plus paracetamol compared with paracetamol plus codeine (Breivik *et al* 1999). Combined treatment with 2 g paracetamol and 75 mg diclofenac provided clinically only a minor advantage over monotherapy with paracetamol or diclofenac with respect to postoperative analgesia or the incidence of side effects in adult tonsillectomy patients (Hiller *et al* 2004). This would suggest that a minimum of 100 mg diclofenac is necessary when combined with paracetamol.

Analgesic activity of paracetamol and NSAIDs was assessed in mice, using the writing test (abdominal constriction after acetic acid intraperitoneal injection). The isobolographic analysis of the various combinations of NSAIDs and paracetamol resulted in synergistic interactions (Miranda *et al* 2006). However, further studies to determine the clinical utility and safety of paracetamol/NSAID combinations as analgesic therapy for common conditions associated with mild to moderate pain are warranted (Altman 2004).

10. Strategy of Pharmacotherapy of Acute Orofacial Pain

As stated at the beginning of this chapter, the aim of drug therapy of acute orofacial pain is to relieve pain at maximum efficacy with minimum side effects. The medical history of the patient is the foremost consideration when choosing an analgesic. These aspects have been extensively discussed above. When efficacy, side effects and cost are balanced, the evidence supports an oral analgesic treatment schedule that begins with paracetamol 500 mg for mild to moderate orofacial pain. Naproxen 500 mg or ibuprofen 400 mg are efficient alternatives for short-term therapy; the safest conventional NSAID in terms of GI side effects is ibuprofen in doses of 400 mg. Higher doses may offer somewhat greater analgesia but with more adverse effects. Other NSAIDs have failed to demonstrate consistently greater efficacy or safety than ibuprofen (Sachs 2005). Although naproxen has been associated with some increase in CV effects it has consistently emerged as the safest NSAID in most studies when CV risks are considered (Juni *et al* 2005; Kearney *et al* 2006; McGettigan and Henry 2006; Antman *et al* 2007) and may be combined with a proton pump inhibitor as needed (Lai *et al* 2005; Morgner *et al* 2007), providing excellent analgesia and GI safety. It is important to appreciate that data are constantly accumulating and the evidence for risk–benefit ratios in individual drugs must be regularly reviewed by clinicians.

For moderate to severe pain not responding to paracetamol, and when ibuprofen or naproxen are contraindicated, the use of narcotics combined with paracetamol is indicated. The combination of paracetamol 500 mg plus oxycodone 5 mg gives good analgesia with minimal side effects. COX-2 inhibitors provide analgesia equal to traditional NSAIDs for many painful conditions, but lack a better safety profile in acute pain treatment and are significantly more expensive (Sachs 2005).

The possibility of preemptive analgesia, i.e. when the analgesics are administered before surgery, has been advocated (Savage and Henry 2004), but the evidence is unclear, and the efficacy of analgesics provided after surgery is probably the same. On the whole in the dental field this is a somewhat academic debate, taking into consideration that the patient is usually anaesthetized with a local anaesthetic that outlasts the surgery.

Sometimes a patient prefers a certain analgesic because 'it works better for him/her', and unless the drug requested is contraindicated we tend not to argue with patients' preferences. One should consider that males and females may differ in their response to NSAIDs and indeed females enjoy less analgesia with ibuprofen than do males (Walker and Carmody 1998). Also, given the fact that patients may differ genetically in their response to analgesics the patient may actually be right (Lotsch and Geisslinger 2006). On the whole the strategy described above is a good starting point when pain severity is our main lead. However, the patient's age, medical background and habits, such as smoking or alcohol consumption, and adverse drug interactions are foremost considerations in order to minimize side effects (Haas 1999). Table 15.1 summarizes the initial and maintenance doses and common medical contraindications for the common single formulation of non-opioid analgesics. Table 15.2 provides assistance for the management of acute orofacial pain that takes into consideration both pain severity and patient's medical background.

References

ADAPT (2006) Cardiovascular and cerebrovascular events in the randomized, controlled Alzheimer's Disease Anti-inflammatory Prevention Trial (ADAPT). *PLoS Clin Trials* **1**(7):e33.

Altman RD (2004) A rationale for combining acetaminophen and NSAIDs for mild-to-moderate pain. *Clin Exp Rheumatol* **22**(1): 110–117.

Andersohn F, Suissa S, Garbe E (2006) Use of first- and second-generation cyclooxygenase-2-selective nonsteroidal antiinflammatory drugs and risk of acute myocardial infarction. *Circulation* **113**(16):1950–1957.

Antman EM, Bennett JS, Daugherty A, *et al* (2007) Use of nonsteroidal antiinflammatory drugs: an update for clinicians: a scientific statement from the American Heart Association. *Circulation* **115**(12):1634–1642.

Arkinstall W, Sandler A, Goughnour B, *et al* (1995) Efficacy of controlled-release codeine in chronic non-malignant pain: a randomized, placebo-controlled clinical trial. *Pain* **62**(2): 169–178.

Ballou LR, Botting RM, Goorha S, *et al* (2000) Nociception in cyclooxygenase isozyme-deficient mice. *Proc Natl Acad Sci USA* **97**(18):10272–10276.

Bannwarth B, Berenbaum F (2005) Clinical pharmacology of lumiracoxib, a second-generation cyclooxygenase 2 selective inhibitor. *Expert Opin Investig Drugs* **14**(4):521–533.

Barden J, Edwards JE, McQuay HJ, *et al* (2003) Single dose oral celecoxib for postoperative pain. *Cochrane Database Syst Rev* (2): CD004233.

Barden J, Edwards J, Moore A, *et al* (2004) Single dose oral paracetamol (acetaminophen) for postoperative pain. *Cochrane Database Syst Rev* (1):CD004602.

Barden J, Edwards J, Moore RA, *et al* (2005) Single dose oral rofecoxib for postoperative pain. *Cochrane Database Syst Rev* (1): CD004604.

Bertolini A, Ottani A, Sandrini M (2001) Dual acting anti-inflammatory drugs: a reappraisal. *Pharmacol Res* **44**(6): 437–450.

Bianchi Porro G, Ardizzone S, Petrillo M, *et al* (1996) Endoscopic assessment of the effects of dipyrone (metamizol) in comparison to paracetamol and placebo on the gastric and duodenal mucosa of healthy adult volunteers. *Digestion* **57**(3): 186–190.

Bigby M (2001) Rates of cutaneous reactions to drugs. *Arch Dermatol* **137**(6):765–770.

Bjornsson GA, Haanaes HR, Skoglund LA (2003) A randomized, double-blind crossover trial of paracetamol 1000 mg four times daily vs ibuprofen 600 mg: effect on swelling and other postoperative events after third molar surgery. *Br J Clin Pharmacol* **55**(4):405–412.

Bombardier C, Laine L, Reicin A, *et al* (2000) Comparison of upper gastrointestinal toxicity of rofecoxib and naproxen in patients with rheumatoid arthritis. VIGOR Study Group. *N Engl J Med* **343**(21):1520–1528.

Brater DC, Harris C, Redfern JS, *et al* (2001) Renal effects of COX-2-selective inhibitors. *Am J Nephrol* **21**(1):1–15.

Breivik H (2003) Appropriate and responsible use of opioids in chronic non-cancer pain. *Eur J Pain* **7**(5):379–380.

Breivik EK, Barkvoll P, Skovlund E (1999) Combining diclofenac with acetaminophen or acetaminophen-codeine after oral surgery: a randomized, double-blind single-dose study. *Clin Pharmacol Ther* **66**(6):625–635.

Bresalier RS, Sandler RS, Quan H, *et al* (2005) Cardiovascular events associated with rofecoxib in a colorectal adenoma chemoprevention trial. *N Engl J Med* **352**(11):1092–1102.

Brogden RN (1986) Pyrazolone derivatives. *Drugs* **32**(Suppl 4):60–70.

Brophy JM (2005) Cardiovascular risk associated with celecoxib. *N Engl J Med* **352**(25):2648–2650; author reply 2648–2650.

Bruera E, Belzile M, Pituskin E, *et al* (1998) Randomized, double-blind, cross-over trial comparing safety and efficacy of oral controlled-release oxycodone with controlled-release morphine in patients with cancer pain. *J Clin Oncol* **16**(10): 3222–3229.

Brune K (2004) Safety of anti-inflammatory treatment–new ways of thinking. *Rheumatology (Oxford)* **43**(Suppl 1):i16–i20.

Buzzi MG, Sakas DE, Moskowitz MA (1989) Indomethacin and acetylsalicylic acid block neurogenic plasma protein extravasation in rat dura mater. *Eur J Pharmacol* **165** (2–3):251–258.

Camu F, Shi L, Vanlersberghe C (2003) The role of COX-2 inhibitors in pain modulation. *Drugs* **63**(Suppl 1):1–7.

Capone ML, Tacconelli S, Sciulli MG, *et al* (2004) Clinical pharmacology of platelet, monocyte, and vascular cyclooxygenase inhibition by naproxen and low-dose aspirin in healthy subjects. *Circulation* **109**(12):1468–1471.

Capone ML, Sciulli MG, Tacconelli S, *et al* (2005) Pharmacodynamic interaction of naproxen with low-dose aspirin in healthy subjects. *J Am Coll Cardiol* **45**(8):1295–1301.

Carlsson KH, Jurna I (1987) Central analgesic effect of paracetamol manifested by depression of nociceptive activity in thalamic neurones of the rat. *Neurosci Lett* **77**(3):339–343.

Carlsson KH, Helmreich J, Jurna I (1986) Activation of inhibition from the periaqueductal grey matter mediates central analgesic effect of metamizol (dipyrone). *Pain* **27**(3):373–390.

Carlsson KH, Monzel W, Jurna I (1988) Depression by morphine and the non-opioid analgesic agents, metamizol (dipyrone), lysine acetylsalicylate, and paracetamol, of activity in rat thalamus neurones evoked by electrical stimulation of nociceptive afferents. *Pain* **32**(3):313–326.

Cashman JN (1996) The mechanisms of action of NSAIDs in analgesia. *Drugs* **52**(Suppl 5):13–23.

Castellano AE, Micieli G, Bellantonio P, *et al* (1998) Indomethacin increases the effect of isosorbide dinitrate on cerebral hemodynamic in migraine patients: pathogenetic and therapeutic implications. *Cephalalgia* **18**(9):622–630.

Catella-Lawson F, Reilly MP, Kapoor SC, *et al* (2001) Cyclooxygenase inhibitors and the antiplatelet effects of aspirin. *N Engl J Med* **345**(25):1809–1817.

Celik G, Pasaoglu G, Bavbek S, *et al* (2005) Tolerability of selective cyclooxygenase inhibitor, celecoxib, in patients with analgesic intolerance. *J Asthma* **42**(2):127–131.

Chan VS (2004) A mechanistic perspective on the specificity and extent of COX-2 inhibition in pregnancy. *Drug Saf* **27**(7):421–426.

Chandrasekharan NV, Dai H, Roos KL, *et al* (2002) COX-3, a cyclooxygenase-1 variant inhibited by acetaminophen and other analgesic/antipyretic drugs: cloning, structure, and expression. *Proc Natl Acad Sci U S A* **99**(21):13926–13931.

Chang DJ, Desjardins PJ, Chen E, *et al* (2002) Comparison of the analgesic efficacy of rofecoxib and enteric-coated diclofenac sodium in the treatment of postoperative dental pain: a randomized, placebo-controlled clinical trial. *Clin Ther* **24**(4): 490–503.

Chang DJ, Desjardins PJ, King TR, *et al* (2004) The analgesic efficacy of etoricoxib compared with oxycodone/acetaminophen in an acute postoperative pain model: a randomized, double-blind clinical trial. *Anesth Analg* **99**(3): 807–815, table of contents.

Chang DJ, Bird SR, Bohidar NR, *et al* (2005) Analgesic efficacy of rofecoxib compared with codeine/acetaminophen using a model of acute dental pain. *Oral Surg Oral Med Oral Pathol Oral Radiol Endod* **100**(4):e74–e80.

Charlier C, Michaux C (2003) Dual inhibition of cyclooxygenase-2 (COX-2) and 5-lipoxygenase (5-LOX) as a new strategy to provide safer non-steroidal anti-inflammatory drugs. *Eur J Med Chem* **38**(7-8):645–659.

Christie PE, Tagari P, Ford-Hutchinson AW, *et al* (1991) Urinary leukotriene E4 concentrations increase after aspirin challenge in aspirin-sensitive asthmatic subjects. *Am Rev Respir Dis* **143** (5 Pt 1):1025–1029.

Clarke RJ, Mayo G, Price P, *et al* (1991) Suppression of thromboxane A2 but not of systemic prostacyclin by controlled-release aspirin. *N Engl J Med* **325**(16):1137–1141.

Cleland LG, James MJ (2006) Marine oils for antiinflammatory effect – time to take stock. *J Rheumatol* **33**(2):207–209.

Cochrane DJ, Jarvis B, Keating GM (2002) Etoricoxib. *Drugs* **62**(18):2637–2651; discussion 2652–2653.

Collett BJ (1998) Opioid tolerance: the clinical perspective. *Br J Anaesth* **81**(1):58–68.

Collins SL, Moore RA, McQuay HJ, *et al* (2000a) Single dose oral ibuprofen and diclofenac for postoperative pain. *Cochrane Database Syst Rev* (2):CD001548.

Collins SL, Edwards JE, Moore RA, *et al* (2000b) Single dose dextropropoxyphene, alone and with paracetamol (acetaminophen), for postoperative pain. *Cochrane Database Syst Rev* (2):CD001440.

Crofford LJ, Lipsky PE, Brooks P, *et al* (2000) Basic biology and clinical application of specific cyclooxygenase-2 inhibitors. *Arthritis Rheum* **43**(1):4–13.

Czerniawska-Mysik G, Szczeklik A (1981) Idiosyncrasy to pyrazolone drugs. *Allergy* **36**(6):381–384.

Daniels SE, Desjardins PJ, Talwalker S, *et al* (2002) The analgesic efficacy of valdecoxib vs. oxycodone/acetaminophen after oral surgery. *J Am Dent Assoc* **133**(5):611–621; quiz 625.

Desjardins PJ, Mehlisch DR, Chang DJ, *et al* (2005) The time to onset and overall analgesic efficacy of rofecoxib 50 mg: a meta-analysis of 13 randomized clinical trials. *Clin J Pain* **21**(3):241–250.

Dinchuk JE, Car BD, Focht RJ, *et al* (1995) Renal abnormalities and an altered inflammatory response in mice lacking cyclooxygenase II. *Nature* **378**(6555):406–409.

Dionne RA, Berthold CW (2001) Therapeutic uses of non-steroidal anti-inflammatory drugs in dentistry. *Crit Rev Oral Biol Med* **12**(4):315–330.

Doyle G, Jayawardena S, Ashraf E, *et al* (2002) Efficacy and tolerability of nonprescription ibuprofen versus celecoxib for dental pain. *J Clin Pharmacol* **42**(8):912–919.

Eccles M, Freemantle N, Mason J (1998) North of England evidence based guideline development project: summary guideline for non-steroidal anti-inflammatory drugs versus basic analgesia in treating the pain of degenerative arthritis. The North of England Non-Steroidal Anti-

Inflammatory Drug Guideline Development Group. *BMJ* **317** (7157):526–530.

Edwards JE, McQuay HJ (2002) Dipyrone and agranulocytosis: what is the risk? *Lancet* **360**(9344):1438.

Edwards JE, Moore RA, McQuay HJ (2000) Single dose oxycodone and oxycodone plus paracetamol (acetaminophen) for acute postoperative pain. *Cochrane Database Syst Rev* (4): CD002763.

Edwards JE, Meseguer F, Faura CC, et al (2001) Single-dose dipyrone for acute postoperative pain. *Cochrane Database Syst Rev* (3):CD003227.

Edwards JE, McQuay HJ, Moore RA (2002) Combination analgesic efficacy: individual patient data meta-analysis of single-dose oral tramadol plus acetaminophen in acute postoperative pain. *J Pain Symptom Manage* **23**(2):121–130.

Eisenberg E, Berkey CS, Carr DB, et al (1994) Efficacy and safety of nonsteroidal antiinflammatory drugs for cancer pain: a meta-analysis. *J Clin Oncol* **12**(12):2756–2765.

Eisenberg E, McNicol ED, Carr DB (2005) Efficacy and safety of opioid agonists in the treatment of neuropathic pain of nonmalignant origin: systematic review and meta-analysis of randomized controlled trials. *JAMA* **293**(24):3043–3052.

Eldor A, Zylber-Katz E, Levy M (1984) The effect of oral administration of dipyrone on the capacity of blood platelets to synthesize thromboxane A2 in man. *Eur J Clin Pharmacol* **26**(2):171–176.

Evans JM, McGregor E, McMahon AD, et al (1995) Non-steroidal anti-inflammatory drugs and hospitalization for acute renal failure. *QJM* **88**(8):551–557.

Feigen LP, King LW, Ray J, et al (1981) Differential effects of ibuprofen and indomethacin in the regional circulation of the dog. *J Pharmacol Exp Ther* **219**(3):679–684.

Finnerup NB, Otto M, McQuay HJ, et al (2005) Algorithm for neuropathic pain treatment: an evidence based proposal. *Pain* **118**(3):289–305.

Fitzgerald GA (2004) Coxibs and cardiovascular disease. *N Engl J Med* **351**(17):1709–1711.

FitzGerald GA, Patrono C (2001) The coxibs, selective inhibitors of cyclooxygenase-2. *N Engl J Med* **345**(6):433–442.

Flower R, Gryglewski R, Herbaczynska-Cedro K, et al (1972) Effects of anti-inflammatory drugs on prostaglandin biosynthesis. *Nat New Biol* **238**(82):104–106.

Forbes JA, Beaver WT, Jones KF, et al (1992) Analgesic efficacy of bromfenac, ibuprofen, and aspirin in postoperative oral surgery pain. *Clin Pharmacol Ther* **51**(3):343–352.

Fricke J, Varkalis J, Zwillich S, et al (2002) Valdecoxib is more efficacious than rofecoxib in relieving pain associated with oral surgery. *Am J Ther* **9**(2):89–97.

Fricke JR Jr, Hewitt DJ, Jordan DM, et al (2004) A double-blind placebo-controlled comparison of tramadol/acetaminophen and tramadol in patients with postoperative dental pain. *Pain* **109**(3):250–257.

Fu JY, Masferrer JL, Seibert K, et al (1990) The induction and suppression of prostaglandin H2 synthase (cyclooxygenase) in human monocytes. *J Biol Chem* **265**(28):16737–16740.

Funk CD (2001) Prostaglandins and leukotrienes: advances in eicosanoid biology. *Science* **294**(5548):1871–1875.

Furberg CD, Psaty BM, FitzGerald GA (2005) Parecoxib, valdecoxib, and cardiovascular risk. *Circulation* **111**(3):249.

Gadisseur AP, Van Der Meer FJ, Rosendaal FR (2003) Sustained intake of paracetamol (acetaminophen) during oral anticoagulant therapy with coumarins does not cause clinically important INR changes: a randomized double-blind clinical trial. *J Thromb Haemost* **1**(4):714–717.

Gaston GW, Mallow RD, Frank JE (1986) Comparison of etodolac, aspirin and placebo for pain after oral surgery. *Pharmacotherapy* **6**(5):199–205.

Gaziano JM, Gibson CM (2006) Potential for drug-drug interactions in patients taking analgesics for mild-to-moderate pain and low-dose aspirin for cardioprotection. *Am J Cardiol* **97**(9A):23–29.

Gerstenfeld LC, Thiede M, Seibert K, et al (2003) Differential inhibition of fracture healing by non-selective and cyclooxygenase-2 selective non-steroidal anti-inflammatory drugs. *J Orthop Res* **21**(4):670–675.

Glasser DL, Burroughs SH (2003) Valdecoxib-induced toxic epidermal necrolysis in a patient allergic to sulfa drugs. *Pharmacotherapy* **23**(4):551–553.

Gobetti JP (1992) Controlling dental pain. *J Am Dent Assoc* **123**(6):47–52.

Gotzsche PC (2005) Musculoskeletal disorders. Non-steroidal anti-inflammatory drugs. *Clin Evid* (14):1498–1505.

Gourlay G (2002) *Clinical Pharmacology of Opioids in the Treatment of Pain.* Seattle: IASP Press.

Gourlay GK, Cherry DA, Cousins MJ (1986) A comparative study of the efficacy and pharmacokinetics of oral methadone and morphine in the treatment of severe pain in patients with cancer. *Pain* **25**(3):297–312.

Graham DJ (2006) COX-2 inhibitors, other NSAIDs, and cardiovascular risk: the seduction of common sense. *JAMA* **296**:1653–1656.

Graham DJ, Campen D, Hui R, et al (2005) Risk of acute myocardial infarction and sudden cardiac death in patients treated with cyclo-oxygenase 2 selective and non-selective non-steroidal anti-inflammatory drugs: nested case-control study. *Lancet* **365**(9458):475–481.

Graham DY, Smith JL (1986) Aspirin and the stomach. *Ann Intern Med* **104**(3):390–398.

Graham GG, Scott KF (2005) Mechanism of action of paracetamol. *Am J Ther* **12**(1):46–55.

Grosser T, Fries S, FitzGerald GA (2006) Biological basis for the cardiovascular consequences of COX-2 inhibition: therapeutic challenges and opportunities. *J Clin Invest* **116**(1):4–15.

Haas DA (1999) Adverse drug interactions in dental practice: interactions associated with analgesics, Part III in a series. *J Am Dent Assoc* **130**(3):397–407.

Harder AT, An YH (2003) The mechanisms of the inhibitory effects of nonsteroidal anti-inflammatory drugs on bone healing: a concise review. *J Clin Pharmacol* **43**(8):807–815.

Hawkey CJ (1999) COX-2 inhibitors. *Lancet* **353**(9149):307–314.

Hawkey CJ, Karrasch JA, Szczepanski L, et al (1998) Omeprazole compared with misoprostol for ulcers associated with nonsteroidal antiinflammatory drugs. Omeprazole versus Misoprostol for NSAID-induced Ulcer Management (OMNIUM) Study Group. *N Engl J Med* **338**(11):727–734.

Heerdink ER, Leufkens HG, Herings RM, et al (1998) NSAIDs associated with increased risk of congestive heart failure in elderly patients taking diuretics. *Arch Intern Med* **158**(10): 1108–1112.

Helin-Salmivaara A, Virtanen A, Vesalainen R, et al (2006) NSAID use and the risk of hospitalization for first myocardial infarction in the general population: a nationwide case-control study from Finland. *Eur Heart J* **27**(14):1657–1663.

Hempenstall K, Nurmikko TJ, Johnson RW, et al (2005) Analgesic therapy in postherpetic neuralgia: a quantitative systematic review. *PLoS Med* **2**(7):e164.

Henman MC, Leach GD, Naylor IL (1979) Production of prostaglandin-like materials by rat tail skin in response to injury [proceedings]. *Br J Pharmacol* **66**(3):448P.

Henry D, McGettigan P (2003) Epidemiology overview of gastrointestinal and renal toxicity of NSAIDs. *Int J Clin Pract Suppl* (135):43–49.

Henry D, Lim LL, Garcia Rodriguez LA, et al (1996) Variability in risk of gastrointestinal complications with individual non-steroidal anti-inflammatory drugs: results of a collaborative meta-analysis. *Bmj* **312**(7046):1563–1566.

Henry D, Page J, Whyte I, et al (1997) Consumption of non-steroidal anti-inflammatory drugs and the development of functional renal impairment in elderly subjects. Results of a case-control study. *Br J Clin Pharmacol* **44**(1):85–90.

Hernandez-Diaz S, Garcia-Rodriguez LA (2001) Epidemiologic assessment of the safety of conventional nonsteroidal anti-inflammatory drugs. *Am J Med* **110**(Suppl 3A):20S–27S.

Hersh EV, Levin LM, Cooper SA, et al (2000) Ibuprofen liquigel for oral surgery pain. Clin Ther 22(11):1306–1318.

Hiller A, Silvanto M, Savolainen S, et al (2004) Propacetamol and diclofenac alone and in combination for analgesia after elective tonsillectomy. Acta Anaesthesiol Scand 48(9):1185–1189.

Hinz B, Brune K (2004) Pain and osteoarthritis: new drugs and mechanisms. Curr Opin Rheumatol 16(5):628–633.

Hippisley-Cox J, Coupland C (2005) Risk of myocardial infarction in patients taking cyclo-oxygenase-2 inhibitors or conventional non-steroidal anti-inflammatory drugs: population based nested case-control analysis. BMJ 330(7504):1366.

Huber MA, Terezhalmy GT (2006) The use of COX-2 inhibitors for acute dental pain: A second look. J Am Dent Assoc 137(4): 480–487.

Huskisson EC, Woolf DL, Balme HW, et al (1976) Four new anti-inflammatory drugs: responses and variations. BMJ 1(6017): 1048–1049.

Hutton CE (1983) The effectiveness of 100 and 200 mg etodolac (Ultradol), aspirin, and placebo in patients with pain following oral surgery. Oral Surg Oral Med Oral Pathol 56(6):575–580.

Hyllested M, Jones S, Pedersen JL, et al (2002) Comparative effect of paracetamol, NSAIDs or their combination in postoperative pain management: a qualitative review. Br J Anaesth 88 (2):199–214.

Ichikawa H, Sugimoto T (2002) The co-expression of ASIC3 with calcitonin gene-related peptide and parvalbumin in the rat trigeminal ganglion. Brain Res 943(2):287–291.

International Agranulocytosis and Aplastic Anemia Study (1986) Risks of agranulocytosis and aplastic anemia. A first report of their relation to drug use with special reference to analgesics. JAMA 256(13):1749–1757.

Israel E, Fischer AR, Rosenberg MA, et al (1993) The pivotal role of 5-lipoxygenase products in the reaction of aspirin-sensitive asthmatics to aspirin. Am Rev Respir Dis 148(6 Pt 1):1447–1451.

Jensen MK, Thomsen AB, Hojsted J (2006) 10-year follow-up of chronic non-malignant pain patients: Opioid use, health related quality of life and health care utilization. Eur J Pain 10(5): 423–433.

Johnson AG (1998) NSAIDs and blood pressure. Clinical importance for older patients. Drugs Aging 12(1):17–27.

Johnson AG, Nguyen TV, Day RO (1994) Do nonsteroidal anti-inflammatory drugs affect blood pressure? A meta-analysis. Ann Intern Med 121(4):289–300.

Juhlin L (1981) Recurrent urticaria: clinical investigation of 330 patients. Br J Dermatol 104(4):369–381.

Julius D, Basbaum AI (2001) Molecular mechanisms of nociception. Nature 413(6852):203–210.

Juni P, Nartey L, Reichenbach S, et al (2004) Risk of cardiovascular events and rofecoxib: cumulative meta-analysis. Lancet 364(9450):2021–2029.

Juni P, Reichenbach S, Egger M (2005) COX 2 inhibitors, traditional NSAIDs, and the heart. BMJ 330(7504):1342–1343.

Kalso E, Allan L, Dellemijn PL, et al (2003) Recommendations for using opioids in chronic non-cancer pain. Eur J Pain 7(5): 381–386.

Karakaya G, Kalyoncu AF (2002) Metamizole intolerance and bronchial asthma. Allergol Immunopathol (Madr) 30(5):267–272.

Katori M, Majima M (2000) Cyclooxygenase-2: its rich diversity of roles and possible application of its selective inhibitors. Inflamm Res 49(8):367–392.

Kearney PM, Baigent C, Godwin J, et al (2006) Do selective cyclo-oxygenase-2 inhibitors and traditional non-steroidal anti-inflammatory drugs increase the risk of atherothrombosis? Meta-analysis of randomised trials. BMJ 332(7553):1302–1308.

Kellstein D, Ott D, Jayawardene S, et al (2004) Analgesic efficacy of a single dose of lumiracoxib compared with rofecoxib, celecoxib and placebo in the treatment of post-operative dental pain. Int J Clin Pract 58(3):244–250.

Kellstein DE, Waksman JA, Furey SA, et al (1999) The safety profile of nonprescription ibuprofen in multiple-dose use: a meta-analysis. J Clin Pharmacol 39(5):520–532.

Kessler W, Kirchhoff C, Reeh PW, et al (1992) Excitation of cutaneous afferent nerve endings in vitro by a combination of inflammatory mediators and conditioning effect of substance P. Exp Brain Res 91(3):467–476.

Khan AA, Brahim JS, Rowan JS, et al (2002) In vivo selectivity of a selective cyclooxygenase 2 inhibitor in the oral surgery model. Clin Pharmacol Ther 72(1):44–49.

Khan KN, Stanfield KM, Harris RK, et al (2001) Expression of cyclooxygenase-2 in the macula densa of human kidney in hypertension, congestive heart failure, and diabetic nephropathy. Ren Fail 23(3-4):321–330.

Kido MA, Muroya H, Yamaza T, et al (2003) Vanilloid receptor expression in the rat tongue and palate. J Dent Res 82(5): 393–397.

Kim H, Neubert JK, San Miguel A, et al (2004) Genetic influence on variability in human acute experimental pain sensitivity associated with gender, ethnicity and psychological temperament. Pain 109(3):488–496.

Lai KC, Chu KM, Hui WM, et al (2005) Celecoxib compared with lansoprazole and naproxen to prevent gastrointestinal ulcer complications. Am J Med 118(11):1271–1278.

Langenbach R, Morham SG, Tiano HF, et al (1995) Prostaglandin synthase 1 gene disruption in mice reduces arachidonic acid-induced inflammation and indomethacin-induced gastric ulceration. Cell 83(3):483–492.

Lanza FL (1998) A guideline for the treatment and prevention of NSAID-induced ulcers. Members of the Ad Hoc Committee on Practice Parameters of the American College of Gastroenterology. Am J Gastroenterol 93(11):2037–2046.

Lanza FL, Royer GL Jr, Nelson RS (1980) Endoscopic evaluation of the effects of aspirin, buffered aspirin, and enteric-coated aspirin on gastric and duodenal mucosa. N Engl J Med 303(3): 136–138.

Larkai EN, Smith JL, Lidsky MD, et al (1987) Gastroduodenal mucosa and dyspeptic symptoms in arthritic patients during chronic nonsteroidal anti-inflammatory drug use. Am J Gastroenterol 82(11):1153–1158.

Lee M, Cryer B, Feldman M (1994) Dose effects of aspirin on gastric prostaglandins and stomach mucosal injury. Ann Intern Med 120(3):184–189.

Leese PT, Talwalker S, Kent JD, et al (2002) Valdecoxib does not impair platelet function. Am J Emerg Med 20(4):275–281.

Levy M (2000) Hypersensitivity to pyrazolones. Thorax 55 (Suppl 2):S72–S74.

Li DK, Liu L, Odouli R (2003) Exposure to non-steroidal anti-inflammatory drugs during pregnancy and risk of miscarriage: population based cohort study. BMJ 327(7411):368.

Libert F, Bonnefont J, Bourinet E, et al (2004) Acetaminophen: a central analgesic drug that involves a spinal tropisetron-sensitive, non-5-HT(3) receptor-mediated effect. Mol Pharmacol 66(3):728–734.

Longstreth GF (1995) Epidemiology of hospitalization for acute upper gastrointestinal hemorrhage: a population-based study. Am J Gastroenterol 90(2):206–210.

Lotsch J, Geisslinger G (2006) Current evidence for a genetic modulation of the response to analgesics. Pain 121(1-2):1–5.

McAdam BF, Catella-Lawson F, Mardini IA, et al (1999) Systemic biosynthesis of prostacyclin by cyclooxygenase (COX)-2: the human pharmacology of a selective inhibitor of COX-2. Proc Natl Acad Sci USA 96(1):272–277.

McGettigan P, Henry D (2006) Cardiovascular risk and inhibition of cyclooxygenase: a systematic review of the observational studies of selective and nonselective inhibitors of cyclooxygenase 2. JAMA 296(13):1633–1644.

Macleod AG, Ashford B, Voltz M, et al (2002) Paracetamol versus paracetamol-codeine in the treatment of post-operative dental pain: a randomized, double-blind, prospective trial. Aust Dent J 47(2):147–151.

McNicol E, Strassels SA, Goudas L, et al (2005) NSAIDS or paracetamol, alone or combined with opioids, for cancer pain. Cochrane Database Syst Rev (1):CD005180.

McQuay H, Edwards J (2003) Meta-analysis of single dose oral tramadol plus acetaminophen in acute postoperative pain. *Eur J Anaesthesiol Suppl* **28**:19–22.

Maier C, Hildebrandt J, Klinger R, *et al* (2002) Morphine responsiveness, efficacy and tolerability in patients with chronic non-tumor associated pain - results of a double-blind placebo-controlled trial (MONTAS). *Pain* **97**(3):223–233.

Majerus PW (1983) Arachidonate metabolism in vascular disorders. *J Clin Invest* **72**(5):1521–1525.

Malmstrom K, Fricke JR, Kotey P, *et al* (2002) A comparison of rofecoxib versus celecoxib in treating pain after dental surgery: a single-center, randomized, double-blind, placebo- and active-comparator-controlled, parallel-group, single-dose study using the dental impaction pain model. *Clin Ther* **24**(10):1549–1560.

Malmstrom K, Kotey P, Coughlin H, *et al* (2004a) A randomized, double-blind, parallel-group study comparing the analgesic effect of etoricoxib to placebo, naproxen sodium, and acetaminophen with codeine using the dental impaction pain model. *Clin J Pain* **20**(3):147–155.

Malmstrom K, Sapre A, Couglin H, *et al* (2004b) Etoricoxib in acute pain associated with dental surgery: a randomized, double-blind, placebo- and active comparator-controlled dose-ranging study. *Clin Ther* **26**(5):667–679.

Malmstrom K, Ang J, Fricke JR, *et al* (2005) The analgesic effect of etoricoxib relative to that of cetaminophen analgesics: a randomized, controlled single-dose study in acute dental impaction pain. *Curr Med Res Opin* **21**(1):141–149.

Mamdani M, Juurlink DN, Lee DS, *et al* (2004) Cyclo-oxygenase-2 inhibitors versus non-selective non-steroidal anti-inflammatory drugs and congestive heart failure outcomes in elderly patients: a population-based cohort study. *Lancet* **363**(9423):1751–1756.

Mamet J, Baron A, Lazdunski M, *et al* (2002) Proinflammatory mediators, stimulators of sensory neuron excitability via the expression of acid-sensing ion channels. *J Neurosci* **22**(24):10662–10670.

Mamet J, Lazdunski M, Voilley N (2003) How nerve growth factor drives physiological and inflammatory expressions of acid-sensing ion channel 3 in sensory neurons. *J Biol Chem* **278**(49):48907–48913.

Maroon JC, Bost JW (2006) Omega-3 fatty acids (fish oil) as an anti-inflammatory: an alternative to nonsteroidal anti-inflammatory drugs for discogenic pain. *Surg Neurol* **65**(4):326–331.

Martel RR, Klicius J (1982) Comparison in rats of the anti-inflammatory and gastric irritant effects of etodolac with several clinically effective anti-inflammatory drugs. *Agents Actions* **12**(3):295–297.

Martin HA, Basbaum AI, Kwiat GC, *et al* (1987) Leukotriene and prostaglandin sensitization of cutaneous high-threshold C- and A-delta mechanonociceptors in the hairy skin of rat hindlimbs. *Neuroscience* **22**(2):651–659.

Martin-Garcia C, Hinojosa M, Berges P, *et al* (2002) Safety of a cyclooxygenase-2 inhibitor in patients with aspirin-sensitive asthma. *Chest* **121**(6):1812–1817.

Martin-Garcia C, Hinojosa M, Berges P, *et al* (2003) Celecoxib, a highly selective COX-2 inhibitor, is safe in aspirin-induced asthma patients. *J Investig Allergol Clin Immunol* **13**(1):20–25.

Mason L, Edwards JE, Moore RA, *et al* (2003) Single-dose oral naproxen for acute postoperative pain: a quantitative systematic review. *BMC Anesthesiol* **3**(1):4.

Mason L, Edwards JE, Moore RA, *et al* (2004) Single dose oral naproxen and naproxen sodium for acute postoperative pain. *Cochrane Database Syst Rev* (4):CD004234.

Micheletto C, Tognella S, Guerriero M, *et al* (2006) Nasal and bronchial tolerability of Rofecoxib in patients with aspirin induced asthma. *Allerg Immunol (Paris)* **38**(1):10–14.

Millan MJ (1999) The induction of pain: an integrative review. *Prog Neurobiol* **57**(1):1–164.

Miranda HF, Puig MM, Prieto JC, *et al* (2006) Synergism between paracetamol and nonsteroidal anti-inflammatory drugs in experimental acute pain. *Pain* **121**(1-2):22–28.

Mizraji M (1990) Clinical response to etodolac in the management of pain. *Eur J Rheumatol Inflamm* **10**(1):35–43.

Moore A, Collins S, Carroll D, *et al* (1997) Paracetamol with and without codeine in acute pain: a quantitative systematic review. *Pain* **70**(2-3):193–201.

Moore A, Collins S, Carroll D, *et al* (2000) Single dose paracetamol (acetaminophen), with and without codeine, for postoperative pain. *Cochrane Database Syst Rev* (2):CD001547.

Moore RA, McQuay HJ (1997) Single-patient data meta-analysis of 3453 postoperative patients: oral tramadol versus placebo, codeine and combination analgesics. *Pain* **69**(3):287–294.

Moore RA, McQuay HJ (2005) Prevalence of opioid adverse events in chronic non-malignant pain: systematic review of randomised trials of oral opioids. *Arthritis Res Ther* **7**(5):R1046–R1051.

Moreau M, Boileau C, Martel-Pelletier J, *et al* (2006) Licofelone reduces progression of structural changes in a canine model of osteoarthritis under curative conditions: effect on protease expression and activity. *J Rheumatol* **33**(6):1176–1183.

Morgner A, Miehlke S, Labenz J (2007) Esomeprazole: prevention and treatment of NSAID-induced symptoms and ulcers. *Expert Opin Pharmacother* **8**(7):975–988.

Morrison BW, Fricke J, Brown J, *et al* (2000) The optimal analgesic dose of rofecoxib: overview of six randomized controlled trials. *J Am Dent Assoc* **131**(12):1729–1737.

Moulin D (1999) *Opioids in Chronic Non-malignant Pain*. Cambridge: Cambridge University Press.

Moulin DE, Iezzi A, Amireh R, *et al* (1996) Randomised trial of oral morphine for chronic non-cancer pain. *Lancet* **347**(8995):143–147.

Murata T, Ushikubi F, Matsuoka T, *et al* (1997) Altered pain perception and inflammatory response in mice lacking prostacyclin receptor. *Nature* **388**(6643):678–682.

Nettis E, Colanardi MC, Ferrannini A, *et al* (2005) Short-term and long-term tolerability of rofecoxib in patients with prior reactions to nonsteroidal anti-inflammatory drugs. *Ann Allergy Asthma Immunol* **94**(1):29–33.

Nielsen GL, Sorensen HT, Larsen H, *et al* (2001) Risk of adverse birth outcome and miscarriage in pregnant users of non-steroidal anti-inflammatory drugs: population based observational study and case-control study. *BMJ* **322**(7281):266–270.

Nikles CJ, Yelland M, Del Mar C, *et al* (2005) The role of paracetamol in chronic pain: an evidence-based approach. *Am J Ther* **12**(1):80–91.

Noda K, Ueda Y, Suzuki K, *et al* (1997) Excitatory effects of algesic compounds on neuronal processes in murine dorsal root ganglion cell culture. *Brain Res* **751**(2):348–351.

Norholt SE (1998) Treatment of acute pain following removal of mandibular third molars. Use of the dental pain model in pharmacological research and development of a comparable animal model. *Int J Oral Maxillofac Surg* **27**(Suppl 1):1–41.

Norman RJ, Wu R (2004) The potential danger of COX-2 inhibitors. *Fertil Steril* **81**(3):493–494.

Nussmeier NA, Whelton AA, Brown MT, *et al* (2005) Complications of the COX-2 inhibitors parecoxib and valdecoxib after cardiac surgery. *N Engl J Med* **352**(11):1081–1091.

O'Callaghan J (2001) Evolution of a rational use of opioids in chronic pain. *Euro J Pain* **5**(Suppl A):21–26.

Ormrod D, Wellington K, Wagstaff AJ (2002) Valdecoxib. *Drugs* **62**(14):2059–2071; discussion 2072-2073.

Ott E, Nussmeier NA, Duke PC, *et al* (2003) Efficacy and safety of the cyclooxygenase 2 inhibitors parecoxib and valdecoxib in patients undergoing coronary artery bypass surgery. *J Thorac Cardiovasc Surg* **125**(6):1481–1492.

Ouellet M, Riendeau D, Percival MD (2001) A high level of cyclooxygenase-2 inhibitor selectivity is associated with a reduced interference of platelet cyclooxygenase-1 inactivation by aspirin. *Proc Natl Acad Sci USA* **98**(25):14583–14588.

Page J, Henry D (2000) Consumption of NSAIDs and the development of congestive heart failure in elderly patients: an underrecognized public health problem. *Arch Intern Med* **160**(6): 777–784.

Pareja J, Sjaastad O (1996) Chronic paroxysmal hemicrania and hemicrania continua. Interval between indomethacin administration and response. *Headache* **36**(1):20–23.

Patrono C, Coller B, Dalen JE, *et al* (2001) Platelet-active drugs: the relationships among dose, effectiveness, and side effects. *Chest* **119**(1 Suppl):39S–63S.

Perez Gutthann S, Garcia Rodriguez LA, Raiford DS, *et al* (1996) Nonsteroidal anti-inflammatory drugs and the risk of hospitalization for acute renal failure. *Arch Intern Med* **156**(21):2433–2439.

Perrone MR, Artesani MC, Viola M, *et al* (2003) Tolerability of rofecoxib in patients with adverse reactions to nonsteroidal anti-inflammatory drugs: a study of 216 patients and literature review. *Int Arch Allergy Immunol* **132**(1):82–86.

Perry S, Heidrich G (1982) Management of pain during debridement: a survey of U.S. burn units. *Pain* **13**(3):267–280.

Portenoy RK, Foley KM (1986) Chronic use of opioid analgesics in non-malignant pain: report of 38 cases. *Pain* **25**(2):171–186.

Pounder R (1989) Silent peptic ulceration: deadly silence or golden silence? *Gastroenterology* **96**(2 Pt 2 Suppl):626–631.

Price MP, McIlwrath SL, Xie J, *et al* (2001) The DRASIC cation channel contributes to the detection of cutaneous touch and acid stimuli in mice. *Neuron* **32**(6):1071–1083.

Psaty BM, Furberg CD (2005) COX-2 inhibitors—lessons in drug safety. *N Engl J Med* **352**(11):1133–1135.

Quintana A, Raczka E, Giralt MT, *et al* (1983) Effects of aspirin and indomethacin on cerebral circulation in the conscious rat: evidence for a physiological role of endogenous prostaglandins. *Prostaglandins* **25**(4):549–556.

Quintana A, Raczka E, Quintana MA (1988) Effects of indomethacin and diclofenac on cerebral blood flow in hypercapnic conscious rats. *Eur J Pharmacol* **149**(3):385–388.

Raffa RB (2001) Pharmacology of oral combination analgesics: rational therapy for pain. *J Clin Pharm Ther* **26**(4):257–264.

Raja SN, Haythornthwaite JA, Pappagallo M, *et al* (2002) Opioids versus antidepressants in postherpetic neuralgia: a randomized, placebo-controlled trial. *Neurology* **59**(7): 1015–1021.

Riendeau D, Percival MD, Brideau C, *et al* (2001) Etoricoxib (MK-0663): preclinical profile and comparison with other agents that selectively inhibit cyclooxygenase-2. *J Pharmacol Exp Ther* **296**(2):558–566.

Robinson DR (1997) Regulation of prostaglandin synthesis by antiinflammatory drugs. *J Rheumatol Suppl* **47**:32–39.

Romsing J, Moiniche S (2004) A systematic review of COX-2 inhibitors compared with traditional NSAIDs, or different COX-2 inhibitors for post-operative pain. *Acta Anaesthesiol Scand* **48**(5):525–546.

Ross FB, Smith MT (1997) The intrinsic antinociceptive effects of oxycodone appear to be kappa-opioid receptor mediated. *Pain* **73**(2):151–157.

Roszkowski MT, Swift JQ, Hargreaves KM (1997) Effect of NSAID administration on tissue levels of immunoreactive prostaglandin E2, leukotriene B4, and (S)-flurbiprofen following extraction of impacted third molars. *Pain* **73**(3):339–345.

Rueff A, Dray A (1993) Sensitization of peripheral afferent fibres in the in vitro neonatal rat spinal cord-tail by bradykinin and prostaglandins. *Neuroscience* **54**(2):527–535.

Sachs CJ (2005) Oral analgesics for acute nonspecific pain. *Am Fam Physician* **71**(5):913–918.

Samad TA, Moore KA, Sapirstein A, *et al* (2001) Interleukin-1beta-mediated induction of Cox-2 in the CNS contributes to inflammatory pain hypersensitivity. *Nature* **410**(6827):471–475.

Sanchez-Borges M, Caballero-Fonseca F, Capriles-Hulett A (2005) Safety of etoricoxib, a new cyclooxygenase 2 inhibitor, in patients with nonsteroidal anti-inflammatory drug-induced urticaria and angioedema. *Ann Allergy Asthma Immunol* **95**(2): 154–158.

Sanchez S, Martin MJ, Ortiz P, *et al* (2002) Effects of dipyrone on inflammatory infiltration and oxidative metabolism in gastric mucosa: comparison with acetaminophen and diclofenac. *Dig Dis Sci* **47**(6):1389–1398.

Sandhu GK, Heyneman CA (2004) Nephrotoxic potential of selective cyclooxygenase-2 inhibitors. *Ann Pharmacother* **38**(4): 700–704.

Savage MG, Henry MA (2004) Preoperative nonsteroidal anti-inflammatory agents: review of the literature. *Oral Surg Oral Med Oral Pathol Oral Radiol Endod* **98**(2):146–152.

Savage SR (1996) Long-term opioid therapy: assessment of consequences and risks. *J Pain Symptom Manage* **11**(5):274–286.

Schafer AI (1999) Effects of nonsteroidal anti-inflammatory therapy on platelets. *Am J Med* **106**(5B):25S–36S.

Schnitzer TJ, Burmester GR, Mysler E, *et al* (2004) Comparison of lumiracoxib with naproxen and ibuprofen in the Therapeutic Arthritis Research and Gastrointestinal Event Trial (TARGET), reduction in ulcer complications: randomised controlled trial. *Lancet* **364**(9435):665–674.

Schoen RT, Vender RJ (1989) Mechanisms of nonsteroidal anti-inflammatory drug-induced gastric damage. *Am J Med* **86**(4): 449–458.

Schug SA, Gandham N (2006). Opioids: clinical use. In: McMahon SB, Koltzenburg M (eds) *Wall and Melzack's Textbook of Pain*, 5th edn. Philadelphia: Elsevier, pp 443–457.

Schug SA, Zech D, Grond S (1992) Adverse effects of systemic opioid analgesics. *Drug Saf* **7**(3):200–213.

Scott LJ, Perry CM (2000) Tramadol: a review of its use in perioperative pain. *Drugs* **60**(1):139–176.

Settipane RA, Schrank PJ, Simon RA, *et al* (1995) Prevalence of cross-sensitivity with acetaminophen in aspirin-sensitive asthmatic subjects. *J Allergy Clin Immunol* **96**(4):480–485.

Seybold VS, Jia YP, Abrahams LG (2003) Cyclo-oxygenase-2 contributes to central sensitization in rats with peripheral inflammation. *Pain* **105**(1-2):47–55.

Seymour RA, Ward-Booth P, Kelly PJ (1996) Evaluation of different doses of soluble ibuprofen and ibuprofen tablets in postoperative dental pain. *Br J Oral Maxillofac Surg* **34**(1): 110–114.

Shaheen SO, Newson RB, Henderson AJ, *et al* (2005) Prenatal paracetamol exposure and risk of asthma and elevated immunoglobulin E in childhood. *Clin Exp Allergy* **35**(1):18–25.

Silverstein FE, Faich G, Goldstein JL, *et al* (2000) Gastrointestinal toxicity with celecoxib vs nonsteroidal anti-inflammatory drugs for osteoarthritis and rheumatoid arthritis: the CLASS study: A randomized controlled trial. Celecoxib Long-term Arthritis Safety Study. *JAMA* **284**(10):1247–1255.

Sindrup SH, Brosen K (1995) The pharmacogenetics of codeine hypoalgesia. *Pharmacogenetics* **5**(6):335–346.

Singh G, Triadafilopoulos G (1999) Epidemiology of NSAID induced gastrointestinal complications. *J Rheumatol Suppl* **56**:18–24.

Singh G, Ramey DR, Morfeld D, *et al* (1996) Gastrointestinal tract complications of nonsteroidal anti-inflammatory drug treatment in rheumatoid arthritis. A prospective observational cohort study. *Arch Intern Med* **156**(14):1530–1536.

Singh VP, Patil CS, Kulkarni SK (2006) Anti-inflammatory effect of licofelone against various inflammatory challenges. *Fundam Clin Pharmacol* **20**(1):65–71.

Slavik RS, Rhoney DH (1999) Indomethacin: a review of its cerebral blood flow effects and potential use for controlling intracranial pressure in traumatic brain injury patients. *Neurol Res* **21**(5):491–499.

Smith WL, Marnett LJ (1991) Prostaglandin endoperoxide synthase: structure and catalysis. *Biochim Biophys Acta* **1083**(1):1–17.

Smith WL, Meade EA, DeWitt DL (1994) Interactions of PGH synthase isozymes-1 and -2 with NSAIDs. *Ann N Y Acad Sci* **744**:50–57.

Solomon DH, Schneeweiss S, Glynn RJ, *et al* (2004) Relationship between selective cyclooxygenase-2 inhibitors and acute myocardial infarction in older adults. *Circulation* **109**(17): 2068–2073.

Solomon SD, McMurray JJ, Pfeffer MA, *et al* (2005) Cardiovascular risk associated with celecoxib in a clinical trial for colorectal adenoma prevention. *N Engl J Med* **352**(11):1071–1080.

Solomon DH, Avorn J, Sturmer T, *et al* (2006) Cardiovascular outcomes in new users of coxibs and nonsteroidal antiinflammatory drugs: high-risk subgroups and time course of risk. *Arthritis Rheum* **54**(5):1378–1389.

Southall MD, Vasko MR (2000) Prostaglandin E(2)-mediated sensitization of rat sensory neurons is not altered by nerve growth factor. *Neurosci Lett* **287**(1):33–36.

Spalding WM, Reeves MJ, Whelton A (2007) Thromboembolic cardiovascular risk among arthritis patients using cyclooxygenase-2-selective inhibitor or nonselective cyclooxygenase inhibitor nonsteroidal anti-inflammatory drugs. *Am J Ther* **14**(1):3–12.

Speziale MV, Allen RG, Henderson CR, *et al* (1999) Effects of ibuprofen and indomethacin on the regional circulation in newborn piglets. *Biol Neonate* **76**(4):242–252.

Spink M, Bann S, Glickman R (2005) Clinical implications of cyclo-oxygenase-2 inhibitors for acute dental pain management: benefits and risks. *J Am Dent Assoc* **136**(10):1439–1448.

Steen KH, Issberner U, Reeh PW (1995) Pain due to experimental acidosis in human skin: evidence for non-adapting nociceptor excitation. *Neurosci Lett* **199**(1):29–32.

Steen KH, Steen AE, Kreysel HW, *et al* (1996) Inflammatory mediators potentiate pain induced by experimental tissue acidosis. *Pain* **66**(2-3):163–170.

Stevenson DD, Sanchez-Borges M, Szczeklik A (2001) Classification of allergic and pseudoallergic reactions to drugs that inhibit cyclooxygenase enzymes. *Ann Allergy Asthma Immunol* **87**(3):177–180.

Stichtenoth DO, Frolich JC (2000) COX-2 and the kidneys. *Curr Pharm Des* **6**(17):1737–1753.

Stichtenoth DO, Frolich JC (2003) The second generation of COX-2 inhibitors: what advantages do the newest offer? *Drugs* **63**(1):33–45.

Sutherland SP, Cook SP, McCleskey EW (2000) Chemical mediators of pain due to tissue damage and ischemia. *Prog Brain Res* **129**:21–38.

Szczeklik A (1990) The cyclooxygenase theory of aspirin-induced asthma. *Eur Respir J* **3**(5):588–593.

Szczeklik A, Stevenson DD (1999) Aspirin-induced asthma: advances in pathogenesis and management. *J Allergy Clin Immunol* **104**(1):5–13.

Szczeklik A, Gryglewski RJ, Czerniawska-Mysik G (1977) Clinical patterns of hypersensitivity to nonsteroidal anti-inflammatory drugs and their pathogenesis. *J Allergy Clin Immunol* **60** (5):276–284.

Taiwo YO, Levine JD (1989) Prostaglandin effects after elimination of indirect hyperalgesic mechanisms in the skin of the rat. *Brain Res* **492**(1-2):397–399.

Taiwo YO, Heller PH, Levine JD (1990) Characterization of distinct phospholipases mediating bradykinin and noradrenaline hyperalgesia. *Neuroscience* **39**(2):523–531.

Taylor DW, Barnett HJ, Haynes RB, *et al* (1999) Low-dose and high-dose acetylsalicylic acid for patients undergoing carotid endarterectomy: a randomised controlled trial. ASA and Carotid Endarterectomy (ACE) Trial Collaborators. *Lancet* **353** (9171):2179–2184.

Tegeder I, Pfeilschifter J, Geisslinger G (2001) Cyclooxygenase-independent actions of cyclooxygenase inhibitors. *FASEB J* **15**(12):2057–2072.

Tramer MR, Moore RA, Reynolds DJ, *et al* (2000) Quantitative estimation of rare adverse events which follow a biological progression: a new model applied to chronic NSAID use. *Pain* **85**(1-2):169–182.

Vainio A, Ollila J, Matikainen E, *et al* (1995) Driving ability in cancer patients receiving long-term morphine analgesia. *Lancet* **346**(8976):667–670.

Vane J (1994) Towards a better aspirin. *Nature* **367**(6460):215–216.

Vane JR (1971) Inhibition of prostaglandin synthesis as a mechanism of action for aspirin-like drugs. *Nat New Biol* **231**(25):232–235.

Ventura-Martinez R, Deciga-Campos M, Diaz-Reval MI, *et al* (2004) Peripheral involvement of the nitric oxide-cGMP pathway in the indomethacin-induced antinociception in rat. *Eur J Pharmacol* **503**(1-3):43–48.

Walker JS, Carmody JJ (1998) Experimental pain in healthy human subjects: gender differences in nociception and in response to ibuprofen. *Anesth Analg* **86**(6):1257–1262.

Wallace JL, Devchand PR (2005) Emerging roles for cyclooxygenase-2 in gastrointestinal mucosal defense. *Br J Pharmacol* **145**(3):275–282.

Watkins PB, Kaplowitz N, Slattery JT, *et al* (2006) Aminotransferase elevations in healthy adults receiving 4 grams of acetaminophen daily: a randomized controlled trial. *JAMA* **296**(1):87–93.

Wennmalm A, Carlsson A, Edlund S, *et al* (1984) Central and peripheral haemodynamic effects of non-steroidal anti-inflammatory drugs in man. *Arch Toxicol Suppl* **7**:350–359.

Whelton A, Stout RL, Spilman PS, *et al* (1990) Renal effects of ibuprofen, piroxicam, and sulindac in patients with asymptomatic renal failure. A prospective, randomized, crossover comparison. *Ann Intern Med* **112**(8):568–576.

Whelton A, White WB, Bello AE, *et al* (2002) Effects of celecoxib and rofecoxib on blood pressure and edema in patients > or = 65 years of age with systemic hypertension and osteoarthritis. *Am J Cardiol* **90**(9):959–963.

Winter L Jr, Bass E, Recant B, *et al* (1978) Analgesic activity of ibuprofen (Motrin) in postoperative oral surgical pain. *Oral Surg Oral Med Oral Pathol* **45**(2):159–166.

Wolfe MM, Soll AH (1988) The physiology of gastric acid secretion. *N Engl J Med* **319**(26):1707–1715.

Wolfe MM, Lichtenstein DR, Singh G (1999) Gastrointestinal toxicity of nonsteroidal antiinflammatory drugs. *N Engl J Med* **340**(24):1888–1899.

Wong M, Chowienczyk P, Kirkham B (2005) Cardiovascular issues of COX-2 inhibitors and NSAIDs. *Aust Fam Physician* **34**(11):945–948.

Woolf CJ, Salter MW (2000) Neuronal plasticity: increasing the gain in pain. *Science* **288**(5472):1765–1769.

Yaksh TL, Rudy TA (1978) Narcotic analgesics: CNS sites and mechanisms of action as revealed by intracerebral injection techniques. *Pain* **4**(4):299–359.

Zelenakas K, Fricke JR Jr, Jayawardene S, *et al* (2004) Analgesic efficacy of single oral doses of lumiracoxib and ibuprofen in patients with postoperative dental pain. *Int J Clin Pract* **58**(3): 251–256.

Zembowicz A, Mastalerz L, Setkowicz M, *et al* (2003) Safety of cyclooxygenase 2 inhibitors and increased leukotriene synthesis in chronic idiopathic urticaria with sensitivity to nonsteroidal anti-inflammatory drugs. *Arch Dermatol* **139**(12): 1577–1582.

Zenz M, Strumpf M, Tryba M (1992) Long-term oral opioid therapy in patients with chronic nonmalignant pain. *J Pain Symptom Manage* **7**(2):69–77.

Zhang J, Ding EL, Song Y (2006) Adverse effects of cyclooxygenase 2 inhibitors on renal and arrhythmia events: meta-analysis of randomized trials. *JAMA* **296**:1619–1632.

CHAPTER 16

Pharmacotherapy of chronic orofacial pain

Rafael Benoliel and Yair Sharav

1. Introduction

Treatment of a disorder ideally aims at its ultimate eradication, a goal that currently eludes us in chronic pain. We are, however, able to offer adequate pharmacological management with many patients responding at least partially to therapy, albeit with significant morbidity. Prescription drugs therefore remain a mainstay of pain management; one of the most widely used drug classes in the USA in 2003 was the opioids and their combinations with over 115 million prescriptions (Health 2003). This reflects the epidemiology of persistent pain in the population; individual orofacial pain syndromes are extremely common and have been reviewed in specific chapters.

The comprehensive management of chronic orofacial pain commonly involves the integration of patient education with multiple treatment avenues such as physiotherapy and pharmacotherapy. The indications and choice of drugs (which and when) for the clinical syndromes are described in Chapters 7–11. In this chapter the application and mechanisms of drugs used in the treatment of these syndromes are described (how and why).

2. Treatment Approach

Ideally drug selection is patient-tailored and targeted at the underlying pathophysiological processes (mechanism-based). However, many of the mechanisms involved in chronic pain and the modes of action of the drugs we use are still unclear. Current pain pharmacotherapy is largely the result of clinical observation, at times serendipitous with double-blind randomized controlled trials (RCT) following later. Despite accepted pharmacotherapy guidelines for many of the craniofacial pain syndromes similar conditions are often treated differently across practitioners and approaches depend on training and continuing education activities of the physician (Green *et al* 2002). Moreover gender, age, ethnicity and race of *both* patient and physician will significantly affect treatment approaches (Green *et al* 2002) and substantial evidence needs to be presented to change established practices. Written treatment protocols reliant on evidence-based medicine help overcome treatment bias.

2.1. Drug Prescription and Treatment Plan

Most of the drugs employed for chronic pain have side effects, some affecting quality of life. Combining drugs (usually of different drug classes) is at times indicated and depends on the suspected pain mechanisms, pain control achieved with a single drug and other factors. Drug combinations are often used in the treatment of migraine (Chapter 9), neuropathic pain (Chapter 11) and acute pain (Chapters 5 and 15); specific combinations are therefore discussed in the chapters covering these entities. However, polypharmacy often significantly increases side effects and drug interactions so there must be a clear gain in therapeutic efficacy to justify combinations (see Chapter 15). Additionally treatment approaches to chronic or recurrent pain may be preventive or abortive and depend partly on pain frequency, associated disability and patient preferences. Patients should be aware of the therapeutic aims (e.g. 50% reduction in pain severity or frequency), which are often less ambitious than their own expectations. The management of chronic pain is a long process involving several drug trials over prolonged periods with multiple follow-up visits and these require patient cooperation. Pain diaries are an essential part of the assessment of treatment outcome in terms of pain severity, attack duration and frequency and must be carefully documented.

Because chronic pain is a complex interaction of physical and emotional experiences the practitioner needs to be aware of comorbidities such as depression, anxiety, sleeplessness and drug abuse. Chronic pain management often requires patient referral to medical colleagues for the management of such comorbidities. Many patients will prefer not to take medications due to potential side effects and opt for non-pharmacologic interventions. Some studies show that cognitive behavioural therapy (CBT) is effective in reducing pain experience and promoting coping in individuals with chronic pain; see Chapter 4. As described in Chapter 17 pain patients are increasingly turning to complementary or alternative medicine for the management of pain. Basic knowledge of available modalities in addition to mainstream therapies is advantageous.

2.2. Assessing Drug Effects

Ideally drugs are effective across the widest range of patients, easy to take and with minimal side effects. To assess the efficacy of available drugs clinicians require an easy tool. The results of RCTs are considered reliable evidence as they account for physician bias and the potent effects of placebo and of patient expectation. Relief obtained with any particular drug must be balanced by the effects observed in the placebo arm of the trial; this may be an active drug and not placebo. Additionally because the endpoint of the trial often differs across studies it should be clearly defined; a 50% reduction in pain severity is commonly used. Meta-analyses and systematic reviews of RCTs provide an excellent way in which to assess effects across different populations, medical teams, countries and over time. These are more likely than individual trials to describe the true clinical effect of a drug.

However, the resulting statistics are often difficult to interpret and apply in everyday practice. One way of expressing the efficiency of a drug relative to placebo is the absolute risk reduction, calculated by subtracting placebo response from the observed drug response. The 'number needed to treat' (NNT) is the reciprocal of the absolute risk reduction and indicates the number of patients that need to be treated in order to obtain one with the desired outcome. Less favourable absolute risk reductions and therefore NNTs could result from a high placebo effect. By discounting the effects of the placebo arm the absolute risk reduction and NNT may control for between-study variability and therefore allow comparison of similar drugs tested by different researchers in different centres. At the same time, however, the

NNT may underestimate the clinical effect of the drug; as clinicians we enjoy the positive outcome of the placebo effect inherent in any intervention. It is essential to appreciate that NNTs are not strict rules but another well-based factor to be considered when deciding on the best treatment strategy for our patients. The NNT is extremely useful for comparing several drugs that have been assessed for the same outcome measure in patients with similar conditions. Using NNTs we can rank interventions relative to one another, making it possible to choose a specific drug based on efficacy (see Chapters 10–13 and 17). However, NNTs need to be balanced against adverse events, costs, patient characteristics, expectations and preferences.

For adverse events the NNT becomes the number needed to harm (NNH) that reflects the number of patients treated so that one would suffer the studied side effect. NNTs and NNHs are collected for each RCT on a particular drug and a mean of all these is calculated. Because the error is usually large and much overlap may exist between drugs, NNTs should be given with 95% confidence intervals. NNTs are disease-specific and cannot be compared across diagnoses. NNT (and NNH) must always specify the comparator, the therapeutic outcome and the duration of treatment necessary to achieve that outcome. As clinicians we are therefore searching for drugs with low NNTs and high NNHs, both with compact confidence intervals.

In addition to scientific journals, there are excellent evidence-based databases available (e.g. Bandolier, http://www.jr2.ox.ac.uk/bandolier/index.html; Clinical Evidence, http://www.clinicalevidence.com/ceweb/conditions/index.jsp; Cochrane Collaboration, http://www.cochrane.org/index.htm) although these generally require a subscription. Additionally many professional bodies publish recommendations but specific guidelines for the management of many orofacial pain syndromes are at present lacking.

Animal studies are also used to assess the efficacy of drugs in various pain states, both inflammatory and neuropathic. Often, however, the extrapolation of experimental findings from rodents to humans is disappointing and drugs that were analgesic in rats prove ineffective in humans. Notwithstanding, experimental data from rodent experiments remain the backbone of our understanding of the mechanisms of drugs and the pathophysiology of chronic pain.

3. Systemic Drugs Used in the Management of Chronic Pain

In many cases drugs used in the management of pain are not listed for such use by the US Federal Drug Administration (FDA) or other national agencies controlling drug use. This is termed 'off-label' prescribing and is accepted clinical practice but should always be based on solid evidence. In some countries and institutions off-label usage requires prior approval.

We review the major drug groups commonly employed in the management of chronic orofacial pain: antidepressants, antiepileptic drugs, antihypertensives, muscle relaxants and triptans. Additionally we provide a short overview on cannabinoids, N-methyl-D-aspartate (NMDA) antagonists and neuroleptics in the treatment of pain and headache. The large number of available drugs is impossible to completely review. Even within the drug groups selected for this chapter the detailed pharmacology, drug interactions and adverse effects are within the scope of clinical pharmacology texts that should form part of any practice or specialized clinic. Adverse effects and drug safety, particularly in pregnant and lactating women, are major concerns. We have provided an overview of the prominent side effects for each drug described and have based recommendations for use in pregnancy (see Table 16.1) and breastfeeding on FDA and other recommendations (Wiener and Buhimschi 2004). However, as reports of adverse effects, particularly for the newer drugs, are constantly updated the reader should refer to clinical pharmacology sources for updated information. The widespread use of personal computers allows Internet access to rich databases (e.g. Micromedex, http:www.micromedex. com; Epocrates, http:www2.epocrates.com; RxList, http: www.rxlist.com), some at no cost. These sources provide all necessary information and, in addition, may offer software that examines possible drug interactions.

Several strategies are essential across all the drugs employed in the management of pain. Needless to say the medical status of the patient must be balanced with the pharmacological profile of the intended drug and possible interactions with other drugs must be explored. It is advisable to start therapy at low doses and slowly titrate upwards based on therapeutic response and side effects; this maximizes patient's adherence to therapy and tends to minimize side effects. Drug therapy may often exert progressive effects over a period of weeks or months and specific drugs should not be abandoned early. Careful supervision and scheduled laboratory tests for drug effects (e.g. in carbamazepine therapy) is essential and reassures the patient that he is being competently cared for.

4. Antidepressants (Table 16.2)

Antidepressants are effective for the treatment of neuropathic, musculoskeletal and neurovascular type pains (see Chapters 7, 9–11). For some syndromes these are the drugs of choice: the best evidence of pain relief in traumatic neuropathies is for tricyclic antidepressants (TCA) e.g. amitriptyline with an NNT of 2 (95% confidence interval (CI): 1.7–2.5) (Saarto and Wiffen 2005). There are only limited data on the analgesic effectiveness of selective serotonin-reuptake inhibitors (SSRIs) and selective serotonin-norepinephrine reuptake inhibitors (SNRIs), but they are less effective than the TCAs.

4.1. Tricyclic Antidepressants (TCAs)

The TCAs were initially used for the treatment of depression. The advent of the newer antidepressants (SSRI, SNRI) with reduced side effects has largely shifted the use of TCAs for other problems such as pain. Amitriptyline is probably the most frequently employed TCA in chronic orofacial pain syndromes but the newer SSRIs and SNRIs have been applied with some success in pain medicine. Human and experimental analgesic trials reveal that drugs with mixed serotonin (5-HT)/noradrenaline effects such as imipramine and amitriptyline or SNRIs (e.g. venlafaxine) are superior to the SSRIs, such as fluoxetine or paroxetine (Mochizucki 2004).

Mode of action. At present much of the research relates to TCAs but as the newer drugs are investigated their modes of action may become clearer. The major pharmacological effect of TCAs is inhibition of 5-HT and noradrenaline reuptake. The modes of action of SNRIs in pain are at present unclear but probably involve some of the mechanisms of the TCAs. The importance of 5-HT and noradrenaline pathways in pain modulation suggests that antidepressants act by enhancing descending inhibitory controls. Indeed 5-HT and noradrenaline antagonists and depletion of central 5-HT and noradrenaline will

Table 16.1	Pregnancy Category Definitions (based on US Food and Drug Administration)
Category	**Description**
A	Controlled studies in women fail to demonstrate a risk to the foetus in the first trimester and no evidence of a risk in later trimesters. The possibility of foetal harm appears remote.
B	Animal-reproduction studies *have not* demonstrated a foetal risk but remain unconfirmed in studies in pregnant women, or: Animal-reproduction studies *have shown* adverse effect that was not confirmed in controlled studies in women in the first trimester.
C	Studies in animals have revealed adverse effects on the foetus but there are no controlled studies in women. Drugs should be given only if the potential benefit justifies the potential risk to the foetus.
D	Positive evidence of human foetal risk. Benefits from use in pregnant women may be acceptable despite the risk for life-threatening situations or serious disease.
X	Studies in animals or human beings have demonstrated foetal abnormalities. The risk of the use of the drug in women that are or may become pregnant clearly outweighs any possible benefit.

Table 16.2 Antidepressant Drugs

Drug	Initial Dose (mg)	Target or Max Dose (mg)[a]	Dose Increase (Titration)[a]	Schedule	Food	Pregnancy Category	Breastfeeding	Medical Contraindications	Drug Interactions	Common Side Effects
Amitriptyline	10	35–50	10 mg/wk	Bedtime	—	D	Probably safe	Cardiac Diabetes Epilepsy Glaucoma Hepatic Psychiatric Thyroid Urinary retention	Anticoagulants Antidepressants Antihypertensives Carbamazepine Catecholamines Cimetidine Ergotamine Fluconazole Insulin NSAIDs Sulfonylureas Thyroid hormones Triptans	Weight gain, bloating, constipation, xerostomia, asthenia, dizziness, headache, blurred vision, urinary retention, vision, fatigue, somnolence
Imipramine	12.5	25–50	12.5 mg/wk	Bedtime	—	C	Unknown			
Venlafaxine	37.5	75–150	75 mg/4–7 d	×2–3/d	[IOI][b]	C	Unknown	Cardiac Epilepsy Glaucoma Hepatic, Renal Hypertension Hyperlipidaemia Psychiatric Other than 3rd trimester	Antidepressants Erythromycin Fluconazole NSAIDs Triptans	Hypertension, sweating, constipation, loss of appetite, nausea, xerostomia, asthenia, dizziness, headache, insomnia or somnolence, tremor, nervousness, abnormal ejaculation, impotence
• Venlafaxine-XR	37.5	75–225	75 mg/4–7 d	1/d						
Duloxetine	20–40	60	20 mg/wk	×1–2/d	—	C	Unknown	Epilepsy Glaucoma Other than 3rd trimester Hepatic, Renal Psychiatric	Antidepressants	Sweating, constipation, loss of appetite, nausea, xerostomia, diarrhoea, gastritis, dizziness, insomnia or somnolence, blurred vision, dysuria, fatigue

[a]Rough guideline; clinically titrate therapeutic response versus side effects.

[b][IOI] = to be taken with food.

attenuate the analgesia obtained with TCAs (Gray *et al* 1999; Schreiber *et al* 1999). However, the clinical effects of TCAs appear following a lag of days to weeks and their pharmacological effects occur within hours. It is therefore suggested that the pharmacological mechanisms although important in themselves also induce changes in gene expression, leading to modified formation of neuropeptides and receptors.

Indeed, chronic TCA administration modifies opioid receptor densities and increases endogenous brain opioid levels (Hamon *et al* 1987; Sacerdote *et al* 1987). TCAs therefore enhance endogenous opioid effects (analgesia and neuronal inhibition) and will act synergistically with opioids in providing pain relief (Luccarini *et al* 2004). Additionally, TCAs have an NMDA antagonist effect that makes them useful in pain syndromes with characteristics of central sensitization (Cai and McCaslin 1992). TCAs possess sodium, calcium and potassium channel blocking properties (Ogata *et al* 1989). The sodium channel blocking properties of TCAs are robust; regional application of TCAs has an effect comparable to that of local anaesthetics (Gerner *et al* 2003). This will stabilize neurons, prevent peripheral sensitization and may underlie the mechanisms of peripheral analgesia (Wang *et al* 2004). More recently it has been shown that a number of antidepressants induce an upregulation of γ-aminobutyric acid (GABA) receptor expression in spinal cord (McCarson *et al* 2006).

Other peripheral actions include the ability to block α-adrenergic receptors which may be beneficial in sympathetically maintained pain syndromes. The enhancement of inhibitory GABA and opioid effects are also present peripherally, increasing the analgesic effects of TCAs (Nakashita *et al* 1997). TCAs and other antidepressants have moderate anti-inflammatory actions that would augment analgesia (Abdel-Salam *et al* 2004). Histamine and cholinergic receptor blockade is thought to augment TCAs' analgesic effects but causes many of the observed side effects (Ferjan and Erjavec 1996; Irman-Florjanc and Stanovnik 1998). Amitriptyline is thought to act antagonistically at cephalic blood-vessel 5-HT$_{2B/7}$ receptors; it downregulates 5-HT$_{2B}$ receptors, thus reducing vessel wall reactivity and vasodilatation (Crews *et al* 1983). For many years amitriptyline has therefore been in the front line of migraine prophylaxis; see Chapter 9. Amitriptyline may be superior to other drugs when pain comorbidity includes myalgia, depression or sleeplessness.

Drugs related to the dopaminergic, serotonergic and adrenergic systems such as the antidepressants have been shown to suppress or exacerbate bruxist activity in humans and animals (Winocur *et al* 2003). However, there is insufficient evidence-based data to draw definite conclusions concerning the effects of specific drugs on bruxism.

4.1.1. Amitriptyline

FDA-approved indications are depression and polyneuropathy, but amitriptyline is used extensively off-label for migraine, fibromyalgia, myofascial pain and other chronic pain states.

Efficacy. Amitriptyline is effective in the management of many chronic orofacial pains and chronic tension-type headache. In addition to reducing subjective pain parameters amitriptyline induces a reduction of myofascial tenderness in the affected areas (Bendtsen and Jensen 2000).

Clinical considerations. The analgesic effect of TCAs is independent of their antidepressant actions and may be attained at much lower doses (Sharav *et al* 1987; Max *et al* 1992); 10 mg taken 1–2 hours before bedtime is the recommended initial dose. The long elimination half-life of amitriptyline (10–26 hours) allows for a once-daily schedule. The dose may be increased if necessary at a rate of 10 mg a week to a maximum of 35–50 mg. Chronic administration of 25 mg amitriptyline daily is not associated with significant reductions in patients' processing or task-performing capacity (Veldhuijzen *et al* 2006). Higher doses (>100mg) are prescribed to patients with headache and other chronic pain syndromes but these are accompanied by significant side effects. Additionally the danger of sudden death increases by 40% for 100 mg or more of amitriptyline or other equivalent TCA dose (Ray *et al* 2004). Analgesic effects may be observed at one week but may take up to several weeks and therapy should be continued for 3–6 months before being slowly tapered and discontinued.

Adverse effects. Side effects at low doses are rare and not serious: usually dry mouth, sedation, palpitations, nausea and sweating. Other common effects include bloating, constipation, asthenia, dizziness, headache, blurred vision, fatigue and somnolence. In patients taking 25mg amitriptyline daily for 12 weeks a mean weight gain of 3.2kg has been reported (Berilgen *et al* 2005). Weight control should therefore be an integral part of patient management. Rarely patients may feel anxiety or agitation and the addition of a benzodiazepine resolves this; e.g. 0.5mg clonazepam, 5 mg diazepam or 0.5–1mg of slow-release alprazolam. This combination may, however, increase sedative effects. Possible contraindications for amitriptyline include urinary retention and narrow angle glaucoma. TCAs decrease the convulsive threshold and are therefore problematic in existing epileptic disorder. The use of TCAs with anti-arrhythmics is contraindicated and the presence of cardiovascular disorders requires a medical consultation. In ongoing antidepressant therapy (e.g. SSRIs) or in depressed or suicidal patients TCAs are to be initiated only after consultation with the treating psychiatrist. TCAs possess antihyperglycaemic effects and therefore may alter insulin or other hypoglycaemic drug requirements in diabetics. Carbamazepine induces the metabolism of TCAs and reduces effective plasma concentrations. Thyroid disease and thyroid hormones may interact with TCAs to induce an increase in receptor sensitivity to catecholamines.

TCAs and SSRIs increase the risk of upper gastrointestinal (GI) bleeding (Dalton *et al* 2003). The number of upper GI bleeding episodes in patients on amitriptyline and imipramine was 2.5 and 3.5 times more than expected and the use of TCAs with nonsteroidal anti-inflammatory drugs (NSAIDs) or aspirin increased risk of GI bleeding by 9.6 and 8.3, respectively. SSRI use was associated with a 3.6 increased risk and combined use with NSAIDs or low-dose aspirin increased the risk to 12.2 and 5.2, respectively (Dalton *et al* 2003). Antidepressants without action on the serotonin receptor had no significant effect on the risk of upper GI bleeding. The increased risk disappeared after complete cessation of SSRI use. However, the risks of upper GI bleeding remained increased during periods when *TCAs* were stopped, suggesting that other mechanisms were involved.

Rare but serious side effects reported include myocardial infarction, cerebrovascular accident, orthostatic hypotension and syncope. Rare haematologic events include agranulocytosis, aplastic anaemia, leukopenia, thrombocytopenia or pancytopenia. Similarly decreased liver function and jaundice have been reported rarely.

Amitriptyline is in pregnancy category D (see Table 16.1) and is excreted into milk; however, with low resulting concentrations in breastfed neonates it is probably safe.

4.1.2. Imipramine

Imipramine has been widely used in the treatment of traumatic neuropathies and may be tried when amitriptyline is not tolerated or is ineffective. Treatment may be initiated at 12.5 mg daily (half a tablet) and slowly titrated up to 25–50 mg daily. Side effects with imipramine are similar to those observed with amitriptyline, but with slightly less sedative effects.

4.2. Venlafaxine

Venlafaxine is a structurally novel SNRI antidepressant that is FDA approved for the treatment of depression, generalized anxiety disorder and social phobia.

Efficacy. Venlafaxine-extended release (XR) has shown promise in the prophylaxis of migraine and tension-type headache (Adelman *et al* 2000). Moreover in a double-blind RCT venlafaxine-XR 150 mg provided significant prophylaxis for migraine patients (Ozyalcin *et al* 2005). There are reports of benefit from the use of venlafaxine in patients with painful diabetic neuropathy or neuropathic pain of unknown cause (Kiayias *et al* 2000; Sumpton and Moulin 2001). Venlafaxine-XR at doses ranging 150–225 mg had an NNT of 4.5–5.7 for moderate or 50% relief in painful diabetic neuropathy (Sindrup *et al* 2003; Rowbotham *et al* 2004). Venlafaxine (75 mg) was found to be modestly effective in the treatment of atypical facial pain (Forssell *et al* 2004). No significant correlation was found between venlafaxine serum concentration and treatment response. Analgesia was independent of antidepressive or antianxiety effects and adverse events were equally common in venlafaxine and placebo.

Clinical considerations. To minimize side effects patients are often started on 37.5 mg daily for the first 4–7 days before increasing to 75 mg daily. If necessary the dose may be increased to 150 mg daily after several weeks. Further increases, to a maximum daily dose of 225 mg, may be made at intervals of not less than 4 days. Modified-release (XR) preparations enable once-daily dosing.

Adverse effects. Most frequently reported events with venlafaxine are nausea, headache, insomnia, somnolence, dry mouth, dizziness, constipation, sexual dysfunction (abnormal ejaculation or impotence), asthenia, sweating, tremor and nervousness. Patients, especially the elderly, should be warned of the risk of dizziness or unsteadiness due to orthostatic hypotension. As with other antidepressants, venlafaxine may impair performance of skilled tasks and, if affected, patients should not drive or operate machinery. Venlafaxine should be used with caution in patients with moderate to severe hepatic or renal impairment and dosage adjustment may be necessary. A medical consultation is indicated in patients with a recent history of myocardial infarction or unstable heart disease, or whose condition might be exacerbated by an increase in heart rate. Because of the risk of dose-related hypertension, blood pressure monitoring may be advisable. Loss of appetite and weight loss are commonly reported.

Measurement of serum-cholesterol levels should also be considered with long-term treatment. Venlafaxine should not be used when bleeding disorders are present. Because of an increased risk in patients with a history of hypomania, mania or epilepsy venlafaxine should also be used with caution and be discontinued in any patient with a history of developing a seizure. Patients with raised intraocular pressure or at risk of angle-closure glaucoma should be monitored closely. Patients who develop a rash, urticaria or related allergic reaction with venlafaxine should be referred for medical consultation. Rare but serious side effects reported include hyponatraemia and hepatitis.

Venlafaxine is in pregnancy category C but extreme caution is recommended in the third trimester. Low levels are detectable in about half of breastfed neonates and the exact risk is unknown.

4.3. Duloxetine

Duloxetine is a new generation SNRI that is FDA-approved for the treatment of major depressive disorder and painful diabetic neuropathy. Experimental data suggest that duloxetine has analgesic properties in neuropathic and inflammatory pain states (Bomholt *et al* 2005; Jones *et al* 2005).

Efficacy. Clinical data have clearly shown the effectiveness of duloxetine in the treatment of painful diabetic neuropathy (Goldstein *et al* 2005; Raskin *et al* 2005). In the treatment of depression usual doses are 20–30 mg twice daily or 60 mg once daily.

Clinical considerations. The recommended dose for pain is 60 mg once daily taken irrespective of meal times. In cases where this dose causes considerable side effects a lower starting dose is indicated. It is unclear whether doses higher than 60 mg are more effective but 120 mg has also been successfully employed, albeit with a higher dropout rate due to side effects (Raskin *et al* 2005).

Adverse effects. The incidence of adverse effects in duloxetine therapy has largely been assessed in open studies so the figures are unreliable. Insomnia, headache and sleepiness are common; less frequent nervous system effects include dizziness, blurred vision, somnolence or fatigue, tremor and agitation. GI effects are also relatively common and include loss of appetite, nausea, diarrhoea or constipation, gastritis and dry mouth; less frequently, anorexia and taste changes have been described. Increased day- and night-time sweating may occur. Duloxetine should not be used in patients with hepatic impairment. Dysuria is common but no dosage adjustment is considered necessary in patients with mild to moderate renal impairment. Rare but serious side effects include worsening of depression, suicidal thoughts and even suicide. Duloxetine is in pregnancy category C but extreme caution is recommended in the third trimester. Due to a lack of data the exact risk to breastfed neonates is unknown.

4.4. Bupropion

Bupropion is chemically unrelated to other classes of antidepressants and is widely used as an aid to smoking cessation. Relative to TCAs, it is a weak blocker of neuronal reuptake of 5-HT and noradrenaline. Bupropion also inhibits the neuronal reuptake of dopamine which is thought to augment analgesic effects in experimental neuropathy (Pedersen *et al* 2005). Indeed bupropion in a slow-release formulation seems effective in the treatment of neuropathic pain (Semenchuk *et al* 2001) but has been disappointing in non-neuropathic pain states (Katz *et al* 2005). Dosages of 150 mg twice daily result in pain relief by the second week, whilst antidepressant effects are usually observed after 4 weeks (Semenchuk *et al* 2001).

5. Antiepileptic Drugs (Table 16.3)

The anticonvulsants or antiepileptic drugs (AED) have been extensively employed in the management of neuropathic pain (e.g. trigeminal neuralgia, diabetic and traumatic neuropathy) and more recently in the prophylaxis of neurovascular pains. The AEDs consist of a number of heterogeneous drugs with varied modes of action and most commonly carbamazepine, valproates and clonazepam are specifically employed in the management of orofacial pain. Newer agents assessed for pain include topiramate, gabapentin, pregabalin and lamotrigine and these possess fewer side effects. Experimentally there seems to be no correlation between antiepileptic activity and analgesic efficacy in neuropathic pain, suggesting multimodal mechanisms (Shannon *et al* 2005). Different drugs possess different combinations of these modes of action and specific drugs may be more effective against particular expressions of neuropathic pain (e.g. mechano-hyperalgesia) or may modulate inflammatory components more than others; see Fig. 16.1 (Bianchi *et al* 1995; Fox *et al* 2003). In some cases therefore the combination of two AEDs may offer some benefit. Many of the modes of action of AEDs in pain are common across a wide variety of agents and these are reviewed below.

5.1. Mode of Action

The therapeutic effects of AEDs in headache, orofacial and neuropathic pain are mediated by a reduction in neurogenic inflammation and central trigeminal activation, modulation of central nervous system effects and an enhancement of antinociceptive mechanisms (Cutrer 2001; Soderpalm 2002). At least in part AEDs are analgesic by their ability to suppress neuronal excitability through a number of mechanisms; see Fig. 16.1 (Moshe 2000; Soderpalm 2002). Different AEDs possess varying combinations of these effects and some of the newer drugs may have as yet undiscovered modes of action.

GABA effects. When GABA is released from the presynaptic terminal it binds to at least two postsynaptic receptors. Activation of the GABA-A receptor induces an influx of chloride ions and of GABA-B an inhibition of calcium channels or deactivation of potassium channels (Moshe 2000). This effectively hyperpolarizes the postsynaptic neuron inhibiting activity. Some AEDs are able to facilitate GABA neurotransmission by increasing presynaptic GABA levels and postsynaptic GABA-receptor function. The central analgesic actions of carbamazepine are partially mediated by GABAergic systems in the periaqueductal grey (Foong and Satoh 1984). Valproate is thought to act by increasing brain levels of GABA whilst benzodiazepines and barbiturates enhance postsynaptic GABA-receptor binding.

Sodium (Na) channel blockade. A large number of AEDs act on Na channels, probably via a prolongation in the recovery phase following channel activation. The effect is use- and voltage-dependent (i.e. the number of channels inactivated increases with each additional stimulus and is more pronounced in excited neurons), leading to the modulation of neurotransmitter release. The stepwise blockade of Na channels is an important facet of certain AEDs and limits side effects.

Glutamate (GLU). GLU is a major excitatory neurotransmitter and its release is modulated by presynaptic sodium (Na) and calcium (Ca) channels. Following its release GLU binds to NMDA and non-NMDA receptors (AMPA, kainite, metabotropic) on the postsynaptic membrane. Activation of non-NMDA receptors induces an influx of Na ions and depolarization and excitation of the neuron. This excitation ultimately leads to the activation of NMDA receptors (see Chapters 3, 12) and an influx of Ca ions, leading to further excitation of the

Table 16.3 Anticonvulsant Drugs

Drug	Initial Dose (mg)	Target or Max Dose (mg)[a]	Dose Increase (Titration)[a]	Schedule	Food	Pregnancy Category	Breastfeeding	Medical Contraindications	Drug Interactions	Common Side Effects
Carbamazepine	100–200	1200	100–200mg/2d	×3–4/d	🍽[b]	D	Probably safe	Bone marrow Cardiac Blood disorders Glaucoma	Alcohol Anticoagulants BDZs Ca Ch-Blockers Cimetidine/ Omeprazole Doxycycline Erythromycin OCP SSRI/TCAs Tramadol	Hyper/hypotension, lightheadedness, rash, pruritus, erythematous condition, nausea, vomiting, confusion, dizziness, nystagmus, somnolence, blurred vision, diplopia
• CR-carbamazepine	400	1200	Usually transfer from regular format to equivalent CR dose	×2/d	—					
Oxcarbazepine	300	1200–2400	300–600mg/wk	×3/d	—	C		Bone marrow Hepatic, Renal Psychiatric	Alcohol OCP	Abdominal pain, nausea, vomiting, ataxia, dizziness, headache, nystagmus, somnolence, tremor, diplopia, rhinitis, fatigue
Sod valproate	200–600	1000–2000	200mg/3d	×2/d	🍽	D	Probably safe	Hepatic Urea disorders	Anti-platelets	Alopecia, weight gain, abdominal pain, diarrhoea, loss of appetite, nausea, vomiting, asthenia, ataxia, dizziness, diplopia, headache
Divalproex	250–500	500–1000	250mg/wk	1–2/d						
• Divalproex-ER	500	500–1000	500mg/wk	1/d						

Clonazepam	0.25–0.5	1–4	0.25 mg/wk	Bedtime	—	D	Risk unclear	Hepatic, renal Psychiatric Glaucoma Respiratory	Alcohol	Salivation, ataxia, dizziness, somnolence, depression, respiratory depression
Gabapentin	300	900–2400	300 mg/1–2 d	×3/d	—	C	Probably safe	Renal	AEDs	Oedema, myalgia, ataxia, dizziness, somnolence, tremor, mood swings, hostility, fatigue
Pregabalin	150	300	50 mg/2–3 d	×2–3/d	—	C	Risk unclear		AEDs	Oedema, weight gain, constipation, xerostomia, ataxia, dizziness, somnolence, blurred vision, diplopia
Lamotrigine	25	400–600	25–50 mg/wk	×1–2/d	—	C	Risk unclear	Hepatic, renal Cardiac Bone marrow Psychiatric	AEDs OCP	Rash, nausea, vomiting, ataxia, dizziness, headache, somnolence, blurred vision, diplopia
Topiramate	25	100	25 mg/week	×2/d	—	C	Risk unclear	Hepatic, renal Psychiatric Glaucoma Respiratory	AEDs OCP Digoxin Valproate	Nausea, dizziness, asthenia, ataxia, tremor, paraesthesia, nystagmus, glaucoma, diplopia, nervousness, fatigue

BDZ, benzodiazepines; Ca Ch, calcium channel; SSRI, selective serotonin reuptake inhibitor; TCA, tricyclic antidepressant; AED, antiepileptic drug; ER, extended release; OCP, oral contraceptive pill; CR, controlled release.

[a] Rough guideline; clinically titrate therapeutic response versus side effects.

[b] 🍽 = to be taken with food.

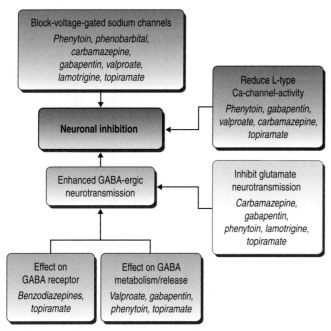

Fig. 16.1 • Anticonvulsants: modes of action.

postsynaptic neuron. GLU exhibits excitotoxic properties by causing membrane depolarization and an influx of Na and Ca. These ionic fluxes, under ischaemic conditions, initiate the cascade of reactions that culminate in neuronal injury and death (Yang *et al* 1998; Leker and Neufeld 2003). The control of GLU release may therefore offer protection from neuronal damage.

AEDs modulate GLU effects directly by blockade of excitatory receptors and alteration of GLU metabolism or its release and indirectly on Na and Ca channels that will affect GLU release. Carbamazepine and phenytoin block NMDA receptors (Moshe 2000) and gabapentin inhibits GLU release in spinal cord (Coderre *et al* 2005). Experimental evidence suggests that inhibition of GLU release by carbamazepine, oxcarbazepine or lamotrigine is probably mediated via Na channel blockade (Waldmeier *et al* 1995; Ambrosio *et al* 2001).

Calcium channel. Blockade of Ca channels modulates neurotransmitter release similar to the effect following Na channel block. AEDs may also act via Ca channels. L-Type Ca channels are involved in the generation of action potentials and in the generation of intracellular Ca signals. At present gabapentin's effects are believed to be mediated primarily via this mechanism.

Effects of chronic therapy. Long-term valproate therapy has been shown to modulate the intracellular pathways strategically involved in the mediation of neurochemical changes and gene expression associated with chronic pain (Li *et al* 2002). These processes lead to long-term neuroplasticity, neuronal sensitivity and activity so that valproic acid may potentially be able to modify these changes. Additionally valproic acid has been shown to induce the neuroprotective gene bcl-2, suggesting that it may be neuroprotective in traumatic neuropathies (Li *et al* 2002). Evidence exists for the neuroprotective

properties of valproic acid, topiramate and lamotrigine in models of ischaemic and traumatic neuronal injuries (Yang *et al* 1998; Li *et al* 2002). Topiramate has demonstrated neuroprotective properties in animal models of epilepsy (Cha *et al* 2002) but not in a peripheral painful mononeuropathy (Bischofs *et al* 2004). In humans, topiramate showed some evidence of encouraging neuroregeneration in diabetic neuropathy (Vinik *et al* 2003) but no further studies have published similar effects. Further research will elucidate the possible role of such mechanisms in the management of chronic pain syndromes.

5.2. Carbamazepine

Carbamazepine is FDA approved for bipolar disorder, acute manic and mixed episodes, epilepsy (partial, generalized, mixed types) and trigeminal neuralgia.

Efficacy. Experimentally carbamazepine elevates pain thresholds in rats (Pinelli *et al* 1997) and suppresses neuronal activity in response to the application of bradykinin to tooth pulp (Satoh and Foong 1983) or spinal nerve injury (Chapman *et al* 1998). Experimental data support the clinical observation that carbamazepine is generally ineffective in orofacial traumatic neuropathies (Idanpaan-Heikkila and Guilbaud 1999). In addition to modes of action described earlier (Fig. 16.1) carbamazepine seems also to exert analgesic effects via the adenosine system (Tomic *et al* 2004).

In orofacial pain carbamazepine is almost exclusively used for trigeminal neuralgia. Rarely a therapeutic trial with carbamazepine is employed in patients with post-traumatic neuropathy that exhibit a prominent lancinating/electrical and paroxysmal quality to their pain. We initiate therapy at 100 mg (half a tablet) in the evening (with food) and increase on alternate days by 100–200 mg in the morning then at midday. In trigeminal neuralgia therapeutic effects are observed at 48–72 hours. Final dose titration is based on response and side effects but may reach 1200 mg/d or more; if side effects are prominent a slower increase in dosage should be performed. When a positive response is observed without serious side effects controlled release (CR) carbamazepine should be initiated at a dose at least equivalent to the standard formulation. CR-carbamazepine has fewer side effects and is taken on a twice-daily schedule with or without food, making it more convenient.

Adverse effects. Side effects such as lightheadedness, confusion, dizziness, vertigo, blurred vision or diplopia, sedation (somnolence), vomiting, nystagmus and nausea are very common and cause 5–20% of patients to request drug cessation. Skin rashes, sometimes pruritic, occur in up to 10% of patients and may be a part of the antiepileptic drug hypersensitivity syndrome. This syndrome, comprising fever, rash, lymphadenopathy and less commonly hepatosplenomegaly and eosinophilia, has been associated with some AEDs including carbamazepine (Knowles *et al* 1999). These reactions usually occur within 30 days and require immediate withdrawal and alternative therapy. Cross-reactivity (75%) may occur with phenobarbital and phenytoin and these drugs should be avoided. Hyper- or hypotension is also commonly reported.

Carbamazepine is a hepatic enzyme inducer and transient elevation in liver enzymes may occur in 5–10% of patients. Carbamazepine therefore induces its own metabolism as well as that of a number of other drugs including some antibacterials (notably doxycycline), anticoagulants and oral contraceptives. Erythromycin may cause substantial elevations of serum carbamazepine levels. Carbamazepine may diminish the activity of warfarin and other coumarins through increased metabolism.

Serious side effects are fortunately rarer but include cardiac arrhythmias, hepatitis, systemic lupus erythematosus, nephrotoxicity, acute renal failure and angioedema. Carbamazepine should be avoided in patients with atrioventricular conduction abnormalities, blood disorders or a history of bone marrow depression. Transient leukopenia is observed in 5% of patients and may become persistent in 2%. Aplastic anaemia is a serious effect that may occur in 1 of 15 000–200 000 cases. Hyponatraemia is observed in 4–22% of carbamazepine-treated cases and requires drug withdrawal; the mechanism is uncertain and may involve direct effects on the kidney or increased secretion of antidiuretic hormone. Mild antimuscarinic properties of carbamazepine suggest that caution be observed in patients with glaucoma or raised intraocular pressure. Scattered punctate lens opacities occur rarely during carbamazepine therapy.

Because of carbamazepine's side effect profile baseline and periodic testing of patients should include liver function, differential blood count, serum electrolytes, serum iron and folic acid, eye examination and renal function. Although the value of such testing has been questioned it is widespread clinical routine. Additionally plasma levels of carbamazepine are monitored to assess patient compliance and adequate drug absorption. No data are available on therapeutic ranges for carbamazepine in the treatment of trigeminal neuralgia (TN) and we generally aim at maintaining therapeutic plasma concentrations as for epilepsy (4–12 µg/mL). Carbamazepine is classified as pregnancy category D and the risk for breastfed babies is probably acceptable.

5.3. Oxcarbazepine

Oxcarbazepine is a derivative of carbamazepine that is FDA-approved for the treatment of partial seizures.

Efficacy. Data from experiments on spinal and trigeminal pain suggest that oxcarbazepine is antinociceptive in inflammatory or neuropathic pain and reduces neuronal activity (Kiguchi *et al* 2004; Jang *et al* 2005). Initial dosage is 600 mg daily by mouth in two divided doses and may be increased thereafter, if necessary, in maximum increments of 600 mg daily at approximately weekly intervals. Maintenance doses are usually in the range of 600–1200

mg daily (up to 2400 mg) and are usually higher than carbamazepine doses for control of TN (Farago 1987); 300 mg of oxcarbazepine is approximately equivalent to 200 mg of carbamazepine (Zakrzewska and Patsalos 1989). Onset of action in TN has been reported to be about 24–48 hours (Farago 1987; Zakrzewska and Patsalos 1989).

Adverse effects. Although adverse events are similar there are indications that oxcarbazepine has significantly less nervous system side effects than carbamazepine. Common side effects include abdominal pain, nausea, vomiting, ataxia, dizziness, headache, nystagmus, somnolence, tremor, diplopia, rhinitis and fatigue

Hypersensitivity reactions such as skin rashes occur less frequently with oxcarbazepine than with carbamazepine but may be serious such as in multiorgan hypersensitivity reaction, Stevens-Johnson syndrome or toxic epidermal necrolysis. Moreover, cross-sensitivity does occur and about 25–30% of patients hypersensitive to carbamazepine may experience such reactions with oxcarbazepine. Dose-related hyponatraemia has also been observed with oxcarbazepine and may even be more common (2.5–29.9%) than with carbamazepine (Zakrzewska and Patsalos 2002). Oxcarbazepine is in pregnancy category C and although probably safe the exact risk to breastfed neonates is unknown.

5.4. Valproate

Valproate is a broad term applied to a group of related compounds including valproic acid, divalproex sodium and sodium valproate. Divalproex sodium is a stable coordination complex comprised of sodium valproate and valproic acid in a 1:1 molar ratio. The group is FDA-approved for the treatment of seizures, acute mania and migraine prophylaxis.

Efficacy. Valproates increase the brain levels of GABA (Loscher 1999). In the trigeminal system valproate decreases both nociceptor-induced activity of second-order neurons (c-fos expression) and meningeal neurogenic inflammation (Cutrer and Moskowitz 1996). Clinical use of valproates also includes the treatment of chronic daily headaches. More rarely we employ valproate as a second or third alternative in the treatment of TN or other neuropathic pain. The formats most frequently used are sodium valproate and divalproex (extended release).

- *Sodium valproate*: The suggested initial oral dose for adults is 600 mg daily in two divided doses. This may be increased by 200 mg every 3 days to a usual range of 1–2 g daily (20–30 mg/kg daily); up to a maximum of 2.5 g daily may be necessary.
- *Valproic acid*: In adults and children an initial daily dose of 15 mg/kg (i.e. 1200 mg/d for an 80-kg adult), increased at one-week intervals by 5–10 mg/kg. Valproic acid may be given in 2–4 divided doses. The maximum recommended dose of valproic acid in the

UK is 30 mg/kg daily, whereas in the USA it is 60 mg/kg daily.

- *Divalproex sodium*: Initial dose is 250mg twice daily; a single 250-mg dose at bedtime may be tried for patients with initial side effects. The usual maximum dose is 1g/day. Extended-release tablets should be initiated with a 500-mg dose once daily for 1 week and may be increased to 1g daily if needed. Divalproex sodium is effective in migraine at 500mg daily, although some patients may need higher doses (Klapper 1997). The extended-release form of divalproex sodium has comparable efficacy to the standard formulation with adverse effect rates comparable to that of placebo (Silberstein and Goadsby 2002).

Adverse effects. Side effects with valproate therapy are very common and are often associated with too high a starting dose, increasing doses too rapidly or concomitant use of other AEDs. The most frequently reported adverse effects are gastrointestinal disturbances (abdominal pain, diarrhoea, loss of appetite, nausea, vomiting) particularly at the start of therapy. These may be minimized by starting with low doses and advising patients to take medication with meals. Enteric-coated formulations are available and may further reduce GI distress; in patients with gastric discomfort adding an antacid (e.g. omeprazole) is helpful.

There may be increased appetite, but long-term (up to 6 years) studies of divalproex use revealed no hepatotoxicity and negligible weight gain (Freitag *et al* 2001). Neurological adverse effects include ataxia, dizziness, diplopia, tremor, sedation, asthenia, ataxia, lethargy and confusion. Less common adverse effects include oedema, headache, reversible prolongation of bleeding time and a dose-dependent thrombocytopenia. Leukopenia or bone marrow depression have been reported.

Elevation of liver enzyme values is common but normally transient and dose-related. Liver dysfunction including hepatic failure and fatality has occasionally been reported, usually in the first few months of treatment and in young children. Baseline testing and routine follow-up of blood counts and liver function is indicated. Life-threatening pancreatitis is a rare but serious adverse event. Valproates are in pregnancy category D and although considered safe low concentrations are found in breastfed neonates.

5.5. Gabapentin

Gabapentin is FDA-approved for use in seizures and postherpetic neuralgia and off-label uses include the treatment of migraine, diabetic neuropathy, TN, SUNCT and cluster headache. Gabapentin is an amino acid structurally related to the inhibitory neurotransmitter GABA. Indeed gabapentin was designed to be a GABA mimetic with increased lipophilicity to enhance nervous system penetration. Despite the structural similarity gabapentin and pregabalin do not have an appreciable effect on GABA receptors although recent findings suggest an effect on presynaptic GABA receptors (Sills 2006). Moreover gabapentin is not converted metabolically into GABA and is not a direct inhibitor of GABA transport (Sills 2006).

Efficacy. Gabapentin is an effective agent for the treatment of experimental neuropathies (Blackburn-Munro and Erichsen 2005; Yasuda *et al* 2005) and reduces post-injury neuronal activity (Chapman *et al* 1998). Gabapentin prevents pain behaviour associated with experimental orofacial pain in rats, suggesting that it may be useful in the treatment of orofacial neuropathies (Christensen *et al* 2001; Grabow and Dougherty 2002). In a rat model of pain following surgical incision, preemptive treatment with gabapentin reduced postoperative allodynia and hyperalgesia; similar effects have been obtained with pregabalin, which suggests that these drugs may be efficient preoperative analgesics (Field *et al* 1997). These studies have formed the basis for human trials showing that gabapentin is a good alternative analgesic in the management of perioperative pain (Pandey *et al* 2005; Turan *et al* 2006). Clinical studies have established that gabapentin is effective for chronic neuropathic pain (Wiffen *et al* 2005b).

Based on available data, it appears that initial target dosage is 900mg; treatment should be started at 300 mg/d and increased by 300mg daily over a period of 3 days, longer if side effects are prohibitive (Backonja and Glanzman 2003). The initiation of gabapentin at low doses is associated with reduced side effects once the maintenance dose is achieved. Additional titration to 1800mg/d is recommended for greater efficacy. Maintenance doses are taken 3 times daily and vary between syndromes: 900–3600mg/d for diabetic neuropathy, up to 2400mg/d for migraine prophylaxis and up to 1800 mg/d for postherpetic neuralgia. However, the effective dose should be individualized according to patient response and tolerability.

Adverse effects. Many of the side effects occur within 3 days of initiating therapy but usually subside with continued use of gabapentin. The most commonly reported adverse effects are somnolence, dizziness, ataxia and fatigue. Visual disturbances, tremor, weight gain, dyspepsia, amnesia, weakness and paraesthesia occur less frequently. Mood swings and hostility have also been reported.

More rarely, seizure, altered liver function tests, erythema multiforme, Stevens-Johnson syndrome, myalgia, headache, oedema, nausea and vomiting have been reported. Gabapentin is in pregnancy category C and although probably safe the exact risk to breastfed neonates is unknown.

5.6. Pregabalin

Pregabalin is an analogue of the inhibitory neurotransmitter GABA and is FDA-approved for diabetic peripheral neuropathy and postherpetic neuralgia.

Efficacy. In preclinical models it has shown activity as an analgesic agent in neuropathic and inflammatory states (Houghton *et al* 1998; Field *et al* 1999). Clinically, pregabalin is efficacious for the treatment of postherpetic neuralgia and diabetic neuropathy with relatively few side effects (Freynhagen *et al* 2005; Richter *et al* 2005). Initial dosage for the treatment of painful diabetic peripheral neuropathy or postherpetic neuralgia is 50 mg three times daily or 75 mg twice daily. Based on efficacy and tolerability this may be increased to 100 mg three times a day within 1 week. Patients may be maintained on 75–150 mg twice daily or 50–100 mg three times a day. In patients who do not experience adequate pain relief following 2–4 weeks of treatment with 300 mg/d and are tolerating pregabalin, dosage may be increased up to 300 mg two times a day, or 200 mg three times a day for a trial period. Pregabalin has shown efficacy in postoperative dental pain; a single dose of 300 mg is significantly analgesic (Hill *et al* 2001). Based on duration of analgesia, a dose interval of every 6 hours is suggested.

Adverse effects. The most common adverse effects include mild to moderate dizziness and somnolence; confusion, headache, amnesia, ataxia and weakness are less frequent. Other common adverse effects include constipation, dry mouth and vomiting. Visual disturbances (blurred vision, diplopia), dose-dependent peripheral oedema and weight gain have been reported. A modest and transient elevation of hepatic enzymes and occasionally a drop in the platelet count may be observed. Myopathy secondary to muscle damage and accompanied by increases in plasma creatinine kinase is a rare complication. Pregabalin is in pregnancy category C and although probably safe the exact risk to breastfed neonates is unknown.

5.7. Clonazepam

Clonazepam is a benzodiazepine with anticonvulsant properties and is FDA-approved for panic disorder and seizures.

Efficacy. Clinical effectiveness of clonazepam has been demonstrated in myofascial pain (Harkins *et al* 1991; Fishbain *et al* 2000) and in some neuropathic pain disorders (Wiffen *et al* 2005a). We primarily use clonazepam in patients with myofascial pain not responsive to amitriptyline, in post-traumatic pain cases that present with panic symptoms and for burning mouth syndrome (BMS); see Chapter 11. Clonazepam may be useful as mono- or add-on therapy for muscular disorders and more rarely to supplement therapy in TN. We initiate therapy at 0.25 mg at night and increase to 0.5–1 mg/d in one or two doses, according to side effects and response. Rarely patients may benefit from higher doses but side effects are usually severe. Treatment should be discontinued slowly by decreasing the dose every 3 days. For BMS patients a possible topical effect suggests that a 1 mg tablet be sucked and not swallowed, thus avoiding side effects associated with systemic therapy (Gremeau-Richard *et al* 2004).

Alternatively if the sedative/hypnotic and anti-panic effects are needed, the tablets may be sucked and subsequently swallowed.

Adverse effects. The most common adverse effect occurring in about half of cases is drowsiness or somnolence, particularly at the start of therapy. Muscle weakness, ataxia and slurred speech may occur. Excessive salivation, dizziness and respiratory depression have been reported. Although the relationship between psychiatric depression and benzodiazepine use is unclear, clonazepam should probably be avoided in depressed patients (Patten and Love 1994). Clonazepam is in pregnancy category D with insufficient evidence to rule out risk for breastfed neonates.

5.8. Topiramate

Topiramate is FDA-approved in the management of seizures, Lennox-Gastaut syndrome (a severe form of childhood epilepsy usually refractory to medical management) and migraine prophylaxis. Topiramate's pharmacologic profile includes all the modes of action discussed earlier in addition to mild inhibition of carbonic anhydrase and of kainite, leading to enhanced neuronal stability.

Efficacy. In animal models of neuropathic pain topiramate is an effective analgesic (Bischofs *et al* 2004; Wieczorkiewicz-Plaza *et al* 2004). Specifically topiramate has dose-dependent and rapid inhibitory effects on trigeminovascular nociceptive neurons (Storer and Goadsby 2004). Clinically topiramate has been successfully applied to the treatment of a variety of pain syndromes (see Chong and Libretto 2003). These include TN (Zvartau-Hind *et al* 2000), diabetic neuropathy (Carroll *et al* 2004; Raskin *et al* 2004), migraine and other headaches (Storey *et al* 2001; Mathew *et al* 2002). Topiramate is therefore a useful alternative in the treatment of chronic orofacial pain. The recommended total daily dose of topiramate in migraine prophylaxis is 100 mg/d in two divided doses with a slow titration schedule over a period of 4 weeks.

Adverse effects. Dose-related adverse events in adults include dizziness, fatigue, nervousness, concentration difficulties, confusion, depression, language problems, anxiety or nervousness. Paraesthesia, asthenia, ataxia, tremor and mood problems are also common. Nausea, abdominal pain and anorexia have been reported.

Topiramate inhibits some isoenzymes of carbonic anhydrase and may induce renal tubular acidosis. Therefore in addition to assessment of renal function (particularly in the elderly), serum bicarbonate levels should be assessed at baseline and periodically during treatment. Topiramate is therefore contraindicated in conditions or therapies that predispose to acidosis such as renal disease, severe respiratory disorders, status epilepticus, diarrhoea, surgery, ketogenic diet or drugs. Ocular side effects include diplopia and nystagmus. Moreover a syndrome consisting of acute myopia associated with secondary angle closure glaucoma has been reported in patients receiving topiramate within 1 month of initiating therapy. The primary treatment to reverse symptoms is discontinuation of topiramate as rapidly as possible. Other serious but rare side effects include pyrexia, pancreatitis, anaemia or leukopenia, hepatitis, liver failure, nephrolithiasis and dyspnoea. Topiramate is in pregnancy category D with insufficient evidence to rule out risk for breastfed neonates.

5.9. Lamotrigine

Lamotrigine is a new generation AED structurally unrelated to other drugs in its class and is FDA-approved for bipolar disorder, Lennox-Gastaut syndrome and seizures.

Efficacy. Studies have confirmed that lamotrigine is analgesic in experimental (Shannon *et al* 2005) and various clinical neuropathic pain states (Eisenberg *et al* 2005). In TN refractory to standard medical therapy adding 400 mg lamotrigine was superior to placebo (Zakrzewska *et al* 1997). However, experimental data suggest that lamotrigine may be inferior to gabapentin in the management of traumatic trigeminal neuropathies (Christensen *et al* 2001). The target dose for the treatment of neuropathic pain is somewhat higher than that employed for seizure control and may reach 400–600 mg. To minimize side effects initial dose should be 25 mg/d and increased very slowly, reaching the target in 7 weeks or more. Dose increase is dependent on side effects and therapeutic response observed.

Adverse effects. Most side effects of lamotrigine are dose-related and commonly include dizziness, nausea or vomiting, sedation, headache, visual disturbances (blurred vision, diplopia) and ataxia. Maculopapular and erythematous rashes have been reported with therapeutic doses of lamotrigine, serious in 1.1% and non-serious in 7–10%. This side effect is related to higher starting doses, and is also possibly more common in patients below the age of 16 years, where the maximum dose is exceeded or the dose is increased at a faster rate than recommended. Any sign of skin rash mandates cessation of lamotrigine to avoid increases in severity; toxic epidermal necrolysis and Stevens-Johnson syndrome have been reported. Rarely cardiovascular (ECG changes) and bone marrow suppression with leukopenia, anaemia or thrombocytopenia have been observed. Other rare but serious events include hepatic necrosis or liver failure, amnesia, seizure and angioedema. Anticonvulsant hypersensitivity syndrome has been associated with lamotrigine therapy. Lamotrigine is in pregnancy category C and insufficient evidence is available to rule out risk for breastfed neonates.

6. Antihypertensives (Table 16.4)

6.1. β-Adrenergic Receptor Blockers: Propranolol

Propranolol is a non-cardioselective β-blocker that is FDA-approved for a number of cardiovascular conditions (e.g. angina pectoris, cardiac dysrhythmia, hypertension), essential tremor, migraine and pheochromocytoma. The beta-adrenergic blockers (β-blockers) were originally introduced for the treatment of cardiac arrhythmias and angina pectoris. Serendipitous observation led to their application in the treatment of hypertension and migraine. Propranolol does not possess intrinsic sympathomimetic activity.

6.1.1. Mode of Action

Sympathetic hyperactivity in regional and generalized muscle disorders such as fibromyalgia suggests that β-blockers may be useful therapeutic agents (see Chapter 7). Experimental inhibition of catechol-*O*-methyltransferase (COMT), an enzyme that metabolizes catecholamines, leads to increased measures of inflammatory pain in rodents (Nackley *et al* 2007). Administration of propranolol reversed this effect, suggesting that β-blockers may have a role in the management of pain that is modulated by sympathetic hyperactivity. Experimental data demonstrate that propranolol can reduce serotonin-induced masseter muscle pain (Ernberg *et al* 2000). Pindolol, also a nonselective β-blocker, was shown to be effective in the management of fibromyalgia; however, the study was not placebo controlled (Wood *et al* 2005). Early data suggest that propranolol may be useful in masticatory myofascial pain but no controlled trials have been published (Bhalang *et al* 2004).

The exact role of vasodilatation in neurovascular pain is questionable and propranolol does not constrict cerebral arteries; β-blockers therefore probably act via additional mechanisms (Tvedskov *et al* 2004). Beta-blockers seem to exert some of their therapeutic effects in migraine via actions at sites in the central nervous system (CNS) intimately involved with nociception (locus coeruleus, thalamus). Propranolol has a high affinity for 5-HT binding sites in the CNS and antagonizes 5-HT$_{1A}$ and 5-HT$_{2B}$ receptors, thus reducing neuronal hyperexcitability. The production of nitric oxide is inhibited by β-blockers (β-2 action). Nitric oxide is intimately associated with the pathophysiology of neurovascular craniofacial pain such as cluster and migraine headache (see Chapters 9 and 10). The membrane-stabilizing properties of propranolol result in neuronal stability. This may be related to inhibition of kainite-induced currents and is synergistic with NMDA blockers (Silberstein and Goadsby 2002).

There are indications that β-blockers exert their effect via the central catecholaminergic system. Inhibition of β1-mediated noradrenaline release leads to reduced central catecholaminergic hyperexcitability and may be a possible mode of action for propranolol (Ablad and Dahlof 1986). The reduction is delayed and parallels that often observed clinically in the prophylactic treatment of migraine with propranolol. Migraineurs exhibit an enhanced centrally mediated secretion of epinephrine after exposure to light, which returns to normal after

Table 16.4 Antihypertensive Drugs

Drug	Initial Dose (mg)	Target or Max Dose (mg)[a]	Dose Increase (Titration)[a]	Schedule	Pregnancy Category	Breastfeeding	Medical Contraindications	Drug Interactions	Common Side Effects
Propranolol • Propranolol-SR	40–80 80	240 160–240	40 mg/wk 80 mg/1–2wks	×2–3/d 1/d	C	Risk unclear	Asthma Cardiovascular Diabetics Hepatic, Renal Hyperlipidemia PVD	Anticoagulants Antiarrhythmics Ca Ch blockers Cimetidine Epinephrine NSAIDs Thyroid hor. Triptans	Arrhythmias, dermatitis, pruritus, rash, loss of appetite, nausea, vomiting, sleepiness, paraesthesia, depression, dyspnoea, wheezing
Verapamil • Verapamil-SR	120 120	120–480 120–480	40–80 mg/1–2 wks 120 mg/1–2 wks	×2–3/d ×1–2/d	C	Risk unclear	Cardiovascular Hepatic, renal	Antiarrhythmics Antiplatelets Beta blockers Carbamazepine Cimetidine	Oedema, hypotension, constipation, nausea, dizziness, headache

Ca Ch, calcium channel; NSAIDs, nonsteroidal anti-inflammatory drugs; PVD, peripheral vascular disease; SR, slow release; hor, hormone.
[a] Rough guideline; clinically titrate therapeutic response versus side effects.

treatment with propranolol (Stoica and Enulescu 1990). This finding therefore supports that migraineurs with signs of central catecholaminergic hyperexcitability will respond well to propranolol.

Cortical potentials in response to various stimuli are abnormal in migraineurs relative to controls, but are normalized following 3–4 months of treatment with propranolol (Sandor *et al* 2000). Increased thalamocortical activity in response to superior sagittal sinus stimulation is inhibited by β-blockers through β1 adrenoceptor antagonist actions (Shields and Goadsby 2005). No effect of propranolol on experimental neurogenic inflammation has been found (Akerman *et al* 2001). In summary these studies suggest that propranolol may act primarily within the CNS.

Efficacy. The positive effect of β-blockers in migraine and neurovascular orofacial pain has been repeatedly shown; see Chapter 9. Propranolol may be prescribed in sustained release format, although the standard formulation is often used initially as trial therapy. For the prophylaxis of neurovascular pain (e.g. neurovascular orofacial pain, migraine) an initial dose of 40–80 mg daily is often used in 2–3 doses. The dose can be increased at weekly intervals up to 240 mg daily if needed. Most often we transfer patients to the slow-release formula, usually 80–160 mg daily in a single dose.

Adverse effects. Fatigue, dizziness and coldness of the extremities, dermatitis and pruritic rashes are common and troublesome side effects experienced with β-blockers. The most frequent and serious adverse effects are related to their β-adrenergic blocking activity and include heart failure, hypotension, heart block and bradycardia. Use of β-blockers in cardiovascular patients requires a medical consultation and monitoring. Bronchospasm with dyspnoea or wheezing is a serious side effect and nonselective β-blockers, such as propranolol, are therefore contraindicated in asthma; atenolol, a cardioselective β-blocker, is a possible alternative in these cases. Paraesthesia, peripheral neuropathy, arthralgia and myopathies, including muscle cramps, have been reported. Adverse gastrointestinal effects include nausea and vomiting, diarrhoea, loss of appetite, constipation and abdominal cramping. Propranolol also commonly causes sleepiness and depression.

Beta-blockers interfere with carbohydrate and lipid metabolism and can produce hypo- or hyperglycaemia, as well as changes in blood concentrations of triglycerides and cholesterol. The β-blockers can reduce the response to insulin and oral hypoglycaemics through their effects on pancreatic β-receptors; their use is therefore contraindicated in diabetics. Blockade of peripheral β-receptors interferes with the effects of sympathomimetics; patients on β-blockers, especially nonselective β-blockers, may develop elevated blood pressure if they are given adrenaline. The bronchodilator effects of adrenaline are also inhibited. Propranolol is in pregnancy category C and is considered safe for breastfed neonates.

6.2. Calcium Antagonists: Verapamil and Flunarizine

Ca-channel antagonists such as verapamil and flunarizine are FDA-approved for angina, hypertension and supraventricular tachycardia.

6.2.1. Mode of Action

The mechanisms underlying the effect of Ca antagonists in neurovascular pain are unclear. Flunarizine inhibits the synthesis and release of nitric oxide (involved in the pathophysiology of headaches) in perivascular neurons (Ayajiki *et al* 1997). Ca antagonists may inhibit the release of substance P (SP) and calcitonin gene-related peptide (CGRP) (Asakura *et al* 2000). Both SP and CGRP are involved in nociceptive transmission and in neurogenic inflammation and CGRP antagonists have been shown to be highly effective in migraine treatment (Olesen *et al* 2004).

Efficacy. At present there is insufficient evidence to support verapamil as a first-line drug for migraine but it may be considered when other first-line prophylactics have been ineffective. However, verapamil is a drug of choice in the prophylaxis of cluster headache and is usually effective at doses between 200 and 480 mg, although occasionally higher doses are needed (Blau and Engel 2004). Flunarizine at a dose of 5–10 mg daily has proven highly effective in the prophylaxis of migraine and is usually considered when β-blockers are contraindicated or ineffective (Andersson and Vinge 1990).

Adverse effects. Cardiac effects include bradycardia, atrioventricular block, worsening heart failure and transient asystole. Rarely these may induce angina or myocardial infarction. Cardiac effects are particularly severe in patients with hypertrophic cardiomyopathies. The most troublesome non-cardiac adverse effect is constipation. Nausea may occur but is less frequent. Other adverse effects include hypotension, dizziness, flushing, headaches, fatigue, dyspnoea and peripheral oedema and rarely syncope. There have been reports of skin reactions and some cases of abnormal liver function and hepatotoxicity. Gingival hyperplasia is reported as in other Ca-channel blockers. Verapamil is in pregnancy category C and is considered safe in breastfed neonates. For flunarizine there are insufficient data available.

7. Muscle Relaxants (Table 16.5)

The 'muscle relaxants' are a heterogeneous group of drugs whose therapeutic use is based on their ability to prevent or alleviate increased muscle tone and activity. Some of these drugs, however, possess additional modes of action that may be important in the management of pain. Benzodiazepines are sometimes used based on their putative muscle-relaxing properties although they decrease

Drug	Initial Dose (mg)	Target or Max Dose (mg)[a]	Dose Increase (Titration)[a]	Schedule	Pregnancy Category	Breastfeeding	Medical Contraindications	Drug Interactions	Common Side Effects
Cyclobenzaprine	5–10	30–60	<3 wks total treatment	×3/d	B	Unknown	Cardiovascular Epilepsy Glaucoma Hepatic Hyperthyroidism Urinary retention	Alcohol Antidepressants	Dysgeusia, constipation, dyspepsia, nausea, xerostomia, confusion, dizziness, headache, somnolence, blurred vision, nervousness
Baclofen	5–15	30–60	5 mg/3 d	×3/d	C	Safe	CVA Epilepsy Psychiatric Renal	Alcohol Antidepressants	Constipation, nausea, vomiting, asthenia, dizziness, headache, somnolence

Table 16.5 Muscle Relaxant Drugs

CVA, cerebrovascular accident.
[a]Rough guideline; clinically titrate therapeutic response versus side effects.

muscle tone at doses that produce unacceptable side effects. However, there is evidence for short-term benzodiazepine efficacy for acute muscular conditions such as low back pain (van Tulder et al 2003). Cyclobenzaprine is considered of significant therapeutic value for painful muscular conditions (Chou et al 2004) and is recommended for similar orofacial pain syndromes. Other muscle relaxants have been proven effective in experimental masticatory muscle pain (Svensson et al 2003). Baclofen has shown efficacy in trigeminal neuralgia.

7.1. Cyclobenzaprine

Cyclobenzaprine is a centrally acting skeletal muscle relaxant, related to the TCAs. It is FDA-approved for skeletal spasticity and is often used as an adjunct in the symptomatic treatment of painful muscle spasm associated with musculoskeletal conditions.

7.1.1. Mode of Action

Cyclobenzaprine acts mainly at the brainstem to decrease tonic somatic motor activity influencing both α and γ motor systems but additional activity at spinal cord sites may be involved. Effects begin within 1 hour of an oral dose; the effects of a single dose have been reported to last as long as 12–24 hours. No specific antinociceptive properties are associated with cyclobenzaprine.

Efficacy. Whether cyclobenzaprine is superior to other drugs for the management of acute myofascial strain is unclear and it usually adds more side effects with little therapeutic gain (Turturro et al 2003). For neck pain, however, mixed results are obtained (Peloso et al 2005). There are no extensive studies on the use of cyclobenzaprine in the management of painful orofacial musculoskeletal conditions. A recent study on patients with orofacial myofascial pain compared the effect of adding therapy with clonazepam, cyclobenzaprine or placebo to a universally applied self-care and patient education programme (Herman et al 2002). The results suggest that cyclobenzaprine is superior to both placebo and clonazepam when added to self-care and education for the management of jaw pain upon awakening. In this study cyclobenzaprine (10 mg/d) failed to significantly improve sleep in the short term but this may have been due to the relatively low dose employed. The usual dose is 5–10 mg three times daily and treatment for more than 2–3 weeks is not recommended.

A meta-analysis concluded that in the short term, cyclobenzaprine at 10–60 mg daily (median 30 mg daily) improves low back pain (Browning et al 2001). Moderate improvement was observed in the first 4 days of treatment and gradually declined with time. There was some evidence of continued improvement at two weeks. Cyclobenzaprine has modest benefits in fibromyalgia: patients reported overall improvement and moderate reductions in individual symptoms particularly sleep (Tofferi *et al* 2004). In most musculoskeletal conditions cyclobenzaprine seems to provide short-term benefit.

Adverse effects. Side effects are common, at least one occurring in 53% of patients, and are similar to those observed with TCAs. Common side effects include dysgeusia, constipation, dyspepsia, nausea, xerostomia, confusion, dizziness, headache, somnolence, blurred vision and nervousness. Particular care should be exercised in the elderly where cyclobenzaprine may induce hallucinations. Additionally there are some rare but serious side effects such as cardiac dysrhythmia, hepatitis and anaphylaxis. Cyclobenzaprine is in pregnancy category B but risk to breastfed neonates is unknown.

7.2. Baclofen

Baclofen is a derivative of GABA that is FDA-approved for the treatment of spasticity but does not appear to possess conventional analgesic activity (Terrence *et al* 1985).

7.2.1. Mode of Action

Baclofen acts specifically at the spinal end of the upper motor neurons to cause muscle relaxation. It inhibits both monosynaptic and polysynaptic reflexes at the spinal level probably by effects on the afferent terminal, but may also affect supraspinal sites. Baclofen increases the stimulus threshold for inducing reflexes, increases the latency between stimulus and reflex and decreases the amplitude of the muscle response. In the trigeminal nucleus baclofen depresses excitatory transmission and facilitates segmental inhibition, most probably via GABA-B receptor actions (Fromm *et al* 1992).

Efficacy. Experimentally baclofen demonstrates antinociceptive properties in neuropathies of sciatic and trigeminal nerves (Idanpaan-Heikkila and Guilbaud 1999; Santos Tde *et al* 1999) and in humans is effective intrathecally for intractable pain of the lower back and/or lower extremities (Zuniga *et al* 2000). Modest doses of baclofen (15–40 mg/d) have also been successfully employed in open trials for the treatment of cluster headache and migraine (Freitag 2003; Hering-Hanit and Gadoth 2000). Baclofen relieves pain in facial postherpetic neuralgia and potentiates opioid analgesia (Fromm 1994; Zuniga *et al* 2000). At doses ranging between 30 and 80 mg/d baclofen has proven efficacy in patients with trigeminal neuralgia (Fromm *et al* 1980; Fromm and Terrence 1987) and appears to enhance the effectiveness of carbamazepine and phenytoin (Fromm *et al* 1984). Baclofen is mainly used as add-on therapy when side effects prevent the increase of carbamazepine, but also as single therapy of trigeminal neuralgia. We initiate therapy at 5 mg (half a tablet) daily in the evening and increase to 15 mg in three doses within 3 days. Dose escalation is continued by 5 mg per dose every 3 days till either there is a positive response or prohibitive side effects.

Adverse effects. Common side effects reported with baclofen include constipation, nausea, vomiting, asthenia, dizziness, headache and somnolence. It is extremely important to inform the patient that abrupt discontinuation of baclofen may produce severe side effects including seizures, hallucinations, paranoia, delusions, psychosis, anxiety, confusion and agitation (Terrence and Fromm 1981). Dosage should be reduced gradually over at least 10–14 days, or longer if symptoms occur. Baclofen is in pregnancy category C and is considered safe to use while breastfeeding.

8. Triptans

Because of the highly specific actions of triptans in neurovascular headaches the clinical aspects of triptan use have been discussed in Chapters 9 and 10. The triptans are agonists of 5-HT$_1$ receptors located at trigeminal and vascular sites. Triptans are in pregnancy category C. While sumatriptan is probably safe in breastfed neonates, the exact risk of zolmitriptan and rizatriptan is unknown.

8.1. Mode of Action

There are a number of sites of action for the antimigraine effect of the triptans (Saxen and Tfelt-Hansen 2006). Peripherally triptans cause vasoconstriction, a 5HT$_{1B}$ receptor postjunctional effect (de Hoon *et al* 2000). Triptans also diminish trigeminal neuropeptide release (5-HT$_{1D}$, 5-HT$_{2B}$ and 5-HT$_7$ effects) and block trigeminal-induced dural plasma-protein extravasation (Jennings *et al* 2004; Ahn and Basbaum 2005). However, antimigraine efficacy is not dependent on this action as other drugs with a specific effect on extravasation are ineffective in migraine (Saxen and Tfelt-Hansen 2006). Centrally triptans inhibit transmission in the trigeminal nucleus caudalis (effects on 5-HT$_{1B}$, 5-HT$_{1D}$, 5-HT$_{1F}$), reducing afferent stimulation of second-order neurons, possibly by blocking the action of CGRP (Storer *et al* 2001; Donaldson *et al* 2002). In clinical trials, abortive therapy with triptans results in relief of pain and symptoms, as well as a concomitant reduction in the jugular levels of CGRP, which usually increase during migraine episodes. In the periaqueductal grey (PAG), triptans induce selective inhibition of trigeminovascular nociceptive afferent input (Bartsch *et al* 2004). This occurs for dural but not facial nociceptors and raises an interesting question on whether triptans will be as effective in facial neurovascular pains (e.g. NVOP) as they are in migraine. In addition to inhibitory effects on the trigeminal nucleus, triptans seem to activate descending pain modulatory pathways augmenting analgesia (Cumberbatch *et al* 1997; Bartsch *et al* 2004). However, this effect is dependent on the inherent ability of individual drugs to penetrate the blood–brain barrier (BBB), which is low for some triptans. Alternatively the BBB is disrupted during migraine, allowing triptan penetration (Ahn and Basbaum

2005). In animal models early administration of triptans blocks the development of central sensitization (Burstein and Jakubowski 2004).

9. Cannabinoids

Cannabis and its subcompounds, the cannabinoids, have been used in medicine for many years. The best known cannabinoids are the tetrahydro-cannabinoids and their metabolites that induce the major psychoactive effects.

9.1. Mode of Action

Two cannabinoid receptors have been cloned—CB1 located in brain and CB2 expressed peripherally—but there are indications that more receptors are present. Cannabinoid's analgesic effects are mediated largely by activation of the CB1 receptor that probably leads to the inhibition of neuropeptide and inflammatory agent release. Topical cannabinoid receptor agonists reverse sensory hypersensitivity (Guindon and Beaulieu 2006) but supraspinal and particularly spinal sites of action are considered important (Martin *et al* 1996; Calignano *et al* 1998). Systemic CB1 agonists reverse behavioural pain parameters and reduce levels of peptides associated with the initiation and maintenance of pain (Costa *et al* 2004). Anandamide (an endogenous cannabinoid) is able to modulate the release of CGRP from sensory fibres (De Petrocellis *et al* 2000). CB1 receptors in spinal cord are persistently upregulated following experimental neuropathy, offering a good target for analgesia (Farquhar-Smith *et al* 2000; Lim *et al* 2003). Combinations of CBN with opioids reveal synergistic effects in animal pain models, suggesting a useful clinical application (Yesilyurt *et al* 2003; Cichewicz 2004). In the trigeminal system cannabinoids act as negative modulators of pain transmission peripherally and centrally, suggesting that they may be useful in orofacial pain syndromes (Liang *et al* 2004).

Efficacy. Exogenous cannabinoids are analgesic in models of persistent inflammatory (Jaggar *et al* 1998), neuropathic (Herzberg *et al* 1997) and cancer pain (Kehl *et al* 2003). In humans cannabinoids have analgesic, muscle relaxant and appetite stimulant effects and reduce intraocular pressure. Synthetic cannabinoids are available for the control of chemotherapy-induced nausea and vomiting. Anecdotal reports exist of benefit from cannabinoids in a variety of disorders including glaucoma, multiple sclerosis and wasting in patients with AIDS and malignant neoplasms.

Cannabinoids have been shown to be efficacious in various pain states and reports indicate that over a third of chronic pain patients have used herbal cannabinoids for symptom relief (Clark *et al* 2005; Ware and Beaulieu 2005). Acute states tested include experimental (Naef *et al* 2003) and postoperative (Buggy *et al* 2003) pain with inconsistent results. In chronic neuropathic pain

syndromes (including secondary to multiple sclerosis) cannabinoids were effective analgesics (Karst *et al* 2003; Berman *et al* 2004; Rog *et al* 2005). There are indications that cannabinoids may be useful in headaches (Evans and Ramadan 2004).

Adverse effects. Common side effects of cannabinoids include dry mouth, euphoria, delusions and sedation. The psychoactive effects of cannabinoids often induce addiction and dependence. As pharmacological (i.e. side effects, addiction), cultural and legal obstacles are overcome cannabinoids will no doubt become an integral part of pain medicine; efforts are in process to delineate guidelines for their use in chronic pain.

10. NMDA Receptor Antagonists

The role of the NMDA receptor in chronic pain mechanisms makes it an attractive therapeutic target. Clinically available NMDA receptor antagonists include ketamine and dextromethorphan. Ketamine is largely used as an anaesthetic and trials of subanaesthetic doses reveal effective analgesia in orofacial pain, glossopharyngeal neuralgia and other neuropathic pains (Mathisen *et al* 1995; Felsby *et al* 1996; Eide and Stubhaug 1997). However, since ketamine is associated with severe side effects these limit clinical use.

10.1. Dextromethorphan

Dextromethorphan is used extensively as an antitussive and acts by elevating the cough threshold in the cough centre located in the medulla oblongata.

10.1.1. Mode of Action

In vitro studies have shown that dextromethorphan is a moderate- to low-affinity noncompetitive NMDA receptor antagonist. In addition, dextromethorphan has been shown to inhibit NMDA-induced convulsions and attenuate hypoglycaemic neuronal injury. Dextromethorphan may play an important role in conditions of glutamate excitotoxicity such as amyotrophic lateral sclerosis because of its ability to suppress the overactivity of the glutamate system in the CNS. NMDA antagonists are, however, accompanied by severe side effects and drugs with reduced receptor affinity such as dextromethorphan have been tested for pain.

Efficacy. In humans, dextromethorphan is analgesic but is still accompanied by limiting side effects (Carlsson *et al* 2004). Dextromethorphan is efficacious in diabetic neuropathy but not postherpetic neuralgia (Nelson *et al* 1997; Sang *et al* 2002). The efficacy of dextromethorphan in preemptive and perioperative analgesia is inconsistent but may reduce opioid requirements (Weinbroum *et al* 2003; Duedahl *et al* 2006). Animal experiments reveal opioid analgesic enhancing effects of dextromethorphan

(Redwine and Trujillo 2003) and synergism with amitriptyline (Sawynok and Reid 2003), suggesting that dextromethorphan may be useful as add-on therapy (Katz 2000). Onset of pain relief with dextromethorphan following oral surgery was found to be delayed and therefore requires careful scheduling (Gordon *et al* 1999).

Dextromethorphan was tried in a crossover RCT for a mixed group of patients ($n = 19$) with trigeminal neuropathy, anaesthesia dolorosa and TN (Gilron *et al* 2000). Dosage of dextromethorphan was 120 mg/d titrated to a maximum of 920 mg/d. In patients with possible trigeminal neuropathy and anaesthesia dolorosa, dextromethorphan decreased pain by a non-significant mean of 2–4%. Two patients with TN had more pain during dextromethorphan treatment than during placebo (lorazepam) treatment although there were extreme fluctuations that do not allow definite conclusions. Dextromethorphan therefore shows negligible analgesic efficacy in trigeminal neuropathies and needs further investigation for TN.

At present dextromethorphan-enhancing effects are employed in morphine combinations that seem efficacious in postoperative pain; the optimal dosage was 60 mg dextromethorphan with 60 mg of morphine (Caruso 2000). In doses of 41 and 80 mg daily dextromethorphan was ineffective in the management of neuropathic pain (McQuay *et al* 1994). Median tolerated dose effective in diabetic neuropathy was 400 mg/d of dextromethorphan (Sang *et al* 2002) and single doses of 270 mg dextromethorphan were effective in traumatic neuropathies (Carlsson *et al* 2004). In contrast the usual adult dose of dextromethorphan for cough suppression is 10–20 mg every 4 hours or 30 mg every 6–8 hours.

Adverse effects. In antitussive doses adverse effects with dextromethorphan are rare and may include dizziness and gastrointestinal disturbances. Higher doses are associated with drowsiness, fatigue, confusion, depression, visual disturbances and nausea. NMDA antagonists will no doubt play an important role in the management of chronic pain but at present are limited by the side effect profile (Sang 2000).

11. Neuroleptics

Antipsychotic drugs (neuroleptics) and antiemetics (some of which are neuroleptics) have long been used for the treatment of acute migraine (Siow *et al* 2005). Neuroleptics affect the 5-HT, dopamine and acetyl choline systems in the CNS. Interestingly they relieve both nausea and headache; the most convincing evidence is for parenteral neuroleptics such as prochlorperazine and droperidol, but these are associated with significant side effects. Of the newer neuroleptics olanzapine has shown promise in the treatment of migraine and cluster headache (Siow *et al* 2005). Research will indicate whether these and further neuroleptic drugs should become part of our drug armamentarium.

12. Long-Term Use of Opioid and Non-opioid Analgesics

Often nonspecific analgesics are combined with prophylactic drugs in the long-term management of chronic pain. In this fashion the analgesics are used less frequently, especially for breakthrough pain, with fewer side effects. The clinical pharmacology of non-opioid and opioid analgesics has been reviewed in Chapter 15.

13. Topical Therapy for the Management of Pain

Targeted peripheral (or topical) analgesics refer to a number of drugs that have a mechanism of action primarily aimed at peripherally modulating pain mechanisms (inflammatory or neuropathic). The analgesics are therefore most effective in conditions with a primarily peripheral component. These drugs are distinct from transdermal analgesics that require effective systemic concentrations accompanied by an increased risk of adverse effects (Argoff 2004).

Topical application aims to induce a high local concentration of the active drug at the affected site with minimal or no systemic absorption. Drug interactions are reduced, which is of benefit to patients on multiple drugs or when specific side effects are problematic (e.g. NSAIDs and gastric ulcers). Moreover local application is easy to use and requires no dose titration commonly needed in systemic therapies (Sawynok 2003). Localized reactions such as rash may occur but are uncommon (Galer 2001) but some topicals (e.g. capsaicin) may induce local pain on application. Topical agents must be able to cross the epithelium or mucosa to induce an effect. The effectiveness of this barrier is dependent on its integrity and age- and disease-related changes. Depending on thickness and keratinization the oral mucosa is up to 10 times more permeable than skin, allowing rapid drug penetration (Padilla *et al* 2000). The effects of saliva will limit the contact time between drug and mucosa and may significantly limit efficacy. Intraorally, the use of topical agents is relatively complex and requires either prolonged isolation of the area or the construction of an intraoral appliance that will allow optimal concentrations for an adequate period (Padilla *et al* 2000). Local application of drugs to facial areas may also be problematic; resultant rashes or dressings may be unsightly. For these reasons there are fewer studies on the use of topical medications for orofacial conditions, but their use is expanding.

There are various commercially available topical analgesics, mostly single drugs but some combinations are available. Many practitioners use single drugs in combination or have these specifically compounded into gels or creams by specialized pharmacies (Ness *et al* 2002). The most commonly used agents are NSAIDs and local anaesthetics, but a wide variety of topical formulations including anticonvulsants, antidepressants, opioids and corticosteroids are in use (Ness *et al* 2002).

13.1. Topical Anaesthetics

Topical anaesthetics (TA) are routinely used in dentistry to attenuate the pain associated with local anaesthetic injections. Moreover TAs are found in creams used for the topical treatment of mouth ulcers and erosive conditions of the oral mucosa. The duration of relief is dependent on the resistance of the carrier to the effects of mechanical movement and saliva. TA mouthwashes are at times integrated into the management of more generalized ulcerative mucosal conditions such as mucositis but provide doubtful benefit.

The use of 5% lidocaine patches for the treatment of postherpetic neuralgia, painful diabetic neuropathy and low back pain is both effective and safe (Argoff *et al* 2004). Only 10% experienced treatment-related adverse effects, mostly local reactions but some cases suffered headache, raised enzyme levels and local burning or paraesthesia. None of the patients demonstrated changes in gross sensory parameters (Argoff *et al* 2004). Lidocaine patches have been tested intraorally with no adverse effects demonstrated and very low plasma levels recorded (Hersh *et al* 1996). Intraoral lidocaine (10–20%) patches provide relatively rapid topical analgesia that may last for up to 45 minutes (Hersh *et al* 1996; Houpt *et al* 1997). A benzocaine patch is effective in reducing the intensity of acute toothache when applied to the periapical mucosa (Hersh *et al* 2003). Topical application of a viscous lidocaine gel significantly alleviates pain in patients who underwent tooth socket curettage for alveolar osteitis (Betts *et al* 1995). These studies suggest that TAs may be successfully employed in the management of painful intraoral syndromes such as neuropathies.

The actions of TAs are mediated by their sodium (Na) channel-blocking properties that inhibit signal transduction. Moreover in injured and inflamed tissue pain and sensitivity are thought partly to occur due to an upregulation in the numbers of Na channels and a reduction in their thresholds. Effective concentrations at the injured site must be balanced with the possible systemic toxicity of TAs that includes CNS and cardiac effects. However, no significant absorption of topical lidocaine mouthwashes was shown even in patients with mucosal breakdown (Elad *et al* 1999).

13.2. Topical Nonsteroidal Anti-inflammatory Drugs

Systemic NSAIDs are extensively used in medicine and dentistry as both analgesics and anti-inflammatory agents but are associated with considerable morbidity and mortality (see Chapter 15). Local delivery reduces plasma drug levels to 5–15% of that observed following systemic administration whilst maintaining high concentrations in the dermis and muscle (Sawynok 2003). In clinical models of cutaneous, neuropathic and muscle pain topical NSAIDs as gel, spray or patch produce effective analgesia with few side effects (Devers and Galer 2000; Galer *et al* 2000, 2004; Argoff 2002; Sawynok 2003) whilst arthritis patients report variable analgesic efficacy (Heyneman *et al* 2000). Adverse events associated with topical NSAIDs occur in 10–15% of patients and are mostly cutaneous: rash or local itching. Systemic effects are rare and tend to occur in patients with a previous history of side effects to systemic NSAIDs (Heyneman *et al* 2000; Sawynok 2003).

In patients with painful TMJs topical diclofenac was as effective as 100 mg oral diclofenac in reducing symptoms (Di Rienzo Businco *et al* 2004). Topical application of 5% ibuprofen (×3/d) was as effective as ibuprofen 400 mg (×3/d) taken orally in relieving post-exercise jaw pain and maximum voluntary occlusal force of TMD patients (Svensson *et al* 1997). At the end of the 3-day trial topical application seemed to offer some advantages over systemic formulation (Svensson *et al* 1997).

Following third molar extraction topical aspirin or acetaminophen had a significant analgesic effect (Moore *et al* 1992). Using the same dental extraction model locally applied ketoprofen (10 mg) is more effective than 10 mg taken orally and is associated with lower plasma levels, suggesting a reduced potential for drug toxicity (Dionne *et al* 1999). A later study with the same experimental model examined flurbiprofen in a slow-release formulation and found that it delayed the onset and lowered the intensity of postoperative pain at doses lower than that usually administered orally (Dionne *et al* 2004).

13.3. Capsaicin

Topical capsaicin has not been extensively used for oral or perioral application. Capsaicin is available as a 0.025 or 0.075% cream and is usually applied sparingly 3 or 4 times daily. A more concentrated cream containing 0.25% capsaicin is available in some countries. Therapeutic response may not be evident for 1–2 weeks for arthritic disorders, or 2–4 weeks for neuralgias.

The major adverse event affecting patient compliance is the extreme and immediate burning sensation capsaicin causes (also a problem in clinical trials where blinding becomes very difficult). Burning may last for up to one week but with repeated applications this effect is reduced.

Capsaicin seems moderately effective in painful diabetic neuropathy and in neuropathic pain but the evidence for efficacy in postherpetic neuralgia is less convincing (Zhang and Li Wan Po 1994; Kingery 1997). In a recent systematic review it was concluded that although topical capsaicin has only poor to moderate efficacy in the treatment of musculoskeletal or neuropathic pain it may be useful in some cases resistant to other modes of therapy or as adjunct therapy (Mason *et al* 2004). A positive effect has also been observed in a heterogeneous group of patients with oral neuropathic pain (Epstein and Marcoe 1994). It was found that trigeminal neuralgia with an intraoral trigger was less responsive to topical therapy than other neuropathic pain. An open trial of capsaicin in patients with traumatic trigeminal dysesthesia demonstrated a positive clinical effect (Canavan *et al* 1994). Capsaicin in a hard candy-like carrier provided only temporary and incomplete relief for patients with mucositis (Berger *et al* 1995). Although thought potentially useful in the management of TMDs (Hersh *et al* 1994) topical application of capsaicin cream (0.025%) to painful TMJs produced no statistically significant influence on pain parameters, muscle and joint sensitivity and maximal mouth opening, when compared to placebo (Winocur *et al* 2000). Capsaicin, or its isomer civamide, has been applied to the nasal mucosa for the prevention of cluster headache with modest effects (Saper *et al* 2002).

Depending on drug concentration capsaicin is able to selectively activate, desensitize or be neurotoxic to small-diameter sensory fibres. Capsaicin's effects are mediated by the vanilloid receptor, a nonselective cation channel present on both C and Aδ fibres. Receptor activation results in an influx of both Na and Ca ions and an action potential. Following capsaicin application substance P is released from both peripheral and central terminals. Repeated application induces desensitization and inhibits SP release and is the basis for its topical therapeutic use (Sawynok 2003).

13.4. Antidepressants

Topical amitriptyline alone or combined with ketamine relieves peripheral neuropathic pain (Lynch *et al* 2003, 2005). Topical application of doxepin significantly relieves chronic neuropathic pain and when mixed with capsaicin the effect was observed significantly earlier (McCleane 2000). In an open, one-dose study doxepin mouth-rinses were shown effective in providing analgesia for patients with mucositis (Epstein *et al* 2001). Some patients reported sedation attributed to systemic absorption but no assays were performed.

The peripheral mode of action of antidepressants is multifactorial (see above under systemic treatment) and includes Na channel blockade and enhancement of opioid effects (Sawynok *et al* 2001).

13.5. Opioids

Topical opioids are being increasingly applied for the relief of pain (Oeltjenbruns and Schafer 2005). Mu receptor agonists are the most potent topical opioid analgesics, δ and κ being less effective (Sawynok 2003). Opioid receptors are present on the peripheral terminals of thinly myelinated and unmyelinated cutaneous sensory fibres

(Coggeshall *et al* 1997). However, peripheral opioid actions are not prominent in normal tissue and appear after the induction of inflammation due to enhanced opioid receptor expression (Zhou *et al* 1998). The analgesic opioid effect precedes these changes and is thought due to the disruption of the perineurial barrier that normally limits access to the nerve (Antonijevic *et al* 1995). The lowered pH at inflammatory sites may also enhance opioid receptor actions (Sawynok 2003). In the presence of inflammation morphine (1 mg) added to a local anaesthetic for dental surgery results in significant improvement of postoperative analgesia (Likar *et al* 1998, 2001). However, application of morphine along the axon (perineurally) or into non-inflamed tissue did not show any reduction in pain scores, underscoring the requirement of an inflammatory process for peripheral opioid effects (Likar *et al* 2001). Since oral surgery procedures are accompanied by an inflammatory reaction, supplemental topical morphine may be of benefit for the relief of postoperative pain (Likar *et al* 1998, 2001). Low doses of morphine administered into the intraligamentary space of a chronically inflamed hyperalgesic tooth produced a dose-related naloxone-reversible analgesia (Dionne *et al* 2001). The effect was significantly higher than in acute inflammation, suggesting that the effects of topical opioids are related to the time-dependent expression of peripheral receptors. However, these results have not been uniform; when morphine was applied locally after third molar surgery it was ineffective in providing analgesia (Moore *et al* 1994).

When administered via intra-articular injection, opioids are effective in the control of joint pain with few systemic side effects (Likar *et al* 1997, 1999). An increased level of opioids in the TMJs of patients with closed lock suggests peripheral upregulation and lends support to the use of intra-articular opioids for TMJ pain (Kajii *et al* 2005). In uncontrolled studies 10 mg of intra-articular morphine injected after arthrocentesis provided excellent pain relief (Kunjur *et al* 2003). However, randomized controlled studies in patients with unilateral TMJ arthralgia/osteoarthritis or after arthroscopy have been inconclusive. Morphine may not be superior to placebo (Bryant *et al* 1999) or bupivacaine (Furst *et al* 2001), no dose-effect relation has been shown (List *et al* 2001), no significant short-term analgesic effect occurs (Furst *et al* 2001; List *et al* 2001) and the magnitude of pain relief is often not clinically relevant at long-term follow-up (List *et al* 2001).

In patients with chemoradiotherapy-induced stomatitis, topical morphine (mouthwash) significantly alleviated pain with a clear dose response (Cerchietti *et al* 2003). No systemically active detectable levels of morphine were found, suggesting that this may be a useful and safe method to alleviate mucositis pain.

13.6. Corticosteroids (Steroids)

Steroids are commonly employed in the symptomatic management of ulcerative mucosal lesions, reducing both pain and lesion size (Lo Muzio *et al* 2001; Hegarty *et al* 2002). Intra-articular injection of steroids has been advocated for the management of inflammatory conditions of the TMJ; in this fashion the systemic side effects may be avoided (Toller 1977; Kopp *et al* 1987; Wenneberg *et al* 1991; Vallon *et al* 2002; Arabshahi *et al* 2005). However, findings of steroid-induced joint damage (El-Hakim *et al* 2005; Schindler *et al* 2005) and the high efficacy of standard arthrocentesis have discouraged the use of intra-articular steroids (see Chapter 8). The available literature suggests therefore that this modality may be useful in the management of TMJ rheumatoid arthritis, for advanced arthritis unresponsive to conservative management or in patients unable to take systemic medication. The potential damage to joint structure must be balanced with the therapeutic effects.

In summary, for specific patients and conditions topically applied drugs are an attractive option in the management of chronic pain.

14. Future

The sequencing of the human genome will allow the systematic research of individual gene function and will eventually radically change clinical practice (Bentley 2004). In the short term, knowledge of the genome will have a profound clinical impact on the diagnostic capability of medical professions (Bell 2004). In animal experiments particular expressions of chronic pain such as heat sensitivity have been directly linked to genetics (Mogil *et al* 2005). In human studies heritability has been reported to account for a large amount of the pain phenotype, e.g. 50% of migraine pain and 40% of carpal tunnel syndrome (Larsson *et al* 1995; Hakim *et al* 2002). The application of advanced molecular biology techniques to the study of pain allows us to examine the genes involved in nociception and the gene polymorphisms associated with pain susceptibility. As the mechanisms of pain are elucidated, an increasing number of proteins with varied functions (receptors, transport, ligands, etc) can be targeted for therapy.

Pharmacogenomics, the science of drug discovery based on knowledge of genes, is based on an understanding of the aetiologic disease mechanisms and enables their prevention. Pharmacogenetics describes the genetic variability in drug metabolism, but often the definitions are used interchangeably (Fagerlund and Braaten 2001). Knowledge of genetically controlled drug toxicity and common adverse drug reactions will ultimately lead to 'individualized medicine' (Evans and Relling 2004). Response variability to analgesic drugs is well established; 6–10% of caucasians, 0–2.3% of Asians and 1.9% of African Americans will exhibit reduced or no pain relief from codeine because of polymorphisms of the cytochrome-P450 enzymes (Fagerlund and Braaten 2001; Flores and Mogil 2001). Polymorphisms of the mu opioid

receptors lead to interindividual differences in responses to pain and its relief by opioid drugs (Uhl *et al* 1999). Such genetically governed interindividual differences are also found in the drug-transport proteins, altering the pharmacokinetics and pharmacodynamics of a variety of drugs and therefore their clinical efficacy.

Gene transfer technology offers the ability to manipulate specific pathways involved in chronic pain (Pohl and Braz 2001). Transplantation of engineered cells and herpesvirus vectors express molecules for an adequate time period and may be useful for pain. Many problems, including potential dangers associated with viral use, control of expression, immune responses and the time course of expression, still must be overcome. Gene therapy is an example of the wide range of delivery methods we may have at our future disposal.

References

Abdel-Salam OM, Baiuomy AR, Arbid MS (2004) Studies on the anti-inflammatory effect of fluoxetine in the rat. *Pharmacol Res* **49**(?):119–131.

Ablad B, Dahlof C (1986) Migraine and beta-blockade: modulation of sympathetic neurotransmission. *Cephalalgia* **6** (Suppl 5):7–13.

Adelman LC, Adelman JU, Von Seggern R, *et al* (2000) Venlafaxine extended release (XR) for the prophylaxis of migraine and tension-type headache: A retrospective study in a clinical setting. *Headache* **40**(7):572–580.

Ahn AH, Basbaum AI (2005) Where do triptans act in the treatment of migraine? *Pain* **115**(1–2):1–4.

Akerman S, Williamson DJ, Hill RG, *et al* (2001) The effect of adrenergic compounds on neurogenic dural vasodilatation. *Eur J Pharmacol* **424**(1):53–58.

Ambrosio AF, Silva AP, Malva JO, *et al* (2001) Inhibition of glutamate release by BIA 2-093 and BIA 2-024, two novel derivatives of carbamazepine, due to blockade of sodium but not calcium channels. *Biochem Pharmacol* **61**(10):1271–1275.

Andersson KE, Vinge E (1990) Beta-adrenoceptor blockers and calcium antagonists in the prophylaxis and treatment of migraine. *Drugs* **39**(3):355–373.

Antonijevic I, Mousa SA, Schafer M, *et al* (1995) Perineurial defect and peripheral opioid analgesia in inflammation. *J Neurosci* **15** (1 Pt 1):165–172.

Arabshahi B, Dewitt EM, Cahill AM, *et al* (2005) Utility of corticosteroid injection for temporomandibular arthritis in children with juvenile idiopathic arthritis. *Arthritis Rheum* **52**(11):3563–3569.

Argoff CE (2002) A review of the use of topical analgesics for myofascial pain. *Curr Pain Headache Rep* **6**(5):375–378.

Argoff CE (2004) Targeted peripheral analgesics therapy for neuropathic pain. *Curr Pain Headache Rep* **8**(3):199–204.

Argoff CE, Galer BS, Jensen MP, *et al* (2004) Effectiveness of the lidocaine patch 5% on pain qualities in three chronic pain states: assessment with the Neuropathic Pain Scale. *Curr Med Res Opin* **20**(Suppl 2):S21–S28.

Asakura K, Kanemasa T, Minagawa K, *et al* (2000) alpha-eudesmol, a P/Q-type Ca(2+) channel blocker, inhibits neurogenic vasodilation and extravasation following electrical stimulation of trigeminal ganglion. *Brain Res* **873**(1):94–101.

Ayajiki K, Okamura T, Toda N (1997) Flunarizine, an anti-migraine agent, impairs nitroxidergic nerve function in cerebral arteries. *Eur J Pharmacol* **329**(1):49–53.

Backonja M, Glanzman RL (2003) Gabapentin dosing for neuropathic pain: evidence from randomized, placebo-controlled clinical trials. *Clin Ther* **25**(1):81–104.

Bartsch T, Knight YE, Goadsby PJ (2004) Activation of 5-HT(1B/1D) receptor in the periaqueductal gray inhibits nociception. *Ann Neurol* **56**(3):371–381.

Bell J (2004) Predicting disease using genomics *Nature* **429** (6990):453–456.

Bendtsen L, Jensen R (2000) Amitriptyline reduces myofascial tenderness in patients with chronic tension-type headache. *Cephalalgia* **20**(6):603–610.

Bentley DR (2004) Genomes for medicine. *Nature* **429**(6990): 440–445.

Berger A, Henderson M, Nadoolman W, *et al* (1995) Oral capsaicin provides temporary relief for oral mucositis pain secondary to chemotherapy/radiation therapy. *J Pain Symptom Manage* **10**(3):243–248.

Berilgen MS, Bulut S, Gonen M, *et al* (2005) Comparison of the effects of amitriptyline and flunarizine on weight gain and serum leptin, C peptide and insulin levels when used as migraine preventive treatment. *Cephalalgia* **25**(11):1048–1053.

Berman JS, Symonds C, Birch R (2004) Efficacy of two cannabis based medicinal extracts for relief of central neuropathic pain from brachial plexus avulsion: results of a randomised controlled trial. *Pain* **112**(3):299–306.

Betts NJ, Makowski G, Shen YH, *et al* (1995) Evaluation of topical viscous 2% lidocaine jelly as an adjunct during the management of alveolar osteitis. *J Oral Maxillofac Surg* **53**(10):1140–1144.

Bhalang K, Light K, Maixner W (2004) Effect of propranolol on TMD and fibromyalgia pain: preliminary findings. The IADR/AADR/CADR- 82nd General Session. Hawaii.

Bianchi M, Rossoni G, Sacerdote P, *et al* (1995) Carbamazepine exerts anti-inflammatory effects in the rat. *Eur J Pharmacol* **294**(1):71–74.

Bischofs S, Zelenka M, Sommer C (2004) Evaluation of topiramate as an anti-hyperalgesic and neuroprotective agent in the peripheral nervous system. *J Peripher Nerv Syst* **9**(2):70–78.

Blackburn-Munro G, Erichsen HK (2005) Antiepileptics and the treatment of neuropathic pain: evidence from animal models. *Curr Pharm Des* **11**(23):2961–2976.

Blau JN, Engel HO (2004) Individualizing treatment with verapamil for cluster headache patients. *Headache* **44**(10): 1013–1018.

Bomholt SF, Mikkelsen JD, Blackburn-Munro G (2005) Antinociceptive effects of the antidepressants amitriptyline, duloxetine, mirtazapine and citalopram in animal models of acute, persistent and neuropathic pain. *Neuropharmacology* **48**(2):252–263.

Browning R, Jackson JL, O'Malley PG (2001) Cyclobenzaprine and back pain: a meta-analysis. *Arch Intern Med* **161**(13):1613–1620.

Bryant CJ, Harrison SD, Hopper C, *et al* (1999) Use of intra-articular morphine for postoperative analgesia following TMJ arthroscopy. *Br J Oral Maxillofac Surg* **37**(5):391–396.

Buggy DJ, Toogood L, Maric S, *et al* (2003) Lack of analgesic efficacy of oral delta-9-tetrahydrocannabinol in postoperative pain. *Pain* **106**(1–2):169–172.

Burstein R, Jakubowski M (2004) Analgesic triptan action in an animal model of intracranial pain: a race against the development of central sensitization. *Ann Neurol* **55**(1):27–36.

Cai Z, McCaslin PP (1992) Amitriptyline, desipramine, cyproheptadine and carbamazepine, in concentrations used therapeutically, reduce kainate- and N-methyl-D-aspartate-induced intracellular Ca2+ levels in neuronal culture. *Eur J Pharmacol* **219**(1):53–57.

Calignano A, La Rana G, Giuffrida A, *et al* (1998) Control of pain initiation by endogenous cannabinoids. *Nature* **394**(6690): 277–281.

Canavan D, Graff-Radford SB, Gratt BM (1994) Traumatic dysesthesia of the trigeminal nerve. *J Orofac Pain* **8**(4):391–396.

Carlsson KC, Hoem NO, Moberg ER, *et al* (2004) Analgesic effect of dextromethorphan in neuropathic pain. *Acta Anaesthesiol Scand* **48**(3):328–336.

Carroll DG, Kline KM, Malnar KF (2004) Role of topiramate for the treatment of painful diabetic peripheral neuropathy. *Pharmacotherapy* **24**(9):1186–1193.

Caruso FS (2000) MorphiDex pharmacokinetic studies and single-dose analgesic efficacy studies in patients with postoperative pain. *J Pain Symptom Manage* **19**(1 Suppl):S31–S36.

Cerchietti LC, Navigante AH, Korte MW, *et al* (2003) Potential utility of the peripheral analgesic properties of morphine in stomatitis-related pain: a pilot study. *Pain* **105**(1–2):265–273.

Cha BH, Silveira DC, Liu X, *et al* (2002) Effect of topiramate following recurrent and prolonged seizures during early development. *Epilepsy Res* **51**(3):217–232.

Chapman V, Suzuki R, Chamarette HL, *et al* (1998) Effects of systemic carbamazepine and gabapentin on spinal neuronal responses in spinal nerve ligated rats. *Pain* **75**(2–3):261–272.

Chong MS, Libretto SE (2003) The rationale and use of topiramate for treating neuropathic pain. *Clin J Pain* **19**(1):59–68.

Chou R, Peterson K, Helfand M (2004) Comparative efficacy and safety of skeletal muscle relaxants for spasticity and musculoskeletal conditions: a systematic review. *J Pain Symptom Manage* **28**(2):140–175.

Christensen D, Gautron M, Guilbaud G, *et al* (2001) Effect of gabapentin and lamotrigine on mechanical allodynia-like behaviour in a rat model of trigeminal neuropathic pain. *Pain* **93**(2):147–153.

Cichewicz DL (2004) Synergistic interactions between cannabinoid and opioid analgesics. *Life Sci* **74**(11):1317–1324.

Clark AJ, Lynch ME, Ware M, *et al* (2005) Guidelines for the use of cannabinoid compounds in chronic pain. *Pain Res Manag* **10** (Suppl A):44A–46A.

Coderre TJ, Kumar N, Lefebvre CD, *et al* (2005) Evidence that gabapentin reduces neuropathic pain by inhibiting the spinal release of glutamate. *J Neurochem* **94**(4):1131–1139.

Coggeshall RE, Zhou S, Carlton SM (1997) Opioid receptors on peripheral sensory axons. *Brain Res* **764**(1–2):126–132.

Costa B, Colleoni M, Conti S, *et al* (2004) Repeated treatment with the synthetic cannabinoid WIN 55,212-2 reduces both hyperalgesia and production of pronociceptive mediators in a rat model of neuropathic pain. *Br J Pharmacol* **141**(1):4–8.

Crews FT, Scott JA, Shorstein NH (1983) Rapid down-regulation of serotonin2 receptor binding during combined administration of tricyclic antidepressant drugs and alpha 2 antagonists. *Neuropharmacology* **22**(10):1203–1209.

Cumberbatch MJ, Hill RG, Hargreaves RJ (1997) Rizatriptan has central antinociceptive effects against durally evoked responses. *Eur J Pharmacol* **328**(1):37–40.

Cutrer FM (2001) Antiepileptic drugs: how they work in headache. Headache **41**(Suppl 1):S3–S10.

Cutrer FM, Moskowitz MA (1996) Wolff Award 1996. The actions of valproate and neurosteroids in a model of trigeminal pain. *Headache* **36**(10):579–585.

Dalton SO, Johansen C, Mellemkjaer L, *et al* (2003) Use of selective serotonin reuptake inhibitors and risk of upper gastrointestinal tract bleeding: a population-based cohort study. *Arch Intern Med* **163**(1):59–64.

de Hoon JN, Willigers JM, Troost J, *et al* (2000) Vascular effects of 5-HT1B/1D-receptor agonists in patients with migraine headaches. *Clin Pharmacol Ther* **68**(4):418–426.

De Petrocellis L, Melck D, Bisogno T, *et al* (2000) Endocannabinoids and fatty acid amides in cancer, inflammation and related disorders. *Chem Phys Lipids* **108**(1–2):191–209.

Devers A, Galer BS (2000) Topical lidocaine patch relieves a variety of neuropathic pain conditions: an open-label study. *Clin J Pain* **16**(3):205–208.

Dionne RA, Gordon SM, Tahara M, *et al* (1999) Analgesic efficacy and pharmacokinetics of ketoprofen administered into a surgical site. *J Clin Pharmacol* **39**(2):131–138.

Dionne RA, Lepinski AM, Gordon SM, *et al* (2001) Analgesic effects of peripherally administered opioids in clinical models of acute and chronic inflammation. *Clin Pharmacol Ther* **70**(1): 66–73.

Dionne RA, Haynes D, Brahim JS, *et al* (2004) Analgesic effect of sustained-release flurbiprofen administered at the site of tissue injury in the oral surgery model. *J Clin Pharmacol* **44**(12):1418–1424.

Di Rienzo Businco L, Di Rienzo Businco A, D'Emilia M, *et al* (2004) Topical versus systemic diclofenac in the treatment of temporomandibular joint dysfunction symptoms. *Acta Otorhinolaryngol Ital* **24**(5):279–283.

Donaldson C, Boers PM, Hoskin KL, *et al* (2002) The role of 5-HT1B and 5-HT1D receptors in the selective inhibitory effect of naratriptan on trigeminovascular neurons. *Neuropharmacology* **42**(3):374–385.

Duedahl TH, Romsing J, Moiniche S, *et al* (2006) A qualitative systematic review of peri-operative dextromethorphan in postoperative pain. *Acta Anaesthesiol Scand* **50**(1):1–13.

Eide PK, Stubhaug A (1997) Relief of glossopharyngeal neuralgia by ketamine-induced N-methyl-aspartate receptor blockade. *Neurosurgery* **41**(2):505–508.

Eisenberg E, Shifrin A, Krivoy N (2005) Lamotrigine for neuropathic pain. *Expert Rev Neurother* **5**(6):729–735.

Elad S, Cohen G, Zylber-Katz E, *et al* (1999) Systemic absorption of lidocaine after topical application for the treatment of oral mucositis in bone marrow transplantation patients. *J Oral Pathol Med* **28**(4):170–172.

El-Hakim IE, Abdel-Hamid IS, Bader A (2005) Tempromandibular joint (TMJ) response to intra-articular dexamethasone injection following mechanical arthropathy: a histological study in rats. *Int J Oral Maxillofac Surg* **34**(3):305–310.

Epstein JB, Marcoe JH (1994) Topical application of capsaicin for treatment of oral neuropathic pain and trigeminal neuralgia. *Oral Surg Oral Med Oral Pathol* **77**(2):135–140.

Epstein JB, Truelove EL, Oien H, *et al* (2001) Oral topical doxepin rinse: analgesic effect in patients with oral mucosal pain due to cancer or cancer therapy. *Oral Oncol* **37**(8):632–637.

Ernberg M, Lundeberg T, Kopp S (2000) Effect of propranolol and granisetron on experimentally induced pain and allodynia/hyperalgesia by intramuscular injection of serotonin into the human masseter muscle. *Pain* **84**(2–3):339–346.

Evans RW, Ramadan NM (2004) Are cannabis-based chemicals helpful in headache? *Headache* **44**(7):726–727.

Evans WE, Relling MV (2004) Moving towards individualized medicine with pharmacogenomics. *Nature* **429**(6990):464–468.

Fagerlund TH, Braaten O (2001) No pain relief from codeine…? An introduction to pharmacogenomics. *Acta Anaesthesiol Scand* **45**(2):140–149.

Farago F (1987) Trigeminal neuralgia: its treatment with two new carbamazepine analogues. *Eur Neurol* **26**(2):73–83.

Farquhar-Smith WP, Egertova M, Bradbury EJ, *et al* (2000) Cannabinoid CB(1) receptor expression in rat spinal cord. *Mol Cell Neurosci* **15**(6):510–521.

Felsby S, Nielsen J, Arendt-Nielsen L, *et al* (1996) NMDA receptor blockade in chronic neuropathic pain: a comparison of ketamine and magnesium chloride. *Pain* **64**(2):283–291.

Ferjan I, Erjavec F (1996) Changes in histamine and serotonin secretion from rat peritoneal mast cells caused by antidepressants. *Inflamm Res* **45**(3):141–144.

Field MJ, Holloman EF, McCleary S, *et al* (1997) Evaluation of gabapentin and S-(+)-3-isobutylgaba in a rat model of postoperative pain. *J Pharmacol Exp Ther* **282**(3):1242–1246.

Field MJ, McCleary S, Hughes J, *et al* (1999) Gabapentin and pregabalin, but not morphine and amitriptyline, block both static and dynamic components of mechanical allodynia induced by streptozocin in the rat. *Pain* **80**(1–2):391–398.

Fishbain DA, Cutler RB, Rosomoff HL, *et al* (2000) Clonazepam open clinical treatment trial for myofascial syndrome associated chronic pain. *Pain Med* **1**(4):332–339.

Flores CM, Mogil JS (2001) The pharmacogenetics of analgesia: toward a genetically-based approach to pain management. *Pharmacogenomics* **2**(3):177–194.

Foong FW, Satoh M (1984) The periaqueductal gray is the site of the antinociceptive action of carbamazepine as related to bradykinin-induced trigeminal pain. *Br J Pharmacol* **83**(2):493–497.

Forssell H, Tasmuth T, Tenovuo O, *et al* (2004) Venlafaxine in the treatment of atypical facial pain: a randomized controlled trial. *J Orofac Pain* **18**(2):131–137.

Fox A, Gentry C, Patel S, *et al* (2003) Comparative activity of the anti-convulsants oxcarbazepine, carbamazepine, lamotrigine and gabapentin in a model of neuropathic pain in the rat and guinea-pig. *Pain* **105**(1–2):355–362.

Freitag FG (2003) Preventative treatment for migraine and tension-type headaches : do drugs having effects on muscle spasm and tone have a role? *CNS Drugs* **17**(6):373–381.

Freitag FG, Diamond S, Diamond ML, *et al* (2001) Divalproex in the long-term treatment of chronic daily headache. *Headache* **41**(3):271–278.

Freynhagen R, Strojek K, Griesing T, *et al* (2005) Efficacy of pregabalin in neuropathic pain evaluated in a 12-week, randomised, double-blind, multicentre, placebo-controlled trial of flexible- and fixed-dose regimens. *Pain* **115**(3):254–263.

Fromm GH (1994) Baclofen as an adjuvant analgesic. *J Pain Symptom Manage* **9**(8):500–509.

Fromm GH, Terrence CF (1987) Comparison of L-baclofen and racemic baclofen in trigeminal neuralgia. *Neurology* **37**(11):1725–1728.

Fromm GH, Terrence CF, Chattha AS, *et al* (1980) Baclofen in trigeminal neuralgia: its effect on the spinal trigeminal nucleus: a pilot study. *Arch Neurol* **37**(12):768–771.

Fromm GH, Terrence CF, Chattha AS (1984) Baclofen in the treatment of trigeminal neuralgia: double-blind study and long-term follow-up. *Ann Neurol* **15**(3):240–244.

Fromm GH, Sato K, Nakata M (1992) The action of GABAB antagonists in the trigeminal nucleus of the rat. *Neuropharmacology* **31**(5):475–480.

Furst IM, Kryshtalskyj B, Weinberg S (2001) The use of intra-articular opioids and bupivacaine for analgesia following temporomandibular joint arthroscopy: a prospective, randomized trial. *J Oral Maxillofac Surg* **59**(9):979–983; discussion 983–984.

Galer BS (2001) Topical medications. In: Loeser JD (ed) *Bonica's Management of Pain*. Philadelphia: Lippincott Williams and Wilkins, pp 1736–1741.

Galer BS, Rowbotham M, Perander J, *et al* (2000) Topical diclofenac patch relieves minor sports injury pain: results of a multicenter controlled clinical trial. *J Pain Symptom Manage* **19**(4):287–294.

Galer BS, Gammaitoni AR, Oleka N, *et al* (2004) Use of the lidocaine patch 5% in reducing intensity of various pain qualities reported by patients with low-back pain. *Curr Med Res Opin* **20**(Suppl 2):S5–S12.

Gerner P, Haderer AE, Mujtaba M, *et al* (2003) Assessment of differential blockade by amitriptyline and its N-methyl derivative in different species by different routes. *Anesthesiology* **98**(6):1484–1490.

Gilron I, Booher SL, Rowan MS, *et al* (2000) A randomized, controlled trial of high-dose dextromethorphan in facial neuralgias. *Neurology* **55**(7):964–971.

Goldstein DJ, Lu Y, Detke MJ, *et al* (2005) Duloxetine vs. placebo in patients with painful diabetic neuropathy. *Pain* **116**(1–2):109–118.

Gordon SM, Dubner R, Dionne RA (1999) Antihyperalgesic effect of the N-methyl-D-aspartate receptor antagonist dextromethorphan in the oral surgery model. *J Clin Pharmacol* **39**(2):139–146.

Grabow TS, Dougherty PM (2002) Gabapentin produces dose-dependent antinociception in the orofacial formalin test in the rat. *Reg Anesth Pain Med* **27**(3):277–283.

Gray AM, Pache DM, Sewell RD (1999) Do alpha2-adrenoceptors play an integral role in the antinociceptive mechanism of action of antidepressant compounds? *Eur J Pharmacol* **378**(2):161–168.

Green CR, Wheeler JR, LaPorte F, *et al* (2002) How well is chronic pain managed? Who does it well? *Pain Med* **3**(1):56–65.

Gremeau-Richard C, Woda A, Navez ML, *et al* (2004) Topical clonazepam in stomatodynia: a randomised placebo-controlled study. *Pain* **108**(1-2):51–57.

Guindon J, Beaulieu P (2006) Antihyperalgesic effects of local injections of anandamide, ibuprofen, rofecoxib and their combinations in a model of neuropathic pain. *Neuropharmacology* **50**(7):814–823.

Hakim AJ, Cherkas L, El Zayat S, et al (2002) The genetic contribution to carpal tunnel syndrome in women: a twin study. *Arthritis Rheum* **47**(3):275–279.

Hamon M, Gozlan H, Bourgoin S, et al (1987) Opioid receptors and neuropeptides in the CNS in rats treated chronically with amoxapine or amitriptyline. *Neuropharmacology* **26**(6):531–539.

Harkins S, Linford J, Cohen J, et al (1991) Administration of clonazepam in the treatment of TMD and associated myofascial pain: a double-blind pilot study. *J Craniomandib Disord* **5**(3):179–186.

Health N (2003) PharmaTrends. Accessed December 2005. Available at: http://www.ndchealth.com/pdf/pharmatrends2002.pdf

Hegarty AM, Hodgson TA, Lewsey JD, et al (2002) Fluticasone propionate spray and betamethasone sodium phosphate mouthrinse: a randomized crossover study for the treatment of symptomatic oral lichen planus. *J Am Acad Dermatol* **47**(2):271–279.

Hering-Hanit R, Gadoth N (2000) Baclofen in cluster headache. *Headache* **40**(1):48–51.

Herman CR, Schiffman EL, Look JO, et al (2002) The effectiveness of adding pharmacologic treatment with clonazepam or cyclobenzaprine to patient education and self-care for the treatment of jaw pain upon awakening: a randomized clinical trial. *J Orofac Pain* **16**(1):64–70.

Hersh EV, Pertes RA, Ochs HA (1994) Topical capsaicin-pharmacology and potential role in the treatment of temporomandibular pain. *J Clin Dent* **5**(2):54–59.

Hersh EV, Houpt MI, Cooper SA, et al (1996) Analgesic efficacy and safety of an intraoral lidocaine patch. *J Am Dent Assoc* **127**(11):1626–1634; quiz 1665–1666.

Hersh EV, DeRossi SS, Ciarrocca KN, et al (2003) Efficacy and tolerability of an intraoral benzocaine patch in the relief of spontaneous toothache pain. *J Clin Dent* **14**(1):1–6.

Herzberg U, Eliav E, Bennett GJ, et al (1997) The analgesic effects of R(+)-WIN 55,212-2 mesylate, a high affinity cannabinoid agonist, in a rat model of neuropathic pain. *Neurosci Lett* **221**(2–3):157–160.

Heyneman CA, Lawless-Liday C, Wall GC (2000) Oral versus topical NSAIDs in rheumatic diseases: a comparison. *Drugs* **60**(3):555–574.

Hill CM, Balkenohl M, Thomas DW, et al (2001) Pregabalin in patients with postoperative dental pain. *Eur J Pain* **5**(2):119–124.

Houghton AK, Lu Y, Westlund KN (1998) S-(+)-3-isobutylgaba and its stereoisomer reduces the amount of inflammation and hyperalgesia in an acute arthritis model in the rat. *J Pharmacol Exp Ther* **285**(2):533–538.

Houpt MI, Heins P, Lamster I, et al (1997) An evaluation of intraoral lidocaine patches in reducing needle-insertion pain. *Compend Contin Educ Dent* **18**(4):309–310,312–314, 316; quiz 318.

Idanpaan-Heikkila JJ, Guilbaud G (1999) Pharmacological studies on a rat model of trigeminal neuropathic pain: baclofen, but not carbamazepine, morphine or tricyclic antidepressants, attenuates the allodynia-like behaviour. *Pain* **79**(2–3):281–290.

Irman-Florjanc T, Stanovnik L (1998) Tricyclic antidepressants change plasma histamine kinetics after its secretion induced by compound 48/80 in the rat. *Inflamm Res* **47**(Suppl 1):S26–S27.

Jaggar SI, Hasnie FS, Sellaturay S, et al (1998) The anti-hyperalgesic actions of the cannabinoid anandamide and the putative CB2 receptor agonist palmitoylethanolamide in visceral and somatic inflammatory pain. *Pain* **76**(1–2):189–199.

Jang Y, Kim ES, Park SS, et al (2005) The suppressive effects of oxcarbazepine on mechanical and cold allodynia in a rat model of neuropathic pain. *Anesth Analg* **101**(3):800–806, table of contents.

Jennings EA, Ryan RM, Christie MJ (2004) Effects of sumatriptan on rat medullary dorsal horn neurons. *Pain* **111**(1–2):30–37.

Jones CK, Peters SC, Shannon HE (2005) Efficacy of duloxetine, a potent and balanced serotonergic and noradrenergic reuptake inhibitor, in inflammatory and acute pain models in rodents. *J Pharmacol Exp Ther* **312**(2):726–732.

Kajii TS, Okamoto T, Yura S, et al (2005) Elevated levels of beta-endorphin in temporomandibular joint synovial lavage fluid of patients with closed lock. *J Orofac Pain* **19**(1):41–46.

Karst M, Salim K, Burstein S, et al (2003) Analgesic effect of the synthetic cannabinoid CT-3 on chronic neuropathic pain: a randomized controlled trial. *Jama* **290**(13):1757–1762.

Katz J, Pennella-Vaughan J, Hetzel RD, et al (2005) A randomized, placebo-controlled trial of bupropion sustained release in chronic low back pain. *J Pain* **6**(10):656–661.

Katz NP (2000) MorphiDex (MS:DM) double-blind, multiple-dose studies in chronic pain patients. *J Pain Symptom Manage* **19** (1 Suppl):S37–S41.

Kehl LJ, Hamamoto DT, Wacnik PW, et al (2003) A cannabinoid agonist differentially attenuates deep tissue hyperalgesia in animal models of cancer and inflammatory muscle pain. *Pain* **103**(1–2):175–186.

Kiayias JA, Vlachou ED, Lakka-Papadodima E (2000) Venlafaxine HCl in the treatment of painful peripheral diabetic neuropathy. *Diabetes Care* **23**(5):699.

Kiguchi S, Imamura T, Ichikawa K, et al (2004) Oxcarbazepine antinociception in animals with inflammatory pain or painful diabetic neuropathy. *Clin Exp Pharmacol Physiol* **31**(1–2):57–64.

Kingery WS (1997) A critical review of controlled clinical trials for peripheral neuropathic pain and complex regional pain syndromes. *Pain* **73**(2):123–139.

Klapper J (1997) Divalproex sodium in migraine prophylaxis: a dose-controlled study. *Cephalalgia* **17**(2):103–108.

Knowles SR, Shapiro LE, Shear NH (1999) Anticonvulsant hypersensitivity syndrome: incidence, prevention and management. *Drug Saf* **21**(6):489–501.

Kopp S, Carlsson GE, Haraldson T, et al (1987) Long-term effect of intra-articular injections of sodium hyaluronate and corticosteroid on temporomandibular joint arthritis. *J Oral Maxillofac Surg* **45**(11):929–935.

Kunjur J, Anand R, Brennan PA, et al (2003) An audit of 405 temporomandibular joint arthrocentesis with intra-articular morphine infusion. *Br J Oral Maxillofac Surg* **41**(1):29–31.

Larsson B, Bille B, Pedersen NL (1995) Genetic influence in headaches: a Swedish twin study. *Headache* **35**(9):513–519.

Leker RR, Neufeld MY (2003) Anti-epileptic drugs as possible neuroprotectants in cerebral ischemia. *Brain Res Brain Res Rev* **42**(3):187–203.

Li X, Ketter TA, Frye MA (2002) Synaptic, intracellular, and neuroprotective mechanisms of anticonvulsants: are they relevant for the treatment and course of bipolar disorders? *J Affect Disord* **69**(1–3):1–14.

Liang YC, Huang CC, Hsu KS (2004) Therapeutic potential of cannabinoids in trigeminal neuralgia. *Curr Drug Targets CNS Neurol Disord* **3**(6):507–514.

Likar R, Schafer M, Paulak F, et al (1997) Intraarticular morphine analgesia in chronic pain patients with osteoarthritis. *Anesth Analg* **84**(6):1313–1317.

Likar R, Sittl R, Gragger K, et al (1998) Peripheral morphine analgesia in dental surgery. *Pain* **76**(1–2):145–150.

Likar R, Kapral S, Steinkellner H, et al (1999) Dose-dependency of intra-articular morphine analgesia. *Br J Anaesth* **83**(2):241–244.

Likar R, Koppert W, Blatnig H, et al (2001) Efficacy of peripheral morphine analgesia in inflamed, non-inflamed and perineural tissue of dental surgery patients. *J Pain Symptom Manage* **21**(4):330–337.

Lim G, Sung B, Ji RR, et al (2003) Upregulation of spinal cannabinoid-1-receptors following nerve injury enhances the effects of Win 55,212-2 on neuropathic pain behaviors in rats. *Pain* **105**(1–2):275–283.

List T, Tegelberg A, Haraldson T, et al (2001) Intra-articular morphine as analgesic in temporomandibular joint arthralgia/osteoarthritis. *Pain* **94**(3):275–282.

Lo Muzio L, della Valle A, Mignogna MD, *et al* (2001) The treatment of oral aphthous ulceration or erosive lichen planus with topical clobetasol propionate in three preparations: a clinical and pilot study on 54 patients. *J Oral Pathol Med* **30**(10):611–617.

Loscher W (1999) Valproate: a reappraisal of its pharmacodynamic properties and mechanisms of action. *Prog Neurobiol* **58**(1):31–59.

Luccarini P, Perrier L, Degoulange C, *et al* (2004) Synergistic antinociceptive effect of amitriptyline and morphine in the rat orofacial formalin test. *Anesthesiology* **100**(3):690–696.

Lynch ME, Clark AJ, Sawynok J (2003) A pilot study examining topical amitriptyline, ketamine, and a combination of both in the treatment of neuropathic pain. *Clin J Pain* **19**(5):323–328.

Lynch ME, Clark AJ, Sawynok J, *et al* (2005) Topical amitriptyline and ketamine in neuropathic pain syndromes: an open-label study. *J Pain* **6**(10):644–649.

McCarson KE, Duric V, Reisman SA, *et al* (2006) GABA(B) receptor function and subunit expression in the rat spinal cord as indicators of stress and the antinociceptive response to antidepressants. *Brain Res* **1068**(1):109–117.

McCleane G (2000) Topical application of doxepin hydrochloride, capsaicin and a combination of both produces analgesia in chronic human neuropathic pain: a randomized, double-blind, placebo-controlled study. *Br J Clin Pharmacol* **49**(6):574–579.

McQuay HJ, Carroll D, Jadad AR, *et al* (1994) Dextromethorphan for the treatment of neuropathic pain: a double-blind randomised controlled crossover trial with integral n-of-1 design. *Pain* **59**(1):127–133.

Martin WJ, Hohmann AG, Walker JM (1996) Suppression of noxious stimulus-evoked activity in the ventral posterolateral nucleus of the thalamus by a cannabinoid agonist: correlation between electrophysiological and antinociceptive effects. *J Neurosci* **16**(20):6601–6611.

Mason L, Moore RA, Derry S, *et al* (2004) Systematic review of topical capsaicin for the treatment of chronic pain. *Bmj* **328**(7446):991.

Mathew NT, Kailasam J, Meadors L (2002) Prophylaxis of migraine, transformed migraine, and cluster headache with topiramate. *Headache* **42**(8):796–803.

Mathisen LC, Skjelbred P, Skoglund LA, *et al* (1995) Effect of ketamine, an NMDA receptor inhibitor, in acute and chronic orofacial pain. *Pain* **61**(2):215–220.

Max MB, Lynch SA, Muir J, *et al* (1992) Effects of desipramine, amitriptyline, and fluoxetine on pain in diabetic neuropathy. *N Engl J Med* **326**(19):1250–1256.

Mochizuki D (2004) Serotonin and noradrenaline reuptake inhibitors in animal models of pain. *Hum Psychopharmacol* **19** (Suppl 1):S15–S19.

Mogil JS, Miermeister F, Seifert F, *et al* (2005) Variable sensitivity to noxious heat is mediated by differential expression of the CGRP gene. *Proc Natl Acad Sci USA* **102**(36):12938–12943.

Moore UJ, Seymour RA, Rawlins MD (1992) The efficacy of locally applied aspirin and acetaminophen in postoperative pain after third molar surgery. *Clin Pharmacol Ther* **52**(3):292–296.

Moore UJ, Seymour RA, Gilroy J, *et al* (1994) The efficacy of locally applied morphine in post-operative pain after bilateral third molar surgery. *Br J Clin Pharmacol* **37**(3):227–230.

Moshe SL (2000) Mechanisms of action of anticonvulsant agents. *Neurology* **55**(5 Suppl 1):S32–S40;discussion S54–S58.

Nackley AG, Tan KS, Fecho K, *et al* (2007) Catechol-O-methyltransferase inhibition increases pain sensitivity through activation of both beta2- and beta3-adrenergic receptors. *Pain* **128**(3):199–208.

Naef M, Curatolo M, Petersen-Felix S, *et al* (2003) The analgesic effect of oral delta-9-tetrahydrocannabinol (THC), morphine, and a THC-morphine combination in healthy subjects under experimental pain conditions. *Pain* **105**(1-2):79–88.

Nakashita M, Sasaki K, Sakai N, *et al* (1997) Effects of tricyclic and tetracyclic antidepressants on the three subtypes of GABA transporter. *Neurosci Res* **29**(1):87–91.

Nelson KA, Park KM, Robinovitz E, *et al* (1997) High-dose oral dextromethorphan versus placebo in painful diabetic neuropathy and postherpetic neuralgia. *Neurology* **48**(5):1212–1218.

Ness TJ, Jones L, Smith H (2002) Use of compounded topical analgesics–results of an Internet survey. *Reg Anesth Pain Med* **27**(3):309–312.

Oeltjenbruns J, Schafer M (2005) Peripheral opioid analgesia: clinical applications. *Curr Pain Headache Rep* **9**(1):36–44.

Ogata N, Yoshii M, Narahashi T (1989) Psychotropic drugs block voltage-gated ion channels in neuroblastoma cells. *Brain Res* **476**(1):140–144.

Olesen J, Diener HC, Husstedt IW, *et al* (2004) Calcitonin gene-related peptide receptor antagonist BIBN 4096 BS for the acute treatment of migraine. *N Engl J Med* **350**(11):1104–1110.

Ozyalcin SN, Talu GK, Kiziltan E, *et al* (2005) The efficacy and safety of venlafaxine in the prophylaxis of migraine. *Headache* **45**(2):144–152.

Padilla M, Clark GT, Merrill RL (2000) Topical medications for orofacial neuropathic pain: a review. *J Am Dent Assoc* **131**(2):184–195.

Pandey CK, Singhal V, Kumar M, *et al* (2005) Gabapentin provides effective postoperative analgesia whether administered pre-emptively or post-incision. *Can J Anaesth* **52**(8):827–831.

Patten SB, Love EJ (1994) Drug-induced depression. Incidence, avoidance and management. *Drug Saf* **10**(3):203–219.

Pedersen LH, Nielsen AN, Blackburn-Munro G (2005) Anti-nociception is selectively enhanced by parallel inhibition of multiple subtypes of monoamine transporters in rat models of persistent and neuropathic pain. *Psychopharmacology (Berl)* **182**(4):551–561.

Peloso P, Gross A, Haines T, *et al* (2005) Medicinal and injection therapies for mechanical neck disorders. *Cochrane Database Syst Rev* (2):CD000319.

Pinelli A, Trivulzio S, Tomasoni L (1997) Effects of carbamazepine treatment on pain threshold values and brain serotonin levels in rats. *Pharmacology* **54**(3):113–117.

Pohl M, Braz J (2001) Gene therapy of pain: emerging strategies and future directions. *Eur J Pharmacol* **429**(1-3):39–48.

Raskin J, Pritchett YL, Wang F, *et al* (2005) A double-blind, randomized multicenter trial comparing duloxetine with placebo in the management of diabetic peripheral neuropathic pain. *Pain Med* **6**(5):346–356.

Raskin P, Donofrio PD, Rosenthal NR, *et al* (2004) Topiramate vs placebo in painful diabetic neuropathy: analgesic and metabolic effects. *Neurology* **63**(5):865–873.

Ray WA, Meredith S, Thapa PB, *et al* (2004) Cyclic antidepressants and the risk of sudden cardiac death. *Clin Pharmacol Ther* **75**(3):234–241.

Redwine KE, Trujillo KA (2003) Effects of NMDA receptor antagonists on acute mu-opioid analgesia in the rat. *Pharmacol Biochem Behav* **76**(2):361–372.

Richter RW, Portenoy R, Sharma U, *et al* (2005) Relief of painful diabetic peripheral neuropathy with pregabalin: a randomized, placebo-controlled trial. *J Pain* **6**(4):253–260.

Rog DJ, Nurmikko TJ, Friede T, *et al* (2005) Randomized, controlled trial of cannabis-based medicine in central pain in multiple sclerosis. *Neurology* **65**(6):812–819.

Rowbotham MC, Goli V, Kunz NR, *et al* (2004) Venlafaxine extended release in the treatment of painful diabetic neuropathy: a double-blind, placebo-controlled study. *Pain* **110**(3):697–706.

Saarto T, Wiffen PJ (2005) Antidepressants for neuropathic pain. *Cochrane Database Syst Rev* (3):CD005454.

Sacerdote P, Brini A, Mantegazza P, *et al* (1987) A role for serotonin and beta-endorphin in the analgesia induced by some tricyclic antidepressant drugs. *Pharmacol Biochem Behav* **26**(1):153–158.

Sandor PS, Afra J, Ambrosini A, *et al* (2000) Prophylactic treatment of migraine with beta-blockers and riboflavin: differential effects on the intensity dependence of auditory evoked cortical potentials. *Headache* **40**(1):30–35.

Sang CN (2000) NMDA-receptor antagonists in neuropathic pain: experimental methods to clinical trials. *J Pain Symptom Manage* **19**(1 Suppl):S21–S25.

Sang CN, Booher S, Gilron I, *et al* (2002) Dextromethorphan and memantine in painful diabetic neuropathy and postherpetic neuralgia: efficacy and dose-response trials. *Anesthesiology* **96**(5):1053–1061.

Santos Tde J, de Castro-Costa CM, Giffoni SD, *et al* (1999) The effect of baclofen on spontaneous and evoked behavioural expression of experimental neuropathic chronic pain. *Arq Neuropsiquiatr* **57**(3B):753–760.

Saper JR, Klapper J, Mathew NT, *et al* (2002) Intranasal civamide for the treatment of episodic cluster headaches. *Arch Neurol* **59**(6):990–994.

Satoh M, Foong FW (1983) A mechanism of carbamazepine-analgesia as shown by bradykinin-induced trigeminal pain. *Brain Res Bull* **10**(3):407–409.

Sawynok J (2003) Topical and peripherally acting analgesics. *Pharmacol Rev* **55**(1):1–20.

Sawynok J, Reid A (2003) Peripheral interactions between dextromethorphan, ketamine and amitriptyline on formalin-evoked behaviors and paw edema in rats. *Pain* **102**(1-2):179–186.

Sawynok J, Esser MJ, Reid AR (2001) Antidepressants as analgesics: an overview of central and peripheral mechanisms of action. *J Psychiatry Neurosci* **26**(1):21–29.

Saxen PR, Tfelt-Hansen P (2006) Triptans, 5-HT1B/1D receptor agonists in the acute treatment of migraine. In: Olesen J, Goadsby PJ, Ramadan NM, *et al* (eds) *The Headaches*, 3rd edn. Philadelphia: Lippincott Williams and Wilkins, pp 469–503.

Schindler C, Paessler L, Eckelt U, *et al* (2005) Severe temporomandibular dysfunction and joint destruction after intra-articular injection of triamcinolone. *J Oral Pathol Med* **34**(3):184–186.

Schreiber S, Backer MM, Pick CG (1999) The antinociceptive effect of venlafaxine in mice is mediated through opioid and adrenergic mechanisms. *Neurosci Lett* **273**(2):85–88.

Semenchuk MR, Sherman S, Davis B (2001) Double-blind, randomized trial of bupropion SR for the treatment of neuropathic pain. *Neurology* **57**(9):1583–1588.

Shannon HE, Eberle EL, Peters SC (2005) Comparison of the effects of anticonvulsant drugs with diverse mechanisms of action in the formalin test in rats. *Neuropharmacology* **48**(7):1012–1020.

Sharav Y, Singer E, Schmidt E, *et al* (1987) The analgesic effect of amitriptyline on chronic facial pain. *Pain* **31**(2):199–209.

Shields KG, Goadsby PJ (2005) Propranolol modulates trigeminovascular responses in thalamic ventroposteromedial nucleus: a role in migraine? *Brain* **128**(Pt 1):86–97.

Silberstein SD, Goadsby PJ (2002) Migraine: preventive treatment. *Cephalalgia* **22**(7):491–512.

Sills GJ (2006) The mechanisms of action of gabapentin and pregabalin. *Curr Opin Pharmacol* **6**(1):108–113.

Sindrup SH, Bach FW, Madsen C, *et al* (2003) Venlafaxine versus imipramine in painful polyneuropathy: a randomized, controlled trial. *Neurology* **60**(8):1284–1289.

Siow HC, Young WB, Silberstein SD (2005) Neuroleptics in headache. *Headache* **45**(4):358–371.

Soderpalm B (2002) Anticonvulsants: aspects of their mechanisms of action. *Eur J Pain 6* (Suppl A):3–9.

Stoica E, Enulescu O (1990) Propranolol corrects the abnormal catecholamine response to light during migraine. *Eur Neurol* **30**(1):19–22.

Storer RJ, Goadsby PJ (2004) Topiramate inhibits trigeminovascular neurons in the cat. *Cephalalgia* **24**(12):1049–1056.

Storer RJ, Akerman S, Connor HE, *et al* (2001) 4991W93, a potent blocker of neurogenic plasma protein extravasation, inhibits trigeminal neurons at 5-hydroxytryptamine (5-HT1B/1D) agonist doses. *Neuropharmacology* **40**(7):911–917.

Storey JR, Calder CS, Hart DE, *et al* (2001) Topiramate in migraine prevention: a double-blind, placebo-controlled study. *Headache* **41**(10):968–975.

Sumpton JE, Moulin DE (2001) Treatment of neuropathic pain with venlafaxine. *Ann Pharmacother* **35**(5):557–559.

Svensson P, Houe L, Arendt-Nielsen L (1997) Effect of systemic versus topical nonsteroidal anti-inflammatory drugs on postexercise jaw-muscle soreness: a placebo-controlled study. *J Orofac Pain* **11**(4):353–362.

Svensson P, Wang K, Arendt-Nielsen L (2003) Effect of muscle relaxants on experimental jaw-muscle pain and jaw-stretch reflexes: a double-blind and placebo-controlled trial. *Eur J Pain* **7**(5):449–456.

Terrence CF, Fromm GH (1981) Complications of baclofen withdrawal. *Arch Neurol* **38**(9):588–589.

Terrence CF, Fromm GH, Tenicela R (1985) Baclofen as an analgesic in chronic peripheral nerve disease. *Eur Neurol* **24**(6):380–385.

Tofferi JK, Jackson JL, O'Malley PG (2004) Treatment of fibromyalgia with cyclobenzaprine: a meta-analysis. *Arthritis Rheum* **51**(1):9–13.

Toller PA (1977) Use and misuse of intra-articular corticosteroids in treatment of temporomandibular joint pain. *Proc R Soc Med* **70**(7):461–463.

Tomic MA, Vuckovic SM, Stepanovic-Petrovic RM, *et al* (2004) The anti-hyperalgesic effects of carbamazepine and oxcarbazepine are attenuated by treatment with adenosine receptor antagonists. *Pain* **111**(3):253–260.

Turan A, White PF, Karamanlioglu B, *et al* (2006) Gabapentin: an alternative to the cyclooxygenase-2 inhibitors for perioperative pain management. *Anesth Analg* **102**(1):175–181.

Turturro MA, Frater CR, D'Amico FJ (2003) Cyclobenzaprine with ibuprofen versus ibuprofen alone in acute myofascial strain: a randomized, double-blind clinical trial. *Ann Emerg Med* **41**(6):818–826.

Tvedskov JF, Thomsen LL, Thomsen LL, *et al* (2004) The effect of propranolol on glyceryltrinitrate-induced headache and arterial response. *Cephalalgia* **24**(12):1076–1087.

Uhl GR, Sora I, Wang Z (1999) The mu opiate receptor as a candidate gene for pain: polymorphisms, variations in expression, nociception, and opiate responses. *Proc Natl Acad Sci USA* **96**(14):7752–7755.

Vallon D, Akerman S, Nilner M, *et al* (2002) Long-term follow-up of intra-articular injections into the temporomandibular joint in patients with rheumatoid arthritis. *Swed Dent J* **26**(4):149–158.

van Tulder MW, Touray T, Furlan AD, *et al* (2003) Muscle relaxants for non-specific low back pain. *Cochrane Database Syst Rev* (2):CD004252.

Veldhuijzen DS, Kenemans JL, van Wijck AJ, *et al* (2006) Acute and subchronic effects of amitriptyline on processing capacity in neuropathic pain patients using visual event-related potentials: preliminary findings. *Psychopharmacology (Berl)* **183**(4):462–470.

Vinik AI, Pittenger GL, Burcus NI, *et al* (2003) Topiramate improves in vitro and in vivo measures of nerve fiber loss in patients with diabetic neuropathy. *J Peripher Nerv Syst* **8**(s1):72–73.

Waldmeier PC, Baumann PA, Wicki P, *et al* (1995) Similar potency of carbamazepine, oxcarbazepine, and lamotrigine in inhibiting the release of glutamate and other neurotransmitters. *Neurology* **45**(10):1907–1913.

Wang GK, Russell C, Wang SY (2004) State-dependent block of voltage-gated Na+channels by amitriptyline via the local anesthetic receptor and its implication for neuropathic pain. *Pain* **110**(1-2):166–174.

Ware M, Beaulieu P (2005) Cannabinoids for the treatment of pain: An update on recent clinical trials. *Pain Res Manag* **10**(Suppl A):27A–30A.

Weinbroum AA, Bender B, Bickels J, *et al* (2003) Preoperative and postoperative dextromethorphan provides sustained reduction in postoperative pain and patient-controlled epidural analgesia requirement: a randomized, placebo-controlled, double-blind study in lower-body bone malignancy-operated patients. *Cancer* **97**(9):2334–2340.

Wenneberg B, Kopp S, Grondahl HG (1991) Long-term effect of intra-articular injections of a glucocorticosteroid into the TMJ: a clinical and radiographic 8-year follow-up. *J Craniomandib Disord* **5**(1):11–18.

Wieczorkiewicz-Plaza A, Plaza P, Maciejewski R, *et al* (2004) Effect of topiramate on mechanical allodynia in neuropathic pain model in rats. *Pol J Pharmacol* **56**(2):275–278.

Wiener CP, Buhimschi C (2004). Drugs for pregnant and lactating women. Churchill Livingstone: New York.

Wiffen P, Collins S, McQuay H, *et al* (2005a) Anticonvulsant drugs for acute and chronic pain. *Cochrane Database Syst Rev* (3): CD001133.

Wiffen PJ, McQuay HJ, Edwards JE, *et al* (2005b) Gabapentin for acute and chronic pain. *Cochrane Database Syst Rev* (3): CD005452.

Winocur E, Gavish A, Halachmi M, *et al* (2000) Topical application of capsaicin for the treatment of localized pain in the temporomandibular joint area. *J Orofac Pain* **14**(1):31–36.

Winocur E, Gavish A, Voikovitch M, *et al* (2003) Drugs and bruxism: a critical review. *J Orofac Pain* **17**(2):99–111.

Wood PB, Kablinger AS, Caldito GS (2005) Open trial of pindolol in the treatment of fibromyalgia. *Ann Pharmacother* **39**(11): 1812–1816.

Yang Y, Shuaib A, Li Q, *et al* (1998) Neuroprotection by delayed administration of topiramate in a rat model of middle cerebral artery embolization. *Brain Res* **804**(2):169–176.

Yasuda T, Miki S, Yoshinaga N, *et al* (2005) Effects of amitriptyline and gabapentin on bilateral hyperalgesia observed in an animal model of unilateral axotomy. *Pain* **115**(1-2):161–170.

Yesilyurt O, Dogrul A, Gul H, *et al* (2003) Topical cannabinoid enhances topical morphine antinociception. *Pain* **105**(1-2): 303–308.

Zakrzewska JM, Patsalos PN (1989) Oxcarbazepine: a new drug in the management of intractable trigeminal neuralgia. *J Neurol Neurosurg Psychiatry* **52**(4):472–476.

Zakrzewska JM, Patsalos PN (2002) Long-term cohort study comparing medical (oxcarbazepine) and surgical management of intractable trigeminal neuralgia. *Pain* **95**(3):259–266.

Zakrzewska JM, Chaudhry Z, Nurmikko TJ, *et al* (1997) Lamotrigine (lamictal) in refractory trigeminal neuralgia: results from a double-blind placebo controlled crossover trial. *Pain* **73**(2):223–230.

Zhang WY, Li Wan Po A (1994) The effectiveness of topically applied capsaicin. A meta-analysis. *Eur J Clin Pharmacol* **46**(6): 517–522.

Zhou L, Zhang Q, Stein C, *et al* (1998) Contribution of opioid receptors on primary afferent versus sympathetic neurons to peripheral opioid analgesia. *J Pharmacol Exp Ther* **286**(2): 1000–1006.

Zuniga RE, Schlicht CR, Abram SE (2000) Intrathecal baclofen is analgesic in patients with chronic pain. *Anesthesiology* **92**(3): 876–880.

Zvartau-Hind M, Din MU, Gilani A, *et al* (2000) Topiramate relieves refractory trigeminal neuralgia in MS patients. *Neurology* **55**(10):1587–1588.

CHAPTER 17

Complementary and alternative medicine

Yair Sharav and Rafael Benoliel

1. Introduction

Complementary and alternative medicine (CAM) has become increasingly popular. In 1990 Americans made an estimated 425 million visits to providers of 'unconventional' therapy; a number that exceeds the 388 million visits to all US primary care physicians in the same year (Eisenberg *et al* 1993). A more recent national survey of CAM use showed an increase in utilization of alternative therapies from 33.8% of the US population in 1990 to 42.1% in 1997 (Eisenberg *et al* 1998). Expenditure, in the United States, for professional alternative medical services was conservatively estimated in 1997 at $21.2 billion, with at least $12.2 billion paid out-of-pocket (Eisenberg *et al* 1998). This figure is apparently growing fast, to a recent estimate of out-of-pocket expenditures of over $34 billion per year in the US for the period 1999–2004 (Herman *et al* 2005). Alternative medicine is used most frequently for chronic conditions including pain and in particular 'back problems' and headache. Surveys of general population samples indicate that symptoms of chronic pain are significant predictors of the use of CAM (Astin 1998). In a recent national survey that included 2055 adults it was found that of those reporting back or neck pain in the past 12 months, 37% had seen a conventional provider and 54% had used complementary therapies to treat their condition (Wolsko *et al* 2003). Chiropractic, massage and relaxation techniques were the most commonly used complementary treatments for back or neck pain. In terms of cost for treatment of painful conditions, CAM therapies that may be considered cost-effective were acupuncture for migraine and manual therapy for neck pain (Herman *et al* 2005).

CAM is often used in situations in which conventional medicine fails to provide adequate relief (Weintraub 2003). Common examples include back and neck pain, arthritis and fibromyalgia. However, contrary to common belief, the majority of alternative medicine users appear to be doing so not because they are dissatisfied with conventional medicine but largely because they find these healthcare alternatives to be more congruent with their own values, beliefs and philosophical orientation towards health and life. Individuals who use CAM are better educated but often less healthy than those who do not use it (Astin 1998).

Additionally, there has been a growing interest in studies of CAM by medical students and physicians all around the world (Visser and Peters 1990; Goldszmidt *et al* 1995; Gracely and O'Connor 1996; Oberbaum *et al* 2003). Thirty years ago not a single CAM course was taught in any American medical school; by 1996, 64% of these schools offered courses in CAM (Wetzel *et al* 1998). The percentage of British medical schools offering courses in CAM increased from 10% in 1995 to 40% in 1997 (Zollman and Vickers 1999). The core curriculum for professional education in pain, published recently by the International Association for the Study of Pain (IASP), includes a chapter on complementary therapies (Charlton 2005).

2. What is Complementary and Alternative Medicine?

CAM therapies are difficult to define and include a broad spectrum of practices and beliefs: e.g. spiritual healing, relaxation techniques, homeopathy, hypnosis, acupuncture, chiropractic manipulation (Charlton 2005). CAM refers usually to medical practices not in conformity with the standards of the medical community (Eisenberg *et al* 1993). This definition is obviously very broad and loose. It is not much improved by utilization of the definition of 'medical interventions not taught widely at US medical schools or generally available at US hospitals' (Eisenberg *et al* 1998). The list of what is considered CAM changes continually; new approaches to healthcare emerge and CAM therapies proven safe and effective become adopted into conventional healthcare.

The widespread use of CAM therapies has intensified the need to evaluate their safety and effectiveness. Some CAM therapies are supported by scientific evidence, but for most, there are key questions that remain unanswered through well-designed scientific studies. These questions include whether these therapies are safe, and whether they work for the diseases or medical conditions for which they are used. In the absence of such evidence for effectiveness, heated debate results each time the introduction of CAM departments into public hospitals or the offering of such services by health organizations is suggested, especially as the standard demanded, in most of these same institutions, for the introduction of a new technology or a new conventional drug is far higher than that demanded from CAM therapy modalities (Glick 2005). Today many patients have access to a large number of websites advertising different therapies. Patients must appreciate, however, that this information must be approached with caution because the evidence often fails to stand up to currently accepted levels of medical scrutiny (Morris and Avorn 2003).

Whilst the gold standard for biomedical research is considered to be the double-blind, randomized, controlled clinical trial (RCT) this is not always easy or feasible for CAM (Eskinazi 1998). In conventional biomedical research, the placebo is often considered to be an ideal control, but because many CAM care systems are multimodal (e.g. change in diet, exercise, spiritual practice and interventions such as herbal therapy and acupuncture — used together), it may be impractical, if not impossible, to control for every aspect of treatment. Other aspects, such as inclusion and exclusion criteria, may impose additional difficulties; CAM systems have considerably different diagnostic definitions from those that apply to classical biomedical research. Additionally the definition of outcome may differ. In CAM, subjective evaluations such as improvement of quality of life, and less interference of the disease with activities of daily living, are often considered more important than objective outcomes (Eskinazi 1998). Moreover, many of the elements of the healthcare encounter that are categorized as incidental (placebo) in the context of drug trials are characteristic (intrinsic) to the complex non-pharmaceutical interventions of CAM (Paterson and Dieppe 2005). Thus the use of placebo or sham-controlled trial designs for a complex CAM intervention will not detect its total characteristic effect and may generate false-negative results (Paterson and Dieppe 2005). The implications derived from these methodological considerations of CAM treatments emphasize the importance of placebo effects as an integral part of their outcome. The placebo effect or phenomenon is discussed next.

3. The Placebo Effect

The attitudes towards placebo have changed dramatically since the introduction of the double-blind RCT (Kaptchuk 1998). In the pre-RCT period the placebo was looked upon as a benevolent deception to comfort and please (hence the name 'placebo', to please) the patient, and sometimes as a diagnostic tool to separate 'imaginary' problems from 'real' ones. It was Beecher in 1955 (Beecher 1955) who explicitly assumed an additive model of placebo effects; the total 'drug' effect is equal to its 'active' effect plus its placebo effect. Therefore, in order to find the 'true' effect of a treatment its results should be subtracted from its placebo effect as derived from an RCT. In the current RCT era, a legitimate therapy must therefore demonstrate an effect greater than a decoy disguised as a real intervention. Thus, the placebo has value only as a comparison marker, and the magnitude of its absolute power has been an incidental question (Kaptchuk 1998).

Yet, the placebo effect is not constant and its power, especially as an analgesic, is context-dependent and can vary in different circumstances (Price 1999; Pollo and Benedetti 2004). Expectation and conditioning are important factors in mediating placebo effects (Montgomery and Kirsch 1997; Price *et al* 1999; Pollo *et al* 2001; De Pascalis *et al* 2002). Thus for example, it was reported that patients after chest surgery received a basal saline infusion under three conditions (Pollo *et al* 2001):

(a) They were told that the drug to be administered is a potent painkiller;
(b) They were told that they may be given either placebo or a pain killer; or
(c) They were told nothing.

All three groups received the same opioid analgesic medication (buprenorphine) but differed in the dose-demand of the drug; the least was requested by those assuming they had a potent painkiller (groups a and b), and the most by those that were told nothing (group c). It was clear from these results that higher expectation for analgesia resulted in a smaller demand for the opioid analgesic (Pollo *et al* 2001). Recently, studies that assessed treatment efficacy after hidden intravenous administration of analgesics, as compared to the same intervention when administered by a physician (open administration), demonstrated that open administration was more effective than the hidden one, and the difference between the two results is considered due to a placebo effect (Colloca *et al* 2004).

Pain is the field in which most of the placebo research has been performed, and its neurobiological mechanisms were made significant when Levine *et al* (1978) showed that placebo analgesia was reversed by the opioid antagonist naloxone, suggesting a role for endogenous opioids. The role of endogenous opioids was further supported by brain imaging studies using positron emission tomography (PET), showing activation in descending opioid-mediated pain-modulating pathways by placebo similar to those demonstrated in response to opioid injections (Petrovic *et al* 2002). Furthermore, functional magnetic resonance imaging (fMRI) studies found brain activation patterns in the prefrontal cortex in anticipation of analgesia following placebo administration (Wager *et al* 2004). For recent reviews of the psychological and neuro-biological mechanisms of the placebo effects see Price *et al* (2005) and Benedetti *et al* (2005).

In alternative medicine, the main question regarding placebo has been whether a given therapy has more than a placebo effect. A recent analysis that reviewed the effect of homeopathy concluded that it is in essence no better than a placebo effect (Shang *et al* 2005). However, just as mainstream medicine ignores the clinical significance of its own placebo (Hrobjartsson and Gotzsche 2001, 2004; Vase *et al* 2002), the placebo effect of unconventional medicine is also ignored, and disregarded except for polemics (Kaptchuk 2002). Thus, according to CAM's thinking the term placebo effect is not an imitation intervention, but the broad mixture of non-specific effects present in the clinical setup. A question of interest is whether the setup of CAM creates more of these 'nonspecific' effects and therefore an 'enhanced' placebo effect. This question, reviewed by Kaptchuk (2002), examines aspects such as patient and practitioner characteristics and the interaction between the two, and concludes that there is scant empirical evidence that any particular type of CAM has an augmented placebo effect. Undoubtedly, mainstream medical interventions possess no less of a placebo effect.

4. CAM and Chronic Facial Pain

Relatively little is known about the prevalence of CAM use to treat chronic facial pain (Myers *et al* 2002). Fourteen out of 63 (22%) women with temporomandibular disorder (TMD), recruited to a study on oral splints, reported on the previous use of CAM therapy. Users were significantly more likely to report work or social disability associated with their facial pain and were more likely to report onset associated with an accident (Raphael *et al* 2003). In a recent survey of 192 patients with documented TMD, it was found that about 36% reported using CAM therapies for TMD although most (96%) used conventional care simultaneously (DeBar *et al* 2003). In general the 'hands-on' CAM therapies (massage, acupuncture, and chiropractic care) were the most satisfactory of the CAM therapies utilized (DeBar *et al* 2003).

In a systematic review on the use of acupuncture as a treatment for TMD three trials met the criteria for inclusion as RCT, and it was concluded that acupuncture might be an effective therapy for TMD although none of the studies controlled for a placebo effect (Ernst and White 1999). Another systematic review by the same group (Ernst and

Pittler 1998) on the effectiveness of acupuncture in treating acute dental pain revealed 16 RCTs, and concluded that acupuncture can alleviate dental pain but more studies are needed to compare its efficacy with conventional methods of analgesia.

Raustia *et al* (1985) compared acupuncture with conservative treatments (counselling, occlusal adjustment, muscle exercises, and occlusal splints) in two parallel groups for 50 subjects with temporomandibular joint (TMJ) dysfunction. The two treatment modalities had similar positive effects on the dysfunction index. Acupuncture was found superior to standard therapy on mouth opening in patients with initial significant limitation of opening; standard therapy was superior when the initial limitation was less marked. In another study, acupuncture was compared to a maxillary occlusal splint or no treatment in 45 patients with myogenous facial pain (Johansson *et al* 1991). Ninety percent of the acupuncture group and 86% of those who received occlusal splints improved, and scored significantly better than the no-treatment group on both the subjective symptoms and objective clinical examination scores, with no significant difference between the two active groups (Johansson *et al* 1991). In a similar study 110 patients with a median 4-year duration of TMDs were allocated to three groups receiving acupuncture, maxillary occlusal splint therapy or no treatment (control group) (List *et al* 1992). Acupuncture and splint therapy were superior to the control group on the pain visual analogue scale (VAS) and clinical dysfunction index, but there was significant reduction in pain frequency only in the acupuncture group. The results in the two treatment groups of the above study were presented separately in a 6-month and 1 year follow-up study (List and Helkimo 1992) performed only on the improved patients. Long-term stability was noted in both groups with no significant difference between the groups for any endpoint. A third study by the same group on 55 out of the original 110 subjects (criteria for selecting these 55 subjects are not clear) found increased thresholds to a pressure algometer applied to the belly of the masseter muscle significantly higher in the treatment groups compared to the non-treated group (List *et al* 1993). This change was maintained in a repeated examination 6 months later. Based on traditional Chinese medicine 7 local acupuncture points and 1 distant point have been recommended for the use of acupuncture in the treatment of TMDs (Rosted 2001). However, both acupuncture and sham acupuncture equally reduced pain evoked by mechanical stimulation of the masseter muscles in myofascial pain patients, and this effect may not be specific to the location of the stimulus as predicted by the classical acupuncture literature (Goddard *et al* 2002).

Myers *et al* (2002) reviewed RCTs of patients who had chronic facial pain and were subjected to a CAM intervention versus a control comparison group. Across studies, results suggested that acupuncture, biofeedback and relaxation were comparable to conservative treatment (for example, an intraoral appliance) and thus warranted further study. Myers *et al* (2002) were unable to comment on other modes of CAM therapy because they could not locate any RCT that tested the effects of other treatments such as homeopathy, massage or chiropractic or herbal remedies on chronic facial pain. One study compared 122 adolescent TMD patients that were divided into three treatment groups: brief information (BI), BI and relaxation training and BI and an occlusal appliance. The groups that used relaxation or an occlusal appliance showed significant improvement but not the group that used BI alone (Wahlund *et al* 2003). Other CAM methods for treating TMD include hypnosis which was effective in decreasing pain frequency, intensity and duration and in improving daily functioning (Simon and Lewis 2000). Analysis suggests that treatment gains were maintained for 6 months after hypnosis treatment and that in addition patients exhibited a significant reduction in medication use.

Conclusion. About a third of patients that we see for chronic facial pain (mostly patients with TMD) are concomitantly utilizing CAM therapy. Acupuncture is the most frequently used mode of therapy, and its effect seems to be comparable to conventionally utilized therapies, such as intraoral splints.

5. CAM and Headaches

A recent survey of CAM utilization by migraine patients in Italy found that about 31% of 481 patients attending a headache clinic reported previous CAM use (Rossi *et al* 2005). Around 40% of patients who used CAM considered it beneficial, but it was less effective for transformed than for episodic migraine (Rossi *et al* 2005). In another survey of 73 headache patients, carried out in New York, it was found that 85% used CAM therapy for their headache, and 60% found it to be beneficial (von Peter *et al* 2002). While it is apparent that there are cultural differences in the rate of CAM utilization for headache, there is no doubt that many patients with headache worldwide seek alternatives to conventional medical therapy. Therapists should be aware of this, especially as more than 60% of patients did not report their CAM treatments to their medical doctors (Rossi *et al* 2005). It is estimated that about 30% of patients do not respond to pharmacological interventions for headache, and among the alternative therapies are behavioural treatments, acupuncture and nutritional therapies (Holroyd and Mauskop 2003). In a meta-analysis of 50 clinical trials (2445 patients, collectively) it was found that both propranolol and relaxation/biofeedback yielded a 43% reduction in migraine headache activity compared to 14% with placebo medication (Holroyd and Penzien 1990). A systematic review of 24 RCT studies examined the effects of CAM therapies (acupuncture, spinal

manipulation, physiotherapy) for non-migrainous headaches (tension-type headache, cervicogenic headache, post-traumatic headache). Evidence from a subset of high-quality studies indicates that some CAM therapies may be useful in the treatment of these conditions (Vernon *et al* 1999). Holroyd *et al* (2001) compared the effects of tricyclic antidepressants with those of stress management on chronic tension-type headache (mean, 26 headache days per month). Four groups were allocated: antidepressants (amitriptyline up to 100mg/d or nortriptyline up to 75mg/d), placebo, stress management (e.g. relaxation, cognitive coping) plus placebo, stress management plus antidepressants. All three active treatments, but not the placebo, yielded improvement in headache activity by the 6-month evaluation, but improvement occurred more rapidly with antidepressants than with stress management. Combined therapy was more likely to produce clinically significant (>50%) reduction in headache index scores (64% of participants) than antidepressants (38%), stress management (35%) or placebo (29%) (Holroyd *et al* 2001).

In a systematic review on acupuncture and headache it was concluded that the existing evidence supports the value of acupuncture for the treatment of idiopathic headache, but that the quality and amount of evidence are not fully convincing (Melchart *et al* 2001). The effect of acupuncture for early (abortive) treatment of migraine was compared to that of sumatriptan (Melchart *et al* 2003). A total of 179 inpatient migraineurs were allocated into three groups: traditional Chinese acupuncture, sumatriptan (6mg subcutaneously) or placebo injection. A full migraine attack was prevented in 21 of 60 patients (35%) by acupuncture, in 21 of 58 (36%) by sumatriptan and 11 of 61 (18%) by placebo; relative risk versus placebo of 0.79 for acupuncture, and 0.78 for sumatriptan were lower than expected, and may be explained by a biased, difficult-to-treat, inpatient migraine patient population. Response to a second intervention in patients who developed a full attack was significantly better with sumatriptan than with acupuncture. In a more recent study by the same group (Linde *et al* 2005), the prophylactic effects of acupuncture and sham acupuncture (superficial needling at non-acupuncture points) compared to a control waiting list group were studied in 302 patients. Acupuncture and sham acupuncture consisted of 12 sessions over 8 weeks, and differences in number of days with headache were compared on diaries from 4 weeks before to 9–12 weeks after randomization. Days with headache were significantly reduced during the period by 2.2 on acupuncture and sham acupuncture as compared to 0.8 on the waiting list. A similar design by the same group (Melchart *et al* 2005) also tested the effect of acupuncture and sham acupuncture on tension-type headache. Acupuncture reduced the number of days with headache by 7.2, sham acupuncture by 6.6 and the waiting list group by 1.5. It was concluded in both studies (Linde *et al* 2005; Melchart *et al* 2005) that acupuncture intervention was more effective than no treatment but not significantly more than sham acupuncture. The effect of acupuncture was tested also in chronic daily headache (CDH) (Coeytaux *et al* 2005). An RCT was carried out on 74 patients that compared medical management provided by neurologists to medical management plus 10 acupuncture treatments. Patients with CDH who received medical treatment only did not improve on their daily pain severity and headache-related quality of life (QoL); patients receiving additional acupuncture were 3.7 times more likely to report less suffering from headaches at 6 weeks. Supplementing medical management with acupuncture resulted in improvement in QoL and the perception by patients that they suffer less from headaches (Coeytaux *et al* 2005).

The cost effectiveness of acupuncture on chronic headache was reported in two recent studies (Vickers *et al* 2004; Wonderling *et al* 2004). In these two studies 401 patients with chronic headache, predominantly migraine, were randomly allocated to receive up to 12 acupuncture treatments or to a control intervention consisting of standard care as offered by the British National Health Service (NHS). Headache score at 12 months, the primary endpoint, was significantly lower in the acupuncture group than in controls (34 and 16% reduction from baseline, respectively). Patients in the acupuncture group significantly experienced 22 fewer days of headache per year than controls, and used 15% less medication (Vickers *et al* 2004). Total costs during the 1-year period of the study were on average higher for the acupuncture group than for the controls (£403 and £217, respectively), because of the acupuncture practitioners' fees. The authors conclude that acupuncture is of benefit for primary-care patients with chronic headache, and improves health-related quality of life at a small additional cost (Wonderling *et al* 2004).

Behavioural modalities of therapy such as biofeedback, relaxation training and cognitive behavioural therapy (CBT) for orofacial pain and headaches are discussed in detail in Chapter 4.

Conclusion. About 30–85% of patients seen in headache clinics are also using CAM therapy. The rate of utilization is cultural-dependent, and where the percentage of CAM use is smaller, the tendency is not to report it to the treating physician. Relaxation/biofeedback treatments yield comparable results with propranolol for migraine prevention, both superior to placebo. Stress management was comparable to antidepressants in controlling headache, but the combination of the two was more effective than each treatment on its own. Acupuncture was effective for treating migraine, but no difference was detected between sham and traditional techniques. Chronic daily headache was likely to respond almost four times more to conventional medications when combined with acupuncture. Acupuncture treatment for headaches is cost effective in terms of improvement of health-related quality of life.

6. Acupuncture: Mode of Action

The use of acupuncture for treatment of pain has become widespread in the past few decades. The introduction of the Gate Control Theory (Melzack and Wall 1965) lent theoretical support for possible pain control by means of an external stimulus applied to the body such as acupuncture. Later investigations have demonstrated that the nervous system, neurotransmitters and endogenous substances respond to needling stimulation (Foster and Sweeney 1987). It has been established that acupuncture analgesia is mediated by opioid peptides produced in the periaqueductal grey, and can be reversed by the opioid antagonist naloxone (Cheng and Pomeranz 1980). The periaqueductal grey and other supraspinal sites of the descending pain modulatory system exert powerful inhibitory effects on the response at the spinal level (Fields and Basbaum 1978; Nicholson and Martelli 2004). Recent evidence shows that acupuncture also increases neuronal nitric acid (NO) expression in the gracile nucleus (Abou-Donia *et al* 2002). NO expression plays an important role in mediating the cardiovascular response to acupuncture, may participate in central autonomic regulation of somatosympathetic reflex activities and could contribute to the therapeutic effects of acupuncture (Nicholson and Martelli 2004).

7. Food Additives

7.1. Omega-3 Fatty Acids

Recently, the effect of omega-3 fatty acids as an anti-inflammatory agent has emerged, with the possibility that they may serve as an alternative to NSAIDs for long-term use (Cleland and James 2006; Maroon and Bost 2006). A search for an alternative safer anti-inflammatory agent became even more important as the concept of 'safe' NSAIDs collapsed (see Chapter 15). Multiple observations have clearly established an increased risk for cardiovascular events associated with use of the new cyclooxygenase (COX)-2-selective, as well as for other non-selective, NSAIDs. This is in addition to the renal, gastrointestinal and other side effects associated with NSAID use.

Fish oils contain long-chain omega-3 eicosapentaenoic acid (EPA) and docosahexaenoic acid that produce competitive inhibition of arachidonic acid (AA) metabolism by COX (Cleland *et al* 2005). EPA is a natural homologue of arachidonic acid, with a structural difference of only one additional double bond (the omega-3 bond). Not surprisingly it is an alternative substrate and inhibitor of AA metabolism by COX (Cleland *et al* 2003). Whereas prostaglandin (P)-GH$_2$ is the COX metabolite of AA, PGH$_3$ is the COX metabolite of EPA. Studies of prostanoid metabolism in the presence of dietary EPA or exogenous EPA added *in vitro* suggest that PGH$_3$ is a poor substrate and an inhibitor of PGE synthase (Hawkes *et al* 1991) and thromboxane (TX)-A synthase (von Schacky *et al* 1985) and a potential substrate without inhibitory effect on PGI synthase. Indeed, the increased PGI_2 synthesis seen with anti-inflammatory doses of fish oils raises the possibility of 'shunting' PGH_2 from blocked PGE synthase and TX synthase to uninhibited PGI synthase (DeCaterina *et al* 1990). Thus, the overall effect of EPA is suppression of PGE_2 synthesis and shifting of the TXA_2/PGI_2 balance in favour of PGI_2. This shift is in contrast with the effects of selective COX-2 inhibitors, which shift the TXA_2/PGI_2 balance in favour of TXA_2 and may cause a 'prothrombotic effect' (see Chapter 15). EPA and docosahexaenoic acid inhibit the activity of both COX-1 and COX-2 with a specificity similar to that for ibuprofen (Lands 1991).

While not suitable for on-demand use, fish oils have a number of advantages over NSAIDs. First, they have not been associated with serious upper gastrointestinal complications (Kremer *et al* 1996). Second, they have been shown to reduce risk for cardiovascular events, including cardiac death, through multiple actions (Kris-Etherton *et al* 2002), in contrast with the increased risk seen with most NSAIDs (Hippisley-Cox and Coupland 2005; Solomon 2005). Third, fish oils have been shown to reduce synthesis of the proinflammatory cytokines tumour necrosis factor (TNF) and interleukin 1 (IL-1) by mononuclear cells (James *et al* 2000; Simopoulos 2002), in contrast to NSAIDs, which can increase synthesis of these cytokines (Demasi *et al* 2003). Thus long-term fish oil treatment may reduce NSAID use and reduce gastrointestinal and cardiovascular events in potential NSAID users.

To date more than 10 randomized control studies have been performed in patients with rheumatoid arthritis (RA), most in patients with disease duration of more than 10 years (Cleland *et al* 2003). The most consistent benefits were reduced morning stiffness and decreased tender joint count, and NSAIDs given on an as required basis could be reduced (Cleland *et al* 2003).

Thus for example, in a double-blind, placebo-controlled, prospective study of fish oil supplementation (Kremer *et al* 1995), active RA patients took either 130 mg/kg/d of omega-3 fatty acids or 9 capsules/day of corn oil while on diclofenac (75 mg twice a day). Placebo diclofenac was substituted at week 18 or 22, and fish oil supplements were continued for another 8 weeks. Patients, who took dietary supplements of fish oil but not of corn oil, exhibited improvements in clinical parameters of disease activity from baseline, including the number of tender joints. These improvements were also associated with significant decreases in levels of IL-1 beta. It was concluded that patients who took fish oil were able to discontinue NSAIDs without experiencing a disease flare-up. Similarly, about 60% of patients with neck or back discogenic pain who ingested a total of 1200 mg/d of omega-3 fatty acids (eicosapentaenoic acid and docosahexaenoic acid) for one month were able to stop taking NSAIDs (Maroon and Bost 2006).

In a long-term, 12-month study 90 patients with active RA were enrolled in a double-blind, randomized study comparing daily supplementations with either 2.6 g of omega-3 or 1.3 g of omega-3 plus 3 g of olive oil, or 6 g of olive oil. Significant improvement in the patient's global evaluation and in the physician's assessment of pain was observed only in those taking 2.6 g/d of omega-3 (Geusens *et al* 1994). Another study conducted in 43 patients with RA showed that 3 g/d of fish oil omega-3 relieved many clinical signs significantly more than soy oil controls. However, the combination of 3 g/d of fish oil and 9.6 mL of olive oil was superior to fish oil alone (Berbert *et al* 2005). The conflicting findings of these two studies may result from the difference in the amount of omega-3 (1.3 and 3 g, respectively) used in combination with the olive oil. The amount of 1.3 g/d is lower than the recommended omega-3 fatty acids dose of about 2.5 g/d for the treatment of adult RA (Cleland *et al* 2003). A recent meta-analysis of the analgesic effects of omega-3 demonstrated its efficacy in reducing joint pain, duration of morning stiffness, number of painful joints and NSAID consumption (Goldberg and Katz 2007). However, further analysis showed that these results were effective only for higher doses (2.7 g/d) taken for at least 3 months.

Significant improvement was noticed under the effects of fish oil and olive oil on the frequency and severity of recurrent migraine in adolescents, although no difference was found between the two treatments (Harel *et al* 2002). Since no additional control (e.g. corn or soy oil) was utilized, these findings are difficult to interpret.

Conclusions. There are not enough data, other than in RA, to recommend the proper clinical utilization (e.g. dose, frequency, duration) of omega-3 for chronic orofacial pain. However, its anti-inflammatory effect, coupled with a high safety profile, should be considered for long-term use in painful arthritis of the TMJ. One should be aware that high quantities are needed (2.5–2.7 g/d), the equivalent of about 6–7 standard capsules per day. In addition, omega-3's antiplatelet and anticoagulant effects should be taken into account when performing oral surgery, particularly in patients on high doses.

7.2. Glucosamine

Glucosamine is a naturally occurring aminomonosaccharide in the human body, biosynthesized from glucose. It is used to form glycosaminoglycan (GAG), a constituent of proteoglycans, itself a component of the extracellular matrix of articular cartilage. Glucosamine sulphate (GS) is regarded as a food supplement and is available in health food and drug stores. Its potential as an adjunctive medication for osteoarthritis (OA) is gaining wide acceptance, and is supported by *in vitro* animal and human studies (Thie *et al* 2001). The biochemical events underlying symptom relief in patients taking GS are partially explained by GS's ability to act as a substrate and stimulant of GAG production within articular cartilage. GS has no analgesic activity and is ineffective against proteolytic enzymes of inflamed tissues and against the biosynthesis of prostaglandins elicited from arachidonic acid or histamine. Thus, studies using chondrocytes isolated and cultured from human osteoarthritic joints found that GS induced a significant dose-dependent increase of proteoglycan synthesis, but did not affect DNA synthesis or chondrocytes production of collagen type II and prostaglandin E_2 (Bassleer et al 1998).

A recent commentary recommends the following: 'Sufficient evidence exists from studies of persons with hip or knee osteoarthritis to support the use of glucosamine as a safe and effective alternative treatment' (Fox et al 2006). The authors continue: 'With the potential harmful effects of chronic NSAID and acetaminophen use and a reluctance to begin chronic narcotic therapy for mild osteoarthritis, glucosamine and possibly chondroitin offer viable, low-cost treatment options or adjuvant medications.' Recommended scheduling is 1500mg of glucosamine daily, either in one or in three divided doses daily, and to continue therapy for at least 4–8 weeks for onset of benefit (Fox et al 2006). On the other hand, the conclusions reached in a recent Cochrane systematic review are more sceptical about the benefit of GS (Towheed et al 2005). Although the overall results suggested the GS was beneficial, analysis of the eight studies with adequate allocation concealment failed to show benefit of glucosamine for pain and function (Towheed et al 2005).

Studies on the effects of GS on the TMJ are scarce, but a recent double-blind RCT compared the effect of 1500mg of GS to 1200mg a day of ibuprofen in patients with OA of the TMJ (Thie et al 2001). It is of special interest since fundamental differences exist between the TMJ and other synovial joints. A major difference is that the articular surface of the TMJ is not cartilage but a dense fibrous connective tissue (also referred to as fibrocartilage) that consists primarily of type I collagen rather than the type II seen in hyaline cartilage. Thie et al (2001) demonstrated in their study that GS and ibuprofen were both effective in reducing pain and improving function with no difference between the two treatments. However, their results are to be interpreted with some caution; no placebo control group was included and the positive response level was set at 20% improvement, a level that may be considered of minimal clinical significance, and probably not different from a placebo effect.

Conclusions. A previous Cochrane review (Towheed et al 2001) with 16 studies showed that glucosamine sulphate taken orally in amounts of 1500mg/d produced a 60% (change from baseline) benefit in pain and increase in function of 33% in osteoarthritis, without side effects. Inclusion of eight new studies in a more recent Cochrane review (Towheed et al 2005), although substantiating the safety of GS, reduces the overall benefit of pain to 28% and function to 21%. At this stage, it is hard to conclude on the benefits of GS in the treatment of osteoarthritis of the TMJ, although its use in dosage of 1500mg/d seems to be safe.

References

Abou-Donia MB, Dechkovskaia AM, Goldstein LB, et al (2002) Sensorimotor deficit and cholinergic changes following coexposure with pyridostigmine bromide and sarin in rats. *Toxicol Sci* **66**(1):148–158.

Astin JA (1998) Why patients use alternative medicine: results of a national study. *JAMA* **279**(19):1548–1553.

Bassleer C, Rovati L, Franchimont P (1998) Stimulation of proteoglycan production by glucosamine sulfate in chondrocytes isolated from human osteoarthritic articular cartilage in vitro. *Osteoarthritis Cartilage* **6**(6):427–434.

Beecher HK (1955) The powerful placebo. *J Am Med Assoc* **159**(17):1602–1606.

Benedetti F, Mayberg HS, Wager TD, et al (2005) Neurobiological mechanisms of the placebo effect. *J Neurosci* **25**(45):10390–10402.

Berbert AA, Kondo CR, Almendra CL, et al (2005) Supplementation of fish oil and olive oil in patients with rheumatoid arthritis. *Nutrition* **21**(2):131–136.

Charlton JE (2005) Complementary therapies. In: Charlton JE (ed) *Core Curriculum for Professional Education in Pain.* Seattle: IASP Press.

Cheng RS, Pomeranz BH (1980) Electroacupuncture analgesia is mediated by stereospecific opiate receptors and is reversed by antagonists of type I receptors. *Life Sci* **26**(8):631–638.

Cleland LG, James MJ (2006) Marine oils for antiinflammatory effect – time to take stock. *J Rheumatol* **33**(2):207–209.

Cleland LG, James MJ, Proudman SM (2003) The role of fish oils in the treatment of rheumatoid arthritis. *Drugs* **63**(9):845–853.

Cleland LG, James MJ, Proudman SM (2005) Fish oil: what the prescriber needs to know. *Arthritis Res Ther* **8**(1):202.

Coeytaux RR, Kaufman JS, Kaptchuk TJ, et al (2005) A randomized, controlled trial of acupuncture for chronic daily headache. *Headache* **45**(9):1113–1123.

Colloca L, Lopiano L, Lanotte M, et al (2004) Overt versus covert treatment for pain, anxiety, and Parkinson's disease. *Lancet Neurol* **3**(11):679–684.

DeBar LL, Vuckovic N, Schneider J, et al (2003) Use of complementary and alternative medicine for temporomandibular disorders. *J Orofac Pain* **17**(3):224–236.

DeCaterina R, Giannessi D, Mazzone A, et al (1990) Vascular prostacyclin is increased in patients ingesting omega-3 polyunsaturated fatty acids before coronary artery bypass graft surgery. *Circulation* **82**(2):428–438.

Demasi M, Cleland LG, Cook-Johnson RJ, et al (2003) Effects of hypoxia on monocyte inflammatory mediator production: Dissociation between changes in cyclooxygenase-2 expression and eicosanoid synthesis. *J Biol Chem* **278**(40):38607–38616.

De Pascalis V, Chiaradia C, Carotenuto E (2002) The contribution of suggestibility and expectation to placebo analgesia phenomenon in an experimental setting. *Pain* **96**(3):393–402.

Eisenberg DM, Kessler RC, Foster C, et al (1993) Unconventional medicine in the United States. Prevalence, costs, and patterns of use. *N Engl J Med* **328**(4):246–252.

Eisenberg DM, Davis RB, Ettner SL, et al (1998) Trends in alternative medicine use in the United States, 1990-1997: results of a follow-up national survey. *JAMA* **280**(18):1569–1575.

Ernst E, Pittler MH (1998) The effectiveness of acupuncture in treating acute dental pain: a systematic review. *Br Dent J* **184**(9): 443–447.

Ernst E, White AR (1999) Acupuncture as a treatment for temporomandibular joint dysfunction: a systematic review of randomized trials. *Arch Otolaryngol Head Neck Surg* **125**(3): 269–272.

Eskinazi D (1998) Methodologic considerations for research in traditional (alternative) medicine. *Oral Surg Oral Med Oral Pathol Oral Radiol Endod* **86**(6):678–681.

Fields HL, Basbaum AI (1978) Brainstem control of spinal pain-transmission neurons. *Annu Rev Physiol* **40**:217–248.

Foster JM, Sweeney BP (1987) The mechanisms of acupuncture analgesia. *Br J Hosp Med* **38**(4):308–312.

Fox BA, Schmitz ED, Wallace R (2006) FPIN's clinical inquiries. Glucosamine and chondroitin for osteoarthritis. *Am Fam Physician* **73**(7):1245–1246.

Geusens P, Wouters C, Nijs J, *et al* (1994) Long-term effect of omega-3 fatty acid supplementation in active rheumatoid arthritis. A 12-month, double-blind, controlled study. *Arthritis Rheum* **37**(6):824–829.

Glick S (2005) CAM–image vs. reality: a personal perspective. *Isr Med Assoc J* **7**(9):604–606.

Goddard G, Karibe H, McNeill C, *et al* (2002) Acupuncture and sham acupuncture reduce muscle pain in myofascial pain patients. *J Orofac Pain* **16**(1):71–76.

Goldberg RJ, Katz J (2007) A meta-analysis of the analgesic effects of omega-3 polyunsaturated fatty acid supplementation for inflammatory joint pain. *Pain* **129**(1-2):210–223.

Goldszmidt M, Levitt C, Duarte-Franco E, *et al* (1995) Complementary health care services: a survey of general practitioners' views. *CMAJ* **153**(1):29–35.

Gracely EJ, O'Connor B (1996) Students' attitudes toward alternative health care. *Acad Med* **71**(2):109–110.

Harel Z, Gascon G, Riggs S, *et al* (2002) Supplementation with omega-3 polyunsaturated fatty acids in the management of recurrent migraines in adolescents. *J Adolesc Health* **31**(2): 154–161.

Hawkes JS, James MJ, Cleland LG (1991) Separation and quantification of PGE3 following derivatization with panacyl bromide by high pressure liquid chromatography with fluorometric detection. *Prostaglandins* **42**(4):355–368.

Herman PM, Craig BM, Caspi O (2005) Is complementary and alternative medicine (CAM) cost-effective? A systematic review. *BMC Complement Altern Med* **5**:11.

Hippisley-Cox J, Coupland C (2005) Risk of myocardial infarction in patients taking cyclo-oxygenase-2 inhibitors or conventional non-steroidal anti-inflammatory drugs: population based nested case-control analysis. *BMJ* **330**(7504):1366.

Holroyd KA, Mauskop A (2003) Complementary and alternative treatments. *Neurology* **60**(Suppl 2):S58–S62.

Holroyd KA, Penzien DB (1990) Pharmacological versus non-pharmacological prophylaxis of recurrent migraine headache: a meta-analytic review of clinical trials. *Pain* **42**(1):1–13.

Holroyd KA, O'Donnell FJ, Stensland M, *et al* (2001) Management of chronic tension-type headache with tricyclic antidepressant medication, stress management therapy, and their combination: a randomized controlled trial. *JAMA* **285**(17): 2208–2215.

Hrobjartsson A, Gotzsche PC (2001) Is the placebo powerless? An analysis of clinical trials comparing placebo with no treatment. *N Engl J Med* **344**(21):1594–1602.

Hrobjartsson A, Gotzsche PC (2004) Is the placebo powerless? Update of a systematic review with 52 new randomized trials comparing placebo with no treatment. *J Intern Med* **256**(2): 91–100.

James MJ, Gibson RA, Cleland LG (2000) Dietary polyunsaturated fatty acids and inflammatory mediator production. *Am J Clin Nutr* **71**(1 Suppl): 343S–348S.

Johansson A, Wenneberg B, Wagersten C, *et al* (1991) Acupuncture in treatment of facial muscular pain. *Acta Odontol Scand* **49**(3):153–158.

Kaptchuk TJ (1998) Powerful placebo: the dark side of the randomised controlled trial. *Lancet* **351**(9117):1722–1725.

Kaptchuk TJ (2002) The placebo effect in alternative medicine: can the performance of a healing ritual have clinical significance? *Ann Intern Med* **136**(11):817–825.

Kremer JM, Lawrence DA, Petrillo GF, *et al* (1995) Effects of high-dose fish oil on rheumatoid arthritis after stopping nonsteroidal antiinflammatory drugs. Clinical and immune correlates. *Arthritis Rheum* **38**(8):1107–1114.

Kremer JM, Malamood H, Maliakkal B, *et al* (1996) Fish oil dietary supplementation for prevention of indomethacin induced gastric and small bowel toxicity in healthy volunteers. *J Rheumatol* **23**(10):1770–1773.

Kris-Etherton PM, Harris WS, Appel LJ (2002) Fish consumption, fish oil, omega-3 fatty acids, and cardiovascular disease. *Circulation* **106**(21): 2747–2757.

Lands WE (1991) Biosynthesis of prostaglandins. *Annu Rev Nutr* **11**:41–60.

Levine JD, Gordon NC, Fields HL (1978) The mechanism of placebo analgesia. *Lancet* **2**(8091):654–657.

Linde K, Streng A, Jurgens S, *et al* (2005) Acupuncture for patients with migraine: a randomized controlled trial. *JAMA* **293**(17): 2118–2125.

List T, Helkimo M (1992) Acupuncture and occlusal splint therapy in the treatment of craniomandibular disorders. II. A 1-year follow-up study. *Acta Odontol Scand* **50**(6):375–385.

List T, Helkimo M, Andersson S, *et al* (1992) Acupuncture and occlusal splint therapy in the treatment of craniomandibular disorders. Part I. A comparative study. *Swed Dent J* **16**(4): 125–141.

List T, Helkimo M, Karlsson R (1993) Pressure pain thresholds in patients with craniomandibular disorders before and after treatment with acupuncture and occlusal splint therapy: a controlled clinical study. *J Orofac Pain* **7**(3): 275–282.

Maroon JC, Bost JW (2006) Omega-3 fatty acids (fish oil) as an anti-inflammatory: an alternative to nonsteroidal anti-inflammatory drugs for discogenic pain. *Surg Neurol* **65**(4): 326–331.

Melchart D, Linde K, Fischer P, *et al* (2001) Acupuncture for idiopathic headache. *Cochrane Database Syst Rev* (1):CD001218.

Melchart D, Thormaehlen J, Hager S, *et al* (2003) Acupuncture versus placebo versus sumatriptan for early treatment of migraine attacks: a randomized controlled trial. *J Intern Med* **253**(2):181–188.

Melchart D, Streng A, Hoppe A, *et al* (2005) Acupuncture in patients with tension-type headache: randomised controlled trial. *BMJ* **331**(7513):376–382.

Melzack R, Wall PD (1965) Pain mechanisms: a new theory. *Science* **150**(699): 971–979.

Montgomery GH, Kirsch I (1997) Classical conditioning and the placebo effect. *Pain* **72**(1-2):107–113.

Morris CA, Avorn J (2003) Internet marketing of herbal products. *JAMA* **290**(11):1505–1509.

Myers CD, White BA, Heft MW (2002) A review of complementary and alternative medicine use for treating chronic facial pain. *J Am Dent Assoc* **133**(9):1189–1196; quiz 1259–1260.

Nicholson K, Martelli MF (2004) The problem of pain. *J Head Trauma Rehabil* **19**(1):2–9.

Oberbaum M, Notzer N, Abramowitz R, *et al* (2003) Attitude of medical students to the introduction of complementary medicine into the medical curriculum in Israel. *Isr Med Assoc J* **5**(2):139–142.

Paterson C, Dieppe P (2005) Characteristic and incidental (placebo) effects in complex interventions such as acupuncture. *BMJ* **330**(7501):1202–1205.

Petrovic P, Kalso E, Petersson KM, *et al* (2002) Placebo and opioid analgesia– imaging a shared neuronal network. *Science* **295**(5560):1737–1740.

Pollo A, Benedetti F (2004) Neural mechanisms of placebo-induced analgesia. In: Price DD, Bushnell MC (eds) *Psychological Methods of Pain Control*. Seattle: IASP Press, pp 171–186.

Pollo A, Amanzio M, Arslanian A, *et al* (2001) Response expectancies in placebo analgesia and their clinical relevance. *Pain* **93**(1):77–84.

Price DD (1999) Placebo analgesia In: Price DD (ed) *Psychological Mechanisms of Pain and Analgesia*. Seattle: IASP Press, pp 155–181.

Price DD, Milling LS, Kirsch I, *et al* (1999) An analysis of factors that contribute to the magnitude of placebo analgesia in an experimental paradigm. *Pain* **83**(2):147–156.

Price DD, Chung K, Robinson ME (2005) Conditioning, expectation and desire for relief in placebo analgesia. *Seminars in Pain Medicine* **3**:15–21.

Raphael KG, Klausner JJ, Nayak S, *et al* (2003) Complementary and alternative therapy use by patients with myofascial temporomandibular disorders. *J Orofac Pain* **17**(1):36–41.

Raustia AM, Pohjola RT, Virtanen KK (1985) Acupuncture compared with stomatognathic treatment for TMJ dysfunction. Part I: A randomized study. *J Prosthet Dent* **54**(4):581–585.

Rossi P, Di Lorenzo G, Malpezzi MG, *et al* (2005) Prevalence, pattern and predictors of use of complementary and alternative medicine (CAM) in migraine patients attending a headache clinic in Italy. *Cephalalgia* **25**(7): 493–506.

Rosted P (2001) Practical recommendations for the use of acupuncture in the treatment of temporomandibular disorders based on the outcome of published controlled studies. *Oral Dis* **7**(2):109–115.

Shang A, Huwiler-Muntener K, Nartey L, *et al* (2005) Are the clinical effects of homoeopathy placebo effects? Comparative study of placebo-controlled trials of homoeopathy and allopathy. *Lancet* **366**(9487):726–732.

Simon EP, Lewis DM (2000) Medical hypnosis for temporomandibular disorders: treatment efficacy and medical utilization outcome. *Oral Surg Oral Med Oral Pathol Oral Radiol Endod* **90**(1):54–63.

Simopoulos AP (2002) Omega-3 fatty acids in inflammation and autoimmune diseases. *J Am Coll Nutr* **21**(6):495–505.

Solomon DH (2005) Selective cyclooxygenase 2 inhibitors and cardiovascular events. *Arthritis Rheum* **52**(7):1968–1978.

Thie NM, Prasad NG, Major PW (2001) Evaluation of glucosamine sulfate compared to ibuprofen for the treatment of temporomandibular joint osteoarthritis: a randomized double blind controlled 3 month clinical trial. *J Rheumatol* **28**(6): 1347–1355.

Towheed TE, Anastassiades TP, Shea B *et al* (2001) Glucosamine therapy for treating osteoarthritis. *Cochrane Database Syst Rev*: CD002946.

Towheed TE, Maxwell L, Anastassiades TP, *et al* (2005) Glucosamine therapy for treating osteoarthritis. *Cochrane Database Syst Rev* (2):CD002946.

Vase L, Riley JL 3rd, Price DD (2002) A comparison of placebo effects in clinical analgesic trials versus studies of placebo analgesia. *Pain* **99**(3):443–452.

Vernon H, McDermaid CS, Hagino C (1999) Systematic review of randomized clinical trials of complementary/alternative therapies in the treatment of tension-type and cervicogenic headache. *Complement Ther Med* **7**(3): 142–155.

Vickers AJ, Rees RW, Zollman CE, *et al* (2004) Acupuncture for chronic headache in primary care: large, pragmatic, randomised trial. *BMJ* **328**(7442):744.

Visser GJ, Peters L (1990) Alternative medicine and general practitioners in The Netherlands: towards acceptance and integration. *Fam Pract* **7**(3):227–232.

von Peter S, Ting W, Scrivani S, *et al* (2002) Survey on the use of complementary and alternative medicine among patients with headache syndromes. *Cephalalgia* **22**(5):395–400.

von Schacky C, Fischer S, Weber PC (1985) Long-term effects of dietary marine omega-3 fatty acids upon plasma and cellular lipids, platelet function, and eicosanoid formation in humans. *J Clin Invest* **76**(4):1626–1631.

Wager TD, Rilling JK, Smith EE, *et al* (2004) Placebo-induced changes in FMRI in the anticipation and experience of pain. *Science* **303**(5661):1162–1167.

Wahlund K, List T, Larsson B (2003) Treatment of temporomandibular disorders among adolescents: a comparison between occlusal appliance, relaxation training, and brief information. *Acta Odontol Scand* **61**(4):203–211.

Weintraub MI (2003) Complementary and alternative methods of treatment of neck pain. *Phys Med Rehabil Clin N Am* **14**(3): 659–674, viii.

Wetzel MS, Eisenberg DM, Kaptchuk TJ (1998) Courses involving complementary and alternative medicine at US medical schools. *JAMA* **280**(9):784–787.

Wolsko PM, Eisenberg DM, Davis RB, *et al* (2003) Patterns and perceptions of care for treatment of back and neck pain: results of a national survey. *Spine* **28**(3):292–297; discussion 298.

Wonderling D, Vickers AJ, Grieve R, *et al* (2004) Cost effectiveness analysis of a randomised trial of acupuncture for chronic headache in primary care. *BMJ* **328**(7442):747.

Zollman C, Vickers A (1999) ABC of complementary medicine. Users and practitioners of complementary medicine. *BMJ* **319**(7213):836–838.

Index